T0363917

Comprehensive Review of Infectious Diseases

2NJDTF662JRXB5MQBK54

Comprehensive Review of Infectious Diseases

Edited by

Andrej Spec, MD, MSCI

Assistant Professor
Division of Infectious Diseases
Washington University in St. Louis School of Medicine
Missouri, United States

Gerome Escota, MD

Assistant Professor of Medicine
Division of Infectious Diseases
Washington University in St. Louis School of Medicine
Missouri, United States

Courtney Chrisler, MD

Assistant Professor
Division of Infectious Diseases
Washington University in St. Louis School of Medicine
Missouri, United States

Bethany Davies, MBBS, MD, FRCPath, MRCP

Senior Lecturer in Infection
Department of Global Health and Infection
Brighton and Sussex Medical School
United Kingdom

ELSEVIER   Edinburgh   London   New York   Oxford   Philadelphia   St Louis   Sydney   2020

© 2020, Elsevier Limited. All rights reserved.

No part of this publication may be reproduced or transmitted in any form or by any means, electronic or mechanical, including photocopying, recording, or any information storage and retrieval system, without permission in writing from the publisher. Details on how to seek permission, further information about the Publisher's permissions policies and our arrangements with organizations such as the Copyright Clearance Center and the Copyright Licensing Agency, can be found at our website: www.elsevier.com/permissions.

This book and the individual contributions contained in it are protected under copyright by the Publisher (other than as may be noted herein).

Notices

Practitioners and researchers must always rely on their own experience and knowledge in evaluating and using any information, methods, compounds or experiments described herein. Because of rapid advances in the medical sciences, in particular, independent verification of diagnoses and drug dosages should be made. To the fullest extent of the law, no responsibility is assumed by Elsevier, authors, editors or contributors for any injury and/or damage to persons or property as a matter of products liability, negligence or otherwise, or from any use or operation of any methods, products, instructions, or ideas contained in the material herein.

Cover images reproduced from:

Michael I. Lewis, Robert J. McKenna, Eds. Medical Management of the Thoracic Surgery Patient. Saunders, 2010. Mucin stain highlights mucinous capsules confirming cryptococcus (red; mucicarmine stain; original magnification 600x).

Mack, Megan, Gregg, Kevin. Diagnosis and Management of Infections in Hospitalized Immunocompromised Patients. Hospital Medicine Clinics, Volume 3, Issue 3, e378-e395. Characteristic appearance of CMV intracytoplasmic inclusions, resembling an owl's eye.

Ramos-e-Silva, Marcia. Dermatologic Clinics 2008. Volume 26, Issue 2 (April), pp 257-269. Paracoccidioidomycosis.

James W., Berger , Elston D., Neuhaus, I. Andrews' Diseases of the Skin 12e. Elsevier, 2016. Cutaneous larva migrans.

Elston D., Ferringer, T., Ko, C.J. et al. Dermatopathology. Elsevier, 2019. Nocardia with Fite stain.

ISBN: 978-0-323-56866-1

Library of Congress Control Number: 2019950904

Content Strategist: Charlotta Kryhl
Content Development Specialist: Kim Benson
Project Manager: Louisa Talbott
Design: Miles Hitchen
Marketing Manager: Michele Milano

Working together to grow libraries in developing countries

www.elsevier.com • www.bookaid.org

Last digit is the print number: 9 8 7 6 5 4 3 2 1

Contents

Foreword

There is no doubt that Infectious Diseases is a wonderful specialty for those interested in clinical practice. ID clinicians span the continuum of medicine from research to individual patient care to public health more than any other clinical specialty. The field is continually enriched by innovation in prevention, diagnosis, and therapy. ID clinicians are widely recognized in many settings as the true medical "detectives," solving diagnostic dilemmas that challenge other doctors. For the individual patient, it is becoming clearer that, for complex infections, care by an ID physician can save lives. The field is constantly challenged by the emergence of new entities or by the re-emergence of old enemies, emboldened by antimicrobial resistance. For these emerging infections, ID clinicians sound the alarm, educate the public, define treatment, and help halt the spread of disease. The experience with HIV infection, which was transformed from a universally fatal infection to a manageable chronic condition in the space of a generation, demonstrates the power of medical science, but also the pace of change. And as the recent experiences with Ebola and Zika have shown us, these emerging infections are truly global and require a well-educated and prepared clinical workforce.

While these are undoubtedly exciting times for an ID clinician, they are also daunting for a trainee interested in ID and for an established clinician who wishes to "catch up" on training that occurred years previously. There is a clear need for resources that will aid clinicians in their learning. Certification (and recertification) examinations are one way that modern societies use to demonstrate expertise. It is for this reason I am delighted to support the talented team of editors and contributors who have put this new study guide together. The editors are all young faculty who have recently completed their training and who understand the practicalities of preparing for examinations. They have assembled an impressive international group of authors, to include both current information but also novel "study aids" and sample questions that will allow for self-testing. This was a daunting challenge and congratulations are due to all involved for such an outstanding outcome. I am sure readers will value their effort and will use the book frequently, both in preparing for examinations or for their own teaching.

Bill Powderly

Thank you for picking up our labor of love. We created this book following a clear vision: a resident matching into an Infectious Disease fellowship, and on that day realizing the immense amount of knowledge they now need to acquire. Infectious disease (ID) is by far the largest field of medicine, comprising all the organ systems, all the stages of life, and the largest number of different diagnoses. All of this is compounded by the fact that ID physicians are frequently called upon to be the "disease detectives" in many hospitals and ferret out diseases that are not infectious in nature. It is a scary realization, but at the same time, it is an invitation to a lifetime of learning. We put together this book for that resident, initially to join them as they embark on their fellowship adventure, and then to be referenced during fellowship training so that when the end of fellowship comes, all pages have been read, lovingly dog-eared and underlined or highlighted (or both), and all the questions read and answered a few times over, all in different stages of their evolution as an ID physician. So, as the fellowship ends, all the studying is done, the fellow is now the attending, and the boards hold no fear for them, because they have long been prepared. That was the vision for this book when we first developed it. We made sure that each chapter is written by experts from all aspects of infectious diseases (including Microbiology and Pharmacology), by rising stars in the field who have recently taken the boards and excelled, and by authors who understand the challenges posed by the complexity of this field of study and practice. Our contributors come from all over the world and this gives our book a richer perspective on infectious diseases.

However, as we progressed through the development, we learned that the book can also be uniquely geared for many other groups. It is a great review for those who are to take the boards, both initial and recertification, and only have a few months to prepare. It is a great resource for those who are not in Infectious Disease but wish to learn more about this complex field; a great resource for hospitalists, residents, and medical students who are looking to get better at this, the most pleomorphic of fields. It is a great book for any healthcare professional who treats infections, which at the end of the day, is every one of us.

As a result, the structure of the book evolved to encompass all of those missions. The book is led by the section on high yield microbiology, not because true microbiology questions are common on boards, but because it forms the basis of the field, and makes the learning of the rest of the topics easier. This is followed by the pharmacology section, so that the agents that we use every day in our practice are discussed. The chapters there make for a good read, but for an even better frequent reference. Then Sections 3 and 4 go deep into the meat of the field of infectious disease, discuss syndromes management, and the bulk of infectious disease. Section 5 is focused on specialty topics such as infection prevention, immunizations for adults, bioterrorism, travel medicine, and so on.

Within each section, each chapter is written as a self-contained entity, containing everything you need to master the subject. That means that many topics are repeated in multiple places as topics overlap, but to borrow from the old Latin saying, *repetitio est mater studiorum*. We learn by hearing the same topics from different angles, and each review of the topic and each new angle will reinforce the knowledge until we fully understand it, and we are ready for the questions.

Speaking of board-style questions, the book is chock-full of them. We chose to dedicate so much time and effort into developing questions, that most of them could not even make it into the book. We wrote so many, that we completely exceeded our page budget, but our overzealous dedication to this form of learning is of great benefit to you, the reader. These questions are available in an electronic format, and we anticipate that they will go a long way toward preparing people for their ID boards, as well as teaching some important pearls along the way.

Last but not least, we want to acknowledge that we have undoubtedly made mistakes. We have also made omissions. ID is an incredibly large field, a complex field, and one that is ever changing. Some things will have been true at the writing of this book, but will fail to be true by the time it is published, and even more so by the time you are reading it. That is inevitable. However, that does not mean we cannot put together a safeguard. Therefore, we implore you, our readers, to help us, and your colleagues studying from this book. If you see a mistake, an omission, or simply have a great mnemonic, please contact us via InfectiousDisease Review@gmail.com. Then, when the next edition is being assembled, all of those individual details will be added to the book, and the contributors will be listed in version 2.

So, let me end this the way we began it. Thank you for picking up this book. It has been a labor of love, and we hope it will help you with your studies.

Andrej Spec
Gerome Escota
Courtney Chrisler
Bethany Davies

List of Contributors

Anand Athavale, MBBS
Clinical Fellow
Infectious Diseases and Geographic Medicine
University of Texas Southwestern Medical Center
Dallas, Texas, United States

John W. Baddley, MD, MSPH
Professor
Medicine
University of Alabama at Birmingham
Alabama, United States;
Professor
Medical Service
Birmingham VA Medical Center
Alabama, United States

Thomas Charles Bailey, MD
Professor of Medicine
Division of Infectious Diseases
Washington University in St. Louis School of Medicine
Missouri, United States

Nicolas Barros, MD
Assistant Professor
Division of Infectious Diseases
Indiana University School of Medicine
Indianapolis, Indiana, United States

Merilda Blanco-Guzman, MD
Assistant Professor
Division of Infectious Diseases
Washington University in St. Louis School of Medicine
Missouri, United States

Andres Bran, MD
Assistant Professor of Clinical Medicine
Department of Medicine
University of Missouri
Columbia, Missouri, United States

Greer Burkholder, MD MSPH
University of Alabama at Birmingham
Alabama, United States

Yvonne Burnett, PharmD
Assistant Professor
Pharmacy Practice
St. Louis College of Pharmacy
Missouri, United States;
Clinical Pharmacy Specialist
Division of Infectious Diseases
Washington University in St. Louis School of Medicine
Missouri, United States

Dominick Cavuoti, DO
Professor
Pathology
University of Texas Southwestern Medical Center
Dallas, Texas, United States

Courtney Chrisler, MD
Assistant Professor
Division of Infectious Diseases
Washington University in St. Louis School of Medicine
Missouri, United States

Aoife Cotter, MB BCh, BAO, PhD
Infectious Diseases Consultant
Mater Misericordiae University Hospital & St Vincent's
    University Hospital
Associate Professor in Medicine University College
Dublin, Ireland

James Cutrell, MD
Associate Professor
Division of Infectious Diseases and Geographic Medicine
Department of Internal Medicine
University of Texas Southwestern Medical Center
Dallas, Texas, United States

Bethany Davies, MBBS, MD, FRCPath, MRCP
Senior Lecturer in Infection
Department of Global Health and Infection
Brighton and Sussex Medical School, University of Sussex
United Kingdom

Blachy Javier Dávila Saldaña, MD
Assistant Professor of Pediatrics
George Washington University School of Medicine and
    Health Science
Washington, District of Columbia, United States;
Attending Physician
Division of Blood and Marrow Transplantation
Children's National Medical Center
Washington, District of Columbia, United States

Latesha E. Elopre, MD, MSPH
Assistant Professor of Medicine
Division of Infectious Diseases
University of Alabama at Birmingham
Alabama, United States

Gerome Escota, MD
Assistant Professor of Medicine
Division of Infectious Diseases
Washington University in St. Louis School of Medicine
Missouri, United States

Alice Chi Eziefula, MBBS, MA, MRCP, MRCPath
Senior Lecturer
Department of Global Health and Infection
Brighton and Sussex Medical School, University of Sussex
United Kingdom

Carlos R. Ferreira, MD
Physician
Medical Genetics Branch
National Human Genome Research Institute
Bethesda, Maryland, United States

Jennifer M. Fitzpatrick, BSc (Hons), BM, MRCP, PhD
Specialty Registrar in Infectious Disease and Microbiology
Brighton and Sussex University Hospitals
Royal Sussex County Hospital
United Kingdom

Alison G. Freifeld, MD
Professor
Division of Infectious Diseases
University of Nebraska Medical Center
Omaha, Nebraska, United States

Ige A. George, MD, MS
Assistant Professor
Division of Infectious Diseases
Washington University in St. Louis School of Medicine
Missouri, United States

Stefan George, BSc, MBChB, MRCP
Doctor
Medicine
Brighton and Sussex University Hospitals NHS Trust
United Kingdom

Ronnie M. Gravett, MD, DTM&H
Clinical Instructor
Division of Infectious Diseases
University of Alabama at Birmingham
Alabama, United States

Yasir Hamad, MBBS
Assistant Professor
Division of Infectious Diseases
Washington University in St. Louis School of Medicine
Missouri, United States

Justin F. Hayes, MD
Assistant Professor
Division of Infectious Diseases
University of Arizona College of Medicine
Tucson, Arizona, United States

Phillip Heaton, PhD, D(ABMM)
Technical Director of Microbiology and Molecular
    Diagnostics
Pathology and Laboratory Medicine
Children's Hospitals and Clinics of Minnesota
Minneapolis, Minnesota, United States

German Henostroza, MD
Associate Professor
Medicine, Infectious Diseases
University of Alabama at Birmingham
Alabama, United States

Kevin Hsueh, MD
Assistant Professor
Division of Infectious Diseases
Washington University in St. Louis School of Medicine
Missouri, United States

Bernadette Johnson, BS
Program Director
Division of Infectious Diseases
University of Alabama at Birmingham
Alabama, United States

**Gill Jones, MBBS, BSc, MSc, MRCP (Infectious
    Diseases), FRCPath**
Consultant in Microbiology and Infectious Diseases
Brighton and Sussex University Hospitals
Royal Sussex County Hospital
United Kingdom

Chris Kosmidis, MD, PhD
Senior Lecturer
Division of Infection, Immunity and Respiratory Medicine
University of Manchester
United Kingdom

Jade Le, MD
Infectious Diseases Specialist
Infectious Care Clinic
Texas Health Physicians Group
Dallas, Texas, United States

Francesca Lee, MD
Assistant Professor
Internal Medicine and Pathology
University of Texas, Southwestern
Dallas, Texas, United States

Rachael A. Lee, MD
Assistant Professor
Medicine, Infectious Diseases
University of Alabama at Birmingham
Alabama, United States;
Assistant Professor
Medicine
Birmingham VA Medical Center
Alabama, United States

Stephen Y. Liang, MD, MPHS
Assistant Professor of Medicine
Division of Infectious Diseases
Washington University in St. Louis School of Medicine
Missouri, United States

Todd P. McCarty, BS, MD
Assistant Professor
Medicine, Infectious Diseases
University of Alabama at Birmingham
Alabama, United States;
Attending Physician
Medicine
Birmingham VA Medical Center
Alabama, United States

Carlos R. Mejia-Chew, MD
Instructor in Medicine
Division of Infectious Diseases
Washington University in St. Louis School of Medicine
Missouri, United States

Alfredo J. Mena Lora, MD, FACP
Clinical Assistant Professor
Department of Medicine
University of Illinois at Chicago
Illinois, United States

Rachel C. Moores, BA, BM BCh, PhD
Consultant in Infectious Diseases and Acute Medicine
Royal Free Hospital
London
United Kingdom

Nabeela Mughal, BSc, MBBS, MRCP (Infectious Diseases), MSc (Microbiology) FRCPath, FHEA, PGCert
Infectious Diseases and Microbiology Consultant
Chelsea and Westminster NHS Foundation Trust
Imperial College Healthcare NHS Trust
Honorary Senior Lecturer
Imperial College London
United Kingdom

Jane A. O'Halloran, MB BcH, BAO, PhD
Assistant Professor
Division of Infectious Diseases
Washington University in St Louis School of Medicine
Missouri, United States

Margaret A. Olsen, PhD, MPH
Professor of Medicine
Division of Infectious Diseases
Washington University in St. Louis School of Medicine
Missouri, United States

Jessica K. Ortwine, PharmD
Infectious Diseases Clinical Pharmacy Specialist
Department of Pharmacy
Parkland Health and Hospital System
Texas, United States;
Clinical Assistant Professor
Department of Internal Medicine
University of Texas Southwestern
Texas, United States

Katie Ovens, MBCHB, DTM&H, MRCP
Specialty Registrar
Genitourinary Medicine
Brighton and Sussex University Hospitals NHS Trust
United Kingdom

Edgar Turner Overton, MD
Professor of Medicine, Division of Infectious Diseases
University of Alabama at Birmingham
Alabama, United States

Shadi Parsaei, DO
Infectious Disease Specialist
Infectious Diseases
Norton Healthcare
Louisville, Kentucky, United States

Morgan A. Pence, PhD, D(ABMM)
Clinical Microbiologist
Laboratory and Pathology
Cook Children's Medical Center
Fort Worth, Texas, United States

Joanna Peters, BSc, MBBS, MSc, MRCP,
FRCPath, DTM&H
Doctor
Consultant
Infection Department
St Mary's Hospital, Imperial College Healthcare Trust
London
United Kingdom

Rachel Presti, MD, PhD
Associate Professor
Division of Infectious Diseases
Washington University in St. Louis School of Medicine
Missouri, United States

James R. Price, FRCPath, PhD, MRCP, MBBS, BSc
(Hons)
Clinical Lecturer in Infectious Diseases and Microbiology
Department of Global Health and Infection
Brighton and Sussex Medical School, University of Sussex
United Kingdom

Laurie Proia, MD
Associate Professor of Medicine
Division of Infectious Diseases
Rush Medical College
Chicago, Illinois, United States

Martha Purcell, BSc (Hons), MSc, MBBS, MRCP
Doctor
Microbiology and Infection Department
Royal Sussex County Hospital
Brighton, United Kingdom

Aadia Rana, MD
Associate Professor of Medicine
Division of Infectious Diseases
University of Alabama at Birmingham
Alabama, United States

Krunal Raval, MD
Second Year Fellow
Infectious Diseases
Barnes-Jewish Hospital
St. Louis, Missouri, United States

David J. Ritchie, PharmD, BCPS
Clinical Pharmacy Specialist, Infectious Diseases
Pharmacy
Barnes-Jewish Hospital
St. Louis, Missouri, United States;
Professor
Pharmacy Practice
St. Louis College of Pharmacy
Missouri, United States

Martin Rodriguez, MD
Professor of Medicine
Department of Medicine, Division of Infectious Diseases
University of Alabama at Birmingham
Alabama, United States

Alberto San Francisco Ramos, MB, MRCP, FRCPath
Doctor
Infectious Diseases and Microbiology
Brighton and Sussex University Hospitals
Royal Sussex County Hospital
United Kingdom

Carlos Santos, MD, MPHS
Associate Professor of Medicine
Division of Infectious Disease
Rush University Medical Center
Chicago, Illinois, United States

Tonya Scardina, PharmD, BCPS, BCIDP
Pharmacy Antimicrobial Stewardship Coordinator
Ann and Robert H. Lurie Children's Hospital of Chicago
Illinois, United States

Ilan S. Schwartz, MD, PhD
Assistant Professor
Division of Infectious Diseases
Department of Medicine
Faculty of Medicine & Dentistry
University of Alberta
Edmonton, Alberta, Canada

Hema Sharma, BM, BSc, MSc, PhD, DTM&H,
MRCP(ID), FRCPath
Doctor
Infectious Diseases, Medical Microbiology and Virology
Infectious Diseases and Medical Microbiology
Royal Free Hospital
London
United Kingdom

Racheol Sierra, MBChB, BSc, MRCP, MSc, FRCPath
Consultant Medical
Microbiology and Infectious Diseases
Western Sussex Hospitals NHS Foundation Trust
Worthing, United Kingdom

Andrej Spec, MD, MSCI
Assistant Professor
Division of Infectious Diseases
Washington University in St. Louis School of Medicine
Missouri, United States

Nicholas Van Wagoner, MD, PhD
Associate Professor
Department of Medicine, Division of Infectious Diseases
University of Alabama at Birmingham
Alabama, United States

Paschalis Vergidis, MD, MSc
Assistant Professor of Medicine
Division of Infectious Diseases
Mayo Clinic
Rochester, Minnesota, United States

Meredith Welch, MD
Assistant Professor
Infectious Diseases
University of Alabama at Birmingham
Alabama, United States

Wesley Willeford, MD
Medical Director of Disease Control
Jefferson County Department of Health
Birmingham, Alabama, United States

James Henry Willig, MD, MSPH
Associate Professor
Department of Medicine, Division of Infectious Diseases
University of Alabama at Birmingham
Alabama, United States

Alexandria Wilson, PharmD, BCPS
Associate Professor
Pharmacy Practice
St. Louis College of Pharmacy
Missouri, United States;
Clinical Pharmacy Specialist, Infectious Diseases
Department of Medicine
Washington University in St. Louis School of Medicine
Missouri, United States

Adrienne D. Workman, MD
Fellow
Infectious Diseases
University of Texas Southwestern Medical Center
Dallas, Texas, United States

Andrea J. Zimmer, MD
Assistant Professor
Division of Infectious Diseases
University of Nebraska Medical Center
Omaha, Nebraska, United States

Introduction to the Board Exam

I. Introduction

The Infectious Disease board exam administered by the American Board of Internal Medicine (ABIM) is the capstone that follows your fellowship training to ensure a minimum level of competency to practice as an Infectious Disease physician. Although not perfect, it is the most objective method of assessing medical knowledge and competency.

A maintenance of recertification (MOC) is scheduled every 10 years after you pass the ABIM exam. The purpose of the MOC exam is to ensure that practicing physicians remain updated with current practices and maintain competence in the field. As of writing, ABIM's new two-year assessment option for MOC is not yet available for Infectious Disease.

II. Content and Structure

- Initial certification: 4 sessions, up to 60 questions each (roughly 240 questions)
- MOC: 3 sessions, up to 60 questions each (roughly >180 questions)

Category	% Questions
Bacterial Diseases	27
HIV	15
Antimicrobial Therapy	9
Viral Diseases	7
Travel and Tropical Medicine	5
Fungi	5
Non-HIV Immunocompromised Host	5
Vaccination	4
Infection Control and Prevention	5
General Internal Medicine, Critical Care, and Surgery	18

III. Format

- The boards are a multiple-choice test, mostly case-based, with a single best answer being present in every case.
- You are expected to make a diagnosis, choose or interpret diagnostic tests, or recommend the best treatment (i.e., from a patient scenario that will provide enough clues to a diagnosis).
- Questions on the underlying pathophysiology (i.e., basic science) of an infectious process are also sometimes asked.
- Clinical images of physical exam findings, radiographs, Gram stains, histopathology, and other features seen on microscopy are very common and high yield in the board exam.
- Expect that some questions will be long and can contain several exposure histories that may or may not be related to the best answer to the question. These often serve as distractors, and differential should be narrowed using epidemiology, lab testing, and incubation periods.

These questions go through a significant vetting process before they are used for scoring. In other words, the first time the question appears on the board exam, they are being used to test their performance, not yours. Exam questions that are too difficult or too easy, or that performed differently from the last time they were used, undergo post-test validation. This process can lead to:

1. Keep the answer/question as is.
2. Change the actual answer from what was originally keyed.
3. Make more than one answer correct (e.g., choice A and B as part of the choices).
4. Make all answers correct (all of the above choice).

These questions are then removed from the question pool and will not be counted to the examinee's score.

Some questions may just be too difficult, or too ambiguous (i.e., impossible to choose the best answer), or require knowledge of very recent data (i.e., from a recent major publication, recent basic science finding, very new antibiotics). These questions are *probably* being pretested and may not count in the end. Pretested questions are determined based on statistical performance criteria before they are included into the actual pool of questions in the next exam cycles. In other words, if the question appears to be impossible, there is a good chance it is not going to count toward your score.

IV. Blueprint

The American Board of Internal Medicine (ABIM) creates and annually updates a blueprint to serve as a guide for examinees on what to expect for the board exam. For more information, you can download the blueprint at: http://www.abim.org/about/exam-information/exam-blueprints.aspx (choose Infectious Disease from the drop-down menu, one for initial certification and for MOC).

We have ensured that this book covers 100% of the topics listed in the blueprint.

V. The Big Day

The test is usually scheduled in the fall (around November) each year. Check https://www.abim.org/certification/exam-information/infectious-disease/exam-content.aspx for more information. There are a few tips to make your exam day go smoothly:

- Make sure to arrive 30 minutes before the start of the exam. You may not be admitted if you arrive after the appointment time.
- Get familiarized with the testing center (i.e., how to get there, parking lot, nearby restaurants) days or weeks before your exam date.
- Remember to bring two valid and current identification cards:
  - Primary: government-issued; has your photograph and signature (e.g., driver's license, passport, state identification cards)
  - Secondary: has either your photograph or your signature (e.g., Social Security card, credit card, ATM card)
  - Note: name on your cards must match the name you provided to ABIM
- All personal items (e.g., cell phone, laptop, tablet, watch, wallet, bag, calculator, pager) are not allowed inside the test center. You will be provided with individual lockers to store them before the start of the exam. The test center, however, will not assume responsibility for any of your personal items. The lockers may be relatively small, so do not bring a book bag, large books, etc.
- You can bring food/drinks; however, test centers will not provide refrigeration or lounge facilities where you can eat, and you cannot bring them in with you to the testing room.
- Other items that are not allowed: jackets/coats, notebooks, pens, or pencils.
  - Do bring a thicker shirt or sweater and put it in your locker. Some of the testing centers can be chilly, and there is no reason to suffer. You can change during session breaks but are not usually allowed to dress and undress in the exam room.
- An erasable notepad and an earphone/headphone will be provided to each examinee for note taking and noise isolation, respectively.
- Essential medical items (e.g., supplies for diabetes, nitroglycerin) can be brought inside the test center, but you will need to submit a request to the ABIM beforehand.
  - If you require such items, it may be wise to contact the specific center where you will be taking the exam ahead of time to ensure that your exam day proceeds smoothly.
- You can raise your hand to notify the exam administrator if you need any assistance, for example, if you need your monitor adjusted or if you need to leave the test center for any reason.
- There are scheduled breaks after each session. Taking these breaks is optional. You can move on to the next session if you opt not to take the break. However, with over 240 questions, burnout is a serious problem. Spacing your day and stretching your muscles, and maybe even fresh air, can go a long way toward making the process easier.
- Contact ABIM for any other questions – details via visit their website https://www.abim.org/contact.aspx.

VI. Passing Score and Passing Rates

- Your score will be reported on a standardized score scale that ranges from 200 to 800.

- A standardized passing score is determined by the ABIM according to a special evidence-based method. This involves dozens of exam raters who give each question a score depending on what they think is the probability that a specialist who is just barely qualified to pass the boards will correctly answer the question. The raters' scores for all the questions are then averaged and a standardized passing score is determined. This score is reviewed every few years to determine its appropriateness. To pass, your standardized score must be equal or greater than the standardized passing score.
- Pass rates for first time takers are:

	2014	2015	2016	2017	2018
Initial certification	88%	94%	98%	97%	98%
MOC	91%	89%	94%	90%	93%

VII. Tips

- Read this book not only once but try to cover as much of it as you can at least twice. Repetition reinforces learning and facilitates memorization of key concepts.
- Preparing for the board exam starts during your first day of fellowship training or even earlier.
- Do not rely on your memory. Write clinical pearls and learning points you get from your attendings, your readings, and lectures. You will find that going through these notes over time will help you not just prepare for the board exam but take care of actual patients.
- If you get a question wrong, or if a concept in this book seems unfamiliar to you, write it down in a separate place, and revisit that often. By doing that, you will create your own high yield study aide.
- As the board exam date nears, create a realistic review schedule that works for you.
- It is important to cover board review questions that mimic the actual exam (such as the ones provided in this book, and the associated online extension). Try answering it on your own. If you do not get the answer correctly, read the explanation that comes after the question and take down notes. Review these notes one more time so that concepts stick in your head.
- Practicing for the exam using the ABIM Certification tutorial acquaints you to how the board exam is actually conducted and what the computer screen would look like. You can access the tutorial here: https://www.abim.org/certification/exam-information/internal-medicine/exam-tutorial.aspx. However, it is near identical to the test you took for Internal Medicine, so if you are short on time, and still familiar with how it looked from that exam, you may not need to devote time to this.
- Know your strengths and weaknesses. Address your weaknesses head on and plan ahead. For example, if you think your knowledge base is poor on infection control and prevention despite your attempts at reviewing it, try to cover this topic one more time a few days before the exam.
- Do not cram! Make sure you have enough time to do second reading. We can't stress this enough.

Resources

More information about the board exam can be found in www. abim.org.

Helpful websites that will give you more tips on how to study for the board exam:

https://knowledgeplus.nejm.org/how-we-help/board-review-study-tips/.

https://knowledgeplus.nejm.org/blog/10-mistakes-studying-for-the-boards/.

https://knowledgeplus.nejm.org/blog/strategies-working-abim-board-questions/.

Abbreviations

AB antibiotic
ABSSSI acute bacterial skin and skin structure infection
ACV aciclovir
ADR adverse drug reaction
AFB acid-fact bacilli
AKI acute kidney injury
ALP alkaline phosphatase
ALT alanine aminotransferase
AmB amphotericin B
ANC absolute neutrophil count
ANS autonomic nervous system
ARDS acute respiratory distress syndrome
ART antiretroviral therapy
ASC antimicrobial stewardship committees
AST antimicrobial susceptibility testing
AST aspartate aminotransferase
AUC area under the curve
BAL bronchoalveolar lavage
BBB blood–brain barrier
BCG Bacille Calmette–Guérin
BHIVA British HIV Association
BMT bone marrow transplantation
BSE bovine spongiform encephalopathy
BSI bloodstream infection
BUN blood urea nitrogen
BV bacterial vaginosis
CAP community-acquired pneumonia
CAUTI catheter-associated urinary tract infections
CBC complete blood count
CF complement fixation
CFU colony forming unit
CIED cardiac implanted electronic device
CJD Creutzfeldt–Jakob disease
CK creatine kinase
CKD chronic kidney disease
CLABSI central line-associated bloodstream infections
CLM cutaneous larva migrans
CMI cell-mediated immunity
CMV cytomegalovirus
CNNA culture-negative neutrocytic ascites
CNS central nervous system
CoNS coagulase-negative staphylococci
CPE cytopathogenic effect
CRAG cryptococcal antigen
CrCl creatinine clearance
CRP C-reactive protein
CRS congenital rubella syndrome
CSF cerebrospinal fluid
CT computed tomography

CVC central venous catheter
CXR chest x-ray
DEET diethyltoluamide
DFA direct fluorescent antibody
DIC disseminated intravascular coagulation
EBV Epstein–Barr virus
ECG electrocardiogram
EIA enzyme-linked immunoassay
EIR entomological inoculation rate
ELISA enzyme-linked immunosorbent assay
EPPs exposure-prone procedures
ERCP endoscopic retrograde cholangiopancreatography
ESR erythrocyte sedimentation rate
EVD external ventricular drain
FBC full blood count
FLQ fluoroquinolones
FVS fetal varicella syndrome
GAS group A streptococcus
GBS group B streptococcus
GCS Glasgow Coma Score
GDH glutamate dehydrogenase
GI gastrointestinal
GNR gram-negative rod
GPR gram-positive rod
GVHD graft versus host disease
H&E hematoxylin and eosin (stain)
HAART highly active antiretroviral therapy
HACEK *Haemophilus, Aggregatibacter, Cardiobacterium, Eikenella corrodens, Kingella*
HAI hospital-acquired infections
HAV hepatitis A virus
HBIG hepatitis B immunoglobulin
HBsAg hepatitis B surface antigen
HBV hepatitis B virus
HCC hepatocellular carcinoma
HCW healthcare worker
HFMD hand, foot, and mouth disease
HHV human herpesvirus
Hib Haemophilus influenzae type b
HIV human immunodeficiency virus
HNIG human normal immunoglobulin
HPLC high-performance liquid chromatography
HPV human papilloma virus
HRT hormone replacement therapy
HSCT hematopoietic stem cell transplantation
HSE herpes simplex encephalitis
HSV herpes simplex virus
HVAC heating, ventilation, and air conditioning
IBS irritable bowel syndrome

ICP intracranial pressure
IDSA Infectious Diseases Society of America
IDU intravenous drug use(r)
IGRA interferon gamma release assay
IM infectious mononucleosis
INR international normalized ratio
IP intraperitoneal
IPV inactivated polio vaccine
IUD intrauterine device
IUFD intrauterine fetal death
IUGR intrauterine growth restriction
IV intravenous
IVDU intravenous drug use/user
IVIG intravenous immunoglobulin
JEV Japanese encephalitis virus
LCMV lymphocytic choriomeningitis virus
LFTs liver function tests
LMWH low molecular weight heparin
LP lumbar puncture
LTBI latent TB infection
LUQ left upper quadrant
LVAD left ventricular assist device
MAC *Mycobacterium avium* complex
MAIC *Mycobacterium avium-intracellulare* complex
MALDI-TOF matrix-assisted laser desorption/ionization
    time of flight
MASCC Multinational Association of Supportive Care in
    Cancer
MCL mucocutaneous leishmaniasis
MCS mechanical circulatory support
MDDR molecular detection of drug resistance
MDR multidrug-resistant
MDRO multidrug-resistant organisms
MDR-TB multidrug-resistant tuberculosis
MERS Middle East respiratory syndrome
MI myocardial infarction
MIC minimum inhibitory concentration
MMR measles. mumps, and rubella (vaccine)
MNBA monomicrobial non-neutrocytic bacterascites
MRI magnetic resonance imaging.
MRSA methicillin-resistant *Staphylococcus aureus*
MSM men who have sex with men
MSSA methicillin-susceptible *Staphylococcus aureus*
MTBC *Mycobacterium tuberculosis* complex
MTCT mother-to-child transmission
NAAT nucleic acid amplification test
NASH nonalcoholic steatohepatitis
NGU nongonococcal urethritis
NNRTI nonnucleoside reverse transcriptase inhibitors
NRTI nucleoside reverse transcriptase inhibitors
NSAIDs nonsteroidal antiinflammatory drugs
NTM nontuberculous mycobacteria
OI opportunistic infection
OPV oral polio vaccine
PCP *Pneumocystis* pneumonia
PCR polymerase chain reaction
PD peritoneal dialysis

PD pharmacodynamic
PET positron emission tomography
PHA polymicrobial bacterascites
PID pelvic inflammatory disease
PIV parainfluenza virus
PJP *Pneumocystis jirovecii* pneumonia
PK pharmacokinetic
PML progressive multifocal leukoencephalopathy
PMN polymorphonuclear leukocyte
PO per os
PPD purified protein derivative
PPH postpartum hemorrhage
PPROM preterm premature rupture of membranes
PrP prion-related protein
PWLH people living with HI infection
RGM rapidly growing mycobacteria
RUQ right upper quadrant
SARS severe acute respiratory syndrome
SCID severe combined immunodeficiency
SCr serum creatinine
SGM slowly growing mycobacteria
SIR standardized infection ratio
SLE systemic lupus erythematosus
SLEV St. Louis encephalitis virus
SOT solid organ transplant
SSI surgical site infection
SSPE subacute sclerosing panencephalitis
SSTI skin and soft tissue infection
STI sexually transmitted infection
SVR sustained virologic response
T liver function test
TAF tenofovir alafenamide
TB tuberculosis
TBM tuberculous meningitis
TDF tenofovir disoproxil fumarate
TDM therapeutic drug monitoring
TEE transesophageal echocardiography
TMP–SMX trimethoprim–sulfamethoxazole
TNF tumor necrosis factor
TSEs transmissible spongiform encephalopathies
TST tuberculin skin test
ULN upper limit of normal
UTI urinary tract infection
UV ultraviolet
VA ventriculo-atrial
VAE ventilator-associated event
VAP ventilator-associated pneumonia
VCL visceral leishmaniasis
VIN vulvar intraepithelial neoplasia
VLM visceral larva migrans
VP ventriculo-peritoneal
VZIG varicella-zoster immunoglobulin
VZV varicella-zoster virus
WCC white cell count
WNV West Nile virus
XDR extensively drug-resistant

1

Bacteriology

MORGAN A. PENCE

Definitions

Aerobe: an organism that lives and grows in the presence of oxygen.

Aerotolerant anaerobe: an organism that shows significantly better growth in the absence of oxygen but may show limited growth in the presence of oxygen (e.g., *Clostridium tertium*, many *Actinomyces* spp.).

Anaerobe: an organism that can live in the absence of oxygen.

Bacillus/bacilli: rod-shaped bacteria (e.g., gram-negative bacilli); not to be confused with the genus *Bacillus*.

Coccus/cocci: spherical/round bacteria.

Coryneform: "club-shaped" or resembling Chinese letters; description of a Gram stain morphology consistent with *Corynebacterium* and related genera.

Diphtheroid: clinical microbiology-speak for coryneform gram-positive rods (*Corynebacterium* and related genera).

Gram-negative: bacteria that do not retain the purple color of the crystal violet in the Gram stain due to the presence of a thin peptidoglycan cell wall; gram-negative bacteria appear pink due to the safranin counter stain.

Gram-positive: bacteria that retain the purple color of the crystal violet in the Gram stain due to the presence of a thick peptidoglycan cell wall.

Gram-variable: bacteria that partially retain the purple color of the crystal violet in the Gram stain; most commonly seen with *Bacillus* spp., *Clostridium* spp., *Acinetobacter* spp., *Streptococcus pneumoniae*.

Microaerophile: an organism that requires a low level of oxygen for growth, increased oxygen may inhibit growth (e.g., *Campylobacter* spp.).

Nonfermenters: gram-negative rods that do not utilize glucose for growth (e.g., *Pseudomonas*, *Achromobacter*, *Acinetobacter*, etc.). *Note:* Nonfermenters are *not* the same as non-lactose-fermenting gram-negative rods (referring to the lack of reaction/lactose utilization on MacConkey or other lactose-containing agar). The two terms are sometimes used interchangeably, which is incorrect.

Obligate aerobe: an organism that grows only in the presence of oxygen (e.g., *Pseudomonas aeruginosa*).

Obligate/strict anaerobe: an organism that grows only in the absence of oxygen (e.g., *Bacteroides fragilis*).

Spirochete: spiral-shaped bacterium; neither gram-positive nor gram-negative.

Gram Stain

- Principal stain used in bacteriology.
- Distinguishes gram-positive bacteria from gram-negative bacteria.

Method

- A portion of a specimen or bacterial growth is applied to a slide and dried.
- Specimen is fixed to slide by methanol (preferred) or heat (can distort morphology).
- Crystal violet is added to the slide.
- Iodine is added and forms a complex with crystal violet that binds to the thick peptidoglycan layer of gram-positive cell walls.
- Acetone-alcohol solution is added, which washes away the crystal violet–iodine complexes in gram-negative cells walls due to thin layer of peptidoglycan.
- Safranin counter-stain is added to stain gram-negative bacteria.
- Slide is viewed on low power to quantitate polymorphonuclear cells (PMNs) and epithelial cells and on high power to quantitate bacteria.

Classification of Bacteria

Classification is based on growth pattern (aerobic vs. anaerobic), Gram stain reaction, and morphology (Figs. 1.1–1.3, Tables 1.1 and 1.2).

Blood Cultures

Collection

- Proper skin preparation/disinfection is essential to prevent contaminated blood cultures.
- One blood culture set is composed of one aerobic bottle and one anaerobic bottle.

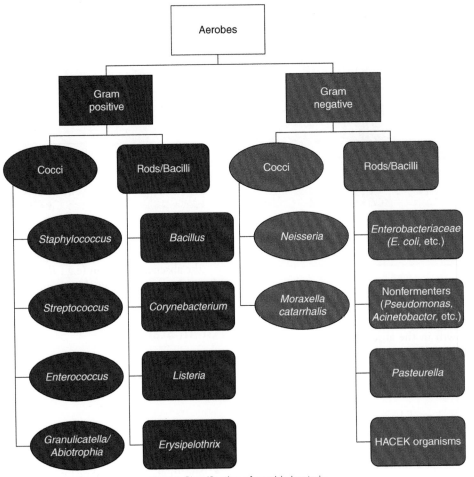

• **Fig. 1.1** Classification of aerobic bacteria.

• Even if anaerobes are low on differential, an anaerobic bottle should still be collected. → Most bacteria grow faster in the anaerobic bottle.
• Collect ≥2 sets from separate sites before administration of antibiotics.
  • Collect up to three blood cultures per day if intermittent bacteremia is suspected (due to undrained abscesses, etc.).

Volume

Volume is the **most important factor** for successful blood cultures.
• Most septic patients have 1–5 CFU/mL in their blood.
• Bacteremia may be missed by drawing too little blood.
• Adults: 20 mL should be collected per set (10 mL per bottle).
• Pediatrics: Weight-based and age-based guidelines exist.
  • Weight-based guidelines recommend collecting 1%–4% of the patient's total blood volume.
  • If pediatric bottles are used, a maximum of 5 mL can be added to each bottle.

Interpretation

• Common contaminants
  • Anaerobic gram-positive cocci.

• *Bacillus.*
• Coagulase-negative staphylococci (not *Staphylococcus lugdunensis*).
• Coryneform gram-positive rods.
• Nonpathogenic *Neisseria.*
• Viridans group streptococci (more likely to be true pathogens in hematology/oncology patients).
• Organisms associated with gastrointestinal neoplasia
  • *Streptococcus gallolyticus, Streptococcus infantarius, Streptococcus alactolyticus, Streptococcus lutetiensis, Streptococcus equinus* (formerly *Streptococcus bovis* group).
  • *Clostridium septicum*
    • Also associated with hematologic malignancy.
    • Swarming morphology on agar.
• Causes of false-negative blood cultures
  • Too little volume collected.
  • Administration of antimicrobials prior to collection.
  • Organism that does not grow in standard blood culture bottles (*Bartonella*, etc.).

Specimens for Bacteriology Culture

• The success of a culture depends on the quality of the specimen submitted!
• Garbage in → garbage out.

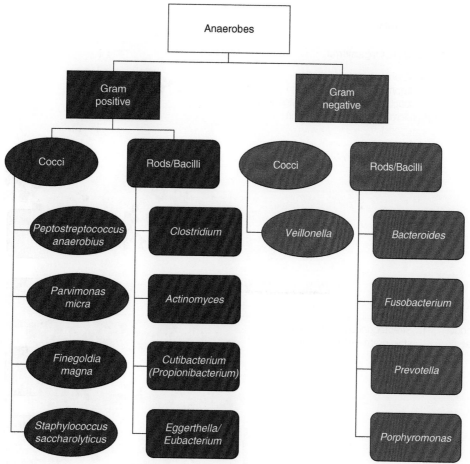

• **Fig. 1.2** Classification of anaerobic bacteria.

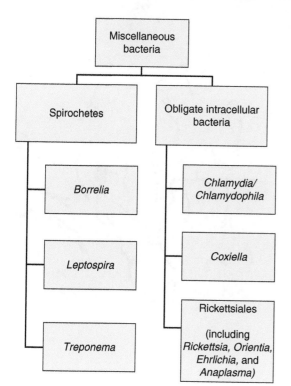

• **Fig. 1.3** Classification of miscellaneous bacteria.

Routine Cultures

- The more specimen, the better!
  - There is a common misconception that the microbiology lab only needs a small amount of specimen.
- Tissues and aspirates/fluids are preferred over swabs.
- If a swab is the only option, a flocked swab, such as the ESwab, is preferred.
  - Traditional rayon swabs only release 3 of every 100 bacteria onto a plate.
- For wound specimens, attention to skin decontamination is critical.
  - Specimens should be taken from the advancing margin of the lesion.
- Do not send superficial swabs of decubitus ulcers.

Anaerobic Cultures

- Sites with normal anaerobic flora are not appropriate for anaerobic culture. Examples include, but are not limited to:
  - Mouth.
  - Throat and nasopharyngeal swabs.
  - Stool.

TABLE 1.1	**Gram Stain Interpretation**	
Gram Stain Result	**Possible Organisms**	**Figures**
Gram-positive cocci in clusters	1. *Staphylococcus* (including *Staphylococcus aureus* and coagulase-negative staphylococci) 2. *Micrococcus* (often found in tetrads) 3. *Aerococcus* 4. *Rothia* (formerly *Stomatococcus*)	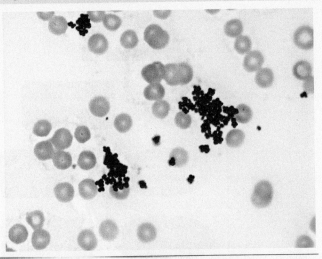
Gram-positive cocci in pairs (lancet-shaped)	1. *Streptococcus pneumoniae* (may stain gram-variable or gram-negative)	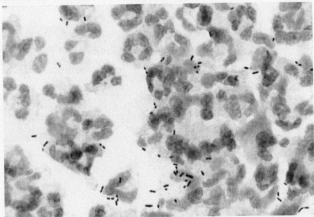
Gram-positive cocci in pairs and chains	1. Viridans group streptococci (including some isolates of *S. pneumoniae*) 2. Beta-hemolytic streptococci (e.g., *Streptococcus pyogenes*) 3. *Enterococcus* 4. *Abiotrophia* and *Granulicatella* (formerly known as nutritionally variant streptococci)	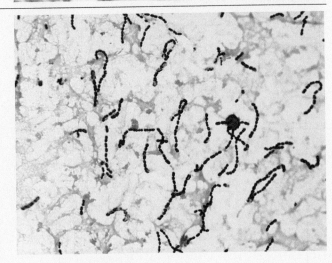

Continued

TABLE 1.1   Gram Stain Interpretation—cont'd

Gram Stain Result	Possible Organisms	Figures
Gram-positive rods – regular	1. *Bacillus* (may be big and boxy, may have spores) 2. *Clostridium* (may be big and boxy, may have spores) 3. *Listeria* (may appear coccobacillary) 4. *Lactobacillus* 5. *Eggerthella*	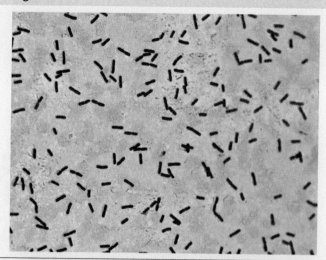
Gram-positive rods – coryneform	1. *Corynebacterium* 2. *Cutibacterium* (formerly *Propionibacterium*) 3. *Actinomyces* (sulfur granules may be seen on histopathology) 4. *Erysipelothrix*	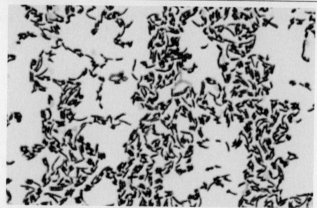
Beaded gram-positive rods	1. *Mycobacterium* 2. *Nocardia* 3. *Actinomyces* (beaded morphology is more commonly seen on histopathology)	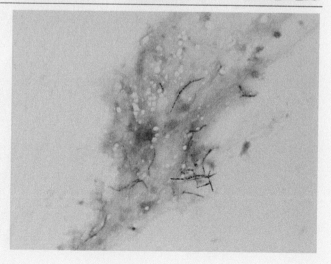

Continued

TABLE 1.1	Gram Stain Interpretation—cont'd	
Gram Stain Result	**Possible Organisms**	**Figures**
Branching, filamentous gram-positive rods	1. *Nocardia* 2. *Streptomyces* 3. *Gordonia* 4. *Tsukamurella*	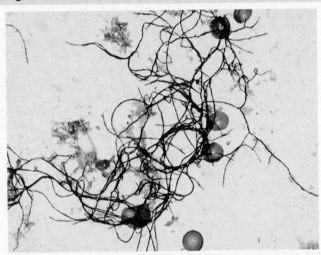
Gram-variable rods	1. *Bacillus* (and related genera: *Paenibacillus*, *Lysinibacillus*) 2. *Clostridium* 3. *Gardnerella vaginalis* 4. Leptotrichia	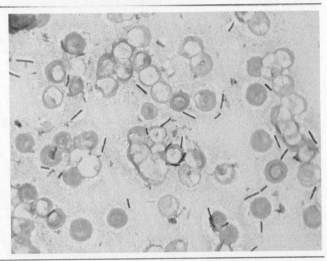
Gram-negative cocci	1. *Veillonella* 2. *Acidaminococcus* 3. *Megasphaera*	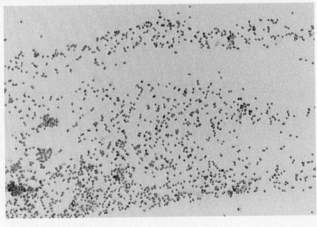

TABLE 1.1   **Gram Stain Interpretation—cont'd**

Gram Stain Result	Possible Organisms	Figures
Gram-negative diplococci	1. *Neisseria* (including *Neisseria meningitidis* and *Neisseria gonorrhoeae*) 2. *Moraxella catarrhalis*	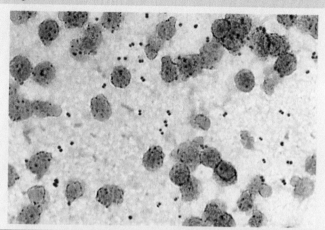
Gram-negative coccobacilli	1. *Haemophilus* 2. *Acinetobacter* (may stain gram-variable) 3. *Aggregatibacter* 4. *Moraxella* 5. *Pasteurella multocida* 6. *Bacteroides* 7. *Francisella tularensis* (tularemia) 8. *Brucella*	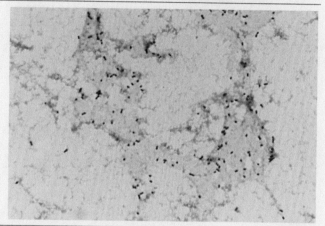
Tiny gram-negative rods/"junky" Gram stain	1. *Francisella tularensis* (tularemia) 2. *Brucella*	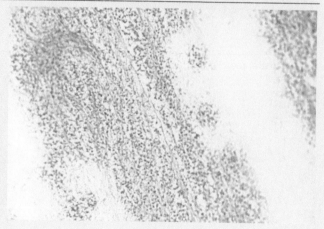

Continued

TABLE 1.1	Gram Stain Interpretation—cont'd	
Gram Stain Result	**Possible Organisms**	**Figures**
Gram-negative rods	1. *Enterobacteriaceae* 2. Nonfermenters (i.e., *Pseudomonas, Achromobacter, Acinetobacter*, etc.) 3. HACEK organisms 4. *Pasteurella* 5. Anaerobic gram-negative rods 6. *Bacillus* (although gram-positive, it can stain gram-variable or gram-negative) 7. *Clostridium* (although gram-positive, it can stain gram-variable or gram-negative)	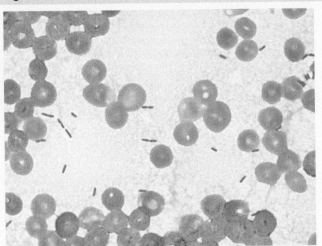
Gram-negative rods – fusiform	1. *Fusobacterium nucleatum* 2. *Leptotrichia* 3. *Capnocytophaga*	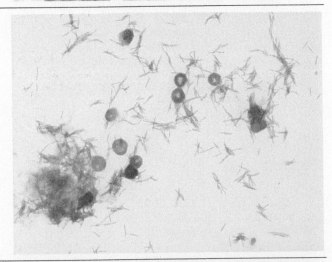
Gram-negative rods – curved	1. *Campylobacter* 2. *Helicobacter* 3. *Arcobacter* 4. *Anaerobiospirillum* 5. *Vibrio* (comma-shaped)	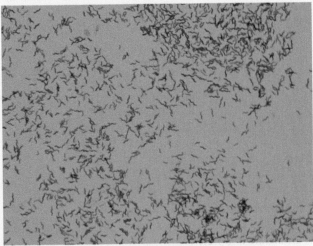

(From Inokuchi R, Ishida T, Maeda J, Nakajima S, Yahagi N, Matsumoto A. *Am J Emerg Med.* 2014;32(7):812e.1.)

HACEK, *Haemophilus, Aggregatibacter, Cardiobacterium, Eikenella corrodens, Kingella.*

TABLE 1.2	Gram Stain Buzzwords
When You Hear This	**Think This**
Gram-negative diplococci – CSF	*Neisseria meningitidis*
Gram-negative diplococci – genital source, urine, joint fluid	*Neisseria gonorrhoeae*
Gram-negative diplococci – respiratory source	*Moraxella catarrhalis*
Big and boxy	*Bacillus* *Clostridium*
Gram-variable	*Acinetobacter* *Bacillus* *Clostridium* *Leptotrichia* *Streptococcus pneumoniae*
Lancet-shaped	*S. pneumoniae*
Seagull-shaped/gull wings	*Campylobacter*
Spores	*Bacillus* and related genera (*Paenibacillus, Lysinibacillus*) *Clostridium*
Tiny gram-negative rods	*Brucella* *Francisella*

TABLE 1.3	Notable Nomenclature Changes/ Reclassifications
Former Name	**Current Name**
Actinobacillus actinomycetemcomitans	*Aggregatibacter actinomycetemcomitans*
Actinobaculum schaalii	*Actinotignum schaalii*
Bacteroides distasonis	*Parabacteroides distasonis*
Clostridium difficile	*Clostridioides difficile*
Enterobacter aerogenes	*Klebsiella aerogenes* (Be careful: intrinsic resistance is still the same as *Enterobacter* spp.)
Enterobacter amnigenus	*Lelliottia amnigena*
Enterobacter gergoviae	*Pluralibacter gergoviae*
Haemophilus aphrophilus	*Aggregatibacter aphrophilus*
Haemophilus segnis	*Aggregatibacter segnis*
Peptostreptococcus spp. (only *Peptostreptococcus* remaining is *P. anaerobius*)	*Anaerococcus* *Atopobium* *Finegoldia magna* *Parvimonas micra* *Peptoniphilus* *Slackia*
Propionibacterium acnes	*Cutibacterium acnes*
Streptococcus "milleri" group (never a confirmed taxonomic name)	*Streptococcus anginosus* group (composed of *S. anginosus, Streptococcus intermedius, Streptococcus constellatus*)

- Superficial wound specimens, including superficial decubitus ulcer specimens.
- Urine (unless collected by suprapubic aspirate).
- Vaginal and cervical swabs.
- The following specimens are acceptable for anaerobic culture:
  - Blood.
  - Deep wounds/abscesses collection by aspirate or surgically.
  - Deep sinus specimens.
  - Sterile body fluids.
  - Tissues.

Anaerobic Transport

- To ensure recovery of anaerobes, specimens submitted for anaerobic culture must be transported to the lab in anaerobic transport:
  - Anaerobic transport vials.
  - Capped syringe with air removed.
  - Tissue specimens that are 1 cm³ or larger can be submitted in a sterile cup.
  - Swabs are not preferred, but if necessary, an anaerobic swab must be used.

Stool Cultures

- Stool must be placed into Cary–Blair or modified Cary–Blair transport media immediately upon passage.

- Stool pathogens begin to die within minutes of passage.
- If raw stool is submitted, sensitivity is decreased, especially for *Shigella* and *Campylobacter*.

Pathogen Associations

Arthropod-Borne Pathogens (Table 1.7)

- Clinically important arthropod vectors include fleas, lice, mites, and ticks.
- Arthropods can transmit a variety of microorganisms, including bacteria, viruses, and parasites.

Biothreat (BT) Agents (Table 1.8)

- Due to the highly infectious nature of these organisms, the clinical microbiology laboratory should be notified when a biothreat agent is suspected. The lab can then take the necessary precautions to prevent exposure of laboratory personnel to the infectious agent.

TABLE 1.4	Routine Bacteriologic Media – Aerobic Cultures		
Media/Primary Use	**What Grows?**		**What Doesn't Grow**
Blood agar/demonstration of hemolysis	Majority of pathogens – gram-positive and gram-negative		• *Haemophilus* • Some *Aggregatibacter* spp. • Some *Neisseria gonorrhoeae* isolates • *Francisella* • *Granulicatella/Abiotrophia* • Organisms that do not grow in routine bacterial cultures (Table 1.14)
Chocolate agar	Almost all organisms, including fastidious organisms Organisms that grow only on chocolate agar: • *Haemophilus* • Some *Aggregatibacter* spp. • Some *N. gonorrhoeae* isolates • *Francisella* • *Granulicatella/Abiotrophia*		• Some *Corynebacterium* do not grow as well on chocolate agar as on blood agar • Organisms that do not grow in routine bacterial cultures (Table 1.14)

MacConkey agar/Lactose-fermentation	Nonfastidious gram-negative rods
	• *Enterobacteriaceae*
	• Most nonfermenters
			• Gram-positive organisms (some *Bacillus* may have breakthrough growth)
			• Fastidious gram-negative organisms, including, but not limited to:
			  • *Brucella*
			  • HACEK organisms
			  • *Francisella*
			  • *Moraxella*
			  • *Neisseria*
			  • *Pasteurella*

- Most clinical labs are "sentinel labs," and it is their job to "recognize, rule out, and refer" any suspected BT agent. If a BT agent cannot be ruled out, the isolate should be sent to the local public health lab.
- Sentinel labs should not attempt to definitively identify suspected BT agents.
  - Suspected BT agents should *not* be subjected to MALDI-TOF or tested on automated identification platforms (see Identification section below).

Important Pathogens in Bite Wounds (Human or Animal)

- Anaerobic oral flora (*Prevotella*, etc.).
- *Eikenella*.
- *Pasteurella*.
- *Staphylococcus intermedius/pseudintermedius*.
- *Streptococcus anginosus* group.

Important Bacterial Pathogens in Culture-Negative Endocarditis

- HACEK organisms (less likely to be culture-negative due to good recovery in current blood culture systems)
  - *Haemophilus*.
  - *Aggregatibacter*.
  - *Cardiobacterium*.
  - *Eikenella corrodens*.
  - *Kingella*.
- *Bartonella*.
- *Brucella*.
- *Chlamydia/Chlamydophila*.
- *Coxiella burnetii*.
- *Legionella*.
- *Mycoplasma*.
- *Tropheryma whipplei*.

Important Pathogens in Cystic Fibrosis Patients

- *Staphylococcus aureus*.
- *Achromobacter* spp.
- *Burkholderia cepacia*.
- *Inquilinus limosus*.
- *Pandoraea* spp.
- *P. aeruginosa*.
- *Stenotrophomonas maltophilia*.
- Other nonfermenters

Important Pathogens in Otitis Media

- Anaerobes.
- *Enterobacteriaceae* (neonates).

TABLE 1.5 Biochemical Characteristics

Biochemical	Positive	Negative
Alpha-hemolysis (greening of the agar)	• Viridans group streptococci (including *Streptococcus pneumoniae*) • Some enterococci	• *Staphylococcus*
Beta-hemolysis	• *Staphylococcus aureus* • Beta-hemolytic streptococci • *Clostridium perfringens* (double zone of hemolysis) • *Aeromonas* • *Escherichia coli* • *Pseudomonas aeruginosa*	• Most coagulase-negative staphylococci • Viridans group streptococci (with the exception of *S. anginosus* group, which can be beta-hemolytic)
Catalase (used primarily for gram-positives)	• *Staphylococcus* • *Bacillus* • *Corynebacterium*	• *Enterococcus* • *Streptococcus* • *Aerococcus* • *Actinomyces* • *Clostridium*
Coagulase	• *S. aureus* • *Staphylococcus intermedius* • *Staphylococcus pseudintermedius* • *Staphylococcus schleiferi*	• All other *Staphylococcus* spp.
Oxidase (gram-negatives)	• *Aeromonas* • *Moraxella* • *Neisseria* • *Pasteurella* • *Plesiomonas shigelloides* • *Pseudomonas* (except *P. luteola* and *P. oryzihabitans*)	• All Enterobacteriaceae except *P. shigelloides* • *Acinetobacter* • *Stenotrophomonas maltophilia*
Indole (gram-negatives)	• *Aeromonas* • *E. coli* • *Morganella morganii* • *Plesiomonas shigelloides* • *Proteus vulgaris* • *Providencia* • *Pasteurella*	• *Acinetobacter* • *Pseudomonas*

- *Haemophilus influenzae.*
- *Moraxella catarrhalis.*
- *P. aeruginosa.*
- *S. aureus.*
- *S. pneumoniae.*
- *S. pyogenes.*

Emerging Pathogens (Table 1.9)

- Several "emerging" pathogens have been reported in recent years.
- While some of the organisms may truly represent emerging pathogens, it is likely that many of the organisms were previously misidentified due to the limitations of biochemical identification methods.

Zoonotic Pathogens (Table 1.10)

- Zoonoses are infections that are naturally transmitted between animals and humans.

- In addition to the bacterial zoonotic pathogens in Table 1.10, many viruses, fungi, and parasites also cause zoonoses.

Gastrointestinal Infections

Foodborne Illness: Bacterial Associations (Table 1.11)

- Many bacteria and bacterial toxins are associated with contaminated or undercooked foods.
- The CDC estimates that there are 48 million cases of foodborne illness each year, resulting in 128,000 hospitalizations and 3,000 deaths.

Stool Pathogens

- Stool culture is the gold standard but is being replaced by culture-independent tests such as antigen testing and molecular testing.
- If using culture, check with performing lab to see which pathogens are being screened.

TABLE 1.6 **Biochemical Buzzwords**

When You Hear This:	Picture This:	Think This:
Gram-negative rod – • Beta-hemolytic • Metallic sheen • Green pigment on MacConkey agar • Oxidase positive	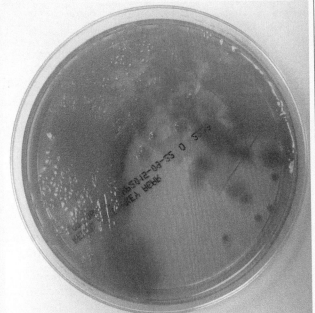 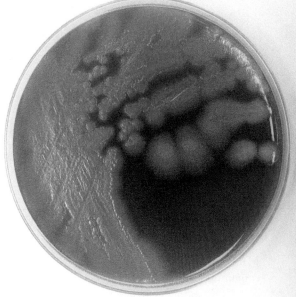	*Pseudomonas aeruginosa*
Gram-negative rod – • Beta-hemolytic • Oxidase negative • Indole positive • Lactose fermenting	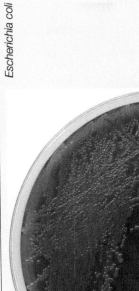 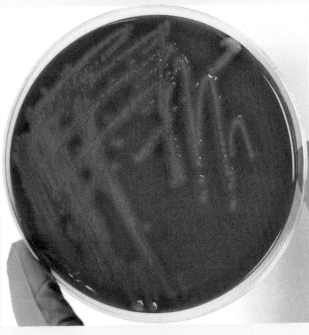	*Escherichia coli*

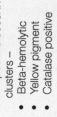

TABLE 1.6 **Biochemical Buzzwords—cont'd**

When You Hear This:	Picture This:	Think This:
Gram-positive cocci in clusters — • Beta-hemolytic • Yellow pigment • Catalase positive	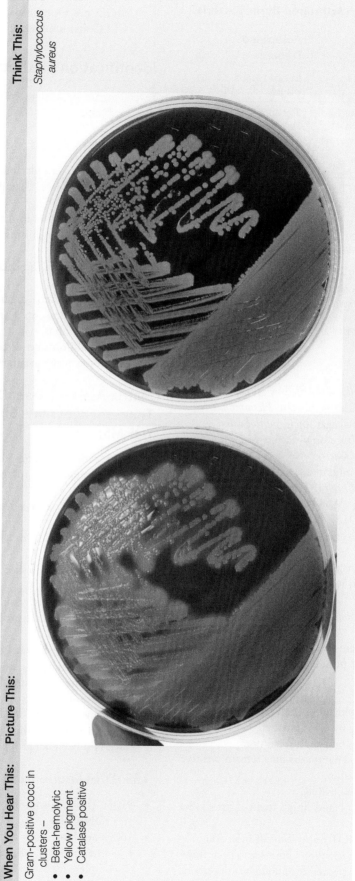	*Staphylococcus aureus*

TABLE 1.7	Associations with Arthropod-Borne Bacteria	
Arthropod	**Associated Pathogens**	**Associated Diseases**
Fleas	*Rickettsia typhi*	Murine typhus
	Yersinia pestis	Plague
Lice	*Bartonella quintana*	Trench fever
	Borrelia recurrentis	Relapsing fever
	Rickettsia prowazekii	Epidemic typhus
Mites	*Rickettsia akari*	Rickettsialpox
	Orientia tsutsugamushi	Scrub typhus
Ticks	*Anaplasma phagocytophilum*	Anaplasmosis
	Borrelia hermsii	Relapsing fever
	Borrelia parkeri	Relapsing fever
	Borrelia turicatae	Relapsing fever
	Ehrlichia spp.	Ehrlichiosis
	Francisella tularensis	Tularemia
	Rickettsia africae	African tick-bite fever
	Rickettsia parkeri	Spotted fovor rickettsiosis
	Rickettsia rickettsii	Rocky Mountain spotted fever

- *Salmonella* and *Shigella* performed by all labs.
- Some labs screen for *Aeromonas* and *Plesiomonas*.
- Some labs add a special agar for *Campylobacter*.
  - *Campylobacter* culture only detects *Campylobacter jejuni* and *Campylobacter coli*.
  - Other species are inhibited.
- Shiga toxin-producing *E. coli* (STEC)
  - Some labs use only MacConkey with sorbitol for detection of *E. coli* O157.
  - Some labs use an enzyme immunoassay to detect all serotypes of STEC.
  - Some labs do both (recommended by CDC).
- Stool must be processed within 30 minutes or placed in transport buffer.
  - *Shigella* and *Campylobacter* begin dying upon passage.
- Antigen testing
  - *Campylobacter* antigen: detects *C. jejuni*, *C. coli*.
  - O157 antigen: poor positive predictive value in low incidence settings.
- PCR/molecular
  - Most common are multiplex gastrointestinal (GI) panels.
  - GI panel targets vary by manufacturer.
  - Increased sensitivity compared to culture.
  - Also detect dead bacteria; results may remain positive 1–4 weeks after infection.
- Shiga-toxin testing (EIA or PCR)
  - Detects Shiga toxin 1 and Shiga toxin 2 associated with STEC.
    - Detection does NOT imply *Shigella* infection.
  - Does not provide information about serotype → however, serotype is only needed for public health reasons → not clinically useful since any serotype can cause hemolytic uremic syndrome (HUS).

- STEC that produce Shiga toxin 2 or Shiga toxins 1 and 2 are more associated with severe disease than STEC that produce only Shiga toxin 1.

Identification Methods

Several organisms have recently undergone significant name changes (Table 1.3).

Biochemical-Based Methods (Tables 1.4, 1.5, 1.6)

- Biochemical methods consist of simple spot tests, such as catalase, oxidase, coagulase, as well as more complex biochemical testing.
- Spot tests allow presumptive identification or identification of certain organisms, such as *S. aureus* and *S. pyogenes*, in minutes.
- For most bacteria, biochemical methods require hours, occasionally days.
- Biochemically-inert organisms (intrinsically or those found in biofilms, etc.) are difficult to identify by biochemical methods.
- Commercial instruments/databases are not up to date with the most recent classification changes or the newest microbes.

Matrix-Assisted Laser Desorption/Ionization Time-of-Flight Mass Spectrometry (MALDI-TOF MS)

- Identification based on protein content → primarily ribosomal proteins due to their relative abundance in the bacterial cell.
- Only a single colony is required for identification.
- Method:
  - Colony is added to a target plate and covered with matrix.
  - Colony/matrix is shot with a laser, which ionizes the proteins.
  - Ionized proteins travel through a vacuum and hit a detector at a rate proportional to their mass/charge ratio.
  - This creates a spectrum or fingerprint, which is compared to a database to determine an identification.
- Fast, accurate identification of aerobes and anaerobes within minutes.
- Second most accurate identification method after sequencing.
  - Much more accurate than biochemical methods for certain bacterial groups.

16S rDNA Sequencing of Bacterial Isolates

- Partial (more common) or complete sequencing of the 16S rDNA gene.
- 16S gene alone is not sufficient for all bacterial genera.
  - Some genera require additional sequencing targets for complete identification.
- Usually limited to reference labs or large academic labs.
- Turnaround time is usually slow.

TABLE 1.8 BT Agents

Organism	Disease	Region/Location	Who's at Risk/Risk Factors	Microbiology Characteristics
Bacillus anthracis *Bacillus cereus* BIOVAR *anthracis*	Anthrax	Worldwide (*B. cereus* BIOVAR *anthracis* reports are limited to Africa)	• Persons who handle animal products • Livestock producers • Veterinarians	• Big and boxy gram-positive rods, often in chains • Catalase positive • Nonhemolytic (*B. cereus* BIOVAR *anthracis* may be slightly beta-hemolytic) • Nonmotile
Brucella	Brucellosis	Worldwide, but especially: • Mexico, South and Central America • The Caribbean • Mediterranean Basin • Eastern Europe • The Middle East	• Eating undercooked meat or raw dairy products • Veterinarians • Abattoir workers • Hunters	• Tiny gram-negative rods • Oxidase positive • Urease positive • May be misidentified as *Ochrobactrum* by MALDI
Burkholderia mallei	Glanders	• Central and South America • Middle East • Asia • Africa	• Veterinarians • Horse caretakers • Abattoir workers	• Gram-negative coccobacilli • Slowly growing • Variable growth on MacConkey agar • Oxidase variable • Colistin resistant
Burkholderia pseudomallei	Melioidosis	• Tropics, especially Southeast Asia and Australia	• Agricultural workers • Persons with open skin wounds, diabetes, or chronic renal disease	• Regular gram-negative rods • Colonies have "cracked/dry earth" appearance • Musty odor (do not actively smell plates!) • Oxidase positive • Colistin resistant • May be misidentified by MALDI as *B. thailandensis*
Francisella tularensis	Tularemia	• North America • Europe • Asia	• Hunters who hunt/skin rabbits, muskrats, prairie dogs • Ticks and deer fly bites • Mowing over a rabbit's nest	• Tiny gram-negative rods • Oxidase negative • Weak catalase-positive • Growth on chocolate agar only (may show breakthrough growth on blood agar)
Yersinia pestis	Plague	• Western United States • South America • Africa • Rare cases in Europe and Asia	• Flea bites • Hunters who hunt/skin rabbits and other rodents	• "Safety-pin"/bipolar staining (Giemsa stain; not commonly seen with Gram stain) • Colonies have "fried egg" appearance • Oxidase negative • Indole negative • Nonlactose fermenter • Nonmotile (25 °C)

TABLE 1.9	**Emerging Bacterial Pathogens**
Pathogen	**Clinical Presentation(s)**
Actinotignum schaalii	UTIs
Corynebacterium propinquum	Respiratory infections, endocarditis
Corynebacterium kroppenstedtii	Breast abscesses
Leptotrichia spp.	Bacteremia in neutropenic patients
Staphylococcus pseudintermedius	Dog bite infections
Staphylococcus lugdunensis	Coagulase-negative *Staphylococcus* with pathogenicity/clinical presentations similar to *S. aureus*

TABLE 1.10	**Bacterial Zoonotic Pathogens**
Animal	**Associated Pathogens**
Birds	*Chlamydia/Chlamydophila psittaci*
Cats	*Bartonella henselae* *Pasteurella* (most commonly *P. multocida*)
Farm animals (cows, sheep, goats, chickens, etc.)	*Bacillus anthracis* *Brucella* *Coxiella burnetii* *Campylobacter* *E. coli* (Shiga toxin producing) *Erysipelothrix rhusiopathiae* *Leptospira* *Salmonella*
Fish	*E. rhusiopathiae* *Streptococcus iniae* *Vibrio*
Dogs	*Campylobacter* (2017 outbreak linked to pet store puppies) *Leptospira* *Pasteurella* (most commonly *P. canis* and *P. multocida*) *Staphylococcus intermedius/ pseudintermedius* (aka the *S. aureus* of dogs)
Leeches	*Aeromonas*
Rabbits	*Francisella tularensis*
Reptiles	*Salmonella*
Rodents	*Leptospira* *Salmonella* (2015–2017 outbreak linked to pet guinea pigs) *Spirillum minus* *Streptobacillus moniliformis* *Yersinia pestis*

Broad-Range PCR/16S Sequencing of Direct Specimens

- For use on sterile specimens when the causative agent is unable to be identified by conditional culture or other diagnostic methods.
  - Can also be used on paraffin-embedded tissues.
  - Options include pan-bacterial, pan-fungal, or pan-AFB.
- Broad range PCR primers are used to amplify bacterial DNA in the specimen, and sequencing is performed to determine the pathogen present.
  - Must be a sterile specimen or normal flora will be amplified.
- Performance:
  - Sensitivity is increased when an organism is seen on stain (Gram stain or pathology stain).
  - Sensitivity is lower than organism-specific PCR/ NAAT tests.
- Slow turnaround time.

Antimicrobial Susceptibility Testing (AST) – Methods

- Kirby Bauer disk diffusion and broth microdilution are the two reference methods for aerobic bacteria.
- Other methods are FDA-approved but not considered reference methods.
- Agar dilution is the reference method for anaerobic bacteria.
  - Due to the demanding methodology and slow turnaround times, anaerobic susceptibility testing is not routinely performed.
  - Susceptibility testing of anaerobes is typically limited to reference laboratories.
- Anaerobic infections are often polymicrobial and treatment is general (rather than targeted as with most aerobic infections), so there is often no need for AST.
- Due to low levels of increasing resistance, AST may be warranted in sterile site infections.
- A nationwide anaerobe antibiogram is available in the Clinical Laboratory Standards Institute (CLSI) M100 document, available for free online.

Kirby Bauer Disk Diffusion (Fig. 1.4)

- Drugs diffuse from impregnated paper disks through the agar, forming a circular gradient.
- The diameter of the zone of inhibition is measured.
- An interpretation (susceptible [S], susceptible-dose dependent [SDD], intermediate [I] or resistant [R]) is assigned based on the zone diameter.

TABLE 1.11	Foodborne Illness: Bacterial Associations
Food	**Organism(s)**
Chitterlings/chitlins	*Yersinia enterocolitica*
Eggs	*Salmonella*
Gravy	*Clostridium perfringens*
Home-canned vegetables and fruits	*Clostridium botulinum*
Honey	*C. botulinum*
Oysters	*Vibrio vulnificus*
Poultry	*Campylobacter* *Salmonella*
Raw milk/cheese	Shiga-toxin producing *Escherichia coli* *Brucella* *Campylobacter* *Coxiella burnetii* *Listeria* *Salmonella*
Rice	*Bacillus cereus*

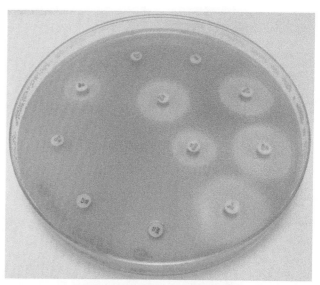

• **Fig. 1.4** Kirby Bauer disk diffusion.

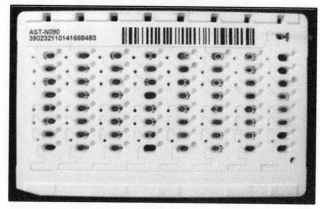

• **Fig. 1.5** Vitek automated susceptibility card.

- No minimum inhibitory concentration (MIC) is given.

Minimum Inhibitory Concentration (MIC) Testing

- The MIC is the lowest concentration of antimicrobial that inhibits bacteria growth *in vitro.*
- Due to testing variabilities, the inherent error of MIC testing is ± one doubling dilution.
  - Thus a reported MIC of 2 µg/mL may actually be 1 µg/mL or 4 µg/mL.

Broth Microdilution

- Antimicrobials are prepared in two-fold dilutions in a 96-well plate.
- The MIC is the lowest concentration of drug that shows inhibition of growth.

Automated Susceptibility Testing (Fig. 1.5)

- May or may not contain two-fold dilutions of antimicrobials.
  - Some instruments only include a few antimicrobial concentrations and use a growth algorithm to determine the MIC.
- Must use FDA breakpoints unless laboratory performs validation testing to utilize CLSI breakpoints.

Gradient Diffusion (Etest, Liofilchem) (Fig. 1.6)

- Hybrid between disk diffusion and broth microdilution.

- Plastic strips are sprayed with an antimicrobial gradient (one antimicrobial per strip).
- Drugs diffuse through the agar.
- The MIC is the value where the ellipse intersects the strip.
- Gradient diffusion strips contain more values than doubling dilutions, but results should be reported in doubling dilutions.
- FDA breakpoints must be used unless the performing laboratory performs validation testing to utilize CLSI breakpoints.

Agar Dilution (Anaerobes Only) (Fig. 1.7)

- Varying concentrations of antimicrobial agents are added to agar plates before solidification.
- Bacteria are resuspended to a standard concentration, and a spot of each isolate is added to a plate of each concentration of antimicrobial.
- The lowest concentration resulting in inhibition of growth is the MIC.

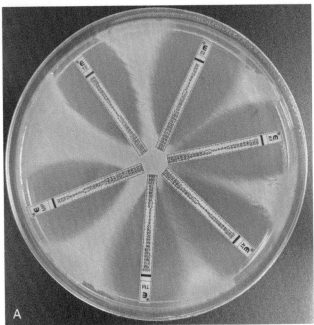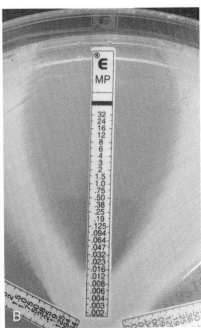

• **Fig. 1.6** Etest.

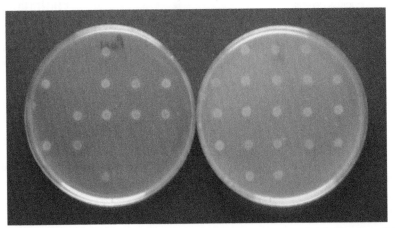

• **Fig. 1.7** Agar dilution: plate with antimicrobial (left) and growth control plate (right). (From Ison CA, Lewis DA. Gonorrhea. In: Morse SA, Holmes KK, Moreland AA, Ballard RC, eds. *Atlas of Sexually Transmitted Diseases and AIDS*. Elsevier; 2010.)

Antimicrobial Susceptibility Testing – Interpretation

Susceptible (S)
- Implies that an isolate will be inhibited by the usually achievable concentration of antimicrobial agent when the dosage recommended to treat the site of infection is used.
- Clinical efficacy is likely.

Susceptible-Dose Dependent (SDD)
- Susceptibility is dependent on the dosing regimen used.
- In order to achieve necessary levels, higher doses, more frequent doses, or both, should be used.
- The drug label should be consulted for recommended doses and adjustment for organ function.

Intermediate (I)
- Implies response rate may be lower than for susceptible isolates.

- Implies clinical efficacy in body sites where the drugs are physiologically concentrated (e.g., fluoroquinolones or trimethoprim–sulfamethoxazole [TMP–SMX] in urine) or when a higher than normal dosage of the drugs can be used.
- Should *not* automatically be interpreted as "do not use."

Resistant (R)
- Implies that an isolate will not be inhibited by the usually achievable concentration of antimicrobial agent when the dosage recommended to treat the site of infection is used.
- Clinical efficacy has not been reliably shown in treatment studies.

Nonsusceptible (NS)
- Category used for isolates for which only a susceptible breakpoint is designated because of absence or rare occurrence of resistant strains.

TABLE 1.12 Intrinsic Resistance

Organism	Intrinsic Resistance
Aerobic gram-negative rods	Clindamycin Vancomycin (rare exceptions)
Non-glucose-fermenting gram-negative rods	Ertapenem
Burkholderia cepacia complex	Ampicillin Piperacillin Ticarcillin Ampicillin/sulbactam Amoxicillin/clavulanate 1st and 2nd-generation cephalosporins Cephamycins Ertapenem Colistin Fosfomycin Note: Isolates of *B. cepacia* complex have chromosomal genes that require mutational changes before leading to resistance for the antimicrobials below. CLSI M100 documents prior to 2019 listed the antimicrobials below as intrinsically resistant, but the 2019 document stated that there is insufficient evidence to determine if isolates that test susceptible *in vitro* will respond *in vivo*. - Piperacillin/tazobactam - 3rd and 4th generation cephalosporins EXCEPT ceftazidime - Aztreonam - Imipenem - Aminoglycosides
Citrobacter freundii complex	Refer to SPICE organisms below
Citrobacter koseri	Ampicillin Piperacillin Ticarcillin
Enterobacter (includes *Klebsiella aerogenes*)	Refer to SPICE organisms below
Escherichia coli	No intrinsic resistance to antimicrobials with activity against gram-negative rods
Klebsiella (not *K. aerogenes*)	Ampicillin Ticarcillin
Proteae (*Proteus, Morganella, Providencia*)	Colistin Nitrofurantoin Tetracyclines/tigecycline May have elevated MICs to imipenem *Also refer to SPICE organisms on the following page
Pseudomonas aeruginosa	Ampicillin Ampicillin/sulbactam 1st- and 2nd-generation cephalosporins Cephamycins Ceftriaxone Ertapenem Trimethoprim–sulfamethoxazole Nitrofurantoin
Salmonella and *Shigella*	1st- and 2nd-generation cephalosporins, cephamycins Aminoglycosides
Serratia marcescens	Nitrofurantoin Colistin *Also refer to SPICE organisms below

Continued

TABLE 1.12	Intrinsic Resistance—cont'd
Organism	**Intrinsic Resistance**
Stenotrophomonas maltophilia	Penicillins Ampicillin/sulbactam Amoxicillin/clavulanate Piperacillin/tazobactam 1st- to 3rd-generation cephalosporins *except* ceftazidime Cephamycins Aztreonam Imipenem Meropenem Ertapenem Aminoglycosides Tetracycline Fosfomycin
Aerobic gram-positive organisms	Colistin Polymyxin B Nalidixic acid
Enterococcus	Cephalosporins Aminoglycosides Clindamycin Trimethoprim–sulfamethoxazole
E. faecalis	Those listed for *Enterococcus*, plus: Quinupristin/dalfopristin
E. casseliflavus and *E. gallinarum*	Those listed for *Enterococcus*, plus: Quinupristin/dalfopristin Vancomycin
Listeria	Cephalosporins

Antimicrobial Resistance Patterns – Intrinsic Resistance (Table 1.12)

Refer to the CLSI M100 document (updated yearly, available for free online) for more information.

SPICE Organisms

- Harbor a chromosomal AmpC beta-lactamase.
- AmpC beta-lactamase results in resistance to penicillins (except piperacillin), ampicillin/sulbactam, amoxicillin/clavulanate, first- and second-generation cephalosporins and cephamycins.
- The *ampC* gene may become de-repressed upon exposure to beta-lactam antimicrobials, which can result in resistance to third-generation cephalosporins, piperacillin/tazobactam, and ertapenem
- The SPICE organisms include:
  - *Serratia* spp.
  - *P. aeruginosa.*
  - Indole-positive proteae (*Proteus vulgaris* group, *Providencia* spp., *Morganella morganii*).
  - *Citrobacter freundii* complex.
  - *Enterobacter* spp.

Colistin-Resistant Bacteria

- Most gram-positive bacteria.
- *Burkholderia.*

- *Inquilinus limosus.*
- *N. gonorrhoeae* and *N. meningitidis.*
- *Pandoraea.*
- *Proteae* (*Proteus, Providencia, Morganella*).
- *Serratia.*

Vancomycin-Resistant Bacteria

- Most gram-negative bacteria.
- *Clostridium innocuum.*
- *Enterococcus gallinarum* and *Enterococcus casseliflavus* (due to chromosomal *vanC*).
- *Erysipelothrix rhusiopathiae.*
- *Lactobacillus* (except *L. acidophilus* and *L. delbrueckii*).
- *Leuconostoc.*
- *Pediococcus.*
- *Weissella.*

Acquired Resistance Mechanisms

Gram-Positive Bacteria

- *mecA, mecC*: encode penicillin binding protein 2a (PBP2a)
  - Responsible for methicillin resistance in staphylococci.
    - *mecA*: most common in United States and worldwide.
    - *mecC*: reported in Europe, rare in the United States.
  - Oxacillin and/or cefoxitin are used as indicator drugs for determining methicillin-susceptible *S. aureus* (MSSA) vs. methicillin-resistant *S. aureus* (MRSA), rather than methicillin.

- Cefoxitin is more sensitive for detection of *mecA*.
- Oxacillin in more sensitive for detection of *mecC*.
- A PBP2a immunochromatographic assay can also be used to determine MSSA vs. MRSA (*mecA* only).
  - Can be performed directly on bacterial colonies.
  - Testing time is approximately 7 minutes.
  - Allows for fast discrimination of MSSA/MRSA while full susceptibility results are pending.
- Methicillin-susceptible staphylococci are susceptible to nafcillin, beta-lactam/inhibitor combinations, cephalosporins, and carbapenems.
- Methicillin-resistant staphylococci are resistant to all beta-lactams with the exception of ceftaroline (and ceftobiprole outside of the United States), which must be tested to determine activity.
- Vancomycin-intermediate *S. aureus* (VISA)
  - Decreased susceptibility to vancomycin.
  - Not an acquired resistance mechanism but not intrinsic either; phenotype is due to gene expression changes in *S. aureus* when exposed to vancomycin.
  - Multiple genomic changes can be responsible for VISA phenotype; most notable is increase in thickness of the cell wall.
- *vanA*, *vanB*: encode cell wall precursors that end with D-alanyl-D-lactate, rather than D-alanyl-D-alanine.
  - Encode vancomycin resistance in enterococci (VRE); rarely reported in *S. aureus* (VRSA).
  - *vanA*: most common in United States, resistant to teicoplanin.
  - *vanB*: susceptible to teicoplanin.

Gram-Negative Bacteria
- Extended spectrum beta-lactamases (ESBLs)
  - Acquired via mobile genetic elements.
  - >900 types/variations discovered.
  - Most ESBLs cause resistance to penicillins, first- to third-generation cephalosporins, and sometimes fourth-generation cephalosporins.
  - High-level expression may cause resistance to ertapenem.
- AmpC beta-lactamases
  - Refer to SPICE organisms on previous page for a list of bacteria with chromosomal AmpC beta-lactamases.
  - AmpC beta-lactamases may also be acquired via mobile genetic elements.
- Carbapenemases
  - Acquired via mobile genetic elements.
  - Cause resistance to most, if not all, beta-lactam antimicrobials.
  - Spectrum depends on the type of carbapenemase.
  - Most common in the United States is *Klebsiella pneumoniae* carbapenemase (KPC), which has been found in *Enterobacteriaceae* as well as nonfermenters.
  - Other carbapenemases:
    - Metallo-beta-lactamases: NDM, IMP, VIM, etc.
    - Oxacillinases: OXA
      - Some remain susceptible to cephalosporins while resistant to carbapenems.
      - May be found on chromosome.

Potential Treatment Options for Resistant Bacteria

MRSA

- Vancomycin.
- Ceftaroline.
- Daptomycin.
- Linezolid.
- Tedizolid.

VRE

- Daptomycin.
- Doxycycline.
- Linezolid.
- Tedizolid.
- Oritavancin.
- Quinupristin-dalfopristin (*E. faecium* only).

Carbapenemase-Producing Organisms

- Ceftazidime/avibactam.
  - No activity against metallo-beta-lactamases.
- Colistin.
- Meropenem/vaborbactam.
  - Limited activity against metallo-beta-lactamases and oxacillinases.
- Tigecycline.

Antimicrobials with Poor CSF Penetration

- Antimicrobials administered by oral route only.
- Beta-lactamase inhibitors (sulbactam, tazobactam, clavulanate).
- First- and second-generation cephalosporins.
- Cephamycins.
- Clindamycin.
- Fluoroquinolones.
- Macrolides.
- Tetracyclines.

Antimicrobials with Anaerobic Coverage

- Ampicillin/penicillin.
  - Recommended only for gram-positive anaerobes.
- Beta-lactam/beta-lactamase inhibitor combinations.
- Cephamycins.
- Carbapenems.
- Clindamycin.
  - Greater than 20% resistance except *Fusobacterium necrophorum/nucleatum*, anaerobic gram-positive cocci, and *Cutibacterium* (*Propionibacterium*) *acnes*.
- Metronidazole.
- Moxifloxacin.
- Tetracycline.

Aerobic Actinomycetes (not to be confused with *Actinomyces*)

- Aerobic actinomycetes are grouped based on similar growth characteristics.
  - Filamentous bacteria found in soil.
  - Not genetically related.
- Gram-positive rods with some form of branching (branching may not occur during all growth phases).
- Typically isolated in fungal cultures (rather than bacterial cultures) due to slow growth rates.
  - If suspected, make sure to order a fungal culture in addition to bacterial cultures.
- Most of the clinically relevant aerobic actinomycetes, with the exception of *Streptomyces*, are positive by modified acid-fast stain due to presence of mycolic acids in their cell wall.
  - The modified acid-fast stain incorporates a sulfuric acid decolorizing step.
  - Aerobic actinomycetes are typically negative when using a traditional acid-fast stain (for *Mycobacterium* spp.), which uses hydrochloric acid as a decolorizer.
- Members of the aerobic actinomycetes include:
  - *Gordonia.*
  - *Nocardia* (see Table 1.13)
    - Most common, clinically important aerobic actinomycete.
    - Causes pulmonary infections, brain abscesses, skin infections in immunocompromised hosts, especially hematology/oncology patients (rare infections in immunocompetent hosts).
    - Colonies are chalky white, dry, and develop an orange pigment with time.
    - Rods are beaded, more delicate than *Streptomyces.*
    - Modified acid-fast positive due to mycolic acids in cell wall.
    - Trimethoprim–sulfamethoxazole is the treatment of choice, but double coverage is often used due to TMP–SMX resistance in certain species.
  - *Rhodococcus.*
  - *Streptomyces* (see Table 1.13)
    - Second most commonly isolated aerobic actinomycete.
    - More commonly recovered as a contaminant than as a pathogen.
    - Thicker rods than *Nocardia.*
    - Modified acid-fast negative.
  - *Tsukamurella.*

Bacteria That Do Not Grow on Routine Culture Media (Table 1.14)

- Although routine bacterial cultures recover the majority of bacterial pathogens, there are notable fastidious pathogens that do grow in routine culture and require specialized testing (Table 1.14).

Acid-Fast Bacilli (AFB)/Mycobacteria (see Chapters 32 and 33)

- Mycobacteria are largely environmental organisms that contain large amounts of mycolic acids in their cell walls.
- During the staining process, mycobacteria are not easily decolorized by acid. →Thus they are known as acid-fast bacilli (AFB).
- AFB are divided into:
  - *Mycobacterium tuberculosis* complex (MTBC).
  - *Mycobacterium leprae.*
  - Nontuberculous mycobacteria (NTM)
    - Also known as mycobacteria other than tuberculosis (MOTT) or atypical mycobacteria.
    - NTM/MOTT is a diverse group of environmental mycobacteria.
      - Vary in their ability to cause disease.
      - Not spread from person-to-person.
    - NTM/MOTT is further divided into:
      - Slowly growing mycobacteria (SGM).
      - Rapidly growing mycobacteria (RGM).

Diagnostic Methods – MTBC

PPD/Mantoux Tuberculin Skin Test (TST)

- 0.1 mL of tuberculin purified protein derivative injected intradermally.
- Read after 48–72 hours.
- Preferred for testing children <5 years of age.
- **Interpreting results**
- Induration ≥5 mm considered positive in:
  - Immunosuppressed patients (including those with HIV, transplant, high-dose prednisone, etc.).
  - A recent contact of a person with TB.
  - Persons with fibrotic changes on chest X-ray consistent with prior TB.
- Induration ≥10 mm considered positive in:
  - Recent immigrants (<5 years) from high-burden countries.
  - IV drug users.
  - Mycobacteriology laboratory personnel.
  - Children <4 years of age.
  - Persons with conditions that place them at high risk.
  - Residents and employees of high-risk congregate settings.
  - Infants, children, and adults exposed to adults in high-risk categories.
- Induration ≥15 mm considered positive in:
  - Any person, including those with no known risk factors.
- False-positives due to:
  - Incorrect administration of test.

TABLE 1.13 Aerobic Actinomycetes

Parameter	Nocardia	Streptomyces
Gram stain		
Modified acid-fast stain		

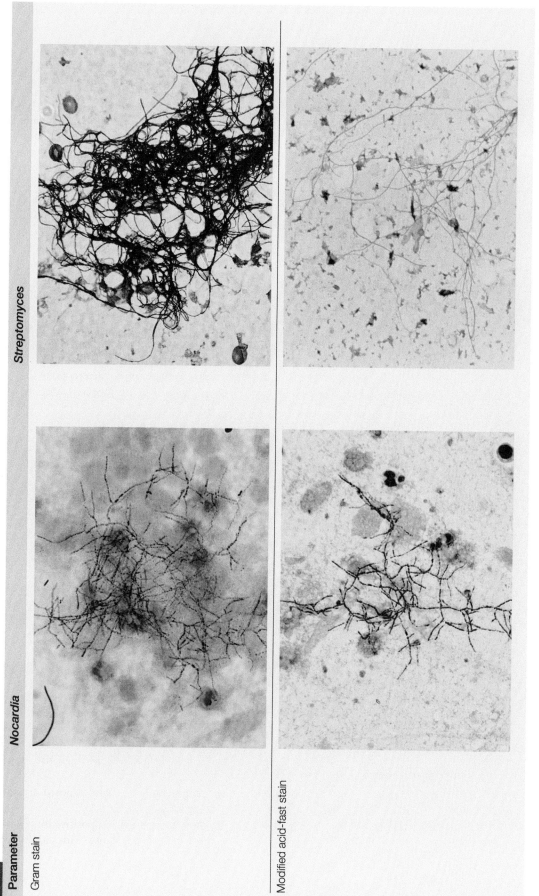

Continued

TABLE 1.13 Aerobic Actinomycetes—cont'd

Parameter	Nocardia	Streptomyces
Colony morphology		

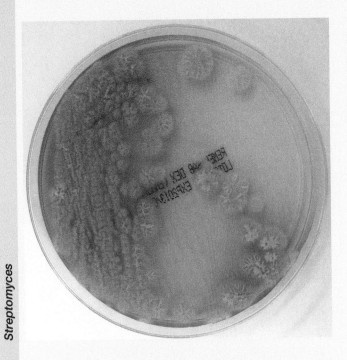

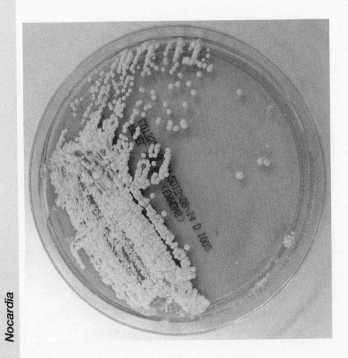

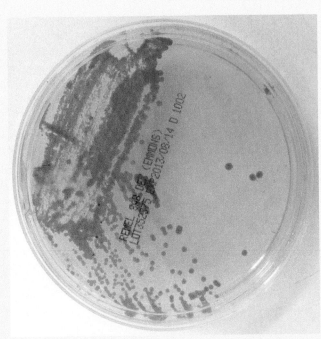

TABLE 1.14 Diagnostic Tests for Bacteria that Do Not Grow on Routine Culture Media

Organism	Test(s) for Diagnosis
Anaplasma phagocytophilum	• PCR/NAAT • Serology – after 2 weeks postinfection
Bartonella	• Serology • PCR/NAAT
Bordetella pertussis/parapertussis	• PCR/NAAT on respiratory specimens

Borrelia burgdorferi	• Serology
	  • Do not test if patient has not been in a Lyme-endemic region due to false-positives
	  • Confirmation by immunoblot
	• PCR/NAAT

Borrelia (relapsing fever-causing)	• Microscopy to look for spirochetes in a blood smear • PCR/NAAT • Serology
Chlamydia trachomatis	• PCR/NAAT • Cell culture • Used primarily for cases of sexual abuse; not all states accept PCR results
Chlamydia/Chlamydophila psittaci	• Serology: IgM and IgG
Chlamydia/Chlamydophila pneumoniae	• PCR/NAAT on respiratory specimens

Coxiella burnetii	• Serology
	  • Phase I > Phase II antibodies indicates past or chronic infection
	  • Phase II > Phase I antibodies indicates acute infection

Ehrlichia	• PCR/NAAT
	• Serology
	  • *E. chaffeensis* only; *E. ewingii* may cross-react
	• Microscopy
	  • Giemsa stain of blood smear may reveal morulae; poor sensitivity

Kingella kingae	• PCR/NAAT of joint fluids for septic arthritis • Culture is typically sufficient for other clinical specimens/presentations (bacteremia, endocarditis, wound infections)
Klebsiella granulomatis	• Visualization of Donovan bodies on tissue crush preparation or biopsy
Haemophilus ducreyi	• Culture on specialized media; only available at select reference labs • <80% sensitive • Rule out syphilis and HSV before testing

Helicobacter pylori	**Noninvasive**
	• Urea breath test
	  • 90%–95% sensitivity and specificity IF bismuth-containing compounds, proton pump inhibitors and antibiotics are stopped 2–4 weeks prior to testing
	• Stool antigen
	  • 90%–95% sensitivity and specificity IF bismuth-containing compounds, proton pump inhibitors, and antibiotics are stopped 2–4 weeks prior to testing
	• Serology
	  • No longer recommended due to lack of utility
	Invasive (performed on duodenal or gastric biopsies)
	• Urease test; also known as the Campylobacter-Like Organism (CLO) test
	  • 90%–95% sensitivity
	  • 95%–100% specificity
	• Histopathology/immunohistochemistry
	• Culture
	  • Requires specialized media
	  • Biopsy must be placed in appropriate transport medium upon collection

Continued

TABLE 1.14 **Diagnostic Tests for Bacteria that Do Not Grow on Routine Culture Media—cont'd**

Organism	Test(s) for Diagnosis
Legionella	• Culture • Requires specialized media • Detects all species • Urine antigen • Detects ONLY *Legionella pneumophila* group 1 • In some regions of the United States, *L. pneumophila* is responsible for less than half of *Legionella* infections • PCR/NAAT on respiratory specimens • Check with lab to determine if PCR detects *L. pneumophila* only or all species. PCRs that detect all species may differentiate *L. pneumophila* but do not differentiate other species
Leptospira	• Culture • Blood and CSF: first week of symptoms • Urine: after 7–10 days of illness • Serology • IgM only: insensitive during first 7–10 days
Mycoplasma genitalium	• PCR/NAAT
Mycoplasma hominis	• PCR/NAAT • Culture on specialized media • Must be transported in *Mycoplasma* transport buffer
Mycoplasma pneumoniae	• PCR/NAAT
Orientia tsutsugamushi	• Serology (CDC) • PCR/NAAT (CDC)
Rickettsia	• Serology
Spirillum minus	• Visualization in blood and infected tissues using Giemsa stain, Wright stain, or darkfield microscopy • Broad-range bacterial PCR/sequencing • 50% of patients have a false-positive nontreponemal syphilis test
Streptobacillus moniliformis	• Culture using enriched liquid media • Broad-range bacterial PCR/sequencing • 50% of patients have a false-positive nontreponemal syphilis test
Treponema pallidum	**Nontreponemal tests: detect antibodies against molecules released by cells damaged by *T. pallidum*** • Rapid plasma reagin (RPR) • High concentrations can cause false-negative "prozone" effect • If test is negative but syphilis is strongly suspected, ask lab to dilute/titer specimen to rule out prozone • False-positive results due to *T. pallidum* subspecies *pertenue* (causative agent of yaws), *Treponema carateum* (causative agent of pinta), *Mycobacterium tuberculosis* (MTB), rickettsial disease • Titer can be used to monitor patient's response to therapy • Venereal Disease Research Laboratory (VDRL) • 30% sensitive, 99% specific **Treponemal tests** • Fluorescent treponemal antibody – absorption (FTA-ABS) • *T. pallidum* particle agglutination (TP-PA) • Once infected, FTA-ABS and TP-PA will remain positive for life • A positive FTA-ABS or TP-PA result does not differentiate between past and active infection • Both tests show cross-reactivity with other *Treponema* species
Tropheryma whipplei	• Histopathology of intestinal biopsy • Periodic acid–Schiff (PAS) stain for foamy macrophages (pathognomonic for Whipple's) • Immunohistochemistry • PCR/NAAT
Ureaplasma	• PCR/NAAT

- Incorrect interpretation.
- Previous BCG vaccination or BCG cancer therapy.
- Infection with NTM/MOTT.
- Hyper-reactive skin.
- False-negatives due to:
  - Incorrect administration of test.
  - Incorrect interpretation.
  - Cutaneous allergy.
  - Recent TB infection (within 8–10 weeks of exposure).
  - Very old TB infection (many years).
  - <6 months of age.
  - Recent live-virus vaccination.
  - Some viral illnesses (e.g., measles, varicella).
  - Overwhelming TB disease.

Interferon-Gamma Release Assays (IGRA)

- Faster turnaround time (~24 h) than TST but more expensive.
- Preferred for:
  - Persons who have received BCG (either as vaccine or cancer therapy).
  - Persons who are unlikely to return for a follow-up reading.
- Measure immune response to MTBC.
  - Patient's blood is incubated with MTB antigens.
  - If infected, T-cells will recognize antigens and release interferon-gamma (IFN-ɣ).
- Two are commercially available in the United States:
  - QuantiFERON-TB Gold (QFT).
    - Detects the amount of IFN-ɣ released.
  - TSPOT.TB
    - Detects the number of IFN-ɣ producing cells.
- Interpreting results:
  - Positive.
  - Negative.
  - Indeterminate/borderline.
- False-positives due to:
  - Infection with NTM/MOTT.
    - Most notably, but not limited to: *Mycobacterium kansasii*, *Mycobacterium marinum*, *Mycobacterium szulgai*.
- False-negatives or indeterminate results due to:
  - >65 years of age.
  - Immunodeficiency.
  - Disseminated tuberculosis.
  - Extrapulmonary tuberculosis.

Cepheid Xpert MTB/RIF PCR

- PCR detection of MTB and rifampin resistance from clinical specimens.
- FDA-approved for sputum.
  - Some labs have validated other sources, such as BAL and CSF.
- Must be used in conjunction with culture.
- MTB/RIF performance (sputum specimens):

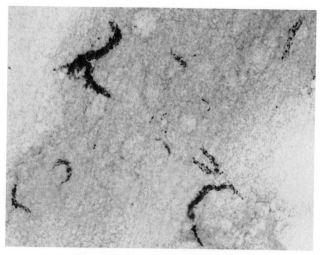

• **Fig. 1.8** Positive Kinyoun acid-fast stain.

- **Smear-positive** specimens: 97%–99% sensitivity, 98%–99% specificity.
- **Smear-negative** specimens: 61%–74% sensitivity, 98%–99% specificity.

Diagnostic Methods – All *Mycobacterium* spp.

Smear Microscopy

- Mycobacteria contain large amounts of mycolic acids in their cell walls.
  - Do not stain well with Gram stain.
  - Stain with carbol fuchsin.
  - Are not readily decolorized by acids after staining → hence, acid-fast.
- Methods
  - Auramine-rhodamine fluorescent stain is used to stain direct specimens.
  - Kinyoun acid-fast stain is used to confirm positive auramine-rhodamine stains and is used to stain positive culture growth (Fig. 1.8).
    - This should not be confused with the modified acid-fast stain, which is used for aerobic actinomycetes.

Culture

- Cultures are inoculated to liquid and solid media.
  - Some species grow better in liquid media; some grow better on solid media.
  - Liquid media is incubated for 6 weeks. Solid media is incubated for 8 weeks.
- Classification: rapidly growing mycobacteria (RGM) vs. slowly growing mycobacteria (SGM) (see Table 1.15).
  - Refers to growth rate from a **dilute specimen** or upon **subculture.**
  - Growth within 7 days → more likely an RGM.
    - *However*, MTBC and other SGM from a high-burden specimen may grow from the original specimen in as little as 3–4 days.

- Growth after 7 days → likely an SGM
  - *However*, RGM from a low-burden specimen may require a week or longer to grow from the original specimen.

Culture Identification Methods

DNA Probes

- For use with positive cultures (broth or solid media).
- Commercially available DNA probes for:
  - MTBC.
  - *Mycobacterium avium-intracellulare* complex (MAIC).
  - *Mycobacterium kansasii.*
  - *Mycobacterium gordonae.*

MALDI-TOF MS

- For use with positive cultures (broth or solid media).
- Requires inactivation and extraction steps to break down mycolic acids and inactivate potential MTBC before performing MALDI-TOF → rest of the process is the same as non-acid-fast bacteria.
- Preparatory/inactivation steps must be performed in biosafety level (BSL) 2+ or BSL 3 laboratory.
- After inactivation, work-up can resume in the routine lab (BSL 2).
- Not all species or subspecies within the MTBC, MAIC, *Mycobacterium abscessus* group, and *M. fortuitum* group can be differentiated.
  - Require sequencing for full identification.

High-Performance Liquid Chromatography (HPLC)

- For use with positive cultures (broth or solid media).
- The makeup of mycolic acids in the cell wall varies by *Mycobacterium* species.
- Mycolic acids are extracted and subjected to HPLC, which creates a profile.
- HPLC profiles are compared to a library and identified based on similarity to the library.
- Cannot differentiate species or subspecies within the MTBC, MAIC, *M. abscessus/chelonae* group, and *M. fortuitum* group.
  - Require sequencing for full identification.
- Previously, HPLC was the most common method of AFB identification, but it is being replaced by MALDI-TOF.

Sequencing

- May be performed on positive cultures or direct specimens (usually a combination of PCR and sequencing).
- Gold standard for diagnosis of mycobacteria but is more technically challenging and has longer turnaround time compared to other methods.
- 16S rRNA gene most commonly used.
  - Additional genes, *rpoB* and *hsp65,* are required for differentiation of certain complexes or closely related species.

- Required for species/subspecies differentiation of MTBC, MAIC, *M. abscessus* group, and *M. fortuitum* group.

Antimicrobial Susceptibility Testing (AST)

- Always performed when MTBC is isolated.
- Typically performed on request for NTM/MOTT.
  - AST may not be needed, depending on the species isolated.
  - SGM
    - MAIC: Only clarithromycin, moxifloxacin, and linezolid have demonstrated *in vitro-in vivo* correlation. Other results do not predict clinical response.
    - *M. kansasii*: Testing is recommended only for clarithromycin and rifampin. Additional second-line drugs may be tested if first-line drugs are resistant.
    - *M. marinum*: Susceptibility breakpoints/interpretive criteria exist for amikacin, ciprofloxacin, clarithromycin, doxycycline, ethambutol, moxifloxacin, rifabutin, rifampin, and trimethoprim–sulfamethoxazole.
    - There are no susceptibility testing breakpoints for other SGM. If tested, *M. kansasii* interpretive criteria may be applied, depending on the performing laboratory.
  - RGM
    - AST results do not correlate with clinical outcomes for pulmonary infections.
    - AST results for aminoglycosides, cefoxitin, and trimethoprim–sulfamethoxazole have been found to correlate with clinical outcomes for extrapulmonary disease.

Agar Proportion

- Agar proportion is the reference method for MTBC susceptibility testing, but it is being replaced by broth methods, which are easier to perform.
- Turnaround time is up to 28–35 days (MTBC).
- Testing is performed using established antimicrobial concentrations:
  - Rifampin: 1 µg/mL.
  - Isoniazid: 0.1 µg/mL and 0.4 µg/mL.
  - Ethambutol: 5 µg/mL.
  - Pyrazinamide: 100 µg/mL.
- Growth on antimicrobial-containing plates is compared to growth on antimicrobial-free plates.
  - If there is ≥1% growth on the antimicrobial-containing plate compared to the antimicrobial-free plate, the isolate is considered resistant to that drug.
- Each antimicrobial is reported as susceptible or resistant. No MIC is determined or reported.

Broth Method

- Microbroth or macrobroth method may be used.
- Microbroth testing.

TABLE 1.15 Rapidly Growing versus Slowly Growing Mycobacteria

Species	Clinical Presentation	Notes
Slowly Growing Mycobacteria (SGM)		
Mycobacterium tuberculosis complex (MTBC)	• Pulmonary disease • Pott's disease	• Airborne isolation precautions required for hospitalized patients • Requires sequencing for accurate species-level identification. *Mycobacterium bovis* is intrinsically resistant to pyrazinamide
Mycobacterium avium-intracellulare complex (MAC/MAIC)	• Pulmonary disease in immunocompromised patients • Lady Windermere syndrome • Hot tub lung • Unilateral cervical lymphadenitis in children	• Requires sequencing for accurate species-level identification
Mycobacterium chimaera	• Infections during open-heart surgery due to contaminated heater–cooler units	• Will be identified as MAC/MAIC by DNA probes, MALDI-TOF MS, and HPLC • Requires sequencing for definitive identification
Mycobacterium gordonae	• Rarely a pathogen • Most cases represent contamination	• Distinctive orange/yellow colonies
Mycobacterium haemophilum	• Cutaneous and bone and joint infections • Unilateral cervical lymphadenitis in children	• Requires incubation at 30–32°C and hemin for growth • If suspicious, alert lab to ensure appropriate culture media is used
Mycobacterium kansasii	• Second most common cause of NTM lung disease in United States • May mimic pulmonary tuberculosis • Extrapulmonary infections are uncommon	• May cause false-positive IGRA
Mycobacterium leprae	• Hansen's disease/leprosy	• Does not grow in culture • Diagnosis made by slit-skin smears or skin scrapings/biopsies
Mycobacterium marinum	• Fish tank granuloma	• Requires incubation at 28–30°C • May cause false-positive IGRA
Mycobacterium szulgai	• Uncommon • May mimic pulmonary tuberculosis	• May cause false-positive IGRA
Mycobacterium ulcerans	• Buruli ulcer	• Very difficult/slow to grow in culture • Requires incubation at 29–33°C • May require 8–12 weeks for growth • If suspicious, alert the lab to ensure appropriate incubation conditions are used, and incubation length is extended
Mycobacterium xenopi	• Pulmonary infection in patients with chronic lung disease • Extrapulmonary is less common	• Thermophile: optimum growth temperature is 42–43°C
Rapidly Growing Mycobacteria (RGM)		
Mycobacterium abscessus group	• Most common RGM • Pulmonary infections, especially in CF patients • Contraindication to lung transplant • Disseminated infection in immunocompromised patients • Soft tissue infections • Otitis media	• Composed of *M. abscessus* subsp. *abscessus*, *M. abscessus* subsp. *bolletii*, *M. abscessus* subsp. *massiliense* • Highly resistant to antimicrobials • *M. abscessus* subsp. *abscessus* may contain an inducible *erm* gene • *M. abscessus* subsp. *bolletii* contains the *erm* gene, resulting in resistance to macrolides • *M. abscessus* subsp. *massiliense* does not contain the *erm* gene • Requires sequencing for accurate subspecies-level identification

Continued

TABLE 1.15	Rapidly Growing versus Slowly Growing Mycobacteria—cont'd	
Species	**Clinical Presentation**	**Notes**
Mycobacterium chelonae	• Localized and disseminated cutaneous infections • The majority of disseminated infections are in immunosuppressed patients, especially patients on systemic corticosteroid therapy • Associated with 2011–2012 outbreak due to contaminated tattoo ink	• Prefers incubation at 28–32°C • Will grow at standard 35–37°C but may show delayed growth
Mycobacterium fortuitum group	• Localized cutaneous infections • Nail salon-acquired furunculosis • Bone and joint infections • CNS infections	• *M. porcinum* is the second most commonly isolated *M. fortuitum* group member (after *M. fortuitum*) • Requires sequencing for accurate species-level identification

- Performed in 96-well plate. Doubling dilutions are used, and an MIC is determined.
- Macrobroth testing
  - Performed with designated concentrations, similar to agar proportion. No MIC is determined or reported.
- Commercial instruments can be used
  - BD BACTEC MGIT.
  - bioMerieux BacT/ALERT.
  - ThermoFisher VersaTREK.
- Turnaround time is up to 12–35 days for SGM and 6–12 days for RGM.

Molecular Detection of Drug Resistance (MDDR) Assay (CDC)

- For use with MTBC only; performed by the CDC.
- Requires positive NAAT/PCR sediment or an isolate.
- Uses PCR combined with sequencing.
- Detection of genetic loci associated with drug resistance to first- and second-line drugs, including:
  - Rifampin.
  - Isoniazid.
  - Pyrazinamide.
  - Ethambutol.
  - Fluoroquinolones.
  - Kanamycin.
  - Amikacin.
  - Capreomycin.
- 2–3 day turnaround time.
- Sensitivity ranges from 55.2% (capreomycin) to 97.1% (rifampin).

- Specificity ranges from 91% (capreomycin) to 99.6% (fluoroquinolones and kanamycin).
- More information can be found at www.cdc.gov/tb/topic/laboratory/mddrusersguide.pdf

Drug-Resistant M. tuberculosis

- Multidrug-resistant (MDR).
  - Resistant to at least the two primary first-line drugs: rifampin and isoniazid.
- Extensively/extreme drug-resistant (XDR)
  - MDR isolate that is also resistant to three or more classes of second-line drugs.

Pathology Stains (Table 1.16)

- Several pathology stains are available to assist with infectious diagnoses in biopsies and tissues.
- In most cases, pathology should not be relied upon as a first-line test and should be used in conjunction with culture and other tests, as applicable.

Further Reading

1. Carroll KC, Pfaller MA, Landry ML, et al. *Manual of Clinical Microbiology.* 12th ed. Sterling, VA: ASM Press; 2019.
2. Procop GW, Koneman EW. *Koneman's Color Atlas and Textbook of Diagnostic Microbiology.* 7th ed. Philadelphia: Wolters Kluwer Press; 2016.
3. Clinical Laboratory Standards Institute M100: Performance Standards for Antimicrobial Susceptibility Testing (published yearly). Free online version: http://em100.edaptivedocs.net/dashboard.aspx.

<table>
<tr><td>TABLE
1.16</td><td>Pathology Stains</td></tr>
</table>

Stain	Image
Giemsa (modified) stain • Enhanced staining of bacteria compared to traditional hematoxylin and eosin (H&E) • Can be difficult to interpret due to nonspecific staining • Used primarily for diagnosis of *Helicobacter* gastritis including *Helicobacter pylori*, *Helicobacter heilmannii*	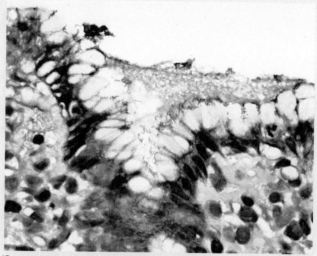 (Courtesy Irene Castaneda-Sanchez, MD.)
H. pylori immunostain • Increased sensitivity and specificity compared to Giemsa • Longer turnaround time and increased cost	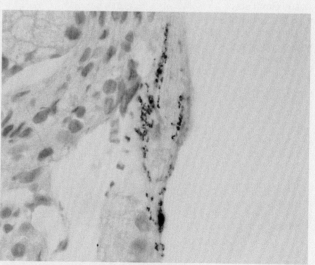 (Courtesy Irene Castaneda-Sanchez, MD.)

Continued

TABLE 1.16 **Pathology Stains—cont'd**

Stain	Image

Periodic acid–Schiff (PAS) stain
- Detects polysaccharides, including mucopolysaccharides
- PAS-positive macrophages in the lamina propria are pathognomonic for Whipple's disease

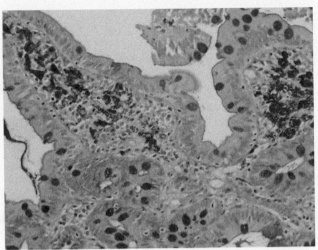

(With permission from Elsevier. The Lancet. From Prof Thomas Marth, et al. *Tropheryma whipplei* infection and Whipple's disease. *Lancet Infect Dis.* 2016;16(3): e13–e22.)

Tissue Gram stain
- Same concept as Gram stain used for cultures with adaptations for staining tissue sections
- Can be difficult to interpret due to nonspecific binding in tissues

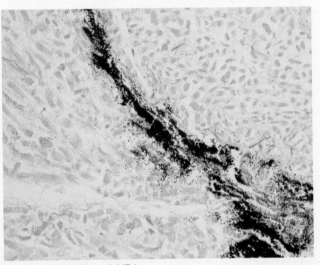

(Courtesy Linda Margraf, MD.)

Continued

TABLE 1.16   Pathology Stains—cont'd

Stain	Image

Warthin–Starry stain
- Silver nitrate stain used for the detection of:
  - Spirochetes (*Treponema*, *Borrelia*, *Leptospira*)
  - *Helicobacter pylori*
  - *Bartonella henselae* (clue for bacillary angiomatosis or bacillary peliosis hepatis)
- Organisms stain dark brown to black against a yellow–gold background
- May be difficult to interpret due to nonspecific staining
- Technically demanding; reproducibility is variable

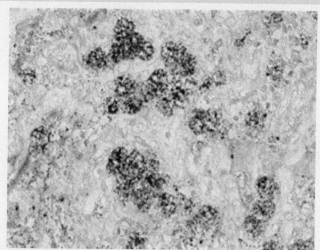

(From Draganova-Tacheva RA, Domsky S. *Clinical Microbiology Newsletter* 2009;31(19):150–152. Fig. 2. © 2009.)

Ziehl–Neelsen/Kinyoun/Fite (AFB stains)
- Mycobacteria stain pink/red
- Ziehl–Neelsen (ZN) and Kinyoun are most commonly used
- Fite stain is used primarily for *M. leprae*, which is frequently decolorized when using ZN or Kinyoun stain
- Fite stain will also stain *Nocardia*
- A negative stain does not rule out mycobacteria

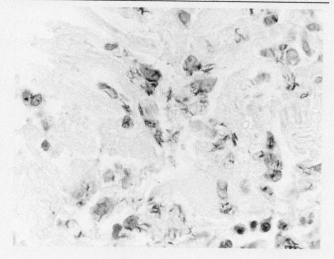

2
Mycology

KRUNAL RAVAL, MORGAN A. PENCE, ANDREJ SPEC

Classification of Medically Important Fungi

- Fungi can be classified in various ways depending on phylogeny or microscopic structure or clinical presentations.
- Following is the classification based on morphologic features into yeast, thermally dimorphic molds (yeast at body temperature and mold at room temperature) and thermally monomorphic molds. This is a widely used classification that does *not* follow true phylogeny of the species, but is the most useful method for laboratory and clinical diagnosis (Fig. 2.1).
- Even though this classification is the most useful one for visual binning of fungi into specific groups (and thus following real life pattern of diagnosis), a culture should always be used for comparison. Even experienced microbiologists and pathologists make mistakes, especially in tissues.
- Throughout the chapter, refer to Fig. 2.1 in order to build a framework of fungal infections.

Definitions

Not all of the following items are important in day-to-day clinical care in patients with fungal infections. However, they are frequently used in many texts, and this list should serve as a reference. The more common and important terms are highlighted. See also Fig. 2.2.

Arthroconidia: a sexual spore formed by the breaking up of a hypha at the point of septation. This is the mechanism that is used by *Coccidioides*.

Basidiospore: a sexual spore formed on a structure known as a basidium, as seen in mushrooms. *Cryptococcus* spp. belong to the group of fungi that form these structures and is thus more closely related to mushrooms than other yeasts such as *Candida* spp.

Blastoconidium: a conidium formed by budding along a hypha, pseudohyphae, or single cells (yeast).

Conidiophore: a specialized hyphal structure that serves as a stalk on which conidia are formed.

Conidia: an asexual propagule that forms on the side or end of the hypha or conidiophore. Microconidia are smaller compared to macroconidia. These are often the infectious particles of many molds, including endemic *Histoplasma.*

Dematiaceous: having structures that are brown or black due to melanotic pigment in the cell walls.

Dermatophyte: fungus with ability to obtain nutrients from keratin and thus infects skin, hair, or nails. This is more of a functional classification than one that represents morphology.

Dimorphic: they exist in mold form at environmental temperatures and in yeast forms (or spherules, for coccidioidomycosis) at body temperatures. This distinction means that *Coccidioides* spp. are not true dimorphic fungi, but they are classified as such in most texts for convenience.

Endemic fungus: fungus commonly found in defined geographical location. Many of these geographic regions are in flux, in part as new areas of endemicity are discovered, in part due to global climate change, and possibly due to other changes in the fungus or ecology that are not yet appreciated.

Fusiform: spindle or "canoe"-shaped conidia. Sometimes referred to as banana-shaped. Most commonly seen in appropriately named *Fusarium* spp.

Hilum: scar of attachment found at the end of conidium.

Hyaline: molds that do not produce pigment and are see through; from the Greek for glass. *Just think of hyaline cartilage, it is see-through.*

Hypha: filamentous structure of fungus.

Hyphomycete: An asexual fungus that produces mycelium that may be colorless (hyaline) or pigmented (dematiaceous).

Mycelium: multiple hyphae together; name used for the whole fungal colony.

Monomorphic: fungus that exist in same morphology at body as well as environmental temperature.

Phialide: a cell that produces and extrudes conidia without tapering or increasing in length with each new conidium.

Pseudohyphae: chain of cells formed by the budding that resembles true hyphae but are constricted at septae.

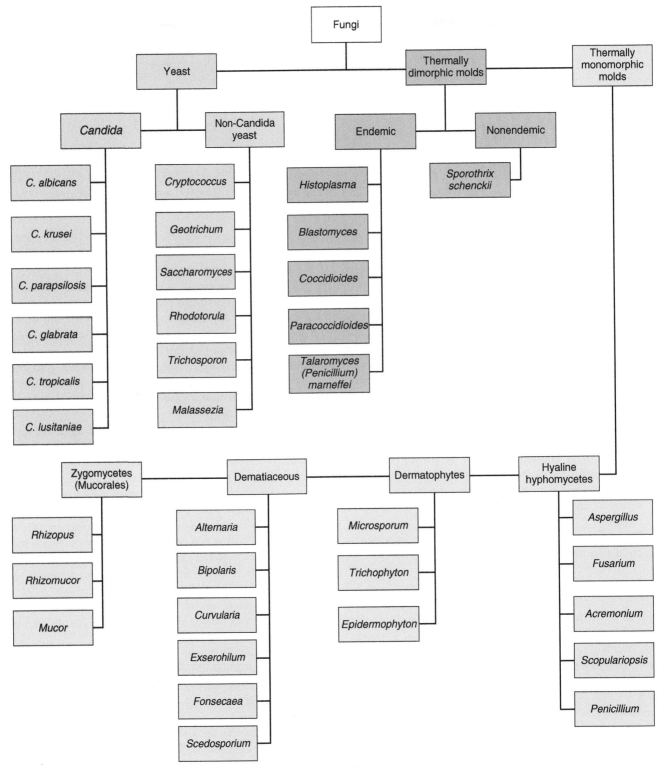

• **Fig. 2.1** Classification of medically important fungi.

This is most commonly seen in *Candida* spp. and can confuse even experienced pathologists and microbiologists (Fig. 2.3).

Sporangium: a closed sac-like structure in which asexual spores are formed by cleavage. Terminology is specific to Zygomycetes.

Sporangiophores: specialized hyphal branch bearing sporangium. Terminology is specific to Zygomycetes.

Rhizoid: root-like structure extending from hyphae.

Yeast: single-celled member of fungi that reproduces with budding.

Zygomycetes: phylum of fungi that have broad irregularly 90 degree/right angle branched hyphae with rare septations. Often described as wavy or ribbon-like.

Zygospore: sexual spore that is characteristic of the Zygomycetes.

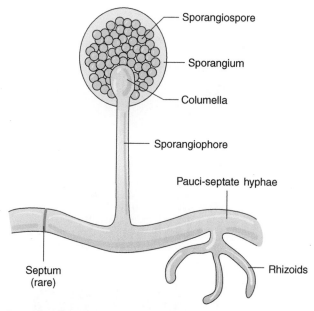

A Sporangiospores
Mucormycete
(*Rhizopus* spp.)

Labels: Sporangiospore, Sporangium, Columella, Sporangiophore, Pauci-septate hyphae, Rhizoids, Septum (rare)

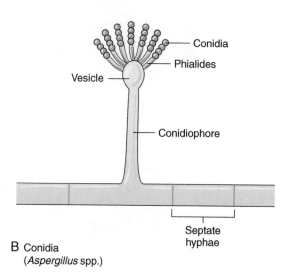

B Conidia
(*Aspergillus* spp.)

Labels: Conidia, Phialides, Vesicle, Conidiophore, Septate hyphae

• **Fig. 2.2** Fungal structures and taxonomy. (From Murray PR, Rosenthal KS, Pfaller MA. *Medical Microbiology*. p. 567–573.e1. Elsevier; 2016.)

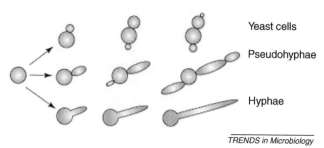

Labels: Yeast cells, Pseudohyphae, Hyphae

TRENDS in Microbiology

• **Fig. 2.3** Hyphae and pseudohyphae. (From Arnaud MB, Costanzo MC, et al. *Trends in Microbiology*. 2009;17(1):295–303.)

Yeast and Yeast-Like Organisms (Table 2.1)

• Most common bloodstream infections with yeast are due to *Candida*. However, they can be distinguished from *Cryptococcus* (the second most common) visually by presence of pseudohyphae and oval shape, where *Cryptococcus* is larger, round, often has a visible capsule, and never forms pseudohyphae.

• The other less common species include *Rhodotorula*, *Malassezia* with different morphology.

• All *Malassezia* spp., other than *M. pachydermatis*, require oil to grow. The specimen needs to be plated with an overlay of olive oil or *tween* to provide the fatty acids that it needs for growth. If clinically suspected, alert the microbiology lab to perform this extra step.

• Tween assimilation test can be performed on the plate. Depending on utilization of tween, it assesses degree of growth and/or reaction (precipitation) of the lipophilic yeasts around the wells

Differences among *Candida* spp.

• *C. albicans, C. tropicalis, C. dubliniensis, C. guilliermondii*: susceptible to fluconazole and echinocandins. These are the prototypical *Candida* spp., and most of the other statements are made as a direct comparison to the most common species, *C. albicans*.

• *C. glabrata*: second most common *Candida* spp. Many of the isolates are resistant to fluconazole, and even those that are sensitive to fluconazole have higher minimum inhibitory concentrations (MIC). Most isolates remain susceptible to echinocandins, but resistance has been reported and appears to be on the rise.

• *C. parapsilosis*: susceptible to fluconazole but increased MIC to echinocandins. Strong biofilm former leading to association with central lines and implantable devices.

• *C. krusei*: intrinsically resistant to fluconazole but susceptible to echinocandins. It also has decreased susceptibility to amphotericin B and flucytosine. Most commonly found in patients with hematologic malignancies, likely due to azole prophylaxis.

• *C. lusitaniae*: resistant to amphotericin B but remains susceptible to fluconazole and echinocandins. Very rare species.

• *C. auris*: an emerging global pathogen that is highly resistant to fluconazole, and many isolates also have shown resistance to amphotericin B and echinocandins (based on tentative breakpoints). Many identification methods can confuse it with *Saccharomyces* spp. or *C. haemulonii*. The identification can be confirmed with matrix-assisted laser desorption/ionization time of flight (MALDI-TOF) or sequencing.

Thermally Dimorphic Molds (Table 2.2)

• Thermally dimorphic molds exist in mold form at environmental temperatures and in yeast forms (or spherules, for coccidioidomycosis) at body temperatures.

TABLE 2.1 Yeast and Yeast-Like Organisms

Fungi	Clinical Features	Microbiologic Features	At-risk Patients or Pearls	Figures
Candida	Bloodstream infection, central-catheter-associated infections, skin infection, and gastrointestinal tract Pneumonia is exceedingly uncommon, and has to be confirmed by biopsy	Round to oval yeast having pseudohyphae with clusters of blastoconidia at the septa	Hematologic malignancy and neutropenia, transplant recipients, central venous catheter, abdominal perforation, parenteral nutrition	10 μm (From Lobo RA, Gershensen DM, Lentz GM, Valea FA. *Comprehensive Gynecology*. 7th ed. Elsevier; 2017.)
Cryptococcus	Meningitis, pneumonia, skin infections, dissemination, and sepsis	Round budding yeast. No hyphae or pseudohyphae	Opportunistic infection in HIV (CD4 <100/μL), transplant recipients, people receiving glucocorticoids, malignancy, liver diseases	10 μm (From Magill AJ, Hill DR, Solomon T, Ryan ET, eds. *Hunter's Tropical Medicine and Emerging Infectious Diseases*. 9th ed. Elsevier; 2013.)
Trichosporon	Bloodstream infection, dissemination, pneumonia	Hyphae (septate), pseudohyphae, barrel-shaped arthroconidia, pleomorphic budding yeast (blastoconidia)	Hematologic malignancy (neutropenia), AIDS, extensive burns, central venous catheter, history of heart valve surgery. Cross reacts with cryptococcal antigen	(From Procop G, Pritt B, eds. *Pathology of Infectious Diseases*. Elsevier; 2015.)
Geotrichum	Bloodstream infection, dissemination, pneumonia	Arthroconidia are unicellular, in chains, rectangle, or barrel shape. True hyphae are also seen	Hematologic malignancy (neutropenia), history of heart valve surgery in immunocompromised host	(From http://thunderhouse4-yuri.blogspot.com/2012/05/geotrichum-candidum.html.)

TABLE 2.1 Yeast and Yeast-Like Organisms—cont'd

Fungi	Clinical Features	Microbiologic Features	At-risk Patients or Pearls	Figures
Rhodotorula	Bloodstream infection, central-catheter associated infections	Unicellular blastoconidia, globose to elongated in shape. No hyphae or pseudohyphae	Usually associated with central lines or indwelling devices in immunocompromised. Growth is usually described as orange, red, or "coral red"	(From Rajmane VS, Rajmane ST, Ghatole MP. *Diagn Microbiol Infect Dis.* 2011;71(4):428-429.)
Saccharomyces	Bloodstream infection, probiotic associated	Unicellular, globose, and ellipsoid to elongated blastoconidia. Multipolar budding	Rarely causes disease (except when associated with probiotic use), but there are cases of *Candida auris* being misidentified as *Saccharomyces*. If not identified by MALDI-TOF, consider *C. auris*	(From Lagoutte D, Nicolas V, Poupon E, et al. *Biomed Pharmacother.* 2008;62(2):99–103.)
Pneumocystis jirovecii	Pneumonia	Round to ovoid, nonbudding with comma-shaped focal thickening on wall	Opportunistic infection causing pneumonia in immunocompromised host, especially HIV (CD4 <200/μL)	(From Long SS, Prober CG, Fischer M. *Principles and Practice of Pediatric Infectious Diseases.* 5th ed. Elsevier; 2018.)

TABLE 2.2 Dimorphic Molds

Fungi	Clinical Features	Microbiologic Features	At-risk Patients or Pearls	Figures
Histoplasma	Pneumonia, reticuloendothelial system (liver, spleen, bone marrow), adrenal glands, dissemination	Small oval budding yeast form at 37°C (2–5 μm). Septate hyphae with round/pear shaped microconidia and large tuberculate macroconidia at 25–30°C Can be confused with *C. glabrata*, which looks similar, has overlapping size, and does not form pseudohyphae	Endemic worldwide but hyperendemic in Mississippi and Ohio river valleys in USA and parts of Latin America Immunocompromised host (malignancy, transplant recipients, AIDS) but can also affect immunocompetent host	10.0 μm (From Kradin RL. *Diagnostic Pathology of Infectious Disease.* 2nd ed. Elsevier; 2018.)
Blastomyces	Pneumonia, bone, skin infection, brain abscess and dissemination	Broad-based budding yeast form at 37°C (7–15 μm). Septate branched hyphae with intercalary or terminal chlamydospores at 25–30°C	Hyperendemic in North America around Mississippi and Ohio river valleys, and the Saint Lawrence Seaway, autochthonous in Africa, South America, and Asia Affects immunocompetent and immunocompromised about equally When thinking of blastomycosis, remember the "B's": Blastomycosis, Broad Based Budding, Breath (pneumonia), Brain, Bone, Body covering (skin) Associated with pseudoepithelioid hyperplasia (biopsies resemble squamous cell cancer)	(From Husain AN. *Thoracic Pathology.* [High-Yield Pathology Series.] Elsevier; 2012.)
Coccidioides	Pneumonia, meningitis, dissemination	Round thick-walled spherules containing endospores at 37°C Septate branched hyphae with thick-walled arthroconidia at 25–30°C	Endemic in Southwestern United States, northern Mexico, Central and South America	(From Husain AN. *Thoracic Pathology.* [High-Yield Pathology Series.] Elsevier; 2012.)
Paracoccidioides	Pneumonia, dissemination	Large round thick-walled yeast (5–50 μm) with budding (ship's-wheel appearance) at 37°C Septate branched hyphae with intercalary or terminal chlamydospores at 25–30°C	Endemic in South America (male and farmer predominance)	(From Ramos-e-Silva M, Saraiva, L do Espirito Santo. *Dermatol Clin.* 2008; 26(2):257–269.)

TABLE 2.2 Dimorphic Molds—cont'd

Fungi	Clinical Features	Microbiologic Features	At-risk Patients or Pearls	Figures
Talaromyces marneffei (previously *Penicillium*)	Dissemination, skin, central nervous system (CNS), and bone	Small oval non-budding yeast form at 37°C Smooth conidiophores with 4–5 terminal metulae, each metula bearing 4–6 phialides at 25–30°C	Endemic in southwest and southern China and Southeast Asia Associated with AIDS Immunocompromised host (malignancy, transplant recipients) Cultures will produce a red diffusible pigment	(Reprinted with permission from Elsevier. The Lancet. From Limper AH, Adenis A, Le T, Harrison TS. Fungal infections in HIV/AIDS. *Lancet Infect Dis.* 2017;17(11):e334–e343.) (Reprinted with permission from Elsevier. The Lancet. From Limper AH, Adenis A, Le T, Harrison TS. Fungal infections in HIV/AIDS. *Lancet Infect Dis.* 2017;17(11):e334–e343.)
Sporothrix	Lymphocutaneous, pneumonia, dissemination	Small fusiform budding yeast form at 37°C Narrow septate hyphae with tapering conidiophores at right angles at 25–30°C	Gardener/farmer. "Rose handler's disease"	(From Rifai N, et al., eds. *Tietz Textbook of Clinical Chemistry and Molecular Diagnostics.* 6th ed. Elsevier; 2018.)
Emmonsia: Considering rapid re-classification this is likely to change	Pneumonia, skin	Large thick-walled budding yeast form at 37°C Septate hyphae with round conidiophores at right angle at 25–30°C	From endemic areas, AIDS (CD4 <100/μL), immunocompromised host (malignancy, transplant recipients)	(From Bottone EJ, *Clinical Microbiology Newsletter.* 2011;33(17):131–134.)

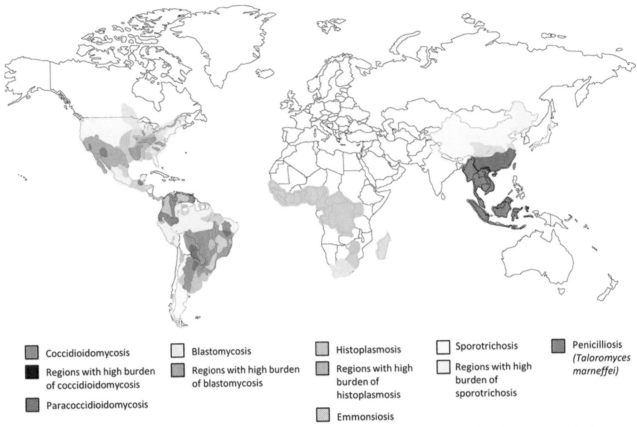

■ Coccidioidomycosis

■ Regions with high burden of coccidioidomycosis

■ Paracoccidioidomycosis

□ Blastomycosis

■ Regions with high burden of blastomycosis

■ Histoplasmosis

■ Regions with high burden of histoplasmosis

□ Sporotrichosis

□ Regions with high burden of sporotrichosis

▨ Emmonsiosis

■ Penicilliosis (*Taloromyces marneffei*)

• **Fig. 2.4** Global distribution of endemic mycosis. (From Lee PP, Lau Y-L. Cellular and molecular defects underlying invasive fungal infections – revelations from endemic mycoses. *Front Immunol.* 2017;8:735.)

• These infections are characterized by long periods of latency and could present decades after exposure.

• Although the endemic mycoses may cause disease in healthy individuals, immunocompromised individuals are at greater risk of severe or disseminated disease.

• Definitive diagnosis of endemic mycosis infection is by growth of the organism in culture. But considering slow growth rate, serology and antigen testing are commonly used.

• Since there is no commensal component to the life cycle of endemic mycoses, all positive cultures represent an infection.

• Many have distributions that are growing and shifting due to environmental change and population shifts (Fig. 2.4).

• Thermally dimorphic molds, when grown in culture, are highly infectious to laboratory personnel. If they are suspected, alert the microbiology lab.

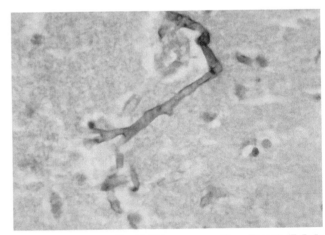

• **Fig. 2.5** Invasive sinusitis with *Rhizomucor* sp. (From Bennett JE, Dolin R, Blaser MJ, eds. *Mandell, Douglas, and Bennett's Principles and Practice of Infectious Diseases*. Updated 8th ed. Elsevier; 2015.)

Zygomycetes Molds

• Mucormycosis is manifested by a variety of different syndromes in humans, particularly in immunocompromised patients and those with diabetes mellitus.

• Devastating rhino-orbital-cerebral and pulmonary infections are the most common syndromes caused by these fungi (Fig. 2.5).

• The genera most commonly found in human infections are *Rhizopus, Mucor,* and *Rhizomucor.*

• *Cunninghamella, Lichtheimia* (formerly *Absidia*), *Saksenaea,* and *Apophysomyces* are genera that are much less commonly implicated in infection.

• Microscopically they have similar structure showing broad nonseptate nonparallel hyphae with unbranched long sporangiophores.

• They can be differentiated morphologically by:

  • *Mucor* spp.: Branched sporangiophores with no rhizoid structure (Fig. 2.6A).

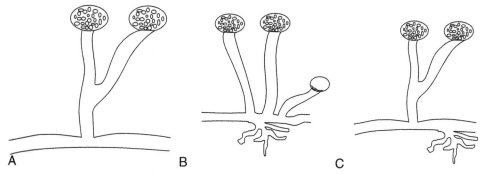

• **Fig. 2.6** The three most common genera of Mucormycetes. (A) *Mucor* spp. (B) *Rhizopus* spp. (C) *Rhizomucor* spp.

TABLE 2.3 Hyaline Hyphomycetes

Fungi	Clinical Features	Microbiologic Features	At-Risk Patients Or Pearls	Figures
Aspergillus	Lung, CNS, sinus, eye, and dissemination	Septate hyphae with conidiophore ending in phialides radiating around vesicle Named after the aspergillum used in church services due to structural similarity	Prolonged neutropenia, use of steroids, immunocompromised host (malignancy, transplant recipients)	(From Yoshida H, Seki M, Umeyama T, et al. *J Infect Chemother*. 2015;21(6):479–481.)
Fusarium	Sinusitis, skin, pneumonia, dissemination	Septate hyphae with canoe-shaped macroconidia It is able to sporulate inside the body, and disseminate through the blood, and will yield positive blood cultures, unlike other hyaline hyphomycetes, which are usually contaminants	Immunocompromised host (malignancy, transplant recipients)	(From Narayanan G, Nath R. *Mayo Clinic Proc*. 2016;91(4):542–543. © 2016.)

• *Rhizopus* spp.: Nonbranching sporangiophore originating from hyphae with rhizoid structure directly below the sporangiophore (Fig. 2.6B).
• *Rhizomucor* spp.: Branching sporangiophore with rhizoid structure away from the origin of the sporangiophore (Fig. 2.6C).
• Patients with uncontrolled DM, hematologic malignancy, transplant recipient (solid or HSCT), iron overload, or chelation are at high risk for mucormycosis.
• Treatment usually includes amphotericin B induction in severe infections.
• Posaconazole or isavuconazole are considered as step-down after induction or for mild/moderate infection.

Hyaline Hyphomycetes (Table 2.3)

• Most common molds in this group are *Aspergillus* and *Fusarium*. Other hyaline hyphomycetes that are frequently seen in cultures (*Penicillium* and *Paecilomyces*).
• Clinical correlation is recommended as hyaline hyphomycetes including *Aspergillus* spp. could represent a contaminant.
• *Aspergillus*
    • It is commonly associated with lung, CNS, sinus involvement in immunocompromised host (Fig. 2.7).
    • In tissue it can be observed in biopsy specimens as narrow (3 to 6 μm wide), septate hyaline hyphae with dichotomous acute angle (45°) branching (Fig. 2.7).

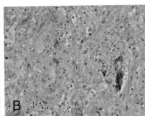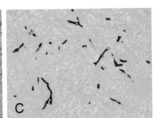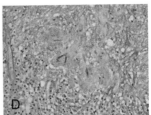

• **Fig. 2.7** Invasive cerebral aspergillosis. (A) Low power demonstrates chronic granulomatous inflammations. (B) At higher power, multinucleated giant cells with empty spaces represent the fungal organisms. (C) Septate fungal hyphae with some branched at right-angles (Gomori methenamine silver stain). (D) Some fungal hyphae are shown within the multinucleated giant cells (periodic acid–Schiff stain). (From Bokhari R, Baeesa S, Al-Maghrabi J, Madani T. Isolated cerebral aspergillosis in immunocompetent patients. *World Neurosurg.* 2014;2(1–2):e325–e333.)

• *Fusarium*
  • It is classically seen during engraftment phase post-stem cell transplant with skin lesions and fevers, and often starts off as a cellulitis surrounding toenails causing onychomycosis due to *Fusarium.* Other sources of initial entry are lungs and sinuses.
  • Varying antifungal "susceptibility" has been observed with *Fusarium* species.
  • *F. oxysporum* has low MICs to amphotericin.
  • *F. solani* and *F. reticulatum* have higher *in vitro* MICs for amphotericin.
  • Empiric treatment prior to species-level identification for fusariosis often includes both amphotericin B and voriconazole.
• In general, for most of the hyaline hyphomycete infection, treatment recommendations include:
  • Amphotericin B for severe cases.
  • Voriconazole/isavuconazole for mild/moderate cases.
• Treatment of choice in most cases of *Aspergillus* is voriconazole.

Dematiaceous Molds (Table 2.4)

• Common pathogens in soil and are commonly associated with traumatic inoculation. They also cause similar diseases as Zygomycetes and hyaline hyphomycetes in patients with hematologic malignancy, hematopoietic stem cell transplant and neutropenia.
• Surgical debridement and antifungal (amphotericin B or voriconazole) are major components of management.
• They can be differentiated in tissue from hyaline hyphomycetes by the use of the Fontana–Mason stain that stains the melanin in dematiaceous molds.
• The most common dematiaceous molds can be remembered as A, B, C, E, but no D. *Alternaria, Bipolaris, Curvularia,* and *Exserohilum.*
• There is debate if *Scedosporium* belongs to the hyaline hyphomycetes or to dematiaceous molds as it does produce a diffusible melanin pigment, but it is not found inside the hyphae in appreciable quantities. It is most commonly classified as dematiaceous.

Amphotericin-Resistant Fungi

• There are a few fungi that could be growing in a patient who is on amphotericin. This makes a good point for board tests.
• They are as follows:
  • *C lusitaniae* (have higher MICs to amphotericin).
  • Some isolates of *C. auris.*
  • Some *Fusarium* spp.
  • *Aspergillus terreus.*
  • Some *Scedosporium apiospermum.*
  • All *Lomentospora (Scedosporium) prolificans.*
  • *Sporothrix schenckii.*
  • *Pseudallescheria boydii.*

Diagnostic Methods

Direct Microscopic Examination

• KOH treatment of clinical specimen can help direct visualization of fungus under microscopy.
• Staining with Calcofluor white and visualizing under florescence increases yield of direct visualization.

Blood Cultures

• Most of the yeasts, including *Candida* spp., are readily recovered from blood.
• Most dimorphic fungi can be found to be positive in blood cultures in disseminated disease, but this is a very slow and insensitive method.
• Thermally monomorphic molds can be isolated from blood. This includes, but is not limited to, *Aspergillus, Scedosporium, Acremonium, Fusarium,* and other Zygomycetes. *Aspergillus* and other hyaline hyphomycetes are rare true bloodstream infections, but the most common mold contaminants. However, due to likelihood of being contamination, clinical correlation and caution must be used while interpreting any blood culture positive for a mold.

| | | TABLE 2.4 Dematiaceous Molds | | |

Fungi	Clinical Features	Microbiologic Features	At-Risk Patients or Pearls	Figures
Alternaria	Traumatic wound infection, dissemination	Dark septate hyphae with alternating septated conidia	Hematologic malignancy, HSCT, and neutropenia	 (From Rifai N, et al., eds. *Tietz Textbook of Clinical Chemistry and Molecular Diagnostics*. 6th ed. Elsevier; 2018.)
Bipolaris	Traumatic wound infection, dissemination	Dark septate hyphae with elongated and septate conidia that taper at both poles (hence "bipolaris")	Hematologic malignancy, HSCT, and neutropenia	 (From Murray PR, Rosenthal KS, Pfaller MA. *Medical Microbiology*. 8th ed. Elsevier; 2016.)
Curvularia	Traumatic wound infection, dissemination	Dark septate hyphae, septate curved conidia	Hematologic malignancy, HSCT, and neutropenia	 (From Rifai N, et al., eds. *Tietz Textbook of Clinical Chemistry and Molecular Diagnostics*. 6th ed. Elsevier; 2018.)
Scedosporium/ Lomentospora	Pneumonia, eye, CNS, skin, dissemination	Septate hyphae with swollen and elongated conidia	Immunocompromised host (malignancy, transplant recipients). Has significant resistances to antifungals and often requires combination therapy	 (From Procop G, Pritt B. *Pathology of Infectious Diseases*. Elsevier; 2015.)
Exserohilum	Phaeohyphomycosis involving skin, soft tissue, CNS, and pulmonary	Dark budding yeast-like cells that eventually produce septate hyphae and flask-shaped conidiogenous cells	Associated with outbreaks due to natural disasters (tornado) and contaminated steroid injection	 (From Rifai N, et al., eds. *Tietz Textbook of Clinical Chemistry and Molecular Diagnostics*. 6th ed. Elsevier; 2018.)

Tissue Cultures

- Most fungi will grow on Emmons modification of Sabouraud's dextrose agar or potato dextrose agar.
- Crushing and processing of tissue prior to plating destroys the mold form, especially in Zygomycetes. If molds are part of the differential, tissue should not be aggressively crushed prior to culture.

Temperature

- Cultures should be incubated at 25°C temperatures to assist in identification of dimorphic molds. Growth at higher temperature is stressful to fungus and results in lower yields.

Time to Positivity

- Varies among different species. Routine fungal cultures are held for 4 weeks.
- *Candida* spp. often grows within 3 days.
- Molds may take up to 4 weeks to grow in culture, however.
- The slow rate of growth leads to a high dependence on serology and antigen testing, as well as empiric therapy.

Stains (Fig. 2.8)

Lactophenol Cotton Blue

- Lactophenol cotton blue is used as mounting fluid and stain to identify fungal structures from colonies on cultures. It has no role in tissue staining.
- Lactic acid acts as a clearing agent and aids in preserving fungal structures while cotton blue works as a stain.
- Most commonly used in labs to microscopically examine fungus cultures.

Calcofluor White Stain (Fig. 2.9)

- Binds to cellulose and chitin and fluoresces when exposed to long wave UV light.
- Useful in screening for almost all fungi.

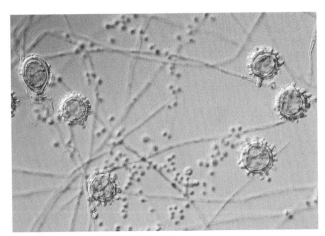

• **Fig. 2.8** Microscopical appearance of *Histoplasma capsulatum* microconidia and macroconidia. (Reprinted with permission from Warnock DW Fungi: Superficial; subcutaneous and systemic mycoses. In Barer MR et al. Medical Microbiology: A Guide to Microbial Infections, 19th edn. Elsevier, 2019.)

Direct Fluorescent Antibody Stain (Fig. 2.10)

- Performed by direct detection of antigen with fluorescently labelled antibody.
- Commonly used for detecting *Pneumocystis jirovecii*.
- The most common technique used is fluorescein-conjugated monoclonal antibody that can visualize both trophic forms and cysts.

Giemsa Stain (Fig. 2.11)

- Typically used for staining malaria and other parasites as well as certain bacteria (*Yersinia* and *Chlamydia*).
- In mycology, it is used in detection of intracellular *Histoplasma capsulatum* in bone marrow or blood smears.

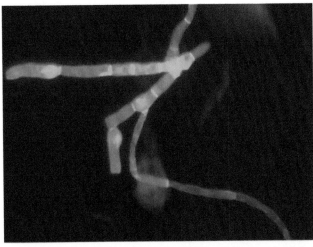

• **Fig. 2.9** *Purpureocillium* (formerly *Paecilomyces*) *lilacinum* in clinical specimens. Sinus specimen with branching septate hyphae (Calcofluor white stain). (Courtesy Anna F. Lau, NIH.)

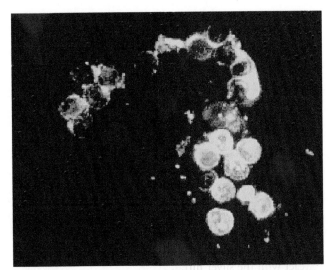

• **Fig. 2.10** *Pneumocystis jirovecii* (bronchoalveolar lavage [BAL]). The direct immunofluorescence test is highly sensitive, revealing green fluorescent-stained organisms and their extracellular products. (Reprinted with permission from Cibas ES and Ducatman BS. Cytology: Diagnostic Principles and Clinical Correlates. 4th edn. Saunders, 2014.)

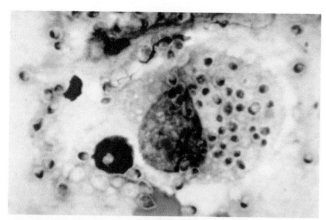

• **Fig. 2.11** Giemsa-stained preparation showing intracellular yeast forms of *Histoplasma capsulatum var. capsulatum.* (Reprinted with permission from Murray PR, Rosenthal KS and Pfaller MA. Medical Microbiology, Elsevier, 2016.)

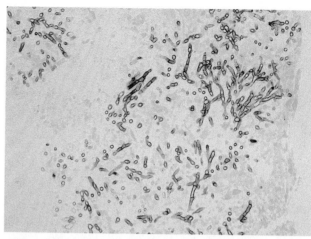

• **Fig. 2.13** GMS stain shows acute angle branching of septate hyphae (×200). (From Husain AN, Chang A. Diagnosis in pediatric transplant biopsies. *Surg Pathol Clin.* 2010;3(3):797–866.)

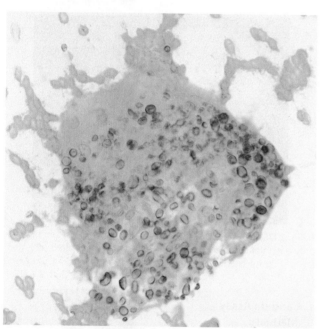

• **Fig. 2.12** Grocott–Gomori methenamine silver (GMS)-stained slide showing round shape and variability in size of yeast forms (GMS stain, ×400). (From Kradin RL. *Diagnostic Pathology of Infectious Disease.* Elsevier; 2018.)

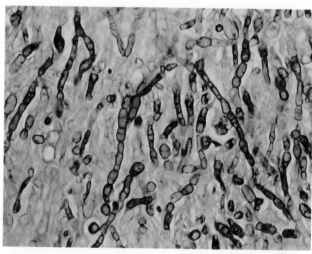

• **Fig. 2.14** Mycelial production of *Coccidioides immitis* with evolving arthroconidia. When exposed to air, *C. immitis* commonly will produce arthroconidia. Narrow, hyaline, branching hyphae could suggest a mycelial pathogen such as *Aspergillus* to the casual observer. Classic *Coccidioides* spherules were present in deeper portions of the nodule. PAS stain, ×1000 magnification. (From Procop G, Pritt B, eds. *Pathology of Infectious Diseases.* Elsevier; 2015.)

Gomori Methenamine Silver Stain (GMS) (Figs. 2.12 and 2.13)

- It is an important diagnostic tool for detecting and identifying fungi in autopsy and biopsy specimens. Arguably the most common and versatile stain when screening for presence of fungus.
- Mucopolysaccharide components of the fungal cell wall react with the silver nitrate, reducing it to metallic silver and thus rendering a brown–black compound.
- Fungi are sharply delineated in black against a pale green background. Inner parts of hyphae are charcoal grey.

Periodic Acid–Schiff Stain (Fig. 2.14)

- It is an effective pan-fungal stain used similarly to GMS.
- Periodic acid attacks carbohydrates containing 1,2-glycol or OH group with the conversion of this group to 1,2-aldehydes, which then react with the fuchsin-sulfurous acid to form the magenta color.
- Identification of fungal elements can be enhanced if a counterstain such as light green is used.

Mucicarmine Stain (Fig. 2.15)

- It is intended for use in the histologic visualization of mucopolysaccharides in the capsule of *Cryptococcus neoformans/gattii.*
- Upon tissues staining, it shows capsule as bright carmine red often with a spiny or scalloped appearance.

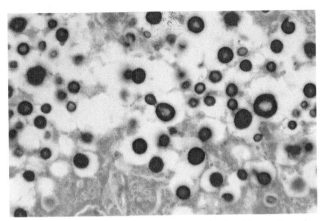

• **Fig. 2.15** *Cryptococcus neoformans* stained with mucicarmine (×1000). (From Murray PR, Rosenthal KS, Pfaller MA. *Medical Microbiology*. Elsevier; 2016.)

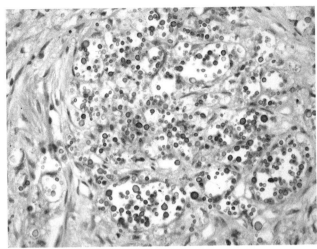

• **Fig. 2.16** Fontana–Masson stain assists in the identification of an "acapsular" variant of *Cryptococcus neoformans* (×400). (From Kradin RL. *Diagnostic Pathology of Infectious Disease*. Elsevier; 2018.)

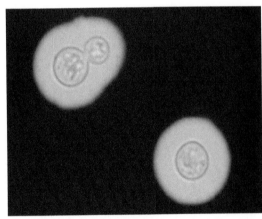

• **Fig. 2.17** India ink staining. Encapsulated yeast seen on India ink preparation of cerebrospinal fluid in a patient with cryptococcal meningitis. (From Perfect JR, et al. Cryptococcosis. *Infect Dis Clin North Am*. 2016;30(1):179–206. Courtesy of JR Perfect, MD, Durham, NC.)

• Useful in distinguishing *Cryptococcus* spp. from other yeast in tissues.
• Can have rare false-negatives in cryptococcal strains that do not form capsules, but these are avirulent and rarely cause disease.
• It can also stain *Rhinosporidium seeberi* and *Blastomyces dermatitidis*.

Fontana–Masson Silver Stain (Fig. 2.16)
• Fontana–Masson is a histochemical technique that oxidizes melanin and melanin-like pigments as it reduces silver giving visible black color.
• It is useful for differentiating fungi that produce melanin, such as *Cryptococcus* spp. and dematiaceous molds from those that do not, such as dimorphic fungi and the hyaline hyphomycetes.
• Fontana–Masson will be positive with capsule-deficient/mucicarmine-negative cryptococci.

India Ink (Fig. 2.17)
• It provides dark background that will highlight hyaline yeast cells and capsular material; important in detecting capsular microorganisms.
• The dye is excluded by the capsule, creating a clear halo around the yeast cell.
• It was predominantly used for identification of *Cryptococcus* in the cerebrospinal fluid specimens. However, since the development of antigen detection, which is easier and carries both a higher sensitivity and specificity, it is largely no longer in use.

Serologies, Antigen, and Molecular Testing

• Serologies and molecular tests are important methods of diagnosing a fungal infection.
• In most cases, they serve to suggest or support fungal diagnoses in appropriate clinical and epidemiologic settings.
• Due to the slow culture times, these tests are often relied on by clinicians more than cultures.

T2Candida Assay
Methods
• T2Candida Panel (T2 Biosystems) is a rapid diagnostic approach that enables sensitive and specific detection of *Candida* directly in whole blood without the need for culture or nucleic acid extraction steps using magnetic resonance.
Interpretation
• In two major studies comparing blood cultures and T2Candida, there was a 98% positive agreement, 100% negative agreement, 91% sensitivity, and 99% specificity.
• Detects candidemia in as low as 1–10 CFU/ml in most candida species.
• More clinical trials needed for further validation.
Use
• The T2Candida Panel utilizes T2MR technology to qualitatively detect five species of *Candida*:
  • *C. albicans*.
  • *C. tropicalis*.
  • *C. parapsilosis*.

- *C. krusei.*
- *C. glabrata.*
- Rarer species will not be diagnosed.

(1,3)-Beta-D-Glucan
Method
- 1,3-Beta-D-glucan, a cell wall component of many fungi, is detected by the beta-D-glucan assay. Routinely used for *Candida* spp. but has significant cross-reactivity.
Interpretation
- Depending on beta-D-glucan concentrations:
  - Negative (range <60 pg/mL).
  - Indeterminate (60–79 pg/mL).
  - Positive (>80 pg/mL).
- In various studies, sensitivity has ranged from 55% to 95%, and the specificity has ranged from 77% to 96%.
- Higher specificity for invasive fungal infections in hematologic malignancies.
Caution
- Similar to galactomannan assay, false-positive can be seen in patients receiving intravenous immunoglobulin (IVIG) and intravenous (IV) penicillin formulations.
- Positive with infections by other fungi, including *Pneumocystis.*
- Sensitivity is much higher if performed on BAL specimens.
Use
- Not specific to single fungal species.
- Useful for detecting candidiasis and invasive aspergillosis in immunocompromised host with appropriate clinical context.
- *Histoplasma* spp. and *Pneumocystis jirovecii* can also yield positive test results.
- Almost always negative in cryptococcosis and Zygomycetes.

Galactomannan Antigen Detection
- Galactomannan is a major polysaccharide constituent of *Aspergillus* cell walls.
Methods
- This diagnostic assay is a double-sandwich ELISA that incorporates the B 1–5 galactofuranose-specific EBA2 monoclonal antibody
Interpretation
- Serum and BAL are only specimens approved to run test.
- OD ≥0.5 is considered positive with sensitivity of 82% and specificity of 81% for diagnosis of invasive aspergillosis. PPV is <50% while NPV is >90%. However, in most clinical situations, the low pretest probability limits the use of this test.
- Clinical context should be considered to determine probability of infection.
Use
- Most useful in diagnosing invasive aspergillosis, especially in high-risk patients with hematologic malignancies.
- Detection in BAL does not differentiate colonization from invasive disease.
- *Fusarium, Penicillium,* and *Histoplasma* yield false-positive results due to presence of galactomannan in their cell walls.

Caution
- Due to presence of cross-reactive antigen, false-positive results can be seen in patients receiving piperacillin/tazobactam or amoxicillin/clavulanate. Test may result positive as long as 5 days after stopping antibiotics. However, the formulations of these antibiotics made after 2010 are almost never positive.
- Antifungal use will yield false-negative results.
- Rarely false-positive results are also noted after receiving IVIG.

Cryptococcal Antigen (CrAg)
- Detects cryptococcal polysaccharides antigen in serum and CSF (cerebrospinal fluid). Highly specific and sensitive for meningoencephalitis and disseminated disease but can be positive in pulmonary disease as well.
Methods
- CrAg is very sensitive and specific.
- Latex agglutination and sandwich ELISA were developed to detect cryptococcal antigen.
- However, a newer lateral flow assay is simpler, cheaper, faster, and more accurate method used widely for detecting antigen.
Use and Interpretation
- CrAg titers loosely correlate with organism burden and prognosis.
- Most common false-negatives are in isolated pulmonary disease.
- Titer should not be followed to assess treatment response, as the capsule polysaccharide can persist for months to years and the decline has not been shown to have an association with outcome or relapse.
Caution
- Rare false-positive results, especially in latex agglutination methods, are seen in *Trichosporon asahii, Rothia* (formerly *Stomatococcus*), and *Capnocytophaga.*

Histoplasma Antigen
Methods
- Detection of *H. capsulatum* galactomannan through EIA.
Use and Interpretation
- Useful in diagnosis of histoplasmosis in patients with a compatible clinical presentation and epidemiologic risk factors.
- Qualitative aspect helps for diagnosis of histoplasmosis.
- Quantitative assay helps ascertain severity, improves reproducibility, and facilitates monitoring antigen clearance during treatment.
- Most commonly performed on urine specimens; however, the test can be performed on blood and CSF. Higher sensitivity in disseminated cases and immunosuppressed patients.
- Highest levels and best performance characteristics are seen in patients with HIV.
- 75% of patient with CNS involvement have a positive CSF antigen.

- 90% of patients with diffuse pulmonary involvement have BAL antigen positive.
  Caution
- False-positive results can be seen with blastomycosis, coccidioidomycosis, talaromycosis, and paracoccidioidomycosis.
- The cross-reactivity with blastomycosis is so high that the urine antigen is often used to diagnose blastomycosis as well as histoplasmosis.
- False-negative tests are common in patients with pulmonary and other localized diseases as well as those that are immunocompetent or have minimal immunosuppression.

Histoplasma Antibodies
Methods
- Complement fixation test using histoplasmin from the yeast and mycelial forms of *H. capsulatum* is more sensitive and widely used.
- Immunodiffusion methods report results as M or H precipitin bands and are more specific.
  Use and Interpretation
- Positive result represents either acute infection or previous infections as elevated antibody titers persist for several years following initial infection.
- M band becomes positive sooner and is seen in most patients with any exposure.
- H band is seen in only fewer than 20% of cases but is very specific for disseminated infection, chronic cavitary pulmonary histoplasmosis, or more severe acute pulmonary histoplasmosis.
- H band clears after 6 months of infection while M band persists for years.
- Presence of both the H and the M band indicates active histoplasmosis.
- Presence of the M band alone indicates early or chronic disease.
- Seroconversion occurs 2–6 weeks after exposure.
- Titer of 1:32 or higher are highly sensitive for acute infection.
- In cases with lower titers, clinical context and epidemiology should be considered before deciding management.
  Caution
- False-positive results can be seen with coccidioidomycosis, blastomycosis, and in some granulomatous diseases like sarcoidosis and tuberculosis.
- False-negative results are seen in immunosuppressed patients.

Blastomyces Antibodies
Methods
- Immunodiffusion assays that measure antibodies to *Blastomyces dermatitidis* A antigen.
  Use and Interpretation
- Cross-reactivity with other endemic mycosis, especially *Histoplasma capsulatum.*
- Poor specificity and sensitivity for blastomycosis along with high degree of cross-reactivity with endemic mycosis, especially *Histoplasma capsulatum* makes it a less useful for diagnosis of blastomycosis. Rarely used in clinical practice.
  Caution
- Cross-reactivity with *Histoplasma capsulatum*, and other mycoses. Poor performance.

Coccidioides Antibodies
Methods
- Enzyme-linked immunoassays (EIA) detecting and measuring IgG and IgM levels.
- Immunodiffusion measures tube precipitin-type antibodies (IgM).
- Complement fixation measures depletion of complement that results after antibodies in a specimen from an infected patient form an immune complex when mixed with a coccidioidal antigen. Detects IgG.
- Test can be performed on serum and CSF.
  Interpretation and Use
- IgM develops within 1 week of clinical presentation and could last for 2–3 months. IgG is detected from 3–6 weeks of clinical presentation and could last up to 2 years.
- EIA is highly sensitive and used as a screening test for coccidioidomycosis.
- Immunodiffusion is highly specific thus making it good confirmatory test after positive EIA.
- CF provides a quantitative measurement of antibodies concentration and should be performed after positive immunodiffusion.
- CF antibody titers of >1:16 are highly predictive of dissemination. Higher titers are predictive of poor prognosis.
- Serial determinations of CF-type antibody titer have prognostic, diagnostic value as well as monitoring response to therapy.
- Positive test result for anticoccidioidal antibodies is usually associated with a recent or active coccidioidal infection. They will return to negative as the infection resolves.
- Detection of antibodies in CSF is highly specific for meningitis.
  Caution
- False-negative test can be seen in early coccidioidal infection.
- False-negative in immunocompromised host including HIV.

Coccidioidal Antigen
- Qualitative and quantitative assay measuring antigen in urine and serum.
- Not used routinely in immunocompetent due to low sensitivity.
- However, in immunocompromised patient with appropriate clinical presentation and negative serologies, antigen test proves beneficial in diagnosis.
- Antigen level serves as surrogate marker of fungal burden in severe disease and can be used to monitor response to therapy.

3

Virology

PHILLIP HEATON

Definitions

Antigenic drift: the accumulation of mutations that result in small changes to a virus over time, thus resulting in an antigenically different virus. Antigenic drift is why the seasonal flu vaccine changes yearly.

Antigenic shift: the phenomenon that occurs when two or more different strains of a virus combine genetic material or reassort their genetic material to form a novel strain. The 2009 H1N1 influenza epidemic is an example of a virus resulting from antigenic shift.

Capsid: the protein coat surrounding and protecting the nucleic acid of a virus.

Cytopathic effect (CPE): structural changes in a host cell due to virus infection.

Envelope: a membrane layer derived from host cell membranes that protects the viral capsid. Though made up of host cell membranes it can have viral proteins and is involved in the virus binding and infecting host cells. It may also be used for immune evasion.

Genotypic assay: sequencing and similar methods that rely on analysis of the nucleic acid sequence to determine a result such as drug susceptibility.

Hemadsorption: adherence of red blood cells to the surface of a cell monolayer. Used to confirm influenza cytopathic effect in cell culture.

IC50: the half maximal inhibitory concentration or 50% inhibitory concentration is the concentration of an antiviral agent that reduces the replication of viruses by 50%. It is one of the ways that phenotypic resistance assays are reported.

Lytic: the main method of viral replication that results in destruction of the infected cell.

Negative-sense: in viral RNA genomes these are strands of RNA that are 3'-5' and require the generation of viral RNA from an RNA polymerase before translation can take place.

Permissive: a cell line that is suitable for virus replication.

Phenotypic assay: an assay that relies on the growth of a virus in the presence of drug to determine susceptibility.

Plaque reduction assay: used to determine the IC_{50} of antiviral drugs. A known amount of virus is challenged with dilutions of a drug and the number of plaques is counted until the number of plaques in the presence of drug is half the number of plaques in wells not containing the drug.

Polymerase chain reaction (PCR): a technique in molecular biology that generates millions of copies of DNA from a single copy.

Positive-sense: in viral RNA genomes these strands serve as mRNA, that is they are 5'-3', and are capable of being translated into proteins. These viruses do not require an RNA polymerase, and naked genome may be infectious although much less so than a virus.

Real-time PCR: a technology based on PCR in which the generation of amplified target is measured in "real time" by the use of fluorescent dyes or probes.

Reverse transcriptase-PCR (RT-PCR): a variation of PCR in which the starting material is RNA that must be first converted to DNA.

Serotype: classification of viruses beyond the species level that is based on the antigens presented by the virus.

Shell vial assay: a cell culture assay that uses slow speed centrifugation to bring the patient sample into contact with the cell monolayer resulting in more rapid viral replication and detection. Virus specific antigen detection is often performed to identify the virus.

Tropism: the specificity of a virus for a host cell or tissue type. Tropism is determined by the ability of proteins on the surface of a virus interacting with proteins on the cell membrane referred to as receptors.

Viremia: the presence of virus in the blood.

Useful Information About Viruses

- A grouping of viruses based on various properties can be seen in Fig. 3.1.
- RNA viruses are more prone to mutations than their DNA counterparts. This is because RNA polymerases have a higher error rate due to the inability to proofread

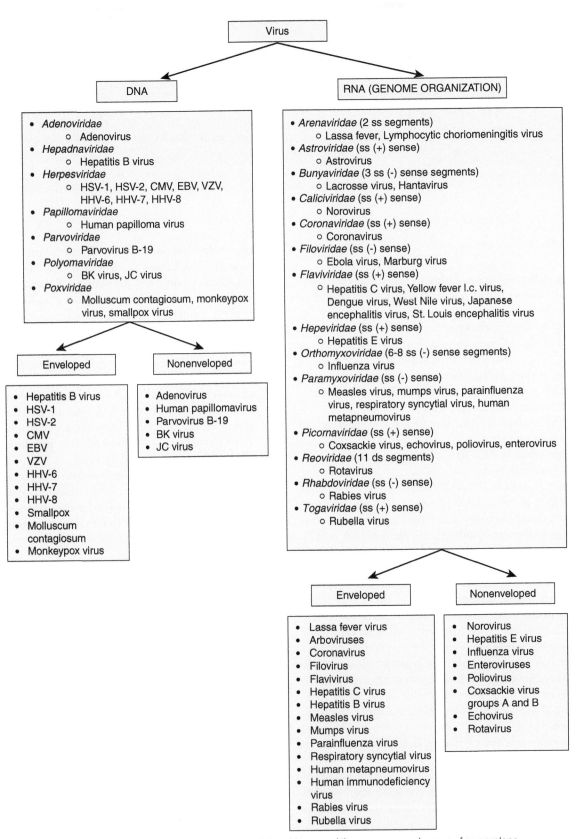

• **Fig. 3.1** Organization of viruses based on nucleic acid type and the presence or absence of an envelope.
Abbreviations: +, positive; −, negative; ss, single-stranded; ds, double-stranded.

TABLE 3.1   Diagnostic Testing Methods in Virology

Test	Description	Caveats
Histology	Useful for detecting viral disease processes in tissues. Specific antibodies and stains can provide specific identification of viruses of interest. Can be useful supplement in viruses that can be PCR-positive without invasive disease	Many viral phenomena are nonspecific. May be limited by the lab's choice of antibodies if thinking of immunohistochemistry
Viral culture	Involves applying the sample to be tested over a monolayer of cells so they may propagate and produce characteristic CPE	Sensitivity and specificity are limited by the lab's available cell lines. Some cultures may take weeks to grow, e.g., cytomegalovirus
NAAT	A general description for any test that amplifies DNA or RNA in a diagnostic assay to detect a pathogen	Issues arrive if the sequence amplified and detected has a mutation. Not always the test of choice as in the case of arboviruses. Does not distinguish between active, replicating virus and residual nucleic acid (see histology)
Antigen testing	Includes both rapid and nonrapid assays. Detects the presence of a viral protein in patient samples	Sensitivity depends on the amount of antigen present. Issues arise in specific cases, such as respiratory viruses where antigen is not shed at a high level in adults
Antibody testing	Detects antibodies made to a specific virus. Most useful if you can demonstrate a four-fold rise in titers over the course of illness	Most useful for epidemiological purposes, though occasionally it may be the test of choice, e.g., arbovirus infection. Occasionally see cross-reaction among viruses

CPE, cytopathogenic effect; *NAAT*, nucleic acid amplification testing.

the RNA it is generating. This is responsible for influenza virus antigenic drift and the ability of HIV to become drug resistant.

- The protein coat or capsid of a virus protects the genome. These are often referred to as icosahedral or helical, which denotes the geometry of virus.
- In general, enveloped viruses are less stable than their nonenveloped counterparts. The envelope is made up of cellular membranes which are sensitive to humidity, detergents, and heat. Nonenveloped viruses are more adaptable to harsh environments.
- Enveloped viruses may escape host immune systems by changing the antigens presented to the host immune system. This is especially true of enveloped RNA viruses as they accumulate mutations in that region of their genome.
- Diagnostic test methods can be found in Table 3.1.
- Viral culture is historically considered the "gold standard" but has been supplanted by real-time PCR and other nucleic acid amplification strategies.
- The biggest advantage of culture is that novel viruses and mutants can be isolated.

Respiratory Viruses (Table 3.2)

Adenovirus

- Nonenveloped virus with double-stranded DNA genome.
- Transmitted by small droplets or larger aerosols.

- Seven species with many serotypes causing a variety of disease. Testing is usually done by culture or NAAT depending on lab capabilities. The source submitted should be based on clinical presentation.
- Other diseases caused by adenovirus:
  - Acute respiratory distress.
  - Acute hemorrhagic conjunctivitis (pink eye, viral conjunctivitis).
  - Hemorrhagic cystitis in children and patients with a bone marrow transplant. It may be seen as a self-limited disease in healthy children.
  - Hepatitis.
  - Sexually transmitted infection resulting in urethritis and conjunctivitis in men and genital ulcers in women.
  - Disseminated disease primarily immunocompromised patients and neonates.
- May be seen as a smudge cell in histopathology (Fig. 3.2).
  - Must use caution as smudge cells are nonspecific.

Respiratory Syncytial Virus (RSV)

- Enveloped virus with a negative-sense single-stranded RNA genome.
- Transmitted by direct contact, large droplets, or fomites.
- There are two subgroups, A and B. Subgroup A is the most pathogenic.
- Causative agent of bronchiolitis in infants and young children. Illness in adults is milder and presents like an

TABLE 3.2	Respiratory Viruses Seasonality, Testing, and Considerations			
Virus	**Seasonality**	**Incubation Time**	**Test Choice (Cx, Ab, Ag, NAAT)[a]**	**Considerations[b]**
Adenovirus	Year round though most prevalent winter through summer	3–10 days	NAAT = Cx = Ag >>> Ab	Culture and NAAT are used most often for testing for adenovirus in other disease presentations
Respiratory syncytial virus (RSV)	Late Fall to Spring with a peak in January	2–8 days	NAAT > Ag > Cx >>> Ab	1. New AAP guidelines on bronchiolitis suggest testing for RSV not necessary due to the number of co-infections and inability to predict disease severity 2. Antigen testing is poor in adults due to the much lower amount of virus shed
Influenza virus	November – March with a peak in the winter months. Influenza A typically shows followed by Influenza B	1–4 days	NAAT ≥ Cx = Ag > >>Ab	1. NAAT may be negative if virus has mutated where the primers and probes bind 2. FDA recently required antigen testing to pass more stringent performance standards. Test is less sensitive in adults than children
Human metapneumovirus	Winter–Spring	3–5 days	NAAT >> Ag > Cx >> Ab	1. Virus is difficult to grow and direct detection lacks sensitivity 2. Almost 100% of kids are infected by age 5
Human coronavirus	Winter–Spring	2–14 days	NAAT	1. NAAT testing is usually part of a larger panel unless performed by CDC or public health labs 2. Serology is for epidemiology purposes
Enterovirus (EV)	Summer–Fall	3–6 days	NAAT >> Cx >>> Ag = Ab	Growth in culture may delay results as it is differentiated from rhinovirus. Differentiation is based on sequencing. Many commercial molecular assays do not distinguish between HRV and EV, but rather base determination on the body site infected, e.g., CSF most likely to be enterovirus than rhinovirus
Rhinovirus (HRV)	Year-round prevalence	1–2 days	NAAT ≥ Cx = Ag	Some NAATs cross-react with enterovirus as rhinovirus is one of the enterovirus species
Parainfluenza virus (PIV)	PIV-1: Fall of each year but peaks in odd numbered years PIV-2: Fall of each year, but can have an every other year periodicity PIV-3: Spring and summer PIV-4: No established seasonality	2–6 days	NAAT ≥ Cx > Ag >> Ab	1. NAAT testing may be a standalone test, but usually part of a larger panel 2. Antigen testing reserved for culture confirmation

[a]*Cx*, culture; *Ab*, serology; *Ag*, antigen detection; *NAAT*, nucleic acid amplification test. When designated with an = sign the choice of test should be based on factors such as the whether the sample type to be tested can be tested by that method and turnaround time.
[b]See sections below for more information.

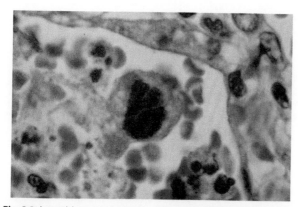

• **Fig. 3.2** Lung biopsy sample showing a smudge cell. Smudge cells in adenovirus infected cells have enlarged nuclei with basophilic inclusions surrounded by a thin layer of cytoplasm. (H&E, ×400.) (From Rhee E.G. and Barouche GH. Adenoviruses. In: Bennett JE, Dolin R, Blaser MJ, eds. *Mandell, Douglas, and Bennett's Principles and Practice of Infectious Diseases.* Updated 8th ed. Elsevier; 2015.)

upper respiratory tract infection with sore throat, nasal congestion, and cough.
• Some evidence that infection when young is linked to asthma later in life.

Influenza Virus

• There are three genera on influenza virus. Influenza A is the most pathogenic and occurs earlier in the season while B happens later in the season and is less pathogenic. Influenza C is typically limited to children.
• Influenza has a segmented genome that allows for swapping or reassortment of RNA segments between strains of viruses that infect other species. This reassortment leads to pandemic strains of influenza.
• Prone to antigenic drift. The machinery responsible for replicating the influenza genome is very error prone leading to changes in the antigens targeted by the flu vaccine. Yearly flu vaccines are needed because of antigenic drift.
• Patients may acquire bacterial pneumonia secondary to influenza infection. The most common causes are *Streptococcus pneumoniae*, *Haemophilus influenzae*, and *Staphylococcus aureus.*
• Drug resistance in influenza:
  • Resistance to M2 channel blockers is due to a mutation in the M2 protein and most influenza A in the United States is resistant. The drugs are not effective for influenza B.
  • Resistance to neuraminidase inhibitors is due to a mutation at the binding site of the neuraminidase protein.
    • Testing for resistance is not normally done unless the patient is immunocompromised. The preferred method is sequencing though some commercial labs offer the neuraminidase inhibition assay.

Human Metapneumovirus (MPV)

• It is an enveloped virus with a single-stranded negative-sense RNA genome.

• Transmission occurs via contaminated surfaces, droplets, and large aerosols.
• Manifests as an upper respiratory tract infection with symptoms similar to other respiratory viruses. Lower respiratory tract infections may mimic RSV and PIV in the form of bronchiolitis and croup.
• Nearly all children are infected by the age of 5.
• Infection with MPV, like RSV and PIV, can disrupt normal eustachian tube function and bacteria clearance giving rise to otitis media.

Coronavirus

• Crown-shaped "corona" virus with a positive-sense RNA genome.
• There are six human coronaviruses (HCoV). Four are distributed worldwide and the other two are severe acute respiratory syndrome (SARS) and Middle East respiratory syndrome (MERS).
• Transmitted by respiratory droplets.

Human Coronaviruses (Worldwide Distribution)
• The endemic viruses include OC43, 229E, NL63, and HKU1 and have a worldwide distribution.
• The peak occurrence of HCoV in the winter months typically presenting as a mild upper respiratory tract infection (URTI) with the rate of occurrence declining in spring.
• Incubation period is 2–5 days based on data obtained on OC43 and 229E.

SARS
• Zoonoses with the reservoir thought to be bats with spread to other animals such as the civet cat, which then transmits the virus to humans.
• Outbreak in 2002–2003 originated in China and resulted in almost 800 deaths.
• No cases have been reported since 2004.

MERS
• First reported infection was in Saudi Arabia in 2012.
• Thought to be transmitted by camels because of the frequency with which it is found in them, but it is uncertain.
• There have been 2,220 deaths since 2012 with 790 deaths associated with MERS CoV.
• No cases have been reported since 2014.

Enterovirus

• The name is derived from the site of replication and not the disease caused by the viruses in this genus.
• Members of *Picornaviridae* family. They are small, non-enveloped viruses with a positive-sense RNA genome.
• Enteroviruses are very stable and persist for long periods of time in part because they are not enveloped.
  • Transmission is typically the fecal–oral route though respiratory transmission is possible.
  • There are 15 species of enterovirus (enterovirus A–L and including rhinovirus A–C), of which 7 infect humans (enterovirus A–D and rhinovirus A–C).

Serotypes from the various species are known to cause a wide array of clinical syndromes (Table 3.3).
- CPE is somewhat indistinguishable from rhinovirus leading to the need for sequencing or specific NAATs for proper identification.
- Because of the similarity to rhinovirus some EV NAATs will cross-react with HRV.
- There are many nonpolio enteroviruses causing a variety of conditions ranging from the common cold to myocarditis and meningitis.

Rhinovirus
- Part of the *Picornaviridae* family and one of over 100 nonpolio enteroviruses.
- Most common cause of the common cold with the highest titers of virus found in the nose "rhino."
  - Accounts for over 50% of cases.
  - Also causes sinusitis and otitis media.

Human Parainfluenza Virus (PIV)
- PIVs are enveloped viruses with a negative-sense RNA genome.
- They are transmitted by respiratory droplets and fomites.
- They account for 75% of cases of viral croup. Other causes include flu, measles, and RSV.
- Imaging demonstrates subglottic stenosis and ballooning of the hypopharynx. It is classically known as the steeple sign (Fig. 3.3).
- Nasopharynx is the ideal source of testing by NAAT and culture.

Viral Gastroenteritis (Table 3.4)

See above for adenovirus.

Astrovirus
- Gets its name from its star-like appearance when viewed with electron microscopy.
- Nonenveloped virus with a single-stranded positive-sense RNA genome.
- Worldwide there is no seasonality, although in the United States it is thought to occur most often during the winter months.
- Transmission occurs via the fecal–oral route usually via contaminated food or water.

Norovirus
- Together with sapovirus are members of the *Caliciviridae* family.
- Nonenveloped with a single-stranded positive-sense RNA genome.
- Most common cause of viral gastroenteritis in the United States.
- Transmission occurs by the fecal–oral route, and infection spreads rapidly.
- Occurs most often in the winter months.

TABLE 3.3	**Illnesses and Their Most Commonly Associated Enterovirus Serotypes**
Virus	**Disease**
Coxsackie A viruses (CV-A)	Herpangina, hand–foot–and–mouth disease (HFMD: CV A6 and A16 most common in the United States), hemorrhagic conjunctivitis (CV A24)
Enterovirus	Acute flaccid paralysis (poliovirus), respiratory illness (EV-D68 outbreak of 2014), hemorrhagic conjunctivitis (EV-70), HFMD (EV-71 is the most common cause worldwide), encephalitis, aseptic meningitis, myositis
Echovirus	Meningitis (EV-13, 18, 30), respiratory illness
Poliovirus	Poliomyelitis
Coxsackie B virus (CV-B)	Myocarditis, herpangina (less frequent than with CV-A)
Rhinovirus	Common cold, otitis media, sinusitis, asthma exacerbation

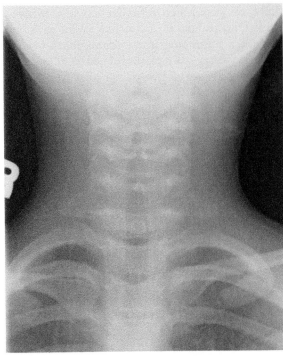

• **Fig. 3.3** Classic subglottic stenosis or "steeple sign" of viral croup seen in cervical radiograph. (Lin HW, Kakarala K, Ostrower ST, Leonard DS. Laryngotracheobronchitis complicated by spontaneous pneumomediastinum. *Int J Pediatr Otorhinolaryngol.* 2010;74:221–224.)

Rotavirus
- Member of the *Reoviridae* family.
- Nonenveloped virus with a genome of 11 segments of double-stranded RNA.

TABLE 3.4 Characteristics of Gastroenteritis Viruses

Virus	Seasonality	Incubation time	Testing[a]	Comments
Norovirus	Fall – Winter	1–2 days	NAAT	Affiliation with cruise ships and close quarters. Exceedingly contagious
Rotavirus	Year round with winter having highest incidence	2 days	Ag ≥ NAAT	NAAT testing is part of larger GI multiplex panels
Sapovirus	Year round	1–2 days	NAAT	
Astrovirus	Year round	1–2 days	NAAT	

[a]NAAT, nucleic acid amplification test; Ag, antigen detection.

- It is the most common cause of infectious diarrhea worldwide with most children having been infected by age 5.
  - Rotavirus is very stable and highly infectious (infectious dose ranges from 1–5 particles). Handwashing and usual sanitation practices are ineffective.
- Transmission is via the fecal–oral route.
- There are currently two vaccines, RotaTeq and Rotarix, approved in the United States.
  - RotaTeq is given at 2, 4, and 6 months.
  - Rotarix is given at 2 and 4 months.

Arboviruses (Table 3.5)

- Just under 90% of arbovirus infections occur in the summer and early fall (September).
- Dengue virus is the most common arbovirus worldwide while West Nile virus is the most common arbovirus in the United States.
  - There are four serotypes of dengue virus, and infection with one serotype does not protect you from the others.
  - Reinfection with a second type of dengue virus causes immunopotentiation, where the robust immune response leads to more severe disease.
- Serology, usually an ELISA, is the test of choice because most arbovirus infections result in only a short window of viremia.
  - Yellow fever and dengue virus are exceptions to the rule.
  - IgM becomes detectable in 1–2 weeks after fever onset and declines over a period of a few months.
  - Paired acute and convalescent sera demonstrating a four-fold rise in IgG titers is suggestive of a recent infection.
  - Plaque reduction neutralization assays (PRNT) may be used by a state public health lab or CDC to identify the specific virus.
    - PRNT takes a standard amount of virus and mixes it with a serial dilution of a patient's serum and allowed to incubate. This mixture is overlaid on to a cell monolayer so the virus has the ability to infect cells. A 50% reduction in plaques compared to serum free virus is the end point of the assay.
- Serologies performed against arboviruses in the same genera such as West Nile, La Crosse, and St. Louis encephalitis virus (all flaviviruses) are cross-reactive. It is virtually impossible to distinguish West Nile and St. Louis encephalitis on routine testing.
- IgM can persist for months or years after infection in some cases.

Hemorrhagic Fever Viruses

- Five virus families (*Flaviviridae*, *Bunyaviridae*, *Arenaviridae*, *Filoviridae*, and *Paramyxoviridae*) are responsible for viral hemorrhagic fever (VHF).
- All viruses are RNA viruses and require an animal or insect host to survive.
  - Humans are not a reservoir for any of the viruses.
- Diagnosis may be made using ELISA, antigen testing, neutralization assays, or NAAT

Ebola Virus
- Member of *Filoviridae* with a single-stranded negative-sense RNA genome.
- Incubation time is 3–21 days.
- Signs and symptoms initially include fever, chills, vomiting, diarrhea, myalgias, and loss of appetite.
  - Rash may occur from the waist up during days 5–7 leading to peeling of the skin.
  - A myriad of symptoms from each organ system occurs such as copious watery diarrhea, vomiting, pericarditis, and uveitis.
  - Hemorrhage occurs within the first 5–7 days after the onset of symptoms though profuse bleeding is not common.
- Case fatality rate averages 50% though ranges from 25% to 90% during various outbreaks.
- Fruit bats are thought to be Ebola's natural host.
- Humans are infected by coming into close contact with infected animals, their bodily fluids, and secretions.
  - Human-to-human transmission is through direct contact with fluids and secretions of infected people.

TABLE 3.5 **Characteristics of Select Arboviruses**

Virus	Vector for Human Transmission	Reservoir	Incubation Time	Disease/Presentation	Geographic Distribution
West Nile virus	*Culex* sp. mosquito	Birds	2–14 days	80% are asymptomatic. Viral meningitis, encephalitis, acute flaccid paralysis	Worldwide
St. Louis encephalitis virus	*Culex* sp. mosquito	Birds	5–15 days	Fever, headache, nausea, malaise Encephalitis, disorientation, stiff neck, and dizziness if there is CNS involvement	North and South America with the majority of cases occurring in the United States
Eastern equine encephalitis virus (EEE)	*Aedes* sp., *Culex* sp., *Coquillettidia* sp.	Birds. Horses are dead-end hosts	4–10 days	Chills, fever, malaise, arthralgia, myalgia. Encephalitis cases could result in coma. 33% of people with EEE die from it	Freshwater hardwood swamps along the Gulf coast and Great Lakes
Western equine encephalitis virus (WEE)	*Culex tarsalis* in the cycle involving birds. *Aedes melanimon* in the black-tailed jackrabbit cycle.	Birds and black-tailed jackrabbits. Horses are dead-end hosts	5–10 days	Ranges from mild febrile illness to encephalitis. 5%–10% of encephalitis cases are fatal	Worldwide though in United States most cases are west of the Mississippi River
Yellow fever virus	*Aedes* sp. (mainly *A. aegypti*)	Monkeys in the tropical rain forest	3–6 days	Fever, myalgias, arthralgias, vomiting, fatigue, and weakness Small portion develop severe disease with fever, jaundice, bleeding, shock, and multiple organ failure	Parts of South and Central America, sub-Saharan Africa, and many Caribbean islands
Dengue virus	*Aedes aegypti, Aedes albopictus*	Humans are the only vertebrate host	4–10 days	Severe headache, retro-orbital pain, muscle and joint pain "break bone fever," and rash Severe dengue 3–7 days after symptoms and can cause severe bleeding, respiratory distress, or organ failure	Worldwide
La Crosse virus	*Aedes triseriatus*	Chipmunks and squirrels. Humans are dead-end hosts.	5–15 days	Fever, headache, nausea, vomiting, fatigue Rarely fatal	Upper Midwest, mid-Atlantic, and southeastern states
Tickborne encephalitis virus	*Ixodes* sp. ticks		4–28 days	Nonspecific flu-like illness in early disease. Second phase of illness results in meningitis or encephalitis	Europe and Asia
Chikungunya virus	*Aedes aegypti* and *Aedes albopictus*	Humans and monkeys	1–12 days	Fever, myalgia, arthralgia, conjunctivitis, nausea, vomiting, rash	Worldwide

TABLE 3.6 Characteristics of Herpesviruses

Virus	Herpesvirus subfamily	Transmission	Incubation Time	Latency	Testing[a]
Herpes simplex virus 1/2 (HHV-1 and HHV-2)	Alpha	Infected secretions	1 day–3 weeks	Dorsal root ganglia HSV-1: trigeminal ganglia HSV-2: sacral ganglia	NAAT > Cx > Ag > Ab
Varicella-zoster virus (HHV-3)	Alpha	Aerosols	10 days–3 weeks	Dorsal root and trigeminal, geniculate, and cranial nerve ganglia	NAAT >> Cx ≥ Ag > Ab
Epstein-Barr virus (HHV-4)	Gamma	Saliva and other body fluids	4–8 weeks	B cells and epithelial cells	Ab > NAAT
Human cytomegalovirus (HHV-5)	Beta	Direct or close contact with infected individual. Found in numerous body fluids	3–12 weeks	Myeloid progenitor cells	NAAT ≥ Cx > Ag = Ab
Human herpesvirus 6 (HHV-6)	Beta	Saliva, droplets, transplant, and vertical transmission	9–10 days	Integrates into the subtelomeric regions of host DNA	NAAT > Ab
Human herpesvirus 7 (HHV-7)	Beta	Saliva, unknown if virus in other fluids plays a role in infection	–	lymphocytes	NAAT though testing often not warranted
Kaposi sarcoma-associated herpesvirus (HHV-8)	Gamma	Sexual transmission, saliva, transplant, and blood transfusion	–	Lymphocytes	NAAT > IHC for LANA

[a]*NAAT*, nucleic acid amplification test; *Cx*, culture; *Ag*, antigen detection; *Ab*, serology; *IHC*, immunohistochemistry. When designated with an = sign the choice of test should be based on factors such as the whether the sample type to be tested can be tested by that method and turnaround time.

- Abnormal lab findings include elevated AST and ALT levels, leukopenia, high or low hematocrit, thrombocytopenia, prolonged prothrombin and partial thromboplastin times, electrolyte imbalances, proteinuria, and increased BUN and creatinine.
- Ebola-specific diagnostic testing includes antigen and antibody detection, NAAT in the form of reverse transcriptase PCR, and real-time reverse transcriptase-PCR. NAAT is used by state health laboratories and some Ebola assessment and treatment centers under an emergency use authorization.
  - Cell culture and the above testing are performed at the CDC.
  - For a complete review of Ebola diagnostics refer to Further Reading (Broadhurst, et al.)
- In addition to Ebola testing blood culture, malaria testing, influenza (if prevalence is high), CBC with differential and platelets, urinalysis, liver function, PT, sodium potassium bicarbonate, BUN, creatinine, and glucose concentrations should be ordered in patients under investigation (PUI) for Ebola.

Herpesviruses (Table 3.6)

- All herpesviruses have a DNA genome and replicate within the nucleus. They cause lifelong infections, and for many PCR positivity is hard to interpret without classic syndromes.

Herpes Simplex Viruses 1 and 2

- Seroprevalence of HSV-1 in the United States was 53.9% in people aged 14–49 from 2005–2010. The seroprevalence of HSV-2 during the same time and in the same demographic was found to be 15.7%.
- HSV-1 and HSV-2 primary infections are followed by a latent period and possible reactivation.
  - Primary infection of HSV-1 is typically thought of as a gingivostomatitis while HSV-2 is typically thought to present as herpes genitalis.
  - HSV-1 is increasingly being transmitted sexually and is indistinguishable from HSV-2 without laboratory testing. The opposite is also true with HSV-2 oral infections occurring with increasing frequency.

- Recurrent disease happens when the virus reactivates and travels along the nerve axon to the oral and genital sites. Recurrent genital disease due to HSV-1 is rarer than HSV-2.
- Infections due to HSV include neonatal herpes, ocular herpes, encephalitis, and viremia. In immunocompromised hosts, can cause a severe fulminant hepatitis that is usually diagnosed with NAAT from the blood.

Diagnostic Testing

- Cell culture
  - CPE develops between 24 hours and one week depending on the viral titer.
- NAAT testing
  - Replacing culture as the gold standard due to its sensitivity and rapid turnaround time.
    - Lesions will remain PCR-positive longer than culture-positive.
  - It is the test of choice for CSF.
  - Non FDA-cleared sources can also be tested (e.g., eye, throat, rectal swab, etc.) provided proper test validation has been performed by the laboratory.
- Antigen detection
  - Detects HSV directly from a patient's specimen using immunofluorescence.
  - Sensitivity varies remarkably based on the quality of the sample submitted.
- Antibody detection
  - Used to detect recent infections if no lesion is present.
  - Only an antibody test that detects antibodies to glycoprotein G can distinguish between HSV-1 and HSV-2.
- Resistance and susceptibility testing
  - Aciclovir mutations typically due to frameshift mutations to the thymidine kinase gene.
  - Can be done using phenotypic or genotypic (sequencing) methods.
    - Plaque reduction assay is the "gold standard" susceptibility test for HSV-1.

Varicella-Zoster Virus (VZV)

- Member of the *Alphaherpesvirinae* subfamily.
- Ubiquitous distribution with infection typically occurring during early childhood prior to the development of a vaccine.
- Primary infection is visualized as chickenpox.
  - Sometimes confused for hand, foot, and mouth disease on presentation due to low incidence.
  - Primary infection can also result in encephalitis. Disseminated infection is possible in immunocompromised hosts (even with reactivation).
  - Congenital VZV possible if infection occurs during the 1st or 2nd trimesters.
    - Results in low birth weight, cicatricial scarring, neurologic defects, limb and digit abnormalities, and death.
  - Reactivation results from decreased T-cell immunity and presents as herpes zoster.

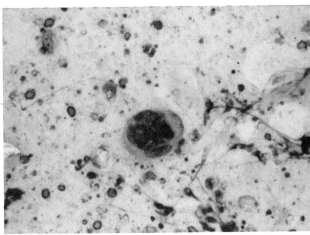

- **Fig. 3.4** Multinucleated giant cell present in a Tzanck smear.

- Occasionally a CNS infection without the vesicular rash occurs.

Diagnostic Testing

Varicella has been found in a variety of specimens including tissue, blood, CSF, and various body fluids.

- Histopathology
  - Tzanck smear (Fig. 3.4)
    - Examine cellular material from the base of a vesicle for the presence of multinucleated giant cells.
    - Lacks specificity as HSV exhibits the same phenomenon.
- Antigen detection
  - DFA used directly from clinical material with antibodies to VZV.
    - Sample must contain cells to perform.
  - Turnaround time is more rapid than culture (~2 hours) and is more sensitive than culture.
- Serology
  - Typically used to determine vaccination status.
- NAAT
  - The most sensitive method for detecting VZV from clinical material and has become the gold standard diagnostic assay.
  - NAAT is the recommended test for detection in CSF.
  - Virus is detectable in crusting lesions when a vesicle is not present.
  - NAAT can be used to detect VZV from a variety of sources.
    - Blood may be most useful in immunocompromised patients in which disseminated zoster is suspected and may not have a characteristic vesicular rash.
    - VZV PCR can be positive in the blood of healthy patients (2%–3%).
- Cell culture
  - Takes up to 2 weeks for CPE to develop due to cell associated nature of the virus and requires confirmation by DFA.
    - Culture turnaround time can be decreased through the use of shell vial assays.

- Susceptibility testing and antiviral resistance
  - Antiviral resistant VZV is not typically seen in immunocompetent hosts, but can be problematic in immunocompromised individuals that have received long courses of aciclovir or one of its analogs.
  - Resistance to aciclovir, valciclovir, penciclovir, and famciclovir are due to mutations in thymidine kinase or the DNA polymerase of VZV.
  - Resistance to foscarnet and cidofovir is due to mutations in the DNA polymerase similar to HSV and CMV.
  - Sequencing is the most common method used, but plaque reduction assays may be used in large institutions or if a novel mutation is suspected.

Epstein–Barr Virus (EBV)

- EBV is a member of the *Gammaherpesvirinae* family also known as human herpesvirus 4 (HHV-4).
- Nearly all individuals will be infected with EBV at some point in their life with nearly 100% of people being seropositive by age 40.
- Transmission from seropositive donors to seronegative recipients is important in the transplant population.
- EBV primary infection often seen as infectious mononucleosis.
- Other forms of disease include:
  - Burkitt lymphoma and nasopharyngeal carcinoma.
  - Post-transplant lymphoproliferative disorder (PTLD) in transplant recipients.
  - Oral hairy leukoplakia in HIV and transplant patients.
    - Latency occurs in B cells and epithelial cells.

Diagnostic Testing

- Serology is the diagnostic test of choice in most cases of EBV infection.
  - Heterophile antibody detection uses red blood cells or latex agglutination to detect antierythrocyte antibodies that are produced as a result of polyclonal B cell expansion seen in mononucleosis.
    - Heterophile antibodies appear about 3 weeks after infection and decline weekly. It is not uncommon for low levels to persist for up to 1 year.
    - Heterophile antibodies may be absent in both adults and children.
    - CMV may cause false-positives.
  - EBV-specific serologic testing is the method of choice to detect EBV infection (Fig. 3.5 and Table 3.7).
    - IgG and IgM antibodies to the viral capsid antigen (VCA), IgG antibody to the early antigen (EA), and IgG to the Epstein–Barr virus nuclear antigen (EBNA) are detected.
    - IgM to VCA appears first followed by IgG antibodies to VCA, then IgG to EA and EBNA-1.
  - EBV does not grow in cells typically used for viral culture.

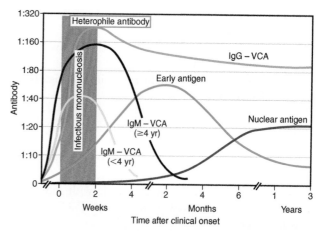

- **Fig. 3.5** Schematic showing the development of EBV antibodies and expression of EBV antigens. IgM to the viral capsid antigen (VCA) is generated early and persists for 4–6 weeks though it may persist for up to 8 weeks in adult patients. IgG antibody levels peak at 2–4 weeks and persist for life. EBNA antibodies take months to generate and remain for life. IgG to early antigen (EA) rises gradually and reaches a peak at 2–3 weeks then declines to undetectable levels by 6 weeks. However, in approximately 15%–20% of cases individuals may have anti-EA IgG that persists for years. (From Kliegman R, Stanton B, Behrman RE, et al., eds. *Nelson Textbook of Pediatrics*. 20th ed. Elsevier; 2016.)

TABLE 3.7	**Interpretation of EBV-Specific Serology**			
Infection	**VCA[a] IgM**	**VCA IgG**	**EA[b] IgG**	**EBNA[c]**
No previous exposure	–	–	–	–
Recent infection	+	+	+	–
Past infection	–	+	–	+

[a]VCA is the viral capsid antigen which makes up the outer protein coat or shell of the virus.
[b]EA or Early Antigen are proteins produced during the early or lytic phase of infection.
[c]EBNA or Epstein-Barr nuclear antigen is a group of proteins that have specific roles in the virus life cycle. Serologic assays target EBNA-1 which maintains the viral genome.

- EBV virus is shed for prolonged periods of time in saliva, up to 6 months. Therefore NAAT testing is not recommended for saliva.
- Immunohistochemistry (IHC) and in situ hybridization (ISH) used to detect virus in tissue.
  - Antibodies are directed to latent membrane protein 1 (LMP1), latent membrane protein 2 (LMP2), EBNA2, and other proteins.
- ISH targeting the noncoding Epstein–Barr virus encoded RNAs (EBER) is considered the gold standard as it is more sensitive than IHC as EBER is produced regardless of the stage of infection or latency of the virus. The function of these transcripts is not fully understood.
- NAAT can be either qualitative or quantitative.

- Quantitative NAAT is useful to obtain viral loads that can be trended.
  - Higher viral loads correlate to an increased probability of PTLD.
  - Changes of 0.5 log represent clinically significant changes in viral titer.

Human Cytomegalovirus (CMV)

- CMV has a worldwide distribution with a seroprevalence of nearly 100% in the elderly population.
- Infections are typically asymptomatic with most children and adults infected at an early age (58.9% after 6 years of age).
- May have a mononucleosis-like illness, but heterophile antibody-negative.
- CMV seen in immunocompetent, critically ill patients is usually due to reactivation and not primary disease.
- Infection in immunocompromised hosts is common and sometimes severe. May be due to either primary infection or reactivation.
  - CMV disease in transplant patients is often related to the transplanted organ, e.g., pneumonia in a lung transplant patient.
  - Late onset CMV disease occurs due to the use of antivirals for prophylaxis and preemptive therapy.
- Congenital CMV disease manifestations vary from hepatosplenomegaly, myocarditis, central nervous system defects, deafness, pneumonitis, and more.

Diagnostic Testing

Historically the gold standard for diagnostic testing has been tissue culture though NAAT has largely replaced it because of its exquisite sensitivity and specificity.

- Histopathology demonstrates large cells with nuclear inclusions that resemble an owl's eye (Fig. 3.6).
  - Histopathology is labor intensive and relatively insensitive compared to other diagnostic methods though sensitivity can be increased with IHC.
  - May correlate better with disease than the more sensitive NAAT testing.
- Serology is used to determine past or present infection in immunocompetent individuals or determine serostatus prior to transplant.
  - Most useful to determine past or present infection in immunocompetent individuals.
  - Also used to determine serostatus prior to transplant.
  - Look for a four-fold rise in IgG titers or the presence of IgM if determining if a patient was infected recently.
- IgM antibody measurement aids in the diagnosis of recent CMV infection.
  - False-positives possible due to rheumatoid factor, cross-reactivity to EBV VCA, and other nonspecific immune complexes.
  - IgM present in only 70% of congenital CMV cases.
- IgG avidity testing aids in determining if someone had a recent or past CMV infection.

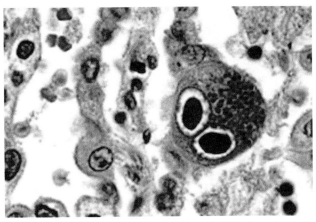

- **Fig. 3.6** Characteristic owl's eye inclusion of CMV. (From Mack M, Gregg K. Diagnosis and management of infections in hospitalized immunocompromised patients. *Hosp Med Clin.* 2014;3(3):e378.)

  - Particularly useful with pregnant women and in transplant recipients.
  - Measures the strength of IgG antibody binding in the presence and absence of a denaturing reagent such as urea. The strength of antibody binding increases over time.
  - ELISA is used to generate optical densities (O.D.) that can be used in the equation: Avidity = O.D. in the presence of urea/O.D. in regular buffer.
    - High avidity is ≥0.6 and suggests an infection at least 3 months prior to testing.
    - Low avidity is ≤0.5 and suggests a recent infection or possibly persistent IgG with low avidity.
      - This result is not as clinically useful as a high avidity result.
- CMV antigenemia is more sensitive than traditional culture but has largely been supplanted by NAAT.
  - Quantifies virus based on the detection of the tegument phosphoprotein pp65.
  - Results are expressed in antigen positive cells per leukocytes examined.
  - Trends should be followed as no hard cutoffs for disease have been uniformly established.
- Cell culture can take 1–4 weeks to become positive though the shell vial culture can decrease the turnaround time to 24 hours.
- NAAT testing has become the standard for diagnosing CMV infection and can be either qualitative or quantitative.
  - Qualitative NAAT testing is most useful for detecting CMV in tissues or rarely encountered samples.
  - Quantitative testing can distinguish between active infection and latency.
    - Higher viral loads correlate with systemic CMV disease while a negative PCR from blood samples has a high negative predictive value for systemic disease.
    - Increases or decreases of 0.5 log or more are considered significant.
    - Increases during antiviral therapy suggest possible drug resistance.

- Off label use of FDA cleared quantitative platforms have been used to test BAL fluid as an aid to diagnose CMV pneumonia in lung transplant patients. Standardization of methodology and more research is needed for meaningful thresholds to be set.

Drug Resistance

- Drug resistance is due to mutations in UL97 (thymidine kinase) or UL54 (DNA polymerase).
  - UL97 mutations confer resistance to ganciclovir.
    - Resistance to ganciclovir is usually the result of prolonged exposure to the drug.
    - 90% of ganciclovir resistance in the transplant setting comes from solid organ transplant patients that are donor (D)-positive, recipient (R)-negative. The percentage of D+/R- cases that develop a ganciclovir-resistant CMV infection ranges from 5%–12%.
    - The rate in people with HIV prior to HAART (highly active antiretroviral therapy) was 20% but is now 5%.
    - The mutations most commonly occurring that confer ganciclovir resistance are those affecting codons 460, 520, and 590–607.
  - UL54 mutations can confer cross-resistance to cidofovir, foscarnet, and ganciclovir.
    - Patients harboring ganciclovir resistance mutations on the *UL54* and *UL97* genes tend to have higher level ganciclovir resistance.
    - UL54 mutations occur much less frequently than UL97 mutations and usually occur following mutations to UL97. Although infrequent, UL54-only mutations can occur, e.g., patient taking cidofovir or foscarnet instead of ganciclovir.
- The plaque reduction assay is considered the gold standard for determining resistance phenotypically. Its area of greatest use is in discovering novel drug resistance mutations as it takes longer than sequencing.
- Sequencing, the standard for detecting known mutations, requires a viral load of approximately 1,000 copies/mL or 581 IU/mL.
  - IU is an abbreviation for international units and is the standard unit of measurement when performing quantitative CMV assays. It is the unit of measure used for the World Health Organization Standard that is used to calibrate FDA cleared and LDT assays.
    - The standard was created due to variations in the performance characteristics of existing quantitative CMV assays which resulted in a wide range of viral loads when one sample was tested by many labs and platforms. Standard material allowed for calibration and more consistent viral load readings between laboratories.
    - 1 IU/mL is between 1.5 and 2.0 copies/mL with the conversion depending upon the assay used by the lab.
- Traditional Sanger sequencing uses a PCR-based template and requires roughly 25% of the virus population to possess the mutation for efficient detection.

- Next Generation Sequencing can sequence directly from a clinical source and detect mutant populations as low as 5%.
  - Minor populations should be viewed carefully and tracked to ensure clinical relevance.

Human Herpesvirus 6 (HHV-6)

- HHV-6 is the causative agent of roseola.
- HHV-6 combined seroprevalence is over 90% by 2 years old with HHV-6B being the most common cause of infection in the United States.
  - HHV-6A is less pathogenic than HHV-6B.
- HHV-6 is capable of integrating into the human chromosomes. Approximately 1% of the population has germline integration of HHV-6 into chromosomal DNA.
- Immunocompromised host infections are typically due to reactivation and may present as disseminated infection, encephalitis, graft vs host disease, post-HSCT acute limbic encephalitis (PALE), as well as a myriad of other symptoms and diseases.
  - There is a large rate of false-positive testing, making diagnosis extremely difficult.
- Quantitative antibody detection via an indirect fluorescent antibody assay is recommended to track and trend titers.
- IgM antibodies are produced during an active infection and persists for 2–3 months following a primary infection.
- NAAT is more sensitive than serology at detecting acute infection.
  - HHV-6 is never detected in plasma or serum samples unless there is active infection or there is chromosomally integrated virus.
  - Quantitative testing allows for trending of viral loads, which is especially useful in immunocompromised patients when attempting to determine whether the patient has an acute infection.

Human Herpesvirus 7 (HHV-7)

- HHV-7 is a member of *Betaherpesvirinae* family and has a seroprevalence is 60%–90%.
- HHV-7 has been found in breast milk, urine, and cervical secretions though it is unknown what role, if any, these play in transmission.
- 5% of roseola cases in immunocompetent patients are cause by HHV-7.
  - Also associated with febrile seizures in pediatric patients.
- NAAT is the test of choice.

Kaposi Sarcoma-Associated Herpesvirus (Human Herpesvirus 8)

- Member of the *Gammaherpesvirinae* family.
- Seroprevalence varies dramatically by geographic location.

- Seroprevalence in Uganda where Kaposi sarcoma is endemic is 50% whereas the United States has a seroprevalence as low as 6%.
- Kaposi sarcoma (KS)
  - Lesions can be seen on skin (Fig. 3.7), in the mouth, and in internal organs.
    - Reddish brown plaques or nodules on skin, organs, and in the mouth.
  - Endemic in Africa.
  - Virus is necessary, but not sufficient for development of KS.
  - There are four forms of KS.
    - African endemic.
      - Occurs primarily in children.
    - Transplant-associated.
    - AIDS-related.
      - Most aggressive form.
      - More common in men that have sex with men.

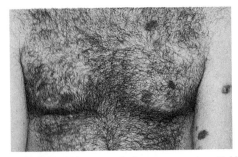

• **Fig. 3.7** Multiple Kaposi sarcoma lesions on a person with HIV. (From Morse SA, Ballard RC, Holmes KK, Moreland AA. *Atlas of Sexually Transmitted Diseases and AIDS*. 4th ed. Elsevier; 2010.)

- Classic KS.
  - Affects older immunocompetent Mediterranean European men.
- Primary effusion lymphoma.
  - Most common in men with HIV.
- Multicentric Castleman's disease.
  - Angiofollicular lymph node hyperplasia.
  - Most common in people with HIV.

Diagnostic Testing

- Immunohistochemistry
  - Uses monoclonal antibodies to the viral protein latency associated nuclear antigen (LANA-1).
- NAAT
  - Most widely used method to test.
  - Available from commercial reference laboratories.

Hepatitis Viruses (Table 3.8)

Hepatitis is covered in detail in Chapter 22.

Hepatitis A Virus (HAV)

- HAV is a nonenveloped virus with a single-stranded positive-sense RNA genome.
- HAV has a worldwide distribution, though it is more predominant in areas with poor sanitation.
- The majority of virus is excreted in feces, though patients can be viremic around the time of illness.
- Diagnostic test of choice is serology to detect IgM antibodies. IgG antibodies and total Ab is not useful as IgG will persist for life.

TABLE 3.8	**Characteristics of Hepatitis Viruses**				
Virus	**Transmission**	**Incubation Time**	**Testing[a]**	**Notes**	
Hepatitis A virus (HAV)	Fecal–oral, blood	15–150 days	Ab > NAAT	IgM Ab detection is the test of choice	
Hepatitis B virus (HBV)	IV drug use, sex, blood exposure (e.g., needlestick), vertical transmission	45–160 days	Ab = Ag = NAAT	10 genotypes	
Hepatitis C virus (HCV)	IV drug use, sex, blood exposure (e.g., needlestick), iatrogenic transmission	14–180 days	NAAT = Ab	7 genotypes. Most common bloodborne infection in the United States	
Hepatitis D virus (HDV)	See HBV though perinatal transmission and sexual transmission is less common than in HBV	30–180 days	Ab only occasionally needed	Requires HBV to replicate	
Hepatitis E virus (HEV)	Fecal–oral, contaminated water primarily	14–60 days	NAAT = Ab		

[a]*NAAT*, nucleic acid amplification test; *Ag*, antigen detection; *Ab*, serology. When designated with an = sign the choice of test should be based on factors such as the whether the sample type to be tested can be tested by that method and turnaround time.

- There is no FDA approved NAAT. Lab developed tests are mainly useful for confirming serology.

Hepatitis B Virus (HBV)

- HBV is an enveloped virus with a circular partially double-stranded DNA genome.
- There are 8 genotypes (A–H) that are well known and two more recent, lesser known genotypes (I and J).
  - B and C are most common genotypes associated with chronic HBV.
  - Genotypes are determined by line probe assay or sequencing of the pre S or S gene.
- HBV is 50–100 times more infectious than HIV.
- HBV serologic progression in acute and chronic HBV infection (Fig. 3.8 and Table 3.9).
- HBsAG is the surface antigen of HBV and indicates the patient is highly contagious.
  - Positive list tests may be repeated to confirm results.
- HBeAg is a protein derived from the translation of RNA from the precore/core portion of the hepatitis B genome and processed.
  - HbeAg is a sign of active viral replication, and positive patients are considered highly infectious.
- Quantitative NAAT can be used with serology in the initial evaluation of a patient or to monitor patients with chronic infection.
- WHO standards exist to account for variability between test methods, which may be helpful for those patients who have test results from different labs.
- Resistance is defined as ≥1 log change in HBV DNA in a compliant patient from their lowest DNA levels that

is confirmed with repeat testing for at least 1 month follow-up.
- Susceptibility testing typically done by sequencing though a commercially available line probe assay is available.
- Mutations in the reverse transcriptase domain of the DNA polymerase confer resistance to nucleotide and nucleoside analogs.
- Genotypic testing involves Sanger or Next Generation Sequencing.
  - Next Generation sequencing platforms can detect minor variant (mutant) populations that may break through during treatment.

Hepatitis C Virus (HCV)

- HCV is a member of the *Flaviviridae* family and has a positive-sense RNA genome.
- There are seven genotypes
  - 1, 2, and 3 are responsible for most infections in the United States.
- Roughly 25% of infected individuals will spontaneously clear their infection while the remaining will have chronic HCV.
- Chronic HCV is due to mutations in the envelope proteins that allow it to go undetected by the host immune system.
- Interleukin 28 variant rs129790860 used to predict response to pegylated interferon and ribavirin therapy. In the era of direct-acting antivirals, this is becoming less relevant.
  - Homozygous CC genotype often leads to a sustained virologic response (SVR)/clearance.

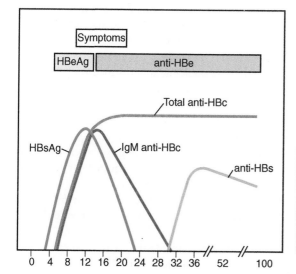 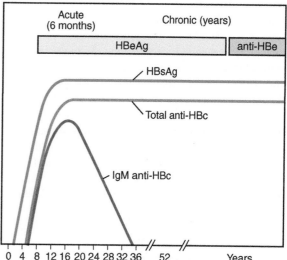

- **Fig. 3.8** Serologic profile of hepatitis B infection. The panel on the left demonstrates acute infection with recovery as evidenced by the drop off of hepatitis B surface antigen (HBsAg) and the production of anti-hepatitis B surface antigen antibodies (anti-HBs). The serologic profile on the right is that of a hepatitis B virus infection that progresses to chronic hepatitis B. The presence of hepatitis B e antigen (HBeAg) and the absence of antibodies to HBeAg is characteristic of active replication. (From Mandell GL, Bennett JE, Dolin R, eds. *Mandell, Douglas, and Bennett's Principles and Practice of Infectious Disease.* 7th ed. Elsevier; 2010.)

TABLE 3.9 Interpretation of Hepatitis B Serology

Interpretation	HBsAg	Anti-HBc	Anti-HBs	HBeAg	Anti-HBe
Acute infection	+	+ Total + IgM	−	+	−
Chronic replicating	+	+ Total − IgM	−	+	−
Chronic, nonreplicating	+	+ Total − IgM	−	−	+
Past infection with recovery	−	+ Total − IgM	+	−	+ or −
Vaccinated	−	− Total − IgM	+	−	−

TABLE 3.10 Interpretation of HCV Serology

Interpretation	Anti-HCV	HCV RNA	Comments
Current infection	+	+	
Past infection	+	−	Could also be a false positive. Consider confirmatory testing with a different assay. If repeat serology is positive most likely a resolved infection
Negative	−	−	If in the acute phase tentatively before seroconversion consider NAAT testing

- Heterozygous C/T tends to have chronic infection more often than SVR.
- Homozygous T/T genotype is associated with chronic infection.
- The amount of fibrosis in liver biopsy, *not* viral load or genotype, is associated with disease progression.
- Serology is recommended for screening. Serology interpretation is listed in Table 3.10.
  - Anti-HCV, if positive, remains positive for life.
- NAAT is useful to diagnose acute infection prior to seroconversion, which can take 4–6 weeks, and for chronic infection to show virus replication and in immunocompromised individuals.
  - NAAT should also be used to follow up a reactive anti-HCV assay.
- Genotyping is useful to determine therapeutic regimen and duration.
  - Genotyping done by sequencing the 5'-untranslated region (UTR), core, and NS5b gene targets.
  - Genotypes 1 and 3 tend to dominate worldwide with genotype 2 also having a worldwide distribution. Genotype 4 is more prevalent in Central sub-Saharan Africa, North Africa, and the Middle East. Genotype 5 is the most prevalent genotype in Southern sub-Saharan Africa. Genotype 6 is seen predominately in Asia, although it is the minority of cases there.

- Genotyping should further divide genotype 1 into 1a and 1b as genotype 1a is more likely to be resistant to simeprevir combination therapy.
- Susceptibility is determined by sequencing.
  - Protease inhibitor resistance due to mutations in *NS3*.
  - Nucleoside inhibitor resistance is due to mutations near the active site.
  - NS5a sequencing is performed on genotypes 1a and 1b.

Hepatitis D Virus (HDV)

- HDV has a circular RNA genome enveloped by HBV surface antigen, which is required for it to become an infectious virion.
- HDV is unable to replicate without HBV, specifically the HBV surface antigen, and the host cell's replication machinery.
- Endemic areas include the Mediterranean, Middle East, Central and Northern Asia, Japan, Taiwan, Greenland, the Horn of Africa and West Africa, the Amazon basin, and \South Pacific Islands.
  - The prevalence of HDV is most likely underestimated because of a lack of testing.
- A diagnosis of HDV is made by detecting total HDV antibodies.

TABLE 3.11 **Characteristics of Retroviruses**

Virus	Transmission	Disease	Test Method	Distribution	Comments
Human immunodeficiency virus 1 (HIV-1) and 2 (HIV-2)	Sex, transfusion, vertical transmission, IV drug use, and transplant	AIDS	Combination of Ab, Ag and NAAT	Worldwide HIV-2 found in West Africa	Transmission from needlestick or percutaneous injury in a healthcare setting is 0.3% (without postexposure prophylaxis) while mucous membrane exposure to infected blood is 0.09%
Human T-cell lymphotropic virus 1 and 2 (HTLV-1, HTLV-2)	Sex, breastfeeding, IV drug use, and blood transfusion	Adult T-cell leukemia/lymphoma and HTLV-1-associated myelopathy/tropical paraparesis	Ab used for screening. Reactive screens must be confirmed	Worldwide. Endemic in Southwest Japan, Caribbean, sub-Saharan Africa, Central and South America, Middle East, and Romania	HTLV-3 and 4 recently discovered

aNAAT, nucleic acid amplification test; *Ag*, antigen detection; *Ab*, serology.

- Though not commercially available some labs have real-time PCR assays to detect and quantify hepatitis D RNA.
  - Can be used to confirm serology and monitor response to therapy.
  - No standards exist for quantitative assays so results are not comparable between laboratories.

Hepatitis E Virus (HEV)

- Member of the *Hepeviridae* family.
- HEV is nonenveloped and has a single-stranded positive-sense RNA genome.
- HEV has a global distribution with an estimated 20 million infections occurring annually, but is most prevalent in East and South Asia.
- Infections are typically self-limited.
- NAAT is the gold standard for diagnosis of acute HEV, though sensitivity is dependent on patient presentation as viremia is highest in the preicteric phase until a week into the icteric phase.
- Serology to detect IgM is preferred for routine diagnosis of HEV in areas of high prevalence though it may be combined with a confirmatory NAAT in areas of low prevalence, such as the United States.

Retroviruses (Table 3.11)

Human Immunodeficiency Virus (HIV) (see Chapters 36–39)

- Member of the *Retroviridae* family and has a single-stranded positive-sense RNA genome.
- Genomes consist of single-stranded RNA that is transcribed into a complementary DNA (cDNA) using the virus's own RNA polymerase once the virus has bound the cell receptor and fused with the host cell membrane.
- The RNA is removed from the cDNA which is then made into double stranded DNA that is eventually incorporated into the cell's DNA via a viral integrase giving rise to a provirus.
- HIV-1 is separated into three groups: M (which has 8 clades/subtypes), N, O.
- Group M accounts for most HIV-1 infections.
- Group O is for outlier and is found primarily in West–Central Africa.
- Group N was discovered by a research team in 1998 after a variant strain of HIV was isolated from a Cameroonian woman who died in 1995. Her serum reacted with simian immunodeficiency virus envelope antigens instead of group M and O antigens This gave rise to group N, which simply stands for neither group M nor O.

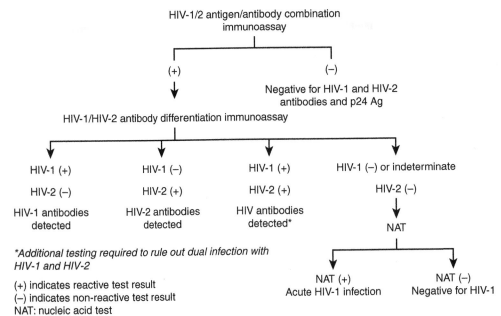

• **Fig. 3.9** CDC recommended laboratory testing algorithm. (From Fordan S, Bennett B, Lee M, Crowe S. Comparative performance of the Geenius™ HIV343 1/HI-2 supplemental test in Florida's public health testing population. *J Clin Virol*. 2017;91(344):79–83.)

• Group N infections are very rare with 19 cases reported to date, 16 of which have been confirmed by sequencing.
• Group P has been discovered and appears to more closely resemble simian immunodeficiency virus from gorillas as opposed to chimpanzees. Extremely rare, accounting for 0.06% of infections.
• HIV-2 is endemic to West Africa but is otherwise similar to HIV-1 in its ability to cause AIDS.
• During replication gp 120 binds the receptor CD4 which is followed by HIV binding either the CXCR4 or CCR5 coreceptors facilitating fusion and entry into the cell.
  • CXCR4 interaction occurs in T-cell tropic viruses while CCR5 occurs in lymphotropic viruses.
  • Maraviroc is only active against viruses that use CCR5 as a coreceptor and which must be determined with a tropism assay.
• Three phases of HIV infection:
  • Acute retroviral syndrome
    • A period of time after initial exposure which sees a rapid rise in viremia and destruction of CD4+ T cells.
    • Lasts 1–2 weeks and presents as a mononucleosis-like syndrome.
    • CD4+ T-cell counts recover and viral load remains steady.
  • Chronic HIV infection (clinical latency)
    • Low-level virus replication occurs and CD4+ T cells depleted slowly.
    • Mean duration is 10 years if patient is not on ART.

• Viral load correlates with CD4+ T-cell rate of decline during this period.
• Acquired immunodeficiency syndrome (AIDS)
  • Defined as a CD4+ T-cell count of below 200 cells/μL.
  • A number of opportunistic infections by viruses, bacteria, fungi, and protozoa as well as other AIDS-defining illnesses are possible.
    • Examples include *Pneumocystis jirovecii* pneumonia, Kaposi' sarcoma, toxoplasmosis involving the brain, and wasting disease.

Diagnostic Testing

• Diagnosis of HIV is made using a combination of serology, antigen detection, and nucleic acid testing (Fig. 3.9). (For more detail see Further Reading, Branson, et al.)
  • The fourth-generation algorithm begins with a screen that detects antibodies to HIV-1 and 2 and the p24 antigen. It shortens the window period from 3 weeks to 2.
  • Samples that are reactive in the initial screening undergo confirmation and differentiation between HIV-1 and HIV-2.
    • Western blots (WB) are still used by some labs to confirm HIV-1. Negative or indeterminate HIV-1 WB are reflexed to test for HIV-2 antibodies.
    • Heterophile antibodies may cause a false-positive screening and HIV-2 confirmation reaction in certain populations, e.g., zookeepers, vet techs, and veterinarians.
  • HIV-1 NAAT may be needed if differentiating assay is indeterminate or nonreactive.

- Point of care testing allows for rapid testing of oral fluid, whole blood, and serum.
  - Sensitivity is lower than laboratory methods, and oral fluid is less sensitive than whole blood or serum.
  - Reactive results must be confirmed by a laboratory method (typically fourth-generation combo assay).
    - Consider retesting if nonreactive and high risk due to the longer window period of some of these assays.
- Qualitative RNA NAATs are useful when patient may fall into the acute phase of infection, especially if considered high risk or when determining the infection status of a neonate.
- Quantitative viral load assay detects and quantifies the amount of HIV-1 RNA present.
  - Can be used similar to qualitative testing as supplement or confirmatory test to serologic screening.
    - The linear range of the real-time RT PCR based assays range from 20–40 copies – 10,000,000 copies/mL.
    - Changes in viral load are considered clinically significant if they are ≥0.5 log.
- HIV-1 susceptibility can be done genotypically or phenotypically.
  - HIV-mutants result from an error-prone polymerase and are selected during therapy.
  - Phenotypic testing measures virus replication in the presence of drugs but is labor intensive and has longer turnaround times, which limits its usefulness in clinical practice.
- Genotypic testing involves sequencing reverse transcriptase and protease genes to determine if there is resistance to nucleoside reverse transcriptase inhibitors (NRTI), nonnucleoside reverse transcriptase inhibitors (NNRTI), protease inhibitors (PI), and integrase inhibitor resistance.
  - Resistance to NRTIs when HIV mutations allow the virus's reverse transcriptase to differentiate between the inhibitor and naturally occurring NTPs.
  - Mutations in the binding site of the RT confer resistance to NNRTIs.
  - Substrate cleft mutations (where a PI binds) are responsible for PI resistance.
  - Integrase inhibitor resistance stems from mutations around the active site of the enzyme.
- The list of mutations responsible for drug resistance is updated by the International Antiviral Society-USA.

Human T-Cell Lymphotropic Virus

- HTLVs 1–4 are members of the *Retroviridae* family and have single-stranded positive-sense genome.
- HTLV-2 has not been definitively associated with a malignancy.
- Serology is the test of choice. Reactive serology requires confirmation and is needed to differentiate HTLV-1 from HTLV-2.
- NAAT testing is reserved for resolving discordant confirmation testing.

Other Viral Agents of Clinical Significance (Table 3.12)

Measles

- Member of the *Paramyxoviridae* family with a single-stranded negative-sense RNA genome.
- Occurs primarily in winter and spring.
- Koplik spots are pathognomonic for measles and occur 2–3 days before the onset of the rash (Fig. 3.10).
  - The rash begins at the hairline on the head and spreads downward over the course of a few days until it reaches the feet as if it has been poured over the head.
- Complications include otitis media, pneumonia, and diarrhea.
  - Complications in immunocompromised patients include Hecht pneumonia, measles inclusion body encephalitis, and death from severe measles without the rash and Koplik spots.
- Subacute sclerosing panencephalitis (SSPE) is a fatal complication of measles that results from persistent measles infection of the CNS.
  - Occurs 7–10 years after measles infection.
- Measles is diagnosed using IgM and IgG serology, NAAT, and viral culture.
  - IgG requires paired acute and convalescent sera. A four-fold rise in titers is needed to be considered recent infection.
  - For NAAT testing a throat swab is needed up to 5 days after rash onset. Urine should be included in the sample collection after day 5.

Mumps

- Member of the *Paramyxoviridae* family. It is enveloped with a single-stranded negative-sense RNA genome.
- Humans are the only known host for mumps virus.
- The decreasing frequency of mumps virus infection has made it more difficult to diagnose clinically.
- Infection involves a prodromal phase followed by nonspecific respiratory symptoms and parotitis and parotid salivary gland swelling.
- Complications include orchitis, oophoritis, mastitis, and meningoencephalitis.
- Real-time PCR, a form of NAAT, is the test of choice. Other test methods include IgM and cell culture though culture is not practical for the lab.

Rubella

- The virus is a member of the *Togaviridae* family. It is enveloped and has a single-stranded positive-sense RNA genome.
- Humans are the only known host with infections occurring more frequently in temperate than tropical climates during late winter and spring.
- Congenital rubella syndrome results in stillbirth, death, deafness, cataracts, and other birth defects acquired from rubella virus infection in utero.

TABLE 3.12	Characteristics of Miscellaneous Viruses			
Virus	**Incubation Time**	**Transmission**	**Clinical Presentation**	**Diagnostic Testing[a]**
Measles	7–18 days	Aerosols, droplets, and fomites	3 Cs – Cough, Coryza, Conjunctivitis – Koplik spots, rash that starts on the forehead and pours down to the trunk and lower extremities	NAAT = Ab > Cx
Mumps	12–18 days	Respiratory droplets and fomites	Nonspecific symptoms, fever, swollen parotid glands	AB > NAAT = Ag = Cx
Rubella	12–23 days	Respiratory droplets and contaminated secretions	Rash is usually the first symptom in children, starting at the face and spreading down to feet Adults may have a prodrome period marked by low grade fever	Ab = Cx > NAAT
Rabies virus	3–8 weeks but could be months	From infected mammals	Initially nondescript flu-like illness with a prickling or itching sensation at the bite site Cerebral dysfunction, agitation, delirium, excitability, hypersalivation as disease progresses	Ag > Ab = NAAT = Cx

[a]*NAAT*, nucleic acid amplification test; *Cx*, culture; *Ag*, antigen detection; *Ab*, serology. When designated with an = sign the choice of test should be based on factors such as the whether the sample type to be tested can be tested by that method and turnaround time.

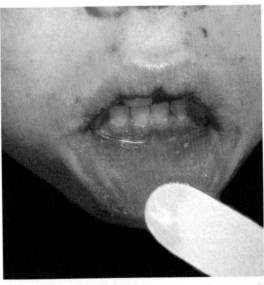

• **Fig. 3.10** Koplik spots are small white spots against an erythematous background that resemble grains of salt. They are pathognomonic for measles. (From Fitzpatrick JE, High WA, Kyle WL. *Urgent Care Dermatology: Symptom-Based Diagnosis.* Elsevier; 2018.)

- Infections that occur prior to 11 weeks are associated with birth defects more often than infections occurring later during gestation.
- Serology used to detect IgM and IgG.
  - IgM ELISAs are positive from day 5–40. The assays are fast and cost-efficient.
- IgG avidity may be used to distinguish recent from past infections though the same can be accomplished

by using paired acute and convalescent sera and looking for a four-fold rise in titers. The latter approach is of little use clinically because of the delay in obtaining convalescent serum.
- NAAT testing is performed on throat swabs and urine. It is the most sensitive assay during the first 5 days of postnatal rubella rash onset.

Rabies
- Member of the *Rhabdoviridae* family with a single-stranded negative-sense RNA genome.
- The mammal responsible for transmission to humans is largely dependent on the location.
  - In the United States common rabid animals are bats, raccoons, skunks, and foxes.
- Diagnosis is made via antigen detection using direct fluorescent antibody detection and is considered the gold standard for determining rabies risk to humans.
  - NAAT and neutralization assays can be used to diagnose human cases of rabies, with NAAT being the more sensitive of the two tests.

Further Reading

1. Centers for Disease Control and Prevention. National Center for Emerging and Zoonotic Infectious Diseases (NCEZID). https://www.cdc.gov/ncezid/index.html.
2. Broadhurst MJ, Brooks TJG, Pollock NR. Diagnosis of Ebola virus disease: past, present, and future. *Clin Microbiol Rev.* 2016;29:773–793.

3. Branson SM, Wesolowski LG, Bennett B, Werner BG, Wrobleski KE, Pentella MA. Laboratory testing for the diagnosis of HIV infection: updated recommendations. Centers for Disease Control and Prevention, Association of Public Health Laboratories, National Center for HIV/AIDS, VH, and TB prevention, Division of HIV/AIDS Prevention. June 27, 2014.

4. Berry M, Gamieldien J, Fielding BC. Identification of new respiratory viruses in the new millennium. *Viruses*. 2015;7:996–1019.

5. Cuthbert JA. Hepatitis A: old and new. *Clin Microbiol Rev*. 2001;14:38–58.

6. Gerlich WH. Medical virology of hepatitis B: how it began and where we are now. *Virol J*. 2013;10:239.

7. Hakki M, Chou S. The biology of cytomegalovirus drug resistance. *Curr Opin Infect Dis*. 2011;24:605–611.

8. Jorgensen JH, Pfaller MA, Carroll KC, et al. *Manual of Clinical Microbiology*. 11th ed. Washington, DC: American Society of Microbiology; 2015.

9. Richman DD, Whitley RJ, Hayden FG. *Clinical Virology*. 4th ed. Washington, DC: American Society of Microbiology; 2017.

10. Royston L, Tapparel C. Rhinoviruses and respiratory enteroviruses: not as simple as ABC. *Viruses*. 2016;8:16.

11. Upadhyayula PS, Yang J, Yue JK, Ciacci JD. Subacute sclerosing panencephalitis of the brainstem as a clinical entity. *Med Sci*. 2017;5:26.

4

Parasitology

ALICE CHI EZIEFULA, MARTHA PURCELL

Overview of Parasitology

Medically important parasites fall into three main classes: unicellular protozoa, multicellular helminths, and ectoparasites. They are usually considered further based on features such as their morphology and their target site within the human host. Life cycles are complex and typically involve significant structural changes between developmental stages. Humans may be infected as an essential, expedient, or accidental host. This chapter addresses the classification, epidemiology, and identification of medically important helminths and protozoa (see Fig. 4.1). Clinical aspects of disease are covered by Chapters 34 and 35.

PROTOZOA (TABLES 4.1–4.3)

- Protozoa are simple unicellular eukaryotic organisms that may be free-living or parasitic. They are commonly classified by movement modality: amebae, ciliates, flagellates, and apicomplexan (nonmotile). Enteric protozoa typically transmit feco-orally whereas blood and tissue protozoa usually require an arthropod vector.
- See Table 4.13 for Identification.
- See also Chapter 34.

Intestinal and Urogenital Amebae, Flagellates, and Ciliates

This section will discuss the amebae, flagellates, and ciliates that parasitize the human urogenital and intestinal tracts.

Overview

- Single-celled, eukaryotic organisms (Table 4.4).
- The organisms associated with human infection have two distinct stages: an active feeding trophozoite form and an infectious, resting cyst form.
  - When environmental conditions do not favor replication, these organisms enter cystic stage.
  - Cysts have thick protective wall and allow transfer to new host via fecal–oral route.

- Excystation occurs under favorable pH and enzymatic conditions within new host.
- Some protozoa which lack a cystic form can also achieve transmission to human hosts.
- Reproduction occurs through asexual multiplication by binary fission.

Epidemiology

- Transmission occurs via fecally contaminated food and water.
- Higher prevalence is associated with poor socioeconomic conditions, poor personal hygiene and sanitation and men who have sex with men (MSM).
- **Chlorination may not clear cysts from water supplies.** Filtration is required.

Identification

- Diagnosis relies largely on laboratory identification by **microscopy** (Fig. 4.2).
  - **Distinct microscopic features are key to diagnosis.**
  - Microscopists must be able to differentiate all species; morphology and characteristics can overlap.
- Immunodiagnostic methods not reliable for intestinal disease.

Molecular Testing of Intestinal and Urogenital Protozoa

- In 2013, FDA approved the first test for simultaneous identification of 11 causes of infectious gastroenteritis, including *Cryptosporidium* spp., *Giardia* spp. and *E. histolytica*.
- FDA has also approved a *T. vaginalis* amplification assay from vaginal/endocervical swabs and urine.
- Several other molecular tests are under development or in clinical trials.

Amebae

Diagnosis

- Trophozoites and cysts are the stages of the amebae used for diagnosis, and both can be found in feces.

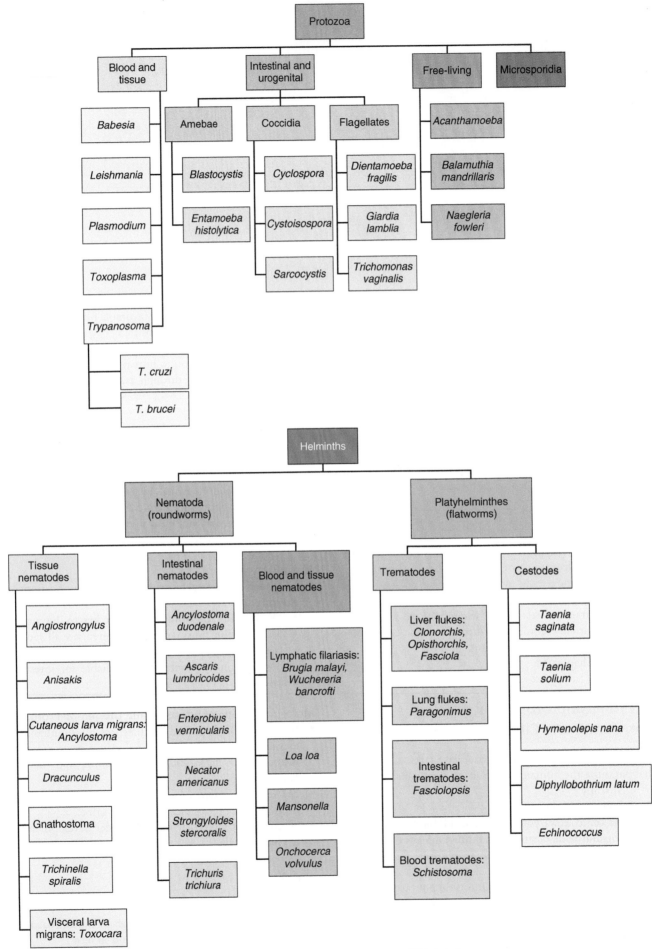

• **Fig. 4.1** Classification of medically important parasites: (A) protozoa; (B) helminths.

TABLE 4.1   Epidemiology of Major Protozoa

Organism	Geographic Distribution	Means of Transmission
Acanthamoeba spp.	Undefined	Water
Babesia spp.	North America, Europe	Tickborne, blood transfusions
Balantidium coli	Worldwide	Zoonosis (pigs), water,[a] fecal–oral
Blastocystis hominis	Unknown	Fecal–oral, water
Cryptosporidium spp.	Worldwide	Water, fecal–oral, zoonosis
Cystoisospora	Worldwide	Fecal–oral, suspected zoonosis
Entamoeba histolytica	Worldwide	Water, fecal–oral, foodborne
Giardia lamblia	Worldwide	Water, fecal–oral, foodborne
Leishmania spp.[b]		Female sandfly, blood transfusion
L. donovani	India, Pakistan, East Africa, China	
L. tropica	Middle East, Central Asia	
L. major	Middle East, India, Pakistan	
L. aethiopica	Ethiopia, Kenya	
L. mexicana	Central America, Texas	
L. amazonensis	South America	
L. chagasi	Latin America	
L. viannia braziliensis	Latin America	
Naegleria spp.	Worldwide	Fresh water, intranasal exposure
Plasmodium spp.	Africa, Asia, South and Central America, Oceania	Female anopheline mosquito, inoculation of infected blood
Sarcocystis spp.	Unknown	Foodborne (meat)
Toxoplasma gondii	Worldwide	Zoonosis (cats), foodborne (meat), blood or organ transplant, congenital
Trichomonas vaginalis	Worldwide	Venereal, during birth (?); nonvenereal, sexually transmitted
Trypanosoma spp.		
T. cruzi	South and Central America	Reduviid bugs
T. brucei gambiense	West Africa	Tsetse fly
T. brucei rhodesiense	East Africa	Tsetse fly

[a]Ingestion of water contaminated with fecal material.
[b]Other *Leishmania* spp. also infect humans but are less common.
From Korpe PS, Ravdin JI, Petri WA. Introduction to protozoal diseases. In: Bennett JE, Dolin R, Blaser MJ, eds. *Mandell, Douglas, and Bennett's Principles and Practice of Infectious Diseases.* Updated 8th ed. Elsevier; 2015.

Microscopy

- Trophozoite motility can be observed in fresh saline mount.
- Cytoplasmic inclusions; erythrocytes in trophozoites and chromatoid bodies in cysts.
- Cysts characteristics are less variable; fresh wet mounts alone may allow speciation.
- Iodine stains of fresh and fixed specimens are recommended for definitive identification of trophozoites and cysts (oil immersion at ×1000).
- Several cysts/trophozoites should be observed for reliability of identification.

- Unidentified organisms should be reported to the appropriate level and a repeat sample requested.

Entamoeba histolytica

Epidemiology

- Geography: **worldwide** distribution, but most prevalent in the tropics. Certain urban areas (Mexico and South America) have an incidence of invasive disease higher than the rest of the world.
- **Risk factors** for higher incidence:
  - LMIC, recent immigrants to industrialized nations.

TABLE 4.2 **Major Clinical Syndromes Caused by Protozoa**

Organism (Disease)	Major Clinical Syndrome
Acanthamoeba spp.	Keratitis, granulomatous amebic encephalitis
Babesia spp. (babesiosis)	Fever, malaise, hepatosplenomegaly, and hemolytic anemia, especially in the asplenic
Balantidium coli (balantidiosis)	Colitis
Blastocystis hominis (blastocystosis)	Diarrhea
Cryptosporidium spp. (cryptosporidiosis)	Self-limiting noninflammatory diarrhea; chronic severe diarrhea in children and immunocompromised adults, and cholangitis in AIDS patients
Cystoisospora spp. (cystoisosporiasis)	Diarrhea
Dientamoeba fragilis	Diarrhea
Entamoeba histolytica (amebiasis)	Diarrhea, colitis, liver abscess
Giardia lamblia (giardiasis)	Noninflammatory diarrhea with malabsorption
Leishmania spp. (cutaneous and visceral leishmaniasis)	Cutaneous or mucosal ulceration; visceral disease with fever, hepatosplenomegaly
Leptomyxida	Granulomatous amebic encephalitis
Naegleria spp.	Meningoencephalitis
Plasmodium spp. (malaria)	Paroxysmal fever, chills, headache, hepatosplenomegaly
Sarcocystis spp.	Myositis, fever
Toxoplasma gondii (toxoplasmosis)	Fever, malaise, lymphadenopathy; chorioretinitis; congenital abnormalities; in immunocompromised host, encephalitis, myocarditis, pneumonitis
Trichomonas vaginalis (trichomoniasis)	Vaginitis, urethritis
Trypanosoma spp. (African sleeping sickness and Chagas disease)	Fever, lymphadenopathy, meningoencephalitis, myocarditis; megaesophagus and megacolon, congestive cardiopathy

AIDS, acquired immunodeficiency syndrome.
From Korpe PS, Ravdin JI, Petri WA. Introduction to protozoal diseases. In: Bennett JE, Dolin R, Blaser MJ, eds. *Mandell, Douglas, and Bennett's Principles and Practice of Infectious Diseases.* Updated 8th ed. Elsevier; 2015.

- MSM, sexual activity that enables fecal–oral transmission.
- The human asymptomatic carrier working as a food handler plays an important role in transmission.
- Statistics: An estimated 500 million people have been infected, of these 50 million had extensive symptoms and 110,000 died. **For every case of invasive disease, there will be 10–20 asymptomatic cyst excreters.**
- Other hosts: the organism can be transmitted from the human reservoir host to other humans, primates, dogs, and cats.
- *E. histolytica, E. dispar, E. moshkovskii,* and *E. bangladeshi* are morphologically identical (on stool microscopy).
  - They are distinguishable with stool antigen or polymerase chain reaction (PCR) testing.
  - Prevalence data that predates these diagnostic innovations may be misleading.
- Pathogenicity

- *E. histolytica* is a pathogenic species; colitis and extraintestinal amebiasis.
  - *E. dispar* is nonpathogenic.
- *E. moshkovskii* was previously thought to be free-living and nonpathogenic, but recent studies indicate infection can cause noninvasive diarrhea.
- *E. bangladeshi:* pathogenicity is undetermined.
- Sexually transmitted amebiasis
  - Related to oral–anal sex or oral–genital sex after anal intercourse, predominately in MSM communities.
  - From 1978 to 1988 in San Francisco the incidence of symptomatic amebiasis among MSM of 20–39 years increased by >1000%.
  - The majority of *E. histolytica* infections are asymptomatic, but people living with HIV may be at higher risk of invasive disease.
- A colonization-blocking vaccine to eliminate *E. histolytica* from the human host has been proposed and is being investigated.

TABLE 4.3 Diagnostic Tests for Clinically Important Protozoa[a]

Disease	Preferred Diagnostic Tests
Amebiasis	
Intestinal	Stool antigen or PCR, serologic tests, colonoscopy
Liver	Ultrasonography or computed tomography, serologic tests, PCR on liver abscess aspiration
Amebic keratitis	Corneal scraping for microscopy and culture
Babesiosis	Giemsa or Wright staining of thin smear, PCR, serology
Cryptosporidiosis	Stool antigen or PCR or acid-fast and auramine-rhodamine staining of fecal samples
Giardiasis	Stool antigen or PCR
Granulomatous amebic encephalitis	Brain biopsy
Leishmaniasis	
Cutaneous and mucocutaneous	PCR, antigen detection, biopsy, touch preparation, culture, serologic tests
Visceral	PCR, antigen detection, bone marrow or splenic aspiration, touch preparation, culture, serologic tests, lymph node biopsy
Malaria	Wright or Giemsa stain of thin and thick blood smear, antigen detection or PCR
Primary amebic meningitis	Cerebrospinal fluid examination, wet mount of CSF for amebic trophozoites, CSF PCR, culture for amebas
Toxoplasmosis	Serologic tests, PCR, Wright–Giemsa stain of tissue, antigen detection
Trichomoniasis	Microscopy, culture, PCR, or antigen detection in genital secretions
Trypanosomiasis	
Chagas disease	Fresh blood or Giemsa-stained smear, PCR, xenodiagnosis; serologic tests for chronic disease
African sleeping sickness	Giemsa-stained blood smear, PCR, serologic tests, CSF examination

CSF, cerebrospinal fluid; PCR, polymerase chain reaction.

[a]See also Table 4.13.

From Korpe PS, Ravdin JI, Petri WA. Introduction to protozoal diseases. In: Bennett JE, Dolin R, Blaser MJ, eds. *Mandell, Douglas, and Bennett's Principles and Practice of Infectious Diseases*. Updated 8th ed. Elsevier; 2015.

Life Cycle

Fig. 4.3 shows the life cycle of *E. histolytica.*

Identification

Intestinal infection usually diagnosed by microscopic examination of feces or endoscopic samples.

- **Samples and microscopy**
  - Feces: trophozoites and cysts (Fig. 4.4).
    - *E. histolytica*: cyst usually 12–15 μm in length; trophozoite >20 μm; range 10–60 μm.
  - Tissue/abscess fluid: trophozoites only.
  - Trophozoites containing ingested erythrocytes can be seen on wet mounts.
  - Often trichrome or iron-hematoxylin stains of fixed specimens are required.
- The challenge is to distinguish pathogenic from nonpathogenic species.
  - *E. histolytica* is **only** confirmed by **trophozoites containing ingested erythrocytes or positive immunoassay**; otherwise reported as *E. histolytica/, E. dispar* group (Fig. 4.4A–B).

- *E. polecki, E. moshkovskii,* and *E. gingivalis* can be confused with E. histolytica.
- *E. hartmanni* can be distinguished from *E. histolytica* due to smaller size cysts and trophozoites (Fig. 4.5).
- **Immunoassays**
  - Can be used to identify genus *Entamoeba* and to differentiate *E. histolytica* from *E. dispar.*
  - These ELISA kits are based on detection of adhesion molecules in fresh stool.
  - These tests are simple, specific, and sensitive.
- **Serologic testing**
  - Useful in diagnosis of extraintestinal disease, in particular amebic liver abscess.
  - Even in presence of true dysenteric disease, results low and difficult to interpret so not recommended for diagnosing intestinal disease.
- **Histology**
  - Trophozoites can be identified within tissues using periodic acid-Schiff staining or hematoxylin and eosin staining.

TABLE 4.4 **Protozoan Infections of the Intestinal and Urogenital Systems of Humans**

Type	Species	Pathogenicity*
Amebae	*Entamoeba histolytica*	+
	Entamoeba dispar	−
	Entamoeba moshkovskii	± Pathogenicity remains controversial; possibly pathogenic in children
	Entamoeba bangladeshi	± Pathogenicity remains controversial; rare, not discussed in text; like *E. moshkovskii*, *E. bangladeshi* resembles *E. histolytica* and *E. dispar*
	Entamoeba hartmanni	−
	Entamoeba coli	−
	Entamoeba polecki	−
	Entamoeba gingivalis†	−
	Endolimax nana	−
	Iodamoeba bütschlii	−
	Blastocystis spp.	± Depends on the subtype(s) present; classification under review
Flagellates	*Dientamoeba fragilis*	+
	Giardia lamblia (duodenalis, intestinalis)	+
	Trichomonas vaginalis	+
	Pentatrichomonas (Trichomonas) hominis	−
	Trichomonas tenax	−
	Chilomastix mesnili	−
	Enteromonas hominis	−
	Retortamonas intestinalis	−
Ciliate	*Balantidium coli*	+

From Garcia LS. Protozoa. In Cohen J, Powderly W, Opal S, eds. *Infectious Diseases*. 4th ed. Elsevier; 2017.

Blastocystis *spp. (Formerly* B. hominis*)*

Epidemiology

- This complex includes many different subtypes/strains and species, all conventionally known as *B. hominis*.
  - Pathogenicity is debated but more likely in immunocompromised individuals.
  - Cysts are found both in the context of symptoms and in asymptomatic individuals.
- High prevalence in stool samples: surveys estimate up to 23% of US population infected, up to 100% of population may be infected in low income countries.
- Studies indicate that **zoonotic transmission** is likely (e.g., pets).
- Cysts can survive up to 19 days in water.

Identification

- Cysts found in stool samples.

- Usually 6–40 μm and contains a large central body (Fig. 4.6).
- Stains employed include D'Antoni's iodine and the trichrome stain.
- Other pathogens must be ruled out first before treating for *Blastocystis* spp.

Flagellates

Diagnosis

- More diverse group than amebae.
- Diagnosed in fecal specimens (*Giardia* spp. and *Dientamoeba fragilis*) and urogenital samples (*Trichomonas vaginalis*).
- **Trophozoite characteristics:** type of motility, shape, number of nuclei, undulating membrane, sucking disk (or adhesive disk), cytostome, spiral groove, number, and location of flagellae.

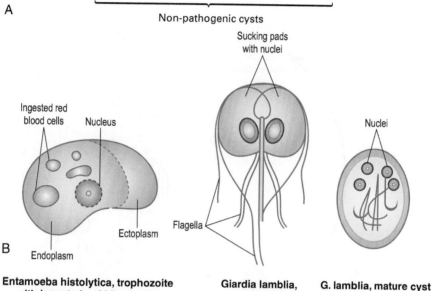

A   Non-pathogenic cysts

Entamoeba histolytica, trophozoite with ingested red blood cells

Giardia lamblia, trophozoite

G. lamblia, mature cyst

B

• **Fig. 4.2** Diagrammatic representation of some intestinal protozoal parasites. (Upper panel from Goering R, Dockrell H, Zuckerman M, Chiodini P. *Mims' Medical Microbiology and Immunology.* 6th ed. Elsevier; 2013. Lower panel from Greenwood D, Slack R, Barer M, Irving W. *Medical Microbiology: A Guide to Microbial Infections: Pathogenesis, Immunity, Laboratory Diagnosis, and Control.* 18th ed. Elsevier; 2012. pp. 642–654.)

- **Cyst characteristics:** shape, size, number and position of nuclei, absence or arrangement of fibrils.
- **Microscopy**
  - Direct or concentrated wet mounts.
  - Iodine-stained mounts.
  - Permanent stains recommended for all samples submitted.

Giardia lamblia (G. duodenalis, G. intestinalis)

Epidemiology
- Zoonotic protozoa that causes disease in range of hosts, including humans.
- **Worldwide** distribution; infection rates of 2%–15% in various countries.
- Viable cysts transmitted via **fecal–oral** route in contaminated food and water.
- A **low infectious dose** is required for infection, cystic stage is small, environmentally and chemically resistant; can survive disinfectant water treatments.
- **Risk factors**
  - Group living in close quarters.
  - **Poor sanitation**; outbreaks have been related to resort/municipal water supplies.
  - MSM: anal/oral sexual practices.

- **Decreased gastric acid production** due to malnutrition/gastrectomy/medication.
- Hikers/campers who drink **stream water** (potential wild/domestic animal reservoirs).
- Common cause of travelers' diarrhea. Visitors to endemic area more likely to be symptomatic.

Life Cycle
The life cycle of *Giardia duodenalis* is shown in Fig. 4.7.

Identification
- **Variable shedding** is demonstrated, so **multiple stool samples** should be examined.
- **Diagnostic methods**
  - Demonstration of cysts in feces (occasionally trophozoites).
    - Typically 11–12 µm in length, oval, 4 nuclei (Figs. 4.8A and B).
  - Permanent stains recommended for definitive diagnosis.
    - Use trichrome and iron-hematoxylin stains.
  - Duodenal aspirates and string test mucous can be examined on wet mounts.
  - Biopsied mucosal tissue: histopathologic methods and trichrome/Giemsa stains.

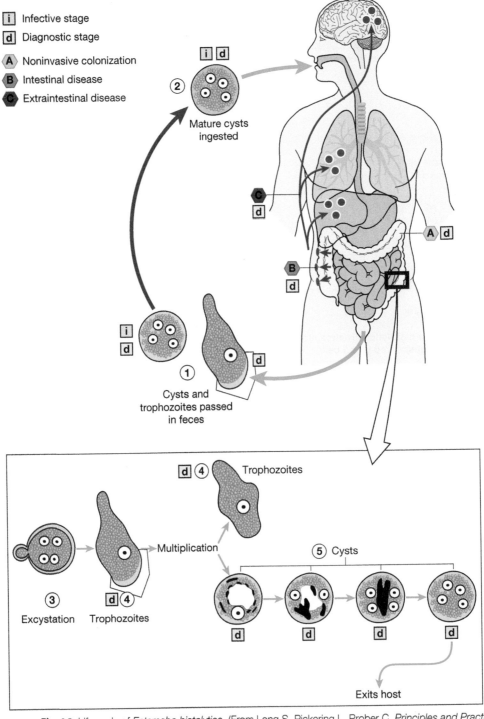

i Infective stage

d Diagnostic stage

A Noninvasive colonization

B Intestinal disease

C Extraintestinal disease

② Mature cysts ingested

① Cysts and trophozoites passed in feces

③ Excystation

④ Trophozoites

Multiplication

④ Trophozoites

⑤ Cysts

Exits host

• **Fig. 4.3** Life cycle of *Entameba histolytica*. (From Long S, Pickering L, Prober C. *Principles and Practice of Pediatric Infectious Diseases*. 5th ed. Elsevier; 2018.)

- Immunoassays
  - Enzyme immunoassay, FA, and immunochromato-graphic flow assays.
  - Results limited to absence or presence of *G. lamblia.*

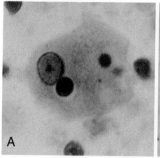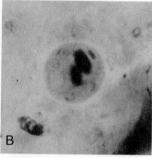

• **Fig. 4.4** (A) *Entamoeba histolytica* trophozoite containing ingested red blood cells. (B) *E. histolytica/E. dispar* cyst. (From Garcia LS. Protozoa. In: Cohen J, Powderly W, Opal S, eds. *Infectious Diseases.* 4th ed. Elsevier; 2017.)

Dientamoeba fragilis

Epidemiology
- Previously thought to bypass gastric acidity by infecting the eggs of *Enterobius* spp.
- Recent studies indicate a cyst form and possible life cycle similar to other intestinal protozoa.
- Infection is self-limiting, and identification is difficult so likely that **infection is under-reported.**
- Some links to irritable bowel syndrome (IBS), allergic colitis, and diarrhea in HIV patients.

Identification
- Variable shedding: requires permanent stains and multiple samples for diagnosis.
- Must be differentiated from *Endolimax nana, Iodamoeba butschlii,* and *E. hartmanni.*
- **Characteristics**
  - Trophozoites can be single or binucleate; 9–12 μm in length.

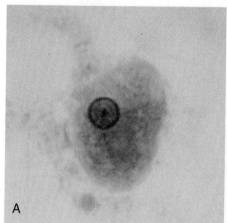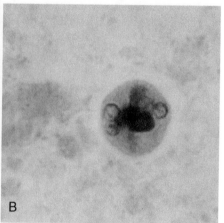

• **Fig. 4.5** *Entamoeba hartmanni.* (A) Trophozoite; (B) cyst containing up to four nuclei and chromatoidal bars with smooth, rounded edges (Trichrome stain). Note: *E. hartmanni* measures smaller than *E. histolytica/E. dispar*; the trophozoite is <12 μm and the cyst is <10 μm). (From Garcia LS. Protozoa. In: Cohen J, Powderly W, Opal S, eds. *Infectious Diseases.* 4th ed. Elsevier; 2017.)

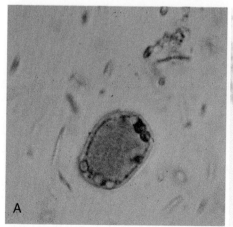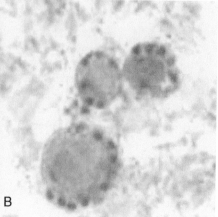

• **Fig. 4.6** *Blastocystis* spp. (A) Central body form with large "empty" area (appears like a vacuole) with multiple nuclei around the edges (D'Antoni's iodine). (B) Three central body forms with the large empty area surrounded by nuclei (Trichrome stain). (From Garcia LS. Protozoa. In: Cohen J, Powderly W, Opal S, eds. *Infectious Diseases.* 4th ed. Elsevier; 2017.)

Giardiasis

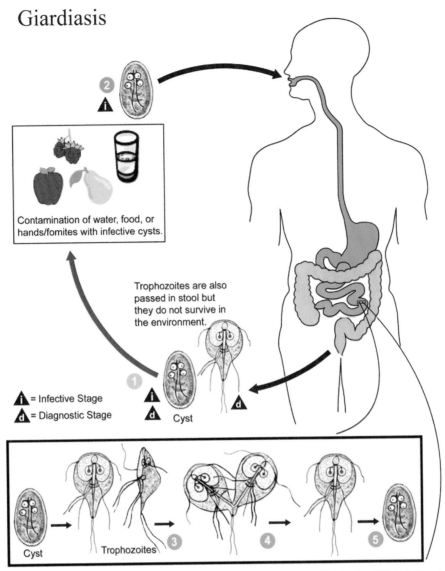

Contamination of water, food, or hands/fomites with infective cysts.

Trophozoites are also passed in stool but they do not survive in the environment.

🛆 **i** = Infective Stage
🛆 **d** = Diagnostic Stage

Cyst

Cyst   Trophozoites

• **Fig. 4.7** Life cycle of *Giardia duodenalis*. (From Rifai N, et al., eds. *Tietz Textbook of Clinical Chemistry and Molecular Diagnostics*. 6th ed. Elsevier; 2018.)

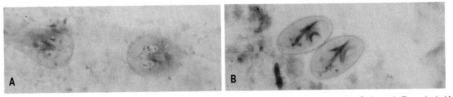

• **Fig. 4.8** *Giardia lamblia*. (A) Trophozoite; (B) cysts. (From Garcia LS. Protozoa. In: Cohen J, Powderly W, Opal S, eds. *Infectious Diseases*. 4th ed. Elsevier; 2017.)

- Nuclei are fragmented and chromatin is in a "tetrad" formation.
- Rare number of cysts.
- Size variation.

Trichomonas vaginalis

See also Chapter 21
- Transmission is via sexual intercourse.
- Identification of asymptomatically infected individuals can prevent further spread.

- Can present as sterile pyuria.

Identification
- Identified by finding motile trophozoites in wet mounts of vaginal fluid, prostatic fluid, fresh urine.
- Trophozoites have a nervous, jerky motion and undulating membrane along half their length.
- Diagnostic methods
  - Saline wet mounts.
  - Stained smear.

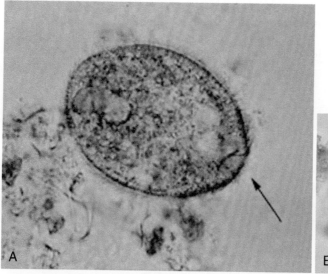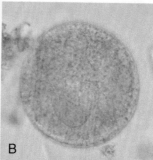

• **Fig. 4.9** *Balantidium coli.* (A) Trophozoite; (B) cyst. (From Suh KN, Kozarsky P, Keystone JS. In: Bennett JE, Dolin R, Blaser MJ. *Mandell, Douglas, and Bennett's Principles and Practice of Infectious Diseases.* Updated 8th ed. Elsevier; 2015.)

• Culture (rapid inoculation onto culture media, growth, and microscopy) is most reliable method.
• Gold standard is nucleic acid amplification.
• Enzyme immunoassay has been developed for ID from vaginal swabs.
• Monoclonal antibodies techniques have been reported as effective.

Ciliates

Balantidium coli

• Transmitted by ingestion of infective cysts in contaminated water or food.
• **Domestic pig** is most important reservoir for human infection.
• Incidence high in areas where pigs are the main domestic animal (New Guinea).
• Epidemics can develop if sanitation and personal hygiene are poor.

Identification

• Trophozoites are easily recognized by large size (40–50 µm), shape and rapid, rotating motion on direct saline mount (Fig. 4.9A).
• Cysts less easily identified but still identifiable by concentration (figure 9b).

Intestinal Coccidia and Microsporidia

• **Opportunistic pathogens**: noted as etiologic agents of **HIV-associated diarrhea** and intestinal disease in other immunocompromised patient groups (organ transplant, chemotherapy recipients).

• Also cause common, worldwide intestinal infections in the immunocompetent.

Identification Overview

• Stool examination by light microscopy is the mainstay of identification.
• Tests for intestinal coccidia and microsporidia may need to be specifically requested.
• See summary in Table 4.5.

Coccidia

• These are obligate intracellular protozoa belonging to the phylum Apicomplexa which infect **small intestine** enterocytes. Species of four genera are pathogenic in humans: *Cryptosporidium, Cyclospora, Cystoisospora,* and *Sarcocystis.*

Cryptosporidium spp

• 14 out of 30 identified species cause disease in humans.
• *C. hominis* is most common in humans.
• Bovine species *C. pestis/C. parvum* most common zoonotic species worldwide.
• Other zoonotic species have been identified in HIV patients and children in resource-poor countries.
  • Moderate public health significance: *C. meleagridis, C. cuniculus, C. felis, C. viatorum.*
  • Minor public health significance – *C. muris, C. parvum, C. andersoni, C. canis, C. suis, C. fayeri, C. ubiquitum.*

Epidemiology

• Geography: detected on **all continents.**

TABLE 4.5 Diagnosis of Intestinal Coccidia and Microsporidia

Microsporidial Species	Intestinal Coccidia			Microsporidia	
	Cryptosporidia	Cyclospora	Cystoisospora	Intestinal	Systemic
Routine Diagnostic Tests					
Light microscopy, stool	+	+	+	+	(+)
Light microscopy, urine, and possibly other body fluids	−	−	−	−	+
Antigen detection, stool	+	−	−	−	−
Molecular detection	+	+	−	+	+
Culture	−	−	−	−	−
Serology	−	−	−	−	−
Biopsy	Intestinal	Intestinal	Intestinal	Intestinal	Infected organ
Morphology of Pathogen					
Staining	AF, IF	AF	AF	Chromotrope, Calcofluor	Chromotrope, Calcofluor, special tissue stains
Size of coccidial oocysts/ microsporidial spores	4–6 μm	8–10 μm	23–33 μm long, 10–19 μm wide	1–3.5 μm	1–3.5 μm
Species identification	Molecular analysis	Molecular analysis	Molecular analysis	Electron microscopy; molecular analysis	Electron microscopy; molecular analysis
Stool Concentration Techniques	FEA	FEA	FEA	−	−

From Garcia LS. Protozoa. In: Cohen J, Powderly W, Opal S, eds. *Infectious Diseases*. 4th ed. Elsevier; 2017.

- Prevalence: 1%–3% industrialized nations, 5%–10% LMIC countries.
  - Sero-epidemiologic studies indicate much higher prevalence, suggesting underdiagnoses or the presence of asymptomatic infection.
    - Transmission: fecal–oral route
      - Humans and animals serve as sources of infectious oocysts.
      - Low infectious dose required: 10 oocysts.
- Risk factors: children under 2 years old, HIV infection, contact with contaminated water/food, contact with infected animals/humans, sexual contacts, nosocomial spread.
- Accounts for 10%–20% of chronic diarrhea in immunocompromised patients with HIV.

Life Cycle

The life cycle of *Cryptosporidium* species is shown in Fig. 4.10.

Identification

- Light microscopy of stool samples:

- Oocysts in fecal smears using **acid-fast staining** or **immunofluorescence** detection (Figs. 4.11A and D).
- Oocyst size measured to distinguish from other coccidian (see Table 4.5).
  - Typically 4–5 μm diameter.
- Concentrating stool samples can increase sensitivity.
- Multiple samples may be needed to improve diagnostic yield.
- **Jejunal biopsies** have demonstrated the presence of cryptosporidia in 10% with negative stool microscopy.
- Stool antigen and PCR-based techniques have improved diagnostic yields but not widely available.
- Cytologic techniques
  - Microscopic examination of duodenal aspirates and intestinal brushings.
- Histologic techniques
  - Basophilic on light microscopy after hematoxylin-eosin staining.
- Serology
  - Predominantly used in epidemiology. IgM/IgG positive within ~2 weeks of symptom onset.

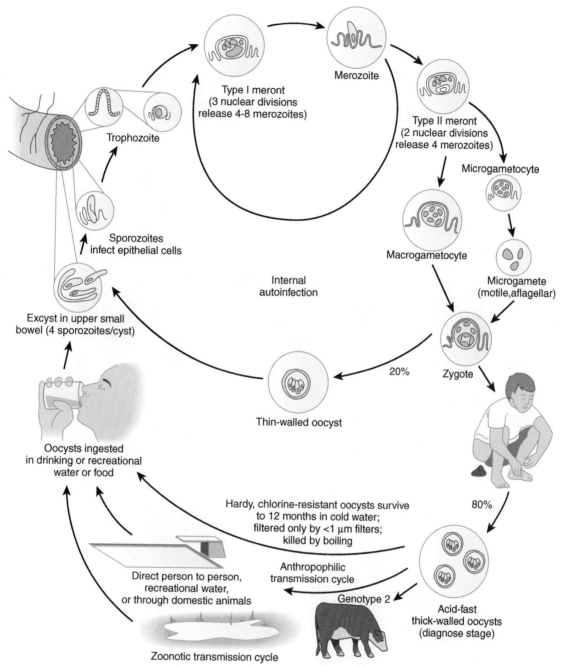

• **Fig. 4.10** Life cycle of *Cryptosporidium* spp. (Redrawn with permission from Kosek M, Alcantara C, Lima AAM, et al. Cryptosporidiosis: an update. *Lancet Infect Dis*. 2001;1:262–269.)

Cyclospora *spp.*

C. cayetanensis
• Previously called cyanobacterium-like bodies.

Epidemiology
• Geography: tropical and subtropical regions.
• Transmission: fecal–oral route via **contaminated fresh fruit and vegetables** from above countries.
  • Outbreaks in USA linked to imported raspberries, basil, snow peas, lettuce, and cilantro.
  • None associated with commercially frozen or canned food to date.

• Oocysts are immature when first shed; they have to sporulate to become infectious, which requires days to weeks, making direct person-to-person transmission unlikely.
• Sporulation is favored by warmth and humidity.

Identification
• Light microscopy of oocysts in wet mounts of fresh stool.
  • May be difficult to detect due to low level of cysts passed.
  • Maximize recovery by examining acid-fast stained smears from stool concentrates using FEA (formalin-ethyl acetate) sedimentation.

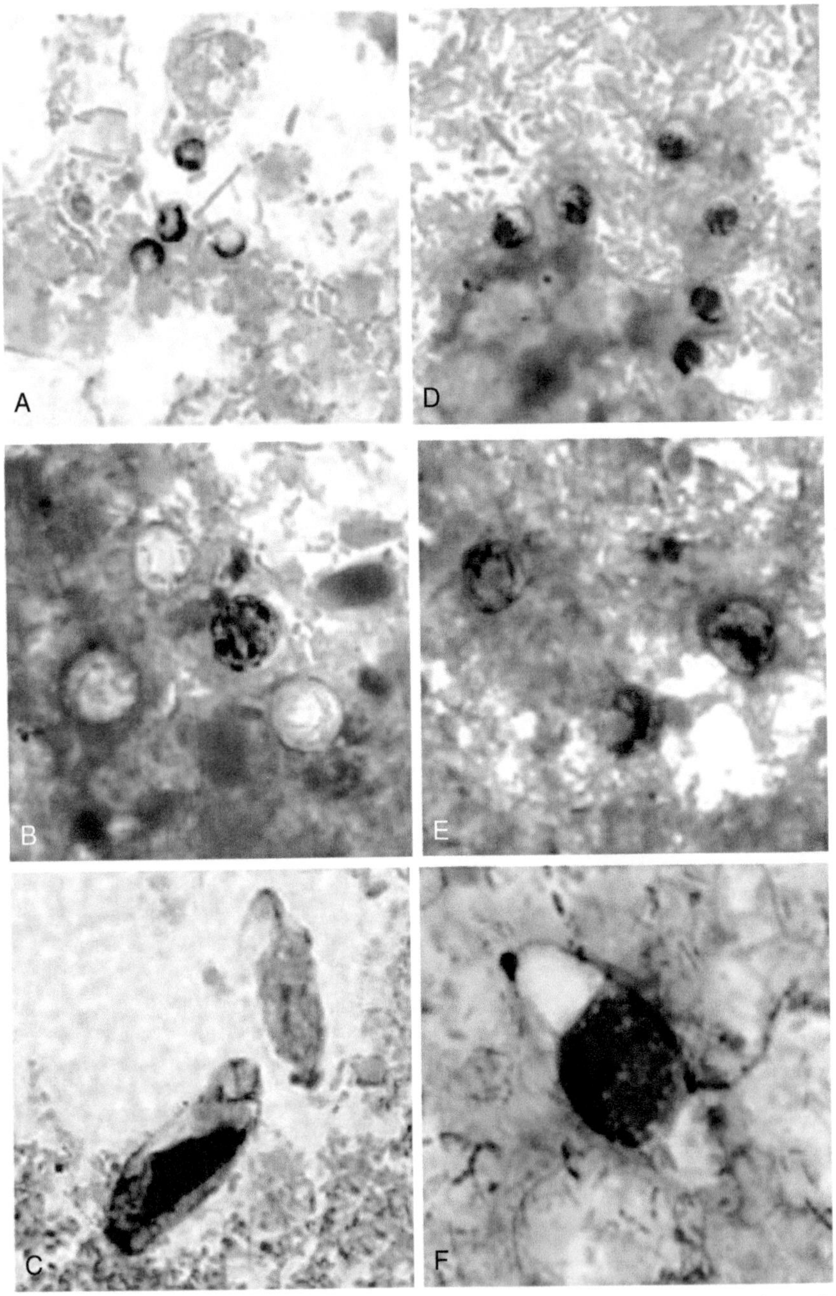

• **Fig. 4.11** Comparison of (A, D) *Cryptosporidium* spp., (B, E) *Cyclospora cayetanensis*, and (C, F) *Cystoisospora belli* stained with modified acid-fast and safranin stains, original magnification ×1000. (From Cama VA, Mathison BA. Infections by intestinal coccidia and *Giardia duodenalis*. *Clin Lab Med*. 2015;35(2): 423–444. © 2015. Fig. 1 Public domain images, courtesy of DPDx, Centers for Disease Control and Prevention, Atlanta, USA.)

• Testing not routinely conducted so needs to be specifically requested.
• Oocysts are variably acid-fast; they appear pink to deep red, many remain unstained (Figs. 4.11B and E).
• *Cyclospora* oocysts are 8–10 μm in diameter.
• They are autofluorescent under UV light (blue/green appearance).
• Molecular PCR-based techniques on stool samples have been described.

Cystoisospora belli

• Formerly known as *Isospora belli*.

• *C. belli* causes cystoisosporiasis (formerly known as isosporiasis).
• Only infects humans.

Epidemiology

• Geography: endemic in parts of Africa, Asia, and South America.
• Typically in patients from developing countries with AIDS and chronic diarrhea.
• Transmission: unknown but thought to be oocyst ingestion from water/food.

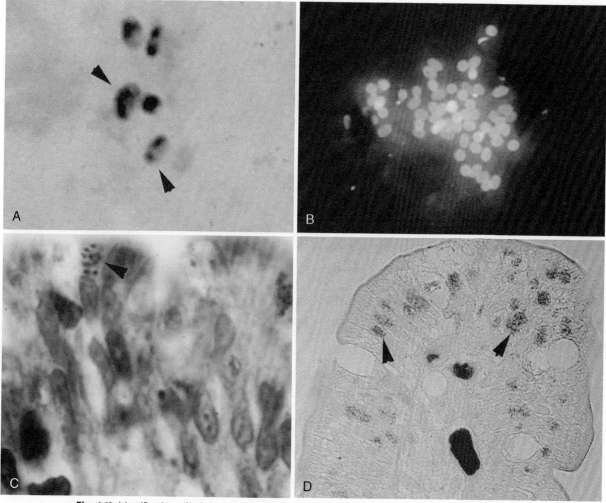

• Fig. 4.12 Identification of microsporidia. (Panels A and C from Bennett JE, Dolin R, Blaser MJ, eds. *Mandell, Douglas, and Bennett's Principles and Practice of Infectious Diseases*. Updated 8th ed. Elsevier; 2015. Panel B courtesy ES Didier, Tulane National Primate Research Center and currently at University of California, Davis. Panel D courtesy D Kotler, St. Lukes-Roosevelt Hospital Center and JM Orenstein, George Washington University School of Medicine, Washington DC.)

- Person-to-person transmission uncommon, likely due to the time required for the immature cyst to sporulate (1–2 days).

Identification

- **Light microscopy** of oocysts in wet mounts of fresh stool or acid-fast stained smears from stool concentrates (Figs. 4.11C and F).
  - 28–30 μm in length.
  - Oocysts are excreted intermittently; may require multiple samples to be examined.
- Histologic examination of small intestine tissue may reveal parasites within enterocytes.

Sarcocystis *spp.*

- *S. hominis* and *S. suihominis* (previously known as *Isospora hominis*)
  - Humans are the definitive host for these species.
  - Cause intestinal sarcocystosis.
- *S. nesbitti*
  - Humans are an accidental, dead-end intermediate host.
  - Causes muscular sarcocystosis.
  - Rare.

Epidemiology

- Acquired by **eating raw meat** from infected cattle/pigs.
- Symptomatic gastrointestinal human infection is rare, but asymptomatic infection has a wide geographic distribution.
- Cases of muscular sarcocystosis are mostly from rural Malaysia.

Identification

- Light microscopy of stool demonstrating oocysts or sporocysts.
  - 10–15 μm; cannot distinguish species.
  - However, shed in small numbers so easily missed.
- Light microscopy of stained muscle biopsy specimens and evidence of myositis or vasculitis.

Microsporidia

- Obligate intracellular, spore-forming eukaryotes: phylum Microsporidia.

TABLE 4.6 Microsporidia That Cause Disease in Humans

Genus and Species	Reported Infections	Animal Hosts[a]
Encephalitozoon		
E. cuniculi[b]	Hepatitis, peritonitis, encephalitis,[c] urethritis, prostatitis, nephritis, sinusitis, keratoconjunctivitis, cystitis, diarrhea,[d] cellulitis, disseminated infection	Mammals (rabbits, rodents, carnivores, primates)
E. hellem[b]	Keratoconjunctivitis,[c] sinusitis, pneumonitis, nephritis, prostatitis, urethritis, cystitis, diarrhea, disseminated infection	Psittacine birds (parrots, lovebirds, parakeets), birds (ostrich, hummingbirds, finches)
E. intestinalis[†]	Diarrhea,[c] intestinal perforation, cholangitis, nephritis, keratoconjunctivitis	Mammals (donkeys, dogs, pigs, cows, goats, primates)
Enterocytozoon		
E. bieneusi	Diarrhea,[c] wasting syndrome, cholangitis, rhinitis, bronchitis	Mammals (pigs, primates, cows, dogs, cats), birds (chickens)
Trachipleistophora		
T. hominis[b]	Myositis, keratoconjunctivitis,[c] sinusitis	Unknown
T. anthropopthera[b]	Encephalitis, disseminated infection, keratitis	Unknown
Pleistophora		
P. ronneafiei	Myositis	Unknown
Pleistophora sp.	Myositis[c]	Fish
Anncaliia		
A. vesicularum	Myositis	Unknown
A. algerae[d]	Keratoconjunctivitis, myositis, skin infection	Mosquitoes
A. connori	Disseminated infection	Unknown
Nosema		
N. ocularum	Keratoconjunctivitis[c]	Unknown
Vittaforma		
V. corneae[†]	Keratoconjunctivitis,[c] urinary tract infection	Unknown
Tubulinosema		
T. acridophagus (and *Tubulinosema* sp.)	Myositis, disseminated infection (skin, liver, peritoneum, lung and retinal involvement)	Insects (*Drosophila melanogaster* and grasshoppers)
Endoreticulatus		
Endoreticulatus sp.	Myositis[‡]	Lepidopteran insects
Microsporidium		
M. africanus	Corneal ulcer[c]	Unknown
M. ceylonensis	Corneal ulcer[c]	Unknown

[a]Animals in which organism has been found other than humans.
[b]Organism can be grown in tissue culture.
[c]Cases reported in immune-competent hosts.
[d]Previously called *Brachiola* and *Nosema*.
From Korpe PS, Ravdin JI, Petri WA. Introduction to protozoal diseases. In: Bennett JE, Dolin R, Blaser MJ, eds. *Mandell, Douglas, and Bennett's Principles and Practice of Infectious Diseases*. Updated 8th ed. Elsevier; 2015.

- More than 190 different genera and 1200 species.
- At least 16 microsporidial species have been identified that can infect humans (see Table 4.6).
- Have been reclassified as fungi; but previously considered to be protozoa, and dealt with by parasitology laboratories.

Epidemiology
- Geography: cases are **globally distributed.**
- Transmission
  - Most likely ingestion of spores.
  - Aerosol transmission has been considered.

- Sources
  - Spores are found in feces, urine, and respiratory secretions.
  - Animals and infected humans are potential sources as well as food, water, and soil.
  - Most frequently seen in **HIV patients** but **emerging pathogen** in organ transplant recipients, chemotherapy recipients, and the immunocompetent (travellers, elderly, children).

Identification (Fig. 4.12)

- **Challenges**: diagnostic stages are **small (1–3.5 μm)**, staining properties can hamper visualization of spores.
- Stool microscopy
  - At least three stool samples should be examined.
  - Light microscopy at ×1000 magnification after chromotrope 2R stain (most specific) or chemofluorescent stain (sensitive but false positives).
  - Differences in spore size can allow tentative genus identification (*Enterocytozoon* 1–1.5 μm and *Encephalitozoon* spp. 2–3 μm).
  - **Electron microscopy or molecular analysis must be used to identify to genus.**
  - Immunofluorescent techniques are promising but not widely available.
- Histologic examination
  - **Duodenal and terminal ileal** tissues may show microsporidial parasites.
    - Biopsies may be indicated for persistent diarrhea in context of immunosuppression.
    - Not more sensitive than stool microscopy as infection may be unevenly distributed.
    - Requires experienced pathologists for reliable identification.
- Cytologic diagnosis
  - Spores have been detected in duodenal aspirates, bile, urine, BAL, CSF, conjunctival scrapings/swabs, sputum, and nasal discharge/nasal scrapings.
  - Patients suspected of disseminated microsporidiosis should have urine sediments examined.
- **Electron microscopy**
  - Considered to be the gold standard.
  - Microsporidial ultrastructure differentiates between most genera.
- Serology
  - Reliable testing of human infection is lacking.
- Cell culture
  - Fastidious and costly.
- Molecular techniques
  - Species-specific and universal microsporidial primers have been developed, as well as oligonucleotide microarrays for detection of four microsporidia.
  - Molecular diagnosis of microsporidia has been performed on a range of samples including fresh/fixed stool, intestinal tissue, and urine.

Free-Living Amebae (Table 4.8)

The free-living amebae known to cause human infections are:

- Super Group Excavata.
  - *Naegleria fowleri.*
- Super Group Amoebozoa.
  - *Acanthamoeba* spp.
  - *Balamuthia mandrillaris.*
  - *Sappinia pedata*: recently identified in brain biopsy of 38-year-old with headache and seizures.
- Defined as amphizoic amebae: these amebae can be free-living or parasitic (Fig. 4.13).
- Cause CNS infections in humans and animals.
- Like *E. histolytica*, they move by producing cytoplasmic bulges (lobopodia).

Naegleria fowleri

- Several species identified so far, but **only *N. fowleri*** causes CNS disease in humans.

Life Cycle

- Transient flagellate state, feeding and dividing trophozoite form, and cystic stage (Figs. 4.13 and 4.14).
- Trophozoites feed on bacteria and multiply by binary fission.
- In unfavorable conditions it converts to a resistant cystic stage.

Epidemiology

- Widely distributed throughout the world and throughout the environment.
- **Thermophilic**: grows at temperatures up to 45 °C.
- **CNS infections in humans associated with summer and aquatic activities**: lakes, ponds, swimming pools, underwater swimming.
- Most commonly affects **children <11 years**, >75% male.

Identification

- Motile amebae can be seen in CSF on light microscopy.
- Giemsa and trichrome stains of CSF smears can aid with delineation of nuclear morphology.
- Trophozoite has a spherical nucleus with a large, central nucleolus and multiple cell organelles (Fig. 4.15).
- Cysts are round with single nucleus with a central dense nucleolus, 7–14 μm.
- Often identified retrospectively using hematoxylin-eosin stained sections.
- Can be **cultured on bacterial-coated agar plates**; flagellates appear within 2–4 hours.
- A real-time PCR assay has been developed to identify DNA in CSF within hours.

Acanthamoeba spp.

- Traditionally grouped within the genus by morphology (see Table 4.7); genotypic grouping (T1–7) now also used.
- Grouping is not related to pathogenicity; species across all groups can cause disease in humans.

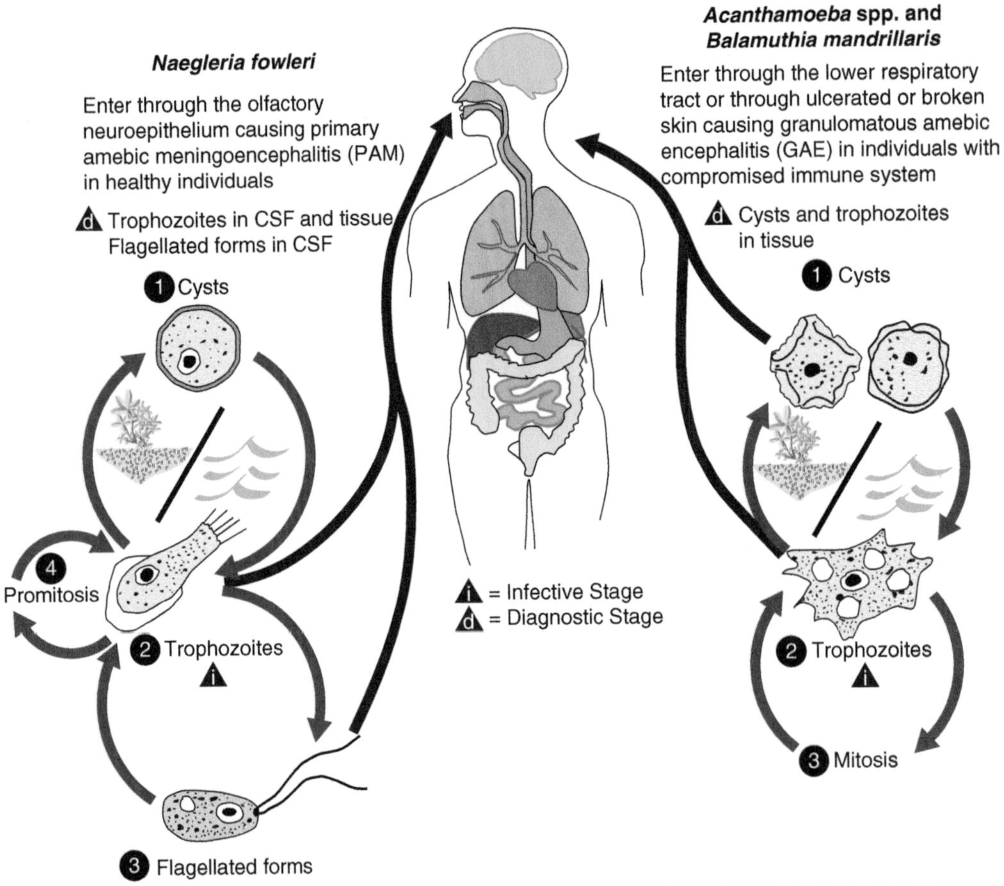

Naegleria fowleri

Enter through the olfactory neuroepithelium causing primary amebic meningoencephalitis (PAM) in healthy individuals

d Trophozoites in CSF and tissue. Flagellated forms in CSF

1 Cysts

4 Promitosis

2 Trophozoites **i**

3 Flagellated forms

Acanthamoeba spp. and Balamuthia mandrillaris

Enter through the lower respiratory tract or through ulcerated or broken skin causing granulomatous amebic encephalitis (GAE) in individuals with compromised immune system

d Cysts and trophozoites in tissue

1 Cysts

2 Trophozoites **i**

3 Mitosis

i = Infective Stage
d = Diagnostic Stage

• **Fig. 4.13** Life cycles of the medically important free-living amebae. (From Bennett JE, Dolin R, Blaser MJ, eds. *Mandell, Douglas, and Bennett's Principles and Practice of Infectious Diseases*. Updated 8th ed. Elsevier; 2015. Courtesy Division of Parasitic Diseases/Centers for Disease Control and Prevention.)

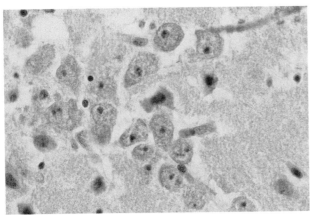

• **Fig. 4.14** *Naegleria fowleri* trophozoite and cyst. (From Rittenhouse Cope J, Yoder JS, Visvesvara GS. Protozoa: Free living amebae. In: Cohen J, Powderly W, Opal S, eds. *Infectious Diseases*. 4th ed. Elsevier; 2017.)

• **_A. castellanii_ complex** (Group II, and Genotype T4) is **most commonly associated with human disease.**

Life Cycle (see Fig. 4.13)
• Feeding and reproducing trophozoite stage and resistant cyst stage.
• Trophozoites are uninucleate, feed on bacteria, and multiply by binary fission.

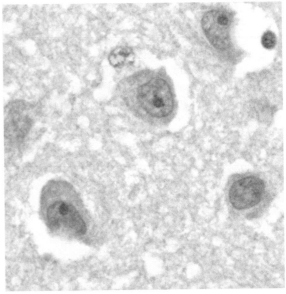

• **Fig. 4.15** Trophozoites of *Naegleria fowleri* in brain tissue. (Courtesy Division of Parasitic Diseases/Centers for Disease Control and Prevention.)

Epidemiology
• Has been isolated from soil, fresh/sea/mineral water, sewage, pools, hot tubs, air conditioning systems, cell cultures, and autopsy specimens.

TABLE 4.7 *Acanthamoeba* Species

Morphologic Group	Trophozoite Size	Cyst Size	Species
Group I	Large, 30–125 µm	16–35 µm	*A. astronyxis, A. comandoni, A. tubiashi A. byersi*
Group II	15–45 µm	18 µm or less	*A. castellanii, A. polyphaga, A. rhysodes, A. hatchetti*
Group III	15–45 µm	Different cyst morphologies and size <18 µm	*A. culbertsoni, A. royreba, A. lenticulata*

- Colonize the biofilm of plumbing systems: public health importance.
- **Keratitis** most common in people who wear **contact lenses** and when contact lens storage and handling involves contaminated water, or **lenses are worn during swimming, showering, or bathing in contaminated water** (Fig. 4.16).
- **CNS infections occur mainly in immunocompromised individuals.**
- Act as hosts for pathogenic bacteria, e.g., *Legionella* spp., *Mycobacterium avium* complex, and *Listeria monocytogenes*.

Identification
- Visual detection in CSF rarely reported.
- Can be cultured from biopsy tissue (brain, skin, lung, cornea) on nutrient agar with layer of gram-negative bacteria at 30°C (cornea/skin) or 37°C (brain/lung).
- Amebae differentiate into cysts after few days' incubation (Fig. 4.17).
  - Amebae: nuclei centrally placed and large densely staining nucleolus, fine granular cytoplasm, and numerous organelles (Fig. 4.17B).
  - Cysts: uninucleate and double-walled: ectocyst (wrinkled, contains protein) and endocyst (stellate, oval, polygonal, contains cellulose) (Fig. 4.17C).
- Identified to genus level based on morphologic appearances of cysts/trophozoites.
- Speciation requires serology, isoenzyme analysis, or DNA profiles.
  - The most reliable technique of identifying species is **sequencing of 18S rDNA.**

Balamuthia mandrillaris

- Molecular studies: only one genotype.
- Life cycle (see Fig. 4.13).
- Irregularly shaped trophozoite, 12–60 µm, uninucleate/binucleate, central nucleolus (Fig. 4.18A).
- Cysts are uninucleate, spherical, 12–30 µm with wavy ectocyst and spherical endocyst (Fig. 4.18B).

Epidemiology
- Has been isolated from soil and biopsy/autopsy samples.

- Serologic studies suggest exposure is more common than disease.
- Infection is more common in Hispanic ethnicity.
- Infection has occurred after transplant from an infected donor.

Identification
- Do not grow on bacteria-coated agar plates.
- Can grow in axenic medium after inoculation of monkey kidney cell culture with brain extract.

Blood and Tissue Protozoa

The genera *Plasmodium*, *Babesia*, *Toxoplasma*, *Leishmania*, and *Trypanosoma* are discussed here. Despite their defined geographical distribution, the diseases caused by this group have a huge socioeconomic impact.

Malaria

Key concepts
- Malaria is caused by the coccidian protozoal parasite: genus *Plasmodium*.
- Transmitted by the *Anopheles* species of mosquito.
- Five *Plasmodium* species that infect humans are known:
  - *P. falciparum*: **most pathogenic; fatal if untreated; no relapses.**
  - *P. vivax*: less pathogenic but can relapse; severe cases are recognized.
  - *P. ovale*: less pathogenic, can relapse, less widespread.
  - *P. malariae*: low pathogenicity, rare, no relapses.
  - *P. knowlesi*: primarily a zoonosis; primate malaria (infects long-tailed and pig-tailed macaques) in Southeast Asia that also infects humans and **can cause severe disease; shortest reproductive cycle.**

Epidemiology
- Malaria is the most damaging parasitic disease affecting mankind; nearly half the world's population is at risk: 212 million cases and 435,000 malaria deaths in 2017.
- **Transmission intensity** is measured as the entomologic inoculation rate (EIR): the number of infectious mosquito bites per person per year.

TABLE 4.8 Summary of Medically Important Free-Living Amebae

	Naegleria fowleri	*Acanthamoeba* spp. (Nonkeratitis Disease)	*Acanthamoeba* spp. (Keratitis)	*Balamuthia mandrillaris*
Disease	Primary amebic meningoencephalitis (PAM)	Granulomatous amebic encephalitis (GAE); cutaneous lesions; sinus infections	Amebic keratitis	GAE; cutaneous lesions; sinus infections
Epidemiology	Most human cases associated with exposure to recreational warm fresh water	Can acquire from soil, water, air	Corneal trauma; poor contact lens hygiene; association with Advanced Medical Optics Complete Moisture Plus	Can acquire from soil, water, air
Groups at risk	Healthy children and young adults, usually male	Immunocompromised individuals	Contact lens wearers (>80% of cases)	Immunocompromised individuals; healthy children and elderly; Hispanics
Signs and symptoms at presentation	Headache, neck stiffness, seizures, coma	Headache, neck stiffness, behavioral changes, coma; sinus disease; skin ulcers	Intense pain, photophobia, tearing; dendriform epitheliopathy (early); stromal ring	Headache, neck stiffness, seizures, hydrocephalus; sinus infection; skin nodules
Clinical course	Prodrome of few days; fulminant disease; without treatment, death occurs within 1–2 weeks	Prodrome of weeks to months; subacute course; acute stage fatal in weeks	Prodrome of days; subacute to chronic keratitis	Prodrome of weeks to months; subacute course; acute stage fatal in weeks
Laboratory diagnosis	CSF wet mount positive for motile amebae; CSF with polymorphonuclear pleocytosis; no cysts seen in brain tissue; PCR from CSF	Amebae rarely seen in CSF wet mount; cysts seen in brain tissue—test by IFA, IIF, or PCR for definitive identification	Corneal scraping or biopsy to find trophozoites or cysts; confocal microscopy	Amebae rarely isolated from CSF, but CSF can have highly elevated protein; cysts seen in brain tissue—test by IFA, IIF, and PCR
Distinct morphologic features	Vesicular nucleus; limacine movement of amebae; flagellate stage; cysts with pores flush at surface	Vesicular nucleus; finger-like pseudopodia projecting from surface; cyst wall with 2 layers and with pores		Vesicular nucleus with single or multiple nucleoli; ameboid and "spider-like" movements in culture; cyst wall with 3 layers
In vitro cultivation	Axenic, bacterized, and defined media; tissue culture cells; optimal growth at ≥37 °C	Axenic, bacterized, and defined media; tissue culture cells; optimal growth at 37°C (CNS isolates) or optimal growth at 30°C (corneal isolates)		Axenic medium; tissue culture cells; optimal growth at 37 °C (bacterized medium not useful)
CT/MRI of head	Nonspecific	Space-occupying or ring-enhancing lesion	Not applicable	Space-occupying or ring-enhancing lesions
Antimicrobial therapy	Intrathecal and intravenous amphotericin B, azoles, rifampin, miltefosine	Pentamidine, azoles, flucytosine, sulfadiazine, miltefosine, amikacin IV and IT, voriconazole	PHMB, chlorhexidine, propamidine, hexamidine, topical and oral voriconazole	Pentamidine, azithromycin, fluconazole, sulfadiazine, flucytosine, miltefosine

CNS, central nervous system; CSF, cerebrospinal fluid; CT, computed tomography; IFA, immunofluorescent antibody staining; IIF, indirect immunofluorescent staining; IT, intrathecal; IV, intravenous; MRI, magnetic resonance imaging; PCR, polymerase chain reaction; PHMB, polyhexamethylene biguanide.
Modified from Visvesvara GS, Moura H, Schuster FL. Pathogenic and opportunistic free-living amoebae: *Acanthamoeba* spp. *Balamuthia mandrillaris*, *Naegleria fowleri*, and *Sappinia diploidea*. *FEMS Immunol Med Microbiol.* 2007;50:1–26.

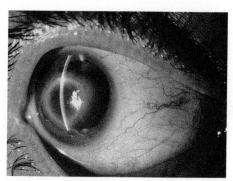

• **Fig. 4.16** *Acanthamoeba* keratitis. (From Visvesvara GS, Roy SL, Maguire JH. Pathogenic and opportunistic free-living amebae. In: Guerrant RL Walker DH, Weller PF, eds. *Tropical Infectious Diseases: Principles, Pathogens and Practice*. 3rd ed. Elsevier; 2011.)

• Most deaths are in children in sub-Saharan Africa (>80%), where there is high transmission intensity (EIR 0.1 to >1000). In Asia, transmission intensity is lower (EIR mainly <1), but population is denser so case incidence is also high.

• Distribution of malaria depends on climatic conditions: development of parasite in the mosquito (sporogony) can **only occur between 16°C and 33°C (61–91°F) and below 2000 m above sea level.**

• Malaria is most prevalent in low resource regions in a vicious cycle of poverty: e.g., it affects fertility, financial productivity, school attendance.

• Geographical distribution (Fig. 4.19)

   • *P. falciparum* is prevalent across all tropical regions, with densest frequencies in sub-Saharan Africa.

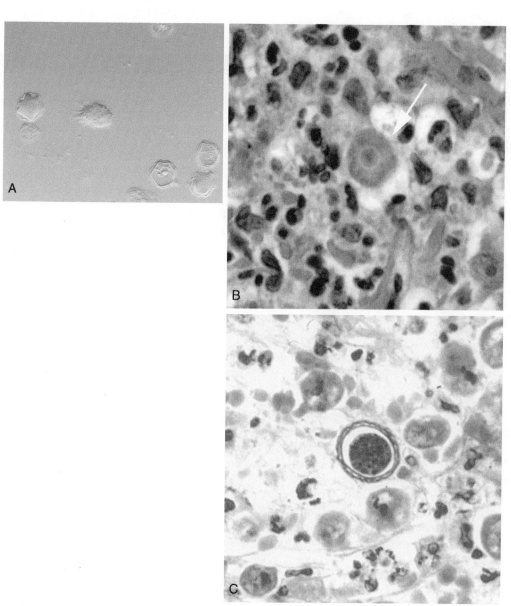

• **Fig. 4.17** (A) *Acanthamoeba castellanii* trophozoite and cyst. (B) *Acanthamoeba castellanii* trophozoite. (C) *Acanthamoeba castellanii* cyst. (Panel A from Rittenhouse Cope J, Yoder JS, Visvesvara GS. Protozoa: Free living amebae. In: Cohen J, Powderly W, Opal S, eds. *Infectious Diseases*. 4th ed. Elsevier; 2017. Panels B and C, courtesy Division of Parasitic Diseases/Centers for Disease Control and Prevention.)

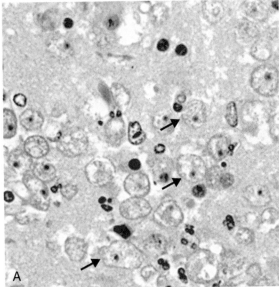

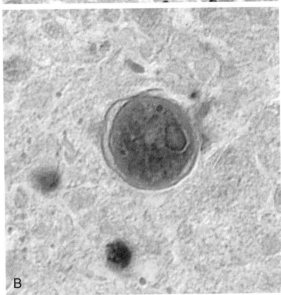

• **Fig. 4.18** *Balamuthia mandrillaris* in brain tissue. (A) Trophozoites; (B) cyst. (Panel A courtesy Division of Parasitic Diseases/Centers for Disease Control and Prevention. Panel B courtesy Division of Parasitic Diseases/Centers for Disease Control and Prevention and the University of Kentucky Hospital, Lexington, Kentucky.)

- *P. vivax* is most prevalent in Asia (~50% of all Asian malaria cases), but also in Central and South America, North Africa, and the Middle East.
  - *P. vivax* is rare in sub-Saharan Africa because the majority of people lack the Duffy blood group antigen (the receptor for *P. vivax* infection). But low levels of *P. vivax* are detected in sub-Saharan Africa, all cases presumably in those who are Duffy antigen-positive.
  - *P. ovale* is mainly prevalent in Africa and Asia.
  - *P. malariae* is currently limited to Southeast Asia.
  - Mixed infections with *P. falciparum* and *P. vivax* are common, especially in Southeast Asia.
- Transmission depends on
  - Mosquito vector factors.
    - Vector longevity.

- Biting habits.
- Rainfall seasonality (mosquitoes depend on rainfall for breeding).
- Human proximity to mosquito breeding sites (swamps, puddles, marshes, rice fields, disused car tires).
- Human infectivity factors
  - During human infection, a small proportion of parasites develop into gametocytes, the infective form for mosquitoes. The gametocyte density in humans enables onward transmission to biting female *Anopheles* mosquitoes.
- Hemoglobinopathies convey a protective effect against severe malaria and occur in balanced polymorphism in malaria endemic areas: heterozygotes are protected from severe disease (e.g., sickle cell disease, G6PD deficiency, thalassemia, and Melanesian ovalocytosis).

CLINICAL PEARL

- Some useful definitions
  - Imported malaria occurs in travelers leaving an endemic area.
  - Airport malaria can occur when infected mosquitoes are transported by plane out of an endemic area.
  - Transfusion malaria is caused by malaria-infected blood and blood products.

Pathogenesis

Life cycle of *Plasmodium* species (Fig. 4.20):

1. Sporozoite injected from female *Anopheles* mosquito mouthparts into human host bloodstream.
2. Multiplies in liver hepatocytes for 5–7 days, forming hepatic schizonts, then released into bloodstream as merozoites.
   - In *P. vivax* and *P. ovale* hypnozoites persist in liver and cause later relapse.
3. Merozoites invade erythrocytes via sialic acid residues.
   - *Pf*Rh5 is an essential parasite ligand.
4. In the erythrocyte, ring-stage trophozoites form and develop into schizonts.
5. Schizonts rupture and release 6–36 merozoites causing proinflammatory cascade
   - Every 48 hours (*P. falciparum, P. vivax*, and *P. ovale*).
   - 24 hours (*P. knowlesi*).
   - 72 hours (*P. knowlesi*).
6. Parasite numbers increase with each erythrocytic cycle.

Virulence factors

- **Cytoadherence**
  - *Pf* schizonts integrate parasite proteins into erythrocyte membrane (e.g., *Pf*EMP1, encoded by the highly variable *VAR* gene family) causing them to **adhere to the vascular endothelium.**
    - They attach to endothelial surface proteins, e.g., CD36, chondroitin sulphate A (CSA, in the placenta) and ICAM-1 (in the brain).

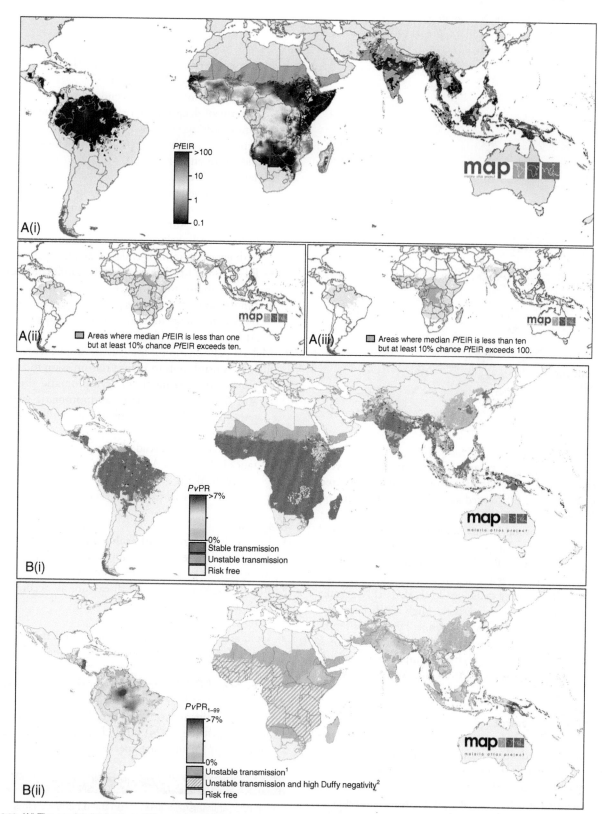

• **Fig. 4.19** (Ai) The spatial distribution of *Plasmodium falciparum* entomological inoculation rate (*pf*EIR) in 2010. Each pixel represents the point estimate (posterior median) *Pf* EIR prediction within the stable limits of transmission. The color scale is logarithmic to allow better differentiation across the heavily positively skewed distribution of values. Areas of unstable transmission (medium grey areas, where *Pf* API < 0.1 per 1,000 pa) or no risk (light grey, where *Pf* API = 0 per 1,000 pa) are also shown. (Aii and Aiii) Indicators of the uncertainty associated with predictions, showing areas with a median prediction less than one or less than ten but where the 90th percentile is at least an order of magnitude larger. (Bi) 2010 spatial limits of vivax malaria risk defined by PvAPI with further medical intelligence, temperature, and aridity masks. Areas were defined as stable (dark grey areas, where PvAPI ≥0.1 per 1000 pa), unstable (medium grey areas, where PvAPI <0.1 per 1000 pa), or no risk (light grey areas, where PvAPI = 0 per 1000 pa). Community surveys of *P. vivax* prevalence conducted between January 1985 and June 2010 are plotted. Survey data are presented as a continuum of light green to red (see map legend), with zero-valued surveys shown in white. (Bii) MBG point estimates of annual mean PvPR1–99 for 2010 within spatial limits of stable vivax malaria transmission, displayed on the same color scale. Areas within stable limits in (Bi) that were predicted with high certainty (>0.9) to have a PvPR1–99 less than 1% were classified as unstable. Areas in which Duffy negativity gene frequency is predicted to exceed 90% are shown in hatching for additional context. (Panel A from Gething PW, Patil AP, Smith DL, et al. A new world malaria map: *Plasmodium falciparum* endemicity in 2010. *Malar J.* 2011;10:378. Panel B from Gething PW, Elyazar IR, Moyes CL, et al. A long neglected world malaria map: *Plasmodium vivax* endemicity in 2010. *PLoS Negl Trop Dis.* 2012;6(9);e1814.)

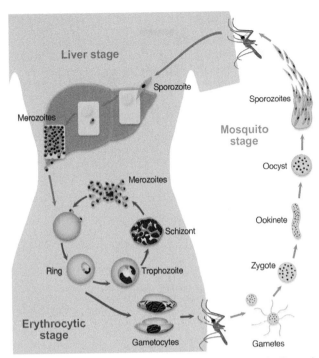

• **Fig. 4.20** Life cycle of *Plasmodium* species. (From *Malaria, Genomic and Personalised Medicine.* Ponts, Le Roch; 2013:1191–1210.)

• Further stickiness, **rosetting with uninfected erythrocytes**, and **auto-agglutination with other infected cells**/platelets further reduce microvascular perfusion (Fig. 4.21).

• Increased **blood-brain barrier permeability** and raised intracranial pressure noted in children with end-stage disease. **Rarely seen in adults.** There is mild generalized increased systemic vascular permeability.

• **Proinflammatory** cytokines TNF, IL-1, IFN-gamma predominate in fatal disease. High TNF correlates with severity, coma, hypoglycemia, hyperparasitemia, and death. Glycosylphosphatidylinositol (GPI) in *P. falciparum* stimulates TNF and lymphotoxin production and upregulates ICAM-1 and VCAM-1 expression in brain.

Prevention and Control

• Vector control: **environmental control** to reduce/clear breeding grounds (biological bacterial larvicides, larvivorous fish); **chemical control** uses pyrethroid or dichlorodiphenyltrichloroethane (DDT) insecticide spraying indoors (indoor residual spraying, IRS), outdoors or in breeding areas. **Insecticide resistance is a major challenge.**

• Reduce vector contact with humans: **insecticide-treated bednets** (ITNs; use associated with huge reduction in child mortality). Challenges: insecticide resistance, distribution and population coverage. Affluent traveler can access: screened windows, air conditioning, protective clothing, repellants (e.g., DEET]).

• Drugs for prevention
  • **Targeted prophylaxis**: intermittent presumptive treatment (IPT) with antimalarials is used for pregnant women (IPTp), children (IPTc), and infants (IPTi) in high endemic areas.
  • Prophylaxis for travelers to endemic areas: depends on patterns of drug resistance, level of transmission, and comorbidities.

• Prompt case management: prompt and effective diagnosis and treatment for cases.

• **Malaria vaccine**
  • Vaccine development challenging because *P. falciparum* genome is highly complex and has highly variable antigenic surface proteins.
  • Cellular and antibody-mediated immunity develops with exposure in high-endemic areas.
  • RTS,S is the first licensed vaccine candidate, based on *Pf* circumsporozoite antigen.
  • Limited efficacy: provides partial protection against *Pf* disease in young children. Use now being piloted in 3 African countries (from 2019).

• Malaria elimination: integrated implementation of malaria control tools to reduce transmission to zero:
  • Considers treatment of symptomatic infections and the large reservoir of asymptomatic (very low parasitemia) infections using molecular detection methods.
  • Crucial to block spread of emerging artemisinin resistance in Southeast Asia and to reduce deaths and morbidity in Africa.
  • New antimalarial drugs in development.

Diagnosis

• Malaria is a **diagnosis of exclusion** in anyone returning from a malaria-endemic country with a fever within 2 months (may persist in liver up to a year).

• Rapid progression to severe disease means accurate diagnosis is urgent.

• Clinical diagnosis is unreliable.

• Gold standard is microscopy: **thick and thin films** for **speciation and quantification** of parasitemia (Figs. 4.22 and 4.23).

• **Presence of *P. falciparum* schizonts denotes severity.**

• Rapid diagnostic tests (RDTs) based on *Pf*HRP2 and *Pf*LDH antigens avert the need for an experienced microscopist (Fig. 4.24) but lack quantification and species (except *Pf*) and stage specificity.

CLINICAL PEARL

• If prior antimalarials taken, need **three negative films over 48 hours** to rule out malaria. Use PCR if suspicion is still high.

Babesiosis

An **emerging tickborne** protozoan parasitic zoonotic disease (see Chapters 30 and 34).

Epidemiology

• Over 100 species that parasitize domestic and wild mammals and birds, in particular cattle.

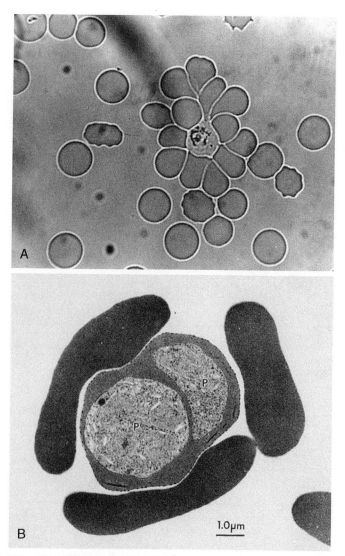

• **Fig. 4.21** Rosetting of infected and uninfected erythrocytes. (A) *P. vivax*; (B) *P. falciparum*. (From Farrar J, et al., eds. *Manson's Tropical Diseases*, 23rd ed. Elsevier; 2014.)

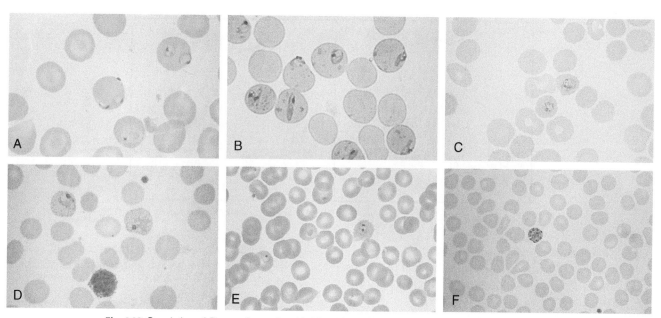

• **Fig. 4.22** Speciation of *Plasmodium* using thin blood films. (From Ferri FF, *Ferri's Color Atlas and Text of Clinical Medicine*. Elsevier; 2009.)

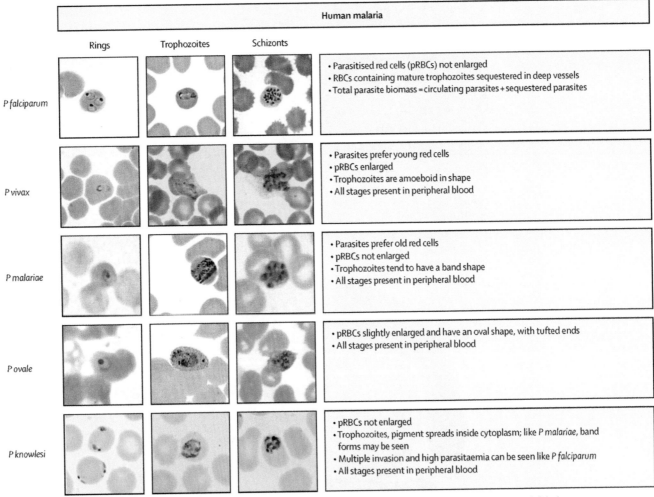

Human malaria

	Rings	Trophozoites	Schizonts	
P falciparum				• Parasitised red cells (pRBCs) not enlarged • RBCs containing mature trophozoites sequestered in deep vessels • Total parasite biomass = circulating parasites + sequestered parasites
P vivax				• Parasites prefer young red cells • pRBCs enlarged • Trophozoites are amoeboid in shape • All stages present in peripheral blood
P malariae				• Parasites prefer old red cells • pRBCs not enlarged • Trophozoites tend to have a band shape • All stages present in peripheral blood
P ovale				• pRBCs slightly enlarged and have an oval shape, with tufted ends • All stages present in peripheral blood
P knowlesi				• pRBCs not enlarged • Trophozoites, pigment spreads inside cytoplasm; like *P malariae*, band forms may be seen • Multiple invasion and high parasitaemia can be seen like *P falciparum* • All stages present in peripheral blood

• **Fig. 4.23** Characteristic microscopic appearances of human malaria. All parasite stages are visible in peripheral blood except *P. falciparum* RBCs containing mature trophozoites where the vast majority are sequestered in deep vessels. Thin blood films were prepared from specimens taken from patients with clinical malaria, stained with modified Field's stain and examined by light microscopy under oil immersion at ×1000 magnification. *P, Plasmodium.* (Reproduced with permission from Elsevier. The Lancet. From Ashley E, et al. Malaria. *Lancet Infect Dis.* 391(10130):1608–1621.)

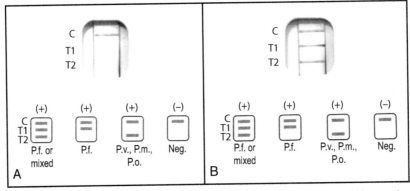

• **Fig. 4.24** Rapid diagnostic tests for malaria. (From Bain B, *Dacie and Lewis Practical Haematology.* 12th ed. Elsevier; 2016.)

• Only a few cause human infection:
  • In America ***B. microti*** causes most cases of babesiosis but also ***B. duncani*** in the northern Pacific coast. The main vector is *Ixodes scapularis.*
  • Majority of cases occur in Connecticut, Massachusetts, New Jersey, New York, Rhode Island, Minnesota, and Wisconsin.

• In Europe ***B. divergens*** is most common, associated with cattle infection, and transmitted via *Ixodes ricinus.*
• Cases also reported from Asia.

Life Cycle (see Fig. 4.25)

1. A tick vector ingests infected blood.

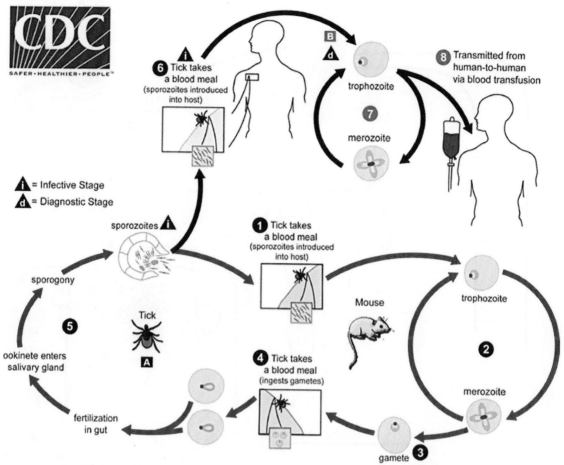

• **Fig. 4.25** *Babesia* life cycle. (From Rifai N, et al., eds. *Tietz Textbook of Clinical Chemistry and Molecular Diagnostics*. 6th ed. Elsevier; 2018. Courtesy of the CDC DPDx: http://www.cdc.gov/dpdx/.)

2. *Babesia* develop into sporozoites in the salivary glands of the vector and are deposited in the skin of host during the vector's blood meal.
3. *Babesia* sporozoites enter erythrocytes and transform into mobile trophozoites.
4. Pear-shaped trophozoites replicate by asynchronous budding to form 2–4 merozoites which can invade other erythrocytes and to form gametocytes, which are infectious to biting tick vector.
   • Humans are practically a dead-end host; little, if any, onward transmission results from ticks feeding on infected people.
   • Human-to-human transmission can occur via blood transfusions.

Identification

• Acute illness: parasites visible in erythrocytes on thin/thick film microscopy.
   • Thin film: Giemsa stain and view under ×100 (Fig. 4.26).
   • Thick film: detects lower levels of parasitemia (*B. bovis*).
   • Basket-shaped and often extracellular merozoites, tetrads in erythrocytes (**Maltese crosses**) and **lack of malaria pigment (hemozoin).**

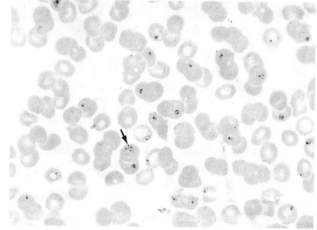

• **Fig. 4.26** *Babesia* species in a thin blood film. (From Gelfand JA, VAanier EG. *Babesia* species. In: Bennett JE, Dolin R, Blaser MJ, eds. *Mandell, Douglas, and Bennett's Principles and Practice of Infectious Diseases*. Updated 8th ed. Elsevier; 2015.)

• Chronic infections: ELISA and IFAT methods against proteins of blood stages.
   • Serologic tests useful in chronic *B. microti* infections with low parasitemia.
• Immunochromatography test (ICT) is a rapid diagnostic device that detects antibodies against a specific antigen; developed for *Babesia* spp. But not available yet.

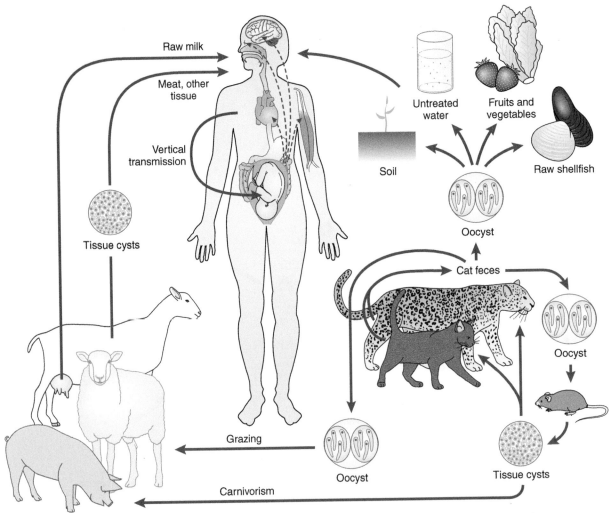

• **Fig. 4.27** Life cycle of *Toxoplasma gondii*. (From Montoya JG, Boothroyd JC, Kovacs JA. *Toxoplasmosis gondii*. In: Bennett JE, Dolin R, Blaser MJ, eds. *Mandell, Douglas, and Bennett's Principles and Practice of Infectious Diseases*. Updated 8th ed. Elsevier; 2015.)

• Molecular methods, e.g., PCR-based methods for acute and chronic stages of infection, are in development.

Toxoplasmosis

• A widespread **zoonotic** infection caused by the coccidian parasite *Toxoplasma gondii*.
• Member of the Apicomplexa subphylum.
• Few, if any, symptoms develop in the acute phase (but **can resemble a mono-like illness**).
• Infection persists throughout life.
• Infection during pregnancy (transmission to the fetus) or in the immunosuppressed can lead to severe clinical manifestations, e.g., neurologic and ophthalmic disease.

Epidemiology
• Estimated that **30% of mankind** infected.
• Transmission usually by oral route.
• Definitive host is felines, including domestic cats but can infect many mammals/birds.

• Geography: highest seroprevalence in Brazil, Central Africa, and Central America.
• Transmission
  • Warm, humid climates and lower altitude favored by parasite.
  • Predominantly foodborne; ingestion of oocysts in unfiltered water or undercooked meat.
  • **Zoonotic** transmission: contact with cat feces or other infected animals.
  • Congenital: **transplacental** route.
  • Rare person-to-person transmission via contaminated transfusions or solid organ transplant.

Life Cycle (Fig. 4.27)
• Life cycle forms: oocysts, tachyzoites (rapid replicators), and the dominant form: bradyzoites (slow replicators).
• **Biphasic cycle**: sexual phase in cats, asexual phase in animals/humans.
  1. Cats ingest cysts from small prey.
  2. Oocysts formed from replication in feline intestine and excreted in feces.

3. Secondary host ingests uncooked meat/water containing cysts.
4. Tachyzoite stage adopted and nucleated cells infected and rupture: symptoms.
5. Tachyzoites sequestered in tissue cells and convert to bradyzoites: chronic infection.

Identification

- Stained tissue and fluid smears may be examined for trophozoites and cysts.
- Diagnosis usually made based on **serologic testing,** often requiring an algorithm for interpretation.
  - IgM
    - Positive within 1 week, positive for >12 months.
    - Lack of specificity is a major problem with *Toxoplasma*-specific IgM.
  - IgG
    - Positive after 2 weeks.
    - First-line testing, typically with EIA.
  - Avidity is the functional affinity of specific IgG.
    - Low avidity typically seen early on, but may persist for months.
    - High avidity is not seen until at least 4 months after infection.
  - The Sabin–Feldman dye test is the reference gold standard.
    - It is a neutralization assay: live organisms are lysed in the presence of a patient's *Toxoplasma*-specific IgG and complement.
      - The requirement for live tachyzoites cultured in animals restricts use to specialist reference laboratories.
    - It is fully quantitative and highly sensitive.
    - It only measures IgG.
  - If IgG and IgM both positive, confirmation required using an alternative test.
- **Maternal infection** diagnosed using serial serology 2 weeks apart; should seroconvert or show an increase in IgG avidity.
- **Fetal diagnosis: PCR for *T. gondii* DNA in amniotic fluid** is most sensitive.
- PCR-based methods also most reliable diagnostic tool for immunosuppressed with likely disseminated disease.

CLINICAL PEARL

- A high avidity IgG result in the 12th–16th weeks of pregnancy excludes an infection acquired during gestation.

Leishmaniasis

Classification

- A group of chronic parasitic infections caused by species of genus *Leishmania*.
- Infection results in three possible clinical syndromes:
  - Visceral leishmaniasis (VL, kala-azar).
  - Mucocutaneous leishmaniasis (MCL).
  - Cutaneous leishmaniasis (CL).

- Belongs to the order Kinetoplastida (flagellated protozoa that possess a kinetoplast).
- Often divided into two geographical groups (Table 4.9):
  - New World *Leishmania* (America).
  - Old World *Leishmania* (Africa, Europe, Asia).

Epidemiology

- Transmission: **Sandflies** (*Phlebotomus* spp.) transmit from animal to human (zoonotic) and human to human (anthroponotic). Approximately 0.2–0.4 million VL and 0.7–1.2 million CL cases per annum.
- Geography (Fig. 4.28)
  - 90% of VL cases in India/Nepal/Bangladesh/Sudan/Ethiopia and Brazil.
  - 90% of CL cases in Brazil/Peru/Algeria/Saudi Arabia/Middle Eastern countries.
- Visceral leishmaniasis:
  - Causes: *L. donovani, L. infantum*, and *L. chagasi.*
  - Population movement, famine, civil war, and climate cause epidemics.
  - Co-infection with HIV common in Africa.
  - Subclinical and self-limiting infections occur frequently with *L. chagasi* and *L. infantum.*
- Cutaneous leishmaniasis:
  - Old World = *L. tropica* causes anthroponotic CL in urban areas. Also *L. major, L. infantum.*
  - New World = *L. mexicana* and *L. brasiliensis* complexes.

Life Cycle

1. **Sandfly vectors** ingest blood containing infected **macrophages** (Fig. 4.29).
2. *Leishmania* live as promastigotes in intestine of the insect.
3. Promastigotes replicate in midgut/hindgut of insect and migrate to oral cavity.
4. New host is infected when bitten and promastigotes penetrate macrophages.
5. Promastigote transforms into a flagellated amastigote and multiplies within macrophages.
6. When host cell ruptures, the amastigotes are phagocytosed by other cells.
7. The organs affected depend on the tropism of the organism (Table 4.9).

Identification

- Standard method = **demonstrate amastigotes in tissue** using **Giemsa** stain (Fig. 4.30).
  - Can also be cultured on suitable media at 26–28 °C (may take 2 weeks to grow).
- Samples
  - For skin lesions: smear from **ulcer edge** or fluid from ulcer, can detect parasites by microscopy in 50%–70% of CL and MCL cases.
  - For VL cases: **bone marrow, lymph node, and splenic aspirates** are samples of choice. Splenic is most sensitive but risk of splenic rupture.

| TABLE 4.9 | Important *Leishmania* Species Affecting Humans |

Subgenus	Complex	Main Pathogenic Species	Main Reservoir	Geographic Distribution	Principal Tropism
Leishmania	*L. donovani*	*L. donovani*	Humans	Indian subcontinent	Viscerotropic
		L. infantum	Dogs	Mediterranean Basin and China	Viscerotropic
		L. chagasi (infantum)	Dogs	Central and South America	Viscerotropic
	L. tropica	*L. tropica*	Humans	Towns in East Mediterranean countries, Middle East, and Central Asia	Dermotropic
	L. major	*L. major*	Birds, gerbils, and other rodents	North and West Africa, the Middle East, and Central Asia	Dermotropic
	L. aethiopica	*L. aethiopica*	Hyraxes	East Africa	Dermotropic
	L. mexicana	*L. mexicana* *L. amazonensis*	Forest rodents and marsupials	North, Central, and South America	Dermotropic
Viannia	*L. braziliensis*	*L. braziliensis*	Edentates, opossums, rodents, and also dogs	South and Central America	Mucotropic
		L. peruviana	Dogs, wild marsupials, and rodents	Peru	Dermotropic
	L. guyanensis	*L. guyanensis*	Sloths and arboreal anteaters	South America	Dermotropic
		L. panamensis	Sloths	Central America and Colombia	Mucotropic

From Garcia LS. Protozoa. In: Cohen J, Powderly W, Opal S, eds. *Infectious Diseases*. 4th ed. Elsevier; 2017.

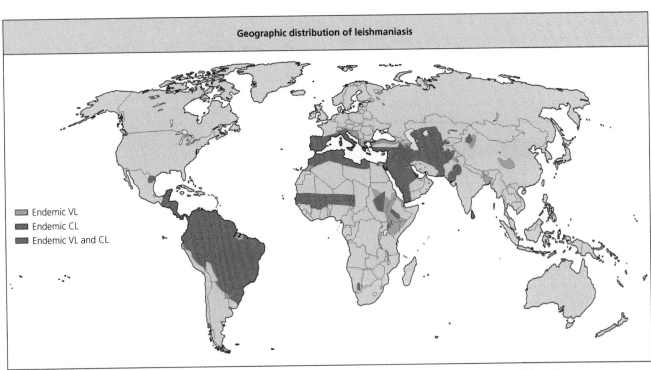

Geographic distribution of leishmaniasis

Endemic VL
Endemic CL
Endemic VL and CL

• **Fig. 4.28** Geographic distribution of leishmaniasis. (From Davidson R. Leishmaniasis. In Cohen J, Powderly W, Opal S, eds. *Infectious Diseases*. 4th ed. Elsevier; 2017.)

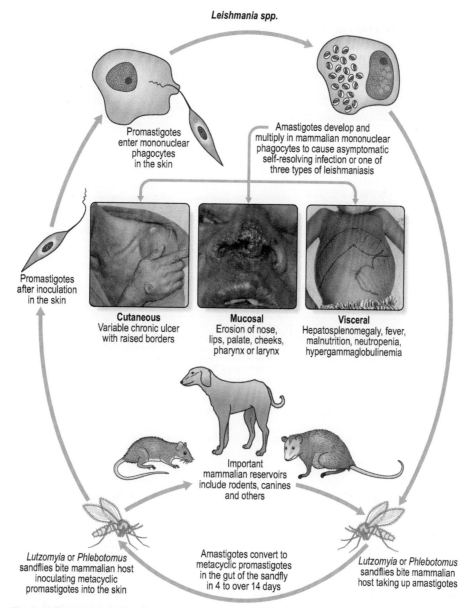

Leishmania spp.

Promastigotes enter mononuclear phagocytes in the skin

Amastigotes develop and multiply in mammalian mononuclear phagocytes to cause asymptomatic self-resolving infection or one of three types of leishmaniasis

Promastigotes after inoculation in the skin

Cutaneous
Variable chronic ulcer with raised borders

Mucosal
Erosion of nose, lips, palate, cheeks, pharynx or larynx

Visceral
Hepatosplenomegaly, fever, malnutrition, neutropenia, hypergammaglobulinemia

Important mammalian reservoirs include rodents, canines and others

Lutzomyia or *Phlebotomus* sandflies bite mammalian host inoculating metacyclic promastigotes into the skin

Amastigotes convert to metacyclic promastigotes in the gut of the sandfly in 4 to over 14 days

Lutzomyia or *Phlebotomus* sandflies bite mammalian host taking up amastigotes

• **Fig. 4.29** The life cycle of *Leishmania* spp. with the different clinical forms in humans. (From Jeronimo SMB, de Queiroz Sousa A, Pearson RD. Leishmaniasis. In: *Tropical Infectious Diseases: Principles, Pathogens and Practice*. Elsevier; 2011.)

- PCR testing of tissue/blood/smears: have higher sensitivity but are not available globally.
- Serology: ELISA, IFAT, and DAT are useful in diagnosis of VL but require trained lab personnel. New RDTs are now becoming available.

Trypanosomiasis

- Infection by hemoflagellate protozoan parasites of the class Kinetoplastida, order Trypanosomatidae, and genus *Trypanosoma*.
- A key diagnostic feature is the **kinetoplast**, which contains mitochondrial DNA.
- Two clinically and geographically distinct conditions (Table 4.10):
  - **American form** = Chagas disease, *T. cruzi*

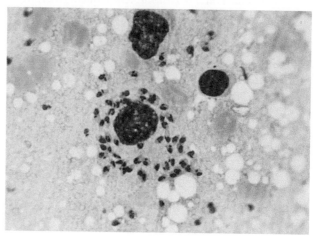

• **Fig. 4.30** *Leishmania infantum* amastigotes in a bone marrow aspirate. (From Davidson R. Leishmaniasis. In: Cohen J, Powderly W, Opal S, eds. *Infectious Diseases*. 4th ed. Elsevier; 2017.)

TABLE 4.10   Key Differences Between Human Trypanosomal Infections.

	West African *T.b. gambiense*	East African *T.b. rhodesiense*
Parasite	*Trypanosoma brucei gambiense*	*Trypanosoma brucei rhodesiense*
Main vectors	*Glossina palpalis* group	*Glossina morsitans* group
Main habitat	Near water	Savanna, cleared bush
Highest incidence	Central African Republic, Democratic Republic of the Congo, South Sudan, north Uganda	South-east Uganda, Tanzania
Main reservoir	Humans, pig, dog	Antelope and cattle
Disease type	Chronic (years)	Acute (months)
Parasitemia	Low	Moderate
Diagnosis	Lymph node aspiration, blood (concentration methods)	Blood
	CSF (lumbar puncture)	CSF (lumbar puncture)
Serology	CATT	None
Treatment		
First stage	Pentamidine	Suramin
Second stage	Nifurtimox-Eflornithine Combination Therapy (NECT)	Melarsoprol
Alternative treatment	(Melarsoprol, Eflornithine)	(Melarsoprol and nifurtimox)
Disease control	Active case search, treatment, tsetse trapping	Tsetse trapping, treatment

Adapted from Pepin J.: African trypanosomiasis. In: Strickland G.T., ed. *Hunter's tropical medicine and emerging infectious diseases*, 8th ed. Philadelphia: Saunders; 2000.643–654.
CATT, Card Agglutination Test for Trypanosomosis.

- **African form** = sleeping sickness, *T. brucei gambiense* (chronic disease) and *T. brucei rhodesiense* (acute severe disease)

African Trypanosomiasis (Sleeping Sickness)

Two forms of human African trypanosomiasis caused by two subspecies of *T. brucei*:

1. *Trypanosoma brucei gambiense*: most common, West Africa, chronic infection
2. *Trypanosoma brucei rhodesiense*: less frequent, East Africa, acute disease.

Epidemiology

- *T.b. gambiense*: endemic in Central West Africa and causes **97% of cases.**
  - Humans are main reservoir: anthroponotic infection.
- *T.b. rhodesiense*: related to safari trips in East Africa, common in travelers.
  - Only 3% of all cases.
  - Wild mammals are main reservoir: a zoonotic infection.
- Disease surveillance and control measures have been successful.

- Estimated 20,000 cases in 2011.

Transmission

- Vector = fly of the genus *Glossina* (**tsetse fly**); **confined to sub-Saharan Africa.**
  - 31 different species of fly transmit the disease.
  - *T.b. gambiense*: transmitted by species favoring **riverine vegetation.**
  - *T.b. rhodesiense*: transmitted by species favoring **savannah.**
- 70% of cases in Democratic Republic of Congo (Fig. 4.31).
- Related to **outdoor activities**: washing clothes, fishing, hunting, and agriculture.

Life Cycle

1. Vector fly ingests blood containing trypanosomes (Fig. 4.31).
2. Parasites transform and multiply in insect midgut and migrate to salivary glands.
3. 2–3 weeks to complete a cycle in the fly.
4. In humans the parasite multiples asexually and spreads to **lymphatic system** and **blood.**
5. Later it invades the **CNS.**

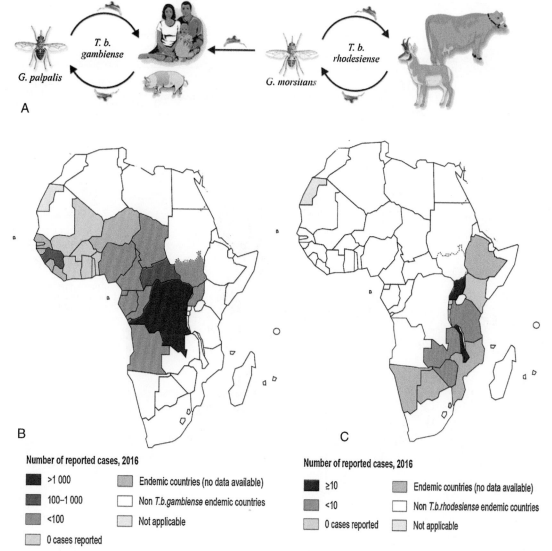

• **Fig. 4.31** The distribution and transmission cycle of human African trypanosomiasis. (Panel A from Kristensson K, et al. African trypanosome infections of the nervous system: parasite entry and effects on sleep and synaptic functions. *Prog Neurobiol.* 2010;91:152–171 with permission from Elsevier. Panels B and C from the WHO Global Health Observatory Map Gallery, 2016, with permission.)

Identification

- Microscopy
  - Repeated microscopic examination of blood, CSF, lymph node, or bone marrow (Fig. 4.32).
  - **More likely to see parasites in acute disease and in *T.b. rhodesiense*.**
  - Concentration methods may help: microhematocrit and miniature anion-exchange centrifugation (m-AECT) and fluorescence microscopy.
  - **Diagnosing late stage disease (CNS) requires CSF examination.**
    - Centrifugation of CSF is recommended.
    - Presence of trypanosomes and WCC >5 per µL are diagnostic (WHO).

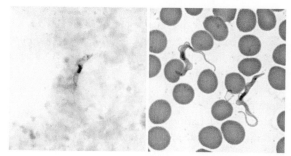

• **Fig. 4.32** *Trypanosoma brucei* sp. trypomastigotes on thick and thin blood films. (From Kliegman R, Stanton B, Behrman RE, et al. *Nelson Textbook of Pediatrics.* 20th ed. Elsevier; 2016.)

- Serologic: card agglutination test (CATT) for *T.b. gambiense* (confirmatory tests needed).
- Molecular: PCR testing only available in reference labs.

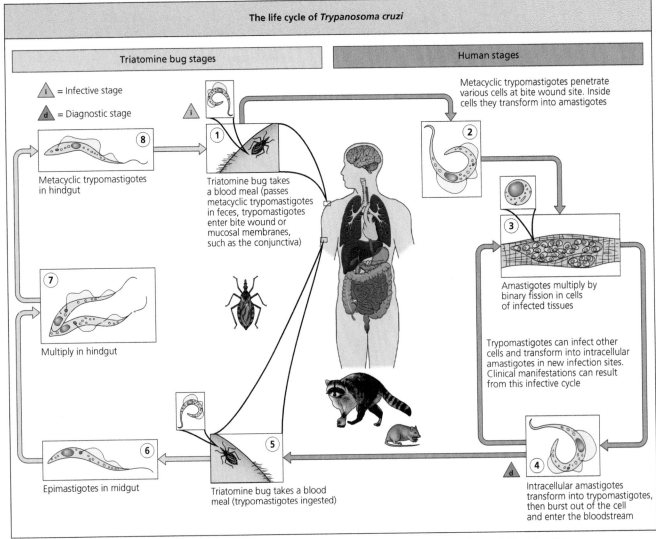

• **Fig. 4.33** Life cycle of *Trypanosoma cruzi*. (From Miles MA. Chagas disease. In: Cohen J, Powderly W, Opal S, eds. *Infectious Diseases*. 4th ed. Elsevier; 2017.)

American Trypanosomiasis (Chagas Disease)

Zoonosis that is endemic in Latin America, caused by *T. cruzi*.

- Classified into six discrete typing units of *T. cruzi* (Tc I – Tc VI) based on geographical associations and clinical manifestations, e.g., Tc I: principal cause of Chagas in countries of north Amazon.

Epidemiology

- Endemic in 21 Latin American countries.
- 6–8 million people are infected and >10,000 deaths per year.
- Disease control has improved greatly in last 20 years due to initiatives in endemic countries.
- Infected people who emigrate from Latin America.
- More than 150 mammal species recorded as infected.

Transmission

- Hemipterous insects of the Reduviidae family (**kissing bugs**): **triatomine bugs.**

- *Triatoma infestans*: main domiciliated vector in Southern Cone countries and Peru.
- *Rhodnius prolixus* + *Triatoma dimidiate*: vectors in northern South America and Central.
- *Panstrongylus megistus*: vector in central and eastern Brazil.
- Many of these vectors are now less widely distributed due to active disease control initiatives.
- Vertical (4%–7% of children to infected mothers), blood transfusion, organ transplant, and oral.

Life Cycle

The life cycle of *Trypanosoma cruzi* is depicted in Fig. 4.33.

Identification

- Acute stage: easy to find parasite in peripheral blood (Fig. 4.34).
  - Fresh blood smear: **parasite observed by direct microscopy** (**Giemsa**-stained thick films can also be used).

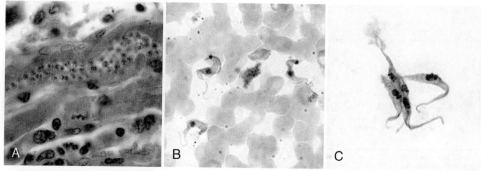

Fig. 4.34 (A) *Trypanosoma cruzi* amastigotes in heart tissue. The section is stained with hematoxylin and eosin (H&E). (B) Three *T. cruzi* trypomastigotes in a thin blood smear stained with Giemsa. (C) *T. cruzi* epimastigotes from culture. Note the location of the kinetoplast anterior to the nucleus. (From Kliegman R, Stanton B, Behrman RE, et al. *Nelson Textbook of Pediatrics*. 20th ed. Elsevier; 2016.)

- Concentration: 3–5 mL blood clotted and centrifuged, supernatant for serologic testing and pellet for microscopy for parasites.
- Microhematocrit technique: 100 µL blood spun in heparinized tube, *T. cruzi* may be observed under microscope in the interface between sera and cells.
- Suspected cases of congenital *T. cruzi* require 6–9 months serologic testing.
- **Chronic stage**: after 2 months, circulating parasite numbers decrease.
- Diagnosis based on serologic testing.
- PCR methods are being developed for use in acute and chronic disease.

HELMINTHS

- **Most common parasitic infection in humans:** over one billion people are infected with at least one helminth species.
- Highest prevalence is in **tropical countries** with poor or inadequate food and water supplies, plentiful invertebrate vectors and poor sanitation allow **food contamination with eggs.**
- Transmitted to humans via food, water, soil, arthropod, and molluscan vectors.
- Found in intestines, liver, lungs, blood, and occasionally brain.
- Helminths include free-living and parasitic worms.
- **Two phyla** (see Fig. 4.1B)
  - Nematoda: roundworms
  - Platyhelminthes: flatworms including Trematoda (flukes) and Cestoda (tapeworms).
- Most detected by identifying the adult worm, eggs, or larvae (Fig. 4.35).

Nematodes (Roundworms)

- Nematodes are nonsegmented, round worms with separate sexes; following mating, the female produces eggs which develop into larvae; these undergo several molts to become a mature adult.

- They are the commonest human parasites; and an individual person may be infected by different species simultaneously and sequentially throughout their life.
- The largest group of nematodes are those that live in the human intestine. Others live or migrate through blood/tissues.

Intestinal Nematodes

Soil Transmitted Helminths (STH) or Nematodes

- Includes *Ascaris lumbricoides*, *Necator americanus*, *Ancylostoma duodenale* and *Trichuris trichiura* (Fig. 4.36).
  - Collectively a possible 2.7 billion people infected worldwide.
  - Transmission: exposure/consumption of contaminated soils.
  - Factors affecting distribution: climate, soil type, customs, sanitation, life cycles.
- *Strongyloides stercoralis*: soil-transmitted, endemic in Africa, South America, and Asia. Prefers warm climates, poor sanitation, and high humidity.
- *Enterobius vermicularis* (**pinworm**): temperate regions, 200 million estimated infections worldwide, acquired in childhood, and high rates in MSM.
- **Life cycles**: see Fig. 4.37.

Ascaris lumbricoides (Roundworm)

1. Can produce 240,000 eggs/day.
   - These are **not immediately infective** – they take 18 days–several weeks in the soil to embryonate and become infective.
2. Eggs are excreted in feces, then ingested, pass to liver, and eventually alveolar sac in lungs.
3. Larvae are coughed up and swallowed and mature in the intestine.
4. Adults usually live in the lumen of the small intestine but **may migrate with heavy worm burden.**
   - Adult worms can live 1–2 years.
   - Both males and females may measure >30cm.
- Ascariasis may also be caused by *Ascaris suum*, found in association with pigs.

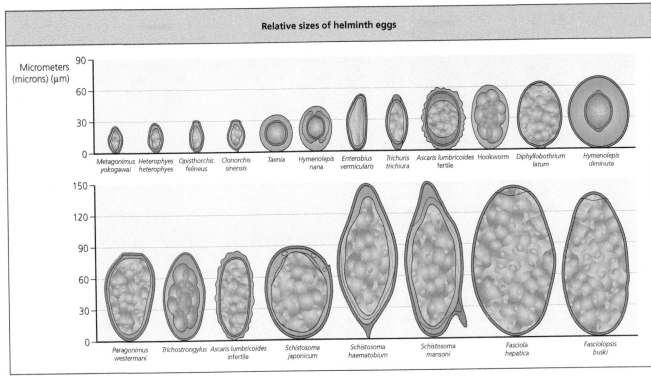

Relative sizes of helminth eggs

- **Fig. 4.35** The relative size of helminth eggs. (From Lindquist HD, Cross JH. Helminths. In Cohen J, Powderly W, Opal S, eds. *Infectious Diseases*. 4th ed. Elsevier; 2017.)

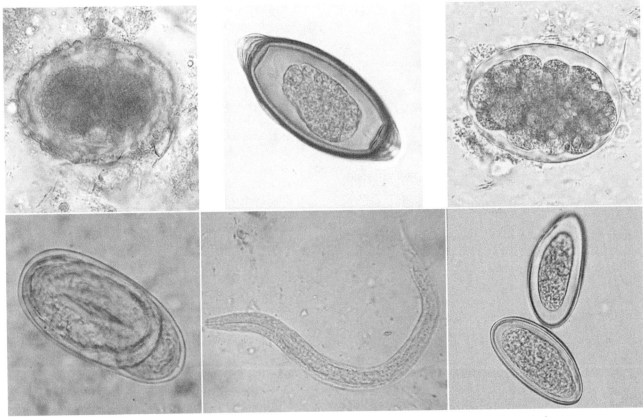

- **Fig. 4.36** Eggs and larvae of common intestinal nematodes. (From Maguire JH. Intestinal nematodes (roundworms). In: Bennett JE, Dolin R, Blaser MJ, eds. *Mandell, Douglas, and Bennett's Principles and Practice of Infectious Diseases*. Updated 8th ed. Elsevier; 2015.)

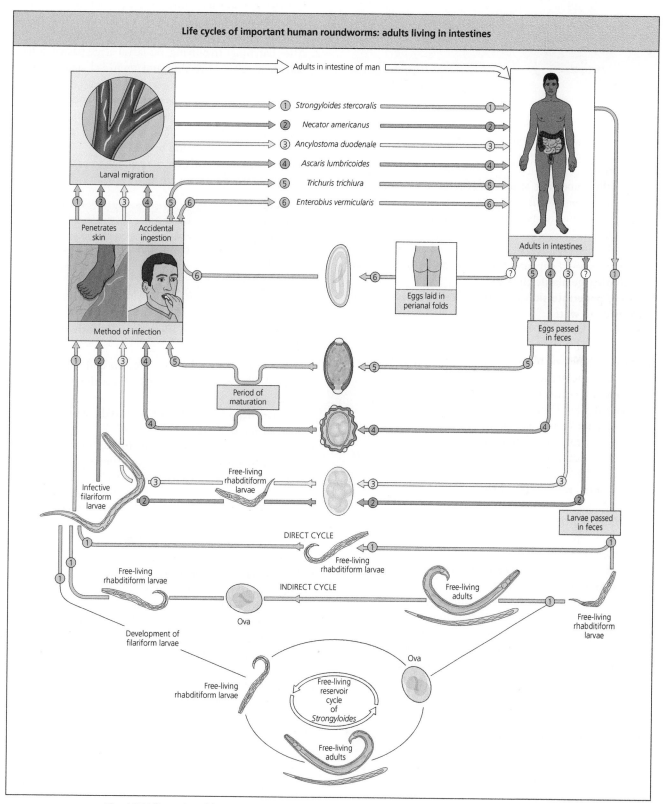

• **Fig. 4.37** Life cycles of important human roundworms. (From Lindquist HD, Cross JH. Helminths. In: Cohen J, Powderly W, Opal S, eds. *Infectious Diseases*. 4th ed. Elsevier; 2017.)

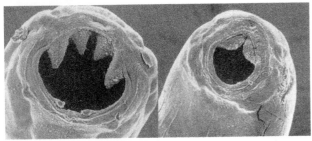

• **Fig. 4.38** Buccal cavities of *Ancylostoma duodenale* (left) and *Necator americanus* (right). (Courtesy Dr. David I. Pritchard. From Hotez PJ, Pritchard DI. Hookworm infection. *Sci Am.* 1995;272:70–74.)

Hookworms

- Clinically important species = *Necator americanus* and *Ancylostoma duodenale*.
1. Females produce eggs, which are excreted with human feces into soil.
2. If conditions warm and moist, larvae are released from eggs.
   - It takes 5–10 days and two molts to become infective third-stage filariform larvae.
3. Larvae **penetrate skin** on human feet/body surfaces or **ingested in water.**
   - Mainly acquired by walking barefoot on contaminated soil.
4. Travel to lungs via bloodstream until pass up pulmonary tree and swallowed.
5. Maturation occurs in intestine in 5 weeks.
   - Females 10–13 mm and males 6–11 mm.
   - Adult hookworms **attach** to the intestinal mucosa using their **cutting apparatus** and suck a plug of tissue into their buccal cavity using negative pressure (Fig. 4.38). They also release **anticlotting agents** and **hydrolytic enzymes, resulting in chronic blood loss.**

Trichuris trichiura (Whipworm)

1. Eggs are deposited in soil via fecal excretion and become infective in 15–30 days.
   - They have a characteristic **barrel-shape** with polar **plugs at each end** (Fig. 4.36).
2. Eggs are swallowed via soil-contaminated food or hands, hatch in intestine, and migrate to colon.
3. Adults reside in large intestine.
   - They anchor themselves to colonic mucosa with one end embedded in the mucosa and the other end free within the lumen (Fig. 4.39B); they feed on fluids, digested tissue, and blood.
   - They measure 3–5 cm and live for ~1 year.

CLINICAL PEARL

- There is no person-to-person transmission of Ascaris, hookworms or, Trichuris as they require an extended time outside the body to complete their life cycle.

Strongyloides stercoralis

- Males and females in free-living life cycle (Fig. 4.40).

- Females only in parasitic cycle ("**parasitic parthenogenetic female worms**").
- Females 1.5–2.5 mm long, esophagus and vulva in posterior third of body.
1. Females deposit eggs on intestinal epithelium.
2. After hatching, free-living 1st larval stage passes in feces and then converts to 2nd and then 3rd stage infective filariform larva.
3. Infective 3rd stage larva **penetrates skin** and enters lung via bloodstream.
4. Passes up pulmonary tree and is swallowed; enters bowel mucosa where maturation occurs.
5. Larvae in soil can also become free-living adults and produce infective filariform larvae.

CLINICAL PEARL

- **Autoinfection:** infective larvae can directly penetrate the lower gut or peri-anal region, leading to a new cycle of infection.
  - This may be uncontrolled in immunocompromised hosts leading to hyperinfection.

Enterobius vermicularis (Pinworm/Threadworm) (Fig. 4.41)

1. Adult worms live in human intestine and mate there.
2. Gravid females migrate at night from the cecum to the anus.
3. Females deposit eggs in perianal folds, which embryonate within 6 hours.
4. Eggs are transferred from anus to mouth under fingernails or become released onto bed sheets.
5. Eggs may remain infective for up to 20 days in humid, cool conditions.
6. After ingestion, it takes 5–6 weeks for larvae to mature.

Capillaria philippinensis (Capillariasis)

- Organism can multiply within intestine.
- Very small worm, female is 2.5–5 mm.
1. Eggs require water for embryonation.
2. Eaten by freshwater fish and develop into infective stage.
3. Then consumed by humans and larvae mature.
4. Females produce young that mature in the intestine; rapid multiplication, infection can be fatal.

Tissue Nematodes

Cutaneous Larva Migrans (CLM)

Epidemiology

- Larvae of hookworm from dogs, e.g., *Ancylostoma braziliensis* and *A. caninum*, cause creeping skin eruption.
- Worldwide but prefers warmer climates.
- Can also cause enteritis in humans (*A. caninum*).

Life Cycle

- Hookworm larvae in skin are unable to continue with life cycle so migrate within the epidermis.

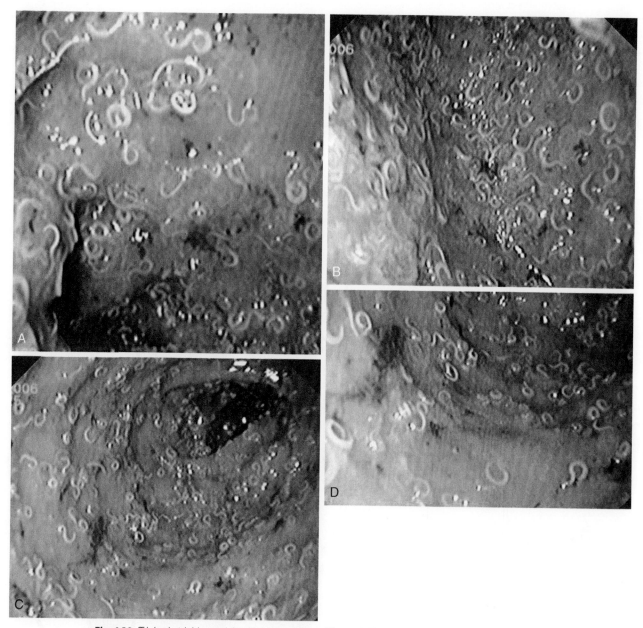

• **Fig. 4.39** *Trichuris trichiura* adult whipworms. (From Khuroo MS, Khuroo MS, Khuroo NS. *Trichuris* dysentery syndrome: a common cause of chronic iron deficiency anemia in adults in an endemic area (with videos). *Gastrointest Endosc.* 2010;71(1):200–204. © 2010.)

• If migrating through skin/subcutaneous tissues, erythematous tracts produced.

Visceral Larva Migrans (VLM)

Epidemiology

• Larvae from *Toxocara* spp. (cat/dog roundworms) cause visceral larva migrans when eggs ingested.
• Occurs worldwide: tropical > temperate areas; rural > urban areas.
• Other risk factors = owning a dog, exposure to public parks and playgrounds, and age <20 years.

Life Cycle

• Humans are **accidental** hosts.
• Infected dogs/cats shed *Toxocara* eggs in their feces.

• These take 2–4 weeks to become infective and may remain so for several years.
• Infection occurs when *Toxocara* spp. larvae hatch after eggs ingested.
• The larvae penetrate the gut wall and are carried via the bloodstream to tissues such as liver, heart, and eyes (ocular larva migrans).
• The host inflammatory response against the migrating larvae causes tissue damage (eosinophilic granulomas).

Neural Larva Migrans

Epidemiology

• *Baylisascaris procyonis*: roundworm of **raccoons**, causes neural larva migrans resulting in severe encephalitis in children and ocular infections in adults.

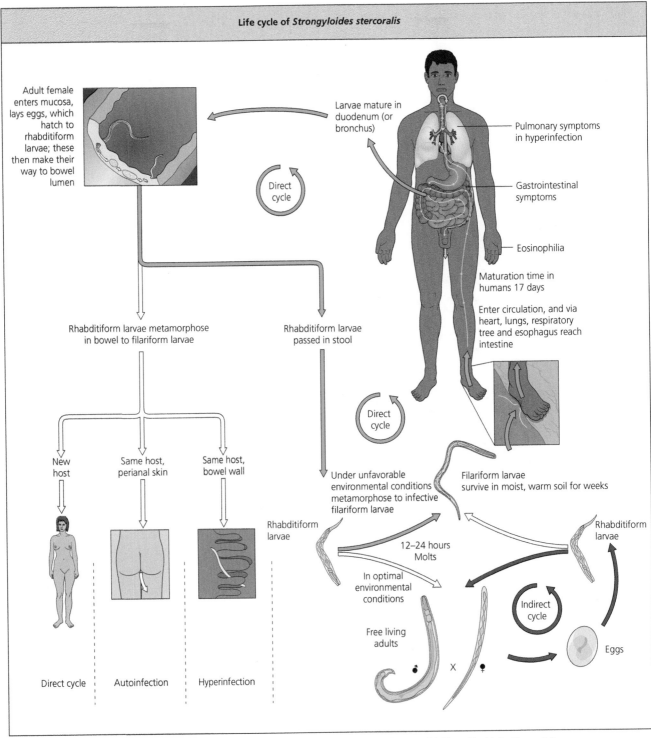

• **Fig. 4.40** Life cycle of *Strongyloides stercoralis*. (From Kelly P, Mutengo M. Parasitical infections of the gastrointestinal tract. In: Cohen J, Powderly W, Opal S. *Infectious Diseases*. 4th ed. Elsevier; 2017.)

• Young children and developmentally disabled persons most at risk as more likely to put **contaminated fingers/soil/objects into mouth.**
• Rare: <25 cases documented in United States; but may be mis-/undiagnosed.

Life Cycle

• Eggs of raccoon nematode *Baylisascariasis procyonis* hatch after ingestion and move through a wide variety of tissues (with **a**

tropism for neural tissue) resulting in **childhood eosinophilic encephalitis**, VLM, and **adult ocular pathology.**
• More damaging than toxocariasis because larvae continue to grow within a human host, wander widely, and do not readily die when compared with *Toxocara*.

Trichinosis

Epidemiology

• *Trichinella spiralis.*

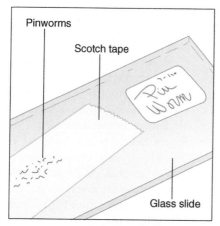 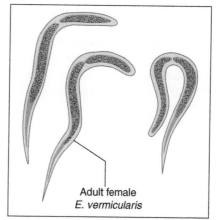

• **Fig. 4.41** Adult *Enterobius vermicularis* worms in the perianal region. (From Buttaravoli PM, Leffler SM. *Minor Emergencies*. 3rd ed. Elsevier; 2012.)

- Other *Trichinella* spp. also implicated in human disease.
- **Worldwide** distribution, especially temperate climates: most common in United States and parts of Europe.
- Transmitted via **eating infected pig/wild animal meat**, other hosts: carnivorous mammals and birds.

Life Cycle
- Acquired by **eating uncooked meat (usually pork)** contaminated with cysts.
- After ingestion larvae emerge from cysts and mature after entering the small bowel mucosa.
- As adults they re-emerge into lumen and reproduce.
  - Females measure 2–4 mm; life span ~4 weeks.
  - New larvae migrate to striated muscle cells via bloodstream where they become cysts (Fig. 4.42).

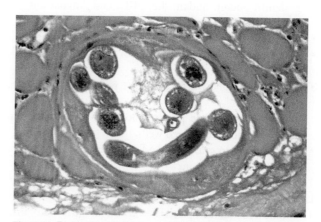

• **Fig. 4.42** *Trichinella spiralis* larvae within a skeletal muscle cell. (From McAdam AJ. Sharpe AH. Infectious diseases. In: Kumar V, ed. *Robbins and Cotran Pathologic Basis of Disease*. 8th ed. Saunders Elsevier; 2009.)

Angiostrongyliasis

Epidemiology
- Caused by molluscan-borne **rat lungworm**: *A. cantonensis*.
- Endemic in rats in Asia, Pacific Islands, Australia, India, Africa, Caribbean, parts of United States.
- Human infection reported mainly in **Taiwan and Thailand**; from **eating snails.**
  - Most prevalent in children in Taiwan and in adult males in Thailand.
  - **Contaminated raw produce** may also be a source of transmission.
- Also *A. costaricensis*: most infections in Costa Rica in children who ingested slugs; rats are also the natural host.

Life Cycle
1. Eggs produced by females mature into larvae, migrate, and are swallowed, then excreted in rat feces.
2. Larvae reintroduced to rat after ingestion of intermediate snail hosts.
3. These larvae are **neurotropic**: they migrate to rat brain where they develop into adult worms, and then to lungs.
4. Humans are incidentally infected after ingestion of snails: eosinophilic meningitis.

- Humans do not transmit either *A. cantonensis* or *A. costaricensis*.

Anisakiasis
- Caused by 3rd stage larvae of *Anisakis simplex* and *Pseudoterranova decipiens*.
- Marine mammals worldwide are natural hosts.
- Acquired by **eating raw saltwater fish/squid.**
  - Eating undercooked/raw/pickled fish containing larvae.
    - High incidence in Japan.
  - **Salmon, herring, cod, mackerel, halibut, red snapper, and squid.**
    - Larvae are grossly visible (2–3 cm) and reside in muscle tissue of fish.
      - May be detected by trained sushi chefs.
- Incidental host, no onward transmission.

Gnathostoma *spp*
- *G. spinigerum* is most commonly isolated in humans.
- Infections commonly reported in **Thailand and Japan**, but also South and Central America and Africa.
- More common in adults.

- Dogs and cats are the first natural hosts and fish/frogs/snakes are second natural hosts.
- Paratenic hosts are ones in which the larvae do not develop further but remain infective, e.g., bird, snake, or frog.
- Humans acquire the infection after:
  - Eating undercooked or raw fish/frogs/poultry/snake meat.
  - Drinking water containing infected *Cyclops*.

Dracunculiasis

Epidemiology
- Caused by *Dracunculus medinensis*.
- Also known as **Guinea worm** disease.
- **Poor communities in rural areas without access to safe drinking water.**
- **Chad, Ethiopia, and Mali** still considered endemic.
  - South Sudan, Sudan, the DRC, and Angola not yet certified as free of transmission by the WHO.
- Mainly age 15–40 years.
- Transmitted via a small crustacean vector (*Cyclops* spp.), which is seasonal.
- Larvae are swallowed in **stagnant water** containing the vector.
  - Examples include ponds, pools in drying riverbeds, and shallow uncovered wells.
- Better access to safe water and education programs have led to near eradication.

Life Cycle
1. Swallowed larvae penetrate through gut wall into abdominal cavity and retroperitoneum (Fig. 4.43).
2. Maturation and copulation occur; males die and adult females migrate through connective tissue toward skin surface.
3. Females induce a blister, usually on the distal leg; this ruptures forming an ulcer.
4. Local discomfort causes the infected human to seek relief by putting leg into cool water.
5. Upon contact, the **female emerges from subcutaneous tissue** (Fig. 4.44), and larvae are released.
   - Females can measure 120 cm long.
6. Transmission: infected copepods are ingested in drinking water by humans.

Blood and Tissue Nematodes (Filarial Infections)

- Nematodes that dwell in the lymphatic, subcutaneous, and cutaneous tissues of humans (Table 4.11).
- Estimated to infect 180 million people worldwide.
- Generally transmitted by arthropods in tropical and subtropical climates.

Lymphatic Filariasis

Epidemiology
- *Wuchereria bancrofti*: endemic in Asia, Africa, Central and South America, Pacific Islands.

- *W. bancrofti* causes 90% of infections.
- Prevalence depends on vector mosquito, climate, human population, sanitation.
  - Most common vector = **culicine mosquito** in urban/suburban areas.
  - *Aedes* mosquito = Pacific Islands vector.
  - *Anopheles* mosquito = Africa vector.
- No known animal reservoirs.
- *Brugia malayi* (rural Asia and Indonesia) and *Brugia timori* (Indonesia) cause filariasis in southern and eastern Asia (Mansonia, *Anopheles*, and *Aedes* vectors). Cats and monkeys can act as reservoirs.
- Worldwide these three filarial species infect an estimated 120 million people.

Life Cycle
1. Microfilariae are produced by adults **between 22:00 h and 02:00 h** at night.
2. Mosquitos take a blood meal at night and infective stage develops in 10–14 days.
3. During next feed: infective stage enter host and can then mature into adults.
4. Cycle begins again, infection can persist for years.

Onchocerciasis (River Blindness)

Epidemiology
- *Onchocerca volvulus*
  - Endemic in 26 countries in Africa.
  - Also endemic in six South/Central American countries.
- Estimated 18 million affected (99% in sub-Saharan Africa): 270,000 blind, 500,000 disabled.
- Vector is the **blackfly** *Simulium damnosum*.
  - Blackfly require **running water** for larval development, so transmission occurs in **close proximity to water sources.**
- Infection is more common in males than females (occupational exposure).

Life Cycle
1. Adults reside in subcutaneous tissues.
   - Females can be 50 cm long.
2. Microfilaria are deposited in skin and then harvested by biting insects.
3. The infective larvae are then passed on during next feeding.
   - Larvae migrate for months before becoming stationary and encapsulated.

Loiasis

Epidemiology
- *Loa loa*: African eye worm.
- Endemic in West and Central Africa.
  - Usually occurs in residents > travelers.
- Vector = deer fly (*Chrysops* spp.).

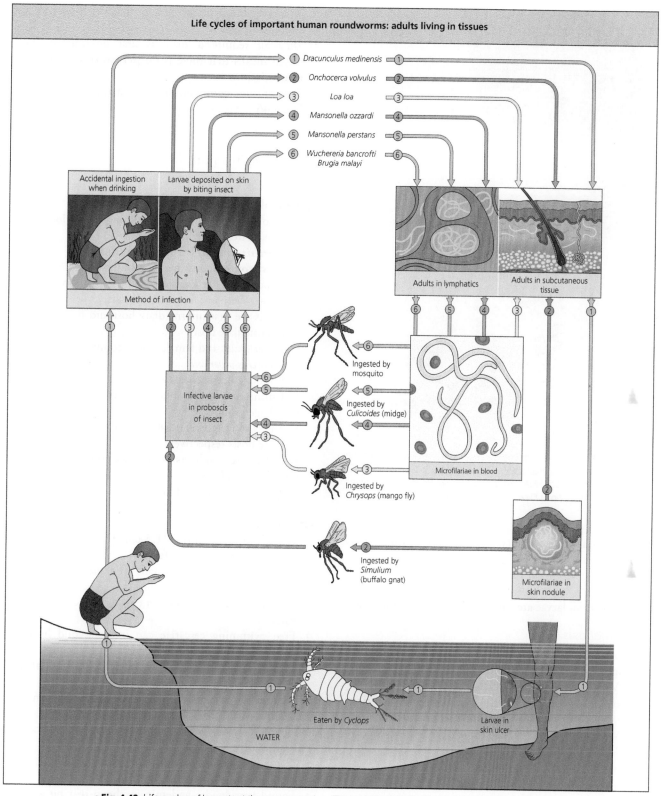

Life cycles of important human roundworms: adults living in tissues

1. *Dracunculus medinensis*
2. *Onchocerca volvulus*
3. *Loa loa*
4. *Mansonella ozzardi*
5. *Mansonella perstans*
6. *Wuchereria bancrofti*
   Brugia malayi

Accidental ingestion when drinking

Larvae deposited on skin by biting insect

Method of infection

Adults in lymphatics

Adults in subcutaneous tissue

Ingested by mosquito

Ingested by *Culicoides* (midge)

Ingested by *Chrysops* (mango fly)

Infective larvae in proboscis of insect

Microfilariae in blood

Ingested by *Simulium* (buffalo gnat)

Microfilariae in skin nodule

Eaten by *Cyclops*

WATER

Larvae in skin ulcer

• **Fig. 4.43** Life cycles of important tissue nematodes. (From Lindquist HD, Cross JH. Helminths. In: Cohen J, Powderly W, Opal S, eds. *Infectious Diseases*. 4th ed. Elsevier; 2017.)

- Breed in canopy of rainforest.
- Day biters, attracted to movement.
- Risk factors: increasing age, bitten during wet season, length of stay in affected areas.
- Monkeys can serve as reservoir.

Life Cycle

- Resides in subcutaneous tissues and even conjunctiva.
  - Adults 3–7 cm, may **migrate.**
- Microfilaria have a diurnal periodicity, which peaks during mid day.

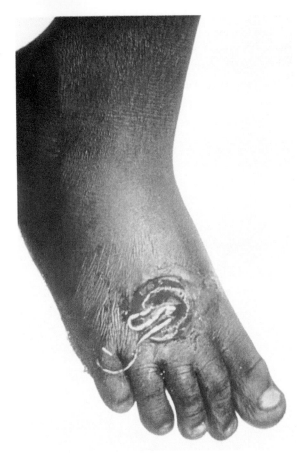

• **Fig. 4.44** Female adult *Dracunculus medinensis* emerging from the skin over the foot. (From KazuraJW. Tissue nematodes. In: Bennett JE, Dolin R, Blaser MJ, eds. *Mandell, Douglas, and Bennett's Principles and Practice of Infectious Diseases*. Updated 8th ed. Elsevier; 2015.)

• *Chrysops* spp. vector ingests microfilaria during blood meal.
• Within the vector the infective larvae develop over 10–13 days.
• At next feed, larvae are passed through bite to humans.

Mansonellosis

• *Mansonella ozzardi*: South America and Caribbean islands.
  • Vectors = midges or blackflies.
• *Mansonella perstans*: Central Africa and South America.
• *Mansonella streptocerca* (streptocerciasis) – tropical forests of West and Central Africa/Uganda.
  • Vector = midges.

Trematodes

• Many infect, but only a few are considered pathogenic (Fig. 4.45).
• Trematodes live in blood vessels, intestines, biliary tract, and lungs.
• They have a dorsoventrally flattened body with bilateral symmetry, i.e., leaf-shaped. They have a complex outer tegument and lack a body cavity.

• There may be great morphologic diversity between developmental stages.
• They all require a snail as first intermediate host, which means that there is **no person-to-person direct transmission.**
• Eggs of some common human trematodes are shown in Fig. 4.46.

Liver/Lung Trematodes

Liver Flukes

Epidemiology
All three of these are transmitted through ingestion of raw/undercooked freshwater fish/crabs.
• *Clonorchis sinensis* (Chinese liver fluke)
  • **Most common**, estimated 7 million people infected.
  • Geography: **Far East**, especially China, South Korea, Japan, Vietnam, far eastern Russia.
  • Snails are first intermediate host and fish are second intermediate host.
  • Older males and females more commonly infected.
• *Opisthorchis viverrini*
  • Endemic in Southeast Asia.
  • Estimated 10 million people infected.
  • All age groups.
  • Snails and freshwater fish are first and second intermediate hosts respectively.
  • Other reservoir hosts = dogs, cats, and other mammals.
• *Opisthorchis felineus*
  • Western Europe and Siberia.

Life Cycles
1. Hermaphroditic worms (1.5 cm) that release eggs into bile ducts and then into feces.
2. Eggs are ingested by snails (*Parafossarulus*, *Thiara*, *Bithynia*).
3. Miracidium is released from egg and develops into cercaria.
4. Free swimming cercariae can infect second host and encyst: fish (cyprinids/carp).
5. **Humans contract infection after ingesting infected fish.**
6. Maturation occurs in bowel/biliary system of human.

Fascioliasis (Sheep Liver Fluke)

Epidemiology
• Caused by *Fasciola hepatica.*
  • Humans are incidental hosts.
• Found worldwide: endemic in **sheep-rearing areas** of the world.
  • Sheep, goats, and cows are the natural hosts.
• Human infection most common in Europe, South America, Middle East.
  • Highest prevalence in **Bolivia and Peru.**
• Infection is acquired by ingestion of water/leafy plants that grow in fresh water.

TABLE 4.11   Parasites Causing Filarial Infections

Parasite	Number of People Infected Worldwide	Associated Disease	Vector	Geographic Distribution	Location of Adult	Location of Microfilariae	Sheathed Microfilariae	Periodicity of Microfilariae
Wuchereria bancrofti	120 million	Lymphatic filariasis	Mosquitoes	Tropics and subtropics worldwide	Lymphatic tissue	Blood	+	Nocturnal (95%) Subperiodic (5%)
Brugia malayi	10 million	Lymphatic filariasis	Mosquitoes	Asia, India, Philippines	Lymphatic tissue	Blood	+	Nocturnal (75%) Subperiodic (25%)
Brugia timori	<0.8 million	Lymphatic filariasis	Mosquitoes	Indonesia, Timor-Leste	Lymphatic tissue	Blood	+	Nocturnal
Loa loa	12 million	Loiasis	Deerflies	Central and West Africa	Subcutaneous tissue	Blood	+	Diurnal
Onchocerca volvulus	39 million	Onchocerciasis	Blackflies	Africa (99%), Americas, Yemen	Subcutaneous tissue	Skin, eye	–	None
Mansonella ozzardi	Unknown	Mansonellosis	Midges, blackflies	South and Central America, Caribbean	Undetermined	Blood	–	None
Mansonella perstans	Unknown	Perstans filariasis	Midges	South and Central America, Africa	Body cavities, mesentery, perirenal tissue	Blood	–	None
Mansonella streptocerca	Unknown	Streptocerciasis	Midges	Africa	Undetermined	Skin	–	None

From Nutman TB. Filarial infections. In: Cohen J, Powderly W, Opal S, eds. *Infectious Diseases.* 4th ed. Elsevier; 2017.

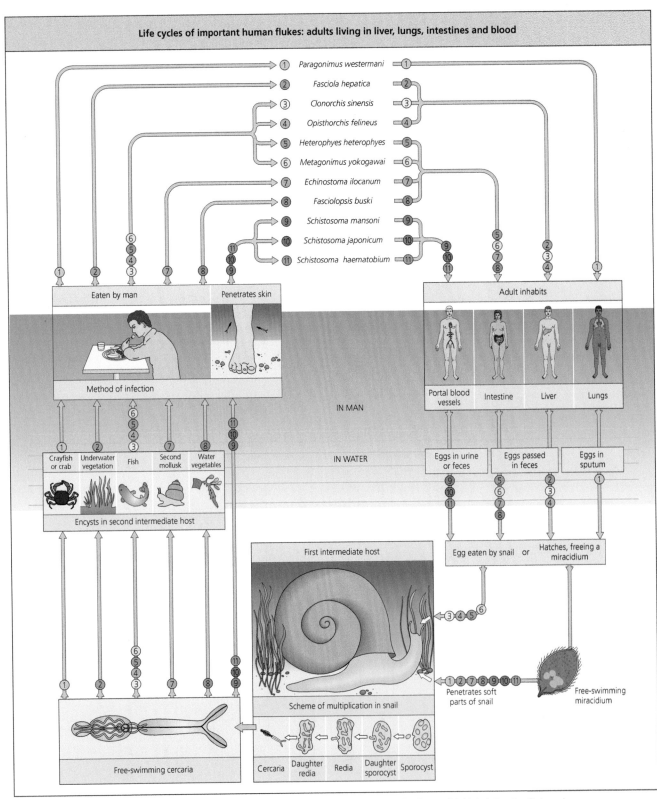

• **Fig. 4.45** Life cycles of important human flukes. (From Lindquist HD, Cross JH. Helminths. In: Cohen J, Powderly W, Opal S, eds. *Infectious Diseases*. 4th ed. Elsevier; 2017.)

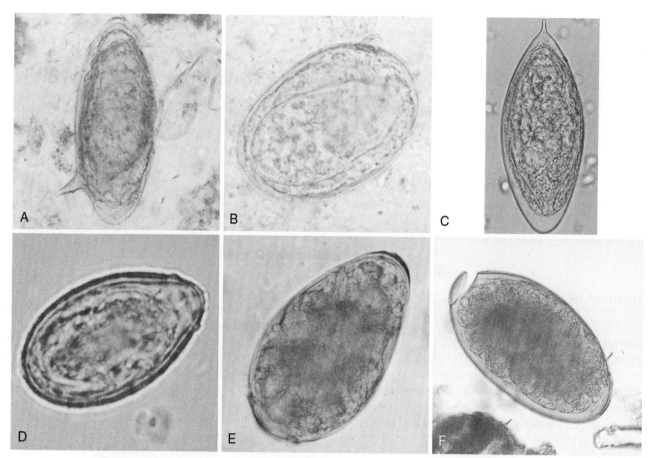

• **Fig. 4.46** Eggs of common human trematodes. (A) *Schistosoma mansoni*. (B) *Schistosoma japonicum*. (C) *Schistosoma haematobium*. (D) *Clonorchis sinensis*. (E) *Paragonimus westermani*. (F) *Fasciola hepatica* (note the partially open operculum). (From Maguire JH. Trematodes. In: Bennett JE, Dolin R, Blaser MJ, eds. *Mandell, Douglas, and Bennett's Principles and Practice of Infectious Diseases*. Updated 8th ed. Elsevier; 2015.)

- **Watercress is commonly implicated with outbreaks of infection.**
- *Fasciola gigantica* is similar in life cycle, pathology, and clinical disease.
  - Occurs predominantly in the tropics and subtropics.
    - Africa, Hawaii, western Pacific, Southeast Asia.

Life Cycle

- *Fasciola hepatica*
  - Large 4 cm worms with a cephalic cone.
  - After ingestion by humans, metacercariae excyst in the duodenum, pass through the gut wall, peritoneum, and liver capsule to reach biliary system where they will release their eggs.
    - Eggs are scanty in number and may not be found in up to 30%.
  - After infection of the intermediate snail host, cercariae are released.
  - In similar fashion to *F. buski*: aquatic vegetation harbor the encysted forms after they leave snails of genus *Lymnaea*.

Lung Fluke

Epidemiology

- *Paragonimus westermani* (oriental lung fluke): can cause serious disease.
- China, Japan, Korea, the Philippines, and Thailand.
- Transmission via **ingestion of seafood (crabs/crayfish)** contaminated with metacercariae.
  - 1st intermediate hosts: snails (*Semisulcospira* sp.).
  - 2nd intermediate hosts: crabs and crayfish.
  - Reservoir hosts: dogs, cats, and other mammals.

Life Cycle

1. Measure about 1.2 cm (coffee-bean shape), live in the **peripheral lungs**, often two together.
2. Eggs are excreted in sputum or feces (after swallowing respiratory secretions).
3. Once in water, a snail acts as intermediate host for replication.
4. Cercariae seek out crustaceans as second hosts and encyst until ingested by humans when excystation occurs.

TABLE 4.12 Characteristic Features of *Schistosoma* Species

Schistosoma sp.	Distribution	Snail Intermediate Host	Location of Adult Worms	Egg Excretion	Egg Morphology Mnemonic (Fig. 4.46)
S. haematobium	Africa and Middle East	Bulinus	Bladder venules	Urine	*S. haematobium* = terminal spine
S. intercalatum	Central and West Africa	Bulinus	Mesenteric venules	Feces	
S. japonicum	Asia Note: reservoir hosts in domestic/wild animals	Oncomelania			*S. japonicum* = looks like the rising sun
S. mansoni	Africa, Middle East, and South America	Biomphalaria			*S. mansoni* = subterminal spine
S. mekongi	Southeast Asia	Neotricula			

Intestinal Trematodes

Fasciolopsis buski (Giant Intestinal Fluke)

Epidemiology

- Largest human intestinal fluke.
- China, Thailand, India, and Bangladesh.
- Pigs act as reservoir hosts, and snails are important vectors.
- The snails release cercariae, which convert to cyst form on plants, e.g., **watercress**, **bamboo**, **water chestnuts.**
- Transmission occurs when these contaminated plants are ingested raw.

Life Cycle

- Largest intestinal fluke: 5–7 cm.
- Similarly to the above liver flukes, eggs pass into feces, miracidium infects snail intermediate, and cercariae leave snail.
- However, the **encysted metacercariae attach to aquatic plant forms and are ingested by humans.**
- After ingestion, the metacercariae excyst and develop into adult flukes.
- Reside in the human intestine, attached to the mucosa, with a life span of about 1 year.

Echinostoma/Heterophyes/Metagonimus

- Cases are mainly reported in Middle East and the Far East (China, Korea, and Japan).
- Transmission occurs in all cases from eating the second intermediate host raw.
  - *Echinostoma* = snails/fish.
  - *Heterophyes/Metagonimus* = fish.

Blood Trematodes

Schistosomiasis (Bilharzia)

Epidemiology

- Mainly tropical and subtropical areas (Table 4.12), estimated 200 million infected people (85% in sub-Saharan Africa).
- Transmission levels are determined by availability of snail hosts and human behaviors.
- Prevalence and intensity of infection (number of eggs excreted in urine/stool) **highest at age 5–15** years.
- Transmission: humans excrete eggs into water, freshwater snails become infected, and during aquatic activity, cercariae from snails infect humans.

Life Cycle

1. The adult parasites reside in the venous blood system.
   - Have separate sexes, oral, and ventral suckers; males: 0.5–2 cm, females 1.5–2.5 cm.
   - Live on average 3–5 years but may survive up to 30 years.
2. Eggs migrate from within the venule, penetrating into the gut or bladder lumen; they are then excreted in urine/feces.
   - Eggs may be swept away in the circulation to other tissues/organs.
3. Miracidia infect suitable snail hosts.
4. Cercariae released from the snails can penetrate human skin.
5. Within humans, larvae migrate to lungs, then the portal vessels where they develop and then pair; the pair then migrates to the intestinal or urogenital venous system.
6. Eggs are produced 4–6 weeks after initial skin penetration by cercariae.

Cestodes (Tapeworms)

- Tapeworms have a head (scolex), which has attachment apparatus (sucker/hooklets).
- The body of the worm is made up of proglottids which are produced by the neck section of the scolex continually. Mature proglottids are hermaphroditic. They become gravid and break free of the adult tapeworm, either passing out intact in feces or releasing eggs after degenerating in the stool.
- Size ranges from large (*D. latum* 2–15 m) to small (*H. nana* 1.5–4 cm).
- They cause human infection either as intestinal tapeworms or as invasive larval cysts (Fig. 4.47).

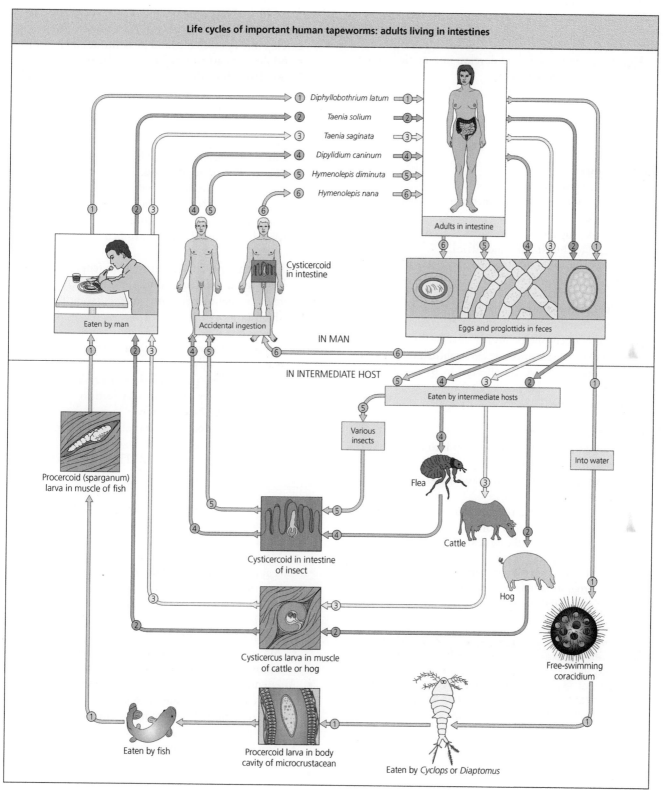

• **Fig. 4.47** Life cycles of important human tapeworms, with adults resident in intestines. (From Lindquist HD, Cross JH. Helminths. In: Cohen J, Powderly W, Opal S, eds. *Infectious Diseases*. 4th ed. Elsevier; 2017.)

Taenia saginata (Beef Tapeworm)

Epidemiology
- Nonpathogenic.
- Worldwide, adults, highest rates in Africa and Asia.

Life Cycle
- Eggs are eaten by cows and develop into cystic larvae in muscles (the cysticercus stage).
- When infected meat is consumed, adult worms develop in the human intestine.
  - Adults usually <5m in length.

Taenia solium (Pork Tapeworm)

Epidemiology
- Can cause cysticercosis.
- Often **source is an asymptomatic carrier within household.**
- Worldwide, highest rates in Mexico, Central and South America, Southwest Asia, and Africa.
- Humans may be both intermediate and definitive host for *T. solium*.

Life Cycle: Cysticercosis
1. The eggs hatch on reaching the acidic stomach environment and oncospheres invade tissues (brain, muscle, skin, eye) causing neurologic and ophthalmic sequelae.
   - The brain and eye are affected in particular due to their immunologic privilege.
   - Cysts can remain dormant for years.

Life Cycle: *T. solium taeniasis*
1. Eggs are eaten by pigs and develop into cystic larvae in muscles (the cysticercus stage).
2. Ingestion of raw or undercooked pork containing the cysticercus stage.
3. Within the intestine, the cysticercus develops over 2 months into an adult tapeworm.
   a. The adult attaches to the small intestine wall with its scolex.
   b. 2–7 m in length.
   c. The adult may survive for years.
4. Gravid proglottids are released (roughly six proglottids per day, with 50,000 eggs per proglottid).
5. Eggs can survive for days–months in the environment.

> **CLINICAL PEARL**
> - People do not get cysticercosis by eating undercooked pork. Eating undercooked pork may result in taeniasis (intestinal tapeworm) if the pork contains larval cysts.

Hymenolepis nana (Dwarf Tapeworm)

Epidemiology
- **Most common tapeworm in North America.**
- Especially seen in children in conditions of poor sanitation.

Life Cycle
- Eggs are immediately infective on being passed in feces.

- Transmission:
  - Ingestion of eggs via contaminated food, water, or hands (Fig. 4.47).
  - Accidental ingestion of an insect intermediate host.
- After ingestion, oncospheres are released from eggs, develop into cysticercoids and then into adult tapeworms.
  - Adults = 15–40 mm length; normal lifespan 4–6 weeks.
- **Internal autoinfection** may allow infection to persist for years.

Diphyllobothrium latum (Fish Tapeworm)

- Largest human tapeworm.
  - Adults may reach up to **30 feet** in length.
  - May survive up to **30 years.**
- Mostly northern hemisphere: decreasing in Scandinavia. Now seen in Siberia, Russia, and Japan.
  - Also reported in Chile/Uganda.
  - May be exported and consumed anywhere in the world.
- Requires intermediate fish/crustacean (copepod) hosts.
  - **Freshwater fish**: e.g., salmon, trout, perch, pike.
- Human = definitive host, reservoirs = bears/dogs/carnivores.
- Transmission:
  - Ingestion of **raw fish** containing the plerocercoid or sparganum stages.
  - **Dried/smoked/pickled fish also a risk.**
- Prolonged or heavy infection may lead to megaloblastic anemia due to **B12 deficiency.**
  - Parasite-mediated dissociation of vitamin B12-intrinsic factor complex in the gut.
  - Uptake and use of vitamin B12 by the adult tapeworm.

Sparganosis

- Infections with migratory **larval stages** of *Spirometra* spp.
- Worldwide but most human cases reported from Southeastern Asia.
  - May occur in North America but rare.
- Cats and dogs are the definitive hosts.
- 1st intermediate host = small crustaceans and 2nd intermediate host = reptiles/amphibians/birds.
- Transmission:
  - Via ingestion of intermediate hosts raw/undercooked.
  - Also reported in southern Asia from using animal tissue as **therapeutic poultices** for wounds or sore eyes.
- After entry into the human GI tract or subcutaneous tissue via contaminated water, aquatic foods and from the use of fresh animals as wound poultices, the organisms migrate causing **tissue and ocular inflammation.**
  - Can live for up to 20 years in a human host.

Echinococcus granulosus

Epidemiology
- Causes cases of cystic echinococcosis (CE) worldwide.
- Highest prevalence: Mediterranean, Central Asia, western China, Siberia, North and East Africa and southern tip of South America.

- Rural grazing areas where dogs ingest raw offal from infected animals.
- Endemic rural areas may have a prevalence of 5%–10%.
- **Dogs** are the definitive hosts; **sheep** are intermediate hosts.
  - Risk factors: herding livestock, owning dogs, proximity to animal slaughter, and poor hygiene.
- Transmission:
  - Accidental consumption via soil/water/food/hands contaminated by dog feces.
  - No human-to-human transmission.
- G1/G2 strain causes most human infections.

Life Cycle

1. Eggs of **dog tapeworms** are ingested by humans.
2. Oncospheres hatch in duodenum and invade tissues.
   - Target organs: liver and lung and less frequently kidney, spleen, brain, heart.
3. Develops into a unilocular hydatid cyst over months to years within tissue.
4. Cyst contains brood capsules within which the protoscolices multiply.
5. If cysts rupture, protoscolices released resulting in dissemination and further cyst formation.
6. Humans are incidental hosts, so the life cycle is not completed.

Echinococcus multilocularis

Epidemiology

- Causes alveolar echinococcosis (AE).
- **Northern hemisphere only.**
  - North America, central continental Europe such as France, Switzerland, Austria, Russia, central Asia, and much of China.
- Definitive hosts are raccoons and **foxes.**
  - **Domestic dogs are another important source.**
    - Intermediate host = rodents.
- Transmission
  - **Accidental consumption via soil/water/food contaminated by carnivore feces.**
  - **Hand-to-mouth transfer of eggs after touching contaminated fur (commonly dog).**

Life Cycle

Larval growth in the liver persists in a proliferative stage, resulting in invasion of surrounding tissues.
- Proliferates indefinitely by exogenous budding.
- Develops multilocular alveolar cysts.
- Resembles a malignancy in appearance.

Identification of Intestinal Pathogens

- Majority of these parasites are in the bowel; stool microscopy is used for diagnosis (simple, cheap, noninvasive).
- Blood, urine, and sputum should also be examined.
- Biopsies are useful for tissue-invading organisms.

- Diagnostic methods are summarized in Tables 4.13 and 4.14.

Specimens and Methods for Diagnosis

Stool and Gastrointestinal Tract Samples

- **Microscopic examination**
  - Wet mount of fresh samples, more than one sample, **ideally three taken every other day.**
    - Soft stool should ideally be examined within 1 hour of passage (may contain both trophozoites and cysts).
    - Formed stool may be kept for up to 1 day and may be refrigerated overnight.
  - Can use iodine stains, but they are better for protozoa than for helminth eggs/larvae.
- **Concentration techniques** are useful because egg concentration can be low: sedimentation technique and formalin-ethyl acetate technique.
- The Kato–Katz technique concentrates stool and uses glycerine to aid visualization and allows estimation of numbers of eggs.
- **Fecal culture**: for hookworms and *Strongyloides* spp. Culture is time-consuming and specialized but can increase diagnostic yield and unlike serology, identifies active (not past) infection.
- **Charcoal culture**: stool mixed with charcoal and water stored on moist filter paper in petri dish for several days. Larvae migrate to charcoal and are removed using a Baermann apparatus (immersed in water for 10–12 hours then drawn off, using rubber tubing, into glass flask for examination).
  - Harada–Mori technique: stool is smeared onto filter paper then stored upright in a tube containing a small volume of water. Water is examined for larvae after 4–10 days.
  - Specific agar plates are available for *Strongyloides* culture.
    - Pinworm, tapeworm, and *lumbricoides* eggs:
- **Perianal swabs** (cotton wool swab in a dry container).
  - Using scotch/cellophane **tape placed on perianal skin,** then placed onto glass slide for examination under microscope.
  - Best obtained in the morning before bathing or defecation.
  - >3 samples on consecutive days before infection excluded.
- Microscopy of duodenal aspirates: *Giardia, Strongyloides, Ascaris,* and flukes.
  - **Peroral string test**: a weighted gelatin capsule containing an absorbent nylon string (Enterotest) is swallowed while the proximal end is held firmly. The free end is attached to the patient's face and then pulled up after **4 hours.** Bile-stained mucus attached to the distal end is examined under a microscope.
  - 90 cm line for children, 140 cm line for adults.

TABLE 4.13   Laboratory Diagnosis of Intestinal Pathogens

Pathogen	Diagnostic Method
Intestinal Protozoa	

Entamoeba histolytica and nonpathogenic ameba (*E. dispar*, *E. hartmanni*, *E. coli*, *Iodamoeba butschlii*, *Endolimax nana*)	1. Fecal microscopy
	  • Wet direct preparations for motile trophozoites
	  • Wet concentrated Lugol's iodine preparations for cysts
	  • Permanent trichrome stained preparations for cysts and trophozoites
	2. Microscopy of liver abscess materials
	  • Permanent trichrome or hematoxylin/eosin-stained preparations
	3. ELISA of fecal specimens to detect galactose-inhibitable lectin antigen
	4. Indirect fluorescent antibody (IFA) test in suspected amebic abscess (and ameboma)
	5. Culture and zymodeme pattern analysis
	6. PCR; often available in reference laboratories
	7. In the absence of ingested red blood cells in *E. histolytica* trophozoites, it is difficult to distinguish this parasite from *E. dispar*. Presence of ingested red blood cells is the definitive diagnostic characteristic for *E. histolytica*.
	8. The IFA test is positive in over 95% of cases after 14 days but should be confirmed by the cellulose acetate precipitin test

Giardia intestinalis	1. Fecal microscopy
	  • Wet iodine or saline preparation for cysts and trophozoites
	  • Permanent trichrome preparations for cysts and trophozoites
	2. String test (enterotest), duodenal aspirate, or biopsy if fecal specimens are negative
	  • Direct wet preparations for motile trophozoites
	  • Permanent trichrome preparations for cysts and trophozoites
	3. ELISA tests to detect antigens in fecal specimens
	4. Indirect immunofluorescence tests for fecal specimens for specific monoclonal antibodies
	5. Direct fluorescence antibody tests (Merifluor DFA) against cell wall antigens
	6. Immunochromatographic assays
	7. Serology (not very useful as cannot distinguish current from past infection)

Blastocystis hominis	1. Fecal microscopy
	  • Wet iodine or saline preparation for cysts
	  • Permanent trichrome preparations for cysts

Dientamoeba fragilis	1. Fecal microscopy • Permanent trichrome stained preparations for trophozoites
Balantidium coli	1. Fecal microscopy • Direct wet iodine or saline preparations (fresh or concentrated specimen)

Cryptosporidium parvum/hominis	1. Fecal microscopy
	  • Direct wet concentrated preparations for cysts
	  • Permanent stained preparations with acid-fast stains (modified Ziehl–Neelsen) or auramine
	2. Immunofluorescence using monoclonal antibodies
	3. Immunochromatographic assays
	4. PCR for species identification (PCR is still principally a reference laboratory technique)
	5. Intestinal biopsy
	  • Permanent stained preparations with hematoxylin/eosin stain or toluidine blue

Cyclospora cayetanensis	1. Fecal microscopy • Permanent stained preparations with acid-fast stains (modified Ziehl–Neelsen) or auramine O (fluorescent)
Isospora belli	1. Fecal microscopy • Permanent stained preparations with acid-fast stains (modified Ziehl–Neelsen) or auramine O (fluorescent)
Nematodes (Roundworms)	
Ascaris lumbricoides	1. Fecal microscopy • Direct or concentrated fecal specimens for ova (embryonated and unembryonated) 2. Macroscopic examination of expelled worms
Ancylostoma duodenale and *Necator americanus* (hookworm)	1. Fecal microscopy • Direct or concentrated (Lugol's iodine-stained preparations) fecal specimens for ova or larvae 2. *Note:* Differentiate hookworm larvae from strongyloides larvae by examining the mouth parts. Hookworm larvae have a long tubular buccal cavity whereas that of strongyloides is shorter. Hookworm is also 3–4 times bigger than strongyloides

TABLE 4.13 Laboratory Diagnosis of Intestinal Pathogens—cont'd

Pathogen	Diagnostic Method
Strongyloides stercoralis	1. Fecal microscopy • Direct or concentrated (Lugol's iodine-stained preparations) fecal specimens for rhabditiform and filariform larvae 2. Fecal culture techniques (agar plate and Baermann) for larvae: useful in light infections 3. Sputum microscopy for larvae in hyperinfections 4. Intestinal biopsy • Hematoxylin and eosin stain
Trichuris trichiura	1. Fecal microscopy • Direct or concentrated wet fecal preparations for ova; adult worms are rarely seen
Enterobius vermicularis	1. Microscopic examination for ova in: • Clear cellulose tape perianal preparations or anal swabs 2. Anal examinations for adult worms 3. *Note:* Eggs or adult worms may be found accidentally in fecal or urine specimens • Specimen collection should be done early in the morning before bathing
Trematodes (Flukes)	
Fasciolopsis buski	1. Fecal microscopy for ova and adult worms in direct preparations 2. *Note:* Adult worms are rarely recovered in fecal preparations
Clonorchis sinensis	1. Fecal/duodenal aspirate microscopy for ova 2. Direct wet preparations and concentrated wet preparations
Heterophyes heterophyes	1. Fecal microscopy for ova and adult worms in direct preparations
Cestodes (Tapeworms)	
Taenia solium	1. Fecal microscopy for ova and proglottids 2. ELISA tests to detect parasite antigens 3. Serologic methods for *T. solium* cysticercosis 4. PCR to differentiate *T. solium* from *T. saginata* 5. *Note: T. solium* and *T. saginata* can be differentiated from gravid proglottids or the scolex recovered after purgation
Taenia saginata	Fecal microscopy for ova and proglottids
Hymenolepis nana	Fecal microscopy for ova
Diphyllobothrium latum	Fecal microscopy for ova or proglottids in wet preparations

From Kelly P, Mutengo M. Parasitical infections of the gastrointestinal tract. In: Cohen J, Powderly W, Opal S. *Infectious Diseases*. 4th ed. Elsevier; 2017.

• Nil by mouth for 12 hours beforehand.
• Flatworms, tapeworm proglottids, and trematodes should be collected and cleaned before microscopic examination. The specimens are fixed in formalin and stained for identification.

Sputum/Bronchoalveolar Lavage

• Process in a Class 1 exhaust protective cabinet in a Containment Level 3 room.
• Possible parasites:
  • *Ascaris lumbricoides, Cryptosporidium* spp., hookworm larvae, *Paragonimus westermani, Strongyloides stercoralis.*
  • Samples should be collected first thing in the morning.
  • Sputum is mixed with NaOH to digest and decontaminate and then centrifuged; **examine pellet for eggs/larvae.**
  • Also examine stool for eggs and consider (lung) tissue sampling for adult worms.

• If *Paragonimus* is suspected, send several sputum samples to look for eggs.

CLINICAL PEARL

• Suspect **Paragonimus infection** in patients with cough, fever and eosinophilia, eosinophilic pleural effusion, ingestion of raw crab/crayfish.

Urine

• Can aid diagnosis of *S. haematobium.*
  • Very few ova present in urine.
  • Number vary throughout the day: highest in urine between 10:00 h and 14:00 h.
  • Terminal portion of urine has highest yield.
  • Send large volume of urine (preferably on ice) and notify lab to be prepared to examine immediately. Centrifuged pellet examined.

TABLE 4.14 **Microscopic Diagnosis of Major Helminth Infections**

Parasite	Microscopic Diagnosis Stage	Microscopic Diagnosis Specimen	Other Methods
Roundworms (Nematodes)			
Intestinal Roundworms			
Ascaris lumbricoides (large intestinal roundworm)	Eggs	Feces	Identification of passed worm
Trichuris trichiura (whipworm)	Eggs	Feces	
Ancylostoma duodenale, Necator americanus (hookworm)	Eggs, larvae	Feces	
Strongyloides stercoralis (threadworm)	Larvae	Feces, duodenal fluid, sputum	Serology*
Enterobius vermicularis (pinworm)	Eggs	Swab of perianal skin; occasionally in feces	Cellophane tape test; identification of adult worms on skin
Tissue Roundworms			
Trichinella spiralis (trichinellosis)	Larvae	Muscle biopsy	Serology*
Dracunculus medinensis (guinea worm)			Identification of emergent adult worm
Wuchereria bancrofti, Brugia malayi (lymphatic filariasis)	Microfilariae	Blood, urine (in setting of chyluria)	Serology, antigen test (blood)
Loa loa (African eye worm)	Microfilariae	Blood	Identification of adult worm in eye, serology
Onchocerca volvulus (river blindness)	Microfilariae	Skin snip	Identification of adult worm in resected nodules
Ancylostoma braziliense, other species (cutaneous larva migrans, creeping eruption)			Inspection of rash
Toxocara canis, Toxocara cati (visceral larva migrans) Baylisascaris procyonis	Larvae	Biopsy of liver, other tissues (usually not necessary)	Serology[a] (preferred)
Flukes (Trematodes)			
Schistosoma mansoni, Schistosoma haematobium, Schistosoma japonicum, Schistosoma mekongi	Eggs	Feces, rectal snips, urine (S. haematobium)	Serology[a], antigen test (serum and urine)
Fasciolopsis buski (intestinal fluke)	Eggs	Feces	
Heterophyes heterophyes (intestinal fluke)	Eggs	Feces	
Metagonimus yokogawai (intestinal fluke)	Eggs	Feces	
Clonorchis sinensis, Opisthorchis spp. (liver fluke)	Eggs	Feces, bile	Serology
Fasciola hepatica (liver fluke)	Eggs	Feces, bile	Serology
Paragonimus spp. (lung fluke)	Eggs	Sputum, feces	Serology*
Tapeworms (Cestodes)			
Intestinal Tapeworms			
Taenia saginata (beef tapeworm)	Eggs	Stool	Identification of passed proglottid (segment)
Hymenolepis nana (dwarf tapeworm)	Eggs	Stool	
Diphyllobothrium latum (fish tapeworm)	Eggs	Stool	Identification of passed proglottid

TABLE 4.14 Microscopic Diagnosis of Major Helminth Infections—cont'd

| Parasite | Microscopic Diagnosis | | Other Methods |
	Stage	Specimen	
Taenia solium (pork tapeworm)	Eggs	Stool	Identification of passed proglottid; stool antigen test; serology
Larval Tapeworms			
Echinococcus granulosus (cystic hydatid disease)	Protoscolices, hooklets	Fluid from cyst	Serology[a], CT, MRI, or ultrasonography can be diagnostic
Echinococcus multilocularis (alveolar hydatid disease)	Larvae	Liver biopsy	Serology
Cysticercus (larval *Taenia solium*)	Larvae	Brain biopsy	Serology[a], CT, or MRI of head can be diagnostic

CT, computed tomography; MRI, magnetic resonance imaging.
[a]Serologic test is available through Division of Parasitic Diseases, Centers for Disease Control and Prevention, Atlanta, GA.
From Maguire JH. Introduction to helminth infections. In: Bennett JE, Dolin R, Blaser MJ. *Mandell, Douglas, and Bennett's Principles and Practice of Infectious Diseases*. Updated 8th ed. Elsevier; 2015.

- Sterile containers without boric acid should be used.
- May also detect microsporidia in urine of immunosuppressed patients.

CLINICAL PEARL

- Either a whole volume urine voided at **noon** or **terminal stream urines** collected over a 24-hour period will give the best results.

Blood

- Microscopy:
  - **Giemsa stain** is recommended for detection and identification of blood parasites.
  - **Thick smears are used for screening**, as the red blood cells have been lysed, and parasites are more concentrated.
  - **Thin smears are useful to identify species** that have been detected on a thick smear.
  - Fluorescent dyes that stain nucleic acid may be useful (e.g., acridine orange in a QBC, quantitative Buffy coat).
  - Parasites that may be detected on a peripheral blood smear include:
- *Plasmodium* spp., *Trypanosoma* spp., microfilaria, *Babesia* spp.
  - Use ×10 objective to screen the entire smear to detect larger parasites such as microfilaria.
  - Use ×100 oil immersion lens for smaller parasites such as malaria.
- Microfilaria
  - A good volume (20 ml) of anticoagulated blood (citrated) should be sent.
  - The time of blood sampling coincides with the peak time of microfilaremia.
    - **Day bloods** (10:00–14:00 h): *Loa loa.*
    - **Night bloods** (22:00–02:00 h): lymphatic filariasis (*W. bancrofti*, *B. malayi*, *B. timori*).

  - **Any time: *Onchocerca*, *Mansonella*.**
- *Plasmodium* spp.
  - WHO recommends that **at least 100 fields are examined,** each containing roughly 20 white blood cells before a thick smear is recorded as negative.
  - US standards recommend at least 300 fields.
  - Quantification of *P. falciparum* is required, usually against red blood cells (rbc).
    - If high parasitemia (e.g., >10%), count 500 rbc.
    - If low parasitemia, count >2000 rbc.
    - Count asexual stages separately from gametocytes.
  - If prior antimalarials taken, need **three negative films over 48 hours** to exclude malaria.

CSF

- An eosinophilic pleocytosis raises suspicion of parasitic infection.
- Examine the centrifuged sediment for microscopic evidence of:
  - *Acanthamoeba* species, *Angiostrongylus cantonensis*, *Balamuthia mandrillaris*, microsporidia: *Encephalitozoon cuniculi*, *Naegleria fowleri*, any nematodes producing VLM (visceral larva migrans), cestodes: *Taenia solium*, *Echinococcus* species.
  - *T. spiralis* larvae have been found in CSF in heavy infections.
  - CSF Containment Level 3 and a safety cabinet are required for the investigation for *N. fowleri*.
- PCR may be available for the diagnosis of free-living amebae at reference laboratories.

Tissue

In most cases, routinely stained hematoxylin and eosin (H&E) sections are suitable for examination for parasitic infection.

- Skeletal muscle.

- Suspected *T. spiralis* infection (trichinosis: myositis, eosinophilia, fever, elevated CK, elevated LDH, and history of ingestion of undercooked game meat).
- Rarely done; ELISA is more reliable and acceptable.
- Sample taken from painful muscle should be sent for:
  - H&E staining as normal for histology.
  - Crushed preparation for low power microscopy may reveal larvae.
  - PCR for molecular identification of species and genotype.
- Biopsy of bladder, reproductive tissue (resected ovary or cervical biopsy), and rectum may be examined histologically for *Schistosomiasis*.

Skin snips

- *Onchocerca volvulus* (suspicion in context of subcutaneous or intramuscular nodules, pruritus, dermatitis and depigmentation, sclerosing keratitis).
- Take 1–2 mg skin snips ×6 (using corneoscleral instrument) from scapulae, iliac crests, and calves.
- Place in saline (in microtiter plates) for up to 24 hours and examine under low power light microscope for microfilariae.
- *Mansonella perstans* (dermatitis, pruritus, lymphadenopathy) microfilariae are also diagnosed in skin snips and distinguishable from *O. volvulus* by their hook-shaped tail.

Fluid from Hydatid Cysts

- *Echinococcus* spp.
  - Should be processed in a Class 1 exhaust protective cabinet in a Containment Level 3 room.

Skin Lesions of Suspected *Leishmania*

- Full-thickness, 2–4 mm diameter punch biopsy taken from edge of lesions.
  - Send for microscopy of impression smears, culture, and PCR as well as in formalin for histology.
  - Samples for culture need specialized media at room temperature (may take up to 3 weeks).
  - Slit-skin smears: from edge of lesion, onto slide, air dried, fixed with methanol, and Giemsa stained.
  - Remember: slit skin smears may also be used for the diagnosis of leprosy.

Bone Marrow and Splenic Aspirates for Suspected *Leishmania*

- Samples should be used to prepare air-dried slides for microscopy, inoculated into culture, and have PCR performed.

CLINICAL PEARL

- **Bone marrow aspirate** is the **preferred** specimen for diagnosis of **Leishmania** infection, even though splenic aspirates are more sensitive. This is due to the **high risk of life-threatening hemorrhage**, even when radiologically guided.

Molecular Tests

- Many tests available, useful when organism not demonstrated on microscopy.
- PCR tests have been developed (PCR assays, quantitative assays, and FISH tests) but may only be available at reference laboratories.
  - UK (via Hospital for Tropical Diseases): *Leishmania*, microsporidia, *E. histolytica*, *Giardia*, *Cryptosporidia*, free living amebae and *Plasmodium* (for detection of subpatent = repeatedly slide-negative malarial infection, mixed infection or *P. knowlesi*).
  - PCR is the **preferred test for microsporidia** infections: more sensitive by 100× than light microscopy; semiquantitative so can provide information on response to treatment; can differentiate between morphologically identical organisms.

Serology and Antigen Tests

- Amebic serology: common test = IFAT. **95% positive in amebic liver abscess**, 75% in amebic colitis.
- Cysticercosis: serum and CSF antibody and antigen testing available.
- **Fascioliasis: serology useful as eggs may not be detected.** Best method in early stages of infection.
- Filariasis: serology is hampered by false positives (hookworm infection commonly, occasionally *Ascaris*) and false negatives; a negative result does not exclude the diagnosis.
- Hydatid disease: also hampered by false positives and negatives. For diagnosis, needs to be compatible with clinical scenario and imaging.
- Visceral and mucocutaneous leishmaniasis: MCL usually positive; VL: **negative serology does not exclude VL especially if HIV co-infection.** DAT (titer >1600 reported as positive) and rK39 tests available. rK39 detects antibodies against *Leishmania donovani* species complex.
- Schistosomiasis: **becomes positive 6 weeks after exposure**; should be requested on patients known to have been exposed to freshwater in endemic areas. Does not distinguish between past (treated) and active infections. False positives with trichinosis.
- Strongyloidiasis: should be requested in the investigation of unexplained eosinophilia or if suggestive clinical picture. Cross-reacts with filarial antibodies.
- Toxocariasis: diagnostic method of choice. May be performed on serum, aqueous and vitreous humor, and CSF. **A negative serum does not exclude ocular *Toxocara* infection.**
- Toxoplasmosis: see section on *Toxoplasma gondii* identification earlier in chapter.
- Trichinosis: reliable test for diagnosis.
- African trypanosomiasis: serologic testing of serum and CSF useful.
- American trypanosomiasis: serologic testing used for chronic infection (symptomatic or screening). May cross-react with *Leishmania* antibodies.

Macroscopic Examination

- Dracunculiasis: characteristic appearance of skin blister and emerging adult worm (see Fig. 4.44).
- Lymphatic filariasis: Doppler ultrasound of inguinal lymph nodes, scrotum, or breast show engorged lymphatic vessels may reveal motile adult worm exhibiting the "**filarial dance**" sign.
- Slit-lamp examination of the eye may reveal *O. volvulus* microfilariae.
- *Loa loa* infection: **Calabar swellings**: 10–20 cm angio-edematous swellings on face and extremities, transient (days to weeks). **Eye worm**: adult worm is seen migrating across the conjunctiva.

Further Reading and Resources

1. CDC: Laboratory Identification of Parasites of Public Health Concern. https://www.cdc.gov/dpdx/az.html.
2. Public Health England: UK Standards for Microbiology Investigations: Investigation of specimens other than blood for parasites. https://assets.publishing.service.gov.uk/government/uploads/system/uploads/attachment_data/file/622944/B_31i5.1.pdf.
3. UK NEQAS Parasitology. http://www.ukneqasmicro.org.uk/parasitology/index.php/ct-menu-item-2.

5

Antibacterials

YVONNE BURNETT, DAVID RITCHIE

Antibacterial Classes and Mechanism of Action

Classification of antibiotics and their basic mechanism of action are set out in Table 5.1. Sites of action are depicted in Fig. 5.1.

ANTIBACTERIAL AGENTS

Cell Wall-Active Agents

Beta-Lactams

Mechanism of Action
- **Inhibit bacterial cell wall synthesis** by binding to penicillin-binding proteins (PBPs) (Fig. 5.2.).
- **Bactericidal.**
  Safety
- Adverse drug reactions (ADRs): gastrointestinal (GI) disturbances and hypersensitivity reactions are the most common adverse events noted. Less common, but serious, events such as electrolyte disorders, interstitial nephritis, seizures, LFT, and hematologic abnormalities may also occur.

> **CLINICAL PEARLS**
> - Beta-lactams do not typically have high oral bioavailability. When treating more serious infections, intravenous (IV) formulations are recommended.

Penicillins

Natural Penicillins
Agents
- Penicillin G.
- Penicillin V.
  Spectrum
- Narrow-spectrum penicillin: good for beta-hemolytic streptococcal and penicillin-susceptible *Streptococcus pneumoniae* infections, some anaerobic infections (*Peptostreptococcus* spp., *Actinomyces* spp.), *Treponema pallidum*, and *Pasteurella multocida*.

- Natural penicillins do not have staphylococcal or gram-negative activity (**with the exception of *P. multocida***).
  Clinical Uses
- **Drug of choice for syphilis, group A streptococcal pharyngitis.**
  Dosing/Therapeutic Drug Monitoring (TDM)
- Penicillin G IV 12–30 million units divided every 4–6 hours, or as a continuous infusion.
- Penicillin V PO 250–500 mg every 6 hours.
- Penicillin G benzathine IM 1.2–2.4 million units administered as a single dose.
- **Requires renal dose adjustment.**
  Safety
- ADRs: similar ADRs to all beta-lactam antibiotics. Hyperkalemia may occur with penicillin G potassium. In this instance, it may be appropriate to utilize penicillin G sodium.
- Contraindications: hypersensitivity to penicillins.
- Drug interactions: no significant drug interactions.
- Monitoring: serum creatinine (SCr), serum electrolytes, complete blood count (CBC); skin for rash/hypersensitivity reactions.

> **CLINICAL PEARLS**
> - The short half-life of natural penicillins mandates frequent dosing or dosing via continuous infusion.
> - IV and IM formulations of penicillin are not interchangeable. IM formulations administered intravenously have been associated with cardiopulmonary arrest and death.

Antistaphylococcal Penicillins
Agents
- Nafcillin.
- Oxacillin.
- Dicloxacillin.
- Flucloxacillin.
  Spectrum
- These penicillins are stable against narrow-spectrum penicillinases.
- Their spectrum is broadened to **include methicillin-susceptible staphylococcal species.**

TABLE 5.1	Basic Mechanisms of Antibiotic Action
Antibiotic Class	**Action**
Disruption of Cell Wall	

β-Lactams
  Penicillins
  Cephalosporins
  Cephamycins
  Carbapenems
  Monobactams
	Bind penicillin binding proteins, enzymes responsible for peptidoglycan synthesis

β-lactamase inhibitors	Bind β-lactamases and prevent enzymatic inactivation of β-lactam
Glycopeptides	Inhibit cross-linkage of peptidoglycan layers
Lipoglycopeptides	Inhibit cross-linkage of peptidoglycan layers and cause disruption of cell membrane potential
Cyclic lipopeptides	Cause depolarization of cytoplasmic membrane, resulting in disruption of ionic concentration gradients
Polymyxins	Inhibit bacterial membranes
Fosfomycin	Inactivates pyruvyl transferase
Inhibition of Protein Synthesis	
Aminoglycosides	Produce premature release of peptide chains from 30S ribosome
Tetracyclines	Prevent polypeptide elongation at 30S ribosome
Glycylcyclines	Bind to 30S ribosome and prevent initiation of protein synthesis
Oxazolidinones	Prevent initiation of protein synthesis at 50S ribosome
MLS Macrolides Clindamycin Streptogramins	Prevent polypeptide elongation at 50S ribosome
Nitrofurans	Reactive intermediates interfere with bacterial ribosomes
Chloramphenicol	Inhibits peptidyl transferase activity in the 50S ribosomal subunit, preventing chain elongation
Inhibition of Nucleic Acid Synthesis	
Fluoroquinolones	Bind α subunit of DNA gyrase
Nitroimidazoles	Disrupt bacteria DNA (cytotoxic compounds produced by reduction of nitro group)
Antimetabolite	
Folate antagonists	Inhibit dihydrofolate reductase and dihydropteroate synthase and disrupt folic acid synthesis

Modified from Murray PR, Rosenthal KS, Pfaller MA. Antibacterial agents. In: *Medical Microbiology*. 8th ed. Elsevier; 2016.

- Agents in this group do not have gram-negative or anaerobic coverage (with the exception of *Peptostreptococcus* spp.).
  Clinical Uses
- **Drug of choice for MSSA infections.**
  Dosing/TDM
- Nafcillin IV 1–2 g every 4 hours.
- Oxacillin IV 1–2 g every 4 hours.
- Dicloxacillin PO 125–500 mg every 6 hours.
- Flucloxacillin PO 500 mg every 6 hours; IV 1–2 g every 4–6 hours.

- No dose adjustments for renal impairment.
- Consider dose reduction in hepatic impairment when using nafcillin or oxacillin.
  Safety
- ADRs: similar ADRs to other beta-lactam antibiotics. **Drug-induced hepatitis** may be more common with oxacillin and flucloxacillin. **Neutropenia** and phlebitis may be more common with nafcillin.
- Contraindications: hypersensitivity.
- Drug interactions: no significant drug interactions.

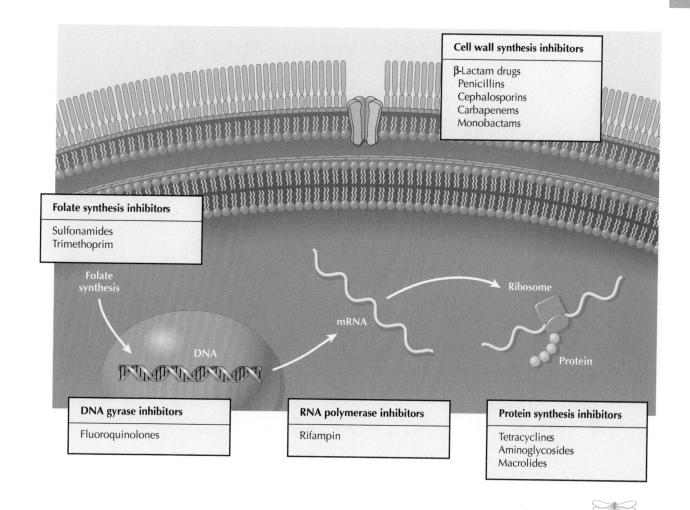

• **Fig. 5.1** Antibiotic sites of action. (From Raffa RB, Rawls SM, Beyzarov EP. Drugs used in infectious disease. In: *Netter's Illustrated Pharmacology.* Updated ed. Elsevier; 2014.)

- Monitoring: SCr, LFTs, serum electrolytes, CBC; skin for rash/hypersensitivity reactions.

CLINICAL PEARLS

- **Antistaphylococcal beta-lactams** are more effective for treatment of MSSA infections than vancomycin and are considered the **drugs of choice** for such infections.
- If ADRs occur with nafcillin or oxacillin, cefazolin is an effective alternative for treating MSSA infections (except meningitis).

Aminopenicillins
Agents
- Amoxicillin.
- Ampicillin.
Spectrum
- Good streptococcal coverage (including beta-hemolytic and *S. pneumoniae*).
- Weak staphylococcal coverage as most staphylococci produce a penicillinase.
- **These agents are active against susceptible strains of enterococci.**
- Aminopenicillins have some gram-negative activity; however, they should only be used based on susceptibility testing.

Clinical Uses. Amoxicillin is the **drug of choice for acute otitis media** and streptococcal pharyngitis. Ampicillin is recommended for ***Listeria monocytogenes*** infections. When treating enterococcal infections, should be combined with an aminoglycoside for bactericidal activity.
Dosing/TDM
- Amoxicillin PO/IV 250–1000 mg every 8–12 hours.
- Ampicillin IV 8–12 g/day divided every 3–6 hours or as a continuous infusion.
- Require renal dose adjustment.
Safety
- ADRs: similar ADRs to all beta-lactam antibiotics.
- Contraindications: hypersensitivity.
- Drug interactions: no significant drug interactions.
- Monitoring: SCr, serum electrolytes, CBC; skin for rash/hypersensitivity reactions.

CLINICAL PEARLS

- Ampicillin is also available PO (usual dose 250–500 mg every 6 hours); however, it has poor bioavailability. When considering switching from IV ampicillin to oral options, PO amoxicillin is preferred due to higher bioavailability, better tolerability, and less frequent administration.

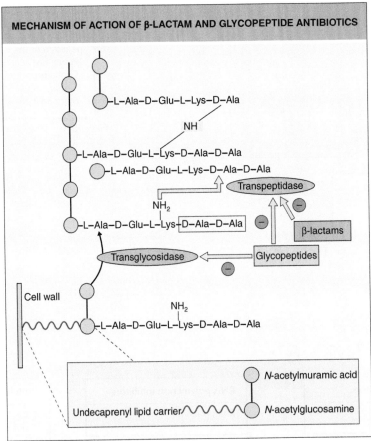

• **Fig. 5.2** Mechanism of action of β-lactam and glycopeptide antibiotics. (From Carley AC, Stratman EJ, Lesher JL, McConnell RC. Antimicrobial drugs. In: Bolognia JL, Schaffer JV, Cerroni L, eds. *Dermatology.* 4th ed. Elsevier; 2018.)

CLINICAL PEARLS—cont'd

• IV ampicillin is only stable for 3 days under refrigerated conditions once mixed. As a result, it is not an ideal drug for outpatient administration.
• The combination of ampicillin 2 g IV every 4 hours and ceftriaxone 2 g IV every 12 hours is effectively used for treatment of endocarditis caused by ampicillin-susceptible enterococci.

Penicillin/Beta-lactamase Inhibitor Combinations

Agents
• Amoxicillin/clavulanate.
• Ampicillin/sulbactam.
• Piperacillin/tazobactam.

Spectrum
• The addition of beta-lactamase inhibitors to these penicillins allows for **broader gram-negative and anaerobic coverage.**
• Amoxicillin/clavulanate, ampicillin/sulbactam: similar spectrum to aminopenicillins, with the addition of **MSSA, enteric gram-negative rods (GNRs),** and anaerobes. The beta-lactamase inhibitor restores activity against MSSA, inhibiting the penicillinase that would otherwise render the penicillin inactive.
• Piperacillin/tazobactam: the broadest spectrum of the penicillins, piperacillin has improved gram-negative coverage, including *Pseudomonas aeruginosa*, as well as *Enterococcus* spp. and anaerobes. The addition of tazobactam provides protection from beta-lactamases, further expanding coverage of anaerobes, GNRs, staphylococci, and enterococci that produce such enzymes.

Mechanism of Action
• These beta-lactamase inhibitors are structurally similar to beta-lactam antibiotics. When co-administered, the beta-lactamase inhibitor binds to beta-lactamase, allowing for the penicillins to be therapeutically active against a wider range of organisms.

Clinical Uses
• Good for **empiric coverage of mixed aerobic and anaerobic infections,** such as intraabdominal infections or diabetic foot infections.
• Aminopenicillin-based combinations: upper and lower **community** respiratory tract infections, urinary tract infections (UTI).
• Piperacillin/tazobactam: empiric therapy for **nosocomial infections,** including nosocomial pneumonia.
• Amoxicillin/clavulanate: first-line **prophylactic antibiotic for dog and cat bites** (especially if cat bite, puncture wound, wound to hand or in immunosuppressed patients).

Dosing/TDM
• Amoxicillin/clavulanate PO 500–125 mg TID or 875–125 mg BID.
• Ampicillin/sulbactam IV 1.5–3 g every 6 hours.

- Piperacillin/tazobactam IV 3.375 g every 6 hours or 4.5 g every 6–8 hours.
- Require renal dose adjustment.

Safety
- ADRs: similar ADRs to all beta-lactam antibiotics.
  - Amoxicillin/clavulanate is associated with **diarrhea.** This is mainly **due to the clavulanate** component, the dose of which is limited to 125 mg in all PO formulations.
  - Aminopenicillin combinations: although rare, **hepatotoxicity** has been reported. Liver function should be monitored in patients with hepatic impairment.
- Contraindications: hypersensitivity.
- Drug interactions
  - Higher rates of acute kidney injury (AKI) have been observed when piperacillin/tazobactam is administered concurrently with vancomycin.
  - Monitoring: SCr, serum electrolytes, LFTs, CBC; skin for hypersensitivity reactions.

CLINICAL PEARLS
- Ampicillin stability issues also apply to use of ampicillin/sulbactam in the outpatient setting.
- Sulbactam alone provides coverage against some *Acinetobacter* spp., and the combination of ampicillin/sulbactam may be used in high doses to treat Acinetobacter infections.
- The beta-lactamase inhibitors in these combination products do not protect against all types of beta-lactamases. Notably, they have poor activity against extended-spectrum beta-lactamase (ESBL) and AmpC beta-lactamase-producing gram-negatives.

Cephalosporins

Cephalosporins are mostly grouped into generations (1 through 4), which are characterized by their spectrum of activity. From generations 1 to 4, gram-negative activity increases with generation, while gram-positive activity (particularly against staphylococci) does not increase. See specific information in each of the generations below regarding coverage and activity. Of note, **cephalosporins do not have activity against enterococci or MRSA (except for ceftaroline).**

First-Generation Cephalosporins
Agents
- Cefazolin.
- Cephalexin.
- Cefadroxil.

Spectrum
- **Good for MSSA and streptococci** with **some enteric GNR** activity. The least gram-negative spectrum of the cephalosporins. **Poor anaerobic activity.** As with other cephalosporins, no enterococcal or MRSA coverage.

Clinical Uses
- Cefazolin is considered equivalent to nafcillin or oxacillin for invasive MSSA infections, except for meningitis.

- Acute bacterial skin and skin structure infections (ABSSSI), MSSA infections, and prophylaxis to prevent surgical site infections.
- Lower UTIs, especially in pregnancy.

Dosing/TDM
- Cefazolin IV 1–2 g every 8 hours.
- Cephalexin PO 250–1000 mg every 6 hours.
- Cefadroxil PO 500 mg every 12 hours.
- Require renal adjustment.

Safety
- ADRs: similar to all beta-lactam antibiotics.
- Contraindications: hypersensitivity.
- Drug interactions: no significant drug interactions.
- Monitoring: SCr, electrolyte abnormalities, CBC; skin for hypersensitivity rash.

CLINICAL PEARLS
- Cefazolin is a therapy of choice for MSSA infections (except meningitis).
- These medications do not cross the blood–brain barrier and should not be used for CNS infections.
- Cefazolin can be conveniently dosed for patients receiving hemodialysis after dialysis on dialysis days, making this a useful option for patients with MSSA bacteremia. Recommended dosing is 2 g if next dialysis expected in 48 hours and 3 g if next dialysis is expected in 72 hours.

Second-Generation Cephalosporins
Agents
- Cefuroxime.
- Cefprozil.
- Cefoxitin.
- Cefotetan.

Spectrum
- Broader gram-negative coverage versus first-generation cephalosporins with moderate gram-positive coverage. Stable to beta-lactamases produced by *Haemophilus influenzae* and *Neisseria gonorrhoeae*. As with other cephalosporins, no enterococcal or MRSA coverage.
- Cefoxitin and cefotetan are classified as **cephamycins** and have anaerobic activity. Can be used for abdominal infections or abdominal surgical prophylaxis. However, there are concerns for increasing rates of *Bacteroides fragilis* resistance, warranting caution if used for treatment of abdominal infections.

Clinical Uses
- Upper respiratory tract infections, community-acquired pneumonia (CAP), gynecologic infections, abdominal surgical prophylaxis (cephamycins).

Dosing/TDM
- Cefotetan IV 1–2 g every 12 hours.
- Cefoxitin IV 1–2 g every 6–8 hours.
- Cefuroxime IV 750–1500 mg every 8–12 hours; PO 250–500 mg every 12 hours.
- Cefprozil PO 500 mg every 12 hours.
- Require renal dose adjustment.

Safety

- ADRs: similar to all beta-lactam antibiotics.
  - **Cefotetan may cause a disulfiram-like reaction** if administered concurrently with alcohol; also may prolong bleeding via vitamin K production inhibition.
- Contraindications: hypersensitivity.
- Drug interactions: no significant drug interactions.
- Monitoring: SCr, LFTs, CBC; skin for hypersensitivity rash.

CLINICAL PEARLS

- Unlike other second-generation cephalosporins, the cephamycins (cefoxitin, cefotetan) are stable to ESBLs *in vitro*. Exercise caution if considering these agents to treat infections due to ESBL-producing organisms as clinical experience is limited.
- Similar to first-generation cephalosporins, second-generation cephalosporins do not readily cross the blood–brain barrier and should not be used for CNS infections.

Third-Generation Cephalosporins

Agents

- Ceftriaxone.
- Cefotaxime.
- Ceftazidime.
- Cefdinir.
- Cefpodoxime.
- Cefixime.

Spectrum

- Broader gram-negative activity (enteric GNRs) vs. first- and second-generation agents. **Generally retain activity against streptococci and MSSA (except for ceftazidime).** Ceftazidime has activity against *P. aeruginosa*.

Clinical Uses

- Lower respiratory tract infections, pyelonephritis, meningitis, gonorrhea, nosocomial infections (ceftazidime), intraabdominal infections (in combination with metronidazole), ABSSSI.

Dosing/TDM

- Cefotaxime IV 1–2 g every 8 hours; IV 2 g every 4 hours for meningitis.
- Ceftriaxone IV 1–2 g every 24 hours; IV 2 g every 12 hours for meningitis; IM 250 mg × 1 dose for gonorrhea.
  - Consider using higher doses of 2–4 g daily for invasive MSSA (methicillin-susceptible *Staphylococcus aureus*) infections.
- Ceftazidime IV 1–2 g every 8 hours.
- Cefdinir PO 300 mg every 12 hours.
- Cefpodoxime PO 100–200 mg every 12 hours.
- Cefixime PO 400 mg daily divided every 12–24 hours.
- Require renal dose adjustment (except for ceftriaxone).

Safety

- ADRs: similar to all other beta-lactam antibiotics.
  - Ceftriaxone: may cause **biliary sludging** leading to hyperbilirubinemia.
  - **Ceftazidime: neurotoxicity** has been reported; patients with renal impairment may be at increased risk.
- Contraindications: hypersensitivity; neonates (ceftriaxone).
- Drug interactions
  - Ceftriaxone can form precipitates with calcium-containing IV medications/solutions in the lungs and kidneys in neonates.
  - Cefdinir: iron salts may decrease serum concentrations by forming insoluble iron–cefdinir complexes; red-appearing, nonbloody stools may develop as a result.
- Monitoring: SCr, LFTs, CBC; skin for hypersensitivity reactions.

CLINICAL PEARLS

- Some third-generation cephalosporins (ceftriaxone, cefotaxime, and ceftazidime) are able to cross the blood–brain barrier, proving them useful in CNS infections.
- Although ceftriaxone does not have appreciable enterococcal activity, the synergistic combination of ampicillin 2 g IV every 4 hours and ceftriaxone 2 g IV every 12 hours is effectively used for treatment of endocarditis caused by ampicillin-susceptible enterococci.
- These agents are not active against AmpC beta-lactamase-producing organisms and have only variable activity against ESBLs.

Fourth-Generation Cephalosporins

Agents

- Cefepime.

Spectrum

- Broad gram-negative coverage, including *P. aeruginosa*; gram-positive spectrum is similar to that of first-generation cephalosporins. **Stable against AmpC** beta-lactamases but not reliable against ESBLs. No anaerobic activity.

Clinical uses

- Nosocomial infections; pneumonia, meningitis, febrile neutropenia.

Dosing/TDM

- Cefepime IV 1–2 g every 8–12 hours; IV 2 g every 8 hours for meningitis or pseudomonal infections.
- Requires renal dose adjustment.

Safety

- ADRs: similar to all other beta-lactams.
  - **Neurotoxicity** has been reported. Elderly patients and those receiving high doses with impaired renal function are at increased risk.
- Contraindications: hypersensitivity.
- Drug interactions: no significant drug interactions.
- Monitoring: SCr, electrolytes, CBC; mental status; skin for hypersensitivity reactions.

CLINICAL PEARLS

- Cefepime is primarily used as empiric therapy for nosocomial infections. When possible, consider de-escalation to narrower-spectrum agents when treating community-acquired infections or when cultures and susceptibilities reveal more susceptible pathogens.
- Like the third-generation cephalosporins, cefepime readily crosses the blood–brain barrier and can be used to treat CNS infections.

Anti-MRSA Cephalosporins

Agents

- Ceftaroline.

Spectrum

- Similar gram-negative activity to third-generation cephalosporins, with expanded gram-positive coverage to **include MRSA.** Good activity against streptococci. **No activity against organisms that produce AmpC beta-lactamases or ESBLs, *P. aeruginosa*, enterococci, or anaerobes.**

Clinical Uses

- FDA-approved for ABSSSI and CAP.

Dosing/TDM

- Ceftaroline IV 600 mg every 12 hours.
  - Off-label dosing of 600 mg every 8 hours is commonly used for invasive MRSA infections, such as MRSA bacteremia and endocarditis.
- Requires renal dose adjustment.

Safety

- ADRs: similar to all other beta-lactams.
  - **Neutropenia** has been noted with longer courses of therapy (> 21 days).
- Contraindications: hypersensitivity.
- Drug interactions: no significant drug interactions.
- Monitoring: SCr, electrolytes, CBC; skin for hypersensitivity.

CLINICAL PEARLS

- Ceftaroline is active against MRSA because it is able to bind to penicillin-binding protein 2a, unlike most other beta-lactams.
- Ceftaroline is classified as a cephalosporin with anti-MRSA activity.
- Because of its MRSA activity, ceftaroline has been utilized to treat invasive infections, such as bacteremia, endocarditis, osteomyelitis, and hospital-acquired pneumonia in the setting of treatment failure and/or drug-resistant pathogens.

Cephalosporin/Beta-lactamase Inhibitor Combinations

Agents

- Ceftolozane/tazobactam.
- Ceftazidime/avibactam.

Spectrum

- Broad gram-negative coverage, including *P. aeruginosa.* Both ceftazidime and ceftolozane are third-generation cephalosporins with antipseudomonal activity and poor gram-positive and anaerobic activity.
- Ceftolozane was developed to target multi-drug-resistant *P. aeruginosa*, and the addition of tazobactam protects against some beta-lactamases.

- **Avibactam** is a **novel beta-lactamase inhibitor,** structurally unrelated to beta-lactams, and **inhibits ESBLs.** It is **also active against many carbapenemases, except metallo-beta-lactamases (MBLs).** Ceftazidime/avibactam has broader Enterobacteriaceae activity versus ceftolozane/tazobactam due to expanded beta-lactamase inhibitory activity.

Clinical Uses

- Multi-drug resistant *psuedomonal* infections, ESBL-producing organisms (especially ceftazidime–avibactam), complicated intraabdominal infections, complicated UTIs.
- Ceftazidime/avibactam is also useful against *Klebsiella pneumoniae* carbapenemase (KPC)-producing carbapenem-resistant Enterobacteriaceae (CRE) infections.

Dosing/TDM

- Ceftolozane/tazobactam IV 1.5 g every 8 hours.
- Ceftazidime/avibactam IV 2.5 g every 8 hours.

Safety

- ADRs: similar to all other beta-lactam antibiotics.
  - Ceftazidime/avibactam: see third-generation cephalosporins.
- Contraindications: hypersensitivity.
- Drug interactions: no significant drug interactions.
- Monitoring: SCr, electrolytes, CBC; skin for hypersensitivity reactions.

CLINICAL PEARLS

- If using for an intraabdominal infection, metronidazole needs to be added for anaerobic coverage. Neither of these agents retain reliable coverage of abdominal anaerobes.
- Confirm susceptibility with the microbiology lab, as resistance may occur.

Carbapenems

Agents

- Ertapenem.
- Meropenem.
- Imipenem/cilastatin.
- Doripenem.

Spectrum

- Broadest gram-negative coverage. Activity against MSSA, streptococci, *P. aeruginosa* (except for ertapenem), *Acinetobacter* spp. (except for ertapenem), AmpC beta-lactamase producing and ESBL-producing Enterobacteriaceae, and anaerobes. Moderate enterococcal activity (except for ertapenem).

Clinical Uses

- Nosocomial infections (not ertapenem if concerned for *P. aeruginosa*), infections due to ESBL-producing organisms, intraabdominal infections, mixed aerobic/anaerobic infections, meningitis (meropenem).

Dosing/TDM

- Ertapenem IV 1 g every 24 hours.
- Meropenem IV 500–2000 mg every 8 hours.
- Imipenem/cilastatin IV 500–1000 mg every 6–8 hours.
- Doripenem IV 500 mg every 8 hours.
- Require renal adjustment.

Safety

- ADRs: similar to all beta-lactam antibiotics.
- Increased risk of seizures; highest with imipenem. May mitigate by appropriate renal dosing and avoiding in patients at high risk for seizures.
- Contraindications: hypersensitivity.
- Drug interactions: may decrease serum concentrations of **valproic acid**; consider alternate therapy as carbapenems may also lower seizure threshold.
- Monitoring: SCr, LFTs, CBC; skin for hypersensitivity reactions.

CLINICAL PEARLS

- Cilastatin is not a beta-lactamase inhibitor but is co-administered with imipenem to **prevent the metabolism of imipenem to a nephrotoxic moiety in the kidneys.**
- Ertapenem is suitable for ESBL infections but not for nosocomial infections where *pseudomonal* coverage is warranted.

Carbapenem/Beta-lactamase Inhibitor Combinations

Agents

- Meropenem/vaborbactam

Spectrum

- See carbapenem section on spectrum. Vaborbactam is a beta-lactamase inhibitor that protects against carbapenemases (**except for MBL**), allowing meropenem to be **active against KPC-producing CRE.**

Clinical Uses

- FDA-approved for complicated UTIs.

Dosing/TDM

- Meropenem/vaborbactam IV 4 g every 8 hours.
- Requires renal adjustment.

Safety

- See carbapenems.

CLINICAL PEARLS

- Meropenem/vaborbactam is best used as a treatment option for documented or suspected infections caused by KPC-producing Enterobacteriaceae, especially when broad additional coverage is also required.

Monobactams

Agents

- Aztreonam (monocyclic beta-lactam antibiotic).

Spectrum

- Activity against *P. aeruginosa* and most GNRs. No appreciable gram-positive or anaerobic activity.

Clinical Uses

- Nosocomial infections in patients with serious beta-lactam allergies.

Dosing/TDM

- Aztreonam IV 1–2 g every 8 hours.
- Requires renal adjustment.

Safety

- ADRs: similar to beta-lactam antibiotics.

- Contraindications: hypersensitivity (see clinical pearls below).
- Drug interactions: no significant drug interactions.
- Monitoring: SCr, LFTs, CBC; skin for hypersensitivity reactions.

CLINICAL PEARLS

- Safe to administer in, and best reserved for, patients with severe beta-lactam allergies. However, if the patient experienced an anaphylactoid reaction to ceftazidime, aztreonam should be avoided, as these agents share the same side chain.
- An inhalational formulation exists for cystic fibrosis patients.

Glycopeptides

Agents

- Vancomycin.
- Teicoplanin

Mechanism of Action

- Prevents crosslinking of peptidoglycan in bacterial cell walls by mimicking terminal D-alanine-D-alanine pentapeptide chains.

Spectrum

- Good for **gram-positive infections:** staphylococci (MSSA and MRSA), streptococci, and enterococci (*E. faecalis* > *E. faecium*). **No gram-negative activity.** Some anaerobic activity against gram-positive anaerobes like *Clostridioides difficile* and *Cutibacterium acnes.*

Clinical Uses

- **Drug of choice for MRSA** infections and empiric treatment for nosocomial infections (IV).
- *C. difficile*-associated diarrhea (PO or PR **only**).
- Surgical prophylaxis in MRSA carriers/implant surgery.
- Peritonitis associated with peritoneal dialysis.

Dosing/TDM

- Vancomycin IV 15–20 mg/kg every 8–12 hours.
  - Requires renal dose adjustment.
- Teicoplanin IV 6–12 mg/kg every 12 hours for 3 doses, then daily.

Therapeutic Drug Monitoring

- Vancomycin
  - Troughs are measured to help **ensure efficacy** (high enough concentrations throughout the dosing interval) as well as to **monitor for toxicity** as higher troughs have been associated with nephrotoxicity (see below).
  - **Trough goals for invasive infections: 15–20 µg/mL.**
  - All troughs should be >10 µg/mL; troughs lower than this may promote resistance and lead to decreased effectiveness.
  - Troughs should be drawn 30 min prior to the next scheduled infusion when the drug concentration is at steady state (after 3–4 doses).
- Teicoplanin
  - Only necessary if prolonged treatment course likely.

- Aim trough ≥20 mg/L but <60 mg/L (>30 mg/L if endocarditis).
- 1st order kinetics, so 50% dose reduction will give 50% reduction in levels.
- Change by increments of 200 mg.
- Vancomycin **PO** 125 or 500 mg every 6 hours (**C. difficile infections only**).

Safety
- ADRs
  - **Nephrotoxicity**: vancomycin-induced nephrotoxicity has been associated with higher troughs and prolonged treatment duration. Caution when using with other nephrotoxic agents. Concurrent administration with piperacillin/tazobactam may also increase risk of acute kidney injury (AKI).
  - Teicoplanin is associated with a lower incidence of nephrotoxicity than vancomycin.
  - Infusion reactions: **red man syndrome** is a **histamine-mediated reaction** related to infusion rate. Patients may become flushed (mainly on trunk and arms), feel warm, and may experience hypotension. Slowing the infusion rate and/or premedicating with diphenhydramine can prevent this effect.
  - Ototoxicity: historically reported with vancomycin and potential association with very high vancomycin levels. Evidence does not clearly support the link between this toxicity and vancomycin use.
- Contraindications: hypersensitivity.
- Drug interactions
  - Caution with use of other nephrotoxic medications.
- Monitoring: SCr, CBC, vancomycin troughs; infusion reactions.

CLINICAL PEARLS

- While vancomycin is active against MSSA, it kills these organisms at a slower rate than antistaphylococcal beta-lactams (nafcillin, oxacillin, cefazolin). If targeting MSSA, an antistaphylococcal beta-lactam is preferred.
- Against staphylococci, a vancomycin MIC of ≤2 mg/L is considered susceptible; however, it may be prudent for patients with serious infections caused by staphylococci with a vancomycin MIC of 2 mg/L to be treated with alternate agents. It has been observed that infections caused by such isolates may have worse outcomes versus those caused by strains having lower vancomycin MICs.
- Timing vancomycin troughs is very important. Before adjusting a vancomycin dose, ensure that the patient has received 3–4 doses and that the trough concentration was drawn on time.
- Oral vancomycin does not have appreciable systemic absorption; however, it achieves very high gut concentrations. Systemic vancomycin will not adequately penetrate the gut. In treating C. difficile-associated diarrhea, vancomycin is given orally or per rectum via enema if the patient has limited gut motility.

Lipoglycopeptides

Agents
- Telavancin.
- Oritavancin.
- Dalbavancin.

Mechanism of Action
- Prevent crosslinking of peptidoglycan in bacterial cell walls by mimicking terminal D-alanine-D-alanine pentapeptide chains. Additionally, lipoglycopeptides disrupt cell membrane potential and alter cell permeability; bactericidal.

Spectrum
- Similar to vancomycin.

Clinical Uses
- ABSSSI and pneumonia (telavancin only).

Dosing/TDM
- Telavancin IV 10 mg/kg every 24 hours.
  - Requires renal dose adjustment.
- Oritavancin IV 1200 mg as a single dose infused over 3 hours.
  - Not studied in creatinine clearance (CrCl) <30 mL/min.
- Dalbavancin IV 1000 mg on day 1 and 500 mg 1 week later OR 1500 mg as a single dose; infuse over 30 minutes.
  - Requires renal dose adjustment.

Safety
- ADRs
  - Telavancin: new onset or worsening **nephrotoxicity; QTc prolongation; taste disturbances**; foamy urine.
  - Long-acting lipoglycopeptides (dalbavancin, oritavancin): nausea, vomiting, diarrhea, and rash reported in clinical trials; infusion reactions (similar to red man syndrome).
  - Oritavancin: cases of osteomyelitis occurrence were reported in clinical trials.
- Contraindications
  - Telavancin
    - Caution in patients with impaired renal function at baseline (CrCl <50) as higher mortality rates have been observed versus vancomycin for treatment of nosocomial pneumonia.
    - **Pregnancy**: patients should have a **negative serum pregnancy test prior to initiating therapy**. Adverse developmental outcomes observed in animal studies. Only use if benefit outweighs the risk.
- Drug interactions
  - Telavancin
    - **May interfere with coagulation testing (aPTT, PT, INR), but *not* anticoagulation medications.** If alternate anticoagulation cannot be utilized, coagulation testing should be timed with telavancin trough concentrations.
    - Increased risk of QT prolongation when given concomitantly with other QTc- prolonging medications

- Oritavancin
  - **Inhibits warfarin metabolism** (increased risk of bleeding); also interferes with PT (24 hours) and aPTT (48 hours) testing: avoid warfarin and heparin during those time periods, respectively.
- Monitoring: SCr, LFTs (long-acting agents) CBC; serum pregnancy test (telavancin); infusion reactions.

CLINICAL PEARLS

- Lipoglycopeptides were developed by modifying the structure of vancomycin and are structurally related to vancomycin. If a patient has a true allergy to vancomycin, these medications may have **cross-reactivity.**
- Oritavancin and dalbavancin
  - Structurally altered to slow elimination; the reason why they are considered **long-acting** lipoglycopeptides.
  - Potential treatment options for patients where compliance may be an issue.
  - Currently only FDA-approved for the treatment of ABSSSI, but their use for more invasive infections (MRSA bacteremia, endocarditis, and osteomyelitis) is being explored.
  - Telavancin has faster bactericidal killing versus vancomycin; may be useful in patients not responding to other MRSA treatments.

Cyclic Lipopeptides

Agents
- Daptomycin.

Mechanism of Action
- **Binds to cell membrane** of gram-positive bacteria causing rapid depolarization due to leakage of intracellular ions resulting in cell death (Fig. 5.3); **bactericidal.**

Spectrum
- Broad gram-positive activity (**MSSA, MRSA, streptococci, and enterococci**). Poor gram-negative and anaerobic activity.

Clinical Uses
- ABSSSI caused by resistant gram-positive organisms; staphylococcal bacteremia or endocarditis; can be used for enterococcal endocarditis.

Dosing/TDM
- Daptomycin IV 4–8 mg/kg every 24 hours.
  - Higher doses of up to 10–12 mg/kg may be appropriate for more invasive and/or resistant infections.
- Requires renal dose adjustment.

Safety
- ADRs
  - **Myopathy/rhabdomyolysis** (risk may be enhanced with concomitant administration of HMG-CoA reductase inhibitors).
  - Eosinophilic pneumonia.
- Contraindications: hypersensitivity.
- Drug interactions
  - **Statins**: may **increase risk of skeletal muscle toxicity**; may consider holding these medications with concomitant daptomycin.

- Monitoring: SCr, CK, muscle pain/weakness.

CLINICAL PEARLS

- Daptomycin is **inactivated by pulmonary surfactant and should not be used to treat pneumonia.**
- Caution in patients with MRSA infection and vancomycin treatment failures, as some isolates with increased vancomycin MICs may also be daptomycin nonsusceptible.
- Synergism with daptomycin and some beta-lactams is being investigated as salvage therapy for some recalcitrant infections.

Polymyxins

Agents
- Colistin (colistimethate).
- Polymyxin B.

Mechanism of Action
- Act as a detergent, binding to and damaging gram-negative bacterial cell membranes resulting in leakage of cellular contents and cell death; bactericidal.

Spectrum
- Gram-negative organisms, including multidrug-resistant *P. aeruginosa*, *Acinetobacter* spp., and *Klebsiella* spp.
- No activity against gram-positive organisms.
- Notable gaps in gram-negative coverage: *Proteus* spp., *Providencia* spp., *Burkholderia* spp., *Serratia* spp., and gram-negative cocci (e.g., *Neisseria* spp.).

Clinical Uses
- Usually **drugs of last resort** for multidrug-resistant gram-negative pathogens.

Dosing/TDM
- Colistin IV 5 mg/kg daily in 2 doses (colistin base activity); dose is based on ideal body weight.
- Requires renal dose adjustment.
- Polymyxin B IV 15,000–25,000 units/kg daily divided in 2 doses.

Safety
- ADRs
  - **Nephrotoxicity: dose-dependent acute renal failure** has been reported. Polymyxin B is thought to be less nephrotoxic versus colistin.
  - **Neurotoxicity**: rare, but may manifest as dizziness, weakness, altered mental status, or paresthesias (especially of the mouth and face). Neuromuscular blockade and fatal respiratory arrest have also been reported.
- Contraindications: hypersensitivity.
- Drug interactions: caution with use of other nephrotoxic medications.
- Monitoring: BUN, SCr; mental status; urine output.

CLINICAL PEARLS

- Because these are **typically last-line agents,** they are often used in combination with other medications. Data suggest that they may be more effective in combination versus monotherapy

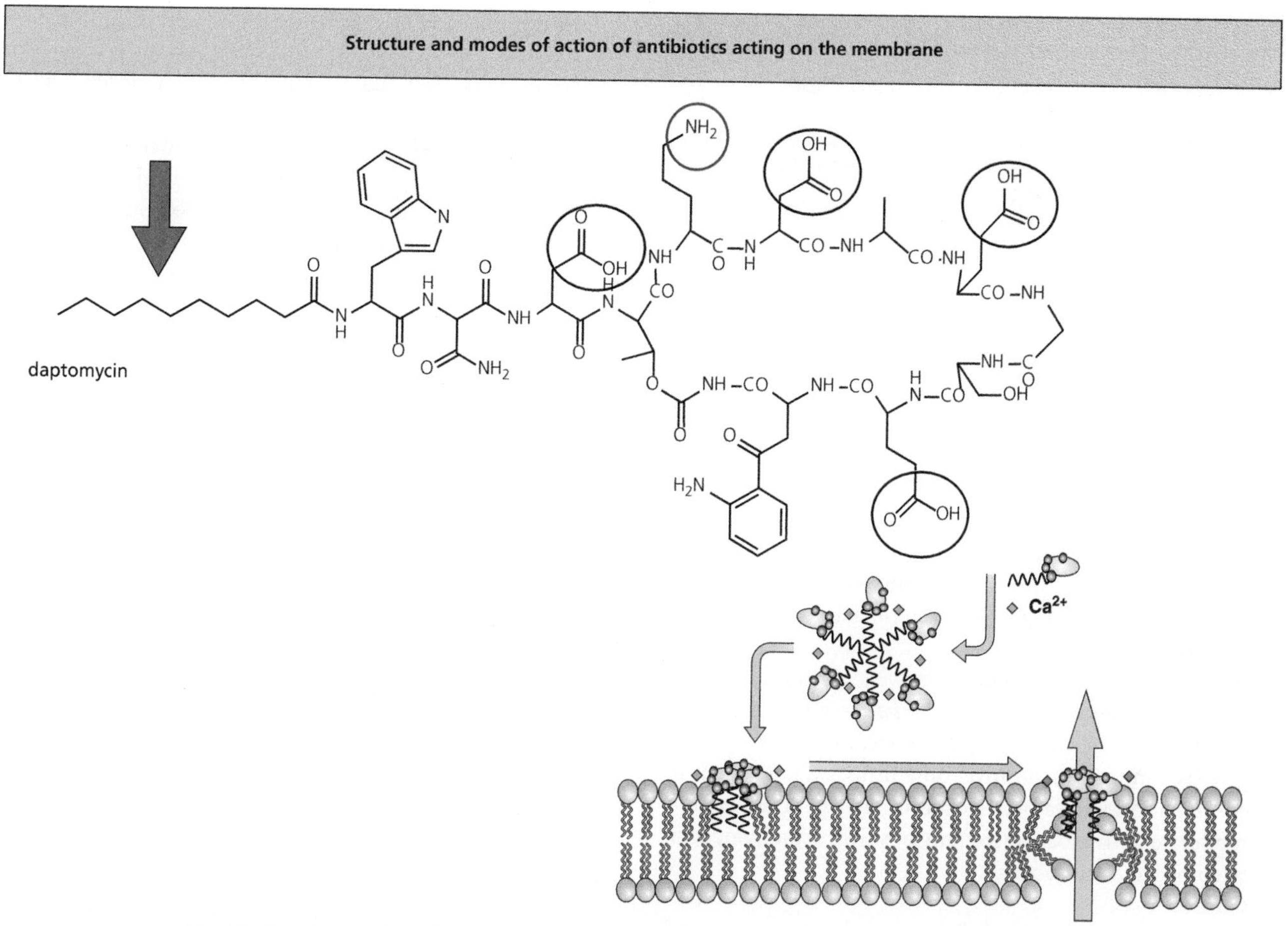

Structure and modes of action of antibiotics acting on the membrane

• **Fig. 5.3** Structure and mechanism of action of daptomycin. (From Van Bambeke F, Glupczynski Y, Mingeot-Leclercq M-P, Tulkens PM. Mechanisms of Action. In: Cohen J, Powderly W, Opal S., eds. *Infectious Diseases*. 3rd ed. Elsevier; 2010.)

CLINICAL PEARLS—cont'd

- Colistin
  - Colistin is a prodrug of the parent compound, colistimethate sodium. Only about 30% of colistimethate is hydrolyzed to colistin after renal elimination. In the United States, it is dosed based in mg of colistin base activity, an estimation of active colistin (400 mg colistimethate = 150 mg colistin base activity).
  - Colistin dosing standards differ by country. The United States doses in mg of colistin base activity. Europe (and most of the rest of the world) doses in international units.
    - 1 mg colistin base activity = 2.7 mg colistimethate = 30,000 units.
    - 1000 units = 80 mg colistimethate = 30 mg colistin base activity.
- Polymyxin B
  - Not eliminated by the kidneys and therefore likely not effective for UTIs. Newer data suggest that adjustment for renal function may not be necessary.
  - Polymyxin B is dosed in mg or international units.
  - 1 mg = 10,000 units.
- Inhaled polymyxins may be utilized to reduce gram-negative colonization, especially in **cystic fibrosis patients.**

Fosfomycin

Mechanism of Action
- Inhibits bacterial cell wall synthesis by inactivating pyruvyl transferase, an enzyme necessary for production of peptidoglycan; bactericidal.

Spectrum
- Good activity against *E. coli, P. aeruginosa, Serratia* spp., *Proteus* spp., *Klebsiella* spp., *Citrobacter* spp., enterococci.
- Poor activity against streptococci and anaerobes.

Clinical Uses
- Uncomplicated cystitis.

Dosing/TDM
- Fosfomycin PO 3 g once.

Safety
- ADRs
  - GI (nausea, vomiting).
- Contraindications: hypersensitivity.
- Drug interactions: no significant drug interactions.
- Monitoring: SCr.

CLINICAL PEARLS

- Only indicated for **uncomplicated UTIs** as bactericidal concentrations are not attained outside of the lower urinary tract; should not be used for pyelonephritis or UTI with sepsis.

CLINICAL PEARLS—cont'd

- Fosfomycin remains active against many ESBL-producing organisms.
- An IV formulation is available for use in some countries against severe gram-negative infections but is not yet available in the United States.

Protein Synthesis Inhibitors

Aminoglycosides

Agents
- Gentamicin.
- Tobramycin.
- Amikacin.
- Streptomycin.

Mechanism of Action
- Inhibit protein synthesis by binding to the bacterial 30S ribosome subunit (Fig. 5.4); bactericidal.

Spectrum
- Active against most gram-negatives, including enteric GNRs, *psuedomonal*, and *Acinetobacter* spp. Poor activity against anaerobes, atypical respiratory tract pathogenesis, and gram-positive organisms. When used in combination with a beta-lactam or glycopeptide, exhibit moderate activity against gram-positives (staphylococci, streptococci, enterococci).

Clinical Uses
- **Serious gram-negative infections**, such as nosocomial pneumonia, sepsis, febrile neutropenia, usually in combination with a beta-lactam.
- **Synergy against gram-positive** organisms for endocarditis, osteomyelitis, and sepsis (primarily gentamicin).
- Combination therapy for drug-resistant mycobacterial infections (streptomycin and amikacin).

Dosing/TDM
- Gentamicin or tobramycin
  - Conventional: IV 3–5 mg/kg daily divided every 8 hours.
    - Peak: 8–10 µg/mL; trough: <1–2 µg/mL.
  - Extended-interval: IV 5–7 mg/kg once daily.
    - Trough: <1 µg/mL.
  - Gram-positive synergy: gentamicin IV 1 mg/kg every 8–12 hours.
    - Peak: 3–4 µg/mL; trough <1 µg/mL.
- Amikacin
  - Conventional: IV 7.5 mg/kg daily day divided every 8 hours.
    - Peak: 25–40 µg/mL; trough: <8 µg/mL.
  - Extended-interval: IV 15–20 mg/kg once daily.
    - Check random level between 6 and 14 hours after infusion and plot on hospital-specific validated nomogram to determine appropriate dosing interval.
    - Trough: <4 µg/mL.
- Require renal dose adjustment.

Safety
- ADRs.
- **Nephrotoxicity:** acute renal failure may develop and is **dose-related.**
  - Mechanism of renal failure is acute tubular necrosis.
  - More likely with multiple-daily dosing than once-daily dosing: consider extended-interval dosing when appropriate.
  - Ensure that adequate troughs are achieved, and correct dosing weight is used to avoid concentration-related injury.
  - Limiting duration of therapy and avoiding concomitant nephrotoxic agents may also help prevent nephrotoxicity.
- **Ototoxicity:** may cause **vestibular** (vertigo, disequilibrium, nausea, vomiting) or **cochlear** (tinnitus, hearing loss) toxicity, which is **usually irreversible.**
  - High peak levels are a risk factor.
  - May even occur with optimal levels and once-daily dosing.
- **Neuromuscular blockade:** higher risk in patients receiving high doses and when given soon after general anesthesia or neuromuscular blockers; may exacerbate muscle weakness with myasthenia gravis.
- Contraindications
  - Caution in patients with concomitant nephrotoxic medications or severely impaired renal function.
- Drug interactions
  - Avoid concomitant use of nephrotoxic medications.
- Monitoring: BUN/SCr; baseline and weekly **audiology exams when on therapy for >2 weeks**; appropriately timed serum concentrations per dosing strategy.

CLINICAL PEARLS

- Toxicity is usually dose-related. Ensure doses are based on the correct body weight and CrCl.
  - Dosing should be based on ideal body weight with two exceptions: obese patients should be dosed on adjusted body weight, and underweight patients should be dosed on total body weight.
- Conventional dosing
  - Loading dose, followed by maintenance dose at intervals determined by renal function and subsequent monitoring of serum levels.
  - Generally preferred versus extended-interval dosing for **patients with CrCl <30 mL/min; pregnant women; patients with burns >20% BSA; patients with ascites.**
  - Measure peak concentration (30 minutes after infusion has completed) and trough concentration (30 minutes prior to next dose).
  - Extended-interval
  - Higher dose is administered at an extended-interval determined by renal function and subsequent monitoring of serum concentrations.
  - Takes advantage of **concentration-dependent killing** with **significant postantibiotic effect**; more convenient dosing/monitoring; potentially safer versus conventional.

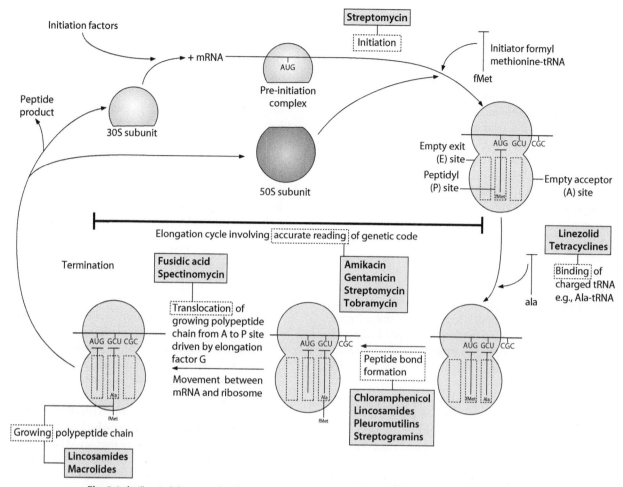

Fig. 5.4 Antibacterial agents that interfere with protein synthesis. (From Chopra I. Modes of action. In: Finch RG, Greenwood D, Norrby SR, Whitley RJ, eds. *Antibiotic and Chemotherapy*. 9th ed. Elsevier; 2010.)

CLINICAL PEARLS—cont'd

- Peaks are not routinely measured, but a pharmacodynamic goal is a peak concentration of at least 10 times the MIC of the pathogen.
- Institution-specific nomograms are used to plot random levels drawn 6–14 hours after infusion to determine dosing interval. Troughs are drawn to monitor clearance, with the goal usually that the **trough is undetectable.**
- Gram-positive synergy
  - As monotherapy, aminoglycosides do not achieve appropriate intracellular concentrations for activity against gram-positive organisms. The addition of gentamicin to penicillin or ampicillin exerts a synergistic killing effect against enterococci, viridans group streptococci, Streptococcus bovis, and staphylococci. This approach to therapy is utilized for endocarditis and infections involving prosthetic material.
  - Note that the dose for synergy is lower than typical aminoglycoside treatment dosing.
  - Streptomycin has also been utilized for this indication.

Tetracyclines and Glycylcyclines

Agents
- Tetracycline.
- Doxycycline.
- Minocycline.
- Tigecycline (glycylcycline).

Mechanism of Action
- Inhibit protein synthesis by binding to bacterial 30S ribosome subunits; **bacteriostatic.**

Spectrum
- Tetracyclines: good activity against atypical respiratory tract pathogens, *Rickettsia* spp., spirochetes, *Plasmodium* spp., staphylococci (including MRSA), *S. pneumoniae*, and *Stenotrophomonas maltophilia* (minocycline). Poor activity against most GNRs, anaerobes, enterococci, and beta-hemolytic streptococci.
- Glycylcycline (tigecycline): Good activity against atypical respiratory tract pathogens, enterococci, staphylococci (including MRSA), *S. pneumoniae*. Covers anaerobes and most GNR (except *P. aeruginosa*, *Proteus* spp., *Providencia* spp.).

Clinical Uses

- Uncomplicated upper/lower respiratory tract infections (sinusitis, bronchitis, CAP).
- Drugs of choice in tickborne diseases.
- Alternate options for ABSSSI, syphilis, bioterrorism (anthrax, plague, tularemia).
- Malaria prophylaxis/treatment (doxycycline).
- Tigecycline: CAP, intraabdominal infections, ABSSSI.

Dosing/TDM

- Tetracycline PO 250–500 mg every 6–12 hours.
  - Requires renal adjustment.
- Doxycycline IV/PO 100 mg every 12 hours.
- Minocycline IV/PO 200 mg × 1 dose followed by 100 mg every 12 hours.
- Tigecycline IV 100 mg × 1 dose followed by 50 mg every 12 hours.
  - Requires hepatic adjustment.

Safety

- ADRs: **photosensitivity**; GI upset (take with a full glass of water); discoloration of developing teeth; tissue hyperpigmentation; intracranial hypertension; vestibular toxicity (minocycline), esophageal ulceration, pancreatitis.
  - Tigecycline: nausea, vomiting, hepatotoxicity, pancreatitis.
  - Increase in all-cause mortality versus comparator-treated patients in meta-analysis of phase III and IV clinical trials. May be increased risk in patients with worsening renal function, complicated infections, or underlying comorbidities.
- Contraindications: **pregnant women and children <8 years old due to teeth discoloration** and concern for accumulation in developing teeth and long tubular bones.
- Drug interactions
  - Warfarin: may increase serum concentrations.
  - Calcium, iron, multivitamins with minerals, antacids, and dairy: tetracyclines chelate with divalent cations, significantly decreasing bioavailability. Separate by at least 2 hours.
  - Tetracycline is a substrate of CYP 3A4; concentrations may be altered with concomitant administration of CYP 3A4 inducers or inhibitors.
- Monitoring: SCr, LFTs.

CLINICAL PEARLS

- PO tetracyclines should be administered on an **empty stomach** to increase total absorption.
- Tigecycline distributes well into tissues; however, bloodstream concentrations are low, making this an inappropriate agent for bloodstream infections.

Oxazolidinones

Agents

- Linezolid.
- Tedizolid.

Mechanism of Action

- Inhibit bacterial protein synthesis by binding to 50S ribosomal subunit and blocking formation of stable 70S complex, preventing translation; bacteriostatic.

Spectrum

- Broad gram-positive coverage including MSSA, MRSA, streptococci, enterococci (including vancomycin-resistant enterococci).
- Moderate coverage against mycobacteria.
- Poor activity against anaerobes and gram-negatives.

Clinical Uses

- Infections caused by resistant gram-positive organisms, including pneumonia, ABSSSI, and UTIs. Tedizolid is only currently FDA-approved for ABSSSI.

Dosing/TDM

- Linezolid IV/PO 600 mg every 12 hours.
- Tedizolid IV/PO 200 mg daily.

Safety

- ADRs
  - **Bone marrow suppression** has been observed, particularly **after ~2 weeks of therapy** with linezolid. **Thrombocytopenia** is most common; however, all cell lines should be monitored. There is not much experience using tedizolid long-term, but a few studies suggest that similar effects may be seen. These effects appear to be **reversible with discontinuation.**
  - **Peripheral and optic neuropathy** have been reported, primarily **after 4 weeks** of therapy. These effects are **potentially irreversible.** If signs of vision impairment or loss are reported, the medication should be discontinued.
  - **Lactic acidosis due to mitochondrial toxicity** may occur. Monitor for nausea, vomiting, unexplained acidosis/low bicarbonate levels with prolonged therapy.
- Contraindications
  - Concurrent use or within 2 weeks of MAO inhibitors.
- Drug interactions
  - Serotonergic medications: linezolid is a mild monoamine oxidase (MAO) inhibitor, and patients are at an increased **risk of serotonin syndrome** when it is administered concomitantly with serotonergic medications, like selective serotonin reuptake inhibitors (SSRIs). Tedizolid has shown minimal to no evidence of MAO inhibition in animal studies.
  - **Tyramine-rich foods** may cause sudden and severe high blood pressure (hypertensive crisis or serotonin syndrome) and should be avoided. Examples include aged cheese, red wine, beer, cured meat, and soy.
- Monitoring: LFTs, CBC; sensory/vision loss and bicarbonate levels with prolonged therapy.

CLINICAL PEARLS

- Linezolid should be avoided for routine treatment of bacteremia due to its primarily bacteriostatic activity.
- When considering linezolid in patients who are taking SSRIs, it is recommended to discontinue the SSRI, if

CLINICAL PEARLS—cont'd

possible. Some SSRIs have relatively long half-lives. The patient may still be at risk for serotonin syndrome as serotonin reuptake is still inhibited for many days after discontinuation. If discontinuation is not feasible, monitor patients for signs and symptoms of serotonin syndrome.

- The use of tedizolid for more severe infections is not well documented; however, once-daily administration, potentially without the MAOI effects of linezolid, makes this agent a potential option. Further studies are needed to evaluate its place in therapy.

Macrolides, Lincosamides, Streptogramins (MLS)

Macrolides

Agents
- Azithromycin.
- Clarithromycin.
- Erythromycin.

Mechanism of Action
- Inhibit bacterial protein synthesis by binding to 50S ribosome subunit; bacteriostatic.

Spectrum
- Active against atypical respiratory tract pathogens, *S. pneumoniae*, *H. influenzae*, *M. catarrhalis*, atypical mycobacteria, *Helicobacter pylori* (clarithromycin), *Chlamydia trachomatis*, *Neisseria gonorrhoeae*, and *S. pyogenes*. **Poor activity against staphylococci, enterococci, enteric GNRs, and anaerobes.**

Clinical Uses
- Upper and lower respiratory tract infections, chlamydia, gonorrhea, atypical mycobacterial infections, and *H. pylori* infections (clarithromycin).

Dosing/TDM
- Azithromycin IV/PO 250–500 mg daily.
- Clarithromycin IV/PO 250–500 mg every 12 hours.
- Requires renal dose adjustment (clarithromycin).

Safety
- ADRs
  - **GI**: significant diarrhea, nausea, and vomiting associated with macrolides; incidence highest with high-dose single-dose regimens
  - **Hepatotoxicity**: hepatic necrosis, failure, and death have occurred with macrolides. Use with caution in patients with preexisting liver disease and discontinue immediately with symptoms of hepatitis.
  - **QTc prolongation and ventricular arrhythmias.**
  - May exacerbate muscle weakness in myasthenia gravis.
- Contraindications
  - History of cholestatic jaundice or hepatic dysfunction with prior macrolide use.
- Drug interactions
  - Metabolized by CYP 3A4 (erythromycin > clarithromycin >> azithromycin); inhibitors may increase serum concentrations.
  - Clarithromycin and erythromycin are **potent CYP 3A4 inhibitors.** May increase concentrations of medications metabolized by CYP 3A4.

- QTc-prolonging agents: may enhance QTc-prolonging effect of QTc-prolonging agents.
- Monitoring: LFTs, SCr, CBC; **QTc.**

CLINICAL PEARLS

- Azithromycin has a relatively long half-life, which is why shorter courses of medication can be administered.
- Erythromycin is still available, but rarely used as an anti-infective. Instead, due to significant GI adverse effects, it is mainly utilized as a gastric motility agent.
- Clarithromycin is used in combination with amoxicillin and a proton pump inhibitor for eradication of *H. pylori* infections.
- There are concerns for increasing rates of macrolide-resistant *S. pneumoniae*. May be suitable for mild to moderate CAP patients managed outpatient, but if more severe pneumonia, choose alternate therapy or add a beta-lactam active against *S. pneumoniae*.

Fidaxomicin

Agents
- Fidaxomicin.

Mechanism of Action
- A macrolide that inhibits ribosomal protein synthesis in *Clostridia* spp.; bactericidal.

Spectrum
- *C. difficile*.

Clinical Uses
- Treatment of *C. difficile*-associated diarrhea.

Dosing/TDM
- Fidaxomicin PO 200 mg every 12 hours.

Safety
- ADRs: GI (nausea, diarrhea, abdominal pain/cramping).
- Contraindications: hypersensitivity.
  - Caution in patients with macrolide allergy.
- Drug interactions: no significant drug interactions.
- Monitoring: no monitoring parameters have been specified.

CLINICAL PEARLS

- Fidaxomicin is a macrolide antibiotic; however, it is not absorbed in the GI tract. It targets *C. difficile* within the gut and spares normal flora.
- As efficacious as oral vancomycin for *C. difficile* treatment but superior in preventing recurrences of *C. difficile* infections.

Lincosamides

Agents
- Clindamycin.

Mechanism of Action
- Inhibits bacterial protein synthesis by binding to 50S ribosomal subunit; bacteriostatic (can be bactericidal at higher concentrations for some pathogens).

Spectrum
- Activity against gram-positive anaerobes (except *C. difficile*), *S. pyogenes*, *S. aureus* (including many MRSA). Less active against gram-negative anaerobes,

including *Bacteroides* spp. Also active against *C. trachomatis, Pneumocystis* spp., *Actinomyces* spp., and *Toxoplasma* spp. Poor activity against enterococci and gram-negative aerobes.

Clinical Uses

- Oral infections/dental prophylaxis, ABSSSI, and intra-abdominal infections.
- **Adjunctive** therapy for **necrotizing fasciitis** or other **toxin-mediated** infections.

Dosing/TDM

- IV clindamycin 600–900 mg every 6–8 hours.
- PO clindamycin 150–450 mg every 6–8 hours.

Safety

- ADRs
  - GI: nausea, vomiting, diarrhea.
  - Can cause severe and potentially fatal *C. difficile*-associated diarrhea and/colitis.
- Contraindications: hypersensitivity
- Drug interactions
  - Minor substrate of CYP 3A4; concentration may be altered if co-administered with a CYP 3A4 inducer or inhibitor.
- Monitoring: LFTs, CBC; signs and symptoms of colitis.

CLINICAL PEARLS

- PO clindamycin has extensive oral bioavailability; however, the oral dose is not equivalent to the IV dose. GI adverse effects (nausea, vomiting, diarrhea) limit the dose of PO clindamycin.
- Concern for cross resistance with strains displaying erythromycin resistance, but test susceptible to clindamycin. Labs should perform a **D-test to confirm clindamycin susceptibility.** If the D-test is positive, clindamycin resistance is inducible in that strain, and clindamycin should not be used.
- Clindamycin can be added to therapy for necrotizing fasciitis or other toxin-mediated infections. Clindamycin plays a role in **decreasing toxin production** because it interrupts translation of bacterial proteins.

Streptogramins

Agents

- Quinupristin/dalfopristin.

Mechanism of Action

- Inhibits bacterial protein synthesis by binding to two different sites on the 50S ribosome subunit; bacteriostatic.

Spectrum

- **Only gram-positive activity,** including resistant organisms, such as staphylococci (including MRSA), *Enterococcus faecium* (including vancomycin-resistant strains), streptococci.
- **No activity against *E. faecalis* or gram-negative organisms.**

Clinical Uses

- Salvage therapy for infections due to MRSA or *E. faecium*.

Dosing/TDM

- Quinupristin/dalfopristin IV 7.5 mg/kg every 8 hours.

Safety

- ADRs: **myalgias and arthralgias (significant)**; phlebitis; hyperbilirubinemia.
- Contraindications: hypersensitivity.
- Drug interactions
  - Inhibits CYP 3A4; may increase concentrations of medications metabolized by CYP 3A4.
  - Will **crystallize** when mixed with normal saline; must be mixed with and lines must be flushed with 5% dextrose in water/other saline-free diluent.
- Monitoring: LFTs and bilirubin, patient complaints of muscle and/or joint pain.

CLINICAL PEARLS

- Due to bacteriostatic activity and significant treatment-limiting adverse effects (myalgias/arthralgias), this agent is generally reserved for definitive therapy only when other treatment options are no longer viable (intolerance or treatment failure).

Nitrofurans

Agents

- Nitrofurantoin.

Mechanism of Action

- Once reduced by bacterial proteins, reactive intermediates interfere with bacterial ribosomes which leads to inhibition of protein synthesis, aerobic energy metabolism, DNA, RNA, and cell wall synthesis; bactericidal.

Spectrum

- Activity against *E. coli, Staphylococcus saprophyticus, Klebsiella* spp., *Citrobacter* spp., enterococci.
- Poor activity against *P. aeruginosa* and *Proteus* spp.

Clinical Uses

- Uncomplicated cystitis; prophylaxis against recurrent uncomplicated UTIs.

Dosing/TDM

- Nitrofurantoin PO 100 mg every 12 hours.

Safety

- ADRs
  - GI (nausea, vomiting).
  - May discolor urine (brown or bright yellow).
  - Two very rare, but serious forms of pulmonary toxicity have been reported: acute pneumonitis (usually resolves with drug discontinuation) and chronic pulmonary fibrosis (may not recover full pulmonary function after discontinuation).
  - Rarely hepatotoxicity, peripheral neuropathy, and optic neuritis have been reported.
- Contraindications
  - Anuria, oliguria, or significant renal impairment; history of cholestatic jaundice or hepatotoxicity with prior use.
- Drug interactions: no significant drug interactions.
- Monitoring: SCr, LFTs.

CLINICAL PEARLS

- Nitrofurantoin is only indicated for **uncomplicated UTIs** as it does not reach bactericidal concentrations outside

CLINICAL PEARLS—cont'd

of the lower urinary tract and should not be used for pyelonephritis or UTI with sepsis.
- Remains active against many ESBL-producing organisms.
- Nitrofurantoin comes in two formulations. One that is administered every 6 hours (Macrodantin) and one that is administered every 12 hours (Macrobid). The dosing above is for Macrobid.
- Both of these medications are only bactericidal when they reach high enough concentrations in the urine. In patients with impaired renal function, there is concern that drug accumulation is insufficient for bactericidal activity. Nitrofurantoin should be avoided in patients with CrCl <50 mL/min, but some data suggest that threshold should be 30 mL/min.

Chloramphenicol

Agents
- Chloramphenicol.

Mechanism of Action
- Inhibits protein synthesis by binding to 50S ribosomal subunit; bacteriostatic.

Spectrum
- Active against aerobic and anaerobic gram-positive and gram-negative bacteria, including enterococci, staphylococci, streptococci, Enterobacteriaceae, and *Burkholderia* spp.; also active against spirochetes, *Rickettsia* spp., and *Chlamydia* spp.; not against *P. aeruginosa* or *Acinetobacter* spp.

Clinical Uses
- Treatment of infections caused by vancomycin-resistant enterococci or multi-drug-resistant gram-negative bacteria.
- May also be used for meningitis caused by *Francisella tularensis* or *Yersinia pestis*.

Dosing/TDM
- Chloramphenicol IV 25 mg/kg every 6 hours, up to a maximum dose of 1000 mg every 6 hours. No renal dosing adjustments are required.
- TDM
  - Peak serum concentrations should be monitored 1 hour postinfusion every 3–4 days.
  - Target peak concentration <25 mg/L.

Safety
- ADRs: idiosyncratic aplastic anemia (occurring in ~1 in 30,000), dose-related bone marrow suppression, and gray baby syndrome may occur.
- Contraindications: hypersensitivity; avoid use in near-term pregnant women due to potential risk for gray baby syndrome.
- Drug interactions: may increase anticoagulant effect of warfarin; rifampin, phenytoin, and phenobarbital may reduce chloramphenicol concentrations.

CLINICAL PEARLS

- Dose reduction is necessary for significant hepatic disease.
- Risk of aplastic anemia is not dose-related; this effect may occur rarely with any formulation of chloramphenicol, including ophthalmic drops.
- Peak concentrations are monitored due to risk of ADRs. Risk of dose-related bone marrow suppression increases with peak concentrations >25 mg/L, and risk of gray baby syndrome appears to increase with peak concentrations >50 mg/L.

Nucleic Acid Synthesis Inhibitors

Fluoroquinolones

Agents
- Ciprofloxacin.
- Levofloxacin.
- Moxifloxacin.
- Delafloxacin.

Mechanism of Action
- Inhibits DNA gyrases (topoisomerase II and IV) which are required for bacterial DNA replication, transcription, repair, and recombination and by promoting breaks in the DNA; bactericidal.

Spectrum
- Ciprofloxacin: enteric GNRs, atypicals (*Mycoplasma pneumoniae*, *Legionella pneumophila*, *Chlamydophila pneumoniae*), *P. aeruginosa*. Poor activity against gram-positive organisms and anaerobes.
- Levofloxacin/moxifloxacin: active against *S. pneumoniae*, enteric GNRs, atypicals, *P. aeruginosa* (levofloxacin only), MSSA (moxifloxacin > levofloxacin), anaerobes (moxifloxacin only). No enterococcal activity.
- **Delafloxacin: broadest in class** covering gram-negatives (including *P. aeruginosa*), gram-positives (streptococci, staphylococci [including MRSA], *E. faecalis*), anaerobes, and atypicals.

Clinical Uses
- UTI (except for moxifloxacin), intraabdominal infections (in combination with other agents), systemic gram-negative infections, pseudomonal infections (when organism is susceptible: ciprofloxacin, levofloxacin, delafloxacin), ABSSSI (not ciprofloxacin), upper/lower respiratory tract infections (not ciprofloxacin).
- Delafloxacin: only FDA-approved for ABSSSI.
- Ciprofloxacin and levofloxacin: **treatment/prophylaxis of bioterrorism agents** (anthrax, plague, tularemia).

Dosing/TDM
- Ciprofloxacin IV 400 mg every 12 hours; PO 500 mg every 12 hours.
  - IV 400 mg every 8 hours or PO 750 mg every 12 hours for *P. aeruginosa*.
- Levofloxacin IV/PO 500 mg daily.
  - IV/PO 750 mg daily for *P. aeruginosa*.

- Moxifloxacin IV/PO 400 mg daily.
- Delafloxacin IV 300 mg every 12 hours; PO 450 mg every 12 hours.
- Require renal dose adjustment (except for moxifloxacin).
  Safety
- ADRs
  - **CNS** effects: dizziness, confusion, hallucinations, seizures, toxic psychosis, insomnia. The elderly and patients with known or suspected CNS disorders may be at increased risk.
  - **Tendinitis and tendon rupture:** rupture of Achilles tendon has been reported most frequently. Most common in elderly patients, especially in the setting of impaired renal function and with combined use of corticosteroids. Discontinue at first sign of tendon pain. May occur up to several months after discontinuation.
  - **Peripheral neuropathy:** may be irreversible: discontinue at first signs of sensory or sensorimotor neuropathy.
  - May exacerbate muscle weakness in myasthenia gravis.
  - QTc prolongation (except delafloxacin); hepatitis; glucose dysregulation; photosensitivity; *C. difficile*-associated diarrhea.
- Contraindications
  - Fluoroquinolones should be reserved for in the setting of acute bacterial sinusitis, acute bacterial exacerbation of chronic bronchitis, or uncomplicated UTI only for patients who have no alternative options due to risk of disabling and potentially serious adverse reactions.
- Drug interactions
  - Calcium, iron, multivitamins with minerals, antacids, dairy: fluoroquinolones chelate with divalent cations, significantly decreasing bioavailability. Separate by at least 2 hours.
  - QTc prolonging agents: may enhance QTc prolonging effect of QTc prolonging agents.
  - Ciprofloxacin is a mild inhibitor of CYP 3A4; may increase concentrations of medications metabolized by CYP 3A4.
- Monitoring: SCr, glucose, LFTs, CBC; EKG; altered mental status; signs and symptoms of tendonitis.

CLINICAL PEARLS

- Antipseudomonal fluoroquinolones: ciprofloxacin, levofloxacin, and delafloxacin.
- Respiratory fluoroquinolones: levofloxacin, moxifloxacin.
- All fluoroquinolones undergo renal elimination, except for moxifloxacin, which is why moxifloxacin is not indicated for UTI treatment.
- Many fluoroquinolones have been introduced and subsequently taken off the market due to adverse effects. While these drugs are often convenient oral options, their use should be reserved for those where alternate options are not available.

Nitroimidazoles

Agents
- Metronidazole, tinidazole.

Mechanism of Action
- Anaerobic bacteria intracellularly reduce metronidazole, which can then bind to and damage bacterial DNA causing cell death; bactericidal.

Spectrum
- Anaerobes (gram-negative and gram-positive), protozoa, and *H. pylori*.
- May have less activity against gram-positive oral anaerobes (*Peptostreptococcus* spp., *Cutibacterium* spp.) and *Actinomyces* spp.
- Poor activity against aerobic bacteria.

Clinical Uses
- Empiric or targeted therapy against abdominal anaerobes, usually in combination with agents covering aerobic organisms.
- Mild–moderate *C. difficile* infections.
- Alternative to amoxicillin in combination treatment of *H. pylori*.
- Vaginal trichomoniasis and GI protozoal infections.

Dosing/TDM
- Metronidazole IV/PO 500 mg every 8 hours.
- Tinidazole PO 2 g once every 24 hours.

Safety
- ADRs
  - GI: **metallic taste**, nausea, vomiting; rare pancreatitis or hepatitis.
  - CNS: headache; potentially reversible **peripheral neuropathy** has been reported with prolonged therapy; rarely seizure or altered mental status.
- Contraindications
  - Pregnant patients (1st trimester).
  - Avoid tinidazole in breast-feeding.
  - **Alcohol**- or propylene-glycol-containing products within 3 days.
  - Disulfiram within 2 weeks.
- Drug interactions
  - Weak inhibitor of CYP 2C9: may increase concentrations of medications metabolized by CYP 2C9.
  - Warfarin: metronidazole inhibits warfarin metabolism (CYP 2C9), increasing anticoagulant effect; **dose reduction of warfarin is usually necessary.**
  - Alcohol: disulfiram-like reaction with consumption of alcohol. Patients should abstain from drinking alcohol while taking metronidazole.
- Monitoring: LFTs, CBC; mental status/sensory loss.

CLINICAL PEARLS

- Often added to therapy to empiric cover for anaerobes. Beware of dual anaerobic coverage with agents like piperacillin/tazobactam and carbapenems.

Antimetabolites

Folate Antagonists

Agents

- Trimethoprim–sulfamethoxazole (TMP–SMX).

Mechanism of Action

- Inhibits DNA synthesis by interfering with the folate biosynthesis pathway; bacteriostatic.

Spectrum

- Good activity against MSSA, MRSA, *Pneumocystis* spp., *Stenotrophomonas* spp., *Listeria* spp.
- Moderate activity against streptococci, enteric GNRs, *Salmonella* spp., *Shigella* spp., *Nocardia* spp.
- Poor activity against *P. aeruginosa*, enterococci, and anaerobes.

Clinical Uses

- Uncomplicated cystitis, UTI prophylaxis, treatment and prophylaxis of *Pneumocystis* pneumonia and treatment of *Toxoplasma* encephalitis, ABSSSIs due to MRSA, CNS infections due to susceptible organisms.

Dosing/TDM

- Oral: every 12 hours; US 1–2 double strength tablets; UK 480–960 mg.
- IV: divided every 6–12 hours; US 8–20 mg (TMP)/kg per day; UK 120 mg/kg per day.
- **Weight-based dosing is based on the trimethoprim component for the US dosing. Dosing in the UK is based on the combined dose of both SMX and TMP.**
- Requires renal dose adjustment.

Safety

- ADRs
  - **Dermatologic:** photosensitivity; SMX component commonly causes nonsevere rash, but can cause life-threatening dermatologic reactions like Stevens–Johnson syndrome and toxic epidermal necrolysis, and should be discontinued at first sign of rash.
  - Hematologic: **bone marrow suppression** can be seen with higher doses (like those used for *Pneumocystis* treatment); **drug-induced thrombocytopenia** has also been reported and usually reverses within 1 week of discontinuation.
  - **Renal:** SMX can cause acute interstitial nephritis and crystalluria; TMP may block creatinine excretion, resulting in increase in SCr without decrease in GFR.
  - **Hyperkalemia:** TMP may act similar to a potassium-sparing diuretic.
- Contraindications
  - Hypersensitivity to sulfa.
  - **Glucose-6-phosphate dehydrogenase deficiency.**
  - **Megaloblastic anemia due to folate deficiency.**
  - History of drug-induced thrombocytopenia with use of sulfonamides or trimethoprim.

- Drug interactions
  - TMP: major substrate of CYP 2C9 and 3A4; inhibits CYP 2C9.
  - Warfarin: inhibits warfarin metabolism (CYP 2C9), increasing anticoagulant effect; dose reduction of warfarin is usually necessary.
  - Monitoring: BUN, SCr, potassium, CBC; **skin for rash.**

CLINICAL PEARLS

- It was previously thought that patients with a sulfa allergy may also have cross-reactivity to other drugs containing a sulfa moiety (e.g., furosemide, hydrochlorothiazide, acetazolamide); however, the likelihood is very low. Sulfasalazine, a nonantibiotic sulfonamide has a similar structure to SMX and may have cross-reactivity.
- Tablets have **high bioavailability** and patients can be converted to PO (nearest tablet size) when tolerating oral medications. Double-strength tablets: 160 mg/800 mg TMP–SMX; single-strength tablets: 80 mg/400 mg TMP–SMX.
- While recommended as empiric therapy for uncomplicated cystitis, *E. coli* resistance rates to TMP–SMX in some areas may be >15%. If resistance is >15–20%, an alternative agent is recommended until susceptibilities can be confirmed, especially if considering treatment of upper UTIs (pyelonephritis) or sepsis with a urinary source.
- To appropriately dilute IV TMP–SMX, large volumes of fluid are required. This factor should be taken into account for patients with fluid restrictions.

SUMMARY TABLES

Special dosing considerations for antibiotics are summarized in Tables 5.2–5.4.

TABLE 5.2 Antibiotics Requiring Renal Dose Adjustment

Aminoglycosides	Glycopeptides
Beta-lactams[a]	Lipoglycopeptides
Colistin	Macrolides (clarithromycin)
Cyclic lipopeptides	Nitrofurantoin
Folate antagonists	Tetracyclines
Fluoroquinolones	

[a]Excludes antistaphylococcal penicillins and ceftriaxone.

TABLE 5.3 Antibiotics with Metabolic Drug Interactions (Interactions with CYP Enzyme System)

	Substrate	Inhibitor
Ciprofloxacin	+	
Clindamycin	+	
Macrolides (erythromycin, clarithromycin)	+	+
Metronidazole		+
Quinupristin/dalfopristin		+
TMP–SMX		+

TABLE 5.4 Dosing Weight and Calculations

Ideal body weight (IBW)	Adjusted (dosing) body weight (ABW)
Male: 50 kg + (2.3 × each inch over 5 ft) Female: 45.5kg + (2.3 × each inch over 5 ft) Underweight patients: TBW < IBW use TBW	IBW + [0.4 × (total body weight (TBW) – IBW)]

Antibiotic Class/Agent	Dosing Weight
Aminoglycosides	IBW[a]
Chloramphenicol[b]	TBW[a]
Colistin	IBW
Daptomycin	TBW[a]
Quinupristin/dalfopristin	TBW
TMP–SMX	TBW[a]
Vancomycin	TBW

[a]Consider use of ABW for obese patients when TBW >120% IBW.
[b]Chloramphenicol maximum dose is 1000 mg every 6 hours.

6

Antimycobacterial Agents

TONYA SCARDINA

Introduction

This chapter provides key summaries regarding spectrum of activity, clinical uses, usual adult dosing, therapeutic drug monitoring (TDM) where applicable, safety, microbiologic activity, and clinical pearls associated with antimycobacterial agents. Medications are listed in alphabetical order. For a more thorough discussion of mycobacterial diseases, see Chapters 32 and 33.

Goals of Therapy

The main goals in treating TB and other mycobacterial infections are to cure the individual, minimize the risk of disability or death, and to reduce spread to other people (for TB). This requires therapy that can eradicate replicating and dormant bacilli while minimizing emergence of resistance and adverse effects (Table 6.1).

- Sole drugs are rarely, if ever, used for treatment of mycobacterial infections and never for TB. Combination therapy is standard and includes multiple drugs to which the bacteria are known, or likely, to be susceptible.
  - Treatment with a single agent may lead to the development of resistance.
  - Additionally, addition of a single agent to a failing regimen may also lead to resistance.

TB Treatment Phases

Treatment regimens for susceptible TB disease all comprise an initial treatment phase followed by a continuation phase.

- Initial treatment (8 weeks)
  - TB bacilli with a high replication rate are killed, reducing the bacillary load significantly.
  - Reduces probability of drug resistance emerging.
    - Related to high replication – mutation rate to first-line anti-TB drugs $= 10^{-7}$ to 10^{-10}.
    - Likelihood of bacilli developing resistance to 2 or more anti-TB drugs = product of the individual mutation rates.

- Continuation phase (4–7 months): kills remaining semi-dormant TB bacilli.

Aminoglycosides

Agents
- Amikacin.
- Kanamycin.
- Streptomycin.

Mechanism of Action
- Inhibit bacterial protein synthesis by irreversibly binding to the bacterial 30S ribosome subunit; **bactericidal**.

Clinical Uses
- Drug-resistant tuberculosis whose isolate has demonstrated or presumed susceptibility to the agents.
  - WHO Group B.
  - SM used to be a first-line agent for the treatment of TB. However, increasing global prevalence of resistance has decreased its overall usefulness.
- Pulmonary *M. avium* complex (MAC)
  - Consider in extensive fibrocavitary pulmonary MAC disease.
  - Patients who have failed prior drug therapy.
  - Macrolide-resistant MAC infection.
- Rifamycin-resistant *M. kansasii* infection.
- *M. chimera* infection.

Dosing/TDM
- Amikacin
  - *M. abscessus*: IV/IM: 10–15 mg/kg daily.
  - *M. tuberculosis* and complicated nontuberculous mycobacteria (NTM): 15 mg/kg daily. Some clinicians prefer 25 mg/kg three times weekly.
  - Nodular or bronchiectatic MAC or treatment durations ≥6 months: 8–10 mg/kg twice to three times weekly.
- Kanamycin

TABLE 6.1 Therapeutic Options for the Treatment of Mycobacterial Infections

First-line Therapies for Tuberculosis

- Isoniazid (INH)
- Rifampin (RIF), [rifapentine – continuation phase only; rifabutin[a] – useful with interactions]
- Pyrazinamide (PZA)
- Ethambutol (EMB)

Second-line Therapies for Tuberculosis[b]

WHO group A	Fluoroquinolones[a] • Moxifloxacin • Levofloxacin
WHO group B	• Injectable aminoglycosides • Streptomycin (SM) • Amikacin[a] • Kanamycin[a] • Capreomycin
WHO group C	Core second-line agents • Ethionamide • Prothionamide • Cycloserine Linezolid
WHO group D	Add-on agents • Para-aminosalicylic acid • Bedaquiline • Carbapenems • Delamanid

Therapeutic Options for _M. leprae_

- Dapsone
- Rifampin
- Clofazimine
- Moxifloxacin
- Minocycline

Therapeutic Options for Nontuberculous Mycobacteria

- Macrolides
- Carbapenems: imipenem/cilastatin, meropenem

[a]Not FDA approved for treatment of TB.
[b]Reserved for drug intolerance or resistant organisms.

- IV/IM: 15 mg/kg daily (maximum dose: 1 gram/day); administered once a day or divided every 12 hours.
  - Peak: 35–45 µg/L.
- Alternative dosing: IV/IM: 25 mg/kg three times weekly.
  - Peak: 65–80 µg/L.
- Streptomycin
  - IV/IM: 15 mg/kg IV/IM daily. Some clinicians prefer 25mg/kg three times weekly.
- **Require renal dose adjustment.**
  Safety
- Adverse drug reactions (ADRs)
  - **Nephrotoxicity**: acute renal failure may develop and is dose related.
  - **Ototoxicity**: may cause vestibular or cochlear toxicity, which may be irreversible. Factors that contribute to ototoxicity include prolonged use of aminoglycosides,

increasing age, preexisting hearing loss, and previous treatment with ototoxic medications. Serial audiogram should be conducted.
  - **Neuromuscular blockade**: greater risk with kanamycin in comparison to amikacin. May cause paralysis and respiratory depression with **myasthenia gravis**.
- Contraindications: caution in patients with concomitant nephrotoxic medications or severely impaired renal function.
- Monitoring: urea + serum creatinine (SCr) obtained weekly or bi-weekly; audiology exams monthly and if eighth nerve toxicity symptoms occur. An audiogram and vestibular testing should be repeated if there are symptoms, weekly serum drug concentrations.

CLINICAL PEARLS

- Aminoglycosides exhibit **concentration-dependent killing**, and thus the area under the concentration-time curve (AUC) is the main pharmacokinetic index to determine their efficacy.
- Due to adverse effects, ensure that renal function is closely monitored and dose adjustments are made based on creatinine clearance.
- Dose should be based on adjusted body weight for obese patients.

Bedaquiline

Mechanism of Action

- Inhibits the activity of mycobacterial ATP synthase by binding to its c subunit, which prevents the bacterium from generating ATP, ultimately leading to cell death; **bactericidal.**

Clinical Uses

- Only active against _M. tuberculosis_.
- Treatment for _M. tuberculosis_ that is **extensively drug-resistant** (resistant to isoniazid, rifampin, fluoroquinolone, and injectable agents).
  - WHO group D2.
- **Only use when an effective regimen cannot otherwise be provided.**

Dosing/TDM

- 400 mg PO daily for 14 days, followed by 200 mg thrice-weekly to complete 24 weeks of therapy (given in combination with at least 3 or 4 other _M. tuberculosis_-susceptible antimicrobials).

Safety

- ADRs
  - May prolong QTc interval. Use with drugs that prolong the QTc interval may cause additive prolongation. Monitor electrocardiograms (ECGs) at baseline and at least 2, 12, and 24 weeks of treatment. Discontinue therapy (and all other QT-prolonging drugs) if patient develops confirmed QTcF interval of >500 ms.

- **Increased risk of death** was seen in the bedaquiline treatment group compared to the placebo treatment group in one placebo-controlled trial.
- Nausea, arthralgia, headache, QTc prolongation, hepatotoxicity.
- Contraindications: none.
- Drug interactions
  - Bedaquiline is a substrate of CYP3A, and thus drugs that induce or inhibit CYP3A can affect exposure of bedaquiline.
  - QT-prolonging agents.
- Monitoring
  - AST, ALT, alkaline phosphatase, bilirubin, and symptoms of **liver dysfunction** (e.g., fatigue, nausea, anorexia, jaundice, dark urine, liver tenderness, and hepatomegaly) at baseline and monthly during therapy, and as needed.
  - Monitor more frequently if patient has underlying hepatic disease or is receiving concomitant drugs.

> **CLINICAL PEARLS**
>
> - Absorption of bedaquiline is enhanced by 95% when it is given with a meal, so bedaquiline should be taken with food.

Capreomycin

Mechanism of Action
- Inhibits bacterial protein synthesis by interacting with the bacterial ribosome.

Clinical Uses
- Only active against *M. tuberculosis*.
- Second line of treatment of *M. tuberculosis* infection in combination with other antituberculous medications.
  - WHO group B.

Dosing
- 15 mg/kg IV/IM. Some clinicians prefer 25 mg/kg three times weekly.

Safety
- ADRs
  - Serious: nephrotoxicity, ototoxicity.
- Contraindications: hypersensitivity to capreomycin or any component of the formulation.
- Drug interactions: capreomycin may cause or enhance **neuromuscular blockade.** Thus caution is recommended if capreomycin is used in conjunction with medications with similar side effects (e.g., colistin/polymyxin B, muscle relaxants, aminoglycosides).
- Monitoring: **audiometric measurements and vestibular function** at baseline and during therapy; renal function at baseline and weekly during therapy; baseline and frequent assessment of serum electrolytes (including calcium, magnesium, and potassium), LFTs.

> **CLINICAL PEARLS**
>
> - Capreomycin may be associated with aminoglycosides due to similar pharmacokinetics and toxicities, but their structures differ; and the spectrum of activity of capreomycin is restricted to mycobacteria.

Carbapenems

Agents
- Imipenem-cilastatin.

Mechanism of Action
- Inhibits bacterial wall synthesis of actively dividing cells by binding to one or more penicillin binding proteins (PBP). Imipenem/cilastatin preferentially binds to PBP2 and PBP1 (transpeptidases implicated in elongation of the bacterial cell wall).

Clinical Uses
- Treatment of *M. fortuitum, M. chelonae, M. abscessus.*
  - >90% of *M. fortuitum* group are susceptible to imipenem; 40–60% of *M. chelonae* or *M. abscessus* are susceptible.
  - Used periodically, may help control symptoms and progression of pulmonary *M. abscessus* infection.
- *M. marinum* are relatively sensitive to imipenem, as are *M. smegmatis* and *M. mucogenicum.*
- WHO group D3 for MDR-TB infections.

Dosing/TDM
- Imipenem-cilastatin IV 500 mg every 6 to 12 hours (used in combination with other antibacterial agents).
- Require renal adjustment.

Safety
- ADRs: seizures, nausea, vomiting, diarrhea, abnormalities in LFTs, neutropenia, eosinophilia, rash.
  - **Increased risk of seizures**; highest with imipenem. May avoid in patients with a history of seizures or develop seizures while prescribed imipenem/cilastatin.
- Contraindications: hypersensitivity.
- Drug interactions: may decrease serum concentrations of **valproic acid**, probably by increasing valproic acid glucuronidation in the liver. Consider alternate therapy as carbapenems may also lower seizure threshold.
  - **Ganciclovir** and imipenem should not be used concomitantly due to risk of seizures.
- Monitoring: SCr, LFTs, complete blood count (CBC), seizures, skin for hypersensitivity reactions.

> **CLINICAL PEARLS**
>
> - In order to reduce the risk of seizures associated with the use of imipenem/cilastatin, it is recommended that **dose adjustments are made among patients with renal impairment.**

Cefoxitin

Mechanism of Action
- Inhibits bacterial wall synthesis of actively dividing cells by binding to one or more penicillin binding proteins (PBP).

Clinical Uses
- Empiric or definitive treatment of *M. abscessus, M. chelonae,* and *M. fortuitum.*
- *M. abscessus* is usually susceptible to cefoxitin, approximately half of *M. fortuitum* isolates are susceptible, and *M. chelonae* is usually resistant.

Dosing/TDM
- Cefoxitin 2 g IV every 4 hours or 3 g IV every 6 hours (maximum dose: 12 g/day).
- Require renal dose adjustment.

Safety
- ADRs: diarrhea, eosinophilia, rash, hemolytic anemia (rare), pancytopenia (rare).
- Contraindications: hypersensitivity.
- Drug interactions: no significant drug interactions.
- Monitoring: SCr, LFTs, CBC; skin for hypersensitivity rash.

CLINICAL PEARLS
- While awaiting further identification and susceptibility results, cefoxitin may be initiated for empiric treatment of rapidly growing mycobacterial infection; typically used in combination with amikacin and macrolides.

Clofazimine

Mechanism of Action
- Unclear.

Clinical Uses
- Combination therapy for lepromatous (multibacillary) leprosy.
- *M. tuberculosis*
  - Not usually recommended for treatment of MDR-TB.
  - Counts as half a drug in a treatment regimen.
  - WHO group C.

Dosing/TDM
- Treatment of multi-bacillary leprosy: clofazimine 50 mg PO daily and 300 mg monthly in combination with daily dapsone and monthly rifampin.
- Treatment of tuberculosis: clofazimine 100–200 mg PO daily.

Safety
- ADRs: abdominal pain, nausea, vomiting, diarrhea, reddish-black or orange **skin discoloration** within a few weeks of starting clofazimine, discoloration in hair, urine, sweat, feces, sputum, and other bodily fluids, reddish-brown corneal and conjunctival discoloration, lymphedema (rare), and exfoliative dermatitis (rare.)
- Contraindications: hypersensitivity.
- Drug interactions: **co-administration with aluminum-magnesium antacid reduces bioavailability** of clofazimine.
- Monitoring: ocular examination, SCr, LFTs.

CLINICAL PEARLS
- Adverse effects related to clofazimine are dose-related and result from its long half-life and tendency to crystallize in fatty tissue. Thus side effects are usually slowly reversible upon discontinuation.
- Clofazimine should be administered with food

Cycloserine

Mechanism of Action
- Competitively inhibiting at least two bacterial enzymes that either supply D-alanine for or incorporate D-alanine into peptide bridges which assist in maintaining the integrity of the bacterial cell wall.

Clinical Uses
- Treatment of active pulmonary or extrapulmonary tuberculosis, in combination with other agents, when treatment with primary tuberculosis therapy has proved inadequate.
- WHO group C.

Dosing/TDM
- *Initial:* 10–15 mg/kg daily (maximum: 1000 mg/day), usually 500–750 mg/day in 2 divided doses. Most clinicians with experience using cycloserine indicate that it is unusual for patients to be able to tolerate this amount. Serum concentrations targeted at 20–35 µg/mL are often useful in determining the optimal dose.

Safety
- ADRs: neurotoxicity (convulsion, somnolence, confusion, tremor, vertigo, drowsiness), elevated LFTs, rash.
- Contraindications: hypersensitivity; epilepsy; depression, severe anxiety, or psychosis; severe renal insufficiency; excessive concurrent use of alcohol.
- Drug interactions: **concomitant use with alcohol is associated with increased risk of seizures**; CNS toxicity may be enhanced with concomitant use with isoniazid.
- Monitoring
  - Renal, hepatic, hematologic tests, and plasma cycloserine concentrations.
  - **Assess neuropsychiatric status at monthly intervals** and more frequently if symptoms occur.

CLINICAL PEARLS

- Some neurotoxic effects may be treated or prevented by **concomitant administration** of 200–300 mg of **pyridoxine** daily or 50 mg of pyridoxine per 250 mg of cycloserine.

Dapsone

Mechanism of Action

- Acts on folic acid synthesis pathway by inhibiting the enzyme dihydropteroate synthase (DHPS).

Clinical Uses

- Treatment of *M. leprae* infection.

Dosing

- 100 mg once daily in combination with one or more other medications active against *M. leprae.*

Safety

- ADRs
  - Common: rash.
  - Serious: **methemoglobinemia, hemolysis,** agranulocytosis, aplastic anemia, hepatotoxicity.
- Contraindications: hypersensitivity to dapsone.
- Drug interactions: rifampin increases the metabolism of dapsone. Probenecid blocks renal excretion of dapsone, resulting in increase in serum levels of dapsone.
- Monitoring: CBC with differential (weekly for the first month, monthly for 6 months, then semiannually), reticulocyte count, and liver function tests; **check G-6-PD levels prior to initiation of dapsone**; monitor for signs of jaundice, hemolysis, or methemoglobinemia.

CLINICAL PEARLS

- Dapsone is **widely distributed throughout all tissues** and concentrates well in the skin, muscle, liver, and kidney. In addition, it crosses the blood–brain-barrier.

Delamanid

Mechanism of Action

A nitro-dihydro-imidazooxazole drug that inhibits mycolic acid synthesis (i.e., cell wall synthesis).

Clinical Uses

- Third-line agent for MDR-TB when WHO-recommended regimens cannot be achieved.
  - WHO group D2.
- XDR-TB in addition to WHO-recommended regimen.
- Conditionally approved in Europe, not FDA approved.

Dosing

- 100 mg twice a day for 24 weeks.
- No levels required.

Safety

- ADRs: rash, nausea, vomiting; QTc prolongation.
- Interactions: QTc-prolonging agents: may enhance QTc-prolonging effect of QTc-prolonging agents.
- Contraindications: pregnancy and breastfeeding; hypersensitivity; hypoalbuminemia.
- Monitoring: baseline and monthly ECGs; serum albumin.

Ethambutol

Mechanism of Action

- Inhibits arabinofuranosyltransferase enzymes that are involved in polymerizing arabinofuranosyl (Araf) residues from DPA into the arabinan components of mycobacterial cell wall arabinogalactan and lipoarabinomannan; bacteriostatic.
- **Least potent first-line TB agent** – included primarily to prevent rifampin resistance emerging in primary isoniazid-resistant infections.

Clinical Uses

- Combination therapy for treatment of tuberculosis.
- Treatment of NTM species including *M. avium* complex, *M. kansasii,* and *M. marinum.*

Dosing/TDM

- Based on lean body weight.
- Treatment of *M. tuberculosis*
  - 15–20 mg/kg daily (maximum dose: 1.6 g),
  - 25-30 mg/kg/dose three times weekly (maximum: 2.4 g),
  - or 35-50 mg/kg/dose twice weekly (maximum dose: 4 g).
- Pulmonary MAC: 25 mg/kg three times weekly or 15 mg/kg daily.
- Nontuberculosis mycobacterium: 15 mg/kg per day.

Safety

- ADRs: **optic neuritis,** peripheral neuritis, nephrotoxicity, rash, liver dysfunction, thrombocytopenia (rare).
- Contraindications: hypersensitivity; optic neuritis (risk vs benefit decision); use in young children, unconscious patients, or any other patient who may be unable to discern and report visual changes.
- Drug interactions: **aluminum hydroxide** may decrease the serum concentration of ethambutol.
- Monitoring: **visual acuity and color discrimination testing:** baseline and monthly throughout treatment period for patients receiving >15 mg/kg daily, SCr, complete metabolic panel.
- Ocular toxicity occurs more frequently in patients receiving treatment for MAC than those being treated for *M. tuberculosis.* In addition, the risk is greater when ethambutol is given on a daily basis versus intermittent administration.

CLINICAL PEARLS

- Ethambutol is primarily excreted through the kidneys and, thus dose adjustment should be made for patient with renal impairment.

Ethionamide

Mechanism of Action
- Interfere with the production of mycolic acids thus disrupting the lipid membrane of mycobacteria.

Clinical Uses
- Core second-line agent for treatment of MDR-TB infection.
  - WHO group C.

Dosing
- 15-20 mg/kg total (usually 250-500 mg once or twice daily) given **in combination** with one or more other medications active against *M. tuberculosis*.

Safety
- ADRs
- Common: gastrointestinal (i.e., nausea, vomiting, abdominal cramps, diarrhea, metallic taste, anorexia).
- Serious: hepatotoxicity, neurologic toxicity (e.g., depression, drowsiness, headache, peripheral neuritis, blurred vision, diplopia) – concurrent use of pyridoxine is suggested, drug rash with eosinophilia and systemic symptoms (DRESS), Stevens–Johnson syndrome (SJS), toxic epidermal necrolysis (TEN).
- Contraindications: hypersensitivity to ethionamide or any component of the formulation; severe hepatic impairment.
- Drug interactions: ethionamide may potentiate neurologic side effects of cycloserine.
- Monitoring: baseline and monthly serum ALT and AST; baseline and periodic ophthalmic exams; periodic blood glucose and TSH.

CLINICAL PEARLS
- In clinical practice, ethionamide and prothionamide are generally regarded as equivalent.

Fluoroquinolones

Agents
- Ciprofloxacin.
- Levofloxacin.
- Moxifloxacin.

Mechanism of Action
- Inhibits DNA gyrase and DNA topoisomerase IV. These two enzymes work together in replication, transcription, recombination, and repair of DNA; **bactericidal.**

Clinical Uses
- Drug-resistant tuberculosis caused by organisms known or presumed to be sensitive, or when first-line agents cannot be used because of intolerance.
  - WHO group A.
- Rifampin-resistant *M. kansasii*.
- *M. chelonae*, *M. abscessus*, and *M. immunogenum* are generally resistant to ciprofloxacin.
- *M. fortuitum* infections.

Dosing/TDM
- Levofloxacin IV/PO 500–1000 mg daily.
- Moxifloxacin IV/PO 400 mg daily.

Safety
- ADRs
  - Fluoroquinolones should be reserved for patients who have no alternative options due to risk of disabling and potentially serious adverse reactions.
  - CNS effects: dizziness, confusion, hallucinations, **seizures**, toxic psychosis, insomnia. Use with caution in patients with known or suspected CNS disorder, or risk factors that may predispose to seizures or lower the seizure threshold.
  - **Tendinitis and tendon rupture**: rupture of Achilles tendon has been reported most frequently. Patients of any age or without preexisting risk factors have experienced these reactions; may occur within hours to weeks after initiation.
  - **Peripheral neuropathy**: may be irreversible – discontinue at first signs of sensory or sensorimotor neuropathy.
  - May exacerbate muscle weakness in myasthenia gravis.
  - **QTc prolongation**, hepatitis, dysglycemia, photosensitivity, *C. difficile*-associated diarrhea.
- Contraindications: hypersensitivity.
- Drug interactions
  - Calcium, iron, multivitamins with minerals, antacids, dairy: **fluoroquinolones chelate with divalent cations, significantly decreasing bioavailability.** These interactions can be minimized by administering the oral quinolone at least 2 hours before, or 6 hours after exposure to the medication/food that contains polyvalent cations.
  - Fluoroquinolones may interact with warfarin; monitor INR (international normalized ratio) and incidence of bleeding.
  - **QTc-prolonging** agents: may enhance QTc-prolonging effect of QTc-prolonging agents.
  - Ciprofloxacin is a mild inhibitor of CYP3A4 – may increase concentrations of medications metabolized by CYP3A4.
- Monitoring: SCr, glucose, LFTs, CBC, ECG, altered mental status, number and type of stools/day for diarrhea, signs and symptoms of tendonitis.

CLINICAL PEARLS
- All fluoroquinolones penetrate well into tissues.
- Moxifloxacin does not undergo renal excretion, and thus would not need to be dose adjusted due to renal impairment.
- Fluoroquinolones usually have a high bioavailability but this may be severely affected by concomitant medications.

Folate Antagonists

Agents
- Trimethoprim–sulfamethoxazole (TMP–SMX)

Mechanism of Action
- Inhibits DNA synthesis by interfering with the folate biosynthesis pathway; **bacteriostatic.**

Clinical Uses
- Cutaneous disease caused by *M. marinum.*
  - May be used as single agent in minimal disease.
- Follow-on combination therapy for infections with *M. fortuitum.*

Dosing/TDM
- Weight-based dosing is based on the trimethoprim component.
- PO TMP–SMX 1–2 double strength (DS) tablets every 12 hours.
- IV TMP–SMX 8–20 mg (TMP)/kg per day divided over 6–12 hours.
- Requires renal dose adjustment.

Safety
- ADRs
  - Common
    - Gastrointestinal: nausea, diarrhea.
    - Renal: acute tubular necrosis, acute interstitial nephritis, crystalluria; TMP may block creatinine excretion, resulting in increase in SCr without decrease in GFR.
  - Serious
    - Dermatologic: photosensitivity, rash, but can cause life-threatening dermatologic reactions like Stevens–Johnson syndrome and toxic epidermal necrolysis.
    - Hematologic: bone marrow suppression.
    - Hepatotoxicity: jaundice, transient elevation of serum alkaline phosphatase, hepatic necrosis (rare).
    - Hyperkalemia: TMP may reversibly impair renal excretion of potassium causing hyperkalemia.
- Contraindications
  - Glucose-6-phosphate dehydrogenase deficiency.
  - History of drug-induced thrombocytopenia with use of sulfonamides or trimethoprim.
  - Hypersensitivity.
  - Megaloblastic anemia due to folate deficiency.
- Drug interactions
  - Warfarin: (attributed to the sulfonamide component of the combination) increases INR.
  - Rifampin: reduces plasma concentration trimethoprim–sulfamethoxazole
  - Dofetilide: TMP may increase the serum concentration of dofetilide.
- Monitoring: BUN (blood urea nitrogen), SCr, potassium, CBC, skin for rash.

CLINICAL PEARLS
- An expanded understanding of allergic mechanisms indicates cross-reactivity between antibiotic sulfonamides and nonantibiotic sulfonamides may not occur, or at the very least this potential is extremely low. In particular, mechanisms of cross-reaction due to antibody production (anaphylaxis) are unlikely to occur with nonantibiotic sulfonamides and antibiotic sulfonamides.

Isoniazid

Mechanism of Action
- Inhibits synthesis of mycolic acids, a critical component of the lipid-rich mycobacterial cell wall.
- **Bactericidal:** concentration-dependent killing.

Clinical Uses
- Treatment of *M. tuberculosis* infection: **CORE DRUG.**
- **In combination with rifampicin, allows short-course regimens with high cure rates.**

Dosing/TDM
- 90% bioavailability.
- Based on lean body weight.
- 5 mg/kg PO daily (maximum of 300 mg daily).
- 15 mg/kg for once/twice/thrice-weekly regimen (maximum dose: 900 mg/dose).
- Metabolism under genetic control: **hepatic acetylation.**
  - Fast acetylators: may require higher dose for same effect.
  - Slow acetylators: higher risk of toxicity (neuro and hepatic).

Safety
- ADRs: hepatotoxicity (1%–2.7%), neurotoxicity (<0.2%), nausea, vomiting, diarrhea, rash (2%), acute pancreatitis (rare), lupus-like syndrome.
- Contraindications: hypersensitivity including drug-induced hepatitis; **acute liver disease**; previous history of hepatic injury during isoniazid therapy; previous severe adverse reaction (drug fever, chills, arthritis) to isoniazid.
- Drug interactions: isoniazid may increase the serum concentration of fosphenytoin; rifampin may enhance the hepatotoxic effect of isoniazid.
- Monitoring: LFTs.

CLINICAL PEARLS
- Isoniazid penetrates well into tissues and body fluids, including CSF.

Linezolid

Mechanism of Action
- Binds to the 50S ribosomal subunit and inhibits bacterial ribosomal protein synthesis.

Clinical Uses
- Second-line therapy for treatment of *M. tuberculosis* infection.
  - WHO group C.
- Severe pulmonary infections with *M. abscessus* (both initial and maintenance therapy).

Dosing
- 300–600 mg once daily.
  - Lower dose tolerated better in longer-term use.

Safety
- ADRs
  - Common: nausea, vomiting, diarrhea.
  - Serious: hypersensitivity (including rash, angioedema, anaphylaxis), **myelosuppression**, **peripheral and optic neuropathy**, lactic acidosis.

- Contraindications: hypersensitivity to linezolid or any component of the formulation; **concurrent use or within 2 weeks of MAO inhibitors.**
- Drug interactions: may enhance the serotonergic effect of selective serotonin reuptake inhibitors and tricyclic antidepressants.
- Monitoring: CBC (weekly) and visual function in patients requiring ≥3 months of therapy or in patients reporting new visual symptoms.

CLINICAL PEARLS

- The same dose can be prescribed when transitioning from intravenous to oral formulation of linezolid due to 100% bioavailability of the oral formulation.

Macrolides

Agents
- Azithromycin.
- Clarithromycin.

Mechanism of Action
- **Inhibit bacterial protein synthesis by binding to 50S ribosome subunit**; bacteriostatic.

Clinical Uses
- Cornerstone of combination treatment for MAC.
- Prophylaxis against MAC.
- Treatment for atypical mycobacterial infections, especially *M. abscessus,* other rapidly growing microbacteria (RGMs), and rifampin-resistant (RR) *M. kansasii.*
- No longer included among the medicines to be used for the treatment of MDR/RR-TB.

Dosing/TDM
- Azithromycin IV/PO.
  - Primary MAC prophylaxis
    - 1200 mg once weekly or 500 mg daily,
    - combined with ethambutol or rifampin for secondary prophylaxis.
  - Treatment of MAC pulmonary disease (nodular/bronchiectatic disease; in combination): 500 mg three times weekly.
  - Treatment of pulmonary MAC (in combination) to treatment for fibrocavitary MAC lung disease or severe nodular/bronchiectatic disease: 250 mg daily.
- Clarithromycin PO 500 mg every 12 hours in combination with other antimycobacterial agents.
- Require renal dose adjustment.

Safety
- ADRs
  - Common
    - **Gastrointestinal:** significant diarrhea, nausea, and vomiting associated with macrolides.
  - Serious
    - **Hepatotoxicity**: hepatic necrosis, failure, and death have occurred with macrolides. Use with caution in patients with preexisting liver disease, and discontinue immediately with symptoms of hepatitis.

- **QTc prolongation** and ventricular arrhythmias.
- May exacerbate muscle weakness in myasthenia gravis.
- Hypersensitivity reaction: eosinophilia, fever, skin eruptions.
- Hematologic toxicity: leukopenia, thrombocytopenia.
- Contraindications
  - History of cholestatic jaundice or hepatic dysfunction with prior macrolide use.
  - Hypersensitivity.
  - Concomitant use with cisapride, pimozide, ergot alkaloids (e.g., ergotamine, dihydroergotamine), or **HMG-CoA reductase inhibitors** extensively metabolized by CYP3A4 (e.g., lovastatin, simvastatin); concomitant use with **colchicine** in patients with renal or hepatic impairment.
- Drug interactions
  - Metabolized by CYP3A4 (erythromycin > clarithromycin > azithromycin); inhibitors may increase serum concentrations.
  - **Clarithromycin is a potent CYP3A4 inhibitor.** Thus it may increase concentrations of medications metabolized by CYP3A4.
  - QTc-prolonging agents: may enhance QTc-prolonging effect of QTc-prolonging agents.
- Monitoring: LFTs, SCr, CBC, QTc.

CLINICAL PEARLS

- Azithromycin has a relatively long half-life, and its elimination is extremely slow.

Para-aminosalicylic Acid (PAS)

Mechanism of Action
- Structurally related to para-aminobenzoic acid (PABA); its mechanism of action is thought to be similar to the sulfonamides, a competitive antagonism with PABA; bacteriostatic.

Clinical Uses
- Treatment of resistant *M. tuberculosis* infection in combination with other antituberculous medications.
  - WHO group D3.

Dosing
- 8–12 g/day (usually 4 g every 8–12 hours) given in combination with one or more other medications active against *M. tuberculosis.*

Safety
- ADRs
  - Common: gastrointestinal irritation (i.e., nausea, vomiting, abdominal cramps, diarrhea), hypothyroidism.
  - Serious: hypersensitivity reaction (i.e., fever, conjunctivitis, rash, and pruritus), hepatitis, neutropenia, agranulocytosis, renal impairment.
- Contraindications: hypersensitivity to aminosalicylic acid or any component of the formulation; severe renal impairment.

- Drug interactions: probenecid increases the serum levels of para-aminosalicylic acid.
- Monitoring: liver function and thyroid function.

CLINICAL PEARLS

- Frequent dosing of para-aminosalicylic acid is needed to maintain sufficient bacteriostatic concentrations.

Pyrazinamide

Mechanism of Action

- Proposed mechanism of action is that pyrazinamide is converted to pyrazinoic acid in susceptible strains of mycobacteria; however, exact mechanism of action has not been elucidated.
- More active in acidic environment (e.g., inside macrophages) and **against dormant/semi-dormant bacilli.**

Clinical Uses

- First-line therapy for treatment of *M. tuberculosis.*

Dosing/TDM

- Widely distributed in tissues including lung and CSF.
  - Based on lean body weight.
  - 20-30 mg/kg by mouth daily (maximum dose: 2 g).
  - 30–40 mg/kg three times per week (maximum dose: 3 g).
  - or 40-60 mg/kg twice weekly (maximum dose: 4 g) to 40-50 mg/kg twice weekly (maximum dose: 4 g).
  - Adjust dose in renal failure (CrCl <30 mL/min).

Safety

- ADRs: **hepatotoxicity**, asymptomatic hyperuricemia, **polyarthralgia** (40% with daily dosing), anorexia, nausea, flushing, rashes, thrombocytopenia (rare).
- Contraindications: hypersensitivity, acute gout, severe hepatic damage.
- Drug interactions: pyrazinamide may decrease the serum concentration of cyclosporin, pyrazinamide may enhance the hepatotoxic effect of rifampin.
- Monitoring: LFTs, serum uric acid.

CLINICAL PEARLS

- Pyrazinamide freely enters the CSF in patients with tuberculous meningitis.
- Monoresistance to pyrazinamide is uncommon; if found, consider whether *M. bovis* is responsible rather than *M. tuberculosis.*

Rifamycins

Agents

- Rifampin.
- Rifabutin.
- Rifapentine.

Mechanism of Action

- Inhibit the beta-subunit of DNA-dependent RNA polymerase, blocking elongating RNA transcript.
- **Bactericidal:** concentration-dependent killing.

Clinical Uses

- **Rifampin is first-line agent for treatment of all forms of tuberculosis** caused by organisms with known or presumed sensitivity to the drug. **Essential component** of all short-course regimens.
- Rifabutin is used as a substitute for rifampin in the treatment of all forms of tuberculosis caused by organisms that are known or presumed to be susceptible to this agent. It is generally reserved for patients who are receiving any medication having unacceptable **interactions** with rifampin or have experienced intolerance to rifampin.
- Rifapentine may be used **once weekly** with isoniazid in special patient populations.
- Treatment of *M. kansasii* and MAC infection.

Dosing/TDM

- Widely distributed including CSF. Concentrates **intracellularly**, especially in polymorphs. Minimal renal excretion.
- Rifampin
  - Tuberculosis, active (PO, IV)
    - Daily therapy: 10 mg/kg per day (maximum: 600 mg/day).
    - Directly observed therapy (DOT): 10 mg/kg (maximum: 600 mg) administered 2 or 3 times/week.
  - Tuberculosis, latent infection (LTBI)
    - 10 mg/kg daily (maximum: 600 mg/day) for 4 months.
- Rifabutin
  - Oral.
  - MAC disease (disseminated) in people with HIV
    - Primary prophylaxis (patients with CD4 count <50 cells/µL) and treatment: 300 mg once daily
  - Tuberculosis: 5 mg/kg daily, usually 300 mg/day
- Rifapentine
  - Rifapentin PO 10-20 mg/kg once weekly.
- Tuberculosis, latent infection (LTBI)
  - Use once weekly for 3 months.
  - **Must be administered under DOT and given in combination with isoniazid** (maximum dose: 900 mg).
    - 25.1 to 32 kg: 600 mg.
    - 32.1 to 50 kg: 750 mg.
    - >50 kg: 900 mg.

Safety

- ADRs: nausea, **rash** (up to 6% with RIF), **hepatotoxicity** (1%–2.7%), hemolytic anemia, leukopenia, **thrombocytopenia** (especially with high-dose therapy), acute renal failure.
- Contraindications: hypersensitivity; concurrent use of many protease inhibitors.
- Drug interactions
  - Inducers of CYP3A4 and CYP2, CYP2C19 and CYPD6 to a lesser extent.
  - **Potency of enzyme inducers: rifampin > rifapentine > rifabutin.**
  - Be mindful of the potential of drug–drug interactions between **macrolide antibiotics, azole anti-fungal agents, caspofungin, oral contraceptives, methadone, protease inhibitors, corticosteroids, and benzodiazepine.**
  - Warfarin: monitor INR, may require 2- to 3-fold dose increase of warfarin.
- Monitoring: SCr/BUN, LFTs, CBC.

CLINICAL PEARLS

- Rifampin achieves extensive distribution into tissues and body fluids, including urine and tears, resulting in an **orange-red discoloration** of these body fluids.
- Rifabutin has a **narrower** induction spectrum and weaker CYP3A4 induction than rifampin.

Tetracyclines and Glycylcyclines

Agents
- Doxycycline.
- Minocycline.
- Tigecycline (glycylcycline).

Mechanism of Action
- Inhibit protein synthesis by binding to bacterial 30S ribosome subunits; **bacteriostatic.**

Clinical Uses
- Treatment of *M. leprae* infection.
- Combination therapy of NTM infections especially RGMs and *M. marinum*.

Dosing/TDM
- Doxycycline IV/PO 100 mg every 12 hours.
- Minocycline IV/PO dosing to *M. leprae*: 100 mg by mouth daily and for *M. marinum*: 100 mg PO every 12 hours.
- Tigecycline IV 100 mg ×1 dose followed by 50 mg every 12 hours.
  - Requires hepatic adjustment.

Safety
- ADRs: photosensitivity, nausea, vomiting, dental staining, tissue hyperpigmentation; vestibular toxicity (minocycline), pill-associated esophagitis (doxycycline), intracranial hypertension (doxycycline).
  - Tigecycline: nausea, vomiting, hepatotoxicity, pancreatitis.
- Contraindications: **pregnant women and children <8 years old** due to teeth discoloration and concern for accumulation in developing teeth and long tubular bones; hypersensitivity.
- Drug interactions
  - **Co-administration of atazanavir** and minocycline may lead to decrease in atazanavir plasma concentrations.
  - Tigecycline may increase serum concentrations of warfarin.
  - Calcium, iron, multivitamins with minerals, antacids, and dairy: **tetracyclines chelate with divalent cations, significantly decreasing bioavailability.** Separate by at least 2 hours.

- Tetracycline is a substrate of CYP3A4; concentrations may be altered with concomitant administration of CYP3A4 inducers or inhibitors.
- Monitoring: SCr, LFTs.

CLINICAL PEARLS

- Documentation of allergenic cross-reactivity between tigecycline and tetracyclines is limited. However, because of similarities in chemical structure and/or pharmacologic actions, the **possibility of cross-sensitivity cannot be ruled out with certainty.**

Further Reading and Resources

1. Centers for Disease Control and Prevention. Core curriculum on tuberculosis: What the clinician should know. Chapter 6: Treatment of tuberculosis disease. https://www.cdc.gov/tb/education/corecurr/pdf/chapter6.pdf.
2. Centers for Disease Control and Prevention. *Treatment of Tuberculosis*, June 2003, https://www.cdc.gov/mmwr/preview/mmwrhtml/rr5211a1.htm.
3. Grayson, M. Lindsay, et al. Kucers' the use of antibiotics: a clinical review of antibacterial, antifungal, antiparasitic, and antiviral drugs. Boca Raton, FL, Taylor & Francis Group, 2018.
4. Griffith DE, Aksamit T, Brown-Elliott BA, et al. An official ATS/IDSA statement: diagnosis, treatment and prevention of non-tuerculous mycobacterial diseases. *Am J Respir Crit Care Med* 2007;175(4):367-416.
5. IDSA (Infectious Diseases Society of America) Guidelines. Treatment of drug-susceptible tuberculosis; and diagnosis, treatment and prevention of NTM disease. https://www.idsociety.org/practice-guideline/practice-guidelines/#/date_na_dt/DESC/0/+/.
6. Lee M, Lee J, Carroll MW, et al. Linezolid for treamtent of chronic extensively drug-resistant tuberculosis. *N Engl J Med* 2012;367(16):1508-18.
7. Lexi-Comp, Inc. (Lexi-Drugs). Lexi-Comp, Inc.; July 17, 2019.
8. Nahid P, Dorman SE, Alipaanh N, et al. Executive Summary: Official American Thoracic Society/Centers for Disease Control and Prevention/Infectious Diseases Society of America Clinical Practice Guidelines: Treatment of Drug-Susceptible Tuberculosis. *Clin Infect Dis* 2016;63(7):853-67.
9. NICE (National Institute for Health and Clinical Excellence) Guidelines: Tuberculosis – clinical diagnosis and management of tuberculosis, and measures for its prevention and control. Clinical guideline [CG117]. https://www.nice.org.uk/guidance/cg117.
10. TB drug monograph: http://www.tbdrugmonographs.co.uk/.
11. WHO (World Health Organization). *Treatment Guidelines for Drug-Resistant Tuberculosis*. Geneva: WHO; 2016.

7
Antifungal Agents

ALEXANDRIA WILSON

Antifungal Pharmacokinetic and Pharmacodynamic Principles

Pharmacokinetics (PK)
- Absorption, distribution, metabolism, excretion – variable, see individual antifungal agents.

Pharmacodynamics (PD)
- Susceptibility
  - Minimum inhibitory concentration (MIC).
  - *Candida albicans* clinical breakpoints for fluconazole.
    - Susceptible MIC <2.
    - Susceptible dose-dependent MIC 4.
    - Resistant MIC >8.
  - Fungicidal.
    - Amphotericin B.
    - Echinocandins (*Candida*).
  - Fungistatic.
    - Azoles.
    - Flucytosine.
    - Echinocandins (*Aspergillus*).
- PD targets
  - Area under the curve (AUC)/MIC.
    - Azoles.
    - Flucytosine.
    - Echinocandins.
  - Maximum concentration (C_{max}):MIC.
    - Amphotericin B.

ANTIFUNGAL CLASSES

Allylamines

Mechanism of Action
- Inhibits squalene epoxidase, leading to decreased ergosterol; see Fig. 7.1 for site of action.

Terbinafine
Spectrum
- Narrow.

Clinical Uses
- Onychomycosis.
- Dermatophytes.
- Sporotrichosis (cutaneous and lymphocutaneous).
Dosing/TDM
- Onychomycosis and dermatophytes: 250 mg PO once daily.
  - Duration
    - Variable, depending upon infection.
    - Typically weeks to months.
    - Onychomycosis of fingernail: 6 weeks.
    - Onychomycosis of toenail: 12 weeks.
- Sporotrichosis: 500 mg PO twice daily for 2–4 weeks following lesion resolution.
Safety
- Adverse drug reactions (ADRs): headache.
- Contraindications: chronic or active liver disease.
- Drug interactions: moderate CYP450 2D6 inhibitor.

> **CLINICAL PEARL**
> - Not for systemic fungal infections.

Polyenes

Agents
- Amphotericin B.
- Nystatin.
Mechanism of Action
- Binds to fungal cell membrane sterols, which increases cell permeability leading to the leakage of intracellular contents; see Fig. 7.1 for site of action.

Amphotericin B
Spectrum
- Wide.
- Yeasts: *Candida* spp. (except *C. lusitaniae* and *C. guilliermondii*) and *Cryptococcus*.
- Molds: *Aspergillus* (except *A. terreus*), *Fusarium*, and *Mucorales*.

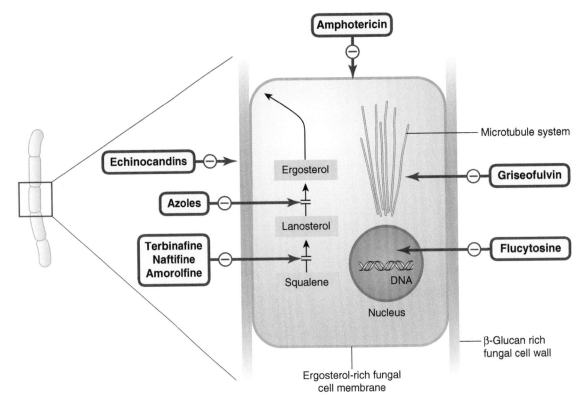

• Fig. 7.1 Sites of action of common antifungal drugs. Fungi are morphologically very diverse organisms, and this diagram of a "typical" fungus is not intended to be technically accurate. The principal sites of action of the main antifungal agents mentioned in this chapter *(in red-bordered boxes)* are indicated as shown. (From Antifungal drugs. In: Rang HP, Ritter JM, Flower RJ, Henderson G. *Rang & Dale's Pharmacology*. 8th ed. Elsevier; 2016.)

- Dimorphic fungi: *Blastomyces, Coccidioides,* and *Histoplasmosis.*
  Clinical Uses
- Recommended agent in clinical treatment guidelines for cryptococcosis, histoplasmosis, coccidioidomycosis, candidiasis, and blastomycosis, especially in severe or disseminated cases.
- Alternative agent for the treatment of aspergillosis.
  Dosing/TDM
- Conventional
  - Amphotericin B deoxycholate 0.5–1 mg/kg daily IV.
  - Lipid formulations (drug is incorporated into phospholipid bilayer membrane).
    - Amphotericin B lipid complex 5 mg/kg daily IV.
    - Liposomal amphotericin B 3–5 mg/kg daily IV.
  Safety
- ADRs
  - Nephrotoxicity.
  - Infusion-related reactions.
  - Potassium and magnesium wasting.
  - Anemia.
  - ADRs are reduced with all lipid formulations compared to the conventional formulation.
- Drug interactions: concomitant nephrotoxic medications.
- Monitoring: Serum creatinine (SCr), potassium, magnesium, hemoglobin (Hgb), hematocrit (Hct).

CLINICAL PEARL

- Conventional amphotericin B deoxycholate is no longer used systemically secondary to high incidence of ADRs.
- May attempt to minimize nephrotoxicity and infusion-related reactions by administering normal saline pre- and post-infusion and administering acetaminophen and diphenhydramine pre-infusion.
- May be the drug of choice for the treatment of a fungal infection in a pregnant woman.

Nystatin
  Spectrum
- *Candida.*
  Clinical Uses
- Oropharyngeal candidiasis.
  Dosing/TDM
- 400,000–600,000 units four times daily: swish and swallow.
  - Retain in mouth as long as possible before swallowing (several minutes).

CLINICAL PEARL

- Not for systemic fungal infections.

Nucleoside Analogs

Mechanism of Action

- Inhibits DNA synthesis by acting as a pyrimidine analog; see Fig. 7.1 for site of action.

Flucytosine

Spectrum
- *Candida* spp. and *Cryptococcus.*

Clinical Uses
- In combination with amphotericin B in the induction phase of treatment for cryptococcal meningitis.

Dosing/TDM
- Dose: 50–150 mg/kg daily PO divided into 4 doses and given every 6 hours.
- TDM: goal peaks (2 hour post-dose) and troughs 30–80 µg/mL.
  - 3–5 days following initiation of therapy.

Safety
- ADRs
  - Bone marrow suppression: leukopenia, thrombocytopenia and/or pancytopenia.
  - Gastrointestinal (GI): nausea, vomiting, diarrhea, abdominal pain.
  - Hepatotoxicity.
- Drug interactions
  - Concomitant nephrotoxic medications may increase flucytosine serum concentration.
- Monitoring
  - CBC, CMP, serum peaks and troughs.

CLINICAL PEARL

- Adjust dose in the setting of renal insufficiency.
- Do not use as monotherapy due to resistance development.

Azoles (Imidazoles and Triazoles)

Mechanism of Action
- Binds 14-alpha demethylase, which inhibits the synthesis of ergosterol from lanosterol during cell membrane production; see Fig. 7.1 for site of action.

Imidazoles

Agents
- Clotrimazole.
- Miconazole.

Spectrum
- *Candida.*

Clinical Uses
- Oropharyngeal candidiasis.

PK/PD
- Nonabsorbed.

Dosing/TDM
- Clotrimazole troches or lozenges 10 mg.
  - Treatment: five times per day.
  - Prophylaxis: three times per day.
- Miconazole buccal tablets 50 mg once daily.
  - Apply to upper gum area.

Safety
- ADRs
  - Clotrimazole: abnormal liver function tests.
  - Miconazole: application site reactions.

CLINICAL PEARL

- Not for systemic treatment.

Triazoles

Agents
- Itraconazole.
- Fluconazole.
- Voriconazole.
- Posaconazole.
- Isavuconazonium sulfate (prodrug of isavuconazole).

Spectrum
- Yeasts
  - *Candida* spp. (except *C. krusei* and some resistance to *C. glabrata*).
  - *Cryptococcus.*
- Molds
  - *Aspergillus* (except fluconazole).
  - *Fusarium* (except fluconazole).
  - Posaconazole and isavuconazonium sulfate have activity against *Mucorales.*
- Dimorphic fungi
  - *Blastomyces.*
  - *Coccidioides.*
  - *Histoplasma.*

Clinical Uses
- Fluconazole is the drug of choice for the consolidation and maintenance phases for the treatment of cryptococcal meningitis, cryptococcal infections at other sites of the body, and fungal urinary tract infections.
- Itraconazole is a recommended treatment for histoplasmosis, blastomycosis, and coccidioidomycosis.
- Voriconazole is the recommended treatment for aspergillosis.

Dosing
- Itraconazole 200–400 mg/day
  - Load: 200 mg PO three times daily for 3 days.
  - Maintenance: 200 mg PO twice daily.
- Fluconazole 100–800 mg/day IV or PO (dose is determined by indication).
- Voriconazole
  - Load: 6 mg/kg IV or 400 mg PO every 12 hours for 2 doses.
  - Maintenance: 4 mg/kg IV or 200 mg PO every 12 hours.

- Posaconazole
  - Suspension: 200–400 mg PO two to four times daily.
  - Delayed release (DR) tablets and IV.
    - Load: 300 mg twice daily for 1 day.
    - Maintenance: 300 mg once daily.
- Isavuconazonium sulfate
  - 1 capsule = 186 mg isavuconazonium sulfate = 100 mg isavuconazole.
    - Load: 372 mg isavuconazonium sulfate PO or IV every 8 hours for 6 doses.
    - Maintenance: 372 mg once daily PO or IV beginning 12–24 hours after last loading dose.

TDM
- Itraconazole
  - Goal 1–10 µg/mL.
  - Sum of itraconazole and major active metabolite hydroxyitraconazole.
  - Trough 7 days following initiation.
  - Once steady state is achieved, clinically significant variations in serum concentration is unlikely.
- Voriconazole
  - Goal trough 1 or 2–5.5 mcg/mL.
  - 5–7 days following initiation.
- Posaconazole suspension (no TDM for DR tabs or IV formulations)
  - Goal treatment trough: >1.25 µg/mL.
  - Goal prophylaxis trough: >0.7 µg/mL.
  - Trough following 7 days of therapy.

Safety
- ADRs
  - All azoles
    - Hepatotoxicity: increased transaminases or hepatitis.
    - GI: nausea, vomiting, diarrhea (especially itraconazole solution).
    - QT prolongation (except isavuconazonium sulfate, which may shorten the QT interval).
  - Itraconazole
    - Heart failure/cardiomyopathy.
  - Voriconazole
    - Central nervous system and visual disturbances.
    - Dermatological: photosensitivity, cutaneous malignancy.
  - Isavuconazole
    - Shorten QT interval.
- Contraindications
  - Avoid IV voriconazole if creatinine clearance (CrCl) <50 due to vehicle cyclodextrin accumulation.
- Drug interactions
  - Proton pump inhibitors, histamine 2-receptor antagonists, and antacids will inhibit the absorption of itraconazole capsules and posaconazole suspension.
  - Cytochrome P450 (CYP) interactions
    - Itraconazole: CYP450 3A4 substrate and inhibitor.
    - Fluconazole: CYP450 2C8/9, 2C19, and 3A4 inhibitor.
    - Voriconazole: CYP450 2C8/9, 2C19, and 3A4 substrate and inhibitor.
    - Posaconazole: CYP450 3A4 inhibitor and p-glycoprotein (p-gp) substrate and inhibitor.
    - Isavuconazole: CYP450 3A4 substrate and inhibitor and p-pg inhibitor.
  - Concomitant agents that prolong QT interval.
- Monitoring: nausea, vomiting, diarrhea, ECG, ALT, AST.

CLINICAL PEARL
- Fluconazole is renally eliminated.
  - Requires dosing adjustments in the setting of renal insufficiency.
  - Appropriate for the treatment of a fungal UTI.
- Itraconazole capsules have poor bioavailability.
- Posaconazole DR oral and IV formulations are not interchangeable with oral suspension.
- Azoles are teratogenic.
- Ketoconazole no longer has a role in the treatment of systemic fungal infections.

Echinocandins

Agents
- Caspofungin.
- Micafungin.
- Anidulafungin.

Mechanism of Action
- Inhibit the synthesis of beta 1,3-D glucan by inhibiting BD synthase, a cell wall component; see Fig. 7.1 for site of action.

Spectrum
- *Candida* spp. (less active against *C. parapsilosis*) and *Aspergillus*.

Clinical Uses
- Echinocandins are recommended for the treatment of candidiasis.

PK/PD
- Good tissue penetration, but negligible concentrations in cerebrospinal fluid.
- Negligible concentrations in urine and not dialyzable.

Dosing/TDM
- Dosing
  - Caspofungin.
    - Load: 70 mg IV once.
    - Maintenance: 50 mg IV once daily.
  - Micafungin 100 mg IV once daily.
  - Anidulafungin.
    - Load: 200 mg IV once.
    - Maintenance: 100 mg IV once daily.

Safety
- ADRs
  - Increased transaminases.
  - Histamine-mediated reactions.
- Drug interactions
  - No CYP450 or p–gp interactions.

- Caspofungin: cyclosporine and inducers.
- Micafungin: sirolimus, nifedipine, and itraconazole.
- Monitoring
  - ALT, AST, alkaline phosphatase, flushing, itching.

CLINICAL PEARL

- Echinocandins are not available in an oral formulation.

Further Reading

1. Kauffman CA, Bustamante B, Chapman SW, Pappas PG. Clinical practice guidelines for the management of sporotrichosis: 2007 update by the Infectious Diseases Society of America. *Clin Infect Dis*. 2007;45(10):1255–1265.
2. Pappas PG, Kauffman CA, Andes DR, et al. Clinical practice guideline for the management of candidiasis: 2016 update by the Infectious Diseases Society of America. *Clin Infect Dis*. 2016;62(4):1–e50.
3. Perfect JR, Dismukes WE, Dromer F, et al. Clinical practice guidelines for the management of cryptococcal disease: 2010 update by the Infectious Diseases Society of America. *Clin Infect Dis*. 2010;50(3):291–322.
4. Wheat LJ, Freifeld AG, Kleiman MB, et al. Clinical Practice guidelines for the management of patients with histoplasmosis: 2007 update by the Infectious Diseases Society of America. *Clin Infect Dis*. 2007;45(7):807–825.
5. Chapman SW, Dismukes WE, Proia LA, et al. Clinical practice guidelines for the management of blastomycosis: 2008 update by the Infectious Diseases Society of America. *Clin Infect Dis*. 2008;46(12):1810–1812.
6. Galgiani JN, Ampel NM, Blair JE. Clinical practice guidelines for the treatment of coccidioidomycosis: 2016 update by the Infectious Diseases Society of America. *Clin Infect Dis*. 2016;63(6):e112–e146.
7. Patterson TF, Thompson III GR, Denning JA, et al. Practice guidelines for the diagnosis and management of aspergillosis: 2016 update by the Infectious Diseases Society of America. *Clin Infect Dis*. 2016;63(4):e1–e60.

8

Antivirals

ANDRES BRAN, JESSICA K. ORTWINE

Antiviral Drugs Against the Herpesviruses (Herpes Simplex Virus, Varicella-Zoster Virus, and Cytomegalovirus)

- Medications are grouped by active agent and prodrug, when available.
- Mechanism of action is summarized in Fig. 8.1.

Acyclic Guanosine Analogs

Aciclovir and Valaciclovir

Spectrum
- Herpes simplex virus 1 and 2 (HSV-1, HSV-2) and varicella-zoster virus (VZV); the acyclic guanosine analogs have a tighter binding affinity to HSV than VZV, and therefore VZV infections require higher doses.

Mechanism of Action
- Competes with deoxyguanosine triphosphate to inhibit viral DNA polymerase and block viral DNA synthesis.

Mechanisms of Resistance
- Most common: low or absent production of viral thymidine kinase (TK).
- Less common: altered TK activity (i.e., selective phosphorylation of thymidine and not aciclovir) or DNA polymerase mutations.

Safety
- Adverse effects
  - Intravenous aciclovir: phlebitis/inflammation upon infusion due to alkaline solution, neurotoxicity manifesting as lethargy, confusion, tremor/myoclonus, agitation, hallucinations, extrapyramidal symptoms and clouding of consciousness, and crystalline nephropathy leading to nephrotoxicity.
    - Dosing based on ideal body weight with appropriate adjustments for renal function minimizes the risk of both neuro- and nephrotoxicity.
    - Maintaining adequate hydration prior to infusion also minimizes risk of nephrotoxicity.
  - Oral aciclovir: rarely causes nausea, diarrhea, rash, and headache.

  - Valaciclovir: well tolerated at recommended doses.
- Drug interactions
- Aciclovir and valaciclovir may increase serum concentrations of zidovudine, leading to increased somnolence and lethargy.
- Concomitant use of aciclovir with other nephrotoxic agents may increase risk for nephrotoxicity.

Other Key Concepts
- Aciclovir oral absorption is poor and should be avoided for the treatment of systemic viral infections.
- Oral administration of the prodrug valaciclovir achieves 3–5 times higher systemic concentrations of aciclovir than administering oral aciclovir and is the preferred oral formulation.

Famciclovir

Spectrum
- Active against HSV-1, HSV-2 and VZV.

Mechanism of Action
- Competes with deoxyguanosine triphosphate to inhibit viral DNA polymerase and block viral DNA synthesis.

Mechanisms of Resistance
- Mutations in viral TK or DNA polymerase.
- HSV isolates resistant to aciclovir due to the absence of TK are also resistant to famciclovir.

Safety
- Adverse effects:
  - Common: headache, nausea, fatigue, and diarrhea.
  - Rare: neutropenia, elevated transaminases, urticarial rash, and confusion.
- Drug interactions: no clinically significant drug interactions.

Ganciclovir and Valganciclovir

Spectrum
- Active against HSV-1, HSV-2, and VZV, but primarily reserved for cytomegalovirus (CMV) infection.

Mechanism of Action
- Competes with deoxyguanosine triphosphate to inhibit viral DNA polymerase and block viral DNA synthesis.

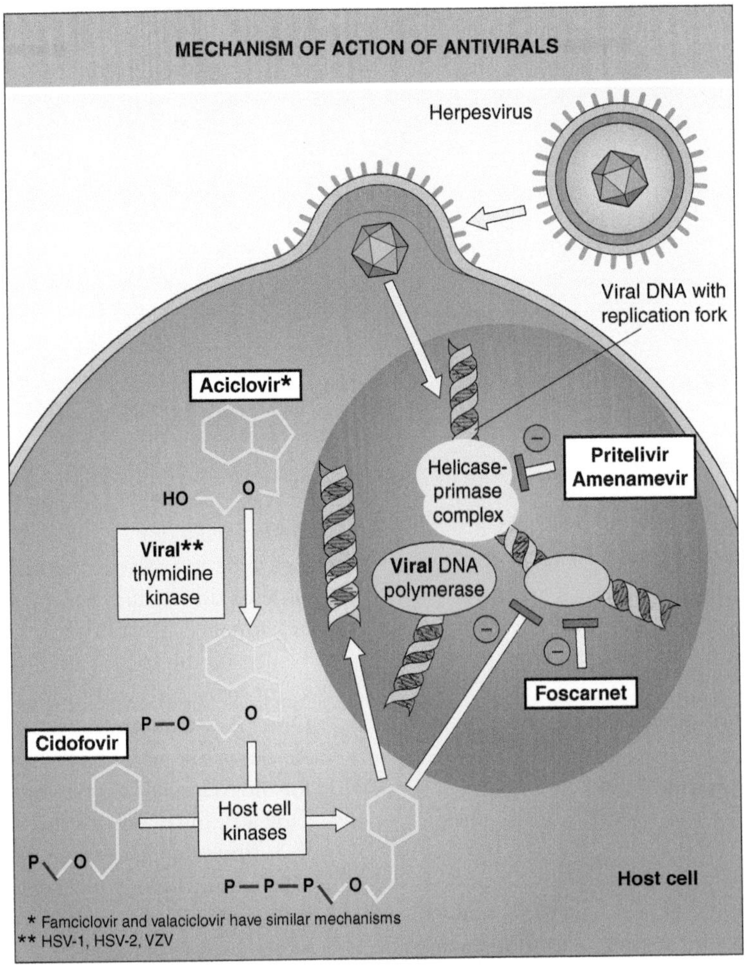

MECHANISM OF ACTION OF ANTIVIRALS

• **Fig. 8.1** Aciclovir is a synthetic purine nucleoside analog (similar in chemical structure to deoxyguanosine) that has a high affinity for HSV-1, HSV-2, and VZV thymidine kinase, which phosphorylates and activates the drug. Human cellular guanylate kinase then phosphorylates aciclovir twice to transform it into aciclovir triphosphate, which blocks viral DNA synthesis by competitively inhibiting and inactivating viral DNA polymerase and by becoming irreversibly incorporated into the viral DNA chain, causing DNA chain termination. Valaciclovir, penciclovir, and famciclovir have similar mechanisms of action. Cidofovir is an acyclic nucleoside phosphate analog of deoxycytosine monophosphate that does not require viral thymidine kinase to become activated but otherwise also has a similar mechanism. Foscarnet, an inorganic pyrophosphate analog, selectively inhibits viral DNA polymerase by blocking its pyrophosphate binding sites. Helicase-primase inhibitors (pritelivir, amenamevir) block DNA unwinding at the replication fork and synthesis of primers during viral replication. These agents have *in vitro* activity against HSV-1/2 and had promising results in early clinical trials, but their development in the United States has been suspended due to potential adverse effects. (From Bolognia JL, Schaffer JV, Cerroni L, eds. *Dermatology.* 4th ed. Elsevier; 2018.)

Mechanisms of Resistance

- *UL97* gene mutation
  - Most common resistance mechanism.
  - Occurs prior to *UL54* gene mutation.
  - Leads to deficiency in viral kinase responsible for ganciclovir phosphorylation/activation.
  - Cidofovir and foscarnet usually retain efficacy.
- *UL54* gene mutation
  - Often clinically observed as co-existing with *UL97* gene mutation.
  - Results in changes to the viral DNA polymerase.
  - Cross-resistance to cidofovir is common, cross-resistance to foscarnet is rare but possible.
  - HSV isolates resistant to aciclovir due to the absence of TK are also resistant to ganciclovir.

Safety

- Adverse effects:
  - Common: neutropenia and thrombocytopenia; often dose-limiting and may be ameliorated by administration of colony-stimulating factor.
  - Rare: headache, confusion, psychosis, anemia, rash, and elevated transaminases.
  - Ganciclovir is considered possibly teratogenic, and breastfeeding should be avoided while receiving either agent.
- Drug interactions:
  - Concomitant administration of either agent with imipenem–cilastatin should be avoided due to the increased risk of seizures.

- Concomitant administration of either agent with zidovudine should be avoided due to an increased risk of hematologic toxicity.
- Renal dysfunction may occur in patients receiving either agent in combination with other known nephrotoxins.

Other Key Concepts

- Oral administration of valganciclovir 900 mg achieves nearly identical serum concentrations to ganciclovir 5 mg/kg IV.

Acyclic Nucleoside Phosphonate Analogs

Cidofovir and Brincidofovir

Spectrum

- Primarily reserved for ganciclovir-resistant CMV infection (*UL97* mutation).
- Effective against HSV and VZV, including aciclovir-resistant isolates.

Mechanism of Action

- Competes with deoxycytidine triphosphate to inhibit viral DNA polymerase and blocks viral DNA synthesis.

Mechanism of Resistance

- Highly ganciclovir-resistant CMV isolates with *UL54* mutations in DNA polymerase show cross-resistance to cidofovir.

Safety

- Adverse effects
  - Common: nephrotoxicity and neutropenia with cidofovir.
  - Administration of probenecid and maintaining adequate hydration minimizes risk of nephrotoxicity.
  - Initiation not recommended if serum creatinine (SCr) >1.5 mg/dL, creatinine clearance (CrCl) ≤55 mL/min or ≥2+ proteinuria.
  - Considered possibly carcinogenic and teratogenic based on animal studies.
  - Brincidofovir is not transported into renal tubular cells and has not been associated with nephrotoxicity.
- Drug interactions: concomitant usage of cidofovir with other nephrotoxins is contraindicated.

Other Key Concepts

- Concomitant administration of cidofovir with probenecid is recommended to prevent rapid renal elimination.

Pyrophosphate Analogs

Foscarnet

Spectrum

- Primarily reserved for ganciclovir-resistant CMV infection (*UL97* and/or certain *UL54* mutations).
- Effective against HSV and VZV, including aciclovir-resistant isolates.

Mechanism of Action

- Inhibits pyrophosphate binding on viral DNA polymerases and suppresses viral replication.

Mechanisms of Resistance

- Can occur secondary to some, but not all, *UL54* mutations.

Safety

- Adverse effects
  - Most common: nephrotoxicity; often dose-limiting and risk may be minimized by ensuring adequate hydration before and during infusion.
  - Frequent
    - Electrolyte abnormalities (hypocalcemia, hypomagnesemia, hypokalemia, hypophosphatemia).
    - CNS effects (dystonia, headache, seizures, tremor, irritability, and hallucinations).
    - Fever, rash, diarrhea, and nausea.
- Drug interactions
  - Concomitant use with other nephrotoxic agents may increase risk for nephrotoxicity.
  - Concomitant use with calcineurin inhibitors (cyclosporine and tacrolimus) may cause neurotoxicity.
  - Concomitant use with zidovudine increases risk for anemia.

CMV Terminase Complex Inhibitor

Letermovir

Spectrum

- Only active against CMV (no activity against any other herpesviruses).

Mechanism of Action

- Inhibits the CMV terminase complex (novel mechanism of action). The function of the terminase complex is to cleave the long DNA chain produced during CMV replication into single units of functional CMV DNA.

Mechanisms of Resistance

- Because of its novel mechanism of action, it is speculated that there should be little to no cross-resistance with current anti-CMV drugs.

Safety

- Adverse effects:
  - Most common
    - Gastrointestinal (GI) upset (nausea, diarrhea, vomiting, and abdominal pain).
    - Peripheral edema, cough, headache and fatigue.
- Drug interactions
  - Concomitant use with statins increases their toxicity.
  - Concomitant use with cyclosporine may increase concentrations of both drugs (close monitoring recommended).

Other Key Concepts

- FDA has only approved it for **prophylaxis** of CMV infection and disease in adult CMV-seropositive recipients of an allogeneic hematopoietic stem cell transplant.
- *In vitro* data suggest that the barrier to resistance is low.
- No dosage adjustment necessary with CrCl >10mL/min.

Antiviral Drugs Against Influenza A and B and Other Respiratory Viruses

Neuraminidase Inhibitors

Oseltamivir

Spectrum
- Treatment and prevention of influenza A and B.

Mechanism of Action
- Binds to viral neuraminidase and prevents the release of new virions from infected cells.

Mechanism of Resistance
- Uncommon, but can occur secondary to neuraminidase mutations.
- More frequent among influenza A.
- Can occur while on therapy.

Safety
- Adverse effects
  - Common: transient nausea, vomiting, and abdominal pain.
  - Rare: abnormal neuropsychiatric events including delirium, abnormal behavior, and hallucinations.
- Drug interactions: no clinically significant drug interactions.

Other Key Concepts
- Treatment should start within 48 hours of disease onset for greatest benefit.
- Treatment after 48 hours is of questionable benefit but is commonly used in hospitalized patients.
- Preferred antiviral for treatment of pregnant women.

Peramivir

Spectrum
- Influenza A and B.

Mechanism of Action
- Binds to viral neuraminidase and prevents the release of new virions from infected cells.

Mechanism of Resistance
- Uncommon, but can occur secondary to neuraminidase mutations.

Safety
- Adverse effects
  - Common: diarrhea, nausea, vomiting, and leukopenia.
  - Rare: serious skin reactions and sporadic, transient neuropsychiatric events including delirium and self-injury.
- Drug interactions: no clinically significant drug interactions.

Other Key Concepts
- Commercially available as intravenous formulation only.
  - FDA approved as one-time dose; however, it has not been studied in severely ill patients, and this regimen should not be used in this population.

Zanamivir

Spectrum
- Treatment and prevention of influenza A and B.

Mechanism of Action
- Binds to viral neuraminidase and prevents the release of new virions from infected cells.

Mechanism of Resistance
- Uncommon, but can occur secondary to neuraminidase mutations.
- Can occur while on therapy.
- May retain activity against some oseltamivir- and peramivir-resistant isolates.

Safety
- Adverse effects: acute bronchospasm, headache, and GI symptoms.
- Drug interactions: no clinically significant drug interactions.

Other Key Concepts
- Commercially available as inhalation only.
- Not recommended for people with breathing problems like asthma or COPD because of the risk for bronchospasm due to route of administration.

Matrix 2 Inhibitors

Amantadine

Spectrum
- Treatment and prevention of influenza A only.

Mechanism of Action
- Blocks the transport of hydrogen ions through the M2 protein channel into the interior of the influenza A virion, preventing viral uncoating and replication.

Mechanism of Resistance
- M2 protein mutations occur commonly during therapy.
- M2 protein mutations confer cross-resistance to rimantadine.

Safety
- Adverse effects
  - Mild neurologic symptoms (anxiety, insomnia, dizziness, headache).
  - GI upset.
- Drug interactions
  - Concomitant use with antihistamines, anticholinergics, and antipsychotics may increase risk for CNS adverse effects.
  - Concomitant use with trimethoprim–sulfamethoxazole or triamterene–hydrochlorothiazide may increase CNS toxicity due to decreased clearance of amantadine.

Other Key Concepts
- Not currently recommended for treatment or prophylaxis of influenza A due to **widespread resistance.**

Rimantadine

Spectrum
- Treatment and prevention of influenza A only.

Mechanism of Action
- Blocks the transport of hydrogen ions through the M2 protein channel into the interior of the influenza A virion, preventing viral uncoating and replication.

Mechanisms of Resistance
- M2 protein mutations occur commonly during therapy.
- Not currently recommended for treatment or prophylaxis of influenza A due to **widespread resistance.**

- M2 protein mutations confer cross-resistance to amantadine.
  Safety
- Adverse effects:
- Uncommon when given for 5-day treatment course, more common when used for longer durations or in elderly patients.
- Mild neurologic symptoms, less severe and frequent than amantadine.
- GI upset.
- Drug interactions
  - Concomitant use with antihistamines, anticholinergics, and antipsychotics may increase risk for CNS adverse effects.
  - Concomitant use with trimethoprim–sulfamethoxazole or triamterene–hydrochlorothiazide may increase CNS toxicity due to decreased clearance of rimantadine.
  Other Key Concepts
- Not currently recommended for treatment or prophylaxis of influenza A due to **widespread resistance**.

Polymerase Inhibitors

Ribavirin

Spectrum
- Broad activity against both DNA and RNA viruses.
- Primarily used for respiratory syncytial virus and hepatitis C.

Mechanisms of Action
- Multiple mechanisms of action, not all well understood.
- Ribavirin monophosphate interferes with synthesis of guanosine triphosphate, leading to a decline in viral protein synthesis.
- Ribavirin triphosphate directly inhibits viral mRNA by interfering with nucleotide binding, leading to decrease viral replication or production of defective virions.

Mechanism of resistance
- Not documented in respiratory viruses.

Safety
- Adverse effects
- Uncommon when given for 5-day treatment course, more common when used for longer durations or in elderly patients.
- Systemic ribavirin: anemia, bilirubinemia, increases in serum iron and uric acid, pruritus, myalgia, rash, nausea, depression, and nervousness.
- Inhaled ribavirin: conjunctival irritation, rash, bronchospasm, and reversible decrease in pulmonary function.
- Drug interactions
  - Concomitant use with didanosine may increase levels of didanosine.
  - Concomitant use with zidovudine or interferon-alpha may increase levels of ribavirin.

Other Key Concepts
- Mutagenic, gonadotoxic, and teratogenic.
- Pregnancy category X.

- Contraception is recommended for at least 6 months after discontinuation of treatment or exposure.
- Healthcare workers that are pregnant should avoid entering the room of a patient receiving inhaled ribavirin.
- Inhaled and oral formulations have similar efficacy for RSV, but inhaled formulation is significantly more expensive.

Antiviral Drugs Against Hepatitis Viruses

Antivirals for Hepatitis B

There are seven FDA-approved drugs to treat chronic HBV infection. Treatment usually consists of **entecavir** or **tenofovir**. Lamivudine, adefovir, and telbivudine are used less often because of development of resistance with chronic use.

Interferons

Spectrum
- HIB, HCV, and HPV (intralesional).

Mechanism of Action
- Binds to host cells' interferon receptors, which causes upregulation of many genes responsible for the production of proteins with antiviral activity.

Safety
- Adverse effects
  - Most common side effect is an **influenza-like syndrome.**
  - At higher doses neurotoxicity (avoid in persons with neuropsychiatric conditions), hepatotoxicity, and retinopathy.

Other Key Concepts
- Cannot be used with decompensated liver disease. Clears HBeAg in about 20%–25% of cases. The "ideal" candidate will be a young patient without cirrhosis, elevated ALT levels, a relatively low HBV DNA level, and with the ability to tolerate its side effects.

Lamivudine[a]

Spectrum
- HBV and HIV.

Mechanism of Action
- Nucleoside analog, triphosphate form inhibits viral polymerase and by competing with dCTP inhibits DNA synthesis.

Mechanisms of Resistance. *YMDD* mutation in the polymerase gene occurs in about 70% of patients with its prolonged use (>5 years) and renders the virus resistant.

Safety
- Adverse effects: lactic acidosis, hepatic steatosis: **severe exacerbation of liver disease** can occur on discontinuance.

Other Key Concepts
- Must exclude co-infection with HIV prior to starting this formulation, dose is lower than HIV dose.

---

[a]In persons co-infected with HIV and HBV it should *only* be used in conjunction with combined antiretroviral therapy to avoid resistance.

Adefovir[a]

Spectrum
- HBV and HIV (at higher doses).

Mechanism of Action
- Inhibits HBV DNA polymerase by competing with dATP.

Mechanisms of Resistance
- Acyclic nucleotide reverse transcriptase inhibitor (adenosine analog), which interferes with HBV viral RNA-dependent DNA polymerase resulting in inhibition of viral replication.

Safety
- Adverse effects
  - Nonadherence or its abrupt discontinuation may lead to liver toxicity as the result of reactivation of HBV replication.
  - Nephrotoxicity and Fanconi-like disorder at higher doses (reason as why not used for HIV).
- Drug interactions: no major interactions reported.

Other Key Concepts
- Effective in the presence of *YMDD* mutation from lamivudine use.

Entecavir[a]

Spectrum
- HBV and HIV.

Mechanism of Action
- Inhibits three activities of the HBV DNA polymerase, including base priming, reverse transcription of the negative strand from the pregenomic mRNA, and synthesis of positive strand HBV DNA. This halts HBV synthesis.

Mechanisms of Resistance
- Requires emergence of *YMDD* mutation and a second mutation in polymerase B, C or D. Resistance mutations in the reverse transcriptase gene of HBV are associated with treatment failure.

Safety
- Adverse effects: lactic acidosis and exacerbation of hepatitis B at discontinuation.

Telbivudine

Spectrum
- HBV.

Mechanism of Action
- Inhibits the activity of HBV viral polymerase.

Mechanisms of Resistance
- Cross-resistant with lamivudine and other l-nucleosides to which HBV may be resistant.
- Lower incidence of resistance when compared to lamivudine.

Safety
- Adverse effects
  - Lactic acidosis, severe hepatomegaly with steatosis, and myopathy.
  - Asymptomatic elevations of CPK reported (7 x ULN).

Other Key Concepts
- Clinical trials have shown it to be more effective than lamivudine or adefovir and less likely to cause resistance.

Tenofovir[a]

Spectrum
- HBV and HIV.

Mechanism of Action
- Inhibits HBV DNA polymerase by competing with dATP.

Mechanisms of Resistance
- Very low incidence of resistance.

Safety
- Adverse effects
  - Osteomalacia and renal toxicity.
  - Severe, acute exacerbation of HB may occur upon discontinuation.
- Drug interactions:
  - Concomitant use of tenofovir alafenamide (TAF) with rifamycins decreases TAF concentrations.

Other Key Concepts
- More effective than lamivudine or adefovir in clinical trials. Tenofovir is active against lamivudine-resistant HBV and generally active against viruses with entecavir-resistant mutations.

Antivirals for Hepatitis C

- The treatment of hepatitis C is a rapidly changing field. Guidelines are being updated almost on an annual basis; low likelihood of being on the boards.
- For treatment indications and treatment in special populations see: http://www.hcvguidelines.org/.
- FDA approved antivirals for hepatitis C are listed in Tables 8.1 and 8.2.
- Goal of treatment is to reduce mortality, progression to end-stage liver disease, and decrease risk for hepatocellular carcinoma. "Cure" is currently defined as undetectable HCV-RNA level at 12 weeks, commonly referred to as sustained virological response or SVR12.
- Be aware of the risk of **hepatitis B reactivation** in patients treated with direct-acting antiviral medications for HCV with current or previous hepatitis B co-infection.

Interferons (in combination with ribavirin)

Refer to interferons in the Antiviral for Hepatitis B and ribavirin in the Antiviral Drugs against Influenza A and B and Other Respiratory Viruses sections.
- Rarely if ever used any more. Direct-acting antivirals (DAAs) are now considered first-line therapy.

Direct Acting Antiviral Agents for HCV (DAAs)

- The main targets of these direct acting antiviral agents are the HCV-encoded nonstructural (NS) proteins that play a vital role in the replication of the virus.

Protease Inhibitors ("... previr")
- Subclass examples: telaprevir,[b] boceprevir,[b] simeprevir, glecaprevir, paritaprevir, voxilaprevir, and grazoprevir.

---

[b]First direct acting antivirals. Used with ribavirin and peginterferon for genotype 1 infection.

TABLE 8.1   FDA-Approved Antivirals for Hepatitis C

Genotype	Ribavirin	NS5a Inhibitors	Protease Inhibitors	RNA Polymerase Inhibitors	Pegylated-Interferon
1a, 1b, 2, 3	±	Declatasvir		Sofosbuvir	
1a, 1b, 4, 5, 6		Ledipasvir		Sofosbuvir	
1, 2, 3, 4, 5, 6		Velpatasvir		Sofosbuvir	
1a, 1b	±	Ombitasvir	Paritaprevir[a] Simeprevir	Dasabuvir	
4	±	Ombitasvir	Paritaprevir[a]		
2, 3, 4, 5, 6	+			Sofosbuvir	±
1, 4	±	Elbasvir	Grazoprevir		

[a]Boost with ritonavir.

TABLE 8.2   FDA-Approved Single-Pill Regimens

Genotype	Ledipasvir/ Sofosbuvir	Dasabuvir/ Ombitasvir/ Paritaprevir/ Ritonavir	Ombitasvir/ Paritaprevir/ Ritonavir	Elbasvir/ Grazoprevir	Sofosbuvir/ Velpatasvir	Sofosbuvir/ Velpatasvir/ Voxilaprevir	Glecaprevir/ Pibrentasvir
1a, 1b, 2, 3							
1a, 1b, 4, 5, 6	+						
1, 2, 3, 4, 5, 6					+	+	+
1a, 1b	+[a]	+					
4			+				
2, 3, 4, 5, 6							
1, 4				+			

[a]In combination with ribavirin.

Mechanism of Action
- Protease inhibitors block the function of the NS3/NS4A protease.
- High potency, low barrier of resistance, multiple drug interactions.

Safety
- Adverse effects: rash, anemia, hyperbilirubinemia.

Other Key Concepts
- Later generation PIs have higher levels of resistance and are pangenotypic.

Nucleos(t)ide Polymerase Inhibitors (NPIs) ("… buvir")
- Subclass examples: sofosbuvir

Mechanism of Action
- They block the function of the NS5B polymerase.
- Moderate-high potency, high barrier of resistance.

Safety
- Adverse effects: mitochondrial toxicity, interactions with HIV antiretrovirals and ribavirin.

Nonnucleoside Polymerase Inhibitors (NNPIs) ("… buvir")
- Subclass examples: dasabuvir.

Mechanism of Action
- They also block the function of the NS5B polymerase.
- Very low barrier of resistance, potency varies depending on genotype.

Safety
- Adverse effects: variable. It may cause pruritus, nausea, asthenia, insomnia, and fatigue (rare).

NS5A inhibitors ("...asvir")

- Class examples: declastavir, elbasvir, ledipasvir, ombitasvir, pibrentasvir, velpatasvir.

  Mechanism of Action
- They block the NS5A protein which has a presumptive role in the organization of the replication complex and in regulating replication. NS5A is also involved in assembly of the viral particle that is released from the host cell.
- High potency, low barrier of resistance.

Other Antivirals

Imiquimod

  Spectrum
- HPV (condyloma acuminatum).

  Mechanism of Action
- Toll-like receptor-7 agonist that activates immune cells. Topical application to the skin is associated with increases in markers for cytokines and immune cells.

  Safety
- Adverse effects: localized skin reactions.

Further Reading

1. Razonable R. Antiviral drugs for viruses other than human immunodeficiency virus. *Mayo Clin Proc.* 2011;86(10):1009–1026.
2. De Clercq E, Li G. Approved antiviral drugs over the past 50 years. *Clin Microb Rev.* 2016;29(3):695–747.
3. Ison M. Antiviral treatments. *Clin Chest Med.* 2017;38(1):139–153.
4. Nováková L, Pavlík J, Chrenková L, Martinec O, Červený L. Current antiviral drugs and their analysis in biological materials – part II: antivirals against hepatitis and HIV viruses. *J Pharm Biomed Anal.* 2017;147:378–399.
5. *Recommendations for Testing, Managing, and Treating Hepatitis C | HCV Guidance [Internet]. Hcvguidelines.org.* 2017. Available from. http://hcvguidelines.org.
6. Marty FM, Ljungman P, Chemaly RF, et al. Letermovir prophylaxis for cytomegalovirus in hematopoietic-cell transplantation. *N Engl J Med.* 2017;377(25):2433–2444.

9

Antiparasitic Agents

TODD P. MCCARTY

ANTIPARASITIC AGENTS

Note: This chapter will not include antibacterial and antifungal agents that also happen to have activity against parasites. Parasites are discussed in more detail in Chapters 34 and 35.

Antimalarial Drugs

Artemisinin Derivatives

- Available drugs: artemether–lumefantrine, artesunate.
- Rapid action, clinical utility extends into severe malaria.
  Spectrum
- All *Plasmodium* spp.
- Retains activity in the setting of multidrug resistance.
- *In vitro* activity against other parasites, however, has not been studied in a clinical setting.
- First-line therapy for severe malaria, in particular *P. falciparum*.
  Mechanism of Action
- Exact mechanism unclear.
- Dependent on the endoperoxide dioxygen bridge.
- Accumulates in multiple compartments of the parasite.
- Cleaved to hydroperoxide, functioning as an oxidizing agent releasing free radicals and reactive metabolites.
- Active on both ring forms and trophozoites.
  Mechanism of Resistance
- Increasing reports of recurrence in Southeast Asia centered around Cambodia.
- *In vitro* resistance noted in clinical isolates.
- Slow clearance of parasitemia should raise the concern for resistant parasites and appears to be related to decreased effect of artemisinin on the immature ring stages.
  Safety
- Adverse effects
  - Generally well tolerated.
  - Gastrointestinal (GI) side effects most common: nausea, vomiting, and/or diarrhea.
  - Hemolysis can occur after IV administration; higher parasite loads increase risk.
    - Termed post-artesunate delayed hemolysis.

  - Occurs more than 7 days after infusion in up to 10%–15% of patients.
  - Self-limited but may require transfusion.
- Neurotoxicity possible based on animal studies, but unclear if possible symptoms in humans related to the drug or severe malaria.
- Urticaria (rare).
- Anaphylaxis (rare).

4-Aminoquinolones

Chloroquine
  Spectrum
- All *Plasmodium* spp., though resistance can occur.
- First-line therapy for malaria in areas of known chloroquine sensitivity.
  Mechanism of Action
- Concentrates in the food vacuole of the *Plasmodium* parasite where it is trapped.
- Accumulation of heme and heme-chloroquine complexes leads to the death of the parasite.
  Mechanism of Resistance
- Decreased chloroquine concentration led by mutations in a transporter gene.
- Found throughout the world in *P. falciparum*, except Central America and Panama Canal.
- Resistance in *P. vivax* is less common, concentrated in SE Asia, likely of a different mechanism.
  Safety
- Adverse effects
  - Well tolerated.
  - Pruritus, in particular of palms, soles, and scalp, is most common.
  - Cardiac and CNS toxicity can occur with parenteral administration, overdose, and very prolonged administration (>5 years).

Mefloquine
  Spectrum
- All *Plasmodium* spp.
- Alternative treatment for malaria treatment.
- Alternative option for malaria prophylaxis in regions with chloroquine resistance.

Mechanism of Action

- Develops complexes with heme molecules that lead to toxicity in the parasite.
- Distinct mechanism from chloroquine.
- *Plasmodium* with chloroquine resistance have increased sensitivity to mefloquine.

Mechanism of Resistance

- *P. falciparum* resistance is most common in Southeast Asia.
- Occurs through increased genetic amplification of *pfmdr1*.

Safety

- Adverse effects
  - Dizziness, diarrhea, and nausea/vomiting are the most frequently reported.
  - Rash and pruritus are infrequently reported.
  - The most serious reported toxicity is neuropsychiatric, most commonly affecting Caucasians and Africans; women more frequently afflicted than men.

Quinine/Quinidine

Spectrum

- Active against all *Plasmodium* spp.
- Active against *Babesia*.
- Alternative therapy for malaria in regions without resistance, typically combined with an oral agent (clindamycin, tetracycline, or doxycycline).

Mechanism of Action

- Unknown.
- Inhibits digestion of hemoglobin and ATPase.

Mechanism of Resistance

- Reported worldwide but prevalence varies.
- Cross-resistance possible with mefloquine.

Safety

- Adverse effects
  - Cinchonism can occur at therapeutic levels, including a combination of tinnitus, deafness, headache, visual disturbances, dysphoria, vomiting, and postural hypotension.
  - Cardiovascular toxicities
    - Postural hypotension.
    - QT prolongation.
    - Syncope.
    - Ventricular arrhythmias related to rapid infusion.
  - Hypoglycemia.

8-Aminoquinolones

Primaquine

Spectrum

- Treatment against *P. vivax* and *P. ovale*.
- Prophylaxis against all *Plasmodium* spp.
- First-line for radical cure of *P. vivax* and *P. ovale*, alternative for malaria prophylaxis in chloroquine-resistant regions.

Mechanism of Action

- Production of oxidative metabolites inhibiting pyrimidine synthesis and disrupting mitochondrial function.

Mechanism of Resistance

- Failures tend to be more related to inadequate knowledge about dosing rather than resistance.

Safety

- Adverse effects
  - GI complaints: nausea, vomiting, abdominal pain, diarrhea.
  - Others: headache, weakness, pruritus, and visual disturbance.
  - Presence of G6PD deficiency can lead to significant hemolysis which can be life-threatening in the setting of <10% enzyme activity.
  - Dose-dependent methemoglobinemia.

Atovaquone

Spectrum

- All *Plasmodium* spp., but lacks activity against liver hypnozoites.
- *Babesia microti*.
- *Toxoplasma gondii*.
- *Cryptosporidium parvum*.
- *Leishmania donovani*.
- *Trichomonas vaginalis*.
- First-line (combined with proguanil) for uncomplicated malaria with *P. falciparum* or unknown species in a region with chloroquine resistance.
- First-line (combined with proguanil) for malaria prophylaxis in chloroquine resistant regions.

Mechanism of Action

- Inhibits electron transport in the cytochrome system.
- Does not cross-react with the human cytochrome system.

Mechanism of Resistance

- Genetic mutations involving the cytochrome b gene.
- Can occur in *Plasmodium* and *Toxoplasma*.

Safety

- Adverse effects
  - Uncommon, generally well tolerated.
  - GI complaints: nausea, vomiting, and diarrhea.
  - Other: fever, headache, elevated LFTs.

Dihydrofolate Reductase Inhibitors

Proguanil

Spectrum

- All *Plasmodium* spp.
- Primary usage as noted above in the atovaquone section.

Mechanism of Action

- Used in combination with atovaquone.
- Metabolites inhibit dihydrofolate reductase.
- Interferes with synthesis of pyrimidines thereby inhibiting nucleic acid replication.
- Also likely has mitochondrial toxicity with atovaquone through an undetermined mechanism.

Mechanism of Resistance

- No specific mechanisms reported.

Safety

- Adverse effects
  - Few, generally well tolerated.
  - Mouth ulcers, dyspepsia, and hair loss all reported.

Pyrimethamine

Spectrum

- Used in combination with a sulfonamide or dapsone.

- Useful in treating *Plasmodium*, *Toxoplasma*, and *Isosporum*.
- First-line treatment for *Toxoplasma*, as part of combination therapy.
  Mechanism of Action
- Blocks pyrimidine production via inhibition of dihydrofolate reductase.
  Mechanism of Resistance
- Mutations in the dihydrofolate reductase gene have led to resistance in *P. falciparum* and *P. vivax*.
  Safety
- Adverse effects
  - Bone marrow suppression, can be avoided with concurrent administration of folinic acid.
  - Rash, typically photosensitive.

Agents for *Leishmania* and Trypanosomiasis

Note: This section will not cover antifungal agents that also have activity against these conditions.

Antimonials
- Available in two forms
  - Sodium stibogluconate (IV or IM).
  - Meglumine antimoniate (IV or IM).
  Spectrum
- *Leishmania*, cutaneous, mucosal, and visceral forms.
- Treatment of choice for cutaneous or mucosal leishmaniasis, alternative therapy for visceral leishmaniasis.
  Mechanism of Action
- Not fully understood, possibilities include
  - Prodrug that affects metabolism and oxidation.
  - Binding of zinc fingers.
  - Inhibitor of *Leishmania* purine metabolism.
  - Host immune system activation.
  Mechanism of Resistance
- Occurs via decreased concentration of the drug in the parasite, but exact mechanism has not been determined.
  Safety
- Adverse effects
  - Pancreatitis, hepatitis.
  - Arthralgias, myalgias.
  - Cardiotoxicity: in particular arrhythmias in patients with a history of cardiovascular disease and ventricular arrhythmias.
- Drug interactions: none known.

Miltefosine
  Spectrum
- All *Leishmania* spp., though response rates are variable.
- Can be used in visceral, mucocutaneous, and cutaneous disease.
- Alternative therapy for all forms of leishmaniasis.
  Mechanism of Action
- Mechanism not fully understood.
- Induces apoptosis of promastigotes and amastigotes.

- Likely via inhibition of phosphatidyl choline production.
  Mechanism of Resistance
- Decreased drug uptake by the organism.
- Increased efflux.
  Safety
- Adverse effects
  - GI complaints: nausea, vomiting, diarrhea.
  - Elevated creatinine.
  - Elevated transaminases.
  - Teratogenic.

Paromomycin
  Spectrum
- All species of *Leishmania*, best response rate for visceral disease.
- *Entamoeba histolytica*.
- *Dientamoeba fragilis*.
- Alternative therapy for visceral leishmaniasis.
- Drug of choice for cyst clearage (luminal disease) in *E. histolytica*; first-line therapy for *D. fragilis*.
  Mechanism of Action
- *Leishmania*: inhibition of parasite mitochondria.
- *Entamoeba* and *Dientamoeba*: clearance of cyst carriage.
  Mechanism of Resistance
- Unclear mechanism, but resistance reported among multiple species of *Leishmania*.
  Safety
- Adverse effects: renal dysfunction, cochlear, and vestibular toxicity.

Benznidazole
  Spectrum
- *Trypanosoma cruzi* as first-line therapy.
  Mechanism of Action
- Unknown.
  Mechanism of Resistance
- Reported, but unclear clinical significance.
  Safety
- Adverse effects
  - Frequent.
  - Peripheral neuropathy and rash most common.
  - Granulocytopenia, requires monitoring.

Eflornithine
  Spectrum
- All stages of *T. brucei gambiense*.
- No activity against *T. brucei rhodesiense*.
- First-line therapy for late disease *T. brucei gambiense* when CNS is involved.
  Mechanism of Action
- Inhibits ornithine decarboxylase.
- Impairs parasite's redox ability and cell division.
  Mechanism of Resistance
- Treatment failures reported, but unclear mechanism.

Safety
Adverse effects
  - Cytopenias are the most common.
  - Seizures possible with high CSF concentrations.
  - Diarrhea in particular with oral therapy.

Melarsoprol
Spectrum Both East and West Africa human trypanosomiasis.
- First line for late disease *T. brucei rhodesiense* with CNS involvement; alternative therapy for late disease *T. brucei gambiense* with CNS involvement.
  Mechanism of Action
- Inhibits trypanothione reductase.
- Leads to reduced redox potential.
  Mechanism of Resistance
- Decreased drug entry through lack of adenosine transporter system.
  Safety
- Adverse effects
  - Encephalopathy, which also has a very high mortality rate.
  - Polyneuropathy.
  - Less common: rash, tremor, abdominal pain, fever.

Nifurtimox
Spectrum
- *Trypanosoma cruzi*.
- In combination with eflornithine to treat *T. brucei gambiense*.
- Second-line agent for *T. cruzi*; can be combined with eflornithine for late disease *T. brucei gambiense* with CNS involvement.
  Mechanism of Action
- Not fully understood.
- Thought to increase oxidative stress.
  Mechanism of Resistance
- Reported but mechanism unknown.
- Clinical significance also not well understood.
  Safety
- Adverse effects
  - Frequent and lead to compliance issues.
  - GI complaints common: nausea, vomiting, diarrhea.
  - CNS complaints: insomnia, paresthesia, seizures.
  - Rashes.

Suramin
Spectrum
- Both East and West Africa human trypanosomiasis.
- Used in the hemolymphatic form; cannot be used in CNS form.
- Onchocerciasis, but should be pre-treated with ivermectin.
- First-line therapy for early stage *T. brucei rhodesiense*; alternative therapy for early stage *T. brucei gambiense*.
  Mechanism of Action
- Unknown.
- Thought to impact redox ability.
  Mechanism of Resistance
- Uncommon and not understood.
  Safety
- Adverse effects
  - Mild proteinuria most common without renal failure.
  - Fever, pruritus, urticaria, stomatitis.
  - Allergic reactions and worsening of ocular lesions with onchocerciasis treatment.

Agents for Other Protozoa

Nitazoxanide
Spectrum
- *Cryptosporidium*.
- *Giardia*.
- *Entamoeba*.
- *Cystoisospora*.
- *Blastocystis*.
- *Microsporidia*.
- Tapeworms and nematodes.
- First-line therapy for cryptosporidiosis (immunocompetent patients) and *Blastocystis*; alternative therapy for giardiasis.
  Mechanism of Action
- Inhibits an oxidoreductase enzyme.
- Impacts energy metabolism.
  Mechanism of Resistance
- Reported in *Giardia*.
- Mechanism unknown.
  Safety
- Adverse effects
  - Studies showed similar AEs to placebo.

Antihelminth Agents

Benzimidazoles

Albendazole
Spectrum
- Tissue and intestinal parasites
  - *Ascaris*.
  - *Echinococcus*.
  - *Necator*.
  - *Ancylostoma*.
  - *Enterobius*.
  - *Trichuris*.
- Neurocysticercosis
  - First-line therapy for cysticercosis, *Echinococcus*, intestinal nematodes (ascariasis, trichuriasis, hookworm, enterobiasis), extraintestinal nematodes (trichinellosis, toxocariasis, cutaneous larva migrans, *Angiostrongylus*, baylisascariasis, gnathostomiasis).
  - Alternative therapy for: clonorchiasis, opisthorchiasis, strongyloidiasis, loaiasis, capillariasis.
  Mechanism of Action
- Binds tubulin preventing polymerization with selectivity for the parasitic version.
- Cell division thereby disrupted and prevents egg hatching.
  Mechanism of Resistance
- Well described in veterinary literature.
- Only recently recognized in human disease, particularly *Wuchereria*, *Trichuris*, and hookworms.
- Mechanism appears to be small alterations to amino-acids in tubulin composition.
  Safety
- Adverse effects

- Unclear if symptoms after single-dose treatment related to the medicine or immune response to dead/dying parasites.
- On extended therapy
  - Elevated transaminases.
  - Alopecia.
  - Potentially irreversible marrow toxicity.

Mebendazole
Spectrum
- Similar to albendazole (and other benzimidazoles).
- First-line therapy for: intestinal nematodes, trichinellosis, visceral larva migrans, and capillariasis.
Mechanism of Action
- Similar to albendazole, but less effective.
- Metabolites do not retain helminthic activity.
Mechanism of Resistance
- Same as albendazole.
Safety
- Adverse effects
  - Abdominal cramps, fatigue, headache, vertigo, nausea.
  - Longer durations: headaches, elevated transaminases, urticarial.
  - Reversible marrow suppression.

Triclabendazole
Spectrum
- *Fasciola*.
- *Paragonimus*.
- First-line therapy for fascioliasis; alternative therapy for paragonimiasis.
Mechanism of Action
- Inhibits microtubule formation.
- Specific to version of microtubules in flukes.
Mechanism of Resistance
- Primarily a veterinary problem at present.
- Mechanism unclear.
Safety
- Adverse effects
  - Generally mild.
  - Abdominal pain, headache, nausea, fatigue.
  - Pain potentially related to expulsion of dead/dying worms via biliary tract.

Other Agents
Ivermectin
Spectrum
- *Onchocerca*.
- *Ascaris*.
- *Enterobius*.
- *Strongyloides*.
- *Wuchereria*.
- *Brugia*.
- *Loa loa*.
- *Mansonella streptocerca, M. ozzardi*.
- *Ancylostoma*.
- *Sarcoptes*.
- Less effective against trichuriasis and hookworms.
- First-line therapy for onchocerciasis, strongyloidiasis.

- Alternative therapy for ascariasis, trichuriasis, enterobius, lymphatic filariasis, cutaneous larva migrans, and gnathostomiasis.
Mechanism of Action
- Activates chloride channels.
- Influx of ions leads to paralysis.
Mechanism of Resistance
- Not well defined.
- Described in veterinary literature first.
- Reports of poor clinical response to treatment.
Safety
- Adverse effects
  - No drug-induced toxicities at recommended therapeutic doses.
  - Post-treatment reactions are possible
    - Postural hypotension.
    - Skin edema, pruritus.
  - Severe complications possible if concurrent *Loa loa* infection when being treated for onchocerciasis (refer to Chapter 35, Intestinal Nematodes).

Diethylcarbamazine (DEC)
Spectrum
- Filariasis.
- Loiasis.
- Larva migrans.
- *Ascaris*.
- First-line therapy for lymphatic filariasis, tropical pulmonary eosinophilia, loaiasis.
Mechanism of Action
- Not well understood.
- No activity noted *in vitro*, pointing toward an alteration host–parasite reaction through unclear means.
Mechanism of Resistance
- Variable response noted, however unclear if this is related to resistance.
Safety
- Adverse effects
  - GI complaints: nausea, anorexia.
  - With infection: inflammation related to killing parasites.
  - With onchocerciasis: Mazzotti reaction: pruritus, fever, arthralgia.

Pyrantel Pamoate
Spectrum
- Hookworm.
- *Ascaris*.
- No activity in trichuriasis.
- Alternative therapy for ascariasis, hookworm.
Mechanism of Action
- Binds acetylcholine receptor of muscle, paralyzing worm.
- Expulsed naturally.

Mechanism of Resistance
- Alteration of receptor binding site.
Safety
- Adverse effects
  - GI complaints: nausea, vomiting, cramping, diarrhea.

Praziquantel
Spectrum
- Trematodes (including *Schistosoma*), except *Fasciola hepatica*.
- Cestodes.
- Used in combination therapy with albendazole for neurocysticercosis and hydatid infection.
- First-line therapy for *Taenia*, *Diphyllobothrium latum*, *Hymenolepis*, schistosomiasis, clonorchiasis, opisthorchiasis, paragonimiasis, *Nanophyetus*, *Metorchis*.

Mechanism of Action
- Disrupts integrity of parasite exterior, impacting ability to adhere to host.
- Complete mechanism incompletely understood.

Mechanism of Resistance
- Reported in *Schistosoma mansoni*, mechanism unclear.
- Could be related to efflux pumps.

Safety
- Adverse effects
  - GI complaints: nausea, vomiting, pain.
  - Dizziness, headache.
  - Likely related to immune response to dying parasites.

Niclosamide
Spectrum
- Adult tapeworms.
- Ineffective against tissue cestodes.
- Alternative therapy for: *Taenia*, *D. latum*, *Hymenolepis*.

Mechanism of Action
- Uncouples oxidative phosphorylation.

Mechanism of Resistance
- Not reported.

Safety
- Adverse effects
  - GI upset, lightheadedness, malaise, pruritus.

Bithionol
Spectrum
- *Fasciola*.
- *Paragonimus*.
- Alternative therapy for fascioliasis, paragonimiasis; usage limited due to side effects.

Mechanism of Action
- Inhibits electron transfer.
- Specific target unique to parasites.

Mechanism of Resistance
- Not reported.

Safety
- Adverse effects
  - GI complaints: anorexia, cramps, nausea, diarrhea.
  - Pruritus.

Further Reading

1. McCarthy JS, Price RN. Antimalarial drugs. In: Bennett JE, Dolin R, Blaser MJ, eds. *Mandell, Douglas, and Bennett's Principles and Practice of Infectious Diseases*. Updated 8th ed. Philadelphia: Elsevier; 2015:495–509.
2. McCarthy JS, Wortmann GW, Kirchhoff LV. Drugs for protozoal infections other than malaria. In: Bennett JE, Dolin R, Blaser MJ, eds. *Mandell, Douglas, and Bennett's Principles and Practice of Infectious Diseases*. Updated 8th ed. Philadelphia: Elsevier; 2015:510–518.
3. McCarthy JS, Moore TA. Drugs for helminths. In: Bennett JE, Dolin R, Blaser MJ, eds. *Mandell, Douglas, and Bennett's Principles and Practice of Infectious Diseases*. Updated 8th ed. Philadelphia: Elsevier; 2015:519–527.
4. Drugs for parasitic infections. *The Medical Letter*. 2013;11(suppl):e1–e31.
5. Kappagoda S, Singh U, Blackburn BG. Antiparasitic therapy. *Mayo Clin Proc*. 2011;86(6):531–583.

10

Fevers and Sepsis

KEVIN HSUEH

FEVERS

Definitions

- **Fever**: a rise in core body temperature, traditionally ≥38°C (100.4°F) when presuming a basal body temperature of 37°C (98.6°F), though this represents significant simplification. Varies greatly in context of the expected basal body temperature of the patient and point of measurement. Technically fevers occur only as part of the *febrile response* as a result of an increased body temperature setpoint, with the term *hyperthermia* applied to temperature elevations by other causes. Colloquially, the term fever is applied broadly to almost all significant body temperature elevations. Fevers are often accompanied by malaise, headache, myalgias, and arthralgias.
  - Febrile response: the inflammatory cascade that occurs in response to an infection of which fever is the most visible sign.
  - Hyperthermia: elevations of body temperature resulting from increases in heat production or decreases in heat dissipation and not as the result of hypothalamic temperature upregulation (Box 10.1).
  - Hyperpyrexia: fevers resulting in extremely elevated body temperatures, exceeding 41.5°C (>106.7°F). Occasionally, severe infections alone can cause hyperpyrexia; however, most often hyperpyrexia occurs in the context of CNS injury (strokes, hemorrhage, trauma).

> **• BOX 10.1 Causes of Hyperthermia**
>
> - Nonexertional heat stroke
> - Exertional heat illness
> - Drug intoxication (stimulants and hallucinogens)
> - Malignant hyperthermia (reaction to inhaled anaesthetics or paralytic agents)
> - Serotonin syndrome
> - Hyperthyroidism/pseudohyperthyroidism
> - Anticholinergic toxicity

- **Fevers of unknown origin (FUO)**: a clinically distinct entity from the common fever, FUOs are fevers whose etiology remains obscure despite a thorough baseline work-up. The approach to FUO is discussed later in this chapter.
- **Febrile neutropenia (FN)**: in the severely neutropenic patient (ANC <500), fever is considered its own infective emergency. In these patients, infections are common, can progress rapidly, and have blunted symptomatology. Risk increases with the degree of immunosuppression. The source of 70%–80% of FN episodes are never determined, with gastrointestinal mucositis or complications of malignancy the primary suspect in most of these cases. Bacteremia occurs in 10%–25% of FN cases. Bacteria are the most common pathogens in cases of FN, though candida and molds do occur, especially with prolonged (≥2 weeks) and profound (ANC <100) neutropenia (Box 10.2).

Epidemiology

- Fever can occur with almost any type of infection – bacterial, viral, fungal, or parasitic.
- Noninfectious insults can trigger the febrile response, causing fevers indistinguishable from infectious fever.
- **Common noninfectious causes of fever**
  - Postsurgical/postprocedural reactions.
  - Drug reactions.
  - Deep vein thromboses and pulmonary emboli.
  - Strokes.
  - Myocardial infarctions.
  - Hemorrhage and hematomas.
  - Malignancies.
  - Transfusion reactions.
- The elderly are less likely to mount fevers, due to impaired thermoregulatory mechanisms and lower basal body temperature.
- Most fever is caused by endogenous pyrogens released as part of the immune response to infection. A few pathogens produce exogenous pyrogens, which can incite fever directly.
  - Exogenous pyrogens.

• **BOX 10.2** **Pathogens in Febrile Neutropenia**

Bacteria

- Coagulase-negative staphylococci
- *Staphylococcus aureus* (MRSA and MSSA)
- Enterococci (including vancomycin-resistant enterococci)
- Viridans group streptococci
- *Streptococcus pneumoniae*
- *Streptococcus pyogenes*
- *Escherichia coli*
- *Klebsiella* spp.
- *Enterobacter* spp.
- *Pseudomonas aeruginosa*
- *Citrobacter* spp.
- *Acinetobacter* spp.
- *Stenotrophomonas* spp.

Fungi

- *Candida* spp.
- *Aspergillus* spp.
- Agents of zygomycosis
- *Fusarium* spp.

Viral

- Respiratory syncytial virus
- Adenovirus
- Coronavirus
- Human metapneumovirus
- Parainfluenza viruses.

- Lipopolysaccharide (LPS): gram-negative rod bacteria.
- Toxic shock syndrome toxin 1 (TSST-1): *Staphylococcus aureus.*
- Streptococcal pyrogenic exotoxins: *Streptococcus pyogenes.*
- Viral infections are by far the most common cause of community onset fevers and rarely require treatment or hospitalization.
- Common causes of fever in the hospitalized patient:
  - Urinary tract infections.
  - Pneumonia.
  - Bloodstream infections.
  - Skin and soft tissue infections.
  - Gastrointestinal infections.

Clinical Approach to Fever

Identification of potential sources is critical in the assessment of the febrile patient, due to the many possible causes of fever.

- **Review of localizing symptoms and signs.** Additional symptomatology and exam findings help localize where an infective source of fever could be.
  - Chills and rigors may indicate potential bacteremia.
  - Dysuria or urinary frequency can point to a urinary tract infection.
  - New cough, sputum, or dyspnea can suggest a respiratory infection such as a viral upper respiratory tract infection or a pneumonia.

- New or worsening localized pain could indicate a potential focus of skin and soft tissue, or musculoskeletal infection.
  - Diarrhea or abdominal pain can suggest gastroenteritis or an intraabdominal infection.
- **Focused testing.** Additional lab work or imaging should be directed by the above examination findings if the symptoms are insufficient to clinch diagnosis alone. For example, blood cultures should be performed if there is suspicion of bacteremia.
- **Assess for noninfectious causes.** Patients without a clear infectious basis for fever should be screened for potential noninfectious causes. Comorbid conditions such as malignancy and vascular events can be causes of fever. Recent surgery or procedures can also cause fever.
- **Review of medications.** Patient medications should be reviewed for drugs that can cause fever. Of concern are antiinfectives, anticonvulsants, and injectable/infusible medications.
- **Screen for signs of sepsis.** Fever is a common symptom in patients who are septic. Hospitalized patients who develop fever should be screened for additional signs of sepsis (see following section on sepsis for more details).

Treatment

Treatment of fever is a controversial topic.

- In the otherwise healthy patient, no clear benefit or harm has been demonstrated from antipyretic therapy.
- Fever can be a critical diagnostic aid, and animal studies have suggested that elevated body temperature can aid response to infection.
- The metabolic demand of increased body temperature can overtax patients with tenuous mental, respiratory, or cardiovascular status.
- The headache, myalgias, arthralgias, and malaise that accompany fever can be distressing to many patients.

Antipyretics

Antipyretics are agents used in the treatment of fever.

- **Acetaminophen.** A mild analgesic, acetaminophen is believed to act as an antipyretic by inhibiting prostaglandin production in the central nervous system. With few side effects and a wide therapeutic margin, acetaminophen is the most commonly used antipyretic.
- **Nonsteroidal antiinflammatory drugs (NSAIDs).** NSAIDS such as ibuprofen and aspirin are potent antipyretics that act by inhibiting prostaglandin production by blocking cyclooxygenase activity centrally and peripherally. Often used alongside acetaminophen, the combination is more potent than each individually.
- **Steroids.** Steroids are extremely potent antipyretics that inhibit both prostaglandin production, as well as endogenous pyrogen production. Rarely used for the explicit purpose of treating fever because of their immunosuppressive effect and numerous side effects such as hyperglycemia, ancillary steroid use can frequently blunt or

block fevers from occurring despite the presence of infections that would normally trigger them.

Direct Cooling

Used primarily in cases of hyperthermia or hyperpyrexia, direct cooling techniques are used to rapidly reduce body temperature.

- Most commonly, cooling blankets or cool baths are used.
- Caution should be taken, due to the risk of paradoxically increasing core body temperature by triggering peripheral vasoconstriction.
- Use of external cooling without the use of antipyretics increases metabolic activity and can tax an already strained patient in the setting of sepsis.

Clinical Approach to a Fever of Unknown Origin (FUO)

- **Characterizing the type of FUO.** The term FUO is frequently used in a host of different scenarios. However, the etiology of fevers is critically influenced by context, as is the urgency of work-up. Thus the first step is to properly identify which category of FUO one is faced with. FUOs generally can be broken down into three overall categories.
  - **Classic FUO**: initially described in the 1960s, classic FUO is defined as fevers occurring over a protracted duration (at least 3 weeks), exceeding 38.3°C (>101.0°F) at least once, and whose etiology remains obscure despite a thorough baseline work-up. The majority of classic FUOs present as low-grade illnesses in patients without known predisposing comorbidities such as malignancy or immunocompromising conditions, and patients are often evaluated in the outpatient setting (Box 10.3).
  - **Nosocomial FUO**: a markedly different entity from classic FUO, nosocomial FUOs present as fevers exceeding 38.3°C (>101.0°F) starting only after a patient is hospitalized and persisting for at least 3 days and that remains obscure despite a thorough baseline work-up. Nosocomial FUOs tend to have more rapid progression and greater systemic symptoms. They correspondingly require a more urgent work-up (Box 10.4).
  - **FUO in the immunocompromised**: illness in immunocompromised patients, such as neutropenic patients and people living with HIV, frequently presents as nonspecific fevers. These are well established predisposing conditions, and work-up and treatment of fever in their context is well established as, for example, febrile neutropenia and illness in the patient living with HIV/AIDS.
- **Confirm/complete a thorough baseline evaluation:** many patients are presumptively diagnosed as having a FUO before a thorough initial work-up has been completed. While an initial work-up should be tailored toward a patient's specific signs and symptoms (if any),

---

• BOX 10.3 Common Causes of Classic FUO

Infectious

- Tuberculosis
- Endocarditis
- Osteomyelitis
- Pneumonia
- Occult abscess (abdominal, dental, perinephric, prostatic, etc.)
- Sinusitis
- Zoonoses (Q-Fever aka *Coxiella burnetii*, Brucellosis, etc.)
- Cytomegalovirus infection
- Epstein–Barr virus (or associated conditions)
- Sexually transmitted infections

Inflammatory/Rheumatologic

- Systemic lupus erythematosus
- Vasculitides (giant cell arteritis, polyarteritis nodosa, Takayasu's, etc.)
- Adult-onset Stills disease
- Inflammatory arthritides (rheumatoid arthritis, psoriatic arthritis, etc.)
- Inflammatory bowel disease (ulcerative colitis, Crohn's disease, etc.)
- Sarcoidosis
- Thyroiditis

Neoplasms

- Lymphomas
- Leukemias
- Solid tumors (colorectal, breast, liver, lung, testicular, kidney, bone, etc.)
- Multiple myeloma

Other

- Drug fevers
- Factitious or self-inflicted injury
- Thromboembolic disease
- Congenital fever disorder

---

there is a general consensus that to meet the definition of FUO a baseline evaluation should include the following (Box 10.5).

Nosocomial FUO, being a more acute phenomenon, is more often due to gross physiologic abnormalities such as clot, embolus, or abscess, and thus thorough imaging is often required prior to concluding that a patient has a FUO.

- **In-depth clinical evaluation**: narrowing down differential diagnoses is critical to the work-up of FUO. Given how broad the possible causes of FUO are and their relative rarity, the likelihood of false-positives is quite high, which is why a "shotgun" approach to diagnostic testing for FUO is generally inadvisable. As a result, the history and physical are central to the work-up of FUO, as they increase the pretesting probability of specific diagnoses, making positive results more appropriately actionable.
- **History**: the most critical component of a diagnostic work-up for FUO is the historical interview, and care should be taken that it is exhaustive. The history allows for detection of localizing symptoms such as pain, discomfort, or functional changes (such as changes in stool

---

• **BOX 10.4** Common Causes of Nosocomial FUO

Infectious

- Pneumonia
- *C. difficile* infection
- Pyelonephritis
- Device-related infections (e.g., line infections)
- Viral illnesses

Vascular

- Venous thromboembolic disease
- Ischemia
- Other embolic disease (such as postop fat emboli)
- Bleeds
- Hematomas

Other

- Drug fevers
- Gouty flare

• **BOX 10.5** Baseline Work-up Needed for FUO

Classic FUO

- Complete history (including travel, sexual, medication, and exposure history)
- Thorough physical exam (including abdominal, musculoskeletal, skin, and oropharyngeal exam)
- Complete blood count with differential
- Basic metabolic panel
- Hepatic function panel
- Urinalysis with microscopy
- Blood cultures (typically at least 3 sets, collected off antibiotic therapy)
- Urine cultures
- HIV screening test
- Chest X-ray

Additional Testing in Nosocomial FUO

- Sinus imaging
- Imaging for DVT and pulmonary embolus
- CT chest/abdomen/pelvis

Other Common Tests as Indicated by History

- Erythrocyte sedimentation rate
- C-Reactive protein level
- Testing for latent tuberculosis
- Blood smears
- Antinuclear antibodies
- Rheumatoid factor

---

frequency or vision). It also allows for identification of risk factors such as family history of illnesses, sick contacts, travel, sexual contacts, wilderness and animal exposures, and occupational exposures. Clinicians should take care to also elicit any history of systemic involvement such as weight loss/gain or fatigue, the duration of symptomatology, and character of the fevers and associated symptoms.

- **Physical**: along with the history, physical signs and localizing symptoms help establish a diagnosis. All systems should be examined; however, notable areas to examine that are often glossed over in more routine exams are the oropharynx and mucosa, anogenital exams, and lymph node chains. These areas are often glossed over on routine exams, but findings such as ulcers, matted nodes, or masses can be critical indications of the source of an FUO (Box 10.6).
- **Focused diagnostic testing**: diagnostic testing should be directed toward any diagnoses that could potentially be associated with the history or exam findings elicited from the patient. If no suggestive findings are identified, then an initial evaluation looking for the more common causes of FUO (e.g., endocarditis, malignancy, autoimmune disease) with blood tests is reasonable, though positive findings should be suspect for false positivity. The decision of whether to initiate more invasive/harmful diagnostic testing should be individualized per patient. It should be recognized that between 25% and 50% of all FUO cases remain without definitive diagnosis despite rigorous work-up and that the fever resolves spontaneously in almost 80% of these cases, with relatively low morbidity and mortality (~3%) for these patients in most case series. Thus a highly aggressive diagnostic stance may put patients at unnecessary risk versus a more patient approach. One way to determine whether or not to be aggressive is through signs of systemic or progressive illness. Signs such as unintentional weight loss, anorexia, or worsening of fever curves can be indicative of a patient who has less time to wait for work-up. In these cases, nonspecific diagnostic imaging is generally chosen, with CT and MRI usually the initial modes chosen, looking for gross physical abnormalities that could indicate a source of inflammation. In patients who still remain undiagnosed despite these exams (and in whom urgent diagnosis is priority), gallium-67 scanning or FDG-PET/CT are generally the last-line of diagnostic imaging used to try to identify a source for febrile illness.

Treatment

In most classic FUO, empiric treatment is generally frowned upon, as benefit is debatable, and use confounds work-up, though it is not uncommon to see providers treat diagnoses that are suspected but not completely confirmed, as long as the treatment is relatively benign (such as treatment for tick-borne illnesses).

In nosocomial FUO, where patients are often more acutely ill, broad-spectrum antibiotics are often initiated, though again there is debate whether or not this is truly warranted or beneficial to the patient. Antibiotics carry not insignificant risk of adverse events, particularly in hospitalized patients where *Clostridioides difficile* is more likely to be acquired. One exception to these general rules is trial discontinuation of drugs that could potentially be causing drug fevers, which should be considered early along with other diagnostic testing.

• BOX 10.6 **Historical and Physical Exam Associations of Common FUO Conditions**

Infectious

- Tuberculosis: history of incarceration, travel to TB-endemic country, close contact with a patient with TB/chronic cough
- Endocarditis: cardiac murmurs, splinter hemorrhages, history of IVDU
- Abscess: historical infections, predisposing conditions such as cavities, diverticulitis
- Zoonoses: exposure to animal carriers or carrier environments, such as through contaminated food or occupational exposure to animals, new or unusual pets

Inflammatory/Rheumatologic

- Systemic lupus erythematosus: malar rash, migratory arthritides, photosensitivity, family history of SLE
- Vasculitides: large artery bruits, abnormal arterial pulses/pressures
- Adult-onset Stills disease: evanescent salmon-colored rash, myalgias, and pharyngitis
- Inflammatory arthritides: joint effusions
- Inflammatory bowel disease: change in stool habits, nodular skin lesions, uveitis
- Sarcoidosis: cough, dyspnea, chest pain

Neoplasms

- Lymphomas: enlarged lymph nodes, B-symptoms
- Leukemias: anemia, easy bruising
- Solid tumors: masses, tenderness
- Multiple myeloma

SEPSIS

Definitions

- **Sepsis**: sepsis is the multisystemic syndrome that can result from significant infection-related inflammatory reactions. Sepsis exists as a spectrum disorder, from a state of mild autonomic and lab abnormalities all the way through multiorgan failure and death. In latter stages the significant metabolic and autonomic abnormalities of sepsis can become self-reinforcing, leading to a vicious cycle of dysfunctional physiologic responses. The clinical definitions of sepsis are currently in significant flux, with different definitions used by separate major organizations.
- **SEPSIS-1**: the first international consensus definition of sepsis, developed in 1991. Academically the SEPSIS-1 criteria are considered obsolete; however, a large amount of literature and policy still refers to part or all of these criteria and thus they remain relevant for now.
  - The **Systemic Inflammatory Response Syndrome (SIRS)**: SIRS is the inflammatory response syndrome that can be caused by infection as well as other insults, such as ischemia and hemorrhage. To count as SIRS, two or more of the following criteria must be met.
    1. Body temperature >38°C (100.4°F) or <36°C (96.8°F).

    2. Heart rate >90 beats/min.
    3. Respiratory rate >20 breaths/min or $PaCO_2$ <32 mmHg (hyperventilation).
    4. White blood cell count >12,000/mm^3 or <4000/mm^3, or band count (immature neutrophils) >10%.
  - Sepsis = SIRS criterion + a proven or probable infective condition. The major criticism of the SEPSIS-1 criteria comes from the concern that the SIRS definition is so broad as to apply to a majority of clinically significant infections, which would imply that all patients with those infections would technically be septic. However, very few of those patients are at risk for severe injury without aggressive intervention, and thus there is concern that this overly broad definition results in excessive medical treatment and takes focus away from patients who would truly benefit from aggressive therapy.
  - **Severe sepsis = Sepsis + organ dysfunction, hypoperfusion, or hypotension.** Examples of organ dysfunction include lactic acidosis, oliguria/acute kidney injury, and altered mental status. Severe sepsis represents a more severely ill subset of septic patients.
  - **Septic shock = Severe sepsis + fluid-refractory hypotension.** Septic shock is the most critically ill subset of septic patients.
- **SEPSIS-3**: the third and most current international consensus definition of sepsis, SEPSIS-3 largely redefines sepsis as the patients previously considered to be having severe sepsis under SEPSIS-1.
  - **Sepsis = Infection causing life-threatening organ dysfunction.** Very similar in principle to the previous SEPSIS-1 concept of "severe sepsis."
    - Research criterion: sepsis = acute increase in the Sequential Organ Failure Assessment (SOFA) score of ≥2 in the context of infection (Box 10.7).
    - Clinical criterion: suspect sepsis if quick Sequential Organ Failure Assessment (qSOFA) score of ≥2 (Box 10.8).
  - **Septic shock** = a subset of sepsis with high mortality due to profound circulatory and metabolic abnormalities. Defined as sepsis with persistent hypotension or requiring vasopressors to maintain a MAP ≥65 mmHg, and a serum lactate >2 mmol/L (18 mg/dL) despite adequate volume resuscitation.

Epidemiology

- Almost all severe infections can result in sepsis; however, most community-acquired sepsis is the result of a very few classes of infection (Box 10.9).
- There are many noninfectious conditions that can mimic the signs and symptoms of sepsis (Box 10.10).
- Common organisms involved in sepsis (Box 10.11).

Clinical Approach to Sepsis

The clinical approach to sepsis has changed radically over the last two decades, in large part due to the efforts of the

• BOX 10.7 Sequential Organ Failure Assessment (SOFA) Score

Score is compiled by adding up all points together.
- PaO_2/FIO_2, mmHg
  - ≥400 = 0 pts
  - <400 = 1 pt
  - <300 = 2 pts
  - <200 (with respiratory support) = 3 pts
  - <100 (with respiratory support) = 4 pts
  - Platelet count, ×10³/mm³
  - ≥150 = 0 pts
  - <150 = 1 pt
  - <100 = 2 pts
  - <50 = 3 pts
  - <20 = 4 pts
- Bilirubin, mg/dL
  - <1.2 = 0 pts
  - 1.2–1.9 = 1 pt
  - 2.0–-5.9 = 2 pts
  - 6.0–11.9 = 3 pts
  - ≥12.0 = 4 pts
- Mean Arterial Pressure/Pressor Requirement (for at least 1 h)
  - MAP ≥70 mmHg = 0 pts
  - MAP <70 mmHg = 1 pt
  - Dopamine <5 µg/kg per min or any dose of dobutamine = 2 pts
  - Dopamine 5.1–15 µg/kg per min or epinephrine ≤0.1 µg/kg per min or norepinephrine ≤0.1 µg/kg per min = 3 pts
  - Dopamine >15 µg/kg/min or epinephrine >0.1 µg/kg per min or norepinephrine >0.1 µg/kg per min = 4 pts
- Glasgow Coma Scale
  - 15 = 0 pts
  - 13–14 = 1 pt
  - 10–12 = 2 pts
  - 6–9 = 3 pts
  - <6 = 4 pts
- Serum creatinine, mg/dL
  - <1.2 = 0 pts
  - 1.2–1.9 = 1 pt
  - 2.0–3.4 = 2 pts
  - 3.5–4.9 = 3 pts
  - >5.0 = 4 pts
- Urine output, mL/day
  - <500 = 3 pts
  - <200 = 4 pts

• BOX 10.8 Quick Sequential Organ Failure Assessment (qSOFA) Score

Score is calculated by the number of applicable items.
- Respiratory rate ≥22 breaths/min
- Altered mentation (equivalent to GCS <15)
- Systolic blood pressure ≤100 mmHg

Surviving Sepsis Campaign (www.survivingsepsis.org), an international venture to reduce the mortality and morbidity of sepsis. Their efforts have been to encourage the protocolization of sepsis treatment around evidence-based interventions. The most recent guidance, published in 2016, focuses on what can be separated into four different aspects

• BOX 10.9 Common Infectious Causes of Sepsis

- Pneumonia
- Urinary tract infections
- Bloodstream infection
- Intraabdominal infection
- Skin and soft tissue infection
- Musculoskeletal infection
- Central nervous system infection

• BOX 10.10 Common Noninfectious Mimics of Sepsis

- Inflammatory bowel disease
- Hypovolemia
- Medication side effect/overdose
- Adrenal insufficiency
- Acute myocardial infarction
- Pulmonary embolus
- Pancreatitis
- Diabetic ketoacidosis
- Small bowel obstruction
- Severe anemia
- Heart failure
- Anaphylaxis
- Systemic lupus erythematosus

of treatment: *initial resuscitation, diagnostic work-up, antimicrobial therapy,* and *continued therapy.*

- **Initial resuscitation:** sepsis represents an infectious emergency. Because it represents a self-reinforcing feedback loop of maladaptive physiologic responses, sepsis can rapidly evolve from moderate to immediately life-threatening illness rapidly. Early and aggressive resuscitation has been shown to reduce absolute risk of death from sepsis by about 10%. The resuscitation guidelines include the following:
  - 30 mL/kg of crystalloid fluid (commonly normal saline) infused within 3 hours of the onset of sepsis.
  - Targeting a mean arterial pressure (MAP) of 65 mmHg if the patient requires vasopressors.
  - Frequent and repeated assessment of vitals (BP, HR, RR, Temp) and other physiologic parameters such as $PaO2$ and urine output.
  - Additional fluid and vasopressors guided toward maintaining hemodynamic status and correcting lactate if abnormal.
- **Diagnostic work-up:** Identifying the infective source of sepsis is a critical component of treatment; however, microbiologic testing can be impaired by antibiotic administration. A critical foundation of the current approach to sepsis is that diagnostic evaluation is important but that it *cannot* be allowed to slow or delay other treatment efforts. Generally the following microbiologic testing should be obtained as quickly as possible once sepsis is recognized, as long as it does not slow the delivery of antibiotics.

> **• BOX 10.11 Common Organisms in Sepsis**
>
> - *Staphylococcus aureus* (MSSA and MRSA)
> - *Escherichia coli*
> - *Streptococcus pneumoniae*
> - *Enterococcus faecalis*
> - *Staphylococcus epidermidis*
> - *Klebsiella pneumoniae*
> - *Pseudomonas aeruginosa*
> - *Bacteroides fragilis*
> - Other streptococci
> - *Serratia marcescens*
> - *Enterobacter cloacae*
> - *Proteus mirabilis*
> - *Candida albicans*

- Blood cultures (two sets). Bacteremia is a common primary or secondary infective cause of sepsis, so blood cultures are almost always warranted in septic patients. While blood cultures have greatest yield prior to antibiotics, treatment should not be delayed in order to accomplish them. In patients who may have line infection as a source, a set of line cultures is also recommended.
- Urinalysis and urine culture. Given that UTIs are one of the most common causes of sepsis, urinary testing is often warranted in septic patients who have any urinary symptoms, or for whom urinary symptoms cannot be properly screened.
- Sputum culture. If the patient is able to provide them, sputum cultures can be invaluable in properly targeting antibiotics in patients who have pneumonia.

Treatment

Antiinfective Treatment

Treatment of the core infection is a critical component of sepsis therapy. Delay in antibiotic therapy after the onset of sepsis has been firmly established to lead to a marked increase in patient mortality, with every hour of additional delay leading to a 7.6% decrease in survival. The approach taken in sepsis patients should include both antimicrobial agent therapy as well as source control if possible.

Antimicrobial Therapy

Rapid antimicrobial therapy is one of the primary aims in the treatment of sepsis, with administration of antibiotics within 1 hour of the onset of sepsis the objective for providers and medical facilities. Treatment regimen should be tailored to broadly cover all likely pathogens. Given the spectrum of bacteria noted in Box 10.8, this generally implies broad coverage for gram-negative bacteria (including *Pseudomonas*) as well as coverage for methicillin-resistant *Staphylococcus aureus* (MRSA). Depending upon the source of infection, however, likely pathogens can vary significantly, as a result the empiric agents recommended for them can vary greatly.

The following are general empiric recommendations of agents and doses applicable to specific sepsis scenarios, though coverage should always be tailored to each patient's specific circumstances. Once specific microbiology and other diagnostic data are obtained, and the patient has stabilized, there can be a narrowing of therapy to a specific target.

Undifferentiated Sepsis
- In cases without a clearly defined source, sepsis coverage in the hospital setting should cover resistant gram-negative bacteria, including *Pseudomonas*, as well as resistant gram-positive bacteria, including MRSA.
  - Resistant gram-negative coverage
    - Cefepime 2 g IV q8h.
    - Piperacillin–tazobactam 4.5 g IV q6h.
    - Meropenem 1 g q8h.
    - Imipenem–cilastatin 500 mg IV q6h.
  - Resistant gram-negative coverage for penicillin-allergic patients
    - Aztreonam 2 g IV q8h.
    - Ciprofloxacin 400 mg IV q8h + aminoglycoside (gentamicin, amikacin, tobramycin).
  - Resistant gram-positive coverage
    - Vancomycin 15 mg/kg IV q8–12h (some practitioners utilize a loading dose of 20 mg/kg for the first dose).
    - Linezolid 600 mg IV q12h.
    - Daptomycin 8–10 mg/kg q24h (note: daptomycin is not active in pulmonary infections).

Pulmonary Focus
- As pulmonary infections are among the most common causes of sepsis, coverage for pulmonary sepsis is largely the same as that for undifferentiated sepsis (except daptomycin should not be used). One notable exception is during influenza season, when community-acquired sepsis can be the result of severe influenza infection. In these circumstances empiric influenza coverage is a reasonable addition to the standard antibacterials.

Urinary Tract Focus
- Urinary sources are common causes of sepsis, and coverage mimics that of undifferentiated sepsis.

Intraabdominal Focus
- In cases where sepsis is due to an intraabdominal focus of infection, gram-negative and anaerobic organisms are the most common pathogens. Additionally, in patients with a recent history of surgery or upper GI perforation, candidiasis is also a possible cause of sepsis.
  - Gram-negative + anaerobic coverage: piperacillin–tazobactam, meropenem, imipenem–cilastatin, cefepime + metronidazole.
  - Candida coverage
    - Micafungin 100 mg IV q24h.
    - Caspofungin 70 mg IV ×1, then 50 mg IV q24h.
    - Anidulafungin 200 mg IV ×1, then 100 mg IV q24h.
    - Fluconazole 800 mg IV ×1, then 400 mg q24h.

Skin and Soft Tissue Infections
- Severe soft tissue infections such as necrotizing fasciitis and gas gangrene can result in sepsis, and in those cases

one concern is for toxin production from such organisms as *Staphylococcus aureus*, *Streptococcus pyogenes*, and *Clostridium perfringens*. Consider adding or utilizing either linezolid or clindamycin to the empiric broad gram-positive and gram-negative coverage.

Risk Factors for Multidrug Resistant Organisms (MDROs)

- Patients who become septic who have risk factors for highly resistant gram-negative pathogens should have two gram-negative agents from different classes used at the same time. These risk factors include such historical elements as recent significant antibiotic exposure (within 90 days), a history of highly resistant gram-negative infection/colonization, neutropenia, mechanical ventilation, and residency in a nursing home.
  - Double gram-negative coverage
    - Antipseudomonal beta-lactam: cefepime, meropenem, or piperacillin–tazobactam, *and*
    - antipseudomonal fluoroquinolone (ciprofloxacin/levofloxacin), *or*
    - an aminoglycoside (gentamicin, tobramycin, amikacin), *or*
    - a polymyxin antibiotic (colistin, polymyxin B).

Source Control

- With the emphasis placed on antimicrobial therapy, it is easy to overlook physical source control as a critical component of antiinfective therapy. Retained sources represent persistent inflammatory foci and markedly reduce the efficacy of antimicrobials in controlling infection. Thus source identification and control should be performed as rapidly as possible. Infected tubes and lines should be removed, abscesses drained, infected bones and tissues debrided.

Continued Therapy

Once initial resuscitation has occurred and the infection evaluated and treated, continued therapy of the patient is tailored to support the patient for as long as it takes antiinfective therapy to bring the patient back from the septic state. Mitigation of end-organ damage while minimizing iatrogenic harm is a particular focus.

- **Maintenance of tissue perfusion**: fluids and vasopressors should be used to maintain target MAP of 65.
- **Prevention of ischemia**: transfusion is recommended only if Hb drops below 7.0, unless there is evidence of myocardial ischemia or hemorrhage.
- **Prevention of bleeding**: platelet transfusions are recommended only if Plt drops below 10,000/mm^3, unless there is high risk of bleeding, where the threshold is 20,000/mm^3.
- **Prevention of lung injury**: controlled ventilatory settings and techniques are recommended to prevent exacerbation of acute respiratory distress syndrome (ARDS) caused by sepsis. Minimizing excessive fluid administration is also recommended for the same purpose.
- **Minimize parenteral nutrition**: early enteral feeding and minimal usage of parenteral nutrition is recommended in order to preserve gut brush-border integrity and minimize the infectious risk posed by parenteral nutrition.

Further Reading

1. Freifeld AG, Bow EJ, Sepkowitz KA, Boeckh MJ, Ito JI, Mullen CA, et al. Clinical practice guideline for the use of antimicrobial agents in neutropenic patients with cancer: 2010 update by the infectious diseases society of America. *Clin Infect Dis*. 2011;52(4):e56–e93.
2. Knockaert DC, Vanderschueren S, Blockmans D. Fever of unknown origin in adults: 40 years on. *J Intern Med*. 2003;253(3):263–275.
3. Singer M, Deutschman CS, Seymour CW, Shankar-Hari M, Annane D, Bauer M, et al. The Third International Consensus Definitions for Sepsis and Septic Shock (Sepsis-3). *JAMA*. 2016;315(8):801–810.
4. Rhodes A, Evans LE, Alhazzani W, Levy MM, Antonelli M, Ferrer R, et al. Surviving sepsis campaign: international guidelines for management of sepsis and septic shock 2016. *Crit Care Med*. 2017;45(3):486.
5. Heffner AC, Horton JM, Marchick MR, Jones AE. Etiology of illness in patients with severe sepsis admitted to the hospital from the emergency department. *Clin Infect Dis*. 2010;50(6):814–820.

11

Head and Neck Infections

MEREDITH WELCH

OPHTHALMIC INFECTIONS

Definitions

Aqueous humor: fluid in the anterior segment.
Chemosis: collection of serous fluid in the conjunctiva; swollen conjunctiva.
Ciliary flush: red ring around the iris.
Conjunctiva: lining of the inside of the eyelid and the globe.
Cornea: transparent covering of the eye. Does not have vasculature, but has many nerve endings.
Hyphema: layering of red blood cells in the anterior chamber.
Hypopyon: layering of inflammatory cells (white blood cells) in the anterior chamber.
Iridocyclitis: inflammation of the anterior uveal tract including the ciliary body.
Keratitis: inflammation of the cornea, usually very painful.
Lens: divides the anterior and posterior segments.
Uvea: includes the iris, ciliary body, and choroid. Very vascular.
Vitreous humor: fluid in the posterior segment.

Anatomy

The anatomy of the eye is shown in Fig. 11.1. Distinguishing signs and symptoms based on anatomical location are listed in Table 11.1.

Conjunctivitis

Definition

- Inflammation of the conjunctiva.

Epidemiology

- Can be from systemic or local introduction of infection.
- Mother-to-child transmission during delivery.
- Sexual transmission.

Microbiology

- **Common viral causes**
  - Adenovirus.
    - Strains 8, 19, and 37 can cause epidemic kerato-conjunctivitis (EKC) which is more fulminant and involves the cornea. EKC is very contagious.
  - Self-limited.
  - Herpes simplex virus (HSV).
- Other viral causes
  - Variola (smallpox), vaccinia, herpes zoster, rubella, rubeola (measles), influenza, EBV.
  - Can get conjunctivitis or preseptal cellulitis as a contact of a patient that received smallpox vaccine or from being vaccinated.
    - Treatment is with vaccinia immunoglobulin and topical trifluridine drops.
  - Picornavirus (enterovirus).
- **Common bacterial causes**
  - *Chlamydia, Neisseria, Staphylococcus aureus, Streptococcus pneumoniae, Haemophilus influenzae.*
- Noninfectious causes
  - Allergic.
  - Chemical.

Clinical Presentation

- Usually a watery, itchy, red eye. Typically is **not painful**, nor does it include significant vision loss.
- Patients may report gritty feeling or feeling of sand in eye.
- Pain would indicate involvement of the cornea and would be called **keratoconjunctivitis.**
  - More purulent discharge is indicative of bacterial conjunctivitis, particularly with *Neisseria*, which is sometimes called hyperacute bacterial conjunctivitis (Fig. 11.2).
- Preauricular lymphadenopathy is usually present in viral conjunctivitis, but may also be present in *Chlamydia* and *Neisseria*.

Chlamydia

- **Leading infectious cause of blindness worldwide.**
- Causes adult inclusion conjunctivitis and trachoma.

Trachoma

- Found in less industrialized countries.
- Serotypes A, B, Ba, and C cause trachoma.
- Trachoma is caused by local inoculation from either contact with secretions or contaminated fomites.
- Starts as conjunctivitis and progresses to eyelid scarring resulting in the eyelid turning inward (entropion) (Fig. 11.3). The eyelashes turn inward (trichiasis) and ulceration of the cornea by abrasions can eventually lead to blindness.

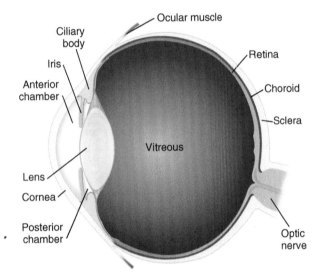

- **Fig. 11.1** Eye anatomy. (From Durand ML. Infectious causes of uveitis. In: Bennett JE, Dolin R, Blaser MJ, eds. *Mandell, Douglas, and Bennett's Principles and Practice of Infectious Diseases*. Updated 8th ed. Elsevier; 2015.)

- Arlt's line: the horizontal line of conjunctival scarring found on the superior eyelid.
- Diagnosis is usually clinical, but PCR is most reliable lab testing. Can send culture and Giemsa stain.
- **Treatment** is directed toward mass treatment.
  - WHO recommends SAFE
    - **S**urgery for trichiasis.
    - **A**ntibiotics for active infection.
    - **F**acial cleanliness.
    - **E**nvironmental improvement.
  - For the patient with active infection:
    - Systemic erythromycin or tetracycline for 3–4 weeks and subsequent topical erythromycin or tetracycline for 6 months.
  - For eradication of the infection in the population WHO recommends
    - Mass treatment (oral azithromycin annually) for at least 3 years if the endemic prevalence of children aged 1–9 years old is >10%.
    - After the 3 years of annual treatment, may discontinue treatment when prevalence is <5% in children aged 1–9 years old.

Adult Inclusion Conjunctivitis

- Chronic follicular conjunctivitis.
- Acquired sexually or via inoculation from contaminated secretions.
- Presents as a red eye with purulent discharge, preauricular lymphadenopathy, and **frequently has a urethritis/cervicitis present.**
- May progress to keratoconjunctivitis.
- Not as likely to lead to scarring and blindness as trachoma.
- **Treatment**
  - Requires systemic treatment (azithromycin) as well as treatment for sexual partners.

TABLE 11.1 **Distinguishing Signs and Symptoms of Eye Infections Based on Anatomical Location**

	Red	Pruritic	Painful	Decreased Visual Acuity	Foreign Body Sensation	Headache	Preauricular Lymphadenopathy
Conjunctivitis	x	x					x (in viral, *Chlamydia*, and *Neisseria*)
Keratitis	x		x	x	x		
Anterior uveitis	x		x	x			
Intermediate and posterior uveitis				x			
Panuveitis	x		x	x			
Endophthalmitis			x	x			
Acute angle closure	x		x	x		x	

Neisseria

- *Neisseria gonorrhoeae.*
- Spread by inoculation from hands to eyes.
- Marked purulent discharge, red eye, swollen eyelid, pre-auricular lymphadenopathy, and chemosis.
- Rapidly progressive if untreated.
- **Treatment**
  - IM ceftriaxone if only conjunctivitis.
  - If cornea involved, would need longer treatment course of ceftriaxone.
  - Concomitant treatment for *Chlamydia* is recommended.
  - Requires frequent flushing of eye to remove inflammation and enzymes harmful to the eye.

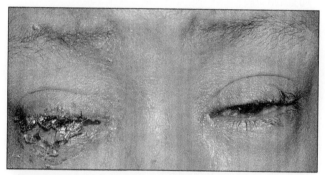

• **Fig. 11.2** Purulent discharge of *Neisseria* conjunctivitis (hyperacute bacterial conjunctivitis). (Courtesy Keith Walter, MD.)

Other Treatment

- Empiric treatment for bacterial conjunctivitis
  - Topical trimethoprim/polymyxin B or bacitracin/polymyxin B.
- Herpes simplex virus (HSV)
  - Refer to ophthalmology.
  - If just conjunctivitis, usually no antiviral is necessary.
  - Need to rule out corneal involvement.
- Varicella-zoster virus (VZV)
  - Refer to ophthalmology.
  - Oral aciclovir or valaciclovir.

Keratitis

- Inflammation of the cornea, which may be infectious or noninfectious.

Epidemiology

- Contact lens use (particularly overnight use or extended-wear lenses).
- Trauma: may be surgical or nonsurgical.
- Diabetes mellitus.
- Immunosuppression.

Microbiology (Table 11.2)

- ***Pseudomonas*** associated with contact lenses (Fig. 11.4).
- Of note, *Neisseria*, *Listeria*, and *Corynebacterium* may invade the intact cornea.

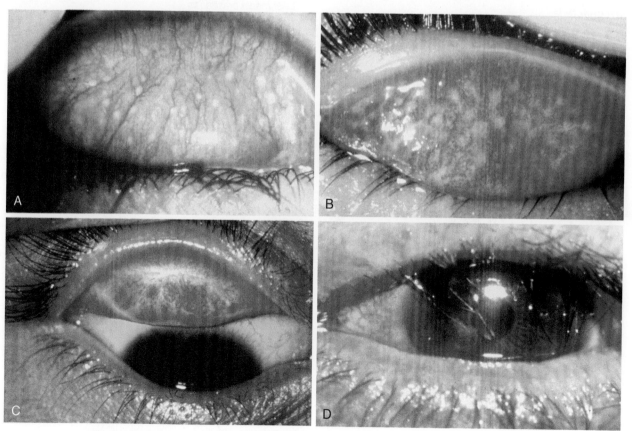

• **Fig. 11.3** Trachoma: (A) follicles; (B) inflammation; (C) trichiasis; (D) conjunctival scarring. (Courtesy International Centre for Eye Health (LSHTM), London.)

TABLE
11.2   **Microbiology of Keratitis**

Bacteria
Gram-Positive Cocci

Staphylococcus aureus
Staphylococcus epidermidis
Streptococcus pneumoniae, S. pyogenes, viridans
   streptococci
Enterococcus faecalis
Peptostreptococcus spp.

Gram-Positive Bacilli

Bacillus coagulans, B. cereus, B. licheniformis
Brevibacillus (Bacillus) brevis, B. (Bacillus) laterosporus
Corynebacterium diphtheriae
Clostridium perfringens, C. tetani

Gram-Negative Coccobacilli

Neisseria gonorrhoeae
Moraxella lacunata, M. nonliquefaciens, M. catarrhalis
Acinetobacter calcoaceticus
Pasteurella multocida

Gram-Negative Bacilli

Pseudomonas aeruginosa, P. stutzeri, P. fluorescens
Burkholderia (Pseudomonas) mallei
Proteus mirabilis
Serratia marcescens
Escherichia coli
Klebsiella pneumoniae
Morganella morganii
Aeromonas hydrophila
Bartonella henselae

Mycobacteria

Mycobacterium tuberculosis, M. chelonae, M. gordonae,
   M. mucogenicum

Actinomycetes

Nocardia spp.

Spirochetes

Treponema pallidum
Borrelia burgdorferi

Viruses

Herpes simplex virus
Varicella-zoster virus
Adenovirus
Vaccinia
Epstein–Barr
Rubeola
Enteroviruses
Coxsackievirus

Fungi

Fusarium spp.
Candida spp.
Aspergillus spp.
Acremonium spp.
Alternaria spp.
Penicillium spp.
Bipolaris spp.
Nosema spp.
Vittaforma (Nosema) corneae
Encephalitozoon spp.

Chlamydia

Chlamydia trachomatis

Parasites

Acanthamoeba polyphaga, A. castellanii
Onchocerca volvulus
Leishmania brasiliensis
Trypanosoma spp.

From Barnes SD, Hallak J, Pavan-Langston D, Azar DT. Microbial conjunctivitis. In: Bennett JE, Dolin R, Blaser MJ, eds. *Mandell, Douglas, and Bennett's Principles and Practice of Infectious Diseases.* Updated 8th ed. Elsevier; 2015.

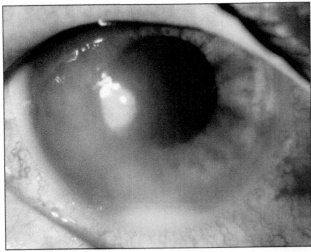

• **Fig. 11.4** *Pseudomonas* keratitis. (From Hong AR, Shute TS, Huang AJW. Bacterial keratitis. In: Mannis MJ, Holland EJ, eds. *Cornea.* 4th ed. Elsevier; 2017.)

Clinical Presentation

- Exquisitely painful eye, with decreased vision, tearing, and corneal edema.
- Has foreign body sensation.
- Fluorescein used to visualize ulcer or infiltrates.
- May have purulent discharge depending on etiology.
- Bacterial keratitis frequently has a white infiltrate or "spot" on the cornea.
- Can rapidly progress.
- Corneal scrapings and culture should be done with PCR as indicated for viral etiology.

Viral Keratitis

HSV 1 and HSV 2
- HSV 1 predominates.
- Most often a result of reactivation from latent disease rather than primary disease.

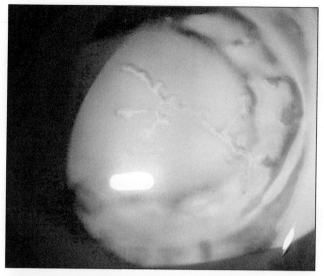

• **Fig. 11.5** Dendritic lesion of HSV keratitis. (From Holland EJ, Schwartz GS, Shah KJ. Herpes simplex keratitis. In: Mannis MJ, Holland EJ, eds. *Cornea.* 4th ed. Elsevier; 2017.)

- Exam reveals dendritic lesions (Fig. 11.5), ciliary flush, and decreased sensation of the cornea.
- May have vesicles on the eyelid.
- Typically unilateral.
- Diagnosis is usually clinical, but scrapings can be sent for PCR.
- **Treatment** is topical antiviral, but may use oral antiviral as well with consideration for oral suppression.
  - Trifluridine, aciclovir, valaciclovir

Varicella

- Can happen before, during, or after a herpes zoster ophthalmicus.
- Complete loss of sensation of cornea is a hallmark for VZV.
- Cornea has dendritic lesions as well.
- Recall Hutchinson's sign.
  - Lesions on tip of nose.
  - Innervated by nasociliary branch of trigeminal nerve.
  - Would require ophthalmic exam as well.
- **Treatment** is topical and oral antivirals.
  - Trifluridine, aciclovir, vaclaciclovir.

Vaccinia and Adenovirus

- Previously outlined under conjunctivitis.

Bacterial Keratitis

- *Neisseria* and *Chlamydia* reviewed previously with conjunctivitis.
- *Nocardia* and *Mycobacterium* associated with surgery (LASIK).
  - *M. chelonae* is most common of the atypical mycobacteria.

Syphilis

- Most often in congenital syphilis.
- Usually presents in teenage years.

- **Treatment**
  - Typically with topical antibiotics, unless etiology warrants a systemic treatment (e.g., syphilis, Lyme, etc.).
  - Common empiric regimen would be topical cephalosporin or vancomycin and topical aminoglycoside.
  - Less severe cases may use topical fluoroquinolone empirically.
  - More severe cases may require systemic antibiotics.

Fungal Keratitis

- *Fusarium, Aspergillus, Candida.*
- *Fusarium* is most common.
- Risk factors include
  - Trauma, immunosuppression, contact lens use, and topical steroid use in eye.
- Usually less suppurative initially, but purulent later in course.
  - Can have hypopyon later.
- **Treatment**
  - Combination of topical and systemic treatment.
  - Natamycin, voriconazole, or amphotericin for molds.
  - Azoles for *Candida.*

Amebic Keratitis

Acanthamoeba

- Is both a trophozoite and a dormant cyst form.
- Associated with **contact lens use** (wearing for prolonged periods) and trauma.
- Was historically associated with the tablets used to make contact solution at home.
- Usually unilateral.
- Clinical features are a red eye, pain, and photophobia.
- Can have a dendritic lesion, so may be mistaken for HSV.
- May have a ring lesion later in course (see Fig. 11.6).
- Calcofluor white stains the trophozoite and the cyst.
- Can plate the scraping on an *E. coli* lawn.
- Topical steroids early on will worsen the disease.
- **Treatment**
  - No consensus on best treatment.
  - Combination treatment.
    - Topical polyhexamethylene guanide *or* chlorhexidine.
    - *Plus* topical propamidine isethionate *or* hexamidine.
- May require keratoplasty.

Uveitis

- Inflammation of the iris, ciliary body, choroid, or retina (Table 11.3)
  - Anterior, intermediate, posterior, and panuveitis.
    - Intermediate: ciliary body and vitreous inflammation.
    - Panuveitis: anterior, posterior, and retina or choroid inflammation.

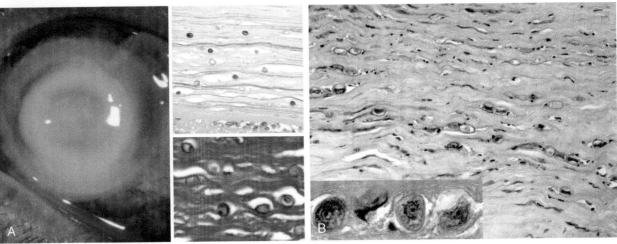

• **Fig. 11.6** Acanthamoeba keratitis. (A) Ring-shaped infiltrate: (top panel) GMS stain with cyst; (bottom panel) PAS stain with cyst. (B) Cyst at higher power. (From Stagner A, Jakoblec FA, Eagle RC, Charles NC. Infections of the eye and its adnexa. In: Kradin RL, ed. *Diagnostic Pathology of Infectious Diseases*. 2nd ed. Elsevier; 2018.)

TABLE 11.3 Classifications of Uveitis

Category	Ocular Findings	Major Infectious Etiologies (%)*
Anterior (iritis, cyclitis, iridocyclitis)	WBCs in aqueous, keratic precipitates, iris nodules, synechiae	Herpes simplex (10%); syphilis (<1%); TB (<1%); Lyme disease (<1%); leprosy (<1%)
Intermediate	WBCs or *snowballs* in the vitreous, pars plana *snow bank*	Lyme disease (<1%)
Posterior (choroiditis, chorioretinitis, retinitis)	Lesions in choroid, retina, or both; vitritis in some	*Toxoplasma* (25%); CMV (12%); ARN (6%); *Toxocara* (3%); syphilis (2%); *Candida* (<1%)
Panuveitis	WBCs in aqueous and vitreous	Syphilis (6%); TB (2%); *Candida* (2%)

ARN, acute retinal necrosis; *CMV,* cytomegalovirus; *TB,* tuberculosis; *WBCs,* white blood cells.
From Durand ML. Infectious causes of uveitis. In: Bennett JE, Dolin R, Blaser MJ, eds. *Mandell, Douglas, and Bennett's Principles and Practice of Infectious Diseases*. Updated 8th ed. Elsevier; 2015.

- Recall the uvea is highly vascular.
- Hematogenous spread or systemic disease is predominant source.
- Most uveitis is from a noninfectious cause.
- Infectious uveitis more commonly implicated in posterior uveitis.

Anterior Uveitis
- Presents as painful red eye with loss of vision.
- HSV is the leading infectious cause.

Intermediate Uveitis
- Loss of vision with floaters.
- Typically painless.
- *Borrelia burgdorferi* is leading infectious cause.
- Exceedingly rare to be infectious.

Posterior Uveitis
- Usually painless loss of vision.
- Higher risk for long-term vision loss.
- *Toxoplasma* is leading infectious cause.

Viral Uveitis

Herpes Simplex Virus (HSV)
- HSV 1 predominates (as in keratitis).
- There is usually a preceding keratitis.
- Reactivation of HSV is mechanism.
- Presentation is usually a unilateral red, painful eye with impaired vision but absence of vesicles.
- Decreased sensation of cornea may be present as in keratitis.
- Diagnosis established by PCR of aqueous humor.

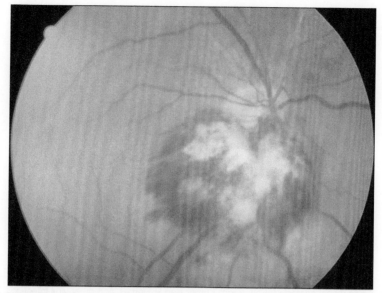

• **Fig. 11.7** CMV retinitis (hemorrhages and inflammation). (From Zamir E. Ocular infections with cytomegalovirus. In: Yanoff M, Duker JS, eds. *Ophthalmology*. 4th ed. Elsevier; 2014.)

- **Treatment**
  - Oral aciclovir, followed by oral suppression.
  - Topical steroids.

Varicella-Zoster Virus (VZV)
- Similar anterior uveitis as in HSV.
- Does not have preceding keratitis.
- Reactivation is mechanism.
- Cause of acute retinal necrosis and leading cause of progressive outer retinal necrosis.
- Diagnosis established by PCR of aqueous humor.
- **Treatment**
  - If retinitis present: IV aciclovir followed by oral aciclovir or valaciclovir.
  - Typically would receive systemic steroids.
  - Intravitreal antivirals as directed by ophthalmology.
  - May require vitrectomy or laser therapy.

Cytomegalovirus (CMV)
- More commonly causes a retinitis.
- Immunosuppressed patient
  - Typically a person with HIV.
- Dilated eye exam reveals retinitis with hemorrhages and flares of inflammation (Fig. 11.7).
- Diagnosis is by clinical appearance but also with PCR of aqueous humor.
- **Treatment**
  - IV ganciclovir
    - Intravitreal antiviral.
    - Oral secondary suppression.
- Topic reviewed further under opportunistic infections in HIV.

Acute Retinal Necrosis (ARN) (Fig. 11.8)
- American Uveitis Society definition
  1. Well demarcated retinal necrosis on peripheral retina.
  2. Rapid progression of necrosis.
  3. Circumferential spread.
  4. Occlusive vasculopathy.
  5. Vitreal and aqueous inflammation.
- **HSV and VZV** are the main causes.
- Occurs in immunocompetent patients.
- Presents as anterior uveitis that progresses to necrosis.
- Very high risk for retinal detachment and blindness.
- **Treatment** as outlined with VZV uveitis.

Progressive Outer Retinal Necrosis (PORN) (Fig. 11.9)
- Retinal necrosis as in ARN **except:**
  - No vasculopathy.
  - Involves the outer retina.
  - Does not have inflammation.
  - **Occurs almost exclusively in immunocompromised patients.**
    - Typically persons with HIV and CD4 <100/μL.
- **VZV is leading cause.**
  - HSV and CMV are other causes.
- Presents as vision loss.
- Very poor prognosis for preserving vision.
- **Treatment**
  - IV antivirals (aciclovir or ganciclovir).
  - Intravitreal antiviral.
  - Systemic steroids usually not needed (unless concerns for IRIS) given lack of inflammation.
  - May require laser therapy and/or vitrectomy.
  - Secondary oral suppression.

Bacterial Uveitis

Syphilis
- Frequently presents as vision loss.
- Can occur at any stage of syphilis.
- Can involve any segment of the eye, but posterior disease and panuveitis predominate.

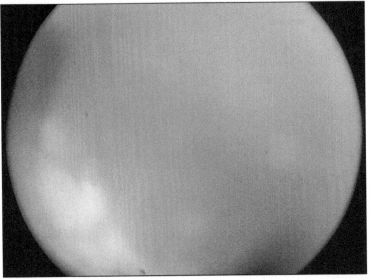

• **Fig. 11.8** Acute retinal necrosis (ARN). (From Kumar Rao P. Herpes and other viral infections. In: Yanoff M, Duker JS, eds. *Ophthalmology.* 4th ed. Elsevier; 2014.)

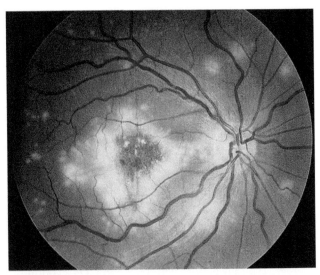

• **Fig. 11.9** Progressive outer retinal necrosis (PORN). (From Kozak I, McCutchan JA, Freeman WR. HIV-associated infections. In: Schachat AP, Wilkinson CP, Hinton DR, Sadda SR, Wiedemann P. *Ryan's Retina.* 6th ed. Elsevier; 2018.)

- Case definition is **ocular disease** (uveitis, panuveitis, diminished visual acuity, blindness, optic neuropathy, interstitial keratitis, anterior uveitis, and retinal vasculitis) **with syphilis of any stage.**
- Requires lumbar puncture and HIV testing.
- Treat as neurosyphilis with aqueous penicillin G.

Bartonella
- *Bartonella henselae.*
- Has ocular involvement as part of cat scratch disease.
- Parinaud's oculoglandular syndrome
  - Result of cat scratch near the eye or self-inoculation near eye.

- Lymphadenopathy of preauricular, submandibular, and cervical nodes along with involvement of lid or conjunctiva.
- Has red eye with watering.
- Treatment is supportive vs oral azithromycin.
- Optic neuritis
  - Can have macular star which is exudate at the macula (not pathognomonic for *Bartonella*).
  - Treatment is prolonged doxycycline and rifampin.

Lyme Disease
- *Borrelia burgdorferi.*
- Ocular disease may occur at any stage of Lyme, but most frequently in later stages.
- Can affect any part of eye, but most frequently causes conjunctivitis in early Lyme.
- Diagnosis is complicated. Use 2-tier testing as for systemic Lyme with ELISA and Western blot.
- Treat as would with systemic disease, and may need topical antiinflammatory agent.

Tuberculosis
- Very uncommon.
- Can infect any part of eye, but most commonly causes uveitis and more specifically a panuveitis.
- Diagnosis is difficult to establish as it is paucibacillary, so unlikely to have positive tissue cultures or acid-fast stains.
  - Relies on appropriate clinical setting and a positive PPD or interferon-gamma release assay.
- Treatment is same as TB meningitis
  - Rifampin, isoniazid, ethambutol, and pyrazinamide.
  - May require systemic steroids.
- Of note, immune reconstitution inflammatory syndrome (IRIS) has been reported in persons with HIV and ocular TB.

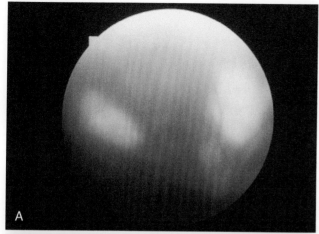
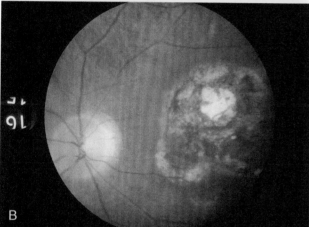
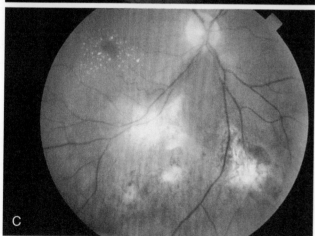

• **Fig. 11.10** Toxoplasmosis chorioretinitis. (Courtesy Dr. Robert Nussenblatt, National Eye Institute, National Institutes of Health, Bethesda, MD; Dr. Claudio Silveira, Erechim, Brazil; and Dr. Rubens Belfort, São Paulo Brazil.)

Parasitic Uveitis

Toxoplasma (Fig. 11.10)

- Occurs in both immunocompetent and immunocompromised patients.
- Can be acutely acquired toxoplasmosis, but can result from latent disease as well as complications later from congenital toxoplasmosis.
- Reactivation usually results in bilateral disease whereas acutely acquired disease is more often unilateral.

- Presents as vision loss. May be painful.
- Usually posterior uveitis or chorioretinitis.
- Very inflammatory posterior segment with necrosis.
- Dilated eye exam typically reveals a white focal lesion with surrounding inflammation. Can have black pigmentation in areas that are healing. May have satellite lesions.
- Diagnosis based on eye exam findings, and can also send PCR of vitreous humor along with serology.
- **Treatment** is as for systemic disease.
  - Pyrimethamine and sulfadiazine with leucovorin.
  - Systemic steroids.
  - May require secondary prophylaxis with TMP/SMX depending on host.

Toxocara

- Mostly found in children.
- Presents as painful loss of vision.
- Causes posterior uveitis, retinitis, or panuveitis.
- Is a result of migrating larvae.
- Serology is not helpful as may be negative if disease only located in eye, or may be positive from a prior exposure.
- Diagnosis is clinical.
- **Treatment** is with vitrectomy and as for visceral larvae migrans with either albendazole or mebendazole and systemic steroids.
- At times may be confused with retinoblastoma. In these cases, vitreal sampling is usually avoided to avoid orbital spread of retinoblastoma.

Endophthalmitis

Definition

- Infection within the globe.

Epidemiology/Microbiology

- Risk factors
  - Instrumentation or trauma of eye.
  - Diabetes mellitus.
  - Injection drug use.
  - Risk factors associated with bacteremia or fungemia.

Diagnosis

- Vitreal Gram stain and cultures.
- Blood cultures.

Treatment

- Outlined in Table 11.4.
- Note echinocandins have poor eye penetration.
- Fluconazole has good eye penetration, but may need voriconazole or amphotericin if concerns for a resistant *Candida*.
- Will require intravitreal treatment, and may require vitrectomy if more fulminant or not responding to therapy.
  - Vitrectomy removes the inflammation (similar to drainage of an abscess)

TABLE 11.4 Endophthalmitis

Category	Microbiology	Clinical Findings	Treatment
Exogenous (Trauma)	*Bacillus*, coagulase-negative staphylococci, *Pseudomonas*, mold	Open globe Fulminant endophthalmitis with *Bacillus*	• Surgical repair and vitrectomy • Systemic and intravitreal vancomycin and ceftazidime • Consider systemic amphotericin
Surgical			
Post-cataract surgery	Coagulase-negative staphylococci, *Staphylococcus aureus*, streptococci, gram-negatives	Pain described as "ache" Vision loss	• Intravitreal vancomycin and ceftazidime
Pseudophakic (Chronic disease post-cataract surgery)	*Cutibacterium acnes* (formerly *Propionibacterium acnes*)	Pain, vision loss, plaque in lens	• Intravitreal vancomycin • Vitrectomy, likely to require lens removal
Intravitreal injection (Macular degeneration treatment)	Coagulase-negative staphylococci and streptococci	Pain and vision loss Hypopyon	• Intravitreal vancomycin and ceftazidime
Bleb-related (Surgical treatment for glaucoma that creates scleral defect)	Streptococci, *Moraxella*, *H. influenzae*	Vision loss, pain, may have red eye Hypopyon	• Intravitreal vancomycin, ceftazidime
Endogenous			
Bacterial	Streptococci, coagulase-negative staphylococci, *S. aureus, Bacillus*	Pain and vision loss May have fever	• Systemic and intravitreal antimicrobials • Fulminant cases require vitrectomy
Fungal	*Candida, Aspergillus*	Vision loss Fluffy vitreal lesions	• Vitrectomy with intravitreal amphotericin or voriconazole • Systemic fluconazole, or voriconazole, or amphotericin

INFECTIONS OF THE HEAD AND NECK

Otitis and Mastoiditis

Definitions

Otitis externa: inflammation of the ear canal.
- Skin flora of external ear that causes infection in moist environment.
- E.g., swimmer's ear.
- Can also occur with disruption of the epithelium such as in eczema.

Malignant otitis externa: otitis externa that invades skull base.
Otitis media: inflammation of the middle ear.
Chronic otitis media: otitis media lasting >3 months.
Mastoiditis: inflammation of the mastoid air cells.
- Complication from otitis media.
- Can invade the bone and CNS.

Epidemiology
- Majority of otitis occurs in children.
- Risk factors

- Diabetes.
- Disruption of the drainage of the Eustachian tube.
- Smoking.

Clinical Features and Treatment (Table 11.5)

Parotitis

Definition
- Inflammation of the parotid gland.
- May be suppurative or nonsuppurative.

Epidemiology
- Elderly and diabetics at higher risk.
- Decreased saliva production poses higher risk.
  - Anticholinergic use, for example.

Microbiology
- Suppurative
  - **S. aureus** predominates.
- Nonsuppurative

TABLE 11.5 Otitis Features and Treatment

	Microbiology	Clinical Findings	Treatment
Otitis externa	Staphylococcus aureus, Pseudomonas	• Ear pain with drainage in canal • May be pruritic	**Topical** • Neomycin/polymyxin/hydrocortisone or • Fluoroquinolone/hydrocortisone
Malignant otitis externa	Pseudomonas	• Severe pain of ear and mastoid with purulent drainage in canal • May have cranial nerve palsy	**Systemic** agent that is **antipseudomonal** • Cefepime, ceftazidime, or piperacillin/tazobactam **Debridement** of necrotic devitalized tissue
Otitis media	Streptococcus pneumoniae, Haemophilus influenzae	• Pain with inflamed bulging TM with purulent fluid in middle ear • May have decreased hearing and fever	**Systemic antibiotic** • Amoxicillin • Amoxicillin/clavulanic acid if not improving • Cephalosporin if PCN allergy • Respiratory fluoroquinolone if severe PCN allergy
Mastoiditis	S. pneumoniae, H. influenzae	• Ear pain, fever, recent or current otitis media	**Systemic** antimicrobials as in otitis media • May require surgical debridement (mastoidectomy)

• Mumps and other viruses.
• Connective tissue disorders such as sarcoidosis.

Clinical Presentation

• Suppurative
  • Typically unilateral.
  • Fulminant presentation.
  • Fever with severe pain and swelling of parotid gland.
  • May be able to "milk" purulence from Stenson's duct.
  • May have obstructing stone.
• Nonsuppurative
  • Typically bilateral.
  • Less fulminant presentation.
  • Prodrome was present prior to the parotitis.

Diagnosis

• Imaging may be helpful (CT vs. ultrasound) to see if drainable abscess.
• Presence of purulence from Stenson's duct.
• Culture and Gram stain of any purulence.
• Serology for viral etiology as indicated.

Treatment

• Suppurative.
• Target S. aureus
  • Vancomycin (or antistaphylococcal beta-lactam if MRSA not suspected) and clindamycin.
  • May require removal of obstructing stone.
• Warm compresses.
• Sialagogues.
• Supportive for viral causes.

Peritonsillar Abscess

Definition

• Abscess located between the capsule of the tonsil and the pharyngeal musculature.
• Sometimes called **quinsy.**

Microbiology

• Streptococci, staphylococci, and anaerobes.

Clinical Features

• Unilateral sore throat with edematous palatine tonsil that may be causing deviation of the uvula.
• Fever.
• Abrupt onset.
• May have drooling or trismus.
• Have to distinguish from epiglottitis and other deep neck space infections.
• Can also lead to a suppurative thrombophlebitis (Lemierre's syndrome).

Diagnosis

• Clinical diagnosis based on a swollen tonsil and uvula that deviates (Fig. 11.11).
• If able, aspiration for Gram stain and culture.
• If concerns for epiglottitis, would avoid aspiration.
• May need imaging (ultrasound vs. contrast CT) if diagnosis is ambiguous.

Treatment

• Airway management and concerns for possible deeper infection are foremost.

- Aspiration or incision and drainage.
  - Gram stain and culture.
- Beta-lactam with beta-lactamase inhibitor (ampicillin/sulbactam, piperacillin/tazobactam).
- Clindamycin also an option.
- May require tonsillectomy.

Ludwig's Angina

Definition

- Bilateral sublingual and submylohyoid space infection.

Epidemiology/Microbiology

- Most are sequelae of odontogenic infection, particularly a molar tooth.
- Odontogenic flora predominate.
  - Polymicrobial oral flora including anaerobes.
  - Streptococci including Group A *Streptococcus*.

Clinical Features

- Rapidly progressing infection of floor of the mouth that is bilateral.
- Fever present and may be toxic.
- Tongue may be markedly swollen and patient may have difficulty swallowing leading to drooling (Fig. 11.12).

Diagnosis/Treatment

- Diagnosis is based on clinical findings and may require CT imaging.
- Treatment is airway protection and prevention of spread to retropharyngeal space or mediastinum.
- Beta-lactam with beta-lactamase inhibitor *or*

- PCN and metronidazole *or*
- Clindamycin.

Vincent's Angina

Definition

- Acute necrotizing ulcerative gingivitis.
- Sometimes called "trench mouth."
  - Term comes from lack of access to dental care or dental hygiene for soldiers during World War I.

Epidemiology

- Gingivitis.
- Smoking.
- Poor oral care.
- Malnutrition.

Microbiology

- Polymicrobial oral flora.
- Anaerobes.

Clinical Features

- Pain with fetid breath.
- Fevers.
- Typically does have regional lymphadenopathy.
- Pseudomembranes with ulcerative gingival lesions (Fig. 11.13).

Diagnosis/Treatment

- Diagnosis is based on clinical appearance.
- Treatment
  - Debridement.
  - PCN or amoxicillin/clavulanic acid or metronidazole.

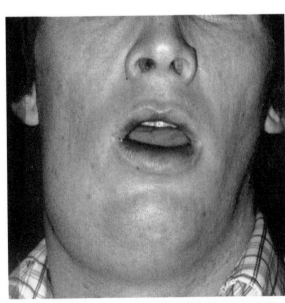

- **Fig. 11.11** Peritonsillar abscess. (From Florin TA, Ludwig S, eds. *Netter's Pediatrics*. Elsevier; 2011.)

- **Fig. 11.12** Ludwig's angina. (From Benko KR. Emergency dental procedures. In: Roberts JR, et al., eds. *Roberts and Hedges' Clinical Procedures in Emergency Medicine and Acute Care*. 7th ed. Elsevier; 2018.)

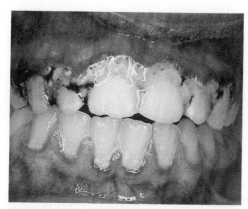

• **Fig. 11.13** Trench mouth. Necrosis and hemorrhage with pseudomembranes of gingiva. (From Martin JM, Baumhardt H, D'Alesio A, Woods K. Oral disorders. In: Zitelli B, McIntire S, Nowalk AJ, eds. *Zitelli and Davis' Atlas of Pediatric Physical Diagnosis.* Elsevier; 2018.)

Lemierre Syndrome

Definition

- Suppurative thrombophlebitis of jugular vein.

Epidemiology/Microbiology

- Typically follows a preceding pharyngitis, but can be related with other oropharyngeal infections such as peritonsillar abscess.
- *Fusobacterium necrophorum* accounts for majority of disease.
- Can be other oral flora including other *Fusobacterium, S. aureus,* and Group A *Streptococcus.*

Clinical Features

- Patients may describe the pharyngitis as "the worst sore throat of my life."
- Usually presents with neck pain and fevers.

- May have other sites of septic emboli, such as pulmonary emboli.

Diagnosis/Treatment

- Imaging diagnoses the suppurative thrombophlebitis (CT with contrast).
- Treatment
  - Beta-lactam/beta-lactamase inhibitor such as ampicillin/sulbactam or piperacillin/tazobactam.
  - Use of anticoagulation is controversial.
  - Historically required jugular vein ligation, but rarely needed now.

Septic Cavernous Sinus Thrombosis

Definition

- Cavernous sinus thrombosis as a result of drainage from infection elsewhere in head or neck.
- Fig. 11.14 shows anatomy.

Microbiology

- Depends on site of infection.
  - Orbit, such as orbital cellulitis or preseptal cellulitis.
  - Sinus (sphenoid or ethmoid more common), otitis.
  - Odontogenic.
- *S. aureus, Streptococcus* (including *S. pneumoniae*), *H. influenzae.*
- Anaerobes if from sinusitis, otitis, or odontogenic source.

Clinical Features

- Headache with fever.
- Cranial nerve III–VI palsy.
  - May have diplopia.
  - Proptosis.
  - Ptosis.

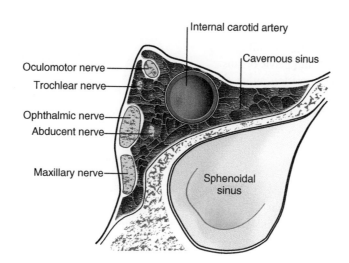

• **Fig. 11.14** Cavernous sinus anatomy, oblique section. (From Tunkell AR. Subdural empyema, epidural abscess, and suppurative intracranial thrombophlebitis. In: Bennett JE, Dolin R, Blaser MJ, eds. *Mandell, Douglas, and Bennett's Principles and Practice of Infectious Diseases.* Updated 8th ed. Elsevier; 2015.)

- Periorbital edema.
- Can lead to vision loss.

Diagnosis

- MRI or MR venography.
- CT if unable to do MRI.

Treatment

- Antibiotics
  - Vancomycin and third- or fourth-generation cephalosporin.
  - Metronidazole if etiology is concerning for anaerobes.
- Surgical
  - May require debridement, particularly if sinusitis present.
- Anticoagulation
  - Controversial.

Cervicofacial Actinomycosis

Epidemiology

- Immunocompetent hosts.
- Diabetes.
- Trauma.
- Dental infections.

Microbiology

- Gram-positive anaerobic branching rod that is normal commensal of oral flora.
- May have "sulfur granules."
  - Sulfur granules are conglomeration of bacteria, but look like sulfur.
- Has molar tooth colony appearance on plates.
- Slower growing and can violate tissue planes.
- Usually infections with *Actinomyces* are polymicrobial.

Clinical Presentation

- Typically presents as a mass or abscess in neck, jaw, or mouth.
- Can invade bone.
- Can be in other anatomical sites as well including lung (empyema necessitans), abdominal, and pelvic organs.
- Usually spread by contiguous local invasion rather than hematogenously.
- Sometimes mistaken for potential malignancy until biopsy results return.
- May not have fevers or systemic symptoms.

Treatment

- First-line treatment is penicillin.
- Duration is prolonged, usually 6–12 months.
- Options for penicillin-allergic patients include doxycycline or clindamycin.
- Surgery may be required for complex abscess or marsupialization of a draining fistula, but first-line treatment would be systemic antibiotics.

DEEP NECK SPACE INFECTIONS

Definition

- Lateral pharyngeal space
  - Base of skull to hyoid.
  - Medial border is the carotid sheath.
- Pretracheal space
  - Esophagus and trachea.
  - Contiguous with mediastinum and carotid sheath.
- Retropharyngeal space
  - Posterior to hypopharynx and esophagus.
  - Extends to mediastinum inferiorly.
- Danger space
  - Between alar fascia and prevertebral fascia
  - Communicates with posterior mediastinum.
- Prevertebral space
  - Spinous process to prevertebral fascia.
- Fig. 11.15 shows anatomy.

Epidemiology/Microbiology

- Odontogenic or oropharyngeal source.
- Polymicrobial but Streptococci predominate.
- Can have *S. aureus*.

Clinical Features

- Fever.
- Toxic.
- Can have dysphagia (particularly with pretracheal).
- Dyspnea.
- Concern is for possible extension into mediastinum.

Diagnosis/Treatment

- Prompt imaging is paramount (CT).
- Treatment
  - Surgical debridement.
  - Many options for antimicrobials, but typically beta-lactam/beta-lactamase inhibitor and possibly vancomycin if concerns for MRSA (i.e., trauma, high risk, colonized).

Osteomyelitis of the Jaw

Definition

- Bone infection of the jaw.

Epidemiology/Microbiology

- Typically some predisposing condition that led to compromised blood supply, and spreads from contiguous site.
  - DM, steroids, radiation, trauma (dental procedure), necrosis from medication.
- Oral flora predominates.
  - Streptococci, *Actinomyces*, *S. aureus*.

Clinical Features

- Jaw pain.

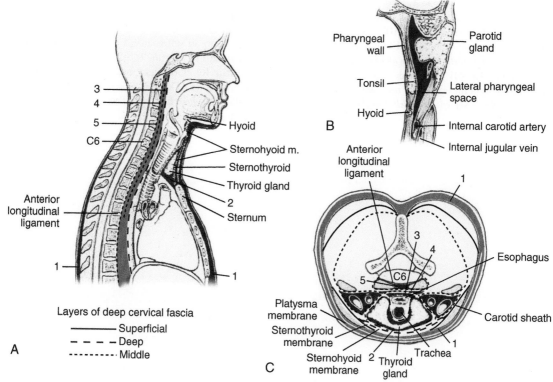

• **Fig. 11.15** Spaces of the neck. (A) Midsagittal section. (B) Coronal section. (C) Cross-section. In all panels: 1, superficial space; 2, pretracheal space; 3, retropharyngeal space; 4, danger space; 5, prevertebral space. (From Chow AW. Infections of the oral cavity, neck, and head. In: Bennett JE, Dolin R, Blaser MJ, eds. *Mandell, Douglas, and Bennett's Principles and Practice of Infectious Diseases*. Updated 8th ed. Elsevier; 2015.)

• Exposed bone.
• Mandible much more common than maxilla given better vascular supply to maxilla.

Treatment

• Surgical debridement of necrotic tissue.
• Directed antimicrobial.
  • Prolonged course usually required.
  • Usually parenteral beta-lactam or beta-lactam/beta-lactamase inhibitor.
  • May need vancomycin if suspicion for MRSA.
• Can consider hyperbaric oxygen as adjunctive treatment, but data is inconclusive for efficacy.

Further Reading

1. Durand ML. Infectious causes of uveitis. In: Bennett JE, Dolin R, Blaser MJ, eds. *Mandell, Douglas, and Bennett's Principles and Practice of Infectious Diseases*. 8th ed. Elsevier; 2015. Updated.
2. Soukiasian S, Baum J. Bacterial conjunctivitis. In: Mannis MJ, Holland EJ, eds. *Cornea*. 4th ed. Elsevier; 2017.
3. Beare NAV, Bastawrous A. Ophthalmology in the tropics and sub-tropics. In: Farrar J, et al., ed. *Manson's Tropical Diseases*. 23rd ed. Elsevier; 2014.
4. Barnes SD, Hallak J, Pavan-Langston D, Azar DT. Microbial keratitis. In: Bennett JE, Dolin R, Blaser MJ, eds. *Mandell, Douglas, and Bennett's Principles and Practice of Infectious Diseases*. 8th ed. Elsevier; 2015. Updated.
5. Hong AR, Shute TS, Huang AJW. Bacterial keratitis. In: Mannis MJ, Holland EJ, eds. *Cornea*. 4th ed. Elsevier; 2017.
6. Holland EJ, Schwartz GS, Shah KJ. Herpes simplex keratitis. In: Mannis MJ, Holland EJ, eds. *Cornea*. 4th ed. Elsevier; 2017.
7. Stagner A, Jakoblec FA, Eagle RC, Charles NC. Infections of the eye and its adnexa. In: Kradin RL, ed. *Diagnostic Pathology of Infectious Disease*. 2nd ed. Elsevier; 2018.
8. Durand ML. Infectious causes of uveitis. In: Bennett JE, Dolin R, Blaser MJ, eds. *Mandell, Douglas, and Bennett's Principles and Practice of Infectious Diseases*. 8th ed. Elsevier; 2015. Updated.
9. Zamir E. Ocular infections with cytomegalovirus. In: Yanoff M, Duker JS, eds. *Ophthalmology*. 4th ed. Elsevier; 2014.
10. Kumar Rao P. Herpes and other viral infections. In: Yanoff M, Duker JS, eds. *Ophthalmology*. 4th ed. Elsevier; 2014.
11. Kozak I, McCutchan JA, Freeman WR. HIV-associated infections. In: Schachat AP, Wilkinson CP, Hinton DR, Sadda SR, Wiedemann P, eds. *Ryan's Retina*. 6th ed. Elsevier; 2018.
12. Montoya JG, Boothroyd JC, Kovacs JA. Toxoplasma gondii. In: Bennett JE, Dolin R, Blaser MJ, eds. *Mandell, Douglas, and Bennett's Principles and Practice of Infectious Diseases*. 8th ed. Elsevier; 2015. Updated.
13. Hills JL. Infections of the head and neck. In: Florin TA, Ludwig S, eds. *Netter's Pediatrics*. Elsevier; 2011.
14. Benko KR. Emergency dental procedures. In: Roberts JR, et al., ed. *Roberts and Hedges' Clinical Procedures in Emergency Medicine and Acute Care*. 7th ed. Elsevier; 2018.

15. Martin JM, Baumhardt H, D'Alesio A, Woods K. Oral disorders. In: Zitelli B, McIntire S, Nowalk AJ, eds. *Zitelli and Davis' Atlas of Pediatric Physical Diagnosis*. Elsevier; 2018.

16. Tunkel AR. Brain abcess. In: Bennett JE, Dolin R, Blaser MJ, eds. *Mandell, Douglas, and Bennett's Principles and Practice of Infectious Diseases*. 8th ed. Elsevier; 2015. Updated.

17. Chow AW. Infections of the oral cavity, neck, and head. In: Bennett JE, Dolin R, Blaser MJ, eds. *Mandell, Douglas, and Bennett's Principles and Practice of Infectious Diseases*. 8th ed. Elsevier; 2015. Updated.

18. Montgomery J, Carroll R, McCollum A. Ocular vaccinia: a consequence of unrecognized contact transmission. *Military Medicine*. 2011;176(6):699–701.

19. Klein JO. Otitis externa, otitis media, and mastoiditis. In: Bennett JE, Dolin R, Blaser MJ, eds. *Mandell, Douglas, and Bennett's Principles and Practice of Infectious Diseases*. 8th ed. Elsevier; 2015. Updated.

12
Central Nervous System Infections

BETHANY DAVIES

MENINGITIS

Definitions

Meningitis: inflammation of the meninges and subarachnoid space, most commonly secondary to infection.
- May be acute, subacute, or chronic.
- Identified by a combination of clinical syndrome and by an abnormal number of white cells in the cerebrospinal fluid (CSF) (see Table 12.1).
- Typically classified by duration of symptom onset and by pathogen.

Meningism: syndrome of headache, photophobia, and neck stiffness due to meningitis.

Acute Bacterial Meningitis

Epidemiology

- Causes significant morbidity and mortality worldwide. Case fatality rate 15%–25%, neurologic sequelae in ~25%.

- Attack rates are substantially higher in resource-poor settings (12/100,000; up to 1000/100,000 during epidemics in the **African "meningitis" belt**; compared with Europe and the United States (0.23/100,000). Mortality is also higher (>50%).
- Pathogen depends on age, immune status, and other risk factors (see Table 12.2).
- Vaccination strategies have altered the epidemiology of community-acquired bacterial meningitis, especially *Haemophilus influenzae* B (HiB) in children, and vaccine serotypes of *Streptococcus pneumoniae*.
- *Listeria* case fatality rates are the highest, at 30%–40%.

Meningococcal Meningitis

- Bimodal distribution: first peak in children under 1-year-old, second in 16–25-year-olds.
- Complement deficiency (especially terminal complement pathway) increases risk of meningococcal infection.
- Meningococcal disease occurs in all countries, but the incidence and serotypes vary (see Fig. 12.1).

CSF Parameters

	Normal	Bacterial	Viral	Tuberculous	Fungal
Opening pressure (cm CSF)	12–20	Raised	Normal/mildly raised	Raised	Raised
Appearance	Clear	Turbid/cloudy	Clear	Clear or cloudy	Clear or cloudy
CSF WCC (cells/uL)	<5	Raised (>100)	Raised (5–100)	Raised (5–500)	Raised (5–500)
Predominant cell type	n/a	PMNs (i.e., neutrophils)	Lymphocytes	Lymphocytes	Lymphocytes
CSF protein (g/L)	0.4	Raised	Mildly raised	Markedly raised	Raised
CSF/plasma glucose ratio	>2/3	Very low	Normal/slightly low	Very low	Low

PMNs, polymorphonuclear leukocytes; WCC, white cell count.

205

TABLE 12.2	Common Pathogens by Age

Age	Common Bacterial Pathogens
<1 month	*Streptococcus agalactiae* (GBS) *Escherichia coli* *Listeria monocytogenes*
<2 years	*Streptococcus pneumoniae* *Neisseria meningitidis* GBS *Haemophilus influenzae* B *E. coli*
2–50 years	*S. pneumoniae* *N. meningitidis*
>50	*S. pneumoniae* *N. meningitidis* *L. monocytogenes* Aerobic gram-negative bacilli
+ Risk Factor	
Relative immunocompromise such as alcohol dependency, diabetes, malignancy, as well as chemotherapy	*Listeria monocytogenes;* aerobic gram-negative bacilli
Basilar skull fracture	*S. pneumoniae, H. influenzae, Streptococcus pyogenes*
Asplenia	All encapsulated bacteria, such as *S. pneumoniae, N. meningitidis,* and *H. influenzae*
Neurosurgical patients	A wider range of bacteria, including *E. coli, Klebsiella* spp., *Pseudomonas aeruginosa,* other *Enterobacteriaceae,* staphylococci, and other streptococci
Strongyloides hyperinfection	Enteric flora such as *Streptococcus bovis* or *E. coli*

Adapted from Brouwer MC, van de Beek D. Acute and chronic meningitis. In: Cohen J, Powderly W, Opal S, eds. *Infectious Diseases*. 4th ed. Elsevier; 2017.

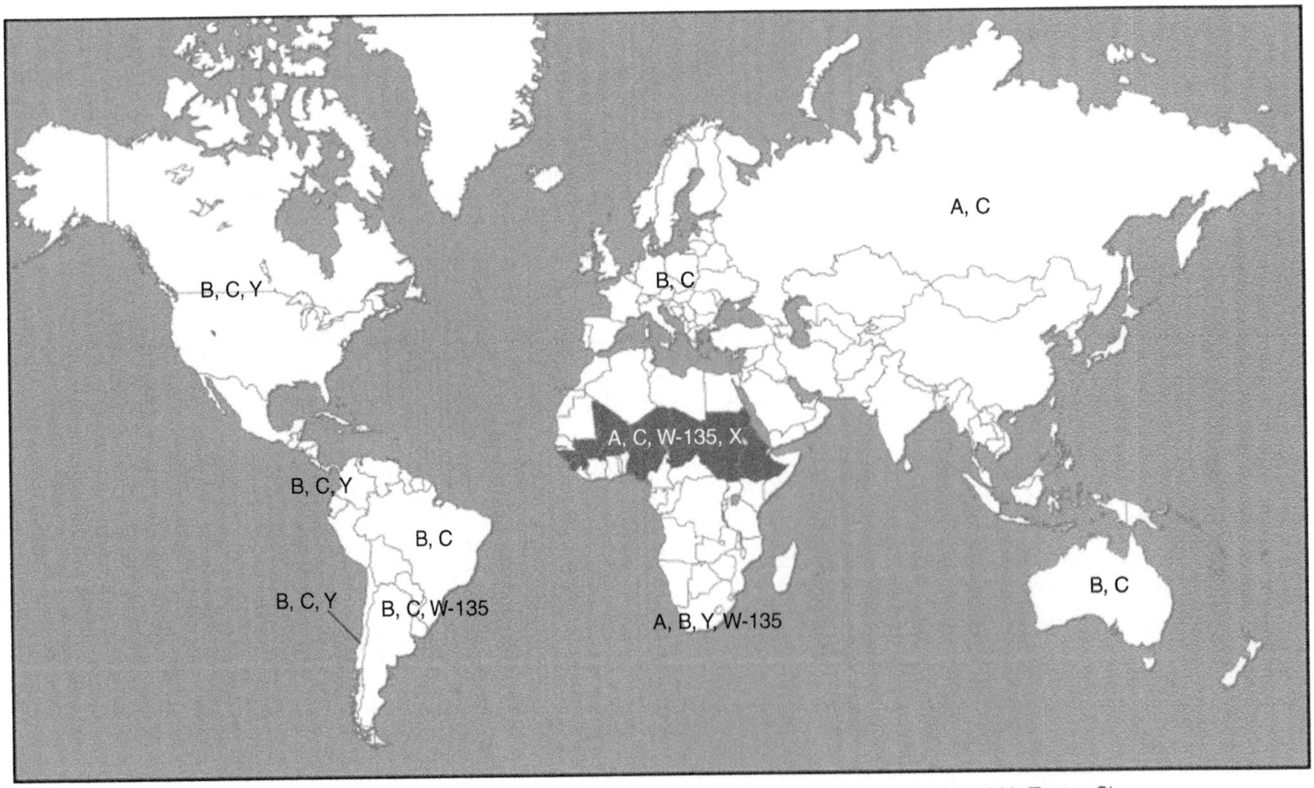

• **Fig. 12.1** Worldwide distribution of major meningococcal serogroups. (From Harrison LH, Trotter CL, Ramsay ME, et al. Global epidemiology of meningococcal disease. *Vaccine*. 2009;27(S2):B51–B63.)

- The meningitis belt of sub-Saharan Africa is associated with large epidemics toward the end of the dry season; and there have been large epidemics of meningococcal disease linked to the annual **Hajj pilgrimage to Mecca** in Saudi Arabia (Fig. 12.2).

Pneumococcal Meningitis

- Often associated with **other foci of pneumococcal infection**, e.g., septic arthritis, pneumonia, endocarditis.
- **Risk factors** include asplenia, alcoholism, chronic renal or liver disease, diabetes mellitus, malignancy, basilar skull fracture (with persistent CSF leak), cochlear implants, HIV.
- High rates of pneumococcal meningitis reflect the burden of pneumococcal infections of all types in the population.

Listeria Meningitis

- CNS infections with *Listeria* may manifest in three ways: meningoencephalitis, cerebritis, or rhombencephalitis.
- Commonest = meningoencephalitis.
  - Neonates, immunocompromised patients, or elderly.
  - Most have a subacute illness so may present with a longer duration of symptoms.
  - There is an **increased risk of seizures and focal neurologic signs.**
- Cerebritis results from direct hematogenous spread into brain parenchyma.
  - Uncommon.
  - May present with fever/headache or with a stroke-like hemiplegia.

- Rhombencephalitis occurs in immunocompetent people.
  - May be associated with contaminated food outbreaks.
  - Biphasic illness with late development of ataxia, nystagmus, and cranial nerve palsies.

Gram-Negative Bacilli Meningitis

1. Neonatal: often associated with neural tube defects or urinary tract infections.
2. Nosocomial: see healthcare-associated meningitis later in this chapter.
3. Spontaneous community-acquired. Gram-negative rods are an infrequent cause of community-acquired meningitis. *Escherichia coli* and *Klebsiella pneumoniae* are the commonest pathogens responsible. May be associated with underlying comorbidities such as diabetes, liver disease, and being elderly. Commonly accompanied by bacteremia, and the patient can have septic shock. Mortality rate high: 40%–80%. (See Box 12.1.)
4. Associated with disseminated **strongyloidiasis** in **hyperinfection syndrome** (see Chapter 35). Bacteria may seed to the meninges during bacteremia associated with larval migration from the bowel; or may be carried by the larvae as they invade through the meninges.

• BOX 12.1 Hypermucoviscous *Klebsiella pneumoniae*

A new hypervirulent strain of *Klebsiella pneumoniae* has emerged:
- Initially in Pacific Rim, now also found in Western countries
- Causes serious life-threatening infection in young, immunocompetent hosts
- Commonly: meningitis, liver abscess, pneumonia, and endophthalmitis
- Can spread metastatically with multiple abscesses
- Hypermucoviscous phenotype with positive "string test" (>5 mm length) (see Fig. 12.3)

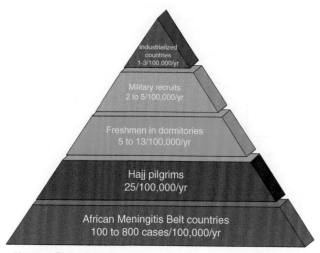

• Fig. 12.2 Risk of meningococcal disease in various settings. (From Wilder-Smith A. Meningococcal disease: risk for international travellers and vaccine strategies. *Travel Med Infect Dis.* 2008;6(4):182–186.)

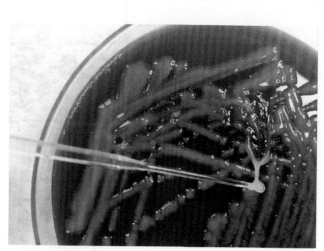

• Fig. 12.3 Positive string-test for hypermucoviscous *Klebsiella pneumoniae*. (Reproduced with permission from Elsevier. The Lancet. From Prokesch BC, TeKippe M, Kim J, Raj P, McElvania TeKippe E, Greenberg D. Primary osteomyelitis caused by hypervirulent *Klebsiella pneumoniae*. Lancet Infect Dis. 2016;16(9): e190–e195.)

Clinical Features

- Classically = fever, headache, neck stiffness, photophobia ± alteration in mental status, with symptom onset <7 days.
- Young children and elderly less likely to present with clear-cut symptoms.
- Infants = fever, irritable, lethargic, and poor feeding; may have bulging fontanelle.
- Petechiae and purpura may be seen with any pathogen but are most commonly seen with *N. meningitidis* (~50%).
- Patients with an underlying basilar skull fracture may have rhinorrhea or otorrhea secondary to a CSF leak.

Diagnosis and Management

- Given high morbidity and mortality, establishing the diagnosis and starting treatment should occur simultaneously in most cases (Fig. 12.4 and Table 12.3).

- Indications for imaging before lumbar puncture (LP)
  - Immunocompromised (IDSA only).
  - History of CNS disease (e.g., stroke, mass lesion) (IDSA only).
  - Focal neurologic signs.
  - Presence of papilledema.
  - Continuous or uncontrolled seizures (plus new onset seizures in IDSA).
  - GCS ≤12.
- LP should also be delayed if the patient has received anticoagulants:
  - 4 h postprophylactic low molecular weight heparin (LMWH).
  - 24 h posttherapeutic LMWH.
  - INR ≥1.4 if on warfarin.
  - **7 days if on clopidogrel.**
  - Platelet count <40 ×10⁹/L if known thrombocytopenia, or if rapidly falling platelet count.
- **No delay for patients on aspirin.**

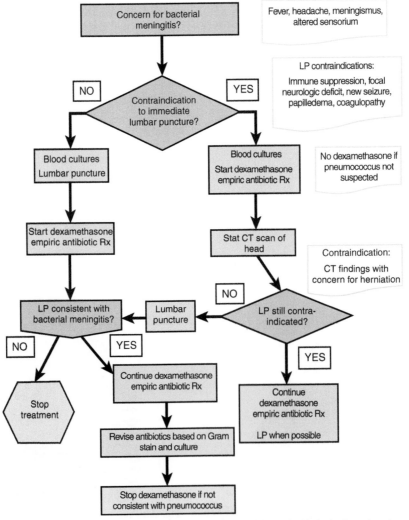

• **Fig. 12.4** Algorithm for early management of suspected bacterial meningitis including when to suspect the diagnosis, when imaging prior to lumbar puncture is appropriate, and when to initiate and discontinue empiric antibiotics and adjuvant dexamethasone. CT, Computed tomography; LP, lumbar puncture; Rx, treatment. (From Parrillo JE, Dellinger RP, *Critical Care Medicine: Principles of Diagnosis and Management in the Adult*. 5th ed. Elsevier; 2019.)

TABLE 12.3   Investigations for Acute Meningitis

	Hematology	Biochemistry	Microbiology	Virology	Other
Bloods	Full blood count Clotting screen	Glucose Renal function Liver function Procalcitonin C-reactive protein	Blood cultures EDTA sample for meningococcal and pneumococcal PCR	Serology save sample	
CSF		Protein Glucose Lactate	Microscopy, culture, and sensitivity Meningococcal and pneumococcal PCR ± Listeria PCR ±16S ribosomal RNA PCR	PCR for HSV-1 + -2, VZV, mumps, and enterovirus	Opening pressure
Throat swab			Bacterial culture	Enterovirus PCR	
Stool				Enterovirus PCR	

HSV, herpes simplex virus; PCR, polymerase chain reaction; VZV, varicella-zoster virus

- Can discuss individual cases with hematology. If LP not possible, review every 12 hours. May still be of diagnostic benefit after several days.

Antibiotics

- Depend on age, likely pathogens, and antibiotic susceptibility.
- Antibiotics need to penetrate into CSF, which may depend on the status of the blood–brain barrier. **Penicillins penetrate poorly when BBB intact,** but penetration enhanced when meninges are inflamed.
- CSF concentrations of β lactams need to exceed the minimum bactericidal concentration by 10–20-fold to achieve maximal effect, and to reduce neurologic sequelae associated with delayed sterilization of the CSF.
- Some combinations of antibiotics may be synergistic, such as ampicillin and gentamicin in *Listeria.*

Empirical Treatment

- If low rates of pneumococcal resistance, **standard treatment is third-generation cephalosporin** (ceftriaxone or cefotaxime).
- As third-generation cephalosporins are inactive in *Listeria* **meningitis, ampicillin should be added** if any risk factors present (immunocompromised, especially cell-mediated; including diabetics or history of alcohol misuse; age >60 years).
- If possibility of high-level ceftriaxone resistance in pneumococci (MIC ≥2 µg/mL), then vancomycin is added. Vancomycin should never be used alone due to concerns about its penetration into CSF in adults.

Pathogen-Specific Treatment

- Table 12.4 details US and UK guidance for antimicrobial choice and duration of treatment once an organism has been identified.

Adjunctive Steroids

- It is routine practice to include **dexamethasone in empirical treatment** for bacterial meningitis.
- Standard adult dosing is 10 mg QID for 4 days.
- Adjunctive dexamethasone attenuates the subarachnoid inflammation associated with antibiotic-induced bacterial lysis.
- Steroids have been shown to reduce severe hearing loss, neurologic sequelae, and case fatality in pneumococcal meningitis, with no increase in adverse effects.
- IDSA guidelines advise steroids should only **be continued** in patients **with evidence of *S. pneumoniae*** (gram-positive diplococci on CSF microscopy, positive CSF, or blood cultures with *S. pneumoniae*).
- UK guidelines advise steroids should be **stopped if a cause other than *S. pneumoniae*** is identified.
- There is no effect on meningococcal outcomes, nor have these benefits been demonstrated in low income countries.

Chemoprophylaxis for Confirmed or Probable Meningococcal Meningitis

- Household or kissing contact in previous 7 days *or*
- Iatrogenic exposure during resuscitation.
- Should be taken within 24 hours.
- Single dose ciprofloxacin.

Rationale

- Most patients with meningococcal infection have acquired the bacteria within the preceding 7 days.
- Eradicating carriage in close contacts may eliminate the original source of meningococcus but is also important as they are at greater risk of infection.
- **Close contacts** have an **attack rate 1000× higher** than the normal attack rate (2–4/1000 population compared with 0.23/100,000).

TABLE 12.4	Pathogen-Specific Treatment				
				Minimum duration of treatment (days)	
Pathogen	1st line	Alternatives	IDSA		UK
Streptococcus pneumoniae	Penicillin G if MIC <0.1 µg/mL; or third-generation cephalosporin ± vancomycin	Chloramphenicol, meropenem, fluoroquinolone	10–14		10–14
Neisseria meningitidis	Penicillin G if MIC <0.1 µg/mL or third-generation cephalosporin	Chloramphenicol, aztreonam, meropenem	7		5
	Will need single dose ciprofloxacin to eliminate throat carriage if not treated with ceftriaxone				
Listeria monocytogenes	Amoxicillin/ampicillin or penicillin G	Trimethoprim–sulfamethoxazole, meropenem	≥21		21
Haemophilus influenzae	Ampicillin if β-lactamase-negative; or third-generation cephalosporin	Chloramphenicol, fluoroquinolone	7		10
Escherichia coli	Third-generation cephalosporin	Meropenem, aztreonam, fluoroquinolone, trimethoprim–sulfamethoxazole, ampicillin	21		21
No identified pathogen	Third-generation cephalosporin		10		

Third-generation cephalosporin = ceftriaxone or cefotaxime. Fluoroquinolone = moxifloxacin or gatifloxacin.

- Even with prophylaxis, this risk persists for at least 6 months.
- Vaccinations may be offered to the index case and contacts.

Outcomes
- 15% of pediatric survivors have severe neurologic sequelae (bilateral severe or profound hearing loss, spasticity/paresis, cognitive problems, seizure disorder).
- Another 20% of children have persisting neurologic impairments causing behavioral, cognitive, and academic difficulties.
- One-third of adult survivors experience long-term mild cognitive impairment, mainly consisting of cognitive slowness. This does not improve with time.

Acute Viral Meningitis

Epidemiology

- **Enterovirus = most commonly identified cause** (90% in countries with established mumps immunization). Enterovirus is found worldwide but incidence varies. Temperate climates have a marked seasonality (summer/autumn) whereas incidence is year round in tropical/subtropical climates.
- Mumps is a common cause in unimmunized populations.
- Arboviruses, HSV-2, and primary HIV infection, also important, as are other herpes viruses.

- Arboviruses include St. Louis encephalitis virus, Eastern equine, Western equine, and West Nile virus (WNV). These have specific geographical areas of endemicity and seasonality.
- HSV infections have a bimodal age distribution, <20 years and >50 years; this may reflect primary infection and reactivation infection respectively.

Clinical Features

Clinical features are not distinctive.
- Enterovirus: plus rash, diarrhea.
- Primary HIV infection: plus malaise, lymphadenopathy, pharyngitis, and maculopapular rash.
- HSV-2 infection: plus genital lesions (85%); may cause recurrent meningitis.
- Lymphocytic choriomeningitis virus (LCMV): occurs in lab personnel, pet owners, or those with rodent-infested living conditions.
- Mumps: plus parotitis (50%).

Diagnosis and Management

- Characterized by lymphocytic pleocytosis in CSF with sterile bacterial cultures.
- **PCR testing for viral nucleic acid in CSF is the test of choice for enteroviruses, herpes viruses, and mumps.**
- PCR of throat and rectal swabs may be useful for enterovirus, influenza, and mycoplasma.

- HIV combined Ag/Ab testing is recommended.
- **Most cases of viral meningitis are treated symptomatically,** with supportive care alone.
- There are some specific antiviral agents available:
  - Aciclovir: no definitive evidence of benefit in use for HSV-2 meningitis but is often used. May speed recovery. May improve outcomes in VZV meningitis.
  - Neuraminidase inhibitors such as oseltamivir: recommended in patients with severe or complicated influenza (confirmed or suspected), including meningitis.
  - Intravenous immunoglobulin (IVIG) may be used in overwhelming neonatal infections with enterovirus.

Chronic Meningitis

- At least **4 weeks** of symptoms, with a CSF pleocytosis.
- Main causes = TB, fungi, Lyme infection, syphilis, and malignancy.

Tuberculous Meningitis (TBM) (see Chapter 32)

- During primary infection or reactivation of latent infection, *Mycobacterium tuberculosis* bacilli enter the bloodstream.
- These seed throughout the brain, meninges, and adjacent bone, establishing scattered tubercles.
- TBM results from the chance rupture of a tubercle into the subarachnoid space.
- TBM is associated with **high frequency of neurologic sequelae and death** even with prompt treatment.

Epidemiology

- The incidence of TBM reflects the incidence and prevalence of TB in the population. 50% have a history of contact with sputum-smear-positive TB.
- High incidence countries: TBM is typically a **postprimary infection in infants and young children,** usually 3–6 months later.
- Low incidence countries: TBM most commonly follows **reactivation** in **adults with immune deficiency** (age, HIV, iatrogenic immunosuppression especially tumor necrosis factor-alpha inhibitors, malignancy). Also need to consider whether immigrant from high incidence country.

Clinical Features

- Insidious, fluctuating onset of headache, fever, anorexia, weight loss.
- Progresses to cranial nerve palsies, confusion, lethargy.
- Then delirium, coma, seizures, worsening focal neurology.

Investigations

- Cannot make or exclude the diagnosis of TBM on clinical features alone.

TABLE 12.5 Thwaites Index for Diagnosis of Adult TBM

Predictive Variable	Score
Age ≥36 years	+2
Blood WCC ≥15 ×10⁶	+4
Number of days of illness ≥6	−5
CSF WCC ≥900 ×10³	+3
CSF % polymorphs ≥75	+4
Total score ≤4 patient has TBM Total score >4, patient has bacterial meningitis	Sensitivity 86% Specificity 79%

Reproduced with permission from Elsevier. The Lancet. Thwaites GE et al. Diagnosis of adult tuberculous meningitis by use of clinical and laboratory features. Lancet 2002;360:1287-92.

TABLE 12.6 Sensitivity and Specificity of Tests for TBM

Test for TBM	Reported Sensitivity/%	Reported Specificity/%
Microscopy for acid-fast bacilli (AFBs) in CSF (Ziehl–Neelsen)	20–80	100
Mycobacterial culture of CSF	71	100
Nucleic acid amplification (can use to confirm but not exclude TBM)	85–95	98

- Five independent variables associated with a diagnosis of TBM were identified in an adult study in Vietnam (Table 12.5).
- Confirmation of TBM increases with volume of CSF examined (minimum 6 mL, ideally 10–15 mL; some units repeat up to 4 daily samples); see Table 12.6.
- Imaging: basal meningeal enhancement, hydrocephalus, tuberculomas, infarcts. **MRI preferred** to CT as better for brain stem and spine.
- **Chest X-ray: 50% of patients with TBM will have changes consistent with active or previous pulmonary tuberculosis.**

Management

- Intensive phase (2 months) of quadruple antituberculous therapy together with dexamethasone (see Table 12.7); followed by maintenance phase (9–12 months) of rifampin/isoniazid (refer to Chapter 6 and Chapter 32 for more details).

TABLE 12.7	CSF Penetration of Antituberculous Drugs	
TBM Drug	**CSF Penetration /%**	
Isoniazid	90–95	Critical agent as bactericidal and excellent CSF penetration
Rifampin	5–25	Penetrates CSF less well but importance shown by higher mortality of RIF-resistant strains
Pyrazinamide	95–100	Penetrates CSF well and reduces total length of treatment
Ethambutol	10–50	Bacteriostatic and penetrates poorly into CNS, even when meninges inflamed. May substitute fluoroquinolone or injectable aminoglycoside

Other Causes of Chronic Meningitis

- Table 12.8 discusses other causes of chronic meningitis, including risk factors, typical clinical features, and recommended treatment regimes.

Neurosurgical Infections

Healthcare-Associated Meningitis

- Develops postneurosurgical procedure; 1.5%–2% infection rate.
- Enterobacteriaceae and *Pseudomonas* spp. account for a greater proportion, as well as *S. aureus* and coagulase-negative staphylococci (80% combined).
- *Candida* spp. implicated in 5% cases.
- Clinical features = new headache, fever, evidence of meningeal irritation, seizures, and/or worsening mental status.

CSF Shunt Infections

- CSF shunts are permanent catheters.
- May be ventriculo-atrial (VA) or ventriculo-peritoneal (VP).
- Incidence of infection 4%–17%.

- Usually indolent infection with CNS or *Cutibacterium* (formerly *Propionibacterium*).

Mechanisms of Shunt Infection

1. Colonization at surgery (70%).
2. Retrograde infection from distal end (VP).
3. Through skin (whether iatrogenic manipulation or erosion).
4. Hematogenous spread (VA).

Clinical Features

- New headache, nausea, lethargy, and/or change in mental status.
- Erythema and tenderness over the tunneled tubing.
- Abdominal pain or peritonitis in a VP shunt.
- Fever, in absence of other cause may be suggestive.

External Ventricular Drain (EVD) Infection

- External ventricular drain = temporary CSF drain.
- EVD infection rate ~ 10.6/1000 catheter days.
- Usually hospital flora.
- Difficult diagnosis as patients usually have impaired conscious level from underlying pathology.
- New or worsening mental status, or new fever and increased CSF white cell count may indicate EVD infection.

Investigations

- CSF cell count and culture are most useful in establishing a diagnosis of healthcare-associated ventriculitis/meningitis, with symptoms of infection.
- **However**:
  - Abnormal CSF cell counts/protein/glucose may not reliably indicate infection.
  - Normal CSF cell counts/protein/glucose may not reliable exclude infection.
- A negative CSF Gram stain does not exclude infection.
- Negative CSF cultures in the setting of prior antibiotic therapy do not exclude infection.
- Need to consider whether positive cultures indicate contamination, colonization, or infection.
- Blood cultures are positive in >90% VA shunt infections.

Management

- Empiric IV antibiotics: **vancomycin (or linezolid) plus meropenem.**
  - Aim vancomycin trough of 15–20.
  - Give for 10–14 days after the last positive culture.
- Intraventricular AB may be considered if there is a poor response to systemic antibiotics.
- Liposomal amphotericin is advised for *Candida* infections.
- **Removal of infected drains/shunts** is recommended.

TABLE 12.8 Differential Diagnosis of Chronic Meningitis

Pathogen	Risk Factors	Associated Clinical Features	Treatment
Brucella spp. See also Chapter 31	Unpasteurized dairy products or contact with infected animals Endemic areas, including the Mediterranean and Middle East	Undulant fever Cranial nerve palsy, especially blurred vision or hearing loss Behavioral change/confusion Serology mainstay of diagnosis Also: blood (15%–70%), CSF (15%) and bone marrow cultures	Any two of: doxycycline, ceftriaxone, rifampicin
Tropheryma whipplei	Gastrointestinal Whipple's	Cognitive impairment, ataxia, ophthalmoplegia, and supranuclear gaze palsy Fever, weight loss, peripheral LNs, and arthralgia CSF PCR	Ceftriaxone followed by trimethoprim–sulfamethoxazole
Cryptococcus spp. See also Chapters 2, 28, 39	Majority have deficient cellular immunity but may occur in previously healthy individuals.	Encephalitis with personality changes, lethargy, memory loss Headache Skin lesions in 10% CSF CRAG-positive >90% CSF culture	Amphotericin B and flucytosine
Coccidioides immitis See also Chapters 2, 28	Endemic areas include SW USA, Central and South America Deficient cellular immunity incl. TNF-α agents and AIDS; African or Filipino ancestry	Persistent headache (75%) Altered mental status, nausea, vomiting, focal neurologic deficits May develop hydrocephalus or cerebral infarctions CSF eosinophils uncommon but highly suggestive CSF culture (15%) – risk to lab staff Serology mainstay of diagnosis. Can compare serum/CSF	Fluconazole (high dose) Can add intrathecal amphotericin B (AmB) Untreated mortality 95% by 2 years
Histoplasma capsulatum See also Chapters 2, 28	Endemic areas include Ohio river valley USA, the Caribbean, and South America Deficient cellular immunity incl. TNF-α agents and AIDS	Fever, fatigue, weight loss Indolent course in immunocompetent Primary investigations = serum and urine antigen testing (75%–100%) Also: blood cultures ×3 should be sent CSF culture (50%) especially if large volume sent, but may take weeks to grow; serology (70%–90%) but delay in developing antibody (Ab) response	Amphotericin B followed by itraconazole
Angiostrongylus cantonensis See also Chapters 4, 35	Rat lung worm Asia and South Pacific Ingestion of infected intermediate hosts: raw or undercooked shellfish and snails, or plants contaminated by these Larvae migrate to CNS, mature into adult worms, which migrate through the brain	Excruciating headache (>90%) Rash with pruritus Paresthesias Peripheral and CSF eosinophilia Serology helpful but not widely available Other causes of an eosinophilic meningitis to consider: gnathostomiasis, baylisascariasis, coccidioidomycosis, Hodgkin lymphoma, adverse drug reactions	No effective treatment Therapeutic LPs may help, as may steroids Self-limiting – 2 months
Borrelia burgdorferi	See Chapter 24		
Treponema pallidum	See Chapter 21		

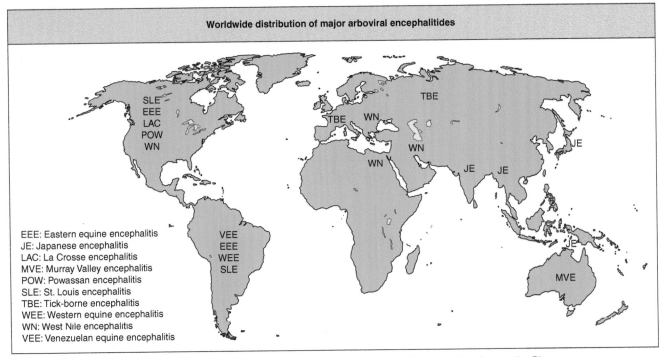

• **Fig. 12.5** Worldwide distribution of major arboviral encephalitides. (Courtesy The Centers for Disease Control and Prevention.)

OTHER CNS INFECTIONS

Encephalitis

Definition

Encephalitis: inflammation of the brain parenchyma, associated with neurologic dysfunction (behavioral changes, altered consciousness, seizures, focal neurology).

- Classically = triad of fever, headache, and altered level of consciousness.

Epidemiology

- Estimated incidence varies: annually approx 1–14/100,000 for all ages.
- Extremes of age at greater risk.
- **50%–70% unexplained.**
- Risk factors to explore include animal contact, immunosuppression, travel, insect contact, recreational activities, vaccination status, occupation, and season.
  - Common causes in UK/US: HSV, VZV, enterovirus.
  - Common causes internationally: rabies, Japanese encephalitis virus (JEV).
  - Common causes in endemic areas: West Nile virus (WNV), tickborne encephalitis virus (TBE), St. Louis encephalitis virus (SLEV) (see Fig. 12.5).

Investigations

- Essential investigations include **MRI and CSF analysis.**
  - CSF PCR is widely available for HSV-1 and -2, VZV, enterovirus, mumps, EBV, CMV, HHV-6 and 7, TB, and toxoplasma. Serum/CSF antibodies may be helpful.
  - CSF analysis: usually lymphocytic, <250 cells/mm^3; normal CSF/serum glucose; moderately elevated protein.
- Also send:
  - Serology for HIV, herpesviruses, arboviruses, Lyme, syphilis.
  - CSF and blood cultures.
  - Peripheral blood smear.
  - Chest X-ray.
  - Throat swab for respiratory virus PCR.
  - Brain biopsy infrequently performed but may have a role in the deteriorating patient.

Neuroimaging

- Some infections have been associated with distinctive neuroimaging findings (Table 12.9).

Management

- All patients should be started with empirical aciclovir (ACV) (untreated HSE case fatality 70%–100%).
- Doxycycline may be added if rickettsial or ehrlichial infection possible.

Key Facts of HSV-1 Encephalitis

- **HSV-1 encephalitis** (HSE) responsible for **~10%** of all encephalitis cases.
- Annual incidence 2–10/million population (estimates have increased since PCR more widely available).
- One-third are due to primary HSV infection, two-thirds result from reactivation of latent infection.

TABLE 12.9   Possible Etiologic Agents of Encephalitis Based on Neuroimaging Findings

Neuroimaging Finding	Possible Infectious Agents
Arteritis and infarctions	Varicella-zoster virus (VZV), Nipah virus, *Rickettsia rickettsia*, *Treponema pallidum*
Calcifications	Cytomegalovirus (cortical), *Toxoplasma gondii* (periventricular), *Taenia solium*
Cerebellar lesions	VZV, Epstein–Barr virus, *Mycoplasma pneumoniae*
Focal lesions in basal ganglia, thalamus and/or brain stem	Epstein–Barr virus, Eastern equine encephalitis virus, Murray Valley encephalitis virus, St. Louis encephalitis virus, Japanese encephalitis virus, West Nile virus (WNV), enterovirus 71, influenzae virus (acute necrotizing encephalopathy), human transmissible spongiform encephalopathies, *Tropheryma whipplei*, *Listeria monocytogenes*
Hydrocephalus	*Mycobacterium tuberculosis*, *Cryptococcus neoformans*, *Coccidioides immitis*, *Histoplasma capsulatum*, *Balamuthia mandrillaris*
Space-occupying lesions	*Toxoplasma gondii*, *Balamuthia mandrillaris*, *Acanthamoeba* spp., *Taenia solium*
Subependymal enhancement	Cytomegalovirus
Temporal and/or frontal lobe involvement	HSV, VZV, HHV-6, WNV, enteroviruses, *Treponema pallidum* (medial lobes)
White matter abnormalities	VZV, cytomegalovirus, Epstein–Barr virus, HHV-6, HIV, Nipah virus, JC virus, measles virus (subacute sclerosing panencephalitis), *Baylisascaris procyonis*, acute disseminated encephalomyelitis

This is not meant to be a comprehensive list to detail all etiologic agents based on neuroimaging findings but to suggest that certain etiologies have been associated with findings on neuroimaging studies.
From Cohen J, Powderly W, Opal S, eds. *Infectious Diseases*. 4th ed. Table 20.5. Elsevier; 2017.

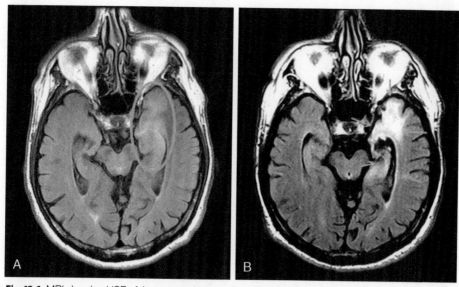

• **Fig. 12.6** MRI showing HSE of the temporal lobes. (From Croll BJ, Dillon ZM, Weaver KR, Greenberg MR. MRI diagnosis of herpes simplex encephalitis in an elderly man with nonspecific symptoms. *Radiol Case Rep*. 2017;12(1):159–160.)

- Investigations: an elevated red cell count in an atraumatic tap is suggestive of HSV-1 infection.
- HSV PCR should be performed on ALL patients with encephalitis. If negative, consider repeating the test 3–7 days later.
- HSE has a predilection for the **temporal lobes** (Fig. 12.6).
- Even with prompt ACV, HSE has an associated mortality of 28%, with severe neurologic sequelae in 20%; **only ~15% completely recover.** The most common residual deficits are dysnomia and impaired new learning.

- Poor outcome more likely in those who are older, sicker at presentation, and when aciclovir treatment is delayed >4 days after symptom onset, or >2 days after admission.
- **Readmission is common** in survivors: for seizure disorder, neuropsychiatric illness, or venous thromboembolism.

Other Causes of Encephalitis

- Table 12.10 discusses other causes of encephalitis, including risk factors, typical clinical features, recommended investigations, and treatment options.

TABLE 12.10 Specific Pathogens Causing Encephalitis

Pathogen	Risk Factors	Presentation and Diagnosis	Treatment
Herpes B virus See also Chapter 31	Infects old world macaques, who are lifelong carriers with asymptomatic shedding of virus. Most animals >2.5 years old are likely to be infected Humans infected by bite/scratch/mucosal contact with oral /genital/ocular fluid, or CNS tissues	**Vesicles develop at site of inoculation, with regional lymphadenopathy.** Followed by flu-like illness, **with paresthesia at inoculation site** Once the virus invades the CNS, neurologic symptoms include diplopia, ataxia, agitation, seizures, ascending paralysis, and coma Investigations: culture and PCR of vesicles and CSF B virus serology MRI (**brain stem encephalitis which spreads over time**)	Valaciclovir recommended (reaches higher serum concentrations than aciclovir) **Untreated case fatality 80%; treated case fatality 20%** **Prophylactic antivirals are recommended for high-risk exposure** No cases reported following post-exposure prophylaxis within 3 days
Japanese encephalitis virus (flavivirus) See also Chapter 30	Distribution: Asia and the Western Pacific Reservoir = **pig** and wading birds Transmitted by *Culex* mosquitoes Primarily in rural agricultural areas Humans = dead-end hosts	Less than 1% develop clinical infection Incubation period (IP) 5–15 days Most frequent in children and nonimmune adults Travelers at risk but low (1 in 150,000 person months of exposure) Typically has **Parkinson's-like syndrome:** mask-like facies, tremor, cogwheel rigidity	Supportive treatment only **Case fatality 20%–30% of encephalitis patients** 30%–50% survivors have persistent neurologic, psychiatric, or cognitive symptoms Prevention: vaccine available
Rabies virus (bullet shaped rhabdovirus) See also Chapter 31	**Bite or mucosal exposure to saliva** of infected mammal 99% cases from domestic dogs Worldwide with some exceptions (bat and terrestrial) Few cases associated with corneal and solid organ transplant	Bite injury (may be unrecognized especially if bat) Incubation period of weeks to months Prodromal flu-like illness Numbness or paresthesia at site of inoculum, progressing to **agitation, hydrophobia, drooling, anxiety, delirium, insomnia, autonomic instability, and coma** 20% "paralytic" rather than "furious" (ascending, Guillain-Barré-like) Death within 2–10 days Serum or CSF antibodies in unvaccinated RT-PCR of saliva or CSF Histology (Negri bodies) of brain tissue Skin biopsy of base of hair follicle with antigen testing of cutaneous nerves	Supportive treatment only **Postexposure prophylaxis with vaccine and rabies immunoglobulin;** ineffective after disease onset
St. Louis encephalitis virus (SLEV) (flavivirus) See also Chapter 30	Reservoir = birds Transmitted by *Culex* mosquitoes Local and regional outbreaks in the United States, Canada, and Mexico; sporadic cases from central and South America	Incubation period 4-21 days Risk of encephalitis is **age-dependent** (1:800 children, 1:85 adults over 60) 4–5 days of flu-like illness with severe headache and meningism, followed by brain stem, cerebellar, and focal cranial nerve deficits. Tremors common: eyelids, tongue, lips, and extremities. Motor and sensory deficits rare. Seizures uncommon. May get **urinary symptoms** Investigations: SLEV specific IgM in CSF or serum	Supportive treatment only **Case fatality 5%-15%, higher in the elderly** Other risk factors for severity include hypertension, diabetes, alcoholism 30%–50% have features persisting for up to 3 years, including sleeplessness, memory loss, irritability, impaired fine motor skills

Tickborne encephalitis (TBE) virus (flavivirus)	Three closely related flavivirus subtypes European, Far Eastern and Siberian with associated endemicity. Transmitted via tick (or less commonly, ingestion of unpasteurized milk). **TBE virus transmitted rapidly after tick attaches; early removal may not prevent encephalitis**	Incubation period 7–14 days. **Biphasic illness**: initial viremia with flu-like and arthralgia symptoms, followed by remission of ~1 week, then CNS symptoms in 20%–30% of patients. May have meningitis, encephalitis, myelitis, or radiculitis. Investigations: detection of viral RNA by PCR and TBEV-specific IgM /IgG in both CSF and serum	Supportive treatment only. **Case fatality varies by subtype** (European 1%–2%, Siberian 8%). Sequelae common (50% still symptomatic at 1 year, 30% with severe impairment). Prevention: effective vaccine available; tick bite avoidance measures
West Nile virus (flavivirus)	Widely distributed globally, including Africa, S Europe, Middle East, Asia, Australia, and the Americas. **NOT in UK (yet!)** Peak in late summer in temperate climates. Main reservoir = birds. Transmitted by mosquitoes. Transmission by blood transfusion, solid organ transplant, and mother-to-baby also possible	Incubation period 3–14 days, **longer if immunosuppressed**. Most infections asymptomatic. 1 in 5 develop fever. 1 in 150 develop CNS disease. Meningitis, encephalitis, or acute flaccid paralysis (damage to anterior horn cells). Serum and CSF for WNV IgM + IgG. Usually detectable 3–8 days after onset, but may persist for >90 days. Compare acute and convalescent samples. Detection of viral RNA in serum, CSF, or tissue by RT-PCR. Other causes of acute flaccid paralysis include poliovirus; nonpolio enteroviruses including coxsackieviruses and echoviruses; Guillain–Barré; transverse myelitis; traumatic neuritis	Supportive treatment only. Case fatality 10% for neuroinvasive infection. Higher if elderly, immunosuppressed, or diabetic. **Many encephalitis survivors (~50%) have persisting neuropsychiatric impairment**
Bartonella henselae See also Chapter 31	Associated with cat scratch (also bite or cat fleas). Worldwide distribution. Occurs in immunocompetent. Predominantly in children, but does occur in adults	Encephalopathy is an infrequent complication of cat scratch disease. More likely in elderly patients. Develops 1–6 weeks after regional tender lymphadenopathy. Typically confusion, seizures, may progress to coma. Normal CT. Abnormal EEG. Histology or PCR of tissue. Serology is unreliable	Treatment: **doxycycline plus rifampin** for 10–14 days. Usually recover within weeks, but neurologic deficits can persist
Acanthamoeba spp. Granulomatous amebic encephalitis (GAE)	Rare. 150 cases reported worldwide. **Majority in immunocompromised: cell-mediated deficiencies**. Found in soil and water, but usually no history of exposure is elicited	Insidious onset of symptoms including personality change, low-grade fever, focal neurology, seizures, hemiparesis, progressing to reduced conscious level and coma. **LP usually contraindicated** due to focal lesions with raised intracranial pressure (ICP). Imaging: **multifocal ring-enhancing lesions throughout brain**, especially temporal and parietal lobes. Diagnosis by brain biopsy: necrotic areas with visible trophozoites and thick-walled cysts on microscopy. Can culture in bacterial lawn on agar, or PCR may be available at reference lab	Most cases fatal. No reliable effective therapy. Suggested treatment: *either* trimethoprim–sulfamethoxazole + rifampin + ketoconazole *or* fluconazole + sulfadiazine + pyrimethamine

Continued

TABLE 12.10 Specific Pathogens Causing Encephalitis—cont'd

Pathogen	Risk Factors	Presentation and Diagnosis	Treatment
Balamuthia mandrillaris: granulomatous amebic encephalitis (GAE)	Rare. 200 cases reported worldwide, especially Central America, S and W USA Risk factors = activities associated with soil exposure, e.g., gardening, agricultural exposure. Organ transplantation has been a source of transmission Occurs in immunocompetent as well as immunocompromised	Progressive, subacute onset May present with initial skin lesion, often trauma-related: up to 2 years before neurologic symptoms (see Fig. 12.7) CNS involvement secondary to thrombotic angiitis, with hemorrhage, infarction, and necrosis Causes focal seizures or motor deficits, cranial nerve palsies, raised ICP, meningeal irritation, and progressive loss of consciousness, leading to coma and death (2–12 weeks) Imaging: multiple discrete lesions, varying in size. Intra-lesional hemorrhage is a useful clue CSF: lymphocytic, high protein, elevated red cell count Microscopy rarely available PCR not widely available Brain biopsy: granulomatous inflammation. May see amebae	Treatment: effective treatment not established Multiple agents for prolonged period, including pentamidine, sulfadiazine, azithromycin, fluconazole, flucytosine, and miltefosine Few survive
Naegleria fowleri: primary amebic meningoencephalitis	Free-living amebae found worldwide in water and soil >30 °C Risk factors = water-related activities where water goes up the nose, e.g., diving, swimming underwater Trophozoites penetrate the nasal mucosa and migrate up the olfactory nerves to the brain	Fulminant, fatal CNS infection Incubation period 5 days Average 5 days from symptom onset to death High fever, severe headache, meningism, smell and taste abnormalities, altered mental status CSF very high pressure (30–60 cmH₂O), with a markedly low glucose, high protein, and polymorph predominance. CSF red cell count also raised Severe cranial hypertension causes herniation and death Trophozoites may be seen in CSF and brain tissue. PCR may be available at national reference laboratories	Effective treatment not established Consider combination of conventional AmB IV and intrathecally, rifampin, fluconazole, miltefosine, and azithromycin

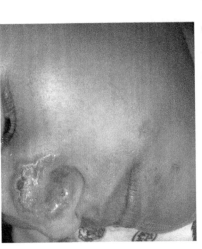

• **Fig. 12.7** *Balamuthia* infection. (Courtesy of Francisco Bravo, MD.)

Brain Abscess

Definition

Brain abscess: focal cerebral infection, beginning as localized cerebritis and developing into a pus-filled cavity.

Etiology of Cerebral Abscesses (Fig. 12.8)

- **Contiguous** spread: usually **single** abscess. Pathogen depends on source of infection, host age, and immune status, and geographical location.
- **Hematogenous** spread: often associated with **multiple** abscesses, seen in middle cerebral artery territory, at grey–white matter interface.

Predisposing Factors (Table 12.11)

Microbiology

- 30%–60% polymicrobial.
- Commonest organisms = **Streptococcus** spp., including **S. milleri** group and viridans group streptococci, **S. aureus**, anaerobes.
- *S. aureus*, Enterobacteriaceae, and *Pseudomonas* common after neurosurgery, trauma, or ear infections.
- Anaerobes often associated with contiguous spread from ENT infections.
- *Nocardia* is associated with cell-mediated immunodeficiency and has a **higher mortality** (30% vs. 10%)
- *Listeria* may cause abscesses, including in brain stem, in immunodeficient patients, especially if on corticosteroids.
- Increased frequency of **Klebsiella pneumoniae** brain abscesses in **Southeast Asia**, especially associated with a primary liver abscess (hypervirulent hypermucoviscous phenotype as discussed above).
- Fungi and protozoa also causative, especially *Aspergillus*, *Taenia solium*, and *Toxoplasma*.
- *Aspergillus* may present with a **stroke-syndrome.**

Clinical Features (Table 12.12)

- Nonspecific, so often a delay in making diagnosis.

Investigation

- **LP usually contraindicated** due to risk of brain stem herniation.
- Blood cultures positive in 15%.
- Microscopy and culture of brain abscess material essential.
  - Yield improved if samples taken before antimicrobials given.
  - **Overall ~2/3 culture-positive.**
- 16S PCR or panfungal PCR useful in culture-negative samples.

Imaging

- **MRI with gadolinium** preferable to CT with contrast. More sensitive plus better views of brain stem.
- Typically = **ring-enhancing lesion**, with thin rim; however, still broad differential, including cancer, infarction. Abscesses are hyperintense on diffusion-weighted MRI.

Management

- Aspiration plus 6–8 weeks of IV ABs.
  - Aspiration is as effective as excision for most cases, but less invasive.
  - Sequential scans are recommended to monitor response to treatment.
  - Radiologic improvement lags behind clinical response.
  - Abnormalities on imaging may persist after successful treatment.
- Empirical AB choice: majority covered by **ceftriaxone plus metronidazole.**
  - If MRSA possible, add vancomycin.
  - If postoperative, add *Pseudomonas* cover with either ceftazidime or meropenem, in addition to MRSA cover.
- Steroids not routinely recommended.

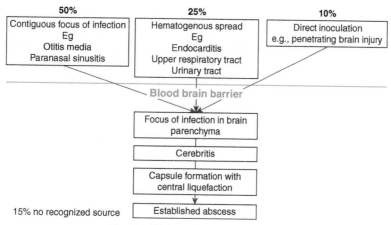

• **Fig. 12.8** Etiology of cerebral abscesses.

TABLE 12.11 **Predisposing Factors for Cerebral Abscesses**

Predisposing Condition	Site
Otitis media or mastoiditis	Temporal lobe Cerebellum
Paranasal sinusitis	Frontal lobe Temporal lobe
Dental infection/manipulation	Frontal lobe
Trauma/neurosurgery	Related to wound
Meningitis	Cerebellum Frontal lobe
Cyanotic heart disease	Middle cerebral artery distribution
Pyogenic lung disease	
Bacterial endocarditis	
Gastrointestinal source	
T-cell deficiency	
Neutropenia	

From Cohen J, Powderly W, Opal S, eds. *Infectious Diseases*. 4th ed. Table 21.1. Elsevier; 2017.

TABLE 12.12 **Clinical Features of Cerebral Abscesses**

Symptom	Frequency (%)
Headache	70
Raised ICP: vomiting, blurred vision, drowsiness, confusion	25
Focal neurologic deficit	50
Seizures	30-50
Fever	50
Triad of fever + headache + focal deficit	<50

Outcomes

- 10% mortality; 50% seizures; 20% significant cognitive impairment.

Subdural Empyema

- Infection between arachnoid and dura mater.
- Complication of sinusitis >> otitis/meningitis/neurosurgical procedure.
- Fever, headache, papilledema, and focal neurologic deficit.
- One-third have periorbital edema and subgaleal abscess.

- Causes rapid deterioration with compression of brain.
- Urgent drainage is mandatory, with prolonged course of IV AB.

Epidural Abscesses

- Infection between dura mater and bone. Spinal and intracranial. **Spinal 9× more common.**

Spinal Epidural Abscess

- Gain access by contiguous spread (e.g., infected disc or psoas muscle); direct inoculation (e.g., epidural anaesthetic); or hematogenous spread. Other risk factors: intravenous drug use, hemodialysis, diabetes mellitus, age 50–70.
- *S. aureus* responsible for two-thirds.
- Spinal cord may be damaged by:
  - Direct compression.
  - Interruption of arterial supply.
  - Thrombosis of veins.
  - Toxin-mediated (bacterial or inflammatory mediators).
- **Clinical features** often nonspecific. Most patients attend several times before diagnosis is made. **Severe localized back pain** (worsened by palpation), **fever, malaise**, neurologic deficit (motor weakness, sensory loss, bladder/bowel dysfunction, paralysis).
- **Investigations**
  - **MRI whole spine** (or CT with contrast). Often extend longitudinally (3–5 segments). Skip lesions (noncontiguous) not common: 9% cases. Majority posterior.
  - Blood cultures ×2.
  - **Aspiration** for microscopy/culture/16S PCR.
- **Management**
  - Consider whether urgent surgical decompression/drainage required.
  - IV ABs as soon as blood cultures taken.
  - Vancomycin plus ceftriaxone.

Intracranial Epidural Abscess

- Related to neurosurgery or extension from otitis media/sinusitis/mastoiditis.
- Pathogens = streptococci, anaerobes, and staphylococci.
- Localized pus with wall of inflammation. No spread caudally as dura mater tightly attached around foramen magnum.
- Management: debridement and IV ABs.

Toxin-Mediated Infection

Tetanus and Botulism

- Table 12.13 compares the main features of tetanus and botulism.

TABLE 12.13   Comparison of the Features of Tetanus and Botulism

	Tetanus	Botulism
Epidemiology	Ubiquitous in soil; also found in animal and human feces **Neonatal:** entry via umbilical stump **Dirty traumatic injury** Risk factors = penetrating, with devitalized tissue, localized ischemia, or foreign body	**Foodborne** ingestion of preformed toxin (usually home preserved goods) **Wound** (intravenous drug user or penetrating wound/compound fracture) **Infant** (95% <6 months old; honey ++)
Mechanism of action	**Blocks inhibitory interneurons** in spinal cord and autonomic nervous system (ANS) See Fig. 12.9	Blocks neurotransmitter release at **peripheral cholinergic** nerve terminals: **neuromuscular junction and ANS.**
Incubation period	~3–21 days	Foodborne: 12–36 hours Wound: ~7.5 days
Clinical features	Generalized tetanus: **tetanic spasms** with trivial external stimuli are sudden, painful, and generalized Lockjaw, risus sardonicus, opisthotonus, abdominal rigidity, apnea **No cognitive deficit** Also: localized, cephalic, and neonatal	Acute onset **bilateral cranial neuropathies** (diplopia, dysphagia, dysarthria); **autonomic** disturbance (dry mouth, fixed or dilated pupils, hypotension) with **descending flaccid paralysis** **No sensory deficit** **No cognitive deficit**
Diagnosis	Baseline serum for **tetanus IgG** (if already positive, NOT compatible with diagnosis of tetanus) **Wound swab or tissue for culture/PCR**	Detection of botulinum toxin in **serum** or fecal specimens Detection and isolation of *C. botulinum* from feces or food samples
Management	Tetanus antitoxin or human normal immunoglobulin, wound debridement and antibiotics; vaccination with tetanus toxoid on recovery	Botulinum antitoxin (neutralize circulating antibody), wound debridement and antibiotics, supportive measures
Mortality and complications	30% mortality Bony fractures, asphyxia, hematomas, rhabdomyolysis	5%–10% mortality due to respiratory paralysis and autonomic dysfunction Most hospitalized for 1–3 months Long-term sequelae variable

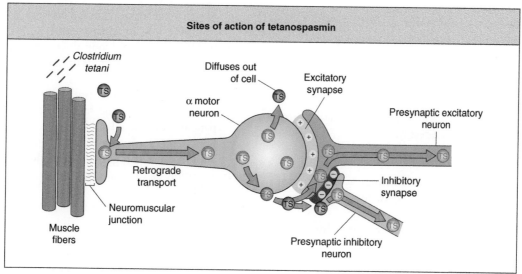

• **Fig. 12.9** Mechanism of action of tetanospasmin. (From Hodowanec A, Bleck TP. Tetanus and botulism. In: Cohen J, Powderly W, Opal S, eds. *Infectious Diseases*. 4th ed. Elsevier; 2017.)

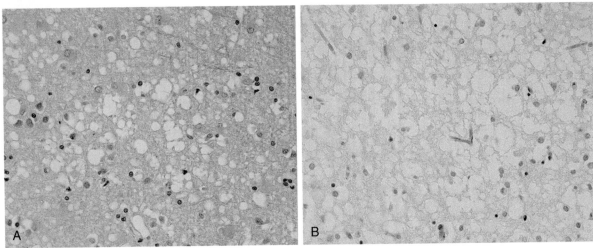

• **Fig. 12.10** Histologic features of spongiform encephalopathy. (A) Confluent spongiform change in deep cortex; (B) severely atrophied, neuron-depleted cortex. (From du Plessis DG. Prion protein disease and neuropathology of prion disease. *Neuroimaging Clin North Am*. 2008;18(1):163–182.)

Transmissible Spongiform Encephalopathies (TSEs)

Transmissible spongiform encephalopathies are a group of infections caused by **prions**, characterized by **severe, irreversible neurologic damage** leading to **progressive dementia and death**. There is characteristic vacuolation of brain tissue (spongiform change, Fig. 12.10A), neuronal loss without inflammation (Fig. 12.10B), and accumulation of an abnormal form of a host cell surface protein.

Prion Protein
- PrP^c: highly conserved cell surface protein, sensitive to protease and detergents.
- **PrP^{sc}: disease-associated isoform**, partially resistant to protease, insoluble in detergents, found aggregated in infected brains.

Human Prion Diseases

Table 12.14 discusses the incidence, etiology, and illness timings of the human prion diseases.

Clinical Features
- Inherited forms: progressive dementia, ataxia, chorea, pyramidal and extrapyramidal signs, myoclonus, pseudobulbar palsy, seizures.
- Classic CJD: **rapidly progressive dementia with myoclonus**, death within 4 months.
  - EEG (characteristic pseudo-periodic sharp wave activity).
  - CSF (14-3-3 protein).
  - MRI (caudate and putamen hyperintensity, cortical ribbon, and thalamic hyperintensity).
- Kuru: progressive cerebellar ataxia with dementia, death within 1 year.
- New variant CJD (vCJD)

- Early: **behavioral and psychiatric** disturbance; sensory symptoms including paresthesia ± pain in limbs; ataxia with unsteady gait.
- Late: hallucinations, paranoia, confabulation, cerebellar signs, chorea, myoclonus, and upper motor neurone signs.
- EEG and 14-3-3 protein not helpful.
- MRI (bilateral pulvinar hyperintensity).
- PrP^{sc} immunostaining on **tonsil biopsy** (100% sensitivity and specificity).

Prevention
- No treatment – all invariably **fatal.**
- Healthcare measures
  - Leukodepletion of blood products.
  - In USA: deferral of blood donors from high risk countries (UK, other European).
  - In UK: deferral of blood donors at higher risk (e.g., recipients of corneal grafts or human pituitary-derived extracts).
  - UK imports plasma derivatives from countries with a low risk of vCJD, and fresh frozen plasma (FFP) for patients born after 1.1.1996.
  - Replacement of cadaveric human growth hormone with recombinant growth hormone (GH).
- Incineration of surgical instruments in confirmed cases of CJD.
- Quarantine of instruments in suspected cases.
- Food chain
  - Cessation of cannibalism.
  - Ban on feeding ruminant-derived protein to other ruminants (interrupt bovine spongiform encephalopathy [BSE] cycle).
  - Specified bovine offal banned from human consumption.
  - Ban on selling UK beef for consumption from animals >30 months old.

TABLE 12.14 Human Prion Diseases

Disease	Incidence	Etiology (Fig. 12.11)	Age of onset or incubation period and duration of illness
Sporadic Creutzfeldt–Jakob disease (CJD)	1 case per 1 million population	Unknown, but hypotheses include somatic mutation or spontaneous conversions of PrP^C into PrP^{Sc}	Age of onset is usually 45–75 years; age of peak onset is 60–65 years; 70% of cases die in under 6 months
Inherited prion disease (Gerstmann–Straussler–Scheinker disease (GSS), fatal familial insomnia (FFI), CJD, PrP systemic amyloidosis)	10%–20% of cases of human prion disease	Autosomal dominant *PRNP* mutation	Onset tends to be earlier in familial CJD compared to sporadic CJD. Can be wide phenotypic variability between and within families
Kuru	>2500 cases among the Fore people in Papua New Guinea	Infection through ritualistic cannibalism	Incubation period 5→40 years; duration of illness 12 months
Iatrogenic CJD	About 500 cases to date	Infections from contaminated human growth hormone, human gonadotropin, depth electrodes, corneal transplants, dura mater grafts, neurosurgical procedures	Incubation periods of cases from human growth hormone 4→40 years; duration of illness 6–18 months
Variant CJD	Over 220 cases in UK and rest of world (greatest risk factor for vCJD is previous residence in the UK or western Europe for ≥6 months between 1980–1996; during peak of BSE crisis)	Infection by BSE-like prions	Mean age of onset 26 years; mean duration of illness 14 months

FFI, fatal familial insomnia; GSS, Gerstmann–Sträussler–Scheinker syndrome; *PRNP*, prion protein gene; PrP^C, normal form of prion protein; PrP^{Sc}, disease-associated isoform of prion protein; BSE, bovine spongiform encephalopathy.
Adapted from Mead S, Collinge J, Tabrizi SJ. Transmissible spongiform encephalopathies of humans and animals. In: Cohen J, Powderly W, Opal S, eds. *Infectious Diseases*. 4th ed. Elsevier; 2017.

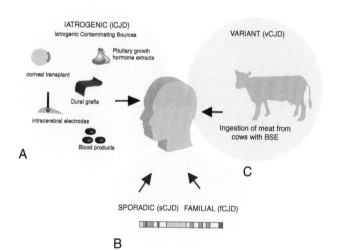

• **Fig. 12.11** Etiology of CJD. (From Venneti S. Prion diseases. *Clin Lab Med.* 2010;30(1):293–309.)

Further Reading and Resources

1. BIA (British Infection Association). British national guidelines on the management of meningitis and encephalitis. https://www.britishinfection.org/guidelines-resources/published-guidelines/.
2. CDC (Centers for Disease Prevention and Control). https://www.cdc.gov/meningitis/clinical-resources.html; https://www.cdc.gov/fungal/index.html.
3. Cohen J, Powderly WG, Opal SM, eds. *Infectious Diseases*. 4th ed. Philadelphia: Elsevier; 2017.
4. IDSA (IDSA Infectious Diseases Society of America). Guidelines. http://www.idsociety.org/Organ_System/#Central%20Nervous%20System%20 (CNS).
5. Public Health England. The green book. https://www.gov.uk/government/collections/immunisation-against-infectious-disease-the-green-book#the-green-book.

13

Respiratory Infections

JUSTIN F. HAYES, JOHN W. BADDLEY

UPPER RESPIRATORY TRACT INFECTIONS

Pharyngitis

- Acute pharyngitis is described as a triad of a sore throat, fever, and pharyngeal inflammation.
- Acute pharyngitis can be a primary disorder, but it can also be the manifestation of a noninfectious disorder (e.g., postnasal drip, thyroiditis, allergies).
- Most cases are due to a virus and are self-limited (Box 13.1).

Treatment

- Since most common cause of pharyngitis is a virus, antibiotics are normally not needed.
- Antibiotics are often prescribed in an effort to prevent complications of group A streptococcal infection (Box 13.2).
- The goal of therapy for group A streptococcus is to decrease time to resolution of symptoms, decrease risk of transmission, and reduce the incidence of suppurative and nonsuppurative complications.
- A 10-day course of penicillin or amoxicillin is recommended for group A streptococcal pharyngitis.

Pertinent Pharyngitis Syndromes

Lemierre's Syndrome

- A rare condition of thrombophlebitis of the internal jugular vein caused most frequently by the gram-negative anaerobe *Fusobacterium necrophorum.*
- Usually follows a normal course of pharyngitis before progressing to fever, lethargy, lateral neck tenderness/edema, and septic emboli (e.g., bilateral nodular lung infiltrates, arthritis).
- Diagnosis confirmed using CT with IV contrast, which demonstrates a filling defect in the internal jugular system (Fig. 13.1).
- First-line treatment is with IV beta-lactamase resistant antibiotics with or without anticoagulation.
- Can be fatal if left untreated.

Diphtheria

- An acute bacterial toxin-mediated infectious disease caused by *Corynebacterium* species that presents with either upper respiratory tract pseudomembrane formation (Fig. 13.2) or cutaneous ulcerative disease.
- **Nonimmune individuals** are at risk for severe respiratory disease and toxin-mediated complications.
- The classic presentation affects the upper respiratory system, leading to clinical manifestations such as a sore throat, low grade fever, and an adherent grayish **pseudomembrane** of the tonsils and pharynx.
- Diagnosis is confirmed with isolation of toxin-producing *Corynebacterium diphtheriae.*
- **Treatment** includes respiratory isolation, **antitoxin administration** in consultation with the CDC, antibiotic treatment, and monitoring for complications.
- **Systemic complications** include myocarditis and delayed peripheral nerve conduction.
- In addition, the pseudomembrane can become dislodged and lead to acute airway obstruction.

• BOX 13.1 Organisms Causing Pharyngitis

Bacteria

Group A streptococcus
    Fusobacterium necrophorum
    Arcanobacterium haemolyticum
    Corynebacterium diphtheriae
    Neisseria gonorrhoeae

Viruses

Rhinovirus
    Coronavirus
    Enteroviruses
    Human immunodeficiency virus (HIV)
    Epstein–Barr virus (EBV)
    Cytomegalovirus (CMV)
    Adenovirus
    Herpes simplex virus (HSV) 1 and 2

> • BOX 13.2 **Complications of Group A Streptococcus Pharyngitis**

Suppurative

Peritonsillar abscess
  Lymphadenitis
  Sinusitis
  Otitis media
  Mastoiditis
  Necrotizing fasciitis
  Toxic shock syndrome

Nonsuppurative

Acute rheumatic fever
  Acute glomerulonephritis

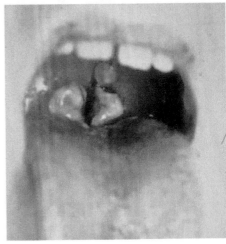

• **Fig. 13.2** Image of a child with diphtheria demonstrating the characteristic membrane. (From Forbes BA. *Clinical Microbiology Newsletter.* 2017;39(5):35–41.)

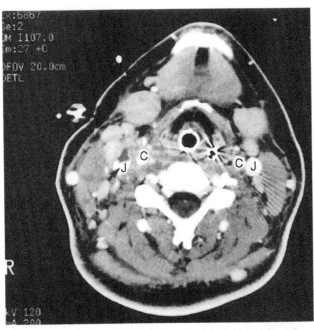

• **Fig. 13.1** Jugular venous thrombosis associated with a right peritonsillar abscess in a young adult. Contrast medium-enhanced axial computed tomographic scan showing a normal right common carotid (*C*) artery but an enlarged right internal jugular vein (*J*) (*arrow*) with a dense or enhancing wall that surrounds the more lucent intraluminal clot. (From Chow AW. Head and neck infections. In; Baddour L, Gorbach SL, eds. *Therapy of Infectious Diseases.* Saunders; 2003.)

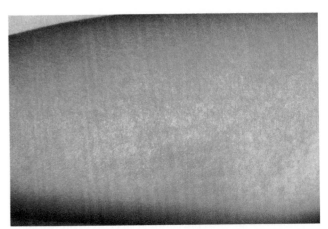

• **Fig. 13.3** Sandpaper-like papules associated with scarlet fever. (Courtesy Centers for Disease Control and Prevention Public Health Image Library. ID#: 5163.)

- Petechiae can appear 1–3 days after the appearance of the rash in a linear distribution along the creases forming Pastia lines.
- Papillae on the tongue become erythematous leading to the **"strawberry tongue"** appearance (Fig. 13.4).
- Treatment with a 10-day course of penicillin or clindamycin (penicillin-allergic patient) is recommended for reduction in transmission and prevention of complications.

Streptococcal Scarlet Fever

- *Streptococcus pyogenes* causes scarlet fever or scarlatina.
- Pharyngitis and scarlet fever tend to peak in the winter and early spring.
- This type of syndrome is caused by the streptococcal **erythrogenic toxin.**
- Classically, the presentation involves the sudden onset of fever, chills, malaise, sore throat before an exanthem appears 12–48 hours later that begins on the trunk and spreads peripherally.
- The remaining skin becomes diffusely erythematous leading to the sunburn appearance of erythroderma (texture is of a sandpaper quality and erythema blanches with pressure) (Fig. 13.3).

Arcanobacterium Haemolyticum

- A nonmotile beta-hemolytic, gram-positive bacillus that causes a small percentage of bacterial pharyngitis cases.
- Has the ability to cause more deep-seated infections, such as meningitis, pneumonia, brain abscess, osteomyelitis, and peritonsillar abscess.
- Peak incidence occurs in patients from the **10- to 30-years-old** age range.
- A rash is present in **25%–50%** of patients and may be urticarial, macular, or maculopapular.
- The rash tends to occur on the trunk and extremities while **sparing** the palms, soles, and face (Fig. 13.5).

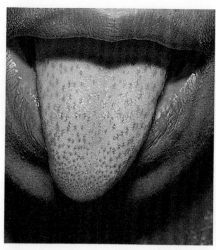

• **Fig. 13.4** Scarlet fever. During the first 1–2 days the tongue has a white coating through which prominent erythematous papillae project – a white strawberry tongue. (From Michaels MG, Williams JV. Infectious diseases. In: Zitelli BJ, McIntire S, Nowalk AJ. *Zitelli and Davis' Atlas of Pediatric Physical Diagnosis.* 7th ed. Elsevier; 2018.)

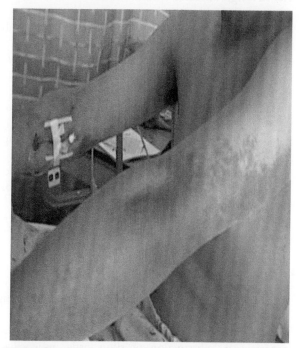

• **Fig. 13.5** Skin rash in a patient with *Arcanobacterium haemolyticum* pharyngitis. (From Kim R, Reboli AC. Other coryneform bacteria and rhodococci. In: Bennett JE, Dolin R, Blaser MJ, eds. *Mandell, Douglas, and Bennett's Principles and Practice of Infectious Diseases.* Updated 8th ed. Elsevier; 2015.)

• First-line treatment is with erythromycin due to increased tolerance of the organism to penicillin.

Infectious Mononucleosis

Clinical syndrome characterized by pharyngitis, fever, lymphadenopathy, and the presence of **atypical lymphocytes** on a peripheral blood smear.

- **Epstein-Barr Virus (EBV)**
  - Establishes lifelong latency in B lymphocytes.
  - Transmitted primarily through exposure to infected saliva.

- Seroprevalence approaches 95% in adults.
- Symptomatic infection tends to peak during adolescence and young adulthood.
- Tends to be a self-limited illness but complications occur, including splenic rupture, encephalitis, autoimmune hemolytic anemia, and mild liver enzyme elevations.
- Diagnosis is made by the appearance of nonspecific heterophile antibodies.
- The presence of IgM viral capsid antigen (VCA) antibodies is closely correlated with acute EBV infection.
- **Cytomegalovirus (CMV)**
  - Clinically overlaps with EBV mononucleosis but tends to be a milder disease.
  - Tends to have less prominent lymphadenopathy.
  - Hepatitis is nearly always present.
  - Isolation of CMV from saliva or urine does not prove infection because asymptomatic shedding is common.
- **Primary HIV infection**
- Causes a febrile illness that resembles mononucleosis.
- **Mucocutaneous ulcerations** and a **rash** are features more common with acute HIV syndrome versus infectious mononucleosis.
- Patients presenting with a negative heterophile antibody mononucleosis-like syndrome should be **screened** for HIV.
- **Toxoplasmosis**
- Causes a syndrome that is characterized by fever and lymphadenopathy.
- Toxoplasmosis usually does **not** cause pharyngitis or hepatitis.
- **Human herpesvirus (HHV) 6 and 7**
- Symptomatic infection is uncommon in adults.
- Occasionally, a mononucleosis-like syndrome with prolonged lymphadenopathy has been described during seroconversion of HHV-6 in adults.

Epiglottitis

Acute Epiglottitis

- Acute epiglottitis is an invasive cellulitis of the epiglottis and its surrounding structures.
- Has the potential to cause abrupt airway obstruction.
- Prior to routine *Haemophilus influenzae* type b conjugate vaccination, the majority of cases occurred in children aged 1 to 4 years old.
- The incidence of epiglottitis has remained stable in the adult population with no identification of a pathogen in the majority of cases.
- The classic clinical presentation is a child who develops fever, irritability, and experiences rapidly progressive respiratory distress with stridor.
- Children affected are classically described as experiencing hoarseness with a **muffled voice.**
- Lateral neck radiographs demonstrate an enlarged epiglottis (**thumbprint sign**, Fig. 13.6) with ballooning of the hypopharynx and prevertebral soft tissue swelling.

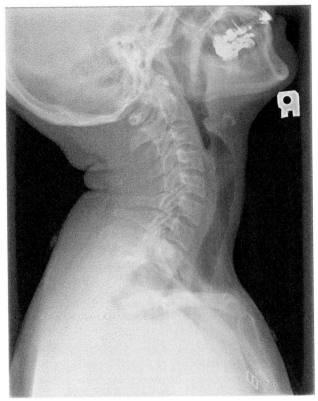

• **Fig. 13.6** Thumbprint sign on lateral radiography of neck. (From Hung TY, Li S, Chen PS, et al. Bedside ultrasonography as a safe and effective tool to diagnose acute epiglottitis. *Am J Emerg Med.* 2011;29(3):359.e1–359.e3.)

• **Diagnosis:** established by visualization of an edematous, cherry-red epiglottis.
• Croup can present in a similar fashion but children tend to be less toxic, experience more frequent episodes of coughing, and have a lack of drooling compared to epiglottitis.

Therapy/Management
• Management of the airway is most important consideration.
• Antibiotic management normally directed at *Streptococcus pneumoniae*, *Haemophilus influenzae*, and occasionally *Staphylococcus aureus*.

Chronic Epiglottitis
• Described as a presentation consisting of mild dysphagia, dysphonia, and/or sore throat.
• Often treated as an outpatient initially with antibiotics.
• Differential diagnosis includes granulomatous disorders, such as tuberculosis, histoplasmosis, coccidioidomycosis, and sarcoidosis.
• Viral etiologies have also been described.
• Diagnosis ultimately relies on direct laryngoscopy and biopsy.
• Treatment is directed at the causative agent or condition.

Sinusitis
• Sinusitis is an inflammatory disorder of the paranasal sinuses (Fig. 13.7).
• Has become one of the most common reasons to see a primary care physician and is responsible for a large number of antibiotic prescriptions.
• Both acute and chronic sinusitis have been described.

Acute Sinusitis
• Most common causes are viral.
• Pathogenesis involves three mechanisms:
  • Obstruction of the sinus ostia,
  • Impairment of the ciliary apparatus,
  • Thickening of sinus secretions.
• *Streptococcus pneumoniae* remains the leading etiology of acute bacterial sinusitis, followed by nontypeable *Haemophilus influenzae* and *Moraxella catarrhalis*.
• **Acute fungal sinusitis** is an invasive infection in immunocompromised hosts.
  • Involves hyphal invasion of blood vessels that results in infarction of the tissues.
  • Infection is usually due to *Aspergillus*, *Mucorales*, *Fusarium*, and occasionally dematiaceous molds.
  • Patients usually present with fever, sinus pain, facial pain, nasal congestion, epistaxis, and sometimes visual disturbances.
  • Aggressive management with both medical therapy and surgical intervention is needed.
• **Nosocomial sinusitis** can be a common presentation in the critical care setting, and consideration for more resistant organisms is needed.
• **Risk factors:** nasal intubation and nasal-enteric feeding.

Chronic Sinusitis
• Defined as signs and symptoms that persist for at least 12 weeks.
• Similar factors as acute sinusitis play a role in the pathogenesis (e.g., obstruction of sinus ostia, mucociliary impairment, and thickening of secretions).
• Bacteria profile may involve other pathogens, such as gram-negative bacilli, MRSA, and anaerobes.
• **Allergic fungal sinusitis** is a distinct entity that is thought to arise from an intense allergic response to chronic fungal colonization.
  • Typically occurs among immunocompetent hosts.
  • Involves noninvasive growth of fungi in areas of compromised mucus drainage.
  • The sinuses contain thick, inspissated mucus that contains eosinophils.
  • Treatment includes both medical (topical and systemic corticosteroids) and surgical interventions.
  • The efficacy of fungal agents is unproven in this disorder.

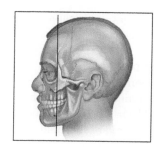

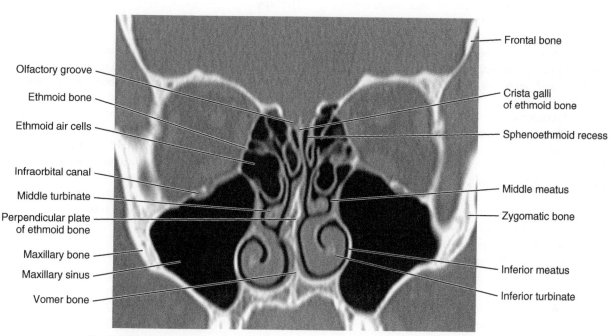

Olfactory groove

Ethmoid bone

Ethmoid air cells

Infraorbital canal

Middle turbinate

Perpendicular plate
of ethmoid bone

Maxillary bone

Maxillary sinus

Vomer bone

Frontal bone

Crista galli
of ethmoid bone

Sphenoethmoid recess

Middle meatus

Zygomatic bone

Inferior meatus

Inferior turbinate

• **Fig. 13.7** Paranasal sinuses: coronal view. (From Lee TC, Mukundan S. *Netter's Correlative Imaging: Neuroanatomy.* Elsevier; 2015.)

Clinical Manifestations of Sinusitis

- Similar to a viral upper respiratory infection (nasal congestion, discharge).
- Bacterial sinusitis tends to have a more persistent course (i.e., symptoms greater than 10 days without improvement).
- Bacterial sinusitis can also have a severe presentation that includes fever with purulent nasal discharge.
- A third presentation of sinusitis due to bacterial infection involves an initial improvement in symptoms with worsening again in the first 10 days of the presentation.
- Patients with chronic sinusitis have persistent symptoms that last for at least 12 weeks and can include facial pain and pressure.

Diagnosis

- Physical exam is limited and diagnosis should be made on clinical grounds.

Therapy

- Since the majority of infections are viral, the treatment for acute sinusitis is mostly supportive (nasal saline irrigation, inhaled corticosteroids, antipyretics).
- Indications for empiric antibiotics (any one of the following):
  - Symptoms lasting ≥10 days.
  - Severe symptoms ≥3–4 days.
  - Double sickening phenomenon (worsening symptoms after a period of improvement).
  - If bacterial sinusitis is diagnosed, amoxicillin–clavulanate is the recommended antimicrobial for use.
  - Doxycycline can be used as an alternative regimen for initial empiric use.
  - Respiratory fluoroquinolones, macrolides, and trimethoprim–sulfamethoxazole can be used but are not recommended for initial empirical therapy.

- Patients presenting with more severe disease or complications of acute sinusitis may require parenteral therapy.

Complications

- Complications occur due to the close proximity of the sinuses to critical structures of the skull and face (Table 13.1).
- Majority of complications occur due to infections of the ethmoid or sphenoid sinuses.
- Fever, altered mental status, and/or focal neurologic deficits should raise concern for complications.
- Immediate surgical intervention is recommended if there is concern for these complications.

Bronchitis

- Acute bronchitis is a clinical syndrome involving a brief, self-limited inflammatory process of large and mid-sized airways with no evidence of pneumonia present.
- Viruses are the most common etiology.
- Bacterial pathogens have been described in a small percentage of cases (e.g., *Mycoplasma pneumoniae*, *Chlamydia pneumoniae*, and *Bordetella pertussis*).

Clinical Manifestations

- Nasal congestion, rhinitis, sore throat, malaise.
- Cough (becomes dominant feature of the illness) of less than 3 weeks' duration.
- Wheezing can also be present.

Diagnosis

- Suspected in an individual with acute respiratory tract illness where cough is the predominant complaint.
- Important to rule out pneumonia.

Therapy

- Since the majority of infections are viral, the treatment of bronchitis is **mostly supportive.**
- **Directed at symptom control**
  - Therapy can be directed at specific pathogen (normally indicated only for pertussis and influenza if proven or suspected).

Acute Exacerbations of Chronic Bronchitis

- Acute exacerbations of chronic bronchitis lead to significant morbidity and mortality.
- In general, more frequent during the winter season.

- Presentation involves an increase in sputum production, worsening dyspnea, and a worsening cough.
- Seen most commonly in patients with chronic lung disease, such as chronic obstructive lung disease and cystic fibrosis.
- Two-thirds of patients with an acute exacerbation have a bacteria or virus or both identified in lower airway secretions.
- *Streptococcus pneumoniae*, *Haemophilus influenzae*, and *Moraxella catarrhalis* are the most common bacterial pathogens isolated.
- Patients that have greater functional impairment and previous antibiotic and corticosteroid use will sometimes have *Pseudomonas aeruginosa* and other Enterobacteriaceae isolated from sputum.

Therapy

- Guidelines have recommended antibiotic therapy if one of the following is present:
  - Presentation with three cardinal symptoms: increased dyspnea, sputum volume, and sputum purulence.
  - Presentation with two of the above cardinal symptoms if increased purulence is one of the symptoms.
  - Presentation with a severe exacerbation that requires mechanical ventilation.
- Therapy normally involves macrolides, second-generation cephalosporins, or fluoroquinolones unless there is concern for *Pseudomonas aeruginosa*.
- Neuraminidase inhibitors should be considered for treatment of suspected influenza infection.

Pertussis

- Pertussis, which is also known as "whooping cough," is a highly contagious respiratory illness caused by the gram-negative coccobacillus *Bordetella pertussis*.
- The organism is fastidious and requires **special media** for culture.
- The incubation period is 1–3 weeks but typically is 7–10 days.
- Pertussis is spread by respiratory droplets.
- In the prevaccine era, it was common in children, but now it is more common in adolescents and adults.
- The classic symptoms are paroxysmal cough, inspiratory whoop, and **post-tussive emesis.**
- Antibiotic treatment given during the early (catarrhal) phase may decrease the duration and severity of cough.
- Specifically, **macrolides** are effective at eradicating *B. pertussis* from the nasopharynx.
- In addition, antibiotic therapy can decrease the spread of the organism to uninfected individuals.
- Childhood vaccination has been highly effective at preventing infection with this organism.
- Routine vaccination with **DTaP** vaccine is performed in the United States.
- Adults aged 19–64 years old should receive a booster administration with the TdaP vaccine.

TABLE 13.1 Complications of Sinusitis	
Intracranial	**Extracranial**
Subdural empyema	Orbital cellulitis
Epidural abscess	Orbital abscess
Brain abscess	Subperiosteal abscess
Meningitis	
Venous sinus thrombosis	

- For **pregnant women,** administration of TdaP to all women between 27–36 weeks gestation is recommended.
- **Postexposure prophylaxis** should be administered to individuals with close contact to a person with pertussis (face-to-face contact within 3 feet of an infected individual).
- The same regimens recommended for treatment should be given for postexposure prophylaxis.

Otitis Media

- Acute otitis media (AOM) is an illness involving middle ear fluid and inflammation of mucosa that lines the middle ear space.
- Peak incidence occurs in the first 3 years of life.
- Strong consideration should be given to patients presenting with fever, pain, and impaired hearing.

Sequelae of Otitis Media
- Hearing loss.
- Cholesteatoma.
- Chronic perforation of tympanic membrane.

Pathogenesis
- Anatomic or physiologic dysfunction of the Eustachian tube appears to play a crucial role.

Microbiology
Bacteria
- *Streptococcus pneumoniae* and *Haemophilus influenzae* consistently demonstrated as pathogens in all age groups.
- *Moraxella catarrhalis* has also been described in mild disease.
- *Staphylococcus aureus* is a rare cause and should be considered in patients with persistent otorrhea after insertion of tympanostomy tubes.
- *Mycoplasma pneumoniae* described in hemorrhagic bullous myringitis but not common.
Viruses
- Viruses may be the initial inciting event that leads to AOM, and co-infections with bacteria have been described.
- Respiratory syncytial virus, influenza, enteroviruses, coronaviruses, and rhinoviruses are the most common viruses described.

Diagnosis
- Diagnosis is made on the basis of the presence of fluid in the middle ear along with signs or symptoms of acute illness with inflammation of the mucosa of the middle ear identified on exam.

Therapy
- Agent chosen should provide coverage against *Streptococcus pneumoniae*, *Haemophilus influenzae*, and *Moraxella catarrhalis* (e.g., amoxicillin).
- Agents active against gram-negative bacilli and MRSA should be considered for the newborn infant, patients with a depressed immune system, and the patient with suppurative complications of chronic otitis media.
- Surgical management is a potential therapeutic option for recurrent episodes of AOM (e.g., myringotomy, adenoidectomy, and placement of tympanostomy tubes).

COMMUNITY RESPIRATORY VIRUSES

- Include many common DNA and RNA viruses that cause respiratory infections.
- In healthy individuals, these viruses usually result in mild to moderate disease but can cause more serious disease in the very young, elderly, and immunocompromised.

Influenza

- Influenza (Fig. 13.8) has been causing recurrent epidemics every 1–3 years for the past 400 years.
- A unique feature of influenza is its ability to alter the **antigenic** properties of the envelope glycoproteins, the hemagglutinin (HA), and neuraminidase (NA).
  - Antigenic **drift** refers to minor modifications (**point mutations**) within HA, NA, or both leading to localized outbreaks.
  - Antigenic **shift** refers to more radical changes in the antigenicity of HA, NA, or both (**segment reassortment**) leading to widespread disease or pandemics.
- The greatest pandemic was in 1918–1919, when 21 million deaths were recorded worldwide.

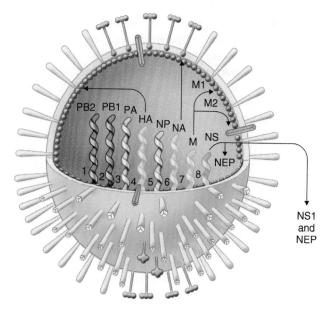

• **Fig. 13.8** Diagram of influenza virus structure. Eight segments of viral RNA are contained within the lipid envelope and matrix (M1) shell. Each codes for one or more proteins that form the virus or regulate its intracellular replication. (Courtesy Dr. Robert G. Webster.)

- In 2009 the H1N1 influenza pandemic demonstrated the risk of severe influenza associated with pregnancy.

Notable Influenza Strains

H1N1	Emerged in 1918
H3N2	Emerged in 1968 (Hong Kong flu)
H5N1	Emerged 2003 in Hong Kong
	Associated with poultry exposure
H7N9	Major outbreak in China. Avian-to-human transmission noted
H7N7	Outbreak in The Netherlands
	Associated with conjunctivitis

- In general, excess mortality has been associated with influenza A/H3N2 and to a lesser extent with influenza A/H1N1.
- Influenza should be suspected in any patient who presents with acute onset of fever, cough, and systemic symptoms, such as myalgias, between fall and spring.
- Fever and cough during a local epidemic are the most predictive findings of influenza infection.

Diagnosis
- Diagnostic testing should only be used when the results will influence clinical decision-making or infection control measures.
- **Rapid influenza diagnostic tests (RIDTs)** are available and work by detecting parts of the virus that stimulate an immune response (i.e., influenza A and B viral nucleoprotein antigens).
- RIDTs provide results within 10–15 minutes but can be variable (i.e., more likely to be a true positive during an influenza outbreak) in sensitivity.
- **RT-PCR** is the preferred confirmatory test and detects the genetic material of the virus (i.e., viral RNA) providing better accuracy than other rapid tests.
- **Empirical treatment** is recommended in patients who present after the onset of fever and cough during influenza season who are at high risk for complications (e.g., young children, adults 65 years of age and older, pregnant women, presence of asthma, heart disease, diabetes, and other comorbidities).
- Empirical treatment is also recommended for severely ill patients who are hospitalized and at high risk for complications of influenza.
  - **Treatment:** Neuraminidase inhibitors (e.g., oseltamivir, zanamivir) are recommended for treatment when initiated in the first 48 hours after symptom onset.
  - Peramivir is a new neuraminidase inhibitor approved for intravenous administration for influenza infection.
- **Secondary bacterial pneumonia** with *Staphylococcus aureus* or *Streptococcus pneumoniae* is a complication of influenza infection.
- **Annual influenza vaccination** is recommended for everyone older than 6 months of age in the United States.

- Inactivated and recombinant influenza vaccines are recommended while the intranasal vaccine is not.
- **Chemoprophylaxis** is recommended in patients
  - Who present within 48 hours of exposure to an infected person.
  - Who are at high risk of developing complications from influenza and have not been vaccinated.
  - Who have been vaccinated within the past 2 weeks.
  - Who are severely immunosuppressed.

Respiratory Syncytial Virus (RSV)

- RSV is a well-recognized cause of morbidity and mortality in immunocompromised individuals.
- Disease can range from a bronchiolitis or mild URI to a more fulminant lower respiratory tract infection (LRTI).
- RSV is a leading cause of viral LRTI in immunocompromised children and adults.
- RSV usually begins with signs and symptoms of a URI, which can progress to bronchiolitis, pneumonitis, and pneumonia.
- Both standard and contact precautions are needed for hospitalized patients with RSV.
- Treatment of RSV must take into consideration the patient's risk of developing more serious disease.
- Ribavirin is a potential treatment option with limited efficacy data.
  - Palivizumab is another option on the market that is a humanized monoclonal antibody designed to reduce RSV infections.

Parainfluenza Virus (PIV)

- PIV are the major causes of croup or laryngotracheobronchitis in young children.
- PIV has also been identified as causing disease in adult immunocompromised patients.
- There is no proven treatment for PIV infection.
- PIV infection has been demonstrated to be a risk factor for airflow decline and a cause of long-term pulmonary complications in hematopoietic stem cell transplant (HSCT) recipients.

Adenovirus (AdV)

- Adenoviruses are DNA viruses that usually cause self-limited disease in normal hosts.
- AdV has been described with respiratory, gastrointestinal, and conjunctival infections.
- AdV can cause end-organ disease and disseminated infections in patients who are recipients of stem cell and solid organ transplants.
- In HSCT recipients, AdV infections have been specifically associated with the following:
  - T-cell depleted graft recipients.
  - Acute graft versus host disease.

- Real-time PCR has been useful for monitoring patients with disseminated AdV infection.
- **Cidofovir** has been shown to be active against all strains of AdV during *in vitro* testing and has been used to treat AdV infections.

Human Metapneumovirus (HMPV)

- Part of the *Paramyxoviridae* family and has been associated with both upper and lower respiratory tract infections in both children and adults.
- Serious disease is reported in immunocompromised individuals, and once pneumonia develops, rapidly progressive pulmonary infiltrates develop along with hypotension and shock.

Radiographic Finding
- Bilateral alveolar and interstitial infiltrates.
- Emphysema and no infiltrates.
- Diffuse alveolar hemorrhage.

Coronavirus

- Coronaviruses normally cause mild respiratory infections in humans but can occasionally lead to more severe infections.
- Coronaviruses also infect many animals and have crossed over to humans (e.g., severe acute respiratory syndrome [SARS] and Middle East respiratory syndrome [MERS]).
- **SARS** was originally identified in Guangdong Province of the People's Republic of China, spread to Hong Kong, and then to the rest of the world.
  - A rapid public health effort was coordinated by the WHO and transmission ceased throughout the world.
  - Infection control work dedicated to contact and droplet spread was used successfully to control the outbreak.
- **MERS** coronavirus was discovered when a man was admitted in 2012 to a hospital in Saudi Arabia with the presentation of acute pneumonia and renal failure.
  - More cases were subsequently discovered in individuals living in or traveling in the Middle East.

LOWER RESPIRATORY TRACT INFECTIONS

Community-Acquired Pneumonia (CAP)

- Pneumonia remains in the top ten most common causes of death and is the most common cause of infection-related mortality.
- History-taking should attempt to define symptoms consistent with pneumonia, the clinical setting in which the pneumonia takes place, deficits in host defense, and potential exposures.

- Fever, cough, sputum production, and dyspnea are the most common symptoms of a pneumonia syndrome.
- Nonrespiratory symptoms like fatigue, malaise, and night sweats may also be a part of the presentation.
  - Community-MRSA pneumonia has been described in previously healthy, younger individuals and has been seen as a postinfluenza infection.
  - Community *Pseudomonas* infections are associated with structural lung disease and repeated COPD (chronic obstructive pulmonary disease) exacerbations that require corticosteroids and/or antibiotics.
- Common and uncommon causes of CAP are listed in Table 13.2.

Diagnosis
- The diagnosis of CAP is based on clinical features and radiographic imaging of the lung.
- Lobar consolidation, cavitation, and large pleural effusions are various radiographic presentations that suggest a bacterial etiology.
- Patchy areas of ground-glass opacities, airspace consolidation, and poorly defined small nodules suggest a viral etiology.
- Fever, cough, pleuritic chest pain, and sputum production are the usual clinical manifestations.
- Recent travel and exposure history may identify possible etiologic agents for pneumonia.
- Diagnostic testing in the setting of CAP is encouraged when identification of a pathogen may change antibiotic management (Box 13.3).
- The yield of sputum cultures can be variable and influenced by the quality of the collection method.
- For *Legionella* the urine antigen test only detects *Legionella pneumophila* serogroup 1.
- For atypical pathogens like *Chlamydophila pneumoniae*, *Legionella species*, and *Mycoplasma pneumoniae*, acute and convalescent-phase serologic testing can be used for diagnosis.

Severe CAP

- Treatment considerations are determined by severity of illness at presentation.
- CURB-65 and pneumonia severity index (PSI) scores have been validated for use in determining initial severity of illness.

TABLE 13.2 Causes of Community-Acquired Pneumonia

Common	Uncommon
Bacteria	**Bacteria**
Streptococcus pneumoniae	Staphylococcus aureus
Legionella spp.	Pseudomonas aeruginosa
Mycoplasma pneumoniae	Mixed anaerobic infections
Chlamydophila pneumoniae	Moraxella catarrhalis
	Escherichia coli
	Klebsiella pneumoniae
	Francisella tularensis

• BOX 13.3 Recommendations for Blood and Sputum Testing for CAP

Blood and sputum cultures should be considered for the following:
- Admission to the ICU
- Cavitary infiltrates
- Leukopenia
- Alcohol abuse
- Advanced liver disease
- Asplenia
- Positive pneumococcal urine antigen test
- Pleural effusion

Sputum cultures without blood cultures for the following
- Failed outpatient antibiotic therapy
- Patients with structural or obstructive lung disease
- Patients who have a positive *Legionella* urine antigen test

---

• BOX 13.4 Criteria for Major and Minor CAP

Major
- Invasive mechanical ventilation
- Septic shock requiring vasopressors

Minor
- Respiratory rate >30 breaths/minute
- PaO_2/FiO_2 <250
- Multilobar infiltrates
- Confusion
- Uremia
- Leukopenia
- Thrombocytopenia
- Hypotension requiring aggressive fluid resuscitation
- Hypothermia

- Admission to the ICU is **required** for patients
  - Requiring vasopressors,
  - Requiring intubation due to respiratory failure.
- Admission is **recommended** for patients with at least three of the minor criteria (Box 13.4).

Nonsevere CAP

- Severity of illness scores like CURB-65 and PSI can be used for risk stratification.
- The ability of the patient to take oral medications and to have access to outpatient resources and support are important variables for deciding whether to treat as an outpatient or inpatient.

Treatment
- Treatment is directed at the most likely pathogen(s) and severity of illness (Table 13.3).

Atypical Pneumonias

- Originally described in a small group of patients that had a mild upper respiratory tract illness followed by a pneumonia.
- *Mycoplasma pneumoniae, Chlamydophila pneumoniae, Legionella* species, and respiratory viruses are the most frequent pathogens described.

Mycoplasma Pneumoniae

- Can account for 10%–30% of the cases of CAP but usually in patients well enough to be treated as outpatients.
- The majority of cases occur in people younger than 40 years old and has specifically been described in younger individuals at military bases, boarding schools, and colleges.
- Increase in incidence in late summer and early fall.
- Classically, presents as URI with constitutional symptoms that then progresses to a lower respiratory tract infection.

- Sore throat is often the initial finding.
- About a third of patients may present with ear findings.
- **Bullous myringitis** (Fig. 13.9) has been associated with mycoplasmal infection but is a rare finding.
- There have also been extrapulmonary findings classically described with mycoplasmal infection (e.g., central nervous system, renal, skin, blood).
- **Radiographic findings** can be more extensive than the physical exam would indicate.
- Lower lobe unilateral or bilateral patchy infiltrates in one or more segments in bronchial or peribronchial distribution have been described.

Chlamydophila Pneumoniae (see Chapter 31)

- Has emerged as an important cause of atypical pneumonia.
- Is often seen with other pathogens.
- Sore throat and URI symptoms usually progress to pneumonia in most clinical presentations.
- A cough may begin days to weeks after initial manifestations.
- *Chlamydophila pneumoniae* has also been associated with **extrapulmonary** infections (e.g., otitis media, sinusitis, pericarditis, myocarditis, and endocarditis).

Legionella

Recognized as major cause of atypical pneumonia syndrome and a cause of severe CAP.

Acquisition from water sources.

Legionella pneumophila causes over 90% of *Legionella* pneumonia with most of those cases caused by **serogroup 1**.

- **Risk factors**
  - Smoking.
  - Immunosuppression.
  - Chronic lung disease.
  - Alcoholism.
  - Exposure to hot tubs.
- People may initially present with milder disease involving malaise, nonproductive cough, and myalgias, but this

TABLE 13.3 Characterization of Likely Pathogens for CAP Based on Severity of Illness With Associated Recommended Treatment Regimens

Outpatient	Inpatient (non-ICU)	Inpatient (ICU)
Mycoplasma pneumoniae *Moraxella catarrhalis* *Haemophilus influenzae* *Chlamydophila pneumoniae* Respiratory viruses **Recommended treatment** Macrolide or doxycycline if no chronic comorbidities Respiratory fluoroquinolone or beta-lactam plus macrolide if patient has chronic comorbidities or received antibiotics within the last 3 months	*Streptococcus pneumoniae* *Legionella* spp. Mycoplasma pneumoniae *Chlamydophila pneumoniae* Haemophilus influenzae Aspiration (e.g., gram-negative enteric pathogens, oral anaerobes) Respiratory viruses (e.g., influenza, RSV, parainfluenza, adenovirus) **Recommended treatment** A respiratory fluoroquinolone or a beta-lactam (preference is for cefotaxime, ceftriaxone, ampicillin, ertapenem) plus a macrolide	*Streptococcus pneumoniae* *Staphylococcus aureus* *Legionella* spp. Gram-negative bacilli *Haemophilus influenzae* **Recommended treatment** Same as non-ICU patients with the following exceptions: If *Pseudomonas* is a concern, need to add pseudomonal coverage If MRSA infection is a concern, need to add vancomycin or linezolid

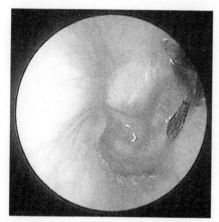

• **Fig. 13.9** Bullous myringitis. The deep ear canal and tympanic membrane are acutely inflamed. A large bulla is seen over the posterior tympanic membrane. (From Brant JA, Ruckenstein MJ. Infections of the external ear. In: Flint PW, et al. *Cummings Otolaryngology*. 6th ed. Elsevier; 2015.)

can rapidly progress to more severe pulmonary symptoms with high fevers.
• **Relative bradycardia** is a classic association with *Legionella* pneumonia.
• **Extrapulmonary manifestations**
  • Mental status changes.
  • Diarrhea.
  • Rash.
  • Hyponatremia.
  • Hypophosphatemia.
  • Elevated liver enzyme levels.
  • Elevated creatinine levels.
  • **Extrapulmonary infection** due to *Legionella* is unusual but normally involves the heart if it occurs (e.g., myocarditis, pericarditis).

Radiographic Findings
• Patchy interstitial or nodular infiltrates that rapidly progress have been described.

Nosocomial Pneumonia

• **Nosocomial pneumonia** refers to a pneumonia that was not incubating at the time of hospital admission and presents 48 hours or more after admission.
• **Healthcare-associated pneumonia (HCAP)** is a term that has also been used and refers to pneumonias acquired within 90 days of infection at a hospital, pneumonias that occur in individuals that reside in a nursing home or long-term care facility, or pneumonias that develop in patients who have received parenteral antibiotic therapy, chemotherapy, or wound care within 30 days of the pneumonia.

Ventilator-Associated Pneumonia/Hospital-Acquired Pneumonia

• **Ventilator-associated pneumonia (VAP)** refers to a pneumonia that develops 48 hours or more after endotracheal intubation.
• **Hospital-acquired pneumonia (HAP)** refers to a pneumonia that develops 48 hours or more after admission to a hospital.
• VAP/HAP have been shown to extend the duration of mechanical ventilation and intensive care unit length of stay.
• There is concern for multidrug-resistant pathogens (MDR) as the etiology of respiratory infections in these individuals (Box 13.5).
• The diagnosis of HAP and VAP is difficult due to atypical clinical signs of pneumonia in hospitalized patients as well as the large differential of noninfectious etiologies of respiratory complications in these susceptible patients (e.g., pulmonary edema, acute respiratory distress syndrome, hypersensitivity reactions, and pulmonary embolism).

Radiography
• Alveolar infiltrates and air bronchograms are the most sensitive radiographic patterns for proven VAP but lack specificity.

• BOX 13.5   Risk Factors for MDR Ventilator-Associated Pneumonia

- Prior intravenous antibiotic use within 90 days (VAP and HAP)
- Septic shock at time of VAP
- Acute respiratory distress syndrome preceding VAP
- 5 or more days of hospitalization prior to the occurrence of VAP
- Acute renal replacement therapy prior to VAP onset

Diagnosis

- Sputum examination and/or bronchoscopy with a bronchoalveolar culture can help confirm clinical suspicion of HAP/VAP.

Treatment

- Empirical coverage for HAP/VAP should be informed by local pathogen data and susceptibility patterns at the institution.
- Empiric coverage for *Staphylococcus aureus*, *Pseudomonas aeruginosa*, and other gram-negative bacilli is recommended.

MRSA Coverage

- If the patient is being managed in a unit where >10%–20% of *S. aureus* isolates are methicillin-resistant or the patient possesses risk factors for MDR pathogens, MRSA coverage should be provided.

Pseudomonal Coverage

- If the patient is being managed in a unit where >10% of isolates are resistant to an agent being considered for monotherapy or the patient possesses risk factors for MDR pathogens, two anti-pseudomonal agents should be prescribed empirically.
- Ultimately, antibiotic selection should be narrowed to avoid harmful side effects, minimize population-level antibiotic resistance, and decrease costs.
- Seven days is the usual duration of therapy for HAP or VAP but can be adjusted depending on clinical circumstances and complicating factors (i.e., empyema, lung abscess, bacteremia).

Chronic Pneumonia

- A pulmonary parenchymal process that can be infectious or noninfectious.
- The syndrome is present for weeks or months and involves abnormal chest radiography and pulmonary symptoms such as dyspnea and cough.
- A detailed history, including age, gender, epidemiologic exposures, occupational, and travel history, is important for the formation of a differential diagnosis for chronic pneumonia syndromes.
- Pancytopenia can be a clue to a disseminated infection in a chronic pneumonia syndrome, but radiographic patterns are usually the most helpful for elucidating a differential diagnosis.

TABLE 13.4   Causes of Chronic Pneumonia

Infectious	Noninfectious
Bacteria	Neoplasia
Mixed aerobic and anaerobic bacteria	Cystic fibrosis
Actinomyces spp.	Sarcoidosis
Burkholderia pseudomallei	Amyloidosis
Nocardia spp.	Vasculitis
Rhodococcus equi	Drugs
Mycobacteria	Radiation
Mycobacterium abscessus	Recurrent pulmonary emboli
Mycobacterium avium complex	Bronchial obstruction
Mycobacterium kansasii	Pulmonary infiltration with eosinophilia syndrome
Mycobacterium tuberculosis	Pneumoconiosis
Parasites	
Dirofilaria	
Echinococcus granulosus	
Filaria	
Paragonimus westermani	
Fungi	
Aspergillus spp.	
Blastomyces dermatitidis	
Coccidioides spp.	
Cryptococcus spp.	
Histoplasma capsulatum	
Scedosporium spp.	
Sporothrix schenckii	

- Infectious and non-infectious causes of chronic pneumonia are listed in Table 13.4.

Radiography

- Radiographic patterns described:
  - Patchy infiltrates.
  - Cavitation.
  - Nodular disease.
  - Diffuse pulmonary infiltration and fibrosis.

Diagnosis

- A good sputum sample can be helpful for diagnosis, but if this is not possible, a more invasive procedure, such as bronchoscopy and/or lung biopsy, may be necessary.
- Serologic testing may be helpful in the setting of chronic pneumonia.

Pulmonary Nocardiosis

- *Nocardia* is a genus of aerobic actinomycetes responsible for localized or disseminated infections in animals and humans.
- Infections have become more common in humans due to an increasing immunocompromised host population as well as an improvement in identification and detection of *Nocardia* species in the laboratory.

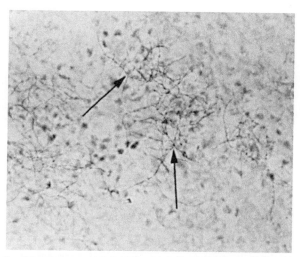

• **Fig. 13.10** Appearance of *Nocardia asteroides* and *Nocardia brasiliensis* (*arrows*) in a properly decolorized acid-fast smear. Organisms appear as fragmented bacilli with stain concentrated in a beaded fashion along portions of the filaments (×160). (From Harik N, Jacobs RF. Nocardia. In: Cherry J, et al. *Feigin and Cherry's Textbook of Pediatric Infectious Diseases.* 8th ed. Elsevier; 2018.)

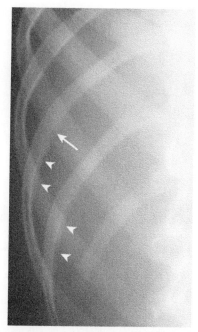

• **Fig. 13.11** Actinomycosis: cavitary nodule. Frontal chest radiograph exposing a dominant cavity right apical nodule with internal opacity (*arrow*), and small surrounding nodules (*arrowheads*). (Courtesy Michael Gotway MD.)

- Pulmonary disease is the most common manifestation of infection due to inhalation from exposures in the environment.
- Symptoms can occur in a subacute or chronic fashion and include dyspnea, nonproductive cough, hemoptysis, as well as fever.
- Radiologic manifestations include ill-defined nodules (occasionally cavitary lesions), reticulonodular or diffuse pulmonary infiltrates, and pleural effusions.
- Respiratory secretions should be obtained to diagnose the infection, and smears will typically demonstrate gram-positive, beaded, fine right-angle branching filaments that are usually weakly acid-fast (Fig. 13.10).
- Growth of *Nocardia* can occur in the range of 48 hours to 14 days.
- Antibiotic therapy is usually effective but can also require surgical drainage or debridement in certain situations.
- **Sulfonamides** have been the mainstay of therapy, and trimethoprim–sulfamethoxazole is the first-line drug used.
- In most instances, two agents are often needed empirically.
- In general, there is no fixed duration of therapy, but patients with pulmonary nocardiosis without CNS involvement are usually treated for a minimum of 6 months.

Pulmonary Actinomycosis

- Can cause subacute to chronic pulmonary infections.
- Follows aspiration of oropharyngeal contents.
- **Periodontal disease** and poor dentition are risk factors.
- Patients look chronically ill but not toxic.
- Fever may be absent and many patients with this infection experience weight loss, fatigue for weeks to months prior to diagnosis.

- Patients eventually develop a productive cough and pleuritic chest pain, while hemoptysis is unusual.
- **Direct extension** of a cavity or mass through an interlobar fissure is the classic imaging finding (Fig. 13.11).
- In advanced disease, actinomycosis can invade anatomic barriers leading to empyema, mediastinitis, pericarditis, and vertebral osteomyelitis.
- Prolonged antimicrobial therapy is the mainstay of therapy, and **penicillin** is the first-line agent.

Melioidosis

- In endemic areas such as **Southeast Asia** and northern **Australia**, melioidosis is a common cause of CAP.
- The etiologic agent is *Burkholderia pseudomallei*, and it is found in soil, vegetation, and water throughout tropical regions.
- It is an aerobic gram-negative bacillus that grows readily on routine culture media.
- Typhoons and heavy rainfall are risk factors for acute pneumonia.
- Diabetes, kidney disease, and alcoholism are additional risk factors for the disease.
- High fever, dyspnea, purulent sputum production, and hemoptysis are manifestations of the disease.
- Associated bacteremia is common.
- Chest imaging normally demonstrates diffuse miliary nodules, which may expand and cavitate (Fig. 13.12).
- The chronic pneumonia syndrome is milder and manifests after a period of latency.
- *B. pseudomallei* is not susceptible to traditional CAP agents but tends to be susceptible to carbapenems, ceftazidime, and trimethoprim–sulfamethoxazole.

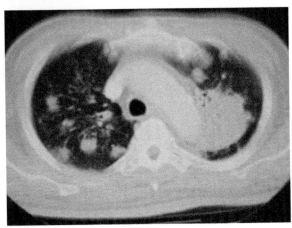

• **Fig. 13.12** A 60-year-old man with underlying diabetes mellitus presented with pyrexia and dyspnea. Plain radiography showed left upper lobe consolidation. Axial CT image showed bilateral multiple lung nodules and segmental consolidation in the left upper lobe. The patient recovered with appropriate treatment, and resolution of the pulmonary findings was seen on repeat imaging. Sputum culture isolated *B. pseudomallei.* (From Lim KS, Chong VH. Radiological manifestations of melioidosis. *Clin Radiol.* 2010;65(1):66–72.)

• Treatment is initially by the intravenous route before transition to oral trimethoprim–sulfamethoxazole for at least 3 months.

Rhodococcus

• *Rhodococcus equi* is a pleomorphic gram-positive coccobacillus that is known for a distinct **salmon-pink color** when grown in culture (Fig. 13.13).
• Associated with exposure to **horses.**
• Occasionally described as a localizing infection in normal hosts but is most commonly seen as an opportunistic pathogen in immunocompromised hosts.
• The majority of cases seen are due to a pulmonary infection.
• Lung manifestations are nodules, cavitation, pleural effusion, and abscesses.
• In immunocompromised hosts, *R. equi* should be considered in the differential diagnosis for **cavitary** lung lesions along with nocardiosis and mycobacterial disease.
• Typically, immunocompromised hosts should be treated with two-drug intravenous therapy with eventual transition to oral therapy once the patient is clinically stable.
• Treatment usually lasts for 6 months or longer.

Mycobacterial Pneumonia

Pulmonary Tuberculosis (see Chapter 32)

• *Mycobacterium tuberculosis* is one of the top 10 causes of death worldwide.
• Infection is typically due to inhalation of droplet nuclei that can travel long distances and reach the terminal air passages.

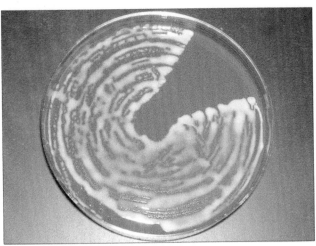

• **Fig. 13.13** Coalescent, mucoid, pink-tinged *Rhodococcus equi* colonies on chocolate agar plate. (Reproduced with permission from Elsevier. The Lancet. From Yamshchikov AV, et al. *Rhodococcus equi* infection. *Lancet Infect Dis.* 2010;10(5):350–359.)

Children

• Pulmonary tuberculosis (TB) usually begins in the midlung zones but can develop anywhere.
• Once tuberculin conversion occurs, fever and occasionally erythema nodosum or keratoconjunctivitis can occur.
• Symptomatic in children less than the age of 5 years, this is often due to extensive lymphadenitis as well as a tendency for progressive **lymphohematogenous dissemination.**
• Can often see miliary and meningeal TB in the very young.

Adults

• **Primary infection** in adults can occur without signs and symptoms, can produce a more typical primary complex, or can result in eventual chronic pulmonary TB.
• **Postprimary pulmonary TB** tends to be asymmetrical and characterized by caseation, fibrosis, and often cavity formation.
• Fever, chills, weight loss, night sweats, anorexia are the classic symptoms described.

Pathogenesis

• Inflammatory response can produce an alveolar exudate, and if this process accelerates, caseous necrosis takes place eventually, leading to formation of granulation tissue and fibrosis.
• Healing can take place, but the caseation can liquefy and drain into the bronchial tree.

Diagnosis

• Radiographic patterns can provide strong evidence of TB, but a positive sputum smear will provide additional evidence.
• An early morning sputum sample is best for accurate diagnosis.

- In total, three specimens in a 24-hour period are recommended.
- Nucleic acid amplification tests (NAATs) allow for direct detection of *M. tuberculosis* in clinical specimens and possess a sensitivity and specificity that approaches culture.
- NAATs can provide a rapid distinction between *M. tuberculosis* and nontuberculous mycobacterial species in the setting of a positive sputum smear sample.
- Negative tuberculin skin tests and interferon gamma release assays can be negative during active disease and should not be used for diagnosis of pulmonary TB.
- Granuloma formation on histology can provide presumptive evidence for a diagnosis but is not specific for *M. tuberculosis* infection.

Radiography
- Subapical-posterior upper lobe cavitary disease (most common).
- Lower lobe disease.
- Less common but seen in adults infected with HIV and in the elderly.

Treatment for Active Pulmonary TB
- In **drug-susceptible TB**, treatment regimen consists of an intensive phase of four-drug therapy for 2 months (isoniazid, rifampin, ethambutol, and pyrazinamide) and then transition to isoniazid and rifampin for an additional 4 months of continuation therapy.
- Pyridoxine (vitamin B6) should be given with isoniazid to all patients who are at risk of neuropathy.
- Chest radiograph should be done at initiation of treatment to assess for cavitation.
- Sputum specimens should be collected at the 1st and 2nd months of treatment to assess for response to treatment.
  #### Reasons for Extending Length of Therapy
- Positive sputum cultures at 2 months into treatment.
- Cavitary lesions on initial chest film.
- In **drug-resistant TB**, treatment requires additional medications for a longer duration of therapy.

Nontuberculous Mycobacteria (see Chapter 33)

- Chronic pulmonary disease is the most common clinical manifestation of nontuberculous mycobacteria (NTM) infections.
- *Mycobacterium avium–intracellulare* complex (MAC), *Mycobacterium kansasii*, *Mycobacterium fortuitum*, and *Mycobacterium abscessus* are the most frequent NTM pathogens causing pulmonary disease.
- Chronic cough is common and constitutional symptoms are prevalent with advancing NTM disease.
- Infections with NTM have been associated with chronic obstructive lung disease and bronchiectasis.
- *M. kansasii* has a similar presentation as TB.
- *M. abscessus* pulmonary infections have been associated with increased mortality in cystic fibrosis patients.

- *M. fortuitum* is similar to *M. abscessus* infections but has been specifically associated with infection in patients with a history of gastroesophageal reflux disease and vomiting.

Diagnosis
- Diagnosis can be difficult due to the fact that NTM species can colonize the respiratory tract.
- For diagnostic purposes, more than one positive culture specimen is generally necessary.
- In addition to microbiology, patient should also meet clinical criteria (e.g., pulmonary symptoms, nodular or cavitary infiltrates on chest radiograph, and/or multifocal bronchiectasis on chest imaging).

Radiographic Presentations
- Fibrocavitary disease.
- Nodular/bronchiectatic disease.
- Hypersensitivity-like disease.

Treatment
MAC
- A macrolide, ethambutol, and a rifamycin recommended for first-line therapy.
- Three-times weekly (intermittent) therapy is allowed for patients presenting with MAC disease that fit into nodular/bronchiectatic category.
- Daily therapy recommended for cavitary disease.
- Injectable aminoglycosides are a consideration in cavitary disease and should be used in more severe disease and in macrolide-resistant infections.
- The goal of therapy is sputum conversion to negative along with symptomatic, clinical, and radiographic improvement.
- Treatment for at least 12 months is normally required.
  #### *M. kansasii*
- A daily regimen of rifampin, ethambutol, isoniazid has been recommended for *M. kansasii* infections. Eighteen months is usually required.
  #### *M. abscessus*
- More **resistance** encountered to antituberculosis drugs than other NTM species.
- Antibiotic susceptibility testing of all clinically significant isolates is recommended.
- Some isolates can acquire **mutational resistance** to clarithromycin and amikacin because the isolates have only one copy of the gene.
- Periodic administration of multidrug therapy, including a macrolide and one or more parenteral agents or a combination of parenteral agents over several months, may help control disease and limit progression of *M. abscessus* lung infections.
- Injectable aminoglycosides, linezolid, cefoxitin, and clofazimine are potential parenteral agents for use in therapy.
- Surgical resection may be considered if disease is more limited.

M. fortuitum

- Isolates are usually susceptible to multiple oral agents, including macrolides, quinolones, doxycycline, minocycline, and sulfonamides.
- Amikacin, cefoxitin, and imipenem are parenteral agents that can be used for therapy.
- Isolates contain an inducible erythromycin methylase gene that confers resistance to macrolides, and macrolides should be used with caution.
- For pulmonary infections, at least two agents with *in vitro* activity against the clinical isolate should be given for a minimum of 12 months.

Pleural Infections

- Pleural infections are normally seen with pneumonia.
- Pleural infections are also postoperative complications.

Diagnosis

- Determining etiology requires analysis of the pleural fluid.
- Thoracentesis can be performed to determine characteristics of the fluid.
- It is the standard to obtain cell count and differential, pH, protein, lactate dehydrogenase (LDH), and glucose.
- If *Mycobacterium tuberculosis* is suspected as a cause of the pleural effusion, can send a pleural fluid sample for adenosine deaminase testing or DNA amplification testing.
- Can determine whether the pleural effusion is transudative or exudative by using Light's criteria.
- If one of the following is present, fluid is defined as an exudate:
  - Pleural fluid protein/serum protein ratio greater than 0.5.
  - Pleural fluid LDH/serum LDH ratio greater than 0.6.
  - Pleural fluid LDH greater than two-thirds the upper limits of the laboratory's normal serum LDH.
- Pleural infections are divided into 3 stages:
  - **Exudative stage**
    - Thin, free-flowing fluid with low numbers of neutrophils present.
    - pH >7.2.
    - Lactate dehydrogenase (LDH) <1000 IU/L.
    - Normal glucose higher than 60 mg/dL.
    - Negative cultures.
  - **Fibropurulent stage**
    - Increasing numbers of neutrophils and fibrin deposition.
    - pH and glucose begin to fall.
    - LDH level increases.
  - **Organizing stage**
    - Fibroblast formation and scarring take place producing a pleural peel that entraps and encases the lung.

Microbiology

- Has changed from being predominantly *Streptococcus pneumoniae* in the preantibiotic era to the **Streptococcus anginosus** group (**milleri**) being more common today.
- **MRSA** and **gram-negative bacilli** can be the causes of hospital-acquired pleural effusions.

Chronic Empyemas

- May erode the chest wall and present with a spontaneous draining abscess called **empyema necessitans** (seen with TB and actinomycosis, Fig. 13.14).
- Pleural effusions can sometimes present resulting from subdiaphragmatic rupture due to amebic etiology, such as *Entamoeba histolytica* (anchovy paste or chocolate appearance to the pleural fluid has been described).

Noninfectious Etiologies of Pleural Effusions

- Rheumatoid arthritis.
- Heart failure.
- Malignancy.
- Postpericardiotomy syndrome.
- Pancreatitis.

Treatment

- Treatment should be directed at CAP and nosocomial pathogens.
- Treatment of infected pleural effusions generally involves a combination of antibiotics and drainage management.
- Prolonged therapy is usually necessary and depends on resolution of effusion.

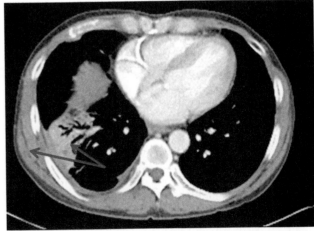

• **Fig. 13.14** Axial computed tomography image demonstrating a 3 × 2.5 cm chest wall mass with limited surrounding inflammatory changes at the level of the 11th rib and minimal right lower lobe parenchymal changes. (From Atay S, Banki F, Floyd C. *Empyema necessitans* caused by actinomycosis: a case report. *Int J Surg Case Rep.* 2016;23:182–185.)

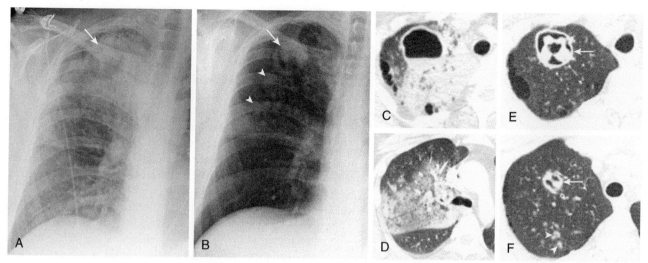

• **Fig. 13.15** Actinomycosis: cavitary nodule. (A) Frontal chest radiograph shows right upper lobe consolidation and a poorly defined nodular opacity (*arrow*). (B) Frontal chest radiograph 2 weeks following (A) shows resolution of the right upper lobe consolidation, now exposing a dominant cavitary right apical nodule with internal opacity (*arrow*) and small surrounding nodules (*arrowheads*). (C and D) Axial chest CT displayed in lung windows performed within 1 day of the presenting chest radiograph (A) shows the right apical opacity as a cavitary nodule with an internal air–fluid level; surrounding ground-glass opacity and consolidation are present, as seen on the chest radiograph (A). (E and F) Chest CT displayed in lung windows performed the same day as B shows the dominant right apical opacity with complex internal architecture (*arrows*) and confirms small surrounding nodules. Biopsy of this lesion recovered *Actinomyces israelii*. (Courtesy Michael Gotway, MD.)

Lung Abscess

- Lung abscess (Fig. 13.15) results when infection causes necrosis of the lung parenchyma leading to eventual cavity formation with a resultant fluid collection.
- Lung abscesses led to far worse outcomes in the pre-antibiotic era, including death, but outcomes became better with the availability of penicillins.
- Today, most patients respond to prolonged antibiotic therapy.
- Lung abscesses are thought to arise from aspiration of oral anaerobic flora and occur in patients with **risk factors for aspiration** (e.g., alcoholism, seizures, stroke, drug overdose).
- Foreign bodies and compression from an enlarging lymph node are less common causes of a lung abscess.
- Patients who present with lung abscesses normally have poor dentition with gingivitis.
- Patients present with constellation of symptoms, including fever, chills, cough with purulent sputum production, and malaise (Box 13.6).
- Weight loss can also occur and be profound.
- Diagnosis is usually made by radiography with films demonstrating a lung cavity with an **air–fluid level.**
- The cavity wall tends to be thick and irregular with a surrounding pulmonary infiltrate.
- Lung abscesses are typically unilateral and occur most frequently in the **posterior segment of the right upper lobe**, followed by the posterior segment of the left upper lobe, and then followed by the superior segments of the lower lobes.

• BOX 13.6 Characteristics of Lung Abscess for Classification

- The causative organism(s) (e.g., anaerobic bacteria, *S. aureus*)
- Presence of a foul odor to expectorated sputum (putrid abscess)
- Duration of symptoms prior to abscess (acute, subacute, chronic)
- Presence or absence of associated conditions (e.g., lung cancer, immunosuppression)

- Foul-smelling sputum in patients with this presentation is assumed to be a polymicrobial anaerobic infection.
- Routine cultures normally demonstrate normal respiratory flora.
- **Differential diagnosis of lung abscess/cavitary lesions** (Table 13.5).

Therapy
- Empiric therapy often consists of broad-spectrum coverage due to polymicrobial infection being assumed.
- Over the years, clindamycin has shown superiority over penicillins for the treatment of anaerobic lung abscess due to production of penicillinases by the common offending organisms.
- Patients are often treated for 6–8 weeks, although there is no agreed-upon recommendation for duration of therapy.
- Clinical improvement demonstrated on chest films can be used to guide duration of therapy.
- Surgical intervention is reserved for patients who do not respond to standard medical therapy.

TABLE 13.5 Differential Diagnosis for Cavitary Lung Lesions

Infectious	Noninfectious
Bacteria	Neoplasms
Oral anaerobes	Pulmonary infarction
Staphylococcus aureus	Vasculitis
Klebsiella pneumoniae	Airway disease
Pseudomonas aeruginosa	Sarcoidosis
Group A streptococcus	
Streptococcus anginosus group	
Nocardia	
Rhodococcus equi	
Actinomyces	
Mycobacteria	
Mycobacterium tuberculosis	
NTM species	
Fungi	
Histoplasma	
Blastomyces	
Coccidioides	
Aspergillus	
Cryptococcus	
Mucorales	
Parasites	
Paragonimus westermani	
Entamoeba histolytica	
Echinococcus	
Septic pulmonary embolism (e.g., endocarditis, Lemierre's syndrome)	

Aspiration Pneumonia

- Aspiration is defined as inhalation of foreign material into the airways that extends beyond the vocal cords.
- Aspiration can be silent with recurrent episodes of micro-aspiration, or it can be a single symptomatic episode of macroaspiration.
- Aspiration pneumonia is an infectious process secondary to an aspiration event.
- **Neurologic disease, altered level of consciousness, and altered swallowing mechanics** are significant risk factors for aspiration.
- Elderly patients, nursing home residents, and patients with esophageal or gastrointestinal disorders are also at a higher level of risk for aspiration.
- The presentation can involve a mild cough or can be an acute process with a more fulminant pneumonitis leading to respiratory failure.
- Aspiration is a disease of exclusion, in which other causes of respiratory failure must be considered, such as pulmonary edema, pulmonary embolism, and community/hospital-acquired pneumonia.
- Radiographic imaging for aspiration pneumonia normally shows findings in dependent portions of the lung.

Treatment
- Normally supportive care.
- Prophylactic use of antibiotics in patients with suspected or witnessed aspiration is not recommended.
- Empirical antibiotic therapy should be considered, however, if the patient fails to respond within 48 hours.

14
Bacteremia and Central Line-Associated Bloodstream Infections

COURTNEY CHRISLER

Definitions

Bacteremia: presence of bacteria in the blood.
- **Primary**: associated with intravascular devices, including central venous catheters (CVCs).
- **Secondary**: related to infections at other sites, including GI/GU tracts, lung, skin/soft tissue, etc.

Community-acquired bacteremia: detected as an outpatient or <48 hours into hospital stay.

Nosocomially-acquired bacteremia: detected >48 hours into hospital stay.

Transient bacteremia: may occur with toothbrushing, dental work, etc., but is typically asymptomatic and self-limited.

Pseudobacteremia: positive blood cultures because of contamination by skin or environmental flora.
- Not representative of true infection.
- Common bacteria detected in contaminated cultures may include:
  - Coagulase-negative staphylococci,
  - *Cutibacterium* (formerly known as *Propionibacterium*) *acnes*.
  - *Corynebacterium* spp. (except *Corynebacterium striatum*, *Corynebacterium jeikeium*).
  - *Bacillus* spp. (except anthrax).

Bloodstream infection (BSI): true infection with a pathogen (bacteria, fungi) detected in the blood.

Central line-associated bloodstream infection (CLABSI): BSI in a patient who had a CVC present within 48 hours of demonstration of BSI and, based on clinical assessment, deemed not to be caused by alternative focus of infection.
- Used for National Healthcare Safety Network (NHSN) surveillance.

Catheter-related bloodstream infection (CRBSI): more stringent category of CLABSI with quantitative culture data and/or differential time-to-positivity (DTP) analysis that supports implication of the catheter as the primary site of infection. (See section below.)

- Definition utilized in the Infectious Diseases Society of America (IDSA) guidelines regarding catheter-associated infections.
- Less pragmatic standard as not all microbiology labs perform quantitative cultures or DTP analysis.

Sepsis: severe infection associated with dysregulated host-response with organ dysfunction (see Chapter 10).

Epidemiology

Depends on source of infection, host risk factors, healthcare exposures.
- **Risk factors for bacteremia**
  - **Age**: very young/old.
  - **Comorbidities**: diabetes, chronic obstructive pulmonary disease (COPD), malignancy, cirrhosis, chronic kidney disease (CKD), alcohol abuse, vaccination status.
  - **Immunocompromised states**: use of steroids or other immunosuppressive medications, neutropenia, hematopoietic stem cell (HSCT) or solid-organ (SOT) transplant, splenectomy, HIV.
  - **Disruption of protective barriers**: intravenous catheter, intravenous drug use (IVDU), burns, wounds, recent surgery or procedure, trauma.
- **Common causes of bacteremia**
  - Top three causes of bacteremia = *Escherichia coli*, *Staphylococcus aureus*, *Enterococcus* spp.
  - Some common and important causes of BSIs are highlighted below; see other chapters for more detailed pathogen-related information.

Gram-Positive BSI

- Risk factors: intravenous catheters, IVDU, skin/soft-tissue infections, prosthetic devices, some GI/GU infections.
- Nosocomial bacteremia is more likely to be caused by gram-positive organisms (*S. aureus*, coagulase-negative staphylococci) because of the prevalence of CVCs.

TABLE 14.1   Common Pathogens Associated With Bloodstream Infections

Gram-positives	Gram-negatives
Staphylococcus aureus	Escherichia coli
Enterococcus spp.	Pseudomonas aeruginosa
Streptococcus pneumoniae	Klebsiella spp.
Coagulase-negative staphylococci	Enterobacter spp.
Streptococcus pyogenes (group A)	Proteus spp.
Streptococcus agalactiae (group B)	Salmonella spp.
Viridans-group streptococci	Stenotrophomonas maltophilia
Listeria monocytogenes	Acinetobacter spp.
Peptostreptococcus spp.	Neisseria spp.
Clostridium perfringens	Haemophilus influenzae

- *Staphylococcus aureus* is the second most common cause of bacteremia overall and is increasingly prevalent with the rise in IVDU.
  - *S. aureus* should never be treated as a blood culture contaminant.
  - Can have high mortality (MRSA>MSSA).
- **Metastatic sites of infection** are common, especially in the setting of high-grade bacteremia, so a careful history and physical examination and other investigations should be undertaken to determine the extent of infection.
- Common complications:
  - Endocarditis.
  - Spinal infections, including osteomyelitis/discitis/epidural abscess.
  - Infection of intravascular devices, grafts, other prosthetic materials.
  - Necrotizing pneumonia and/or septic emboli to the lung.
  - Septic arthritis and osteomyelitis.
  - Brain abscess/meningitis.
  - Skin, intramuscular, and visceral abscesses.
  - Septic thrombophlebitis, assorted other embolic phenomena (liver, spleen, extremities).
- Infection relapse and treatment failure are not uncommon; careful attention to assessment management is required.
- **Enterococcal BSI** typically arises from GI/GU sources, i.e., gut translocation or perforation, diverticular disease, biliary tract disease, complicated UTI, etc.
  - *Enterococcus* spp. cause a significant proportion of cases of infective **endocarditis**, so consideration for echocardiography is warranted.

- **Streptococcus pneumoniae BSI** more common in very young and elderly patients, unvaccinated patients, those with underlying comorbid conditions, including alcoholism, COPD, cardiovascular disease, chronic liver disease, CSF leak, CKD, diabetes, immunosuppression (SOT, HSCT, HIV, immunosuppressive medications).
- Patients with pneumococcal bacteremia should be screened for HIV.
- Most commonly related to sinopulmonary disease and/or meningitis but can be caused by a variety of other syndromes.
- Austrian's syndrome: triad of pneumococcal endocarditis, meningitis, and pneumonia.
- **Coagulase-negative staphylococcal** bacteremia is typically associated with the presence of intravenous catheters and prosthetic devices, but positive blood cultures should be interpreted carefully; coagulase-negative staphylococci are a common cause of pseudobacteremia.

Gram-Negative BSI

- Risk factors: **immunocompromise** (HSCT, SOT, use of glucocorticoids, etc.), various **comorbidities** (malignancy, DM, COPD, ESRD, chronic liver disease) conditions, **nosocomial** exposures.
- Increasing incidence of antimicrobial resistance, in some settings, can make antibiotic management challenging; for some multidrug resistant organisms, combination therapy may be required.
- *E. coli* is the most common cause of bacteremia.
  - Most often secondary to complicated **UTI** but is also commonly caused by GI pathology.
  - Enterobacteriaceae, including *E. coli*, are also important causes of bacteremic pneumonia.
- *Klebsiella* **spp.** are usually associated with a GI/GU source, including liver abscess, other hepatobiliary pathology, and UTI.
- *Pseudomonas* **spp.** are particularly important causes of bacteremia in patients with **neutropenia** or **burns.**
  - Sources may include the lung, GI/GU tracts, skin/soft tissues, and indwelling lines or drains.

Clinical Presentation and Initial Assessment

- **Fever** is the most common presenting symptom for patients with BSI but may be absent, especially in the elderly and immunocompromised, and in those with infections caused by low-virulence pathogens.
- **Localizing signs and symptoms** can be important clues to the underlying cause of the BSI and help guide empiric therapy.
- A comprehensive history and physical examination should be performed and should include inspection of indwelling catheters and implanted devices.

- Signs and symptoms of **septic shock** should provoke urgent evaluation and prompt initiation of supportive care and antibiotic therapy (see Chapter 10).
- **qSOFA-2** score is a quick sepsis-screening tool. One point is awarded for each of the following:
  - Hypotension (SBP <100mmHg), tachypnea (RR ≥22), altered mental status (GCS <15).
  - Scores ≥2 predict higher mortality and prolonged ICU stay.
- If bacteremia is suspected, at least **two sets of blood cultures** should be drawn, at the same time, from separate sites.
  - Blood cultures should be drawn prior to antibiotics, if at all possible.
  - Careful attention to aseptic technique should be taken to avoid contamination of the sample, blood culture bottle, and intravenous line (if applicable).
  - If CLABSI is a consideration, one blood culture set should be drawn from the catheter and the other should be drawn from the periphery.
  - Both bottles should be filled with the same volume (at least 10 mL, but preferably 20 mL).
- Once cultures are positive, rapid, nonculture-based, molecular techniques (FISH, MALDI-TOF, microarrays) may be able to assist in species level identification before cultures have had enough time for adequate growth for the organism to be identified by traditional methods.
- **Empiric antibiotic therapy** should be administered based on Gram stain results and speciation (if available), clinical suspicion of most-likely pathogens, the patient's risk factors and past history of infections (particularly if there is a history of infections with multidrug resistant organisms), and local antimicrobial susceptibility information.
- Additional **imaging and diagnostics** may be indicated depending on suspected sites of infection and/or organism identified.
- **Echocardiography** is often indicated for evaluation of a patient with bacteremia to evaluate for evidence of infective endocarditis.
  - Recommended for all patients with *S. aureus* bacteremia.
  - Should be performed for all patients with signs/symptoms of endocarditis and/or those with persistent bacteremia with organisms known to have propensity to cause endocarditis (*Enterococci*, viridans group streptococci, etc.).

Treatment

- Antibiotic therapy should be **targeted** as species and susceptibility information become available.
- **Duration of therapy** depends on pathogen and underlying syndrome/extent of infection. (See individual syndrome chapters for recommendations regarding treatment duration; CLABSI is discussed broadly below.)

- Most patients will need IV therapy, but in selected cases (i.e., short-lived bacteremia with pansusceptible *E. coli* from pyelonephritis), oral therapy may be an option.
- **Source control** is crucial (abscess drainage, intravenous device removal, valve replacement, wound debridement, etc.) to clearing infection quickly and definitively.

S. aureus BSI

- Requires specific attention given the potential gravity of its often-associated complications.
- It is necessary to determine if the patient has uncomplicated vs. complicated bacteremia, both to decide on duration of antibiotic therapy and to assess for any additional needed procedural interventions.
- Cornerstones of management for *S. aureus* BSI are similar to management for any BSI:
  - Appropriate antibiotic selection and dosing.
  - Assessment for/management of metastatic sites of infection, including any needed source control measures.
  - Echocardiography to exclude infective endocarditis.
  - Repeat blood cultures to document clearance.
  - Appropriate antibiotic duration and follow-up.
- **Duration of therapy is typically 4 weeks**, at minimum, but selected patients may be candidates for shorter or longer courses of therapy.
  - Uncomplicated bacteremia can be managed with 2 weeks of IV antibiotics, but the criteria are stringent and require patients to have all of the below:
    - A defined and removable focus of infection that is removed.
    - No metastatic sites of infection.
    - No evidence of infective endocarditis via transesophageal echocardiogram.
    - No indwelling prosthetic devices.
    - Defervescence in 2–3 days.
    - Clearance of blood cultures within 2–4 days of removal of focus of infection and initiation of appropriate antibiotics.
  - Complicated bacteremia, especially those patients with endocarditis or vertebral osteomyelitis, etc., require longer courses of therapy, i.e., 6–8 weeks.
  - Chronic suppressive antibiotics may need to be considered for patients who have retained infected prosthetic materials.
- Not all antistaphylococcal agents are appropriate for management of *S. aureus* bacteremia; parenteral agents are preferred.
- Recommended agents: MSSA (nafcillin, oxacillin, cefazolin); MRSA (vancomycin, daptomycin).

Central Line-Associated Bloodstream Infections (CLABSI)

- Central line-associated bloodstream infections (CLABSIs) are the most common cause of nosocomially-acquired BSI.

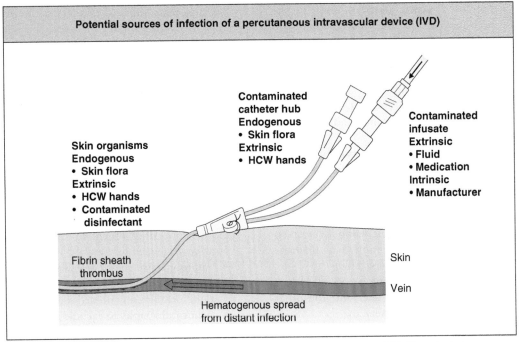

• **Fig. 14.1** Potential sources of infection of a percutaneous intravascular device (IVD). These include contiguous skin flora, contamination of the catheter hub and lumen, contamination of infusate and hematogenous colonization of the IVD from distant, unrelated sites of infection. *HCW,* healthcare worker. From Crnich CJ, Maki DG. *Clin Infect Dis.* 2002;34(9):1232–1242.8. © The University of Chicago Press.

• Catheter-related factors that increase for BSI:
  • Type of catheter: peripheral IV < peripherally inserted central catheter (PICC) < tunneled CVC < nontunneled CVC.
  • Site of CVC: subclavian < internal jugular < femoral CVC.
  • Longer duration of presence of catheter.
  • Urgent insertion of catheter.
  • Submaximal barrier precautions/antiseptic technique at time of insertion of catheter.
  • Skin condition at catheter insertion site.

Pathogenesis (see Fig. 14.1)
• **Skin colonization** is the most common cause of CLABSI. Skin flora migrate down the catheter tract through the insertion site, colonizing the intracutaneous and intravascular portion of the catheter.
• **Intraluminal and/or hub contamination** is a more likely cause of CLABSI in catheters that have been in place >2 weeks.
• **Hematogenous seeding** occurs when BSI from a secondary site seeds the catheter, resulting in biofilm formation.
• **Infusate contamination** is rare but can occur after administration of contaminated infusate or additives.

Microbiology
• Important gram-positives: coagulase-negative staphylococci, *S. aureus,* enterococci.
• Important gram-negatives: *Pseudomonas* spp., *Klebsiella* spp., *Enterobacter* spp.

• *Candida* spp. are also important causes of CLABSIs (see Chapter 27), particularly in patients on total parenteral nutrition and nosocomial settings.

Clinical Presentation and Diagnosis
Clinical manifestations are generally the same as for any BSI, but patients may have other local signs of inflammation or infection. Patients do not need to have external signs of infection at the catheter site to have a CLABSI.
• **Phlebitis**: inflammation of vein resulting in local clot formation; often presents with induration or erythema along tract of a catheterized or recently catheterized vein.
• Supportive care, including NSAIDs and ice packs, may be useful.
• Anticoagulation and catheter removal are warranted for deep venous thromboses.
• **Exit-site infection**: infection of the skin around the catheter site without purulent drainage at the entry site or systemic signs of illness.
• **Tunnel infection**: infection along the subcutaneous tract of the catheter, resulting in tenderness, erythema, induration, and/or purulence at the catheter insertion site.
• **Pocket infection**: infected fluid collection in the pocket of an implanted device; presents with fluctuance, tenderness, erythema, and sometimes spontaneous purulent drainage.
• Patients may also report worsening fevers, chills, other symptoms that start abruptly after catheter infusion as bacteria are flushed into their bloodstreams from the catheter apparatus.

Diagnosis

- At least **two sets of blood cultures** should be drawn, at the same time, from separate sites.
- Not all microbiology labs perform quantitative cultures or routinely report DTP, but suggested criteria from the IDSA for CRBSI include:
  - **Confirmed CRBSI**
    - Peripheral culture and catheter tip culture both positive for the same organism.
    - Peripheral culture and catheter lumen culture both positive for same organism with either:
      - Quantitative cultures showing ≥3-fold higher CFU from the catheter.
      - Delay to positivity (DTP) showing that the catheter culture is positive 2 hours before the peripheral culture.
  - **Possible CRBSI**
    - Quantitative cultures from two different lumens of the same catheter positive for the same organism with ≥3-fold differential in CFU between lumens.
    - One positive blood culture from a catheter without positive peripheral cultures, especially if the catheter culture was positive for a common colonizer or contaminant like coagulase-negative *Staphylococcus* spp., may not signify true infection, but based on the clinical scenario, repeat blood cultures and initiation of antibiotics may be warranted while awaiting further data.
      - Catheter colonization is a risk factor for developing true infection.

Treatment

- Treatment involves systemic **antimicrobials** and at least consideration of need for **catheter removal.**
- A patient's IV access limitations, severity of illness, and identified pathogen type typically dictate the feasibility and necessity of catheter removal.
- **Antibiotic therapy** should be directed at the isolated pathogen and susceptibility results once available, but empiric therapy is often needed.
  - CLABSIs most commonly involve gram-positive organisms, including *S. aureus* and coagulase-negative staphylococci, so empiric therapy should include an agent with activity for both (i.e., vancomycin, daptomycin, etc.)
  - Need for empiric coverage for gram-negative organisms depends on individual patient history and disease severity (i.e., nosocomial exposures, neutropenia, clinical instability, etc.).
  - Empiric antifungal may be warranted for patients at high risk for candidemia.
  - Total parenteral nutrition, HSCT transplant, prolonged use of broad-spectrum antibiotics, colonization with *Candida* at multiple sites, femoral catheterization.
  - Antibiotic selection should ultimately be tailored based on culture and susceptibility results.

- Repeat blood cultures are needed to document clearance of bacteremia.
- Definitive antibiotic course duration begins on the date of the first negative blood culture.
- Antibiotic duration depends on pathogen, catheter retention or removal, and extent of infection.
  - *S. aureus*: discussed above; if isolated CLABSI without any complicating factors, negative TEE, rapid improvement on antibiotics, and the catheter was removed, can consider 2 weeks of therapy.
  - Coagulase-negative staphylococci: catheter removed: 5–7 days, catheter retained: 10–14 days.
  - Uncomplicated other CLABSI: generally 2 weeks of appropriate therapy; see IDSA guidelines for selected pathogen-related recommendations.
  - *Candida* spp. requires at least 2 weeks of therapy but also exclusion of other metastatic sites of infection, with evaluation for endovascular and intraocular disease (see Chapter 27).
- Antibiotic or alcohol lock therapy: may be useful as an adjunct with systemic antibiotics if attempting line salvage.

Catheter Removal

- **Catheter removal** is generally preferred, but catheter salvage may be attempted in some specific circumstances, depending on pathogen, severity of illness, and especially if IV access options are limited.
- Catheter removal is generally indicated for those patients with:
  - Severe sepsis or hemodynamic instability.
  - Endocarditis or evidence of other metastatic infection (septic emboli, osteomyelitis, etc.).
  - Persistent bacteremia >72 hours after initiation of appropriate antimicrobial therapy.
  - Tunnel or pocket infection.
  - Suppurative thrombophlebitis.
  - Infection with *S. aureus*, *P. aeruginosa*, fungi, mycobacteria, and some low virulence Gram-positive organisms (*Micrococcus* spp., *Cutibacterium* (*Propionibacterium*) *acnes*, *Bacillus* spp.).
  - Short-term catheters (<14 days) should also be removed for enterococcal and non-*Pseudomonas* gram-negative infections.
  - If a catheter is retained and bacteremia relapses, catheter removal should be reconsidered, and assessment for other foci of infection should be undertaken.

Prevention

- Incidence of CLABSIs can be reduced by:
- Avoiding line contamination by using appropriate hand hygiene, aseptic technique at times of catheter manipulation, barrier precautions at time of catheter insertion, and by performing appropriate catheter care.
- Limiting duration of catheter presence and removing the catheter as soon as possible.

- Use of antimicrobial-impregnated catheters in some select circumstances (i.e., in an ICU with CLABSI rates that are above average).

Further Reading

1. Liu C, Bayer A, Cosgrove E, et al. Clinical Practice Guidelines by the Infectious Diseases Society of America for the treatment of methicillin-resistant *Staphylococcus aureus* infections in adults and children. *Clin Infect Dis.* 52(3):e55. https://doi.org/10.1093/cid/ciq146.

2. Kern W. Infections associated with intravascular lines and grafts. In: Cohen J, Powderly W, Opal S, eds. *Infectious Diseases.* 4th ed. Philadelphia: Elsevier; 2017.

3. Mermel LA, Allon M, Bouza E, et al. Clinical practice guidelines for the diagnosis and management of intravascular catheter-related infection: 2009 Update by the Infectious Diseases Society of America. *Clin Infect Dis.* 2009;49(1):1–45.

15

Cardiac and Cardiac Device Infections

MERILDA BLANCO-GUZMAN

INFECTIONS INVOLVING CARDIAC STRUCTURES

Endocarditis

Definitions

Endocarditis: inflammation of the endocardial surface of the heart.
- **Left- vs. right-sided endocarditis:** right-sided endocarditis is typically associated with intravenous drug use or catheter related bloodstream infections. Right-sided infective endocarditis (IE) vegetations tend to have lower bacterial density. Most common complications in right-sided IE are septic thrombophlebitis and septic pulmonary embolism.
- **Cardiac implanted electronic device (CIED)-related endocarditis:** can have isolated vegetations of the device wires, cardiac valves, or both. Most commonly occur within a year of implantation or device exchanges.
- **Native vs. prosthetic valve endocarditis:** although the pathogenic mechanisms are similar, epidemiology of infection and management differ according to presence or absence of prosthetic valves.
- **Acute vs. subacute endocarditis:** acute endocarditis occurs in a period of 3–10 days with rapid evolution of symptoms. Subacute endocarditis presents insidiously with constitutional symptoms such as fatigue, exertional limitation, night sweats, weight loss, and low-grade fevers. Virulence of the causative organism is responsible for these syndromes.

Epidemiology and Etiology

- IE incidence is high with an associated in-hospital mortality of 10%–25%.
- The epidemiology of the disease has changed over time to reflect the increased use of implanted cardiac devices,

IV catheters for infusions and hemodialysis, prosthetic valves, and intravenous drug use. In developed countries, the organisms causing IE have changed from oral streptococci to predominantly staphylococci. In developing countries with high prevalence of rheumatic heart disease, streptococci continue to predominate as cause of IE.
- Infections are the most common cause of endocarditis. Gram-positive bacteria are the predominant group responsible for IE. Among gram-negatives, the HACEK group (*Haemophilus*, *Aggregatibacter*, *Cardiobacterium*, *Eikenella*, and *Kingella*) accounts for 5%–10% of community acquired IE cases. Most common agents of IE are listed in Box 15.1.
- In 15% of the cases the etiology of IE can not be determined by blood cultures. This is more commonly due to antimicrobial administration prior to obtaining cultures or due to the presence of fastidious or intracellular organisms. Box 15.2 lists agents of culture-negative endocarditis. Noninfectious causes of endocarditis are listed in Box 15.3.

Clinical Presentation

- Fever in a patient with risk factors is the most common presentation of IE. See Box 15.4 for a list of cardiac and noncardiac risk factors for IE.
- A new cardiac murmur is noted in 85% of the patients.
- Presentation is variable and can include chills, anorexia, weight loss, malaise, arthralgias, and night sweats.
- Patients may present with fever and complications from IE such as heart failure, stroke, intracerebral hemorrhage, septic emboli to the pulmonary or systemic circulation, or metastatic infection.
- Cutaneous/ocular manifestations are supportive of the diagnosis but are only present in a minority of patients. These include:
  - Splinter hemorrhages: nonblanching linear red-brown lesions under the nail bed.

• BOX 15.1 **Common Causes of Infective Endocarditis**

Bacteria

- Oral streptococci (viridans group streptococci)
- *Streptococcus bovis*
- Staphylococci (*S. aureus* and coagulase-negative staphylococci)
- Enterococci
- *Enterobacteriaceae*

Fungi

- *Candida* spp.

• BOX 15.2 **Causes of Culture-Negative Endocarditis**

- *Coxiella burnetii*
- *Bartonella* spp.
- *Brucella* spp.
- *Legionella* spp.
- *Mycoplasma* spp.
- *Tropheryma whipplei*
- *Abiotrophia* spp.
- *Cutibacterium acnes*

• BOX 15.3 **Noninfectious Causes of Endocarditis**

- Acute rheumatic fever
- Libman–Sacks endocarditis
- Rheumatoid arthritis
- Marantic endocarditis
- Löeffler's endocarditis

• BOX 15.4 **Risk Factors for Infective Endocarditis**

Cardiac

- Prior IE
- Presence of prosthetic valve or implanted device
- Congenital heart disease
- Valvular abnormalities

Noncardiac

- Intravenous drug use
- Indwelling IV lines
- Immunosuppression
- Recent dental or surgical procedure associated with bacteremia

- Janeway lesions: nontender macules on the palms and soles.
- Osler nodes: tender subcutaneous violaceous nodules on the finger and toe pads.
- Roth spots: retinal hemorrhagic lesions with pale centers.
- See Figs. 15.1–15.3 for clinical manifestations of IE.

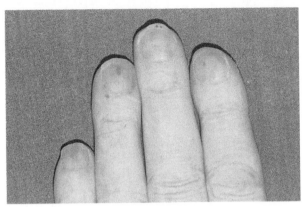

• **Fig. 15.1** Splinter hemorrhage in the ring finger and older, fading splinter in the index finger of a patient with IE. (From Epstein O, Perkin GD, Cookson J, Watt I, Rakhit R, Robins A, Hornet G. The heart and cardiovascular system. *Clinical Examination*. 4th ed. Elsevier; 2008.)

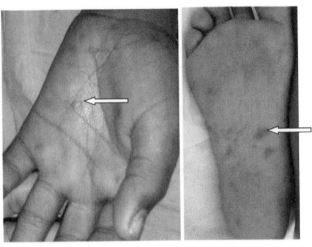

• **Fig. 15.2** Janeway lesions. Small macular lesions on palms and soles (*arrows*). (From Dash N, Verna S. Janeway lesion: a forgotten entity. *J Pediatr*. 2016;172: 218–218e1.)

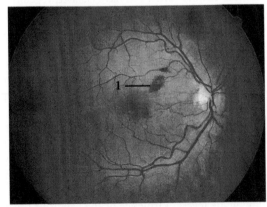

• **Fig. 15.3** Roth spots. A classic Roth spot, or white-centered hemorrhage is present within the superotemporal arcade (marked as 1). (From Olsen TW. Retina. In: Palay D, Krachmer J, eds. *Primary Care Ophthalmology*. 2nd ed. Elsevier; 2005.)

- Vascular phenomena: arterial emboli, septic pulmonary infarcts, mycotic aneurysm, conjunctival hemorrhage, or Janeway lesions.
- Immunologic phenomena: glomerulonephritis, Osler nodes, Roth spots, and rheumatoid factor.

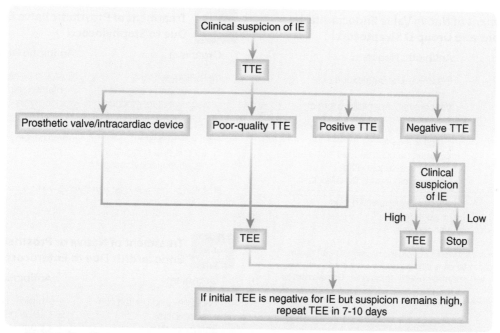

- **Fig. 15.4** Algorithm for the role of echocardiography in the diagnosis of infective endocarditis. (From Habib G, Hoen B, Tornos P, et al. for the ESC committee for practice guidelines. Guidelines on the prevention, diagnosis and treatment of infective endocarditis: the task force on the prevention, diagnosis and treatment of infective endocarditis of the European Society of Cardiology. *Eur Heart J*. 2009;30:2369–413.)

Diagnosis

- Nonspecific laboratory findings include elevated ESR and CRP, positive rheumatoid factor, anemia, and leukocytosis.
- The cornerstone for the diagnosis of IE are blood cultures. At least three sets of blood cultures from different sites should be obtained, with the first and last samples drawn at least 1 hour apart.
- Serologies and molecular testing for Q fever and *Bartonella* should be considered depending on the patient's exposures.
- Echocardiogram should be done in all patients suspected of IE. See Fig. 15.4 for an algorithm on the use of echocardiography in the diagnosis of endocarditis.
- Other imaging modalities include cardiac computed tomography (CT), positron emission tomography (PET), or magnetic resonance imaging (MRI), but these are not yet well established for the diagnosis of IE.
- Accepted criteria for the diagnosis of IE are the modified Duke criteria. The criteria and definitions of IE are summarized in Boxes 15.5 and 15.6.

Treatment

- After obtaining adequate blood cultures, patients with high suspicion for IE should be started on empiric antimicrobial therapy. This should be directed to the most common organisms based on the suspected source. IV bactericidal agents should be used.
- Once the organism has been identified on culture, therapy should be targeted. Treatment regimens and duration for some organisms will differ in patients with native valve

• BOX 15.5 Modified Duke Criteria for the Diagnosis of IE

Major Criteria

- Typical organism for IE in two separate blood cultures
- Positive blood culture or phase I IgG for *Coxiella burnetii* titer ≥1:800
- Endocardial involvement
- Echocardiogram suggestive of IE

Minor criteria

- Predisposing heart condition or IVDU
- Fever (temperature >38 °C)
- Vascular phenomena
- Immunologic phenomena
- Blood culture that does fulfill major criteria

• BOX 15.6 Definition of IE According to the Modified Duke Criteria

Definite IE

- Pathologic criteria
  - Microorganisms demonstrated on culture or pathologic exam of vegetation or intracardiac abscess
- Clinical criteria
  - Two major criteria
  - One major criterion and three minor criteria
  - Five minor criteria

Possible IE

- One major and One minor criterion
- Three minor criteria

TABLE 15.1 Treatment of Native Valve Endocarditis by Viridans and Group D Streptococci

Organism	Antibiotic Regimen
Penicillin MIC[a] <0.12 µg/mL	Penicillin G or ceftriaxone *plus* gentamicin Vancomycin if penicillin allergic
Penicillin MIC[a] 0.12–0.5 µg/mL	Penicillin G *plus* gentamicin for the first 2 weeks Ceftriaxone can be used alone if the isolate is susceptible Vancomycin if penicillin allergic
Penicillin MIC >0.5 µg/mL[b]	Ampicillin or penicillin *plus* gentamicin Vancomycin

[a]Duration of treatment is 4 weeks. For organisms with MIC <0.12 µg/mL, a 2-week regimen can be done if no cardiac or extra cardiac abscess, no renal disease, and no infection with *Abiotrophia, Granulicatella* or *Gemella* spp.
[b]Duration of treatment is 4–6 weeks.

TABLE 15.2 Treatment of Prosthetic Valve Endocarditis by Viridans and Group D Streptococci

Organism	Antibiotic Regimen
Penicillin[a] MIC <0.12 µg/mL	Penicillin G or ceftriaxone ±gentamicin for first 2 weeks Vancomycin if penicillin allergic
Penicillin[a] MIC ≥0.12 µg/mL	Penicillin G or ceftriaxone *plus* gentamicin Vancomycin if penicillin allergic

[a]Duration of treatment is 6 weeks. For organisms with MIC <0.12 µg/mL, the addition of gentamicin does not improve cure rates and should be used with caution.

TABLE 15.3 Treatment of Native Valve Endocarditis Due to Staphylococci

Organism	Antibiotic regimen
Methicillin-sensitive *S. aureus* and coagulase-negative staphylococci[a]	Oxacillin or nafcillin Cefazolin Vancomycin if penicillin allergic
Methicillin-resistant *S. aureus* and coagulase-negative staphylococci[a]	Vancomycin

[a]Duration of treatment is 6 weeks. For treatment of brain abscesses due to methicillin-susceptible organisms, nafcillin should be used over cefazolin.

TABLE 15.4 Treatment of Prosthetic Valve Endocarditis Due to Staphylococci

Organism	Antibiotic Regimen
Methicillin-sensitive *S. aureus* and coagulase-negative staphylococci[a]	Oxacillin or nafcillin *plus* rifampin *plus* gentamicin Vancomycin if penicillin allergic
Methicillin-resistant *S. aureus* and coagulase-negative staphylococci[a]	Vancomycin *plus* rifampin *plus* gentamicin

[a]Duration of treatment is ≥6 weeks with 2 weeks of gentamicin.

TABLE 15.5 Treatment of Native or Prosthetic Valve Endocarditis Due to Enterococci

Organism	Antibiotic Regimen
Penicillin- and gentamicin-susceptible Enterococci[a]	Ampicillin or penicillin G *plus* gentamicin Or ampicillin *plus* ceftriaxone
Penicillin-susceptible and gentamicin-resistant[a]	Ampicillin *plus* ceftriaxone
Vancomycin- and aminoglycoside-susceptible, penicillin-resistant[a]	Vancomycin *plus* gentamicin
Vancomycin-, ampicillin-, and aminoglycoside-resistant[b]	Linezolid or daptomycin

[a]Duration of treatment is 6 weeks. For penicillin- and gentamicin-susceptible enterococcus in patients with NVE and symptoms <3 months duration can be shortened to 4 weeks.
[b]Duration of treatment is ≥6 weeks.

TABLE 15.6 Treatment of Native or Prosthetic Valve Endocarditis Due to HACEK Organisms

Organism	Antibiotic Regimen
HACEK organisms	Ceftriaxone OR ampicillin OR ciprofloxacin[a]

[a]Ceftriaxone is preferred therapy. Duration of treatment is 4 weeks.

endocarditis is >80%. The guideline recommended initial treatment is amphotericin B, although clinical experience with echinocandins is growing. After completion of initial parenteral therapy, life-long suppression with an oral azole is reasonable.

- Fungal endocarditis is a standalone indication for valvular surgery. Other indications for valvular surgery in IE are presented in Box 15.7.

Prevention

- Cardiac conditions and procedures with indication for IE antimicrobial prophylaxis are listed in Boxes 15.8 and 15.9.

(NVE) vs. prosthetic valve (PVE) endocarditis. See Tables 15.1 to 15.7 for targeted antimicrobial therapy for viridans and group D streptococci, staphylococci, enterococci, HACEK, and culture-negative IE in NVE and PVE.

- Despite aggressive combination therapy with surgical and medical management, the mortality for fungal

TABLE 15.7	Guide to the Treatment of Culture-Negative Endocarditis
Presentation	**Antibiotic Regimen**
NVE with acute clinical symptoms	Vancomycin *plus* cefepime
NVE with subacute clinical symptoms	Vancomycin *plus* ampicillin–sulbactam
PVE within a year of valve surgery	Vancomycin *plus* rifampin *plus* gentamicin *plus* cefepime
PVE after a year of valve surgery	Vancomycin *plus* ceftriaxone

Duration of therapy is ≥6 weeks.

• BOX 15.7 Recommendations for Early Valve Surgery

Left-sided IE

- Acute heart failure
- Fungal endocarditis
- IE due to highly resistant organisms
- Heart block, annular or aortic abscess, penetrating lesions
- Bacteremia >5 days despite adequate antibiotics and no other sites of infection
- Severe valvular regurgitation and mobile vegetations >10 mm
- PVE with recurrent emboli despite appropriate antibiotic treatment
- Relapsing PVE

Right-sided IE (repair preferred over replacement if feasible)

- Severe tricuspid valve (TV) regurgitation with right heart failure unresponsive to medical therapy
- Persistent infection with difficult to treat organisms
- TV vegetations >20 mm
- Recurrent PE despite adequate antimicrobial therapy

- Although antimicrobial prophylaxis is not recommended for gastrointestinal (GI) or genitourinary (GU) procedures, in patients with an active GI or GU infection who will undergo GI or GU tract manipulation and have one of the cardiac conditions in Box 15.9, treatment with an adequate antibiotic agent is recommended.

Pericarditis

Definitions

Pericarditis: inflammatory disease of the pericardium.

- The pathologic changes of acute pericarditis are non-specific inflammation with cellular infiltration and fibrin deposition.
- **Recurrent pericarditis** is a syndrome in which acute pericarditis recurs after the agent inciting the initial

• BOX 15.8 Cardiac Conditions Requiring Prophylaxis

- Prosthetic heart valves
- Previous IE
- Congenital heart disease
  - Unrepaired cyanotic defect
  - Repaired defect with prosthetic material or device during the first 6 months postrepair
  - Repaired defect with residual defect adjacent to prosthetic material or device
- Cardiac transplantation with residual valvulopathy

• BOX 15.9 Procedures Requiring IE Prophylaxis

- All dental procedures with manipulation of gingival tissue, perforation of the mucosa, or the periapical region of teeth
- Procedures involving surgery in the respiratory mucosa (tonsillectomy, bronchoscopic biopsy)
- Procedures on infected skin, skin structures, or musculoskeletal tissue

---

attack is resolved or inactive. This syndrome can be seen in up to 15%–30% of patients with acute pericarditis.

- **Constrictive pericarditis** occurs when there is significant scarring and loss of the elasticity of the pericardial sac.
- **Cardiac tamponade** occurs when fluid accumulates in the pericardial sac under pressure resulting in hemodynamic instability.

Epidemiology and Etiology

- Although autopsy series have reported an incidence of pericarditis of 2%–6%, the clinical diagnosis is only reported in 0.1% of hospitalized patients.
- Pericarditis can be due to infectious or noninfectious etiologies. Most commonly pericarditis is due to viral infection or idiopathic.
  - The most common noninfectious causes of pericarditis are **malignancy, uremia, and connective tissue disease.** Other causes include Dressler syndrome (postmyocardial infarction [MI] pericarditis), medications (e.g., penicillin, doxorubicin, hydralazine, minoxidil, etc.), radiation, trauma, and aortic dissection with pericardial leak.
  - Infectious causes of pericarditis include viral, bacterial, fungal, and parasitic agents.
    - Most common infectious causes are viral such as **Coxsackie A and B**, **echovirus 8**, **adenovirus**, and human immunodeficiency virus (**HIV**).
    - In the developing world, **tuberculosis** is an important cause of acute and constrictive pericarditis.
    - *Histoplasma capsulatum* is the most common cause of fungal pericarditis with incidences of up to 6% noted during large outbreaks with disseminated histoplasmosis.

- Pericarditis due to parasites is rare but has been reported with *Toxoplasma gondii*, *Entamoeba histolytica*, *Echinococcus granulosus*, and *Schistosoma* spp.

Clinical Presentation

- **Acute sharp substernal chest pain** that worsens with inspiration and when lying down and is alleviated with sitting and leaning forward is the most common symptom on presentation.
- A **pericardial friction rub** is a characteristic exam finding.
- If associated with pericardial tamponade, pulsus paradoxus may be present.
- In cases of viral pericarditis, patients will present with fever and recent upper respiratory or GI symptoms.
- Bacterial pericarditis is accompanied by severe systemic infections, or local infections involving the head and neck, chest/mediastinum.
- Tuberculous pericarditis is insidious and is usually accompanied by constitutional symptoms. Chest pain may or may not be a significant feature.

Diagnosis

- Echocardiogram (ECG) is the mainstay for the diagnosis. It will show evidence of pericardial effusion and/or findings suggestive of early tamponade.
- ECG will show diffuse ST segment elevation with an upward concave movement and without reciprocal ST segment depression, and PR segment depression in the limb leads (Fig. 15.5). Electrical alternans may be present in patients with large effusions.

- CXR may show enlargement of the cardiac silhouette.
- Patients with isolated pericarditis may have slight elevations in their cardiac biomarkers.
- In patients suspected to have viral pericarditis, viral testing of nasopharyngeal swabs or stool may be performed. Antibody testing with convalescent sera can also demonstrate a viral etiology.
- If pericardiocentesis or pericardiotomy is done, fluid or pericardial tissue can be used for cell studies, culture, and molecular and polymerase chain reaction (PCR) testing for the suspected etiologies.

Treatment

- In the absence of a particular cause, the mainstay of treatment is with antiinflammatory agents. High-dose aspirin, nonsteroidal antiinflammatory drugs (NSAIDs) or colchicine are the preferred drugs. NSAIDs should be avoided if there is a component of myocarditis, as they have worsened outcomes in animal models.
- Corticosteroids are used in pericarditis due to systemic inflammatory conditions.
  - These are also used in patients with idiopathic pericarditis who fail to respond to the preferred antiinflammatory agents or who have contraindications for them.
  - Corticosteroids are no longer routinely recommended in the management of tuberculous pericarditis. Selected patients with tuberculous pericarditis with high inflammatory cells or markers in pericardial fluid or with early signs of constrictive pericarditis may still benefit from steroid therapy.

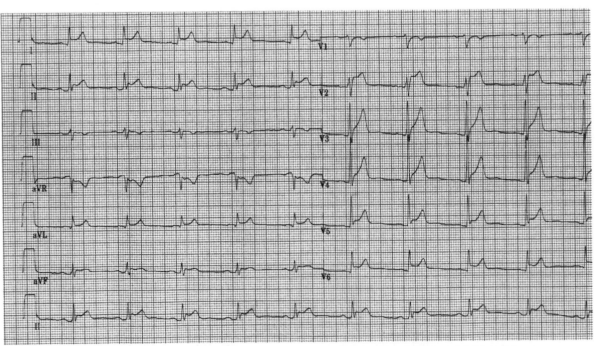

• **Fig. 15.5** ECG showing typical findings of pericarditis with diffuse PR depressions and ST elevation. (From Foerg F, Gardner Z. *Hosp Med Clin*. 2015;4,(2):205–215. Data from ECGPedia. CardioNetworks Foundation. Available at: http://en.ecgpedia.org/wiki/File:ECG000026.jpg; with permission.)

- Emergent pericardiocentesis should be performed in patients with cardiac tamponade.
  - Bacterial, tuberculous, and fungal pericardial effusions also require drainage as they are more likely to result in hemodynamic complications and require control of the source.
  - Pericardiocentesis is also recommended in patients with persistent effusion after more than 1 week of treatment with antiinflammatory therapies.
- Patients with specific bacterial or fungal causes of pericarditis should receive directed antimicrobial therapy for the causal organism.

Myocarditis

Definitions

Myocarditis: inflammatory disease of the myocardium.
- The histopathology of the disease will vary depending on the etiologic agent, host response, and course of illness.
- **Acute myocarditis** has a wide spectrum of presentations, ranging from an asymptomatic illness to severe myocardial dysfunction and death. Pathologic changes can go from reversible inflammatory findings to fulminant myocardial necrosis.
- **Chronic myocarditis** is commonly associated with subacute deterioration of cardiac function with histologic evidence of myocardial lymphocytic infiltration.

Epidemiology and Etiology

- Approximately 10% of new onset unexplained cardiomyopathy can be attributed to myocarditis. Myocarditis can be of infectious or noninfectious etiologies.
  - **Infectious:** occurs through a variety of mechanisms including direct cytopathic injury (e.g., Coxsackie virus), through the effect of bacterial toxins on the myocardium (e.g., *Corynebacterium diphtheriae*), secondary to the immune response to the infectious agent (e.g., Chagas disease, see Chapter 34), or from cellular injury due to vascular inflammation (e.g., parvovirus).
    - In developed countries, viral diseases are the most common infectious cause of myocarditis. Recent studies using molecular techniques have identified **parvovirus B19** and **human herpesvirus-6 (HHV-6)** as the most prevalent agents. Additional high yield infectious causes of myocarditis are listed in Table 15.8.
  - **Noninfectious** systemic conditions associated with myocarditis are listed in Box 15.10.

Clinical Presentation

- Clinical symptoms are nonspecific and may include fever, fatigue, malaise, chest pain, dyspnea, and palpitations.
- Physical exam may reveal tachycardia, muffled heart sounds, transient murmurs, or ventricular gallops. In more severe cases, signs of congestive heart failure (CHF) are present.
- Friction rubs are uncommon but can be present if the pericardium is involved.
- There should be a high index of suspicion for myocarditis in any patient presenting with new onset of CHF or malignant arrhythmias that are otherwise unexplained in the setting of an acute febrile illness.

Diagnosis

- **Endomyocardial biopsy** (EMB) is the gold standard for the diagnosis of myocarditis.
  - EMB is only recommended for cases where the results of biopsy may alter the treatment course.
  - It should be considered in patients with rapidly progressive cardiomyopathy refractory to conventional therapeutic management or an unexplained cardiomyopathy (not due to ischemic, familial, toxin, or valvular-related) that is associated with progressive conduction system disease or life-threatening ventricular arrhythmias. It should also be done when cardiovascular signs or symptoms develop in a patient

TABLE 15.8 Selected Infectious Causes of Myocarditis

Industrialized countries	Viruses: parvovirus B19, human herpesvirus 6, Coxsackie virus A and B, influenza A and B, hepatitis B and C Bacteria: *Corynebacterium diphtheriae*, *Borrelia* spp.
Developing countries	Viruses: mumps, rubella, dengue, chikungunya, polio, Ebola, and yellow fever Bacteria: *Leptospira* spp., *Salmonella* spp. Parasites: *Trypanosoma cruzi*, *Trypanosoma gambiense*, *Trichinella spiralis*
Immunocompromised hosts	Viruses: human immunodeficiency virus, cytomegalovirus, Epstein–Barr virus, varicella-zoster virus, adenovirus, parvovirus Fungi: *Candida* spp., *Cryptococcus* Parasites: *Toxoplasma gondii*, *Trypanosoma cruzi*

BOX 15.10 Noninfectious Causes of Myocarditis

- Connective tissue disorders
- Inflammatory/infiltrative conditions
- Hypersensitivity reactions
- Cardiotoxins
- Endocrinopathies
- Radiation

with a systemic disease known to cause left ventricular dysfunction.

- The Dallas criteria are histologic criteria used for the definition of myocarditis on EMB, but these have been limited by their low diagnostic accuracy. The World Health Organization (WHO) has developed new diagnostic definitions based on the combination of the histologic criteria with immunologic and immunohistochemical data, with improvement in diagnostic accuracy up to 70%. This can be further improved by the use of molecular and PCR techniques on biopsy tissue.
- Echocardiogram is recommended in the initial evaluation of all patients suspected of having myocarditis. It can show cardiac dysfunction of varying degrees with focal wall motion abnormalities. Left ventricular (LV) dilation and right ventricular (RV) dysfunction are rare findings.
- Nuclear myocardial imaging and cardiac MRI are noninvasive diagnostic techniques for myocarditis. MRI findings associated with the diagnosis of myocarditis include focal myocardial enhancement associated with regional wall motion abnormalities. Later in the course there can be global enhancement followed by return to normal within 90 days.
- ECG is nonspecific and can show focal ST segment elevations or T wave inversions. AV node or intraventricular conduction defects are suggestive of widespread cardiac involvement or can point to specific etiologies such as Lyme myocarditis.
- Cardiac biomarkers will be elevated, and in contrast to ischemic cardiac injury in which CPK levels trend down at 72 hours, they may remain elevated for up to a week in myocarditis.

Treatment

- Supportive care for the management of LV dysfunction and conduction abnormalities is the mainstay of treatment. This may include the use of diuretic, angiotensin-converting enzyme (ACE) inhibitors, beta blockers, and antiarrhythmic agents. Patients with fulminant myocarditis may require inotropic and vasopressor support and will occasionally require mechanical circulatory support with ventricular assist devices.
- Avoidance of exercise is suggested given worsened histologic findings in exercising patients with viral myocarditis.
- Routine antiviral therapy for myocarditis is not recommended but can be used when the agent is directed to a particular viral diagnosis.
- If a pathogen is identified, directed antimicrobial therapy should be instituted.
- Numerous trials have evaluated the use of immunomodulators such as interferon-beta (IFN-β), intravenous immunoglobulin (IVIG), and immunosuppressants. Interferon beta has been shown to improve recovery of cardiac function at 6 months.

Rheumatic Fever

Definitions

- **Acute rheumatic fever (ARF)** is an autoimmune non-suppurative condition resulting from an inflammatory response to group A streptococcal (GAS) infection.
  - Although the disease is self-limited, patients who recover from ARF are more prone to additional episodes following streptococcal infections.
- Inflammation of the cardiac valves during ARF can evolve to a chronic and progressive damage of the valvular tissue known as rheumatic heart disease.

Epidemiology and Etiology

- ARF is now rarely seen in industrialized nations but continues to be the most common cause of acquired heart disease in childhood globally, mainly due to high incidences in developing countries. Factors associated to its incidence in low-income countries include overcrowding, poor sanitation, and difficulties with medical access.

Clinical Presentation

- ARF features will present after 1–5 weeks of a prior GAS infection.
- Most common symptoms on presentation are **fever** and **arthritis** (75% of cases). Arthritis in ARF is migratory, asymmetric, polyarticular and affects mainly large joints.
- **Carditis** can be present with involvement of pericardium, myocardium, or endocardium. Acute valvulitis most often affects the mitral valve and is associated with mitral regurgitation and a Carey Coombs murmur (short, mid-diastolic rumble, best heard at the apex). Other common cardiac findings are tachycardia and heart block.
- **Choreiform movements** in ARF involve mostly the upper body, worsen with purposeful action, and disappear during sleep.
- **Erythema marginatum** is a pink serpiginous rash that begins as a macule and clears centrally.
- **Subcutaneous nodules** appear predominantly on bony surfaces and tendons, are painless, and are strongly associated with the presence of severe carditis.

Diagnosis

- **Jones criteria** are used for the diagnosis of ARF. Two major manifestations of ARF or one major and two minor are required for the diagnosis, with additional evidence of a recent prior streptococcal infection. These are listed in Box 15.11.
- In developing countries with high prevalence of ARF Jones criteria have been modified to increase their sensitivity. In these settings, monoarthritis is also included as a major manifestation. Monoarthralgia and lower cutoff values for fever (38°C instead of 38.5°C) and

inflammatory markers (ESR >30 instead of 60 mm/h) are included as additional minor manifestations.

- Evidence of a recent streptococcal infection can be demonstrated by positive throat swabs/cultures, rapid antigen test, or positive antistreptococcal serology (antistreptolysin O, anti-DNAase B, antihyaluronidase). Within 2 months of infection, 80% of patients will have a positive antistreptolysin O.
- Echocardiogram is helpful in evaluation of subclinical carditis and rheumatic heart disease.

Treatment

- Treatment is aimed at eliminating any active infection, treating heart failure, and decreasing inflammation.
- With acute rheumatic fever, antibiotic treatment aimed at eradication of GAS should be provided, whether or not pharyngitis is present at the time of diagnosis.
- Heart failure in ARF will require typical medical management with diuretics, ACE inhibitors, etc.
- **Aspirin and NSAIDS** are the cornerstone of antiinflammatory therapy. They result in symptomatic improvement in 1–3 days.
- Steroids are used if there is failure to respond to salicylates or in the presence of severe carditis.
- All antiinflammatories should be tapered to avoid rebound of symptoms.
- For severe chorea, **carbamazepine or valproate** have been used successfully.
- ARF will resolve spontaneously within 12 weeks. After the initial episode resolves, follow up is required for administration of adequate antimicrobial prophylaxis and monitoring for the development of rheumatic heart disease.
- Secondary prophylaxis of rheumatic fever can be done with **benzathine Penicillin G** every 3–4 weeks, Penicillin V twice daily, sulfadiazine once daily, or with a macrolide in penicillin/sulfa allergic patients. The duration of secondary prophylaxis with these agents is summarized in Box 15.12.

• BOX 15.11 Jones Criteria for the Diagnosis of Rheumatic Fever

Major Manifestations

- Carditis
- Polyarthritis
- Sydenham chorea
- Erythema marginatum
- Subcutaneous nodules

Minor Manifestations

- Arthralgia
- Fever
- Elevated ESR/CRP
- Prolonged PR interval

CARDIAC DEVICE-RELATED INFECTION

Cardiac Implanted Electronic Device (CIED)-Related Infections

Definitions

- **Cardiac implanted electronic device (CIED)** is a term inclusive of **pacemakers** and **cardioverter defibrillators.** Infections related to these devices can involve the device pocket or endocarditis involving the device wires or valvular structures.

Epidemiology and Etiology

- The rates of CIED-related infection have continued to climb over the past several decades despite completely prepectoral implantation techniques and smaller devices. This is likely due to higher implantation rates, implantation in patients with more advanced age, and larger number of comorbidities.
- The pathogenesis of CIED infections is more commonly secondary to introduction of skin flora at the time of device implantation, exchange, or manipulation. Secondary hematogenous infection due to bacteremia from a distant source is another mechanism of infection but not as common as primary local infection. Biofilm formation has a significant role in the pathogenesis of CIED-related infections.
- Gram-positive skin organisms, predominantly **coagulase-negative staphylococci** and *S. aureus*, account for approximately 75% of all CIED infections. The remainder are due to other gram-positives (*Corynebacterium* spp., *Cutibacterium acnes*), gram-negatives (*Pseudomonas* spp.), *Candida* spp., and polymicrobial infections.
- Risk factors associated with CIED infection are diabetes mellitus, heart failure, chronic kidney disease, recent generator exchange, oral anticoagulation, fever within 24 hours of device implantation, and lack of antimicrobial prophylaxis use.

• BOX 15.12 Duration of Secondary Prophylaxis for Rheumatic Fever

- RF with carditis and residual valvular disease
  10 years or until age 40 (consider lifelong)[a]
- RF with carditis but no residual heart disease
  10 years or until age 21[a]
- RF without carditis
  5 years or until age 21[a]

[a]The longer interval of the two should be chosen for treatment duration.

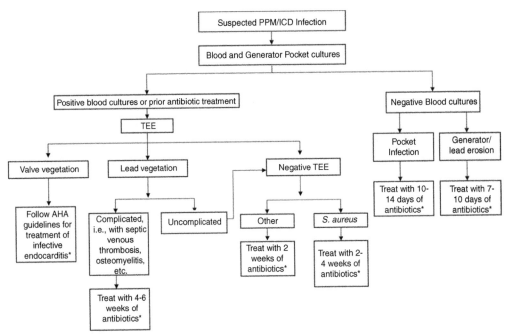

• **Fig. 15.6** Management of permanent pacemaker (PPM) and implantable cardioverter defibrillator (ICD) infections. (From Sohail MR, Uslan DZ, Khan AH, et al. Management and outcome of permanent pacemaker and implantable cardioverter defibrillator infections. *J Am Coll Cardiol*. 2007;49(18):1851–1859.)

Clinical Presentation

• Clinical presentation will vary according to the site of infection of the CIED. Common clinical presentations are local signs of inflammation over the device pocket, device erosion with drainage, fever, and occult bacteremia with no local signs over the device or with findings for endocarditis.

Diagnosis

• All patients with suspected CIED infection should have at least two sets of blood cultures done prior to initiation of antimicrobial therapy.
• Patients with positive blood cultures or with negative blood cultures after receiving antimicrobials should undergo echocardiographic evaluation with transesophageal echocardiography (TEE) to rule out infection of CIED wires or valvular endocarditis. TEE should also be done in all patients suspected of having CIED-related endocarditis.
• When the device is explanted, samples for culture should be obtained from the pocket and leads.
• A combined diagnostic and management algorithm for CIED infections is presented in Fig. 15.6.

Treatment

• Complete removal of all hardware is the recommended treatment for patients with demonstrated CIED infection or device erosion, including cases of pocket infection without systemic symptoms. This is due to high relapse rates with device retention.
• When complete removal of the device is not achievable, as much as possible should be removed and antimicrobial suppression should be considered after an initial course of antimicrobials.
• Empiric antimicrobial therapy is directed at the most common causative organisms. Vancomycin is the typical drug of choice. Once culture data are available, therapy should be targeted to the isolated organism(s).
• See Fig. 15.6 for details on duration of therapy for management of CIED infections.
• See Fig. 15.7 for the algorithm on timing of CIED reimplantation after extraction due to CIED infection.

Mechanical Circulatory Support Device-Related Infections

Definitions

• **Mechanical circulatory support devices (MCS)** include durable **left ventricular assist devices (LVADs)**, right ventricular assist devices (RVADs), biventricular assist devices (BiVADs), and total artificial hearts (TAH).
• LVADs are the most commonly used MCS device and are frequently associated with device-related infections.
• LVADs can be implanted with a goal of bridge to transplantation or as destination therapy in patients who are not candidates for transplantation.
• Fig. 15.8 shows the components of an LVAD and the different pump flow modalities.

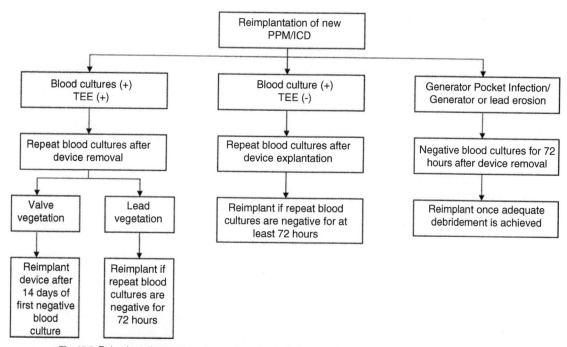

• **Fig. 15.7** Reimplantation strategy for cardioverter defibrillator and pacemaker infections. (From Van Hoff R, Friedman H. Implantable cardioverter defibrillator and pacemaker infections. *Hosp Med Clin.* 2015;4(2):150–162. Original from Sohail MR, Uslan DZ, Khan AH, et al. Management and outcome of permanent pacemaker and implantable cardioverter defibrillator infections. *J Am Coll Cardiol.* 2007;49(18):1851–1859.)

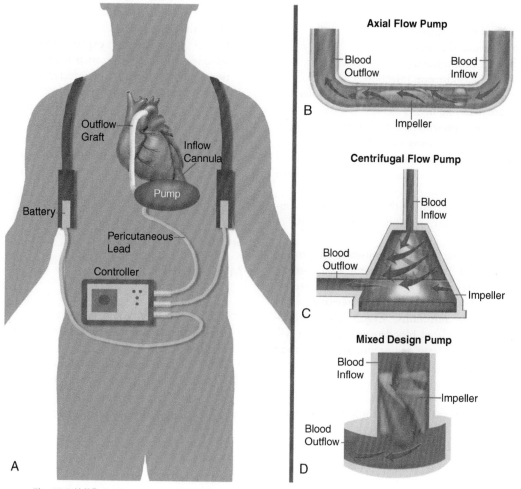

• **Fig. 15.8** LVAD system components (A) and features of continuous flow axial (B), centrifugal (C), and mixed design pumps (D). (From Mancini D, Colombo P. Left ventricular assist devices. *J Am Coll Cardiol.* 2016;65(23):2542–2555.)

Epidemiology and Etiology

- Infection is the fourth most common cause of death within a year after LVAD implant.
- The pathogenesis of LVAD infections can be secondary to introduction of skin flora at the time of device implantation, ascending infection through the driveline exit site, or secondary hematogenous infection due to bacteremia from another source. Biofilm formation has a significant role in the pathogenesis of LVAD infections.
- Most commonly encountered organisms are gram-positives, with **coagulase-negative staphylococci**, *S. aureus,* and *Enterococcus* spp. being responsible for over 50% of all initial infections. The predominant gram-negative organisms are the Enterobacteriaceae and *Pseudomonas aeruginosa.* Candida is the most common fungal pathogen and candidemia in these patients has been associated with mortality rates of over 25%.
- Previously reported risk factors associated to LVAD infections include diabetes, large BMI, elevated creatinine, depression, and driveline trauma.

Clinical Presentation

- Clinical presentation will depend on the infected LVAD site. LVAD-related infections can include:
  - Driveline exit site with or without involvement of the tunnel.
  - Pocket.
  - LVAD-related mediastinitis.
  - Pump or cannula infections.
  - LVAD-related endocarditis.
  - LVAD-related bloodstream infection.
- Frequently patients will go on to develop infection involving more than one site.
- The most common presentation is driveline infection. Patients will have local signs of inflammation at the driveline exit site or tunnel, purulent drainage or fluid collections, plus/minus bacteremia, and systemic signs of infection.
- Pocket infections can present with local signs of inflammation over the pocket, erosion, draining sinus, or bloodstream infection.
- Mediastinitis related to the LVAD is usually seen in the postoperative period. Patients will present with systemic symptoms such as fever, chest pain, drainage from sternal wounds, unexplained leukocytosis, or bacteremia.
- Pump and cannula infections, LVAD-related endocarditis, and LVAD-related bloodstream infection will invariably present with fever or systemic symptoms and bacteremia.

Diagnosis

- At least two sets of blood cultures should be performed on patients suspected of LVAD-related infection.
- Patients with drainage at the driveline exit site should have sterile aspirate obtained for gram stain and routine cultures.

- In patients with bacteremia of unclear source or suspicion for pocket infection, additional imaging with ultrasound, CT of the chest and abdomen, or nuclear imaging should be done to evaluate for fluid collections or inflammatory changes of the LVAD components or pocket. In bacteremic patients, echocardiogram should also be obtained to rule out LVAD-related endocarditis.
- If the LVAD is removed due to infection, cultures should be obtained from the inflow and outflow cannula, internal pump (through saline instillation), pocket, and other concerning LVAD surfaces.

Treatment

- Different to other device-related infections, source control through device removal/exchange is not always feasible for LVADs due to the patient's comorbidities, as well as the complexity and high risk of the surgical procedure.
- Due to the presence of biofilms in infections associated with the device, infections managed with device retention will require long-term antimicrobial suppression after an initial course of antimicrobial therapy. Antimicrobial suppression is extended usually until heart transplant for patients being bridged or lifelong for patients on destination therapy.
- The exception to the need for chronic antimicrobial suppression are superficial driveline infections that respond well to initial antimicrobial therapy and immobilization of the driveline.
- Even if the device is not explanted, surgical interventions aimed at source control, such as drainage of fluid collections and debridement of infected or necrotic tissue, is recommended whenever possible.
- Duration of initial antimicrobial therapy will vary depending on the site of infection and response to treatment. Initial empiric antimicrobials are directed at the most common organisms but final choice of antimicrobials should be targeted to the organisms on culture.

INFECTION INVOLVING THE MEDIASTINUM

Mediastinitis

Definitions

- **Mediastinitis**: infection involving the structures of the mediastinum.
- Box 15.13 shows the criteria from the Centers for Disease Control (CDC) for the definition of mediastinitis.

Epidemiology and Etiology

- Mediastinitis is rarely a primary infection. More commonly it is the result of extension of infection from another space.

BOX 15.13 CDC Definition of Mediastinitis

- One of these criteria
  - Organisms cultured from mediastinal tissue or fluid
  - Gross anatomical or histopathologic evidence of mediastinitis
  - Fever, chest pain, or sternal instability
- Plus one of the following
  - Purulence from mediastinal area
  - Mediastinal widening on imaging

- In the past, the most common causes of mediastinitis were esophageal rupture or extension of infections from the oropharynx or neck. Now, most cases of mediastinitis are related to infection of the site after cardiothoracic surgery. Less commonly mediastinitis can be associated to extension of pneumonia, pancreatitis, subphrenic or epidural abscesses.
- The causative organisms in mediastinitis will be dependent on the associated entity and whether it is postoperative or not. Postoperative mediastinitis is more commonly associated with **coagulase-negative staphylococci** and **S. aureus**. Mediastinitis associated with oropharyngeal and neck infections are usually polymicrobial and include oral anaerobes, gram-positives, and gram-negatives.

Clinical Presentation

- Postoperative mediastinitis will usually present within 30 days postsurgery.
- Local signs include purulence from the sternal wound, wound dehiscence, and sternal instability. Fever and leukocytosis are also frequent clinical presentations.

Diagnosis

- When mediastinitis is suspected based on the clinical presentation, radiographic imaging with CT may show evidence of sternal wire displacement, sternal disruption, free gas, or fluid collections in the mediastinum, which are highly suggestive of the diagnosis.
- Wound exploration and samples for cultures are needed to definitely establish the diagnosis and direct therapy.

Treatment

- Surgical intervention with removal of infected sternal plates and wires, debridement of tissue necrosis, and irrigation of surrounding soft tissue is recommended when feasible. Techniques utilized for closure after debridement include primary closure with rewiring and drainage placement, negative pressure wound therapy (Wound Vac), and primary or delayed flap closures.
- Targeted antimicrobial therapy should be instituted upon culture result. The duration of antimicrobials will be variable and depend on extent of infection, ability of source control with surgery, and clinical/radiographic response.

Further Reading

1. Baddour LM, Wilson WR, Bayer AS, Fowler Jr VG, Tleyjeh IM, Rybak MJ, et al. Infective endocarditis in adults: diagnosis, antimicrobial therapy, and management of complications: a scientific statement for healthcare professionals from the American Heart Association. *Circulation*. 2015;132(15):1435–1486.
2. Wilson W, Taubert KA, Gewitz M, Lockhart PB, Baddour LM, Levison M, et al. Prevention of infective endocarditis: guidelines from the American Heart Association: a guideline from the American Heart Association Rheumatic Fever, Endocarditis, and Kawasaki Disease Committee, Council on Cardiovascular Disease in the Young, and the Council on Clinical Cardiology, Council on Cardiovascular Surgery and Anesthesia, and the Quality of Care and Outcomes Research Interdisciplinary Working Group. *Circulation*. 2007;116(15):1736–1754.
3. Gerber MA, Baltimore RS, Eaton CB, Gewitz M, Rowley AH, Shulman ST, et al. Prevention of rheumatic fever and diagnosis and treatment of acute streptococcal pharyngitis: a scientific statement from the American Heart Association Rheumatic Fever, Endocarditis, and Kawasaki Disease Committee of the Council on Cardiovascular Disease in the Young, the Interdisciplinary Council on Functional Genomics and Translational Biology, and the Interdisciplinary Council on Quality of Care and Outcomes Research: endorsed by the American Academy of Pediatrics. *Circulation*. 2009;119(11):1541–1551.
4. Baddour LM, Epstein AE, Erickson CC, Knight BP, Levison ME, Lockhart PB, et al. Update on cardiovascular implantable electronic device infections and their management: a scientific statement from the American Heart Association. *Circulation*. 2010;121(3):458–477.
5. Kusne S, Mooney M, Danziger-Isakov L, Kaan A, Lund LH, Lyster H, et al. An ISHLT consensus document for prevention and management strategies for mechanical circulatory support infection. *J Heart Lung Transplant*. 2017;36(10):1137–1153.

16
Gastrointestinal Infections

NABEELA MUGHAL

Definitions

Gastroenteritis: a rapid-onset diarrheal illness, lasting less than 2 weeks, with diarrhea three or more times a day or at least 200 g of stool which is either viral or bacterial in etiology.

Diarrhea: loose or watery stools passed at least three times in 24 hours which can be acute, chronic, or persistent.

- Acute: lasting less than 14 days often due to either viral or bacterial pathogens.
- Persistent: lasting between 14 and 29 days.
- Chronic: lasting greater than 30 days, may be due to parasites, and noninfectious etiology should be excluded
- Small bowel diarrhea: often watery, associated with crampy abdominal pain and of large volume with bloating and gas. Accompanying fever and blood or inflammatory cells in the stool are rare.
- Large bowel diarrhea: small volume painful stools which occur often with blood, mucus, and inflammatory cells found in the stools and an accompanying fever.

Risk Factors for Gastroenteritis

Foodborne

- A thorough food exposure history should be undertaken to elicit the possible causative organisms, with timing of symptoms in relation to food consumption noted (see Table 16.1).
- Consumption of raw or undercooked meat products or unpasteurized milk or dairy products.
- Consumption of raw fish/shellfish or undercooked eggs.

Exposure-Related

- It is important to ascertain if other members of the family or household have symptoms as this may be indicative of an outbreak situation where more than two cases are suggestive of a common food source or exposure.

- Travel history is also important to ascertain certain pathogens, including travel to resource-poor settings, a cruise, or exposure to recreational water facilities such as pools, lakes, brackish or salty water.
- Occupational exposure, such as food handlers, chefs, or laboratory workers.
- Healthcare exposure, including recent courses of antibiotics.
- Animal contacts, including pets, farms, and zoos, including young poultry.
- Contact with reptiles even though they may be pets and other household pets with diarrhea.
- Institutionalized individuals such as patients in long-term care facilities/prisons.
- Childcare facilities.

Host-Related

- Young children and elderly.
- Immunosuppressed patients.
- Men who have sex with men.
- Ano-genital, oral-anal, or digital-anal contact.
- Hemochromatosis or hemoglobinopathy.

Clinical Presentation (see also Table 16.2)

- Fever in the absence of diarrhea is often suggestive of enteric fever especially when accompanied by epidemiologic risk factors such as travel history or exposure to known contacts of enteric fever.
- Evaluation for dehydration and electrolyte imbalance following diarrhea losses is paramount as this increases the risk of death and life-threatening illness, especially in the young and elderly.
- Assessment should also include review of extraintestinal and postinfectious manifestations of diarrhea illness (see Table 16.3).

Red Flag Symptoms of Gastroenteritis Requiring Urgent Investigation

- Persistent stool for >1 week.
- Fever.
- Bloody diarrhea.

TABLE 16.1 **Differential Diagnosis for Gastroenteritis In Adults**

Incubation Period	Pathogen	Duration of Illness	Food Risk Factors	Type of Diarrhea
1–6 hours	Staphylococcal aureus Bacillus cereus	24–48 hours	Preformed toxin in unrefrigerated foods	Watery diarrhea; prominent vomiting
24–48 hours	Norovirus, rotavirus	48–72 hours	Molluscs and shellfish, leafy vegetables, fruit such as melon and raspberries, sandwiches, seasonal vomiting virus	Watery diarrhea; prominent vomiting; may have fever
8–16 hours	Clostridium perfringens	24–48 hours	Meat, poultry, canned foods	Watery diarrhea
10–16 hours	Enteric viruses (rotavirus, enteric adenovirus, astrovirus, sapovirus)	2–9 days	Fecally contaminated food or water	Watery diarrhea
24 hours	Listeria monocytogenes	Variable	Processed/delicatessen meats, hot dogs, soft cheese, pâtés, and fruit	Watery diarrhea
1–3 days	Enterotoxigenic Escherichia coli	2–3 days	Fecally contaminated food or water	Watery diarrhea
1–3 days	Nontyphoidal Salmonella	1–7 days	Poultry, eggs, and egg products, fresh produce, meat, fish, unpasteurized milk or juice	Inflammatory diarrhea with fever, mucus, or bloody stools
1–3 days	Campylobacter spp.	5–14 days	Poultry, meat, unpasteurized milk	Inflammatory diarrhea with fever, mucus, or bloody stools
1–3 days	Shigella spp.	2–3 days	Raw vegetables, MSM activity	Inflammatory diarrhea with fever, mucus, or bloody stools
1–3 days	Vibrio parahaemolyticus	3 days	Raw seafood and shellfish	Inflammatory diarrhea with fever, mucus, or bloody stools
1–8 days	Enterohemorrhagic E. coli	1 week	Ground beef and other meat, fresh produce, unpasteurized milk and juice	Inflammatory diarrhea with fever, mucus, or bloody stools
4–6 days	Yersinia spp.	1–3 weeks	Pork or pork products, untreated water	Inflammatory diarrhea with fever, mucus, or bloody stools
7–14 days	Giardia lamblia	Days to weeks	Fecally contaminated food or water	Watery diarrhea
1–11 days	Cyclospora cayetanensis	May remit and relapse over a few weeks	Herbs and berries	Watery diarrhea
2–28 days	Cryptosporidium parvum	May remit and relapse over a few weeks	Vegetables, fruit, unpasteurized milk	Watery diarrhea
N/A	Clostridioides difficile	Varies but can be up to 10–14 days or longer	Antibiotic associated colitis, proton pump inhibitors	Watery or inflammatory diarrhea with fever, mucus, or bloody stools

- Severe abdominal pain.
- Signs and symptoms of dehydration such as tachycardia/hypotension/confusion/decreased urine output.
- Weight loss.
- Recent hospital stay or recent antibiotic exposure.
- Pregnant.
- Over 65 years.
- Diabetic or living with HIV or immunocompromised.

TABLE 16.2   Clinical Features and Differential Diagnosis

Clinical Feature	Pathogens
Persistent or chronic diarrhea	*Cryptosporidium* spp., *Giardia lamblia*, *Cyclospora cayetanensis*, *Cystoisospora belli*, and *Entamoeba histolytica*
Bloody stool	STEC, *Shigella*, *Salmonella*, *Campylobacter*, *Entamoeba histolytica*, noncholera *Vibrio* species, *Yersinia*, *Balantidium coli*, *Plesiomonas*
Fever	Viral, bacterial, and parasitic infections Higher temperatures are suggestive of bacterial etiology, such as *Salmonella* or *E. histolytica*
Abdominal pain	STEC, *Salmonella*, *Shigella*, *Campylobacter*, *Yersinia*, noncholera *Vibrio* species, *Clostridioides difficile*
Persistent abdominal pain and fever	*Yersinia enterocolitica* and *Yersinia pseudotuberculosis*, may mimic appendicitis
Nausea and vomiting lasting ≤24 hours	Ingestion of *Staphylococcus aureus* enterotoxin or *Bacillus cereus* (short-incubation emetic syndrome)
Vomiting and non-bloody diarrhea lasting 2–3 days or less	Norovirus (low-grade fever usually present during the first 24 hours in 40% if infectious)
Diarrhea and abdominal cramping lasting 1–2 days	Ingestion of *Clostridium perfringens* or *B. cereus* (long-incubation emetic syndrome)

Adapted from IDSA Practice Guidelines for the Diagnosis and Management of Infectious Diarrhea, 2017.

TABLE 16.3   Extraintestinal and Postinfectious Manifestations of Gastroenteritis

Manifestation	Pathogen
Aortitis, osteomyelitis, deep tissue infection	*Salmonella*, *Yersinia*
Intestinal perforation	*Salmonella*, including *Salmonella Typhi*, *Shigella*, *Campylobacter*, *Yersinia*, *Entamoeba histolytica*
Postinfectious irritable bowel	*Campylobacter*, *Salmonella*, *Shigella*, STEC, *Giardia*
Hemolytic anemia	*Campylobacter*, *Yersinia*
Immunoglobulin A nephropathy	*Campylobacter*
Glomerulonephritis	*Shigella*, *Campylobacter*, *Yersinia*
Hemolytic uremic syndrome	STEC, *Shigella dysenteriae* serotype 1
Erythema nodosum	*Yersinia*, *Campylobacter*, *Salmonella*, *Shigella*
Reactive arthritis	*Salmonella*, *Shigella*, *Campylobacter*, *Yersinia*, rarely *Giardia*, and *Cyclospora cayetanensis*
Meningitis	*Listeria*, *Salmonella* (infants ≤3 months of age are at high risk)
Guillain–Barré syndrome	*Campylobacter*

Indications for Antibiotic Use

- Most infections are mild and self-limiting and very rarely require antibiotics.
- Oral hydration support should be offered.
- For more severe cases, extraintestinal infections (see Table 16.3), and in immunocompromised patients, the elderly, or young children, antimicrobial therapy is warranted).
- Antibiotics can be started after appropriate stool or blood culture specimens have been sent.
- Immunosuppressed patients who are systemically unwell with fever or bloody diarrhea or abdominal pain.
- Children <3 months of age.
- Returning travelers with a temperature >38.5° and/or with signs of sepsis.
- Antibiotics are not indicated in cases of suspected Shiga toxin or *E. coli* 0157.

- Empiric antibiotic therapy includes either a fluoroquinolone or azithromycin based on local epidemiology and resistance patterns in adults and a third generation cephalosporin in those <3months of age.
- Once an isolate has been cultured, antibiotics should be reviewed, modified, or stopped based on available susceptibilities.
- Close attention should be paid to oral or intravenous hydration in more severe cases.
- Ancillary treatment such as antiemetics can be considered although antimotility agents are strongly discouraged in cases of infectious diarrhea, especially in those <18 years of age.

VIRAL GASTROENTERITIS

Epidemiology

- Viral gastroenteritis peaks in winter and spring.

Clinical Features

- Nausea.
- Diarrhea.

- High frequency of vomiting.
- Incubation period of 24–60 hours.
- Short duration of symptoms 12–60 hours.
- Norovirus lasts on average 2 days.
- Rotavirus lasts 3–8 days.
- Weight loss and fatigue occur occasionally, rarely respiratory symptoms.
- Diffuse abdominal pain with voluntary guarding on examination.
- Fever >38°C in half of patients.

A small percentage of patients (<10%) have signs of dehydration with dry mucous membranes and reduced skin turgor and hypotension.

Investigations and Diagnosis

Viral gastroenteritis usually lasts less than a week and is a self-limiting illness not often requiring confirmation unless causing an outbreak, hospitalization, or red flag symptoms.

- Stool cultures for microscopy and culture are negative.
- Feces negative for leucocytes, occult blood, and lactoferrin.
- Serum white cell count normal or elevated.
- Electrolytes are normal unless there are clinical signs of dehydration.
- Stool testing with commercially available enzyme immunoassays (EIA) for norovirus, adenovirus, and rotavirus can be performed.
- Stool polymerase chain reaction (PCR) testing for viral causes is highly specific and sensitive.

Treatment and Management

- No antiviral medication is indicated.
- Empiric antibiotics are not indicated if the etiology is viral gastroenteritis.
- Supportive oral rehydration is sufficient unless there are signs of volume depletion, in which case oral rehydrating solutions (ORS) or intravenous supplementation can be provided with normal saline or Ringers lactate solution.
- In patients <65 years, 1–2 days of an antimotility agent such as loperamide can be used as adjunctive therapy; however, it should not be used in bloody diarrhea, patients >65 years, or in abdominal distension, as there is a risk of paralytic ileus.
- Antiemetics can be used for 1–2 days if required to allow oral rehydration in patients unable to keep down oral fluids.

Specific Causes of Viral Gastroenteritis

Norovirus

Epidemiology

- Is a nonenveloped RNA virus from the Caliciviradae family which includes *Sapovirus.*
- Multiple different genotypes exist, which are indistinguishable clinically despite differing receptors, genetic recombination, and sequences.
- Commonest cause of gastroenteritis worldwide (Fig. 16.1) and often known as "winter vomiting virus" due to seasonal prevalence. It was first described in Norwalk, Ohio, causing an outbreak in 1968.

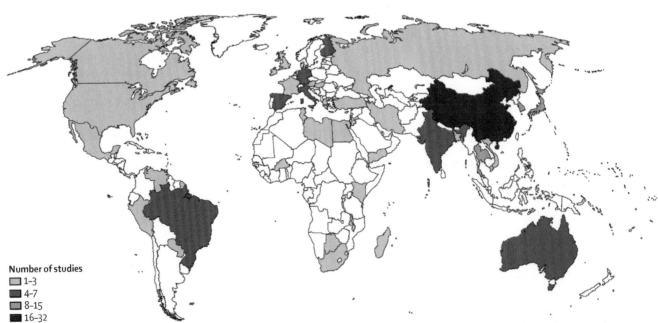

Number of studies
- 1–3
- 4–7
- 8–15
- 16–32

• **Fig. 16.1** Map of norovirus across the world. (Reprinted with permission from Elsevier. The Lancet. Ahmed SM, et al. Global prevalence of norovirus in cases of gastroenteritis: a systematic review and meta-analysis. *Lancet Infect Dis.* 2014;14(8):725–730.)

- Although antibody prevalence rises throughout childhood, re-infection can occur, and there is no lasting immunity due to re-infection with a diversity of strains.

Transmission

- Spread by the feco-oral route from person to person.
- Virus can be spread via aerosols in vomitus, contaminated food and water, and fomite contamination of surfaces.
- Incubation period is 24–48 hours.
- Shedding in the stool following an illness occurs over 24–48 hours but can be as long as 4 weeks and several months in the immunocompromised, but transmission is often among symptomatic individuals, and nosocomial transmission causing outbreaks is common.

Outbreaks

- Due to the stability of norovirus in the surroundings, it is able to resist killing by chlorine and alcohol, freezing and temperature up to 60°C, hence causing outbreaks both in the community and healthcare setting.

Clinical Manifestations

Although symptomatic and asymptomatic infection can occur, systemic symptoms include:
- Vomiting.
- Watery diarrhea, nonbloody and nonbilious, 4–8 stools over 24-hour period.
- Fever in 50% of cases.
- Malaise.
- Headache.
- Abdominal pain.
- Patients are at risk of dehydration.
- White cell count can be elevated or normal with lymphopenia often present.
- Short duration of illness of 48–72 hours with complete recovery, although this can be prolonged in immunocompromised patients with continued watery diarrhea, shedding for longer than 48 hours and up to several months, and histopathologic changes of disorganization and flattening of intestinal epithelium.

Investigations and Diagnosis

- Norovirus infection is often diagnosed clinically although laboratory antigen detection by enzyme immunoassays

EIA or PCR tests can be useful in an outbreak setting to confirm the diagnosis initially.
- Although EIA has a lower sensitivity and specificity than PCR, it is often widely utilized, and positive results of both PCR and ELISA testing should be interpreted in the clinical and epidemiologic setting.

Management

- Treatment consists of supportive measures as described for all viral gastroenteritis causes.

Infection Prevention and Control

- Patients should be isolated in single rooms wherever possible or cohorted in bays with a risk assessment carried out with regard to colonization or infection with other pathogens.
- Healthcare workers should carry out hand washing with soap and water as norovirus is resistant to killing with alcohol-based disinfection alone.
- Individuals should be excluded from work for 48–72 hours after symptom resolution and until they have formed stools.
- Food handlers should also be excluded until 48–72 hours after symptom resolution and until they have formed stools.
- Surface decontamination in hospital settings should be done in accordance with local guidelines and must include a bleach-based cleaning regimen

Adenovirus

- Spread by the feco-oral route and can be transmitted in virus present in vomit.
- Longer incubation period of 10 days and symptoms can last for 2 weeks with enteric adenovirus serotypes 40 and 41.
- It is an uncommon cause of gastroenteritis, especially in children in temperate areas, and vomiting is often absent.
- Outbreaks in nurseries and pediatric units, with prolonged diarrhea and low grade fever, can occur.

Rotavirus

- Mean duration of symptoms for 3–8 days and occurs in children aged 6 months to 2 years.
- It can occasionally cause diarrhea in the elderly.
- Often year-round in tropical climates and in the winter months in temperate areas.
- Vomiting is less of a prominent feature than in norovirus, although it can be difficult to distinguish between them.

Sapovirus

- Occurs year round, affecting toddlers and babies but does not often lead to outbreaks like norovirus.

• BOX 16.1 **Key Facts**

The following Kaplan criteria should raise the suspicion of norovirus as the cause of an outbreak:
- Two or more cases with a common source or exposure and a short incubation period of 24–48 hours and duration of illness of 12–60 hours.
- Stool cultures negative for bacterial pathogens.
- Vomiting as the predominant symptom in more than half the cases.

- Causes diarrhea and vomiting, generally without accompanying fever.

BACTERIAL GASTROINTESTINAL INFECTIONS

The incidence of bacterial gastroenteritis is far less than viral gastroenteritis and varies from country to country, depending on rural versus urban settings and the immunosuppressive risk factors of the individual. However, the CDC through FoodNet has collated the incidence within the United States.

The incidence per 100,000 cases of culture-confirmed cases of diarrhea in 2016 on FoodNet include:

- *Salmonella*: 15.4
- *Campylobacter*: 11.8
- *Shigella*: 4.6
- Shiga toxin-producing *E. coli*: 2.8
- *Vibrio*: 0.45
- *Yersinia*: 0.42
- *Listeria*: 0.26

This differs to the UK, where *Campylobacter* spp. is the most common cause, with an incidence of 4.6 per 100,000 cases in the community.

Specific Causes of Bacterial Gastroenteritis

Escherichia coli

- *E. coli* are usually found as normal bacteria in the gut; however, they can become pathogenic and cause bacterial gastroenteritis.
- Pathogenic forms include:
  - Enterotoxigenic *E. coli* (ETEC).
  - Enteropathogenic *E. coli* (EPEC).
  - Enterohemorrhagic *E. coli* (EHEC, also called Shiga toxin-producing *E. coli* or STEC).
  - Enteroinvasive *E. coli* (EIEC).
  - Enteroaggregative *E. coli* (EAEC or EAggEc).
- *Although E. coli* can be identified from culture, pathogenic strains require further testing at the reference laboratory.

Enterotoxigenic E. coli (ETEC)

- A cause of dehydrating diarrhea especially in the developing world in those <2 years due to its ability to survive in water and food and presence of heat-stable and heat-labile toxins.
- Causes watery diarrhea in returning travelers with nausea but no vomiting and symptoms lasting as long as 5 days.

Enteropathogenic E. coli (EPEC)

- Diarrhea is often seen in those <6 months of age in the developing world, although infrequently in adults, and is often seen sporadically or in outbreak settings.
- Severe diarrhea can result in dehydration and malnutrition.

Enterohemorrhagic E. coli (EHEC, also called Shiga toxin-producing E. coli or STEC)

- Incubation period of 1–4 days.
- Symptoms are due to *E. coli* O157:H7 or *E. coli* O104:H4 (STEC).
- Often cause bloody diarrhea; abdominal tenderness with a lack of fever.
- Raised white cell count.
- May lead to outbreaks.
- EHEC is a rare cause of pseudomembranous colitis when culture negative for *C. difficile.*
- Can cause hemolytic uremic syndrome (HUS) with renal failure, thrombocytopenia, and microangiopathic anemia 5–10 days after diarrhea.
- HUS can be seen with both *E. coli* O157 and non-O157 strains.
- HUS can occur in 6%–9% of EHEC infections, with the majority in those <10 years of age.
- Long-term sequelae with renal failure and hypertension are seen in 39% of HUS.
- Neurologic symptoms, including motor deficits and seizure, with fever can be seen in 4%.
- Stool culture on sorbitol MacConkey (SMAC) agar can detect *E. coli* O157 infection in first 6 days of infection with bloody diarrhea.
- Culture as well as toxin detection are important in the management and tracing of an outbreak.
- Treatment with supportive measures and the avoidance of antimotility agents to reduce the risk of complications is important.
- Antibiotic therapy increases the risk of developing HUS in EHEC infections by about 25% and should be avoided, especially in young children while a diagnostic test is pending.

Enteroinvasive E. coli (EIEC)

- Disease is relatively rare and closely related to *Shigella*.
- Often watery diarrhea and very rarely progresses to bloody diarrhea.

Enteroaggregative E. coli (EAEC or EAggEc)

- Often seen in the immunocompromised.
- Can cause persistent diarrhea in people with HIV.
- Affects young children more frequently.
- Treatment with antibiotics often results in eradication.

Campylobacter

Definition

- *Campylobacter* is a Gram-negative organism (Fig. 16.2) that belongs to the Enterobacteriales family and was first named as a genus in 1973, having previously been known as a *Vibrio*-type organism and associated in the early twentieth century as a cause of abortion in cattle and sheep.

Epidemiology

- Seen worldwide and a leading cause of gastroenteritis, including the Arctic and temperate areas.

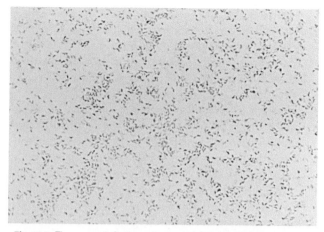

• **Fig. 16.2** Fine-curved, S-shaped, or spiral, lightly staining gram-negative appearance of *Campylobacter jejuni* in pure culture (×1000). (From Alios BN, Jovine NM, Blaser MJ. *Campylobacter jejuni* and related species. Bennett JE, Dolin R, Blaser MJ, eds. *Mandell, Douglas, and Bennett's Principles and Practice of Infectious Diseases*. Updated 8th ed. Elsevier; 2015.)

- *Campylobacter jejuni* is the commonest cause of *Campylobacter*-associated diarrhea.
- Commonly seen in children and then a second peak occurs in adults.

Transmission

- Associated with cross-contamination of food as it is found as a normal commensal in the gastrointestinal tract of many wild and domestic animals, including poultry and birds.
- Food handlers should adhere to good hand hygiene to prevent cross-transmission during preparation, and meat should be cooked to high temperatures (170°F for breast and 180°F for thighs).
- In some studies 48% of *Campylobacter* infections are contracted from poultry, travel-related infection 9%, water 8%, with a large reservoir of unknown infection at 24%.
- Transmission can occur from eating undercooked meat or cross-contamination of food from infected raw meat.
- *Campylobacter* is found contaminating many natural and fresh water sources and is able to survive many weeks at temperatures below 15°C, hence swimming in or drinking contaminated water poses an infection risk.
- Purified and treated water and pasteurized milk are important measures to reduce the infection risk.
- Direct transmission from infected animals, pets, or animal carcasses can occur and hand washing should be encouraged especially for children and vulnerable adults visiting farms or zoos.
- Person-to-person transmission is rare but can occur in the setting of nursery staff working with children who are infected.
- Sexual transmission especially in men who have sex with men has been documented.
- Increased infection in patients is observed in those with reduced gastric acidity such as achlorhydria or proton pump use.

Clinical Features

- Incubation period 3 days (mean 1–7).
- *Campylobacter* can affect either the large or small bowel and hence can cause both watery and bloody diarrhea.
- A prodrome with fevers, rigors, and dizziness can occur in one-third of patients prior to the gastrointestinal symptoms, and such patients go on to suffer increased severity of disease.
- Abdominal pain, which is often abrupt, severe, cramping, colicky, and periumbilical, is often but not always accompanied by diarrhea; diarrhea is often self-limiting and lasts for a mean of 7 days.
- Abdominal pain may radiate to the right iliac fossa in time, mimicking appendicitis and can persist even after diarrhea has settled.
- Nausea and vomiting is seen in 15%–25% of patients.
- A small percentage of patients, 0.1%–1%, can go on to develop a bacteremia and are more susceptible if immunosuppressed.
- Hypogammaglobulinemic patients have more severe disease and prolonged infection due to a lack of humoral immune system.
- Following infection, asymptomatic shedding can occur for up to 38 days, but retesting is not necessarily required in the absence of symptoms and chronic carriage may occur with relapse in 5%–10% of patients and recurrent infections and bacteremia in immunosuppressed individuals who can go on to have long-term carriage.

Complications

- *Campylobacter* infection has been linked with post-infectious sequelae: *Guillain-Barré* disease and reactive arthritis.
  - Reactive arthritis is seen in only 2.6% of patients and does not relate to the severity of illness but is often associated with the presence of HLAB27. It can begin 1–2 weeks after infection, affecting the small joints, wrists, knees, and ankles and can last for several weeks and up to 6 months. It has a good prognosis and usually responds to nonsteroidal therapy.
  - *Guillain–Barré* syndrome (GBS), an acute immune-mediated polyneuropathy following *Campylobacter jejuni* infection, can occur 1–2 weeks after an infection and is linked to *Campylobacter* infection in 3%–40% of cases.
    - The incidence of GBS is 100-fold higher following *C. jejuni* infection compared to the general population and 1 in 1000 people in the United States go on to develop it, as a result of antibody formation that cross-reacts with GM1 ganglioside, present in peripheral nerve myelin.
  - A similar variant syndrome of GBS, called Miller–Fischer, has also been linked to *C. jejuni* infection.
  - Colitis, which can mimic acute inflammatory bowel disease (IBD), can be seen with *Campylobacter* infections, and it may play a role in the pathogenesis of IBD. Infection usually affects the jejunum and ileum and can go on to affect the cecum and colon.

Investigations and Diagnosis

- Gram stains of stool show beautiful characteristic gull-shaped curved gram-negative rods.
- In reactive arthritis and GBS, stool cultures will be culture-negative, and serology should be sent for the detection of *C. jejuni* antibodies, and complement fixation tests or ELISA can be used.

Treatment and Management

Campylobacter infections are often self-limiting, and it is important to be aware of antimicrobial resistance. Treatment can reduce symptom duration by 1.3 days and is indicated in the following circumstances:

- Immunosuppressed individuals, elderly, and pregnant patients.
- Severe disease with fever, bloody diarrhea, symptoms lasting longer than one week or relapsing symptoms, and extraintestinal disease.
- In uncomplicated *Campylobacter* infection, unless resistance is suspected, ciprofloxacin or levofloxacin or azithromycin can be used for 3 days or until symptoms and signs have improved.
- For those who are immunosuppressed or have severe disease, 7–14 days of therapy should be advised.
- In the United States, ciprofloxacin resistance rates range from 20% to 27%.
- Macrolides can also be utilized, and resistance rates worldwide are <5% with the exception of Thailand and Ireland, where higher rates have been reported.
- Severe infections including bacteremia and in patients unable to tolerate oral medication, carbapenem therapy with an aminoglycoside can be utilized.

Salmonella

Definition

Salmonella are motile gram-negative bacilli that belong to the Enterobacteriales family. Known to cause:

- Gastroenteritis with nontyphoidal *Salmonella* spp.
- Enteric fever (*Salmonella Typhi* and *Salmonella Paratyphi*).
- Bacteremia and endovascular infections.
- Osteomyelitis and deep seated metastatic abscesses.
- Asymptomatic carriage.

Epidemiology

- Nontyphoidal *Salmonella* causes inflammatory diarrhea worldwide.
- *Salmonella Enteritidis* and *Salmonella Typhimurium* are the commonest cause of gastroenteritis.
- The highest incidence of diseases is seen in Asia where 4 per 100 cases of gastroenteritis are due to *Salmonella* infection.
- Second only to norovirus, nontyphoidal *Salmonella* infections result in the greatest number of cases of gastroenteritis in the United States and account for the largest number of hospitalized cases and deaths.
- There is seasonal variation with peaks of infection in summer and autumn.

Transmission

- Feco-oral route; ingestion of poultry, eggs, and meat products, including fresh produce.
- Transovarial transmission can occur from infected hens to intact egg shells, and these can subsequently result in infection.
- Contaminated infant milk formula has also been implicated.
- Contact with animals colonized with *Salmonella* spp. (snakes, iguanas, lizards, frogs, and turtles in particular); also with pets such as mice, hamsters, and rats as well as cats, dogs, chickens, and ducklings.
- Petting farms and zoos allowing contact with animals.
- Travel overseas and poor food and water hygiene can put individuals at risk of contracting *Salmonella* infection.

Clinical Features

- Incubation period of 8–72 hours following ingestion of contaminated water and food depending on the bacterial inoculum.
- Severity of symptoms relates to the bacterial dose, with increased severity of disease being seen with higher bacterial dose; symptoms may be very mild and asymptomatic carriage can also occur.
- Diarrhea resolves in 4–7 days with abdominal pain; nausea, vomiting, and fever usually resolves in 48–72 hours.
- Bloody stool can be seen in children, although there are no distinguishing features compared to other forms of gastroenteritis.
- Less than 5% of gastroenteritis cases with nontyphoidal *Salmonella* go on to develop bacteremia.
- Bacteremia can give rise to mycotic aneurysms, abscesses, and osteomyelitis, infective endocarditis, and endovascular infection.
- Achlorhydria, inflammatory bowel disease, and sickle cell disease may be associated with more severe infection

Investigations and Diagnosis

- Stool cultures, which require 48–72 hours incubation, should be sent.
- Blood cultures should be taken if the patient continues to be febrile especially if still febrile by the time cultures return as they may be bacteremic.

Treatment and Management

- *Salmonella* gastroenteritis is usually self-limiting and does not require treatment for immunecompetent patients between 12 and 50 years of age where the risks of antibiotic therapy and potentially prolonging carriage outweigh the benefit.
- It is important to provide supportive advice for the patient regarding oral hydration.
- Antibiotic therapy is also not indicated for bloody diarrhea alone.
- It is notifiable to the local health protection unit.
- Indications for treatment include risk of severity of invasive disease as gauged by:

- Immunosuppressive state (organ transplant, in receipt of steroids or immunosuppressants, lymphoproliferative disease, cancer sickle cell disease and other hemoglobinopathies, cancer, cirrhosis, and disorders of the reticuloendothelial system).
- People with HIV who are at risk of invasive disease and recurrent bacteremia due impaired cellular immunity.
- Aged over 50 years, where due to atherosclerotic disease they have a high risk (10%) of endovascular infection if bacteremia develops.
- Younger than 12 months, infants have a high risk of neurologic infection and mortality and often may not appear unwell.
- Stools greater than 9–10/day.
- Persistent fever.
- Hospital admission.
- Cardiac or other valvular disease.

Antibiotic Treatment

This should be guided by antimicrobial sensitivity where possible due to increasing antimicrobial resistance, and where there has been a molecular diagnosis of *Salmonella* infection, this should be followed up with culture for sensitivities

- Quinolones such as ciprofloxacin or levofloxacin, which have good intracellular and tissue penetration.
- Third-generation cephalosporins such as ceftriaxone.
- Azithromycin, which has good intracellular cover.
- Trimethoprim–sulfamethoxazole if unable to tolerate quinolones or cephalosporins.
- In the United States 0.4% of isolates have been reported as ciprofloxacin-resistant versus 3.6%–5% in Europe.
- Ceftriaxone resistance in the United States is 2.4% versus in UK 1.4% for cefotaxime.
- 3–7 days if they have severe gastrointestinal disease and are not bacteremic.
- 3–14 days if they are at risk of endovascular or joint complications and are being treated due to age associated risk factors for bacteremia.
- As *Salmonella* can persist in the reticuloendothelial infection, immunosuppressed patients can have difficulties clearing the infection and should be treated for a prolonged period of time, bacteremia and metastatic infection should be suspected and investigated, and an infectious diseases consult should be sought.
- 14 days of therapy as a minimum to prevent infection relapsing or persisting.
- 2–6 weeks may be required in people with HIV for gastroenteritis.

Asymptomatic Carriage

- Compared to other serotypes, *Salmonella typhimurium* is cleared quickly and has less carriage.
- Following symptomatic infection versus asymptomatic infection, excretion can continue for a prolonged period.
- Shedding can be intermittent, and hence several cultures may be required to detect carriage.
- Shedding can continue for up to 5 weeks.
- Previous short-course antibiotic therapy does not reduce the risk of carriage and may prolong shedding.

Chronic Carriage

Definition: Continued shedding for over a year with a previously positive stool one month after symptom resolution and repeated positive cultures, seen in 0.6%–2% of individuals and tends to affect:

- Women.
- Older adults.
- Young children.
- Biliary tract abnormalities such as gallstones.

Prolonged treatment with antibiotics for clearance can be attempted if needed due to HIV disease, immunosuppressive state for the patient or family member, or occupational requirements.

- Quinolones if tolerated for up to 4–6 weeks, *or*
- Amoxicillin or ampicillin for 6 weeks, *or*
- Trimethoprim–sulphamethoxazole for 3 months.
- Antibiotic therapy and a cholecystectomy may be required in some cases although neither the antibiotic therapy nor the cholecystectomy can guarantee eradication.
- Follow up cultures 6 months after completing therapy may be useful to review successful eradication.

Food Handlers and Healthcare Workers

- Advice should be sought from their local occupational health advisor and policies followed.
- Individuals may be permitted back to work 48 hours after symptom resolution, and as long as good hand hygiene is adhered to, they pose a minimal risk as they are only likely to be shedding intermittently.
- Some employers may insist on one or more culture-negative stool samples 48 hours apart before permitting employees back to work.

Enteric Fever or Typhoid

Enteric fever or typhoid is caused by *Salmonella enterica* serotype *Typhi* or *Salmonella enterica* serotype *Paratyphi* A, B, or C, which cause fever and abdominal pain. Enteric fever refers to both typhoid and paratyphoid fever, and "typhoid" and enteric fever are terms that are often used interchangeably.

Epidemiology

Humans are the only known reservoir for infection, and transmission occurs through the feco-oral route, through direct contact with an infected individual, or indirect contact through food or water.

- Enteric fever is relatively common in impoverished areas of the world, although under-reported, and hence the true prevalence is not known.
- It is seen in Southeast Asia and West and East Africa with rates >100 per 100,000 of the population while the north and south of Africa have a variable rate, and some countries report rates <5/100,000.
- *S. Paratyphi A* is uncommon in Africa but prevalent in Southeast Asia, and in general *S. Typhi* is a more common cause of enteric fever, although the two can not necessarily be clinically distinguished.

- Enteric fever tends to affect young children and adults rather than the elderly.
- Often seen in returning travelers outside of endemic regions, and antibiotic resistance is often encountered
- Chronic carriage occurs with shedding in the urine or stool for >12 months after an acute infection, and rates range from 1%–6%. It is seen more frequently in women, and while rare in the urine, it can be due to stones, prostatic hyperplasia, or concurrent *Schistosoma* infection. The commonest carriage, however, is due to biliary tree infection and the presence of stones.

Clinical Features of Enteric Fever

- Progression of symptoms occurs step-wise over a series of weeks.
  - Week 1: Fevers >40°C with bacteremia are common with chills while rigors are rarer and bradycardia with pulse temperature dissociation can be seen.
  - Week 2: abdominal pain occurs with "rose spots," which are faint salmon-colored spots that transiently appear (Fig. 16.3).
  - Week 3: abdominal perforation secondary to necrosis and lymphatic hyperplasia of Peyer's patches (uncommon in those <5 years of age), hepatosplenomegaly, intestinal bleeding, and secondary bacteremia are common, and septic shock with altered consciousness can result.
- Constipation can often be seen, especially in adults in about 30% early on whereas diarrhea is commoner in children and in those with HIV.
- Resolution of infection is often seen in a few weeks to months without antibiotic therapy (causes fever of unknown origin), although death can sometimes result from severe infection.
- Extraintestinal manifestations can include headache in 44%–94% of cases, "typhoid encephalopathy," altered sleep pattern, myelitis, acute psychosis, signs of upper motor neurone disease, ataxia, and parkinsonism; however, meningitis and focal neurologic infections are rare.
- Seeding as a result of bacteremia to the cardiovascular, hepatobiliary, respiratory, genitourinary, and musculoskeletal system are infrequently observed, although cough and arthralgia with myalgia occur more frequently.
- Laboratory investigations often show a leucopenia with anemia, especially in adults, while a leucocytosis is seen in children or adults with intestinal perforation.

Diagnosis

- Blood and stool cultures should be requested.
- Blood cultures are positive in 40%–80%.
- Stool culture positivity is 30%–40%.
- Bone marrow may have additional yield >90% in more complicated cases or if unresponsive to treatment and can remain positive for >5 days after antibiotic initiation.
- Serology using the Widal test which detects anti-*S. Typhi* antibodies requires an acute and convalescent sample to demonstrate a 4-fold rise and has limited utility.

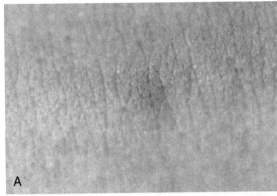
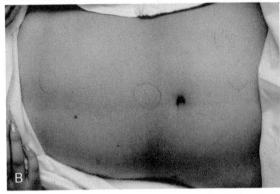

• **Fig. 16.3** Rose spots. (A) A rose spot in a volunteer with experimental typhoid fever. (B) Small clusters of rose spots are usually located on the abdomen. (Reprinted with permission from Elsevier. The Lancet. From Huang DB, DuPont HL. Problem pathogens: extra-intestinal complications of *Salmonella enterica* serotype Typhi infection. *Lancet Infect Dis.* 2005;5:341–348.)

- Antibiotic susceptibility testing is important as increased resistance to fluoroquinolones and third-generation cephalosporin is seen in South Asia.

Treatment

Antibiotic Treatment for Enteric Fever

- Antibiotic resistance is prevalent worldwide with many strains now multidrug resistant to ampicillin, trimethoprim–sulfamethoxazole, and chloramphenicol and is especially seen in South Asia with increasing resistance seen to fluoroquinolones.
- Most strains remain sensitive to ceftriaxone and azithromycin.
- Empiric therapy includes treatment with only one drug and depends on the suspicion of antibiotic resistance and severity of disease.
- For severe disease, parenteral therapy with ceftriaxone is recommended as resistance is rare, and once symptoms have improved, patients can be changed to an oral agent with susceptibility data if available, which have a quicker time to defervescence (10–14 days are advised as shorter course can result in a risk of relapse).
- In nonsevere disease and if no fluoroquinolone resistance is suspected, ciprofloxacin, which is bactericidal and concentrated intracellularly as well as in the bile, can be used, resulting in a rapid clearance of intracellular bacteria and are more effective than beta-lactams.

- Alternatives include azithromycin, ampicillin, trimethoprim–sulfamethoxazole, and chloramphenicol.
- Azithromycin in particular is associated with quicker time to defervescence, lower rates of post-treatment fecal carriage, and greater clinical cure rates in multidrug resistant strains when given for 5 days.
- In uncomplicated cases the time to defervescence is usually 4–6 days, and fevers in this period are not uncommon and do not necessarily suggest failure of therapy.
- Relapse usually occurs 2–3 weeks after resolution of the fever and is dependent on the choice of antimicrobial, usually necessitating treatment with further antibiotics.
- Eradication for long-term carriage can be attempted in patients where onward transmission is a concern, such as food handlers, and up to 4 weeks of ciprofloxacin can be used, although patients should be closely monitored to ensure that they do not develop antibiotic-associated diarrhea.

Shigella

Definition

- *Shigella* are nonmotile gram-negative facultative anaerobic organisms which belong to Enterobacteriales family.
- There are four species of *Shigella*: *S. s. dysenteriae* (serogroup A), *S. flexneri* (serogroup B), *S. boydii* (serogroup C), and *S. sonnei* (serogroup D).

Epidemiology

- In the United States, the incidence of *Shigella* was 6.59/100,000 cases in 2008 and is the third commonest cause of gastroenteritis after *Salmonella* and *Campylobacter* infections.

Transmission

- Humans are the only known host and reservoir.
- Transmission can also occur from infected water and food and is spread feco-orally.
- Sexual transmission among men who have sex with men is also very prevalent, and antimicrobial drug resistance, especially azithromycin, is a concern.
- Outbreaks in daycare centers and among institutionalized patients or among crowded populations can occur.

Clinical Features (Fig. 16.4)

- *Shigella* invade the colonic mucosa cells causing abscess formation and mucosal ulceration.
- It is also able to spread from cell to cell and produces enterotoxins; the virulence plasmid-encoded ShET2 (produced by all four species), chromosomally encoded ShET1 (produced by *S. flexneri* 2a) and Shiga toxin (*Stx*) produced by *S. dysenteriae*.
- These toxins result in the loss of water and solutes.
- **Hemolytic uremic syndrome** is seen in 8% of children with *S. dysenteriae* infection, mediated by *Stx* toxin.
- Incubation period 3 days (range 1–7).
- Abdominal pain, watery diarrhea, which proceeds to bloody diarrhea 35%–55% and mucus 70%–80%, fever, and vomiting.

- Disease is self-limiting to about 7 days.
- Shedding post-infection can be for up to 6 weeks and the duration of asymptomatic shedding is unknown.
- Complications include bacteremia (1%–7%) HUS, reactive arthritis, leukemoid reaction, neurologic symptoms, hyponatremia, hypovolemia.

Investigations and Diagnosis

- The best yield is from mucus stool, and stool rather than rectal swabs in turn yield better results.
- White and red blood cells can be seen on microscopy of the stool.
- PCR testing can be performed.
- Antimicrobial susceptibilities must be tested even if detected through molecular methods as there are significant concerns regarding resistance and are likely due to plasmid transfer.

Treatment and Management

- In Asia and Africa fluoroquinolone resistance is 20%–30%, quinolone (nalidixic acid) and trimethoprim–sulphamethoxazole is 65%–85%.
- Antibiotics can decrease the duration of shedding and hence onward transmission as well as symptom duration of fever and diarrhea by 2 days.
- Most infections are self-limiting and antibiotic treatment is not indicated unless patients have the following risk factors:
- Immunosuppressed, including people with HIV.
- Bacteremia or extraintestinal disease.
- Food handlers, healthcare, residential home residents or workers, and nursery staff at risk of passing on the infection to others.

  Antibiotic choice should be based on patient demographics and likely local resistance profile.
- Patients without risk factors can be given a fluoroquinolone.
- Patients with risk factors can be empirically given ceftriaxone pending sensitivities.
- Fluoroquinolones should be given for 3 days and up to 5–7 days in HIV patients or those with *S. dysenteriae* infection.

Yersinia

Definition

- Yersiniosis, caused by *Yersinia enterocolitica*, is a zoonotic infection and can be isolated from wild and domestic animals although the majority of isolates are nonpathogenic.

Epidemiology

- Seen more in resource-rich settings than resource-poor.
- *Yersinia enterocolitica* is seen in the United States compared with *Y. pseudotuberculosis*, which is largely found in Europe.

Transmission

- Associated with unpasteurized milk, undercooked meat especially pork, water contaminated with feces; pigs are a frequently identified source of infection.

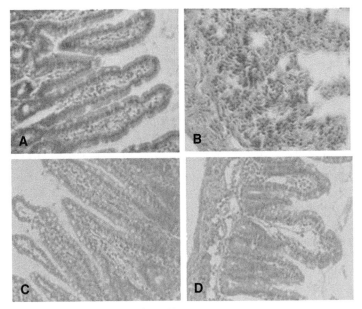

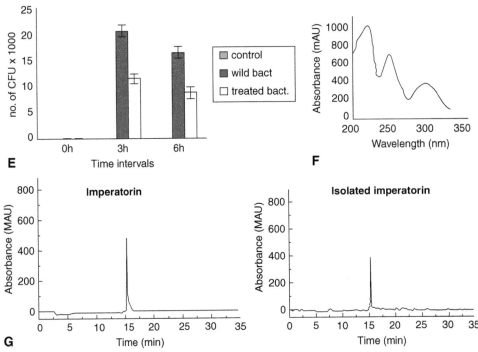

• **Fig. 16.4** Histology of rat ileal loop and intracellular bacterial count in infected rat ileal loop. (A) Control – showing normal architecture of rat intestinal mucosa. (B) Loop infected with *Shigella dysenteriae* showing shortening of villus, edema of villi, ulceration, and inflammatory infiltration of hemorrhagic exudates in the luminal surface of the mucosa. (C) Loop infected with AEAM-treated *S. dysenteriae* showing normal architecture with minimal inflammatory lesions. (D) Loop incubated with AEAM alone showing normal architecture. (E) Intracellular bacterial count in infected rat ileal loop. Intracellular bacterial count of ileal loop was decreased by 46% in case of AEAM treated *S. dysenteriae* infected loop when compared to wild *S. dysenteriae* infection. (F) and (G) UV-visible spectral and HPLC analysis of isolated imperatorin aqueous extract of Aegle marmelos; (F) shows UV spectrum of AEAM with three absorption peak at 219, 254 and 302 nm; (G) HPLC which shows a peak at 254 nm (retention time – 14.51 min). (From Raja SB, et al. Imperatorin a furocoumarin inhibits periplasmic Cu–Zn SOD of *Shigella dysenteriae* thereby modulates its resistance towards phagocytosis during host–pathogen interaction. *Biomed Pharmacother.* 2011;65(8):560–568.)

• BOX 16.2 Key Facts

- Patients may often present with pharyngitis in 20% which is not seen in other causes of gastroenteritis.
- Throat cultures may also yield positive growth for *Y. enterocolitica.*
- Localization of pain to the right lower quadrant can be a diagnostic clue.
- Although *Yersinia* does not cause thyroiditis it shares antigens that resemble TSH and hence cross-react with antibodies in Graves disease.

- After ingestion, the organism proliferates in the lymphoid tissue of the small intestine where it may cause hyperemia, neutrophil infiltration, and ulceration.

Clinical Features

- 1–14 days incubation period.
- Disseminated infection due to hematogenous spread can lead to metastatic abscess formation in the liver and spleen; other complications: mesenteric adenitis, terminal ileitis, pseudoappendicitis.
- Post-infectious immunologic sequelae (e.g., reactive arthritis and erythema nodosum).

Investigations and Diagnosis

- Stool cultures can be set up and isolates should be referred to a reference laboratory, as biotyping and/or serotyping are necessary to establish pathogenicity.
- Mesenteric lymph nodes, pharyngeal exudates, peritoneal fluid, or blood and throat cultures can also be cultured.

Treatment and Management

- There are **no** controlled trials that indicate that antimicrobial treatment of acute, uncomplicated yersiniosis is beneficial.
- Unless the patient has severe disease or has an underlying comorbid illness, antibiotics are not recommended.
- Treatment of enterocolitis in adults if indicated is with fluoroquinolone.
- Septicemia should be treated with IV ceftriaxone or ciprofloxacin if susceptible.

Vibrio

Definition

- *Vibrio* species are natural inhabitants of brackish and salt water worldwide.

Epidemiology

The diarrhea-causing species most frequently isolated are
- *Vibrio cholerae* (the causative agent of cholera).
- *Vibrio parahaemolyticus.*
- *Vibrio vulnificus,* which can cause diarrhea, but has been isolated from the blood and tissues of septic patients (especially those with liver disease).

Vibrio cholerae

- Strains of *V. cholerae* O1 are the etiologic agents of epidemic cholera.
  - *V. cholerae* O1 has two biotypes: classical and El Tor.
  - *V. cholerae* O1 can also be subdivided into three serotypes: Ogawa, Inaba, and Hikojima.
- In 1993, a new cholera-causing serogroup, *V. cholerae* O139 Bengal, emerged in southern India and spread to several countries in the Asian continent and the Americas.

Transmission

- Feco-oral.
- Cholera outbreaks are most often associated with contaminated water and contaminated food, particularly undercooked or raw seafood.
- *V. cholerae* O1 and O139 are producers of the cholera toxin (CT), unlike *V. cholerae* non-O1/non-O139 strains, which only occasionally produce enterotoxin.

Clinical Features

- A cause of profuse watery diarrhea known as "rice water stool."
- Mucus but no blood is present.
- Incubation period: a few hours to a few days.
- Significant hypovolemia and electrolyte abnormalities can occur within a few hours of symptom onset, are the most important sequelae of severe cholera.
- Abdominal discomfort, borborygmi, and vomiting are other common symptoms, particularly in the early phases of disease.

Treatment and Management

- Antibiotics can shorten the duration of diarrhea, reduce the volume of stool losses, and decrease the duration of *V. cholera* shedding.
- Options for cholera include macrolides, fluoroquinolones, and tetracyclines based on local resistance profile.
- Fluid resuscitation is paramount.

Vibrio vulnificas

- Ingestion of shellfish which may give rise to gastroenteritis and cellulitis and bullous lesions (especially in cirrhotic patients).
- Infection can proceed to invasive disease with bacteremia and systemic signs in the immunosuppressed and in those with liver disease or hemochromatosis.
- *V. vulnificus* can be isolated from virtually all oysters harvested in the Chesapeake Bay and the United States Gulf Coast when water temperatures exceed 20ºC.
- There is a high mortality rate with septicemia of over 40%, and this can exceed 90% if patients present with signs of hypotension.
- Patients with a presumptive diagnosis of *V. vulnificus* septicemia should be started immediately on antibiotic therapy and managed aggressively in an intensive care unit.

- A tetracycline plus a third-generation cephalosporin is recommended.
- Fluoroquinolone monotherapy is an alternative.

Fresh Water Pathogens

Aeromonas

- *Aeromonas* is a gram-negative organism able to cause diarrheal illness usually found in fresh water, brackish, and marine environments.
- Although extraintestinal disease can occur with bacteremia, deep seated and wound infections, diarrhea is the commonest manifestation.
- Stool, blood cultures, and wound swabs if indicated should be sent for culture to identify the causative species and susceptibility pattern.
- Most *Aeromonas* infections are self-limiting but antimicrobial therapy along with supportive hydration is indicated in severe diarrhea, septicemia, immunosuppressed patients, and wound infections.
- Therapy options include doxycycline, aminoglycosides, second- and third-generation cephalosporins, carbapenems, chloramphenicol, and trimethoprim–sulfamethoxazole; should be adjusted and guided by susceptibility pattern.

Plesiomonas shigelloides

- Gram-negative infections that occur in water environments causing diarrhea in warm temperatures; contracted from ingestion of raw seafood.
- Incubation is usually less than 48 hours and, although the illness is usually self-limiting, symptoms can be severe and patients may remain symptomatic for up to 4 weeks.
- Individuals who are immunocompromised or have hepatobiliary disease are at increased risk of infection associated with water-related injuries.
- Fluoroquinolone therapy, azithromycin amoxicillin–clavulanic acid can be used or, for more severe cases, ceftriaxone or carbapenem therapy may be indicated.
- 3–5 days therapy is recommended for gastroenteritis symptoms.
- 1–2 weeks for extraintestinal manifestations, dependent on clinical response.

Listeria

- *Listeria* is a pathogen that can affect both neonates and adults irrespective of their immune status, including pregnant women.
- It often presents as invasive disease with bacteremia but can cause gastroenteritis which has a shorter incubation period of 24 hours (although can range from 6 hours to 10 days) versus 11 days (and up to 28 days) for invasive disease.
- *Listeria* accounts for a very small proportion of gastroenteritis cases, about 1%, but is known to cause outbreaks and is more common in the summer.

- Risk factors for acquiring gastroenteritis include consuming unpasteurized milk or products containing unpasteurized milk; other high-risk foods include soft cheeses or pate, prepared salads containing tuna, chicken, or ham, or refrigerated smoked seafood.
- A self-limiting febrile gastroenteritis is often seen with a high attack rate of 50%–100% following ingestion of contaminated food.
- In those who are immunocompromised, over 65 years of age, or pregnant, there is a risk of invasive disease, often resulting in bacteremia and infection of the neonate or loss of fetus in pregnant women.
- Stool cultures, especially in the setting of an outbreak, are indicated, and special media is required as routine laboratory testing does not support its growth and blood cultures if febrile should be undertaken.
- Treatment is not usually indicated in gastroenteritis and has usually fully resolved before the diagnosis can be confirmed.
- In those patients where there is a risk of invasive disease, oral amoxicillin or trimethoprim–sulphamethoxazole can be considered.
- In pregnant women at risk of invasive disease, oral amoxicillin is advised.

Clostridioides (formerly *Clostridium*) *difficile*

- *C. difficile* is a gram-positive anaerobic bacillus that is spore-forming and able to produce toxin.
- *C. difficile* causes an antibiotic associated inflammatory colitis and is the commonest cause of healthcare-associated diarrhea.
- Infection requires spores to be acquired and for the gut microbiota to be disrupted, usually through preceding antibiotic therapy.
- It is not an invasive disease and nontoxin producing strains do not often cause disease but can colonize the gut, and asymptomatic shedders of spores can continue to act as a reservoir for infection.
- *C. difficile* produces two toxins: Toxin A, an enterotoxin and Toxin B, a cytotoxin.
  - Toxin A causes inflammation with intestinal fluid secretion and damage to the mucosa.
  - Toxin B, more potent than toxin A, acts as a virulence factor.
- A hypervirulent strain of *C. difficile* known as NAP1/B1/027 has caused many outbreaks, producing larger quantities of toxin A/B compared to other strains and is associated with a higher rate of recurrence, severe disease, and mortality.
- Neonates and children below 2 years of age have a high rate of asymptomatic carriage and may be protected from disease due to the lack of intestinal receptors.
- Recurrent disease can be due to spore persistence in the gut and can occur 2–8 weeks following therapy for an initial episode with mild, severe, or fulminant disease, and risk factors include age >65 years of age with ongoing antibiotic therapy.

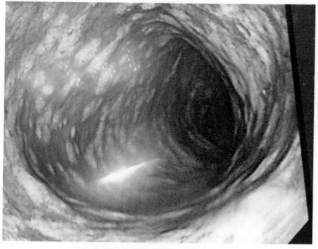

• **Fig. 16.5** *Clostridioides difficile* bowel.

Clinical Manifestations (Fig. 16.5)

- Clinical manifestations include asymptomatic carriage where patients can continue to act as reservoirs of infection for others, colitis, and toxic megacolon, beginning usually within 2 weeks to 1 month following antibiotic therapy and can be classified as:
- Nonsevere: WBC <15000 mL/cell and serum creatinine <1.5 mg/dL.
- Severe: WBC >15000 mL/cell and serum creatinine >1.5 mg/dL.
- Fever >38.5°C can be seen in about 15% of cases accompanied by abdominal pain and cramps along with blood-stained or mucus diarrhea.
- Fulminant colitis: lower abdominal pain and distension with possible toxic megacolon (colonic diameter >7 cm on imaging or >12 cm at the cecum), fever, hypotension, ileus or shock; diarrhea may be a less prominent feature.
- Unusual presentations of *C. difficile* can occasionally include extraintestinal manifestations in the form of reactive arthritis, bacteremia, soft tissue infection, and appendicitis as well as a protein-losing enteropathy or small bowel infection.

Investigations and Diagnosis

- Stool samples for *C. difficile* should be tested using a multi-step algorithm, which involves a glutamate dehydrogenase (GDH) and toxin testing or a nucleic acid amplification test (NAAT) along with GDH and toxin as opposed to toxin on its own. PCR is also commonly used.
- Stool samples from asymptomatic patients should not be tested, and samples from symptomatic patients should not be repeated within 7 days during the same episode of diarrhea as they can remain positive for up to 6 weeks with no test of cure advised through repeat sampling.
- Neonates and children below the age of 2 have a high carriage rate, and stool samples should not be tested for *C. difficile*.
- In children >2 years, samples can be sent for testing if other causes for on-going diarrhea have been excluded.

Management

- Infection prevention and control precautions are key to preventing the onward spread of infection to other patients.
- Reviewing and discontinuing proton pump inhibitors should be encouraged.
- Concomitant antibiotic therapy should be reviewed and de-escalated or discontinued where appropriate due to the ongoing risk of *C. difficile*, and an active antibiotic stewardship program should continue to target antibiotics associated with a higher *C. difficile* risk to prevent further cases.
- Treatment for an initial *C. difficile* episode should include oral vancomycin (which achieves high levels in the colon unlike IV vancomycin which is not excreted into the colon) or fidaxomicin rather than metronidazole (metronidazole leading to greater treatment failures), for 10 days, although metronidazole can be used for mild cases if vancomycin or fidaxomicin are not available.
- In fulminant infection, with hypotension and toxic megacolon, the dose of oral vancomycin can be increased and in the presence of an ileus, rectal vancomycin can be administered along with IV metronidazole, although there is a higher risk of perforation and caution is advised.
- Imaging and an early surgical opinion are advised if there are concerns about severe disease or ongoing or worsening abdominal pain.
- Imaging may show signs of toxic megacolon or bowel perforation in addition to bowel mucosa and sub-mucosa edema, sometimes seen as the "double halo-sign" or "thumb-printing" when edema of the submucosa causes scalloping of the bowel wall.
- If lower GI endoscopy is performed to exclude other causes, pseudomembranes as raised patches of yellow and white, 2 cm in diameter, on the mucosa may be visible (see Fig. 16.5).
- Additional intravenous immunoglobulin (IVIG) may be useful in severe or refractory infection.
- Recurrent infections can be treated with a tapering course of oral vancomycin or fidaxomicin if not used on the first occasion or a course of oral vancomycin if metronidazole is used during the first course.
- Fecal microbiota transplant can be considered for recurrent infections that do not respond to treatment.

PARASITIC CAUSES OF DIARRHEA

This is discussed in greater detail in Chapter 34, Protozoa.

- Patients with persistent diarrhea, which is usually the presence of symptoms for more than 14 days, should be evaluated for a parasitic cause for their symptoms; this should include the persistence of diarrhea in the setting of antibiotic treatment where along with antibiotic resistance, persistent parasites may be a cause.
- A travel history, exposure to contaminated food and water along with any immunosuppression such as HIV are considered risk factors as well as residence in daycare centers.

- Travel to mountainous regions or countries such as Nepal or Russia can result in infections with *Giardia*, *Cyclospora*, or *Cryptosporidium*.
- Men who have sex with men may also pass on parasites such as *Giardia*.
- Parasites can also result in community waterborne outbreaks, and appropriate samples should be sent.
- Weight loss and signs of malabsorption are occasionally observed.
- Stool for culture for bacterial causes of gastroenteritis should be sent along with stools for ova, cysts, and parasites.
- Three consecutive daily samples increase the yield of positivity as parasites can be shed intermittently.
- Special modified acid fast or trichome stains for *Cryptosporidium*, *Cyclospora*, and *Cystoisospora* can be performed in the laboratory.
- Stool antigens for *Giardia* and *Entamoeba* can be additionally requested.

TOXIN-MEDIATED GASTROENTERITIS

Definition

- Gastroenteritis secondary to a preformed toxin or chemical irritant, which presents with sudden onset vomiting and diarrhea within a short period of time following ingestion.

Specific Causes of Toxin-Mediated Disease

Clostridium perfringens
Definition

- *C. perfringens* causes a foodborne toxin-mediated watery diarrheal illness.

Epidemiology

- It is common worldwide and in the United States is the second commonest cause of bacterial gastroenteritis, with around one million cases each year.

Transmission

- *C. perfringens* is associated with undercooked or poorly stored meat products and gravy.
- Infection is caused by *C. perfringens* spores which survive in food, proliferate, and release an enterotoxin.
- *C. perfringens* Type A is often the cause of outbreaks and causes infection through poorly heated food and meat products, as spores survive heating.
- Type C produces hemorrhagic necrosis of the jejunum through a beta toxin known as **enteritis necroticans** or **pigbel disease** following consumption of pork products. The trypsin inhibitors that are found in sweet potatoes may inhibit breakdown of the toxin in the intestines when ingested together with meat products containing *C. perfringens* spores and hence potentiate the infection.

Clinical Features

- Incubation period 6–24 hours (usually 10–12 hours).
- Symptoms include watery diarrhea and crampy abdominal pain; fever and vomiting are rare.
- Pigbel disease (clostridial necrotizing enteritis), known in Papua New Guinea and as "Darmbrand" in Germany, presents with segmental necrosis of the jejunum and ileum, severe abdominal pain, distension, and dilated loops of bowel (Fig. 16.6).
  - *C. perfringens* Type C causes enteritis necroticans and is found in the soil and stools of animals and man.
  - It occurs in children with protein deficiency in the developing world but is rare in the developed world, where it is seen in diabetic patients.
  - "Darmbrand" refers to the appearance of "burnt bowel" and was seen in patients who had previously been starved and then consumed large meals of meat and vegetables following World War II.
  - In Papua New Guinea, an outbreak occurred in 1963, among 17 male patients (both adult and children) after ceremonial fasting on sweet potatoes and inadequately cooked pork contaminated with pig intestines.
  - Patients presented with severe abdominal pain and samples from the meat, stools, and resected intestine segments of affected patients isolated *Clostridium perfringens* Type C.
  - Mortality in children was 50% and subsequently reduced by treating with antisera.
  - The disease was subsequently called "pigbel" due to the abdominal pain following a "pig" feast.
- *C. perfringens* Type A causes gas gangrene in patients with necrotic bowel secondary to food poisoning worldwide.
- *C. perfringens* Types B and D do not cause disease in humans.

Diagnosis and Management

- *C. perfringens* should be clinically suspected when a patient presents with a history of ingesting poorly cooked or stored meat or meat products (8–16 hours after).
- Both stool and food should be tested for toxin and cultured if possible.
- *C. perfringens* infection is often self-limiting and does not require treatment with antibiotics.

Staphylococcal aureus
Epidemiology

- *S. aureus* can be found as a commensal in the nose and skin of some individuals (20%–30% can have persistent carriage) and when shed from food handlers, it can contaminate food, multiplying at room temperatures to form significant amounts of heat stable *S. aureus* enterotoxins (SEs) in meat, eggs, salads, and other food produce such as cakes and sandwiches.
- *S. aureus* forms part of the gut flora and may normally be found in small numbers in feces.

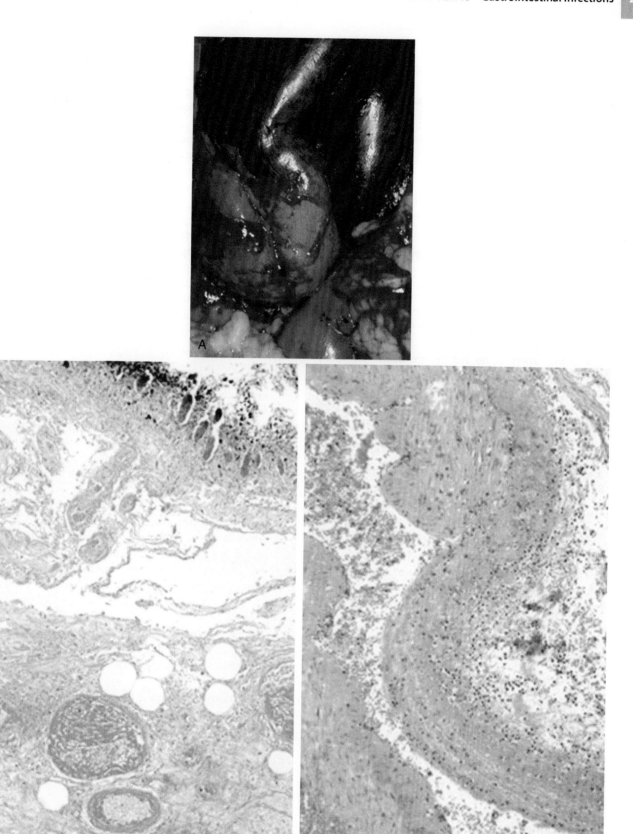

• **Fig. 16.6** Patients with *Clostridium perfringens* necrotizing enterocolitis (also known as pigbel, Darmbrand, or fire belly). (A) Gross photograph shows the necrotic portions of the bowel to the side of viable intestinal loops. (B) Microscopic photograph shows necrosis of the different intestinal layers. (C) Close-up shows mild inflammatory infiltrate for the amount of necrosis. (From Procop G, Pritt B, eds. *Pathology of Infectious Diseases*. Elsevier; 2015.)

Transmission

- Heat stable enterotoxin found in contaminated food products.
- The toxins are relatively stable and may be present in the absence of viable organisms after cooking, pasteurization, or prolonged storage of foodstuffs.
- No person-to-person spread.

Clinical Features

- Vomiting 1–6 hours following ingestion; fever is rare.
- Symptoms usually resolve within 24–48 hours.

Diagnosis/Investigation and Treatment

- This is usually a clinical diagnosis.
- Diagnosis is confirmed by culturing the feces from infected persons as well as from incriminated foods.
- Detection of enterotoxin in feces or vomit is of limited diagnostic value.
- **Treatment:** There is no specific treatment for toxin-mediated *S. aureus* infection other than supportive measures with oral hydration.

Bacillus cereus

Definition

- *Bacillus cereus* is a common cause of food poisoning by ingestion of a toxin rather than infection with living organisms; heat stable emetic toxin-mediated gastroenteritis.

Transmission

- *B. cereus* toxin found in starchy food such as rice.
- Spore formation enables *B. cereus* to survive in the environment for extended periods and withstand extremes of temperature.
- Spores and vegetative bacteria can contaminate food, causing gastrointestinal illness.

Clinical Features

- Symptoms 1–6 hours after ingestion.
- Causes profuse vomiting and nausea; usually self-limiting.
- The diarrheal syndrome due to an enterotoxin, resembles *C. perfringens* food poisoning and causes diarrhea and abdominal pain 8–16 hours after ingestion of the contaminated food following multiplication in the intestine.
- The emetic syndrome caused by a thermostable peptide is associated with the ingestion of rice and pasta-based foods and is characterized by nausea and vomiting 1–5 hours after consumption of the implicated foodstuff.

Diagnosis and Management

- This is usually clinically diagnosed.
- Reference laboratory testing of vomitus and food can demonstrate the presence of toxin.
- Toxin-mediated disease does not require treatment.

Scombroid

Definition

- Food poisoning associated with seafood is known as scombroid poisoning. It is commonly misdiagnosed as a seafood allergy.
- It is due to the incorrect storage of fish above 4°C resulting in bacterial overgrowth and a build up of toxic levels of histamine and other biogenic amines by the bacterial enzyme histidine decarboxylase found in dark fish meat.
- Storing fish at 20°C for 2–3 hours can be enough to result in scombroid poisoning.
- The bacteria responsible are *E. coli*, *Klebsiella* spp., halophilic *Vibrio* species, *Proteus*, *Clostridium*, *Salmonella*, and *Shigella* spp.
- Raw milk contaminated before production of Swiss cheese results in similar bacterial overgrowth and histamine build up.

Transmission

- Poisoning is acquired through seafood consumption, especially consumption of dark meat of finfish from the Scombridae and Scomberesocidae families, such as tuna, mackerel, skip-jack, and bonito; other fish such as dolphin fish, tilapia, salmon, swordfish, trout, sardines, and anchovies have been implicated.
- Histamine is unable to be broken down by refrigeration, freezing, or cooking and can build up at any time before preparation of the fish even if it was stored correctly at the time of being caught.
- Opened cans of tuna pose a similar risk and must be stored in the fridge to prevent poisoning.
- Fish may appear to have "honey-combed" scales and taste "peppery," "bubbly," or "spicy."

Clinical Features

- Symptoms are due to histamine reaction occurring within 1 hour of consumption. The commonest symptoms are:
  - Cutaneous flushing with a feeling of uncomfortable warmth.
  - Urticarial rash on the face and upper torso (Fig. 16.7).
  - Headache.
  - Diarrhea.
- The most serious symptoms, which occur rarely, are bronchospasm, respiratory distress, and cardiac arrhythmias
- Other symptoms include:
  - Perioral burning, itching, or edema.
  - Blurring of vision.
  - Tachycardia and palpitations.
  - Hypotension and dizziness.
- Elderly patients and those taking medication, which prevents the breakdown of histamine such as monoamine oxidase inhibitors or isoniazid, are likely to have more severe and prolonged symptoms as compared with those taking antihistamines.

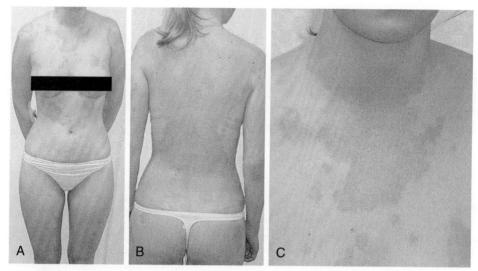

Fig. 16.7 Scombroid rash. (A and B) Widespread erythematous rash predominantly on the face (not shown) and trunk of patient 1. (C) Close-up view of the upper chest area. Note the absence of wheals. (From Jantschitsch C, Kinaciyan T, Manafi M, Safer M, Tanew A. Severe scombroid fish poisoning: an underrecognized dermatologic emergency. *J Am Acad Dermatol.* 2011;65(1):246–247.)

- Symptoms usually resolve within 12–48 hours and are dependent on the amount of fish produce consumed.
- There are no serious sequelae following scombroid poisoning.

Treatment and Management

- Respiratory or cardiac distress should be treated as anaphylaxis in a hospital setting with observation as an in-patient following treatment and resolution of symptoms.
- Moderate to severe symptoms with flushing, edema, itching, and a rash still warrant treatment with antihistamines, H1 (diphenhydramine or hydroxyzine), H2 antihistamines (e.g., ranitidine or cimetidine).
- Milder symptoms can be treated with oral antihistamines.
- Treatment can continue for 24–48 hours to prevent recurrence of symptoms caused by any further absorption of toxin.
- Fluid resuscitation appropriate to the level of dehydration should be administered in the case of severe vomiting or diarrhea.

Ciguatera Poisoning

- This is a foodborne illness that is caused by consumption of reef fish contaminated with multiple toxins, including ciguatera toxin, which arise from dinoflagellates.
- The toxins accumulate in the flesh and organs of affected fish.
- Over 400 fish types can be affected, including barracuda, amberjack, moray eel, and certain types of grouper, snapper, or parrotfish.
- Very rarely nontropical fish such as temperate farm-raised salmon have been affected.

> **• BOX 16.3 Key Facts**
>
> - Fish with ciguatera toxin do not look, smell, or taste any different, unlike with scombroid poisoning.
> - Caribbean ciguatera poisoning is not life-threatening and presents with gastrointestinal symptoms followed by neurologic signs *without* altered mental status.

Transmission

- Ingestion of toxin which is formed by dinoflagellates of the genus *Gambierdiscus*; single-celled algae-like organisms that grow on and around coral reefs.
- The ciguatera neurotoxin is heat-stable, lipid-soluble, and acid-stable and not affected by freezing, cooking, or marinating the affected fish.

Clinical Features

- Ciguatera poisoning can cause a variety of symptoms:
  - Gastrointestinal (diarrhea, abdominal pain, vomiting): occur within 3–6 hours but can occur up to 30 hours after consumption and resolve in 24–48 hours but may take up to 4 days.
  - Neurologic (weakness, paresthesia, headache, vertigo, pruritus, hallucinations): within 3–72 hours after consumption, with abnormalities persisting for several weeks to months (20%).
  - Cardiovascular (bradycardia, hypertension): within a few hours of consumption and resolve in 24–48 hours but may take up to 4 days.

Investigations and Diagnosis

Although ciguatera toxin can be tested for in fish with mouse bioassay and IgG immunoassays, these are not widely accessible and other affected individuals can be used as evidence as well as compatible gastrointestinal and neurologic symptoms following consumption of reef fish.

Treatment and Management

- Ciguatera poisoning should be notified to the local health protection unit and regional poison center to identify the source and affected reef.
- Management should focus on airway, breathing, and circulation support as well as vomiting, diarrhea, pruritus, and neurologic symptoms, which may be reversed with mannitol, gabapentin, amitriptyline, or pregabalin.

Further Reading and Resources

1. Public Health England (PHE). The Green Book. https://gov.uk/government/collections/immunisation-against-infectious-disease-the-green-book#the-green-book. Cholera, ch. 14 (2013); Typhoid, ch. 37 (2015); Rotavirus, ch, 27b (2015).
2. IDSA. 2017 Infectious Diseases Society of America Clinical Practice Guidelines for the Diagnosis and Management of Infectious Diarrhea. *Clin Infect Dis.* 2017;65(12):e45–e80. doi.org/10.1093/cid/cix669.
3. Uptodate. Approaches to the diagnosis and management of patients with gastroenteritis. https://www.uptodate.com/.
4. Public Health England (PHE). UK Standards for Microbiology Investigations: Investigation of Faecal Specimens for Enteric Pathogens (2014). https://www.gov.uk/government/collections/standards-for-microbiology-investigations-smi.
5. World Gastroenterology Organisation (WGO). Guideline for Acute Diarrhoea in Adults and Children – A Global Perspective (2013). http://www.worldgastroenterology.org/guidelines/global-guidelines/acute-diarrhea.
6. Centers for Disease Control and Prevention (CDC). Updated Norovirus Outbreak Management and Disease Prevention Guidelines (2011). https://www.cdc.gov/mmwr/preview/mmwrhtml/rr6003a1.htm.
7. Healthcare Infection Control Practices Advisory Committee (HICPAC). Guideline for the Prevention and Control of Norovirus Gastroenteritis Outbreaks in Healthcare Settings (2011). https://www.cdc.gov/infectioncontrol/pdf/guidelines/norovirus-guidelines.pdf.
8. Norovirus Working Party: Guidelines for the Management of Norovirus Outbreaks in Acute and Community Health and Social Care Settings (2012). https://www.gov.uk/government/publications/norovirus-managing-outbreaks-in-acute-and-community-health-and-social-care-settings.
9. Clinical Practice Guidelines for *Clostridium difficile* Infection in Adults and Children: 2017 Update by the Infectious Diseases Society of America (IDSA) and Society for Healthcare Epidemiology of America (SHEA). *Clin Infect Dis.* 2018;66(7):e1–e48. doi.org/10.1093/cid/cix1085.

17

Peritonitis, Intraabdominal Abscess, Hepatobiliary Infections, Splenic Infections

JAMES R. PRICE

Definitions

Intraabdominal infection: infection of the peritoneal cavity or retroperitoneal space.
Peritonitis: inflammation of the peritoneum, either:
- Not directly related to intraabdominal pathology (**primary**).
- Relating to intraabdominal pathology (**secondary**).
- Persisting or recurring after treatment (**tertiary**).

Intraabdominal abscess: an abscess within the peritoneal cavity, retroperitoneal space, or abdominal viscera.
Cholecystitis: inflammation of the gallbladder.
Cholangitis: inflammation of the biliary tree.
Pancreatitis: inflammation of the pancreas.

Peritonitis

- **Primary peritonitis** (spontaneous bacterial peritonitis): where infection is not directly related to intraabdominal pathology.
- **Secondary peritonitis**: where intraabdominal pathology results in infection.
- **Tertiary peritonitis**: a later stage disease occurring when clinical peritonitis persists or recurs following treated secondary disease.
- **Peritoneal dialysis (PD)-associated peritonitis.**

Primary Peritonitis

Epidemiology

- Associated with liver cirrhosis and ascites.
- Risk factors: concomitant GI bleed, previous peritonitis, and low ascitic protein concentration.

- Three variants:
  - **Culture-negative neutrocytic ascites**, associated with difficult-to-culture organisms (*M. tuberculosis*) and noninfective causes.
  - **Monomicrobial nonneutrocytic bacterascites**, reflecting early bacterial colonization of ascitic fluid (85% progress to infection).
  - **Polymicrobial bacterascites**, usually from traumatic paracentesis.

Microbiology

- Usually **endogenous monomicrobial** infection caused by enteric flora.
- **Anaerobes and yeasts are uncommon** due to bacteriostatic properties in ascites.
- *Streptococcus pneumoniae* associated with HIV and prepubertal girls (ascending infection from genital tract).
- TB and dimorphic fungi in at-risk individuals.

Pathogenesis

- Bacterial spread via lymph, blood, or transmural migration from gastrointestinal (GI) or urogenital tract.
- TB peritonitis usually arises from hematogenous spread or rarely follows rupture of intraabdominal lymph nodes.

Secondary Peritonitis

Microbiology

- Polymicrobial infection
  - Organisms reflect anatomical location of pathology.
- Infrequent
  - *N. gonorrhoeae.*
  - *C. trachomatis.*
  - TB.

- Immunocompromised patients may undergo spontaneous bowel perforation involving opportunistic pathogens (*Strongyloides stercoralis*, cytomegalovirus [CMV]).

Pathogenesis

- Secondary to **intraabdominal mucosal breaches,** which leak organisms/chemicals into the peritoneal cavity, leading to inflammation and infection.

Tertiary Peritonitis

- Uncommon.
- Risk factors: age, underlying etiology, malnutrition, and multidrug-resistant organisms.

Microbiology

- Typically opportunistic and low-virulence organisms (e.g., enterococci, fungi).
- Multidrug resistance more common in nosocomial infection.

Pathogenesis

- Failed source control.
- Inadequate treatment of peritonitis.
- Impaired host response.

PD-Peritonitis

- Commonly complicates PD.
  - One episode per patient per year.
  - ≤70% patients experience first episode within first year.

Microbiology

- Commonly skin organisms (CoNS, *Staphylococcus aureus*, streptococci, diphtheroids).
- **Consider underlying bowel pathology if gram-negative organisms cultured.**

Pathogenesis

- Organism entry via **catheter, exit site**, dialysate fluid, or transmural migration.
- Exit-site and catheter-tunnel infections are major predisposing factors.

Clinical Presentation of Peritonitis

- Acute illness of fever and diffuse abdominal pain.
  - TB = indolent onset.
- PD-peritonitis = generalized abdominal pain, tenderness, and purulent peritoneal fluid. **Fever is infrequent** (10%).
- **Differential diagnosis:** appendicitis, pneumonia, diabetic ketoacidosis, porphyria, familial Mediterranean fever, SLE, uremia.

Diagnosis

- Leukocytosis (neutrophilia).
- Blood cultures and **paracentesis** (see Table 17.1).
- Imaging:
  - AXR = free air in perforation.
  - USS = ascites volume and abscess formation.
  - CT = source or evidence for other cause (e.g., TB and intraabdominal nodes.
- Surgical exploration required when diagnosis is unclear or for targeted biopsy.

Management

Primary Peritonitis

- **Treat empirically** if:
  - Gram stain or culture are positive (regardless of cell count).
    - 40% patients with positive culture and normal counts develop infection.
  - WCC >250 polymorphs/microliter (regardless of culture).
- **Antibiotics**
  - 10–14 days (typically).
    - 5-day courses have been shown to be efficacious.
  - Clinical response usually within 48 hours.
  - IP antibiotics are not effective.

Secondary and Tertiary Peritonitis

- Start empirical treatment immediately after cultures taken.
- Use broad-spectrum agents that penetrate peritoneum (e.g., β-lactams or quinolones).
- Antifungals if yeasts are seen.
- **Follow-up cell counts are useful but not essential.**

PD-Peritonitis

- Treat immediately if:
  - Symptomatic.
  - Peritoneal fluid is cloudy.
- **IP antibiotics are preferred** as infection is localized to the peritoneum (bacteremia is uncommon).
- Peritoneal inflammation increases systemic absorption of IP antibiotics. As levels are potentially variable IV antibiotics are recommended if evidence of systemic infection.
- No regimen is superior.
- Recommended treatment duration is **14–21 days** (or one week after catheter removal).
- Eosinophilic peritonitis is rare and a diagnosis of exclusion.

Prevention

Primary Peritonitis

- Patients who survive primary peritonitis have an **increased one-year probability of recurrence.**
- Antibiotic prophylaxis decreases recurrence in (i) concomitant GI bleed, (ii) pre-liver transplant, (iii) low ascitic protein levels but **does not confer a survival advantage.**

TABLE 17.1   Typical Pre-Treatment Peritoneal Fluid and Blood Culture Results In Peritonitis

	Peritonitis							
	Primary				Secondary	Tertiary	Peritoneal Dialysis (PD)	Tuberculosis (TB)
	Typical	CNNA	MNBA	PBA				
Leucocyte count[a] /µLr	≥250 PMN		<250 PMN		≥250 PMN	≥250 PMN	≥100 total[b] usually >50% PMN	150–4000 total usually lymphocytes
Gram	Variable[c]	Negative	Variable	Usually positive	Variable	Variable	Positive 10%–50%	Negative AAFB smear has low yield
Culture	Positive	Negative	Positive	Positive	Positive	Variable	Positive	Negative <20% culture positive
Organisms	Monomicrobial	Variable	Monomicrobial	Polymicrobial	Polymicrobial	Polymicrobial	Monomicrobial	Monomicrobial
Total protein	<1 g/dL	Variable	Normal	Normal	>1 g/dL	Variable	Variable	>3 g/dL
Glucose	≥2.8 mmol/L	Variable	Normal	Normal	<2.8 mmol/L	Variable	Variable	Low
LDH	Within serum range	Variable	Normal	Normal	>Serum	Variable	Variable	High (>90 U/ml)
Blood culture	75% positive	Negative	Negative	Negative	Negative	Negative	Negative	Negative

[a]Corrected PMN count should be calculated if aspirate is traumatic (bloody) due to entry of excess PMN: 1 PMN subtracted for every 250 RBC/mm³.
[b]Eosinophilia may be seen after tube placement (and rarely in some cases of fungal disease).
[c]Insensitive with high false-positive rate.
[d]Increase bacterial yield (up to 100%) if inoculated early into enrichment media.
CNNA, culture-negative neutrocytic ascites; LDH, lactate dehydrogenase; MNBA, monomicrobial non-neutrocytic bacterascites; PBA, polymicrobial bacterascites; PMN, polymorphonuclear leucocyte.
Note: Lactate and pH are unhelpful.

Secondary and Tertiary Peritonitis
- Preoperative antibiotics reduce peritonitis (30%–50% depending on surgery).
- No evidence to support continuing antibiotics >24 hours after operation (only increases resistance rates).

PD-Peritonitis
- Infection rates reduced by:
  - Prophylactic antibiotics prior to catheter intervention.
  - Training of patients in best technique.
  - Use of disconnect systems with "flush before fill" design.
  - Prompt treatment of exit-site or tunnel infections.
- Daily exit-site mupirocin is recommended by some.
- No evidence for choice of dialysate fluid.

Prognosis
Primary Peritonitis
- Poor prognosis in those with renal impairment, hypothermia, high bilirubin, or low albumin.
- **If poor response, consider complication** (perforation, intraabdominal abscess).

Secondary and Tertiary Peritonitis
- Survival depends on age, comorbidities, duration of illness, primary process, organisms involved.

PD-Peritonitis
- **Low mortality** (1%).
- Recurrent peritonitis, intractable infection (fungal, mycobacterial, *Pseudomonas aeruginosa*), and catheter failure are reasons to discontinue PD.

Inraabdominal Abscesses

Intraperitoneal Abscess
Microbiology
- **Polymicrobial infection** associated with bowel flora.

Pathogenesis
- Complicates intraabdominal disease, trauma, surgery.
- Location relates to site of primary disease.
- **Different pathogens play different roles**

| TABLE 17.2 | **Typical Diagnostic Features and Empirical Treatment of Inraabdominal Abscesses** | | | |

	Blood tests	Imaging	Sampling	Empirical Treatment[a]
Intraperitoneal Pancreas Liver (pyogenic)	Leukocytosis with raised inflammatory markers As above plus abnormal LFTs Blood cultures positive in 50% cases	USS, CT or MRI to identify abscess CXR may reveal a pleural effusion indicating subphrenic abscess	Radiologically guided aspiration for diagnosis confirmation, source control and culture. Also distinguishes pancreatic pseudocysts. Culture should be aerobically and anaerobically	Broad-spectrum IV agents targeting Enterobacteriaceae and anaerobes
Liver (amebic)	Leucocytosis (without eosinophilia) and raised inflammatory markers Abnormal LFTS (raised ALP in 80% cases) Amebic serology positive in up to 99% (negative up to day 7)[b]	USS/MRI most effective If appropriate, consider investigation for secondary cardiac, pulmonary, or CNS infection	Radiologically guided aspiration for microscopy and culture. Large lesions may require repeat aspiration. Brown foul-smelling (anchovy) fluid is characteristic Microscopy (± PCR) of abscess fluid and stool for *E. histolytica*	Metronidazole for hepatic stage plus intraluminal agent (diloxanide, paromomycin, iodoquinol)
Retroperitoneum or psoas muscle	Raised inflammatory markers	CT or MRI most effective	Radiologically guided aspiration for source control and culture but can be technically challenging	Broad spectrum IV agents targeting *S. aureus* and Enterobacteriaceae

[a]Start after blood cultures are taken.
[b]Cannot differentiate acute and previous infection
[c]Concomitant liver abscess and colitis is uncommon so stool microscopy (and PCR) usually negative.
ALP, alkaline phosphatase; CNS, central nervous system; CT, computed tomography; CXR, chest X-ray; IV, intravenous; LFTs, liver function tests; MRI, magnetic resonance imaging; USS, ultrasound scan.

- Coliforms involved in early infection.
- Anaerobes implicated in subsequent abscess formation.

Clinical Presentation
- **Fluctuating fevers**, rigors, and tenderness over affected area.
- Chronic presentations reported.

Diagnosis and Management (see Table 17.2)
- Drainage is fundamental for source control.
  - Percutaneous approach for accessible, avascular, unilocular collections.
  - Surgical intervention for multiple or loculated abscesses.

Prognosis
- Complications include extension of infection, fistula formation, or erosion of major blood vessels.

Pancreatic Abscess

Microbiology
- Commonly **polymicrobial** involving fecal flora.

Pathogenesis
- Complicates

- Pancreatitis (10%).
- Pancreatic penetration by a peptic ulcer.
- Secondary infection of pancreatic pseudocyst.
- Hematogenous seeding.

Clinical Presentation
- Fevers, rigors, and left upper quadrant (LUQ) tenderness.

Diagnosis and Management (see Table 17.2)
- Surgical intervention for local debridement.

Prognosis
- As per intraperitoneal infections.

Pyogenic Liver Abscess

- Most common visceral abscess
  - Incidence = 2.3 per 100,000.
- Associated with:
  - Men.
  - Diabetes.
  - Underlying hepatobiliary/pancreatic disease.
  - Chronic granulomatous disease.
  - Sickle cell anemia.

Microbiology

- Caused by **enteric bacteria,** including *Streptococcus milleri* group (*S. anginosus, S. intermedius, S. constellatus*).
- ***Klebsiella pneumoniae*** is an emerging pathogen (particularly in Asia).
  - Causes community-acquired liver abscess in the absence of hepatobiliary disease.
  - More common in diabetics and immunosuppressed patients with preceding antibiotic use.
  - Virulence associated with capsular serotype K1 causing a hypermucoviscous variant.
  - *Yersinia enterocolitica* and *Candida* spp. can cause disease in immunosuppressed patients.
  - Consider *Burkholderia pseudomallei* (causing melioidosis) in patients from Southeast Asia and Northern Australia.

Pathogenesis

- Bacterial spread from the biliary tree (multiple abscesses), portal vein, adjacent structures, hematogenous seeding, or hepatic trauma.
- The **right lobe** of the liver is commonly involved due to **larger size and greater blood supply** than other lobes.

Clinical Presentation

- Fever with right upper quadrant (RUQ) pain.

Diagnosis and Management (see Table 17.2)

- Treat for at least 1 month.
- Rationalizing antibiotics remains contentious as polymicrobial infection is common.
  - Many advocate broad-spectrum antibiotics despite culture of single sensitive organism.
  - While sampling is important, caution is advised if **hydatid disease** is possible (due to risk of seeding).
    - If appropriate, consider serological testing prior to sampling.
  - Serial imaging recommended to confirm resolution.
- Melioidosis requires intensive therapy followed by prolonged eradication:
  - Intensive therapy
    - ≥2 weeks IV ceftazidime, meropenem, or imipenem.
    - Some add co-trimoxazole, although lack of proven benefit.
  - Eradication therapy (recrudescence/relapse prevention):
    - ≥3 months oral co-trimoxazole (± doxycycline).
    - Alternatives include chloramphenicol and co-amoxiclav.

Prognosis

- Cure rates are >90% with early diagnosis and uncomplicated disease.
- Poor prognosis:
  - Open drainage.
  - Malignancy.

- Anaerobic infection.
- Overall mortality is 2%–12%.

Amebic Liver Abscess

- Most common extraintestinal manifestation (10%) of amebiasis.
- Highest prevalence in countries with suboptimal sanitation.
- **More common in men** (×10) despite equal gender distributions of colonic disease.
- Seen in migrants and travelers to endemic areas (India, Africa, Central and South America).
- **Disease is uncommon in short-term travelers,** but can occur after exposures as short as 4 days.
- Patients with **impaired cell-mediated immunity** are more likely to develop invasive disease.

Microbiology/Pathogenesis

- Caused by ***Entamoeba histolytica*** (protozoa).
- Main reservoir = humans.
- **Feco-oral route** transmission (suboptimal hygiene).
- **Increasing reports of sexual transmission.**
- Protozoa pass from gut into bloodstream and ascend to liver via the portal venous system, **usually affecting the right lobe.**

Clinical Presentation

- Frequently asymptomatic.
- **Symptoms occur 8–20 weeks** after primary infection.
- RUQ pain and fever.
- Jaundice, cough, sweating, and weight loss can be seen.
- **Amebic dysentery occurs in one-third.**

Diagnosis and Management (see Table 17.2)

- Treat with tissue agent followed by intraluminal agent.
- Tissue agents:
  - Metronidazole (7–10 days) or tinidazole (5 days).
    - High cure rate (>90%).
    - Excellent oral bioavailability.
  - Alternative: nitazoxanide (10 days).
- Intraluminal agents (to eliminate intraluminal cysts):
  - Paromomycin (7 days).
  - Diiodohydroxyquin (20 days).
  - Diloxanide furoate (10 days).
  - Availability of these drugs can be limited.
- **Give even if stool microscopy is negative.**
- **Aspiration may not be required** unless large lesion, threat of rupture, or failure of medical treatment.

Prognosis

- Complications
  - Rupture and spread (lungs, heart, brain).
  - Thrombosis of hepatic vein or inferior vena cava.
- Mortality of uncomplicated disease is <1%.

Hydatid Liver Abscess

See Chapter 4, Parasitology, and Chapter 35, Intestinal Nematodes.

Retroperitoneal and Psoas Abscesses

Microbiology

- *S. aureus* and coliforms are typically implicated.
- TB is recognized yet infrequent in developed countries.

Pathogenesis

- Most commonly metastatic spread via blood or lymphatics.
- Other
  - Direct extension from retroperitoneal structures.
  - Intraabdominal sepsis.
  - Traumatic hemorrhage.

Clinical Presentation

- **Challenging to detect clinically** as anatomically deep. Consequently, symptoms may be insidious/nonspecific.
- **Pain on hip flexion suggests psoas muscle involvement.**

Diagnosis and Management (see Table 17.2)

- Investigate source of metastatic spread even if blood cultures are negative.

Prognosis

- Poor prognosis:
  - Delayed or inadequate treatment.
  - Advanced age.
  - Bacteremia.
  - Relapse (15%–36%).
  - Can occur 1 year after infection.
  - Untreated, mortality rates can reach 100%.

Splenic Abscess

- See Splenic Infection.

Hepatobiliary Infection

Epidemiology

- Cholecystitis is almost universally associated with **gallstones** (>90%).
- Acute (or ascending) cholangitis associated with:
  - Gallstones.
  - Preceding intraabdominal surgery.
  - Hepatobiliary tumor.
- Cholangiopathy occurs in untreated people with HIV.

Pathogenesis

- Obstruction is a common feature.
  - Cholecystitis = cystic duct.
- Cholangitis = bile duct.
- Increasing intraductal pressure and impaired blood/lymphatic flow lead to stasis and infection.
- Hematogenous spread is rare.
- Mechanical irritation or recurrent attacks of acute cholecystitis lead to fibrosis, gallbladder thickening, and chronic cholecystitis.

Microbiology

- Commonly intestinal flora (**polymicrobial**).
- **Parasites may obstruct the biliary tree** leading to hepatobiliary infection, such as *Fasciola hepatica*, *Clonorchis sinensis*, *Opisthorchis* spp., and *Ascaris lumbricoides*.

Clinical Presentation

- Acute cholecystitis presents with fever and abdominal pain.
  - Early disease = mild epigastric pain alone.
  - Persistent obstruction = increasingly severe RUQ pain with signs of peritoneal irritation (shoulder tip pain) or pain below the right scapula (**Boas' sign**).
  - Gallbladder palpable in 30%–40%.
  - Positive **Murphy's sign** (pain on deep inspiration at the point of the gallbladder) supports diagnosis.
  - Acute cholangitis presents with **Charcot's triad** (85% cases): high fever, jaundice, and RUQ pain. Additional features of sepsis and confusion (**Reynolds' pentad**) indicates worsening of condition.
  - Chronic cholangitis ranges from asymptomatic to severe abdominal symptoms.
- **Differential diagnosis**: peptic ulcer disease, intestinal obstruction, appendicitis, acute hepatitis, perforated viscus, Fitz-Hugh–Curtis syndrome (perihepatitis secondary to gonorrheal infection), right lower lobe pneumonia, myocardial infarction.

Diagnosis

- Leukocytosis (neutrophilia).
- LFTs are frequently abnormal.
- Blood cultures are positive in one-third of cases of acute cholangitis.
- Radiology
  - Abdominal USS = modality of choice.
  - CT/MRI useful when USS is indeterminate.
  - CXR: gas in gallbladder is diagnostic of emphysematous cholecystitis.

Management

- Empirical antimicrobial treatment should cover polymicrobial infection.
  - Many recommend dual agents with different mechanisms of action.
- Common practice to **treat as polymicrobial infection** even if culture-negative or a single organism is isolated.
- Most cases of acute cholecystitis settle within 4 days.
  - Consider suppurative cholangitis in those patients who fail to defervesce.

- Decompression by ERCP or surgery is often required.
- Cholecystectomy after infection is advocated by some, yet no difference in morbidity between early and delayed surgery.

Prognosis

- Antibiotics do not affect outcome or incidence of complications.
- Complications arise in 10%–15% (see Box 17.1).
- Prompt surgery if:
  - Gangrenous.
  - Emphysematous cholecystitis.
  - Perforation.
  - Abscess formation.
  - Mortality for acute cholecystitis and cholangitis is 10%–30%, increasing in complicated disease.

Pancreatitis

- Pancreatic inflammation can be sudden (acute pancreatitis [AP]) or progressive (chronic pancreatitis [CP]).

Epidemiology

- AP is common.
  - 5–35 per 100,000 population.
  - Incidence increasing due to:
    - Alcohol consumption.
    - Better diagnostics.
- Independent risk factors
  - Age (four-fold increase between ages 25 and 75).
  - Increased abdominal fat (not BMI).
  - Gallstones.
  - Excess alcohol consumption.
  - Smoking.
  - Black ethnicity.

Microbiology

- Primary infections (see Box 17.2).

• BOX 17.1 Complications of Hepatobiliary Infections

- Sepsis
- Gallbladder empyema
- Emphysematous (or gangrenous) cholecystitis (elderly, diabetic men)
- Gallbladder perforation
- Hepatic duct obstruction caused by extrinsic compression from an impacted stone in the cystic duct or Hartmann's pouch of the gallbladder (**Mirizzi's syndrome**)
- Gallstone ileus
- Pericholecystic abscess
- Intraperitoneal abscess
- Cholecystoenteric fistula
- Cholangitis
- Liver abscess
- Pancreatitis
- Bacteremia

- Secondary infections (pancreatic superinfection) include:
  - Pancreatic abscesses.
  - Necrotic infection (enteric bacteria, fungi).

Pathogenesis

- Causes of AP include:
- **Blockage** of biliary tree (gallstones, cancer, strictures).
- **Organisms** and **antimicrobial agents** (see Boxes 17.2 and 17.3).
- Drugs and toxins: **alcohol**, thiazides, sulfasalazine, valproate, aspirin, estrogen, organophosphate poisoning, and venom (via cholinergic stimulation) from brown recluse spider, scorpions, and Gila monster lizard.
- Metabolic: high lipids and calcium.

• BOX 17.2 Infective Organisms Implicated in Pancreatic Infection

Infective Organisms	Causing Acute Pancreatitis	Pancreatic Abscesses Without Acute Pancreatitis
Bacteria	Legionella	Actinomyces spp.
	Leptospira	Mycobacterium avium
	Mycoplasma	Mycobacterium tuberculosis
	Salmonella typhi	Nocardia asteroides
Viruses	Coxsackie	
	CMV	
	HBV	
	HSV	
	Echovirus	
	Mumps	
	VZV	
	HIV	
Fungi	Aspergillus	Candida spp.
		Coccidioides immitis
		Cryptococcus neoformans
		Histoplasma capsulatum
		Paracoccididioides brasiliensis
		Phycomyces
		PCP
Parasites	Ascaris	Clonorchis spp.
	Cryptosporidium	Echinococcus granulosus
	Toxoplasma	Entamoeba histolytica
		Leishmania donovani
		Paragonimus westermani
		Schistosoma hematobium
		Strongyloides stercoralis

BOX 17.3 Antimicrobial Agents Causing Acute Pancreatitis (rare, 0.3%–1.4%)

Type of Antimicrobial	Agents
Antibiotics	Beta-lactams including ampicillin, penicillin, ceftriaxone
	Isoniazid
	Macrolides including erythromycin, clarithromycin, roxithromycin
	Metronidazole
	Nitrofurantoin
	Rifampin
	Sulfonamides including co-trimoxazole
	Tetracyclines
Antivirals	Didanosine
	Interferon/ribavirin
	Nelfinavir
	Ritonavir
Antifungals and others	5-Fluorouracil
	Pentamidine
	Stibogluconate

- Trauma: penetrating injury or post-ERCP.
- Vascular.
- Pregnancy and congenital.
- Specific conditions: renal transplant, α1-antitrypsin deficiency.
- Toxic materials (enzymes, vasoactive substances) injure pancreatic cells leading to increasing vascular permeability and pancreatic swelling.
- Disruption of microcirculation leads to necrosis, which liquefies into collections.
  - Two-thirds remain sterile, developing into pseudocysts.
  - One-third become infected with gut flora (usually >7 days) and develop into abscess.
  - **No correlation between extent of necrosis and risk of infection.**
- Recurrent AP causes CP.

Clinical Presentation

- Acute severe epigastric pain radiating to the back.
- **Secondary infected necrosis should be suspected in those who acutely deteriorate or fail to respond after 7 days.**
- CP = episodic flares with impairment of endocrine and exocrine function (diabetes, malabsorption).
- **Differential diagnosis**: peptic ulcer disease, gallstones, cholangitis, cholecystitis, perforated viscus, intestinal obstruction, mesenteric ischemia, hepatitis.

Diagnosis

- Diagnosis of AP requires two of three criteria:
  - Appropriate history.
  - Elevated serum amylase (or lipase).
  - Characteristic findings on imaging.

- Severity assessment
  - Ranson's criteria.
  - APACHE II.
  - Procalcitonin may have a role in predicting severity and risk of developing infected necrosis.
- Biochemical testing:
  - LFTs (ALT ×3 upper limit of normal = 95% PPV for gallstone pancreatitis).
  - Triglycerides.
  - Calcium.
  - Fasting glucose.
  - β-HCG in premenopausal women.
- Blood culture should be taken if signs of systemic infection (20% develop extrapancreatic infection).
- Imaging:
  - Abdominal USS = inflammation or cyst formation.
  - CT/MRI can diagnosis pancreatitis and identify cause and complications.
    - Pancreatic calcification is common in CP.
    - MRI has a higher sensitivity (compared with CT) to detect early AP.
    - Necrosis will lack contract enhancement.
- Tissue sampling is recommended if:
  - Infected necrosis.
  - Persistent systemic toxicity in the first 7–14 days.
  - Abscess formation.

Management

- Supportive.
- ERCP may be warranted to relieve obstruction.
- **No consensus on prophylactic antimicrobials** (including selective digestive decontamination) due to inconsistencies among trials. Although **currently not recommended,** surveys show that 88% of surgeons in UK/Ireland prescribe preemptive antibiotics in AP.
- Antibiotic use in necrotizing pancreatitis is controversial as identifying infected necrosis can be challenging in a patient already in an inflammatory state.
  - When indicated, the choice should take into account ability to penetrate necrotic tissue at appropriate levels (Table 17.3).
  - Initial studies treated infected necrosis with imipenem, but there is no evidence that other broad-spectrum β-lactams are inferior to carbapenems.
  - Debridement of necrosis is often necessary although the timing is debatable (prompt removal vs. stable patient and demarked tissue).
  - Recurrent pancreatitis frequently requires analgesia and endocrine/exocrine replacement therapy.

Prognosis

- Most patients recover from AP in 3–5 days without complications.
  - 20% will develop severe disease.
- Overall mortality rates are 5%.
  - Increases to 40% in patients with pancreatic necrosis.

TABLE 17.3	**Antimicrobial Penetration Into Necrotic Tissue**	
Agents Reaching MIC to Most Relevant Organisms		**Agents that Poorly Penetrate Necrotic Tissue**
• Cefepime • Ceftazidime • Chloramphenicol • Clindamycin • Doxycycline	• Fluconazole • Fluoroquinolones • Imipenem • Metronidazole	• Aminoglycosides • Ampicillin • Cefoxitin • First-generation cephalosporins

Splenic Infection

Epidemiology

- Abscess is the most common manifestation.
  - Bimodal age distribution (3rd and 6th decade).
    - Associated with infective endocarditis (IE), trauma, sickle cell disease, intravenous drug use (IVDU), immunosuppression.
- Risk factors for other splenic infections relate to pathogen exposure and immunosuppression.

Microbiology

- Splenic abscesses are frequently monomicrobial.
  - Commonly involving *S. aureus*, streptococcal spp., or Enterobacteriaceae.
    - Anaerobes are infrequently isolated.
- *Salmonella*, fungi (*Candida*, *Aspergillus*, mucor) and mycobacteria (TB, atypical) are emerging pathogens in immunosuppressed patients.
  - Melioidosis should be suspected in at-risk patients.
- Nonabscess splenic infection (Table 17.4).

Pathogenesis

- Splenic abscesses develop by:
  - **Hematogenous seeding is most common** (IE, IVDU, rarely genitourinary/gastrointestinal tract, surgical wounds).
  - Splenic infarction (trauma, sickle cell disease).
  - Direct extension of intraabdominal infection.
- Nonabscess infections arise from direct invasion of splenic cells or vasculature.

Clinical Presentation

- Abscesses
  - Fever (95%).
  - Abdominal pain, either generalized or localized to LUQ with radiation to the left shoulder.
  - **Splenomegaly occurs in about 50%.**
- Nonabscess (see Table 17.4).

Diagnosis (see Table 17.4)

- Leukocytosis is common.
- Blood cultures are positive in IE (persistent bacteremia).
- Imaging
  - ≤80% patients with splenic abscess have CXR abnormalities:
    - Raised left hemi-diaphragm.
    - Pleural effusion.
    - Infiltrates.
  - **USS** is a **sensitive** (93%) method to detect splenic abscesses.
  - **Fungal infections have varying appearances:**
    - Wheel within a wheel.
    - Bull's-eye lesion.
    - Uniformly hypoechoic nodules.
    - Multiple small echogenic micro-abscesses.
  - CT/MRI
    - **Abscesses can resemble infarcts**, particularly wedge-shaped abscess seen in patients with septic emboli.
    - TB can appear as LN enlargement, intestinal wall thickening, and ascites.
  - Image-guided FNA for culture and histology is valuable when diagnosis uncertain.

Management

- Antimicrobial agents alone are rarely curative.
  - Broad-spectrum agents should be started after sampling.
  - Optimum route and duration has not been established.
  - **Common practice is to treat for up to 6 weeks with IV therapy.**
  - Consideration for oral switch depends on:
    - Source control.
    - Pathogen(s) identified.
    - Resolution of biochemical abnormalities and radiological response.
- Drainage for culture and source control.
  - Most successful for small (<3.5 cm) solitary lesions.
- Splenectomy remains gold standard for treatment
  - Commonly reserved for large or multiple splenic abscesses and those who fail conservative measures. (See Chapter 45 for management of the asplenic patient).
- Management of other splenic infections will depend on underlying etiology (Table 17.4).

Prognosis

- Complications of splenic abscess include perforation into peritoneum and adjacent organs.
- Complications of nonabscess infections are shown in Table 17.4.
- All-cause mortality is up to 14%, with higher rates in immunosuppressed and untreated.

TABLE 17.4 Summary of Splenic Infections That Classically Do Not Cause Abscess Formation

Condition	Pathogen(s)	Vector	Risk Factors
Infection Affecting Blood Flow			
Schistosomiasis	S. mansoni S. japonicum S. mekongi	Snail	Fresh water exposure in endemic areas
Echinococcosis	See Liver abscess section		
Response to Infection			
Infectious mononucleosis	EBV CMV	Human	More common in adolescence
Hyper-reactive malarial splenomegaly[a]	P. vivax, P. malariae, rare with P. falciparum, P. ovale	Anopheles mosquito	Long-term resident in endemic countries[b]
Trypanosomiasis	T. cruzi causing Chagas disease	Triatomine ("kissing") bug	Long-term resident in Central and South America
	T. brucei complex causing African sleeping sickness	Tsetse fly	Long-term resident in West (T. brucei gambiense) or East (T. brucei rhodesiense) Africa
Brucellosis	B. abortus, B. suis B. melitensis	Cattle, pig, goat, sheep	Exposure to infected animals and unpasteurized dairy product, particularly in Africa and the Middle East
Ehrlichiosis	E. ewingii, E. chaffeensis	Lone star tick	Exposure in endemic areas (USA)
Visceral leishmaniasis (Kala-azar)	L. donovani spp., L. infantum, L. chagasi, rarely, L. amazonensis or L. tropica	Sandfly	Long-term resident in endemic areas, HIV
Mycobacterial granuloma	M. tuberculosis complex including M. tuberculosis, M. africanum, M. orygis, M. bovis, M. microti, M. canettii, M. caprae, M. pinnipedii, M. suricattae, M. mungi	Humans Also found in animal reservoirs (e.g., cattle, badgers)	HIV, immunosuppression, latent TB, homeless, IVDU, resident in endemic area
	M. avium complex including M. avium and M. intracellulare	Ubiquitous in environment	HIV, immunosuppression

[a]Caused by chronic antigen stimulation. Also known as tropical splenomegaly syndrome.
[b]Particularly Eastern Indonesia and Papuan highlands.

Key features	Diagnosis	Treatment	Complications
Katayama fever Eosinophilia	Serology Eggs in feces	Praziquantel	Involvement of other organs
Fever, sore throat, lymphadenopathy	Atypical lymphocytes, heterophile antibodies, serology (± viral load)	Supportive	Splenic rupture Hematological and neurological abnormalities
Massive splenomegaly symptoms relating to size	Blood film,[c] RDT, PCR macroglobulinemia,[d] hypersplenism	Antimalarial therapy (during exposure), splenectomy	Hemolytic anemia, splenic rupture, latent infection, severe malaria
Acute Chagas disease, cardiac, or GI disease	Wet prep or Giemsa stain of blood or other tissue sample in acute disease	Nifurtimox or benznidazole in acute disease, supportive therapy in chronic disease	Bradyarrhythmias Megaesophagus
Chancre, posterior cervical lymphadenopathy (Winterbottom's sign), neurological symptoms	Serology and PCR in chronic disease	Treatment depends on species and stage of disease Melarsoprol, pentamidine, suramin, eflornithine	Side-effects of treatment, high failure rate
Undulant fevers, malodourous perspiration, osteoarticular disease (sacroiliitis), depression	Radiology,[e] culture (blood/bone marrow), serology, or PCR on blood. Die inhibition tests rarely used	Doxycycline plus gentamicin, streptomycin or rifampicin Minimum 6 weeks	Chronic disease
Headache, myalgia, fever	Serology, PCR on blood	Doxycycline Chloramphenicol	Opportunistic infection[f]
Massive splenomegaly, discoloration of skin[g]	Biopsy (spleen, bone marrow, lymph node or liver). Amastigotes may be seen with Wright or Giemsa stain, PCR on tissue	Pentavalent antimony compounds (sodium stibogluconate), liposomal amphotericin, miltefosine	Hemorrhage Secondary infections
Fevers, weight loss, night sweats	Tuberculin skin test, IGRA, sampling, and culture	Standard therapy. MDR-TB requires expert involvement	Disseminated disease, side effects of treatment Compliancy of medication (may require directly observed therapy)
PUO, pulmonary disease in elderly women (Lady Windermere syndrome), lymphadenitis in children	Sampling for culture	Usually 3 agents (macrolide, rifampicin, ethambutol) for 12 months	Side effects of treatment, relapse

[c] Although parasitemia is uncommon.
[d] Overproduction of IgM
[e] Pedro pons sign = preferential erosion of anterior-superior corner of lumbar vertebrae giving parrot beak appearance.
[f] Via tumor-necrosis factor-alpha suppression.
[g] Kala-azar = black fever.
CMV, cytomegalovirus; EBV, Epstein–Barr virus; IGRA, interferon gamma release assay; MDR-TB, multi-drug resistant tuberculosis; PCR, polymerase chain reaction; PUO, pyrexia of unknown origin; RDT, rapid diagnostic test.

Further Reading

1. Bennett JE, Dolin R, Blaser MJ, eds. *Mandell, Douglas, and Bennett's Principles and Practice of Infectious Diseases.* 8th ed. Philadelphia: Elsevier; 2015.

2. Török E, Moran E, Cooke F, eds. *Oxford Handbook of Infectious Diseases and Microbiology.* 2nd ed. Oxford: Oxford University Press; 2017.

Websites
Centers for Disease Control and Prevention, www.cdc.gov
ClinicalKey, www.clinicalKey.com
UpToDate, www.uptodate.com

18

Obstetric and Gynecologic Infections

KATIE OVENS

Lower Genital Tract Infections

Lower genital tract infections affect the vulva, vagina, and cervix (see Tables 18.1 and 18.2). They can be classified by the causative organism or by the affected site.

Bacterial Vaginosis (BV)

Epidemiology

- Commonest cause of an abnormal vaginal discharge.
- More commonly affects African-American women than non-Hispanic white women.

Pathogenesis

- **Alteration in the normal flora of the vagina** from lactobacilli to gram-negative rods (e.g., *Mobiluncus* sp.) and gram-variable rods and cocci (e.g., *Gardnerella vaginalis*, *Prevotella* spp., *Porphyromonas* spp.).
- It is not currently believed to be sexually transmitted.

Clinical Features

- Asymptomatic.
- Malodorous (**fishy**), thin, grey vaginal discharge.
- Pregnancy: may cause miscarriage or preterm labor.

Investigations

- Clinically suspicious odor.
- pH >4.5.
- Microscopy will show:
  1. Clue cells (vaginal epithelial cells with attached coccobacilli) (Fig. 18.1).
  2. Reduced lactobacilli.
  3. Mixed bacterial flora.
- BV is graded using:
  a. Clinical criteria (Amsel's criteria).
  b. Microscopy (Nugent or Hay/Ison criteria).

Management

- General advice
  - Avoid douching.
  - Use soap substitutes.

- **Smoking cessation.**
- No benefit of treating sexual partners.
- Encourage **condom use.**
- **Metronidazole** single dose or 5-7 day course
  - Caution: avoid stat dose if pregnant or breastfeeding.
  - Do not consume alcohol.
- Metronidazole vaginal gel or clindamycin vaginal cream.
  - Caution: clindamycin may weaken condoms.
- Alternatives: oral tinidazole or clindamycin.

Trichomonas Vaginalis (TV)

See Chapter 21, Sexually Transmitted Infections.

Vulvovaginal Candidiasis

Epidemiology

- Very common.
- Higher prevalence with recent antibiotic therapy, immunosuppression, diabetes mellitus, pregnancy, steroid use, hormone replacement therapy (HRT); intrauterine device (IUD), spermicide or condom use, and the combined oral contraceptive pill.

Pathogenesis

- Caused by commensal yeasts entering the vulvo-vaginal mucosa.
- May be caused by:
  - *Candida albicans* (most common) (Fig. 18.2).
  - *Candida glabrata.*
  - *Candida krusei.*
  - *Candida tropicalis.*

Clinical Features

- Asymptomatic.
- Vulvo-vaginal pruritus.
- **White curd-like vaginal discharge.**
- Inflammation.
- Fissures.
- Dysuria and dyspareunia.

TABLE 18.1	**Vulvitis, Vaginitis, and Cervicitis**		
	Vulvitis	**Vaginitis**	**Cervicitis**
Epidemiology	Common	Very common	Common among **sexually active** females
Noninfectious causes	• Vulvar dermatitis • Vulvar intraepithelial neoplasm (associations with human papilloma virus and HIV) • Vulvodynia (may have infective triggers) • Vulvar lichen sclerosis • Vulvar vestibulitis	• Allergy • Atrophic vaginitis • Irritants	• Trauma • Inflammatory conditions • Irritants • Iatrogenic • Malignancy
Infectious causes	• *Candida* spp. • *Trichomonas vaginalis* • Ulcerative causes such as herpes simplex virus or syphilis (not covered in this chapter) • Group B and D streptococcus (more commonly associated with vaginitis)	• Candidiasis • *Trichomonas vaginalis* • Herpes simplex virus (HSV) • Group B and Group D streptococcus • Bacterial vaginosis	• *Chlamydia trachomatis* • *Neisseria gonorrhoeae* • *Mycoplasma genitalium* • Herpes simplex virus • *T. vaginalis* • Streptococci (rare)
Clinical features of infectious causes	• Discharge • **Pruritus** • Vulvar inflammation • Vulvar edema • Vulvodynia	• Vaginal discharge • Dysuria • Vulvodynia, dyspareunia, or abdominal pain • Pruritus • Vaginal inflammation	• May be asymptomatic • Discharge • **Dyspareunia** • **Postcoital or intermenstrual bleeding** • Dysuria • Cervical inflammation • Evidence of pelvic inflammatory disease (PID)
Investigations	• Vulvar swab for MC&S • Vulvar PCR multiplex swab (if ulceration present) • Consider vulvar biopsy (for noninfectious causes such as vulvar intraepithelial neoplasia [VIN]) • Consider sexual health screen	• Sexual health screen • Vaginal pH • Lateral vaginal wall swab for microscopy • Consider high vaginal swab for MC&S • Posterior fornix swab for wet mount microscopy (for *T. vaginalis*) • Consider *Candida* culture	• Pregnancy test • Endocervical/vaginal **microscopy** • Endocervical culture • HSV swab if suspected • Sexual health screen

MC&S, microscopy, culture, and sensitivities; PCR, polymerase chain reaction.

Investigations

- High vaginal swab (anterior fornix).
- Microscopy (wet prep and Gram stain).
- Culture.

Management

- Only treat symptomatic patients.
- Topical azole, e.g., clotrimazole pessary or vaginal cream (however, many other azole and non-azole preparations are available).
  - Be aware that some topical azoles may weaken condoms and diaphragms.
  - In pregnancy: use 7 days topical imidazoles.
- Oral fluconazole or itraconazole (not suitable if pregnant or breastfeeding).
- *Candida krusei* is intrinsically resistant to fluconazole.
- If recurrent, consider host factors.

- Tight glycemic control reduces frequency of infection in those with diabetes.
- Treatment of partners is not recommended.
- Nonpharmacologic
  - Avoid tight underwear.
  - Avoid perfumed products.
  - Use soap substitutes.

Female Pelvic Infections

Pelvic Inflammatory Disease (PID)

Epidemiology

- About 1 million cases/year in the United States.
- Most common in the **younger age groups** (15–25 years) and those with **previous history** of a sexually transmitted infection.

TABLE 18.2	Treatment Options for Vulvovaginal and Cervical Infections		
Pathogen	**Management of uncomplicated infection**	**Pregnancy**	**Partner Notification and Treatment**
Chlamydia trachomatis	1st = Doxycycline (or azithromycin) Alternative: erythromycin or ofloxacin	Azithromycin, erythromycin, or amoxicillin	Required

Neisseria gonorrhoeae	Ceftriaxone IM
	Alternatives:
	• Azithromycin alone if no other alternative option (concerns regarding resistance with the use of macrolides)
	• Azithromycin with either:
	  • Cefixime
	  • Spectinomycin
	  • Gentamicin
	• If sensitivities known then ciprofloxacin can be used
		Ceftriaxone IM
		Alternative:
		• Spectinomycin IM
		• Azithromycin stat if no other alternative
			Required

Mycoplasma genitalium	Doxycycline for 7 days followed by azithromycin for 3 days Alternative: Moxifloxacin	Azithromycin	Required
Herpes simplex virus	Aciclovir Alternatives: • Valaciclovir • Famciclovir	See Fig. 18.2	Not required

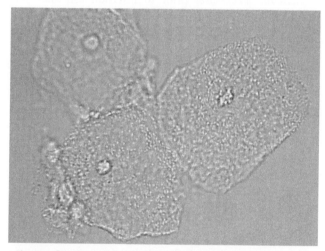

• **Fig. 18.1** Clue cells. The squamous epithelial cells shown have refractile bacteria plastered over their surfaces, a morphologic appearance called clue cells (their appearance is a clue to the diagnosis) and indicative of bacterial vaginosis. Normal vaginal flora includes large gram-positive rods of lactobacilli. Bacterial vaginosis includes gram-negative cocci of *Gardnerella* spp. and small curved rods of *Mobiluncus* spp. Inflammatory cells and infectious agents such as *Candida albicans*, trichomonads, and clue cells of bacterial vaginosis (e.g., *Gardnerella vaginalis*) can be seen on a Pap smear. (From Klatt EC. *Robbins and Cotran Atlas of Pathology*. 3rd ed. Elsevier; 2015.)

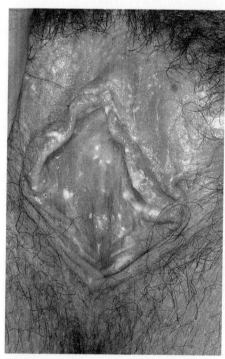

• **Fig. 18.2** *Candida albicans*. (From Dinulos JGH. Fungal infections. In Habif TS, Dinulos JGH, Chapman MS, Zug KA. *Skin Disease: Diagnosis and Treatment*. 4th ed. Elsevier; 2018.)

Pathogenesis

• Less than half of PID cases are caused by *Chlamydia trachomatis* and *Neisseria gonorrhoeae*.
• Other possible causative organisms include:
  • *Gardnerella vaginalis*.
  • *Mycoplasma genitalium*.
  • *Mycoplasma hominis*.
  • *Streptococcus agalactiae*.
  • *Trichomonas vaginalis*.
  • *Ureaplasma urealyticum*.
  • Anaerobic bacteria.

Clinical Features

- Discharge: typically malodorous and purulent.
- Abnormal vaginal bleeding.
- Bilateral pelvic/lower abdominal pain.
- **Deep dyspareunia.**
- Bimanual examination: **adnexal tenderness and cervical motion tenderness.**
- Systemic features
  - Pyrexia.
  - Peritonitis.
  - Sepsis.
  - Fitz-Hugh–Curtis syndrome.
- Can be asymptomatic.

Investigations

- Clinical diagnosis.
- BHCG (to exclude an ectopic pregnancy).
- Bloods, including FBC and CRP/ESR.
- Endocervical or vaginal microscopy.
- Endocervical culture and sensitivities.
- Sexual health screen including *Mycoplasma genitalium* test if possible.

Management

- Exclude differential diagnoses for lower abdominal pain (and consider surgical or gynecology review).
- Empirical antibiotic treatment.
- **Partner notification and treatment of partners** (must both abstain until treatment is completed).
- Multiple outpatient antibiotic regimes available; however, the most common regime in the UK is:
  - IM ceftriaxone stat then 14 days of oral doxycycline and metronidazole.
  - Second line agents include moxifloxacin, ofloxacin and azithromycin +- metronidazole.
  - Avoid quinolones if suspecting gonorrhea.
  - Avoid macrolides if suspecting *Mycoplasma genitalium*.
- If IV required (again multiple regimes are available but the most commonly used UK regime is):
  - IV ceftriaxone and doxycycline followed by oral doxycycline and metronidazole (14 days).
- **Consider admission** for IV antibiotics and surgical review in patients with:
  - Severe disease.
  - Tubo-ovarian abscess.
  - Poor response to oral antibiotics.
  - Pregnancy (can use IV/IM ceftriaxone with IV/oral erythromycin [+ metronidazole]).
- Surgical interventions may be required (e.g., abscess drainage or adhesiolysis).

Intrauterine Device (IUD)-Associated Infections
Definitions

- Early: 0 to 7 days postinsertion.
- Late: 7 days to 3 months postinsertion.

Epidemiology

- **PID following insertion is rare** (<1% in the Mirena coil), but clinicians should have a low threshold for treating for PID.

Pathogenesis

- As per PID, plus:
  - *Fusobacterium.*
  - *Peptostreptococcus.*
  - *Actinomyces* infection.

Clinical Features

- As per PID.

Investigations

- As per PID, plus:
  - β-HCG.
  - Ultrasound (if persistent symptoms).
  - If IUD removed, send for microscopy, culture, and sensitivities (including prolonged culture for *Actinomyces* spp.).

Management

- See PID section.
- Vulvo-vaginal NAAT for *Chlamydia trachomatis* and *Neisseria gonorrhoeae* prior to insertion can allow for infections to be treated before insertion.
- Consider IV antibiotics in severe infection or if symptoms not resolving.
- Limited evidence regarding removal of an IUD in the presence of PID and the risks/benefits need to be assessed on an individual basis. However, **consider removal if:**
  - *Actinomyces* infection (which thrives on foreign bodies).
  - Symptoms not resolving on review at 48-72 hours.
  - Moderate to severe infection.
- Consider emergency contraception if removing an IUD.

Postabortion Sepsis
Epidemiology

- More common after **induced abortion.**
- Rare in spontaneous abortion.

Complications

- Arise due to potential for retained products of conception, plus bladder/bowel injury.
- Associated with:
  - Salpingitis.
  - Peritonitis.
  - Septicemia.
  - High morbidity and mortality.

Pathogenesis

- Most common pathogens: *Escherichia coli*, *Staphylococcus aureus*, *Enterobacter aerogenes*, hemolytic streptococci, *Proteus vulgaris*.

- Other pathogens: anaerobic bacteria (e.g., *Clostridium perfringens*) or fungi. *C. perfringens* is associated with a high mortality.
- Tetanus in induced abortion performed in nonsterile environments.
- Can be caused by a combination of organisms.

Clinical Features

- Fever.
- Vaginal bleeding and loss of birth products.
- Vaginal discharge.
- Abdominal pain.
- Examination: signs of sepsis/septic shock; tender abdomen with evidence of peritonitis; tender bimanual examination; dilated os.

Investigations

- Septic screen.
- βHCG.
- Pelvic ultrasound.
- Consider computed tomography (CT)/magnetic resonance imaging (MRI) abdomen and pelvis.

Management

- Stabilization of the patient if hemodynamically unstable.
- Broad-spectrum antibiotics as per local guidelines and likely causative organism.
  - e.g., Amoxicillin + gentamicin + clindamycin.
- Urgent **surgical evacuation of intrauterine products** (ensure endometrial tissue sent for culture).
- Hysterectomy and bilateral salpingo-oophorectomy may be indicated if there is:
  - Air within the uterine wall.
  - Pelvic crepitations.
  - Discolored uterus/adnexa.
  - *Clostridium* (suspected or proven).
- Consider tetanus vaccine.

Postpartum Endometritis

Definition

- Endometrial infection in the postpartum period (**within 10 days following delivery**).
- Commonest cause of postpartum fever.

Epidemiology

- More common following:
  - **Cesarean section (C-section)** (up to 27% in comparison to 1%–3% of vaginal births).
  - Premature rupture of the membranes.
  - Preterm or postterm delivery.
  - Chorioamnionitis.
  - Prolonged labor.
  - Maternal anemia or diabetes.
  - Multiple vaginal examinations during labor.
  - Bacterial vaginosis.

Pathogenesis

- Transmission of vaginal bacteria into the uterus during delivery.
- **Usually polymicrobial.**
- Associated with multiple organisms
  - Group A and B streptococci.
  - Staphylococci.
  - *Mycoplasma hominis.*
  - Aerobic gram-negative rods.
  - *Neisseria gonorrhoeae* (uncommon).
  - *Chlamydia trachomatis* (uncommon).
  - *Gardnerella vaginalis.*
  - Anaerobic bacteria (e.g., *Bacteroides fragilis*, *Clostridium sordellii*, *Clostridium perfringens*).

Clinical Features

- Fever
  - ≥38.7 °C (0–24 hours following delivery).
  - ≥38.0 °C (24 hours to 10 days postdelivery).
  - Low-grade fever postpartum is common and believed to be physiologic rather than pathologic.
- Malodorous, purulent discharge.
- Abdominal and pelvic pain.
- Uterine bleeding.
- Complications include:
  - Abscess.
  - Toxic shock syndrome.
  - Peritonitis.
  - Sepsis/septic shock.
  - Septic pulmonary emboli.
  - Myometritis.

Investigations

- Septic screen.
- Vulvo-vaginal swabs (including NAAT for *Chlamydia*, *Gonorrhea*, and *Mycoplasma genitalium*).
- Cervical cultures and swabs.
- **Imaging** to identify pelvic collections or retained products of conception.

Management

- IV antibiotics such as:
  - Clindamycin + gentamicin.
- Failure to respond to antibiotic therapy may be due to enterococcal infection, resistant anaerobes, abscess formation, or septic thrombophlebitis.

Chorioamnionitis

Definition

- Inflammation of membranes and placenta due to ascending bacterial infection.
- Also known as intraamniotic infection.

Epidemiology

- 1%–4% of all births; 40%–70% of preterm births.

- Risk factors include:
  - Prolonged membrane rupture (including PPROM [preterm premature rupture of the membranes]).
  - Prolonged labor.
  - Smoking, alcohol, or drug abuse.
  - Multiple digital vaginal exams.
  - Internal monitoring of labor.
  - BV or colonization with group B streptococcus (GBS).
  - Nulliparity.

Pathogenesis

- Usually associated with polymicrobial bacterial infection with membrane rupture
  - **Ureaplasma urealyticum (47%), Mycoplasma hominis (30%)**, *Gardnerella vaginalis* (25%), *Bacteroides* spp. (30%), GBS (15%), *Escherichia coli* (8%).
  - Can occur with intact membranes.
  - Rarely hematogenous in origin.

Clinical Features

- Fever.
- Uterine fundal tenderness.
- Maternal and fetal tachycardia.
- Purulent or foul amniotic fluid.

Complications

- Increased C-sections (2–3×).
- Increased focal infection (endometritis, pelvic abscess, wound infection) (2–4×).
- 10% bacteremia (commonly GBS and *E. coli*).
- Increased PPH (dysfunctional uterine contractions due to inflammation) (2–4×).
- Fetal complications include death, neonatal sepsis, and multiorgan injury with long-term morbidities, including cerebral palsy and neurodevelopmental delay.

Investigations

- Amniotic fluid culture is gold standard, but not much use clinically due to time delay.

Management

- Broad-spectrum IV antibiotics
  - Amoxicillin + gentamicin + metronidazole.
  - Clindamycin + gentamicin in severe penicillin allergy.
  - *or* Co-amoxiclav, piperacillin/tazobactam, cefuroxime + metronidazole.

Urinary Tract Infections (UTI) during Pregnancy

Epidemiology

- Asymptomatic bacteriuria occurs in 2%–10% of pregnancies.
- Acute cystitis occurs in 1-2% of pregnancies.

Pathogenesis

- *Escherichia coli* (most common).
- Other gram-negative bacteria, e.g., *Proteus mirabilis*, and *Klebsiella* spp.
- Gram-positive bacteria, e.g., group B streptococci, *Staphylococcus saprophyticus*, *Staphylococcus aureus*.

Complications

- Asymptomatic bacteriuria and untreated cystitis cause increased maternal and fetal morbidity (odds ratios 1.3–2.2):
  - Pyelonephritis.
  - Pre-eclampsia.
  - Preterm delivery (<37 weeks gestation).
  - Low birthweight (<2.5kg).
  - Increased perinatal mortality.
  - Developmental delay.

Clinical Features

- Asymptomatic.
- Dysuria.
- Urinary frequency.
- Hematuria.
- Suprapubic tenderness.
- Pyrexia.
- Evidence of pyelonephritis.

Investigations

- Septic screen.
- Ultrasound kidney/ureter/bladder.
- Urine microscopy, culture and sensitivities.

Management

- Screen and treat asymptomatic infections.
- If GBS is isolated then prophylactic antibiotics are advised during labor and delivery.
- Treat according to local guidelines. Usually for 7 days.
  - Avoid nitrofurantoin in the 3rd trimester.
  - Avoid trimethoprim if the patient is on a folate antagonist, has used trimethoprim within the previous 12 months, or has a folate deficiency. Although widely used in 2nd and 3rd trimester, manufacturers advise against use in pregnancy.
  - Check sensitive before using amoxicillin due to rates of resistance.
- Antibiotics that are **NOT safe in pregnancy**:
  - Tetracyclines.
  - Sulfonamides.
  - Quinolones.
- Consider admission for parenteral antibiotics and fluid resuscitation if evidence of fever, failure to improve, sepsis, or pyelonephritis.
- Urine MC&S as a **test of cure**.

Other Infections Complicating Pregnancy

Complications of other infections in pregnancy, including herpes simplex virus, varicella-zoster virus, *Listeria*, Chagas disease, and Q fever, are covered in Chapter 20, Infections of Pregnancy.

Further Reading and Resources

1. Centers for Disease Control and Prevention (CDC), www.cdc.gov/.
2. British Association of Sexual Health and HIV (BASSH). Guidelines. Available from: www.bashh.org/guidelines.
3. Mackeen AD, Packard RE, Ota E, Speer L. Antibiotic regimens for postpartum endometritis. *Cochrane Database Syst Rev.* 2015;2:1–88.
4. Smaill FM, Vazquez JC. Antibiotics for asymptomatic bacteriuria in pregnancy. *Cochrane Database Syst Rev.* 2015;8:1–50.
5. NICE (National Institute for Health and Care Excellence). Urinary tract infection (lower) women. Available from: https://cks.nice.org.uk/urinary-tract-infection-lower-women#!scenario:3.

19

Genitourinary Tract Infection

AOIFE COTTER

Definitions and Terminology

Pyuria: 10 leucocytes per microscopic field or 5–10 per high-powered field in centrifuged sample; not indicative of presence or absence of infection.

Significant bacteriuria: 10^5 colony-forming units per mL and in two consecutive samples in women, or a single sample in men.

Asymptomatic bacteriuria: 10^5 colony-forming units per mL of urine. Treat only in the context of pregnancy, or if about to undergo invasive procedure of the genitourinary tract. Some experts treat in the setting of renal transplant especially early after transplant. With the exception of these situations, rarely proceeds to invasive infection.

Catheter-associated asymptomatic bacteriuria: absence of signs and symptoms of urinary tract infection and bacteriuria of 10^5 colony-forming units per mL.

Urinary tract infection (UTI): bacteriuria plus symptoms reflecting site of infection (i.e., lower or upper tract). May be difficult to determine in elderly patients who poorly localize symptoms and may only have delirium.

Cystitis: typical symptoms include: dysuria, urinary frequency, urinary urgency ± objective sign of suprapubic tenderness.

Catheter-associated UTI: signs and symptoms of urinary tract infection and bacteriuria of $>10^3$ colony-forming units per ml associated with a urinary catheter.

Acute pyelonephritis: typical symptoms: flank pain ± dysuria, urinary frequency and urgency; can present with objective signs of fever and renal angle tenderness.

Acute prostatitis: subjective complaint of peroneal or suprapubic pain ± dysuria, urinary frequency and urgency and can present with signs of sepsis including fever, usually significant prostatic tenderness on examination.

Urosepsis: evidence of UTI in association with signs of sepsis including fever, tachycardia, tachypnea, leukocytosis.

Cure: negative cultures on antibiotics.

Persistence: sustained significant bacteriuria of organism causing initial infection after 48 hours or lower levels beyond that time while on treatment.

Recurrences: include relapse or reinfection:

Relapse: bacteria determined to cause initial infection in post-treatment culture.

Reinfection: new infection can occur at any time, easier to identify if infection with different bacteria.

Papillary necrosis: complication of pyelonephritis that can lead to tract obstruction. Risk factors include diabetes mellitus or with obstruction, sickle cell disease.

Intrarenal abscess: typically a complication of bacteremia; also increasingly a recognized complication of ascending infection including pyelonephritis.

Perinephric abscess: a complication of pyelonephritis or bacteremia and pus/infection can extend into perinephric tissue and retroperitoneal space.

Urinary Tract Infection: Pathogenesis

Urinary tract infection (UTI) occurs when (virulent) bacteria overcome host defenses, including urinary tract structural defenses and host immunity.

Mode of Infection

1. **Ascending:** risk factors include sexual activity, spermicide use, catheterization, estrogen deficiency/postmenopausal state, structural abnormality.
2. **Hematogenous:** complication of *Staphylococcus aureus* bacteremia and fungemia with *Candida* species.

Virulence Factors

- *Escherichia coli*: common pathogen with some serogroups particularly implicated. These are termed uropathogenic *E. coli* (UPEC).
- Certain factors facilitate adherence to urinary tract epithelium and evasion of host immune defenses leading to successful invasion and consequent infection.
- Factors on *E. coli* cell surface include:
  - Adhesins: improve adherence to uroepithelium.
    - Filamentous surface structures: fimbriae.
    - Nonfilamentous proteins.
  - Other surface factors: aerobactin; capsular polysaccharide; cytotoxic necrotizing factor type 1; hemolysin; K surface antigen; siderophore receptor.
  - Toxins
    - α-hemolysin.

- Urease: organisms that produce urease split urea into CO_2 and ammonia, causing crystal formation and promoting bacterial adherence and raising pH.
  - Uropathogens that produce urease include *Proteus* spp., *Klebsiella* spp., *Pseudomonas* spp., *Staphylococcus aureus*, *Corynebacterium urealyticum*.

Host Defense

- Bladder and urine
  - Some antibacterial activity.
  - Low pH and osmolality driven by urea inhibit growth.
  - Epithelial cell secretion.
  - Flushing mechanism of bladder.
- Innate immunity
  - Inflammatory response led by cytokine production.
  - TLR4, IL-1β, IL-6, IL-8 implicated.
- Humoral immunity: little role in defense against UTI.
- **Structure**
  - Obstruction to urine outflow increases risk of infection by impairment mechanics of urine flow partially or completely and may be intra- or extrarenal.
  - Vesicoureteric reflux.

Epidemiology and Natural History

- UTI is more common in **women** than men and not infrequently recurs. Within 6 months, 60% of women have a second UTI.
- Men with UTI are considered as complicated UTI until obstruction of the urinary tract is excluded.
- UTI in children may cause significant renal scarring and chronic kidney disease while **UTI in adults rarely impacts renal function** unless there is an additional complication such as obstruction.
- UTI can be associated with **reversible impairment of concentrating ability** of kidney during infection that may **compromise antibiotic levels**/penetration.
- **Asymptomatic bacteriuria** is more frequent than UTI, **increases in prevalence with age** and in certain categories or subpopulations is associated with ascending infection and warrants treatment. In the majority, however, it is benign and does not require treatment.
- **Catheterization** is associated with a **10% risk** of subsequent development of UTI.
- **Risk factors** include:
  - Premenopausal women: frequent sexual intercourse, new partner, failure to void postcoitus, spermicide use, prior infection, diabetes mellitus.
  - Postmenopausal women: estrogen deficiency, incontinence, postvoid residual, catheterization.
  - Men: reduced prostatic secretions in older men, postvoid residual, incontinence, catheterization (Table 19.1).

IDSA Recommendations: Asymptomatic Bacteriuria

- **Screening and treatment advised** in:
  1. Pregnancy.

2. Those undergoing urologic procedure likely to involve mucosal bleeding.

- **No recommendation for solid organ transplant**: some experts advised screening in renal transplants for 6 months post-treatment.
- **Screening not recommended**:
  - Premenopausal women, nonpregnant women.
  - Diabetic women.
  - Elderly subjects living independently.
  - Spinal cord injury.
  - Catheterized subjects (although consider treatment if persistent bacteriuria after catheter removal).
- **Asymptomatic candiduria**:
  - Catheter removal alone is sufficient in 30%–40%.
  - Do not treat in solid organ transplant: previously used to treat but a study demonstrated higher mortality in those treated.
  - Treat if undergoing urologic procedure.
  - Ascending infection can occur in diabetics or obstruction.
  - If treatment indicated: 1 week of fluconazole.

Microbiology (Table 19.2)

- Enterobacteriaceae dominate; anaerobic infection is rare.

Clinical Features

- Symptomatology variably relates to site of infection within the urinary tract.
- Lower tract/cystitis: irritation of urethral and bladder mucosa leading to urinary urgency and frequency and suprapubic discomfort.
- Upper tract/pyelonephritis:
  - Usually associated with fever, rigors, flank pain, ± lower tract symptoms.
  - Flank pain with **radiation to the groin suggests a stone.**
  - More generalized abdominal pain and delirium often observed in elderly patients who are also more likely to have bacteremia and consequent sepsis and shock.
  - In those with urinary catheters, focal symptoms may be few.

Diagnosis

- Rapid dipstick tests
  - Leucocyte esterase.
  - Nitrite: indirect test for presence of bacteria that reduce nitrate to nitrite (i.e., *E. coli*, *Proteus* spp., *Klebsiella* spp., and **not staphylococci or enterococci**).
  - **False-negative tests** can occur if dilute urine, or partial washout from **multiple voids**; however, those with negative leucocyte esterase *and* nitrite are unlikely to have UTI.
- Microscopy
  - For pyuria = 5–10 white cells per high powered field (sensitivity >90%, specificity 70%).
  - Presence of 1 bacterium per high powered field = 10^5 colony forming units (CFU) per mL of urine.

TABLE 19.1   Asymptomatic Bacteriuria and Risk of Infection

Patient Category	Prevalence	Subsequent Infection
Girls	1%–5%	30%
Boys	<1%	–
Women	1%–3%	8%–55%
Pregnancy	2%–10%	20–30-fold risk of pyelonephritis
Men	0.1%	-
Postmenopausal women	3%–9%	-
Elderly women – community	11%–16%	Treatment not associated with subsequent reduction in infection
Elderly women – long-term care	25%–50%	Treatment not associated with subsequent reduction in infection
Elderly men – community	10%	Treatment not associated with subsequent reduction in infection
Elderly men – long-term care	15%–40%	Treatment not associated with subsequent reduction in infection
Diabetes mellitus – women	9%–27%	Treatment not associated with subsequent reduction in infection or hospitalization
Diabetes mellitus – men	4%–19%	–
Spinal cord injury – intermittent self-catheterization	23%–89%	Treatment not associated with subsequent reduction in infection
Short-term catheter	9%–23%	10%–25% but data unclear because of confounding (many patients on antibiotics for other indications) Whether there are benefits of treatment for sustained bacteriuria after catheter removal remains uncertain
Long-term catheter	100%	No difference in outcomes in treated vs. untreated subjects but greater risk of subsequent drug resistance in those exposed to antibiotics

Data from Nicolle LE, Bradley S, Colgan R, Rice JC, Schaeffer A, Hooton TM. Infectious Diseases Society of America Guidelines for the Diagnosis and Treatment of Asymptomatic Bacteriuria in Adults. *Clin Infect Dis*. 2005;40:643–654.

TABLE 19.2   Pathogens Associated With Genitourinary Tract Infection

Enterobacteriaceae	*Escherichia coli*	Majority of uncomplicated UTI, especially outpatients
	Proteus, *Klebsiella*, and *Enterobacter* spp.	
	Resistance increasingly identified in hospital-acquired complicated UTI	Extended spectrum β lactamase Inducible AMP-C β lactamase Carbapenemase-producing Enterobacteriaceae
Other gram-negatives	*Pseudomonas* spp.	
	Acinetobacter spp.	
Gram-positives	*Staphylococcus* spp.	Complication of *S. aureus* bacteremia
	Enterococcus spp.	Complicated UTI
	Corynebacterium urealyticum	
Viruses	Adenovirus	Hemorrhagic cystitis in hematopoietic stem cell transplant recipients
	BK virus	Associated with graft nephropathy in renal transplant recipients

- Absence of bacteria per high powered field = fewer than 10^4 CFU per mL of urine.
- MSU culture: a mid-stream properly collected urine is normally sterile.
- Relating to *Enterobacteriaceae* only (i.e., not staphylococci, fungi, or fastidious organisms) *and* symptomatic subjects.
- >10^5 CFU per mL: 95% have infection.
- But significant proportion of those with infection have <10^4 CFU per mL.
- <10^5 CFU per mL *plus* lower tract symptoms, 33% have infection.
- 10^4–10^5 CFU per mL in an asymptomatic woman is confirmed in second sample in only 5% of cases.
- In men, 10^3 CFU per mL organisms *plus* symptoms suggests infection.
- Catheter specimen threshold is lower at 10^3 CFU per mL.
- False-negative results may be due to contamination of sample by cleaning products, e.g., soap; complete obstruction; infection with a fastidious organism; renal tuberculosis; or diuresis.

Management

Supportive Management

- Hydration.
- Urinary pH.
- Analgesia.
- Prevention of recurrence.

Antimicrobial Management

- Clearance of bacteriuria relates to the urinary concentration of antibiotic.
- Some agents may not achieve clearance of bacteria because the kidney cannot concentrate the antibiotic. In general, penicillins, cephalosporins, and fluoroquinolones (FLQ) can reach appropriate levels in urine, and the first two at least are considered first line in renal impairment.
- Many commonly used antibiotics do not reach adequate serum levels. However, in the context of bacteremia, adequate serum levels of antibiotic must be achieved.
- Response should occur promptly within 48–96 hours. Failure to respond by 72 hours should prompt imaging.
  - **Cure:** negative cultures on antibiotics.
  - **Persistence:** sustained bacteriuria of >10^5 CFU per mL of consistent organism 48 hours after treatment or lower levels beyond that time.
  - **Relapse:** 1–2 weeks after stopping antibiotics usually due to deep-seated kidney bed infection, prostatitis in men, or structural abnormality.
  - **Delayed relapses** probably due to reinfection rather than relapse.

Choice of Agent

- Upper tract – need antibacterial activity in serum – β-lactams, FLQ, trimethoprim–sulfamethoxazole (TMP–SMX), aminoglycosides.

- Lower tract – need antibacterial activity in urine – nitrofurantoin or fosfomycin sufficient.
- Resistance:
  1. 35% isolates from community resistant to amoxicillin.
  2. 20% isolates resistant to TMP–SMX.
  3. Approaching 10% FLQ resistance.
  4. Nitrofurantoin and fosfomycin maintain activity.

Duration

- **Uncomplicated cystitis:**
  - Nitrofurantoin 5 days, TMP–SMX 3 days, *or*
  - Fosfomycin 3 g × 1 dose.
  - FLQ avoided due to risk of ecologic collateral damage.
  - In nursing home resident at risk of further upper tract infection consider 7–10 days.
- **Pyelonephritis:** although 14 days is traditional, 7 days of ciprofloxacin or 5 days with levofloxacin is adequate. One strategy, where local resistance to fluoroquinolone is >10%, is to administer FLQ with one dose of intravenous third-generation cephalosporin while awaiting susceptibility.
  - In men, UTI is considered as complicated infection unless obstruction (anatomical or functional) is excluded.
- **Complex UTI:** more likely to have drug-resistant organism and for that reason probably more likely to relapse or persist. Infected stone or foreign body (e.g., stent) is associated with increased risk of persistence.
  - Consider possibility of drug resistance: e.g., extended spectrum β-lactamase.
  - For lower tract infections with susceptible isolates: TMP–SMX, nitrofurantoin, or fosfomycin.
  - Polycystic disease: TMP–SMX or FLQ will penetrate cyst/closed space.

IDSA Recommendations for Catheter-Associated Urinary Tract Infection and Catheter-Associated Asymptomatic Bacteriuria

Catheter-associated UTI (CA-UTI) is the most common hospital-acquired infection and is characterized by signs and symptoms of lower urinary tract infection associated with ≥10^3 CFU/mL in a catheter specimen or a mid-stream urine in a patient with a recent catheter removal. Catheter-associated asymptomatic bacteriuria (CA-ASB) is determined if there are ≥10^5 CFU/mL and an absence of signs or symptoms of UTI.

Reduce Risk of CA-UTI

- Avoid unnecessary catheterization, e.g., not appropriate to catheterize a patient to manage incontinence.
- Remove catheters as soon as possible.
- If catheter is still required after diagnosis of CA-UTI, it should be replaced to expedite resolution.

Duration of Treatment

- 7 days.
- 10–14 days if slow to respond.

- 5 days of levofloxacin if not severe infection.
- 3 days after catheter removal in premenopausal women with mild lower tract infection.

Relapsing Infection
- Cause includes:
  1. Deep-seated renal parenchymal infection.
  2. Anatomical abnormality, e.g., stone.
  3. Foreign body, e.g., stent.
  4. In male, prostatic infection.
- Consider 6-weeks treatment; 6 weeks of treatment associated with greater cure than second 2-week course. In context of stones, could consider long-term antibiotic.

Recurrent Infection
- Infrequent: 2–3 per year. In young to middle-aged and sexually active, treat each episode discretely. Advise regarding postsex voiding, or consider single-dose prophylactic antibiotic.
- Frequent: long-term chemoprophylaxis decreases incidence of infection but does not totally abolish recurrences.
- **Suggested:**
  - Nitrofurantoin 50-100 mg.
  - TMX-SMX 240-480 mg.

Urinary Tract Infection in Pregnancy

See Chapter 18 for further discussion.

Increased estrogen causes muscle relaxation and reduced tone leading to increased bladder capacity and impaired bladder emptying as well as dilation of the ureters. The gravid uterus can compress ureters and probably also contributes to ascending infection. Trimester-specific alterations in *E. coli* virulence factors are also described.

Management
- Screen for asymptomatic bacteriuria in the 1st and 3rd trimesters.
- With consideration of local resistance rates, treatment options may include amoxicillin, amoxicillin–clavulanate, cephalexin, TMP–SMX, nitrofurantoin.
- **FLQ is usually avoided in pregnancy** as causes arthropathy in animal studies.
- **Trimethoprim is usually avoided in the 1st trimester** although 5 mg folic acid supplements may facilitate use; it should be avoided throughout pregnancy in patients taking folate antagonists.
- TMP–SMX not recommended in the 3rd trimester because of an association with neonatal hemolysis and methemoglobinemia. Increased risk of kernicterus in neonates is not supported by available evidence.
- Nitrofurantoin should be avoided when labor is imminent as it may cause a hemolytic crisis in the neonate.

Lower Tract Infection
- Fosfomycin 3 g × 1 dose.

- Cephalexin 500 mg QDS.
- Nitrofurantoin 100 mg BD; avoid in first trimester and near term due to risk of hemolytic anaemia in neonate.

Upper Tract Infection
- Third-generation cephalosporin: cefotaxime, ceftriaxone, ceftazidime.
- Mild infection:
  - Oral cefixime if mild infection.
  - If earlier in pregnancy, TMP–SMX.
- **Duration:** 14 days aiming for sterile urine.
- **Prophylaxis:** postcoital cephalexin 250 mg or nitrofurantoin 50 mg.

Renal Abscess

Perinephric Abscess
- Relatively uncommon, onset can be subacute (e.g., 2 weeks), and urinalysis can be normal in 40% and culture-negative in 30%. Usually confined to perinephric space by fascia but may spread throughout the retroperitoneum.
- Risk factors: diabetes, renal stones.

Intrarenal Abscess
Hematogenous spread and usually unilateral and cortical in location. Increasingly recognized to occur with ascending infection within both cortex and medulla. Clinical presentation similar to acute pyelonephritis but delayed resolution is typical.

Uncommon Diagnoses

Emphysematous Pyelonephritis
Severe multifocal infection with gas visible within the kidney and retroperitoneal space (Fig. 19.1). Diabetes and obstruction are risk factors. *E. coli*, *Proteus*, and *Citrobacter* species have been implicated. There is significantly high mortality even with antibiotic treatment, and nephrectomy is often required to control infection.

Xanthogranulomatous Pyelonephritis (XGP)
Chronic infection of kidney characterized by granulomatous inflammation and foamy cells (i.e., lipid-laden macrophages) (Fig. 19.2). Risk factors include urinary obstruction, lymphatic obstruction, renal stones, renal ischemia, diabetes mellitus. Complications include retroperitoneal spread and fistula formation. Can present like a renal malignancy.

Size of Abscess and Resolution
- <3 cm likely to respond with antibiotics alone.
- >3–5 cm 92% resolve with antibiotics alone.
- **>5 cm require percutaneous drainage.**

Imaging
- Not all infections require imaging.
- Indications include:
  - Failure to improve within 72 hours.

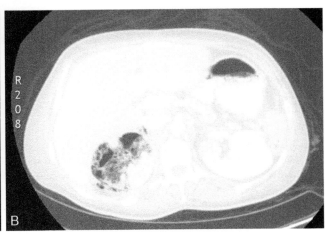

• **Fig. 19.1** Diffuse emphysematous pyelonephritis. (A) and (B) reveal extensive gas within the parenchyma of the right kidney. Gas is also seen in the perinephric space anteriorly and posteriorly (*arrows* in A). (From Zagoria RJ, Dyer R, Brady C. The kidney: diffuse parenchymal abnormalities. In: *Genitourinary Imaging: The Requisites*. Elsevier; 2015.)

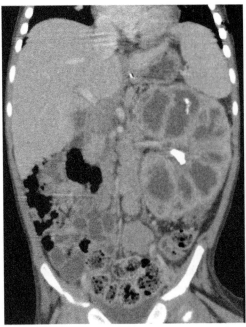
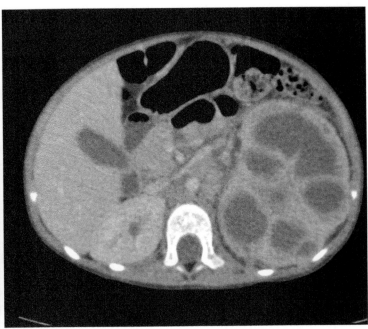

• **Fig. 19.2** Left kidney with xanthogranulomatous pyelonephritis. Lymph node enlargement and a renal calculus are also apparent in addition to global renal enlargement. (From Zugor V, Schott GE, Labanaris AP. Xanthogranulomatous pyelonephritis in childhood: a critical analysis of 10 cases and of the literature. *Urology.* 2007;70(1):157–160.)

- • Immunocompromise.
  - • Diagnosis unclear.
- • Modality
  - • Ultrasound: no radiation dose, noninvasive.
  - • CT: demonstrates stones well.

Epididymitis, Orchitis, Prostatic Infection

Epididymitis

Sexually transmitted infection covered elsewhere (see Chapter 21).

- • Bacterial infection of the epididymis presents with symptoms including scrotal pain and swelling ± lower urinary tract symptoms. In men >35 years, consider bacterial infection with *E. coli* or *Pseudomonas* species. Enterococci are less frequently involved.
- • May have a **history of urologic procedure** including catheterization. Acute or chronic prostatitis and bacteremia during prior urologic procedures are noted risk factors for subsequent development of epididymitis. Insertive anal intercourse is also associated with an increased risk for acute bacterial epididymitis by enteric coliforms.
- • Other less common etiologies:
  - • TB.
  - • Fungal, e.g., blastomycosis.
  - • Brucellosis.

- Iatrogenic: *Mycobacterium bovis* infection associated with recent intravesical therapy with BCG.

Management

- Empiric treatment.
- Scrotal elevation, analgesia, icepacks.
- Expect patient to **improve by day 3** of therapy.
- Failure to resolve should prompt investigation for other less common etiologies, including TB.
- Complications include infarction, abscess, pyocele.

Orchitis

Infection involving the testis with erythema, swelling, and tenderness on examination. Isolated orchitis much less common than epididymitis or prostatitis.

- **Infectious etiology**
  - **Viral**: most cases
    - Majority = **mumps** (15%–30% of postpubertal males with mumps infection; unilateral in 2/3; may result in testicular atrophy; impaired fertility is debatable).
    - Coxsackie B virus and lymphocytic choriomeningitis virus may also result in orchitis.
  - Bacterial
    - Unusual in isolation; usually contiguous spread, may be hematogenous seeding.
    - Patients may be overtly septic with high fevers.
    - *E. coli*, *Klebsiella pneumoniae*, *Pseudomonas aeruginosa*, staphylococci, streptococci, *Brucella* spp., *Mycobacterium tuberculosis*.
  - **Fungal**: blastomycosis.
- **Treatment and complications** as for epididymitis; abscess may need surgical drainage.

Prostatitis

Prostatitis is the most common urologic problem in younger men (<50 years). It can be divided into 4 categories:
1. Acute bacterial prostatitis.
2. Chronic bacterial prostatitis.
3. Chronic prostatic pelvic pain syndrome.
4. Asymptomatic inflammatory prostatitis.

Both acute and chronic prostatitis are associated with bacteriuria, but **tenderness in the prostate is only present in acute prostatitis.**

Some antibiotics poorly penetrate the prostate. Only small, nonprotein-bound, high lipid solubility antibiotic molecules will penetrate the inflamed prostate. **Fluoroquinolones** are preferred option especially in stable patients. Trimethoprim readily enters the prostate but sulfamethoxazole levels are much lower, which is not ideal. Nitrofurantoin poorly penetrates. Tetracyclines and macrolides have limited or no activity against Enterobacteriaceae respectively but achieve fair tissue levels and may have role in context of defined gram-positive infection. Rifampicin has reasonable prostatic penetration. For those patients who are systemically unwell, the inflamed prostate is penetrated by **third-generation cephalosporins** or **piptazobactam**, and the addition of an aminoglycoside offers additional cover in the event of a drug-resistant organism.

Acute Bacterial Prostatitis

- **Features**
  1. **Lower urinary tract symptoms.**
  2. Signs of sepsis, including fever.
  3. Suprapubic tenderness and exquisitely tender prostate on examination.
  4. Organisms similar to epididymitis: *E. coli*, *Pseudomonas* spp., and *Enterococcus* spp.
  5. Known complication of *S. aureus* bacteremia/metastatic *S. aureus* infection.
- **Diagnosis**
  - Mid-stream urine culture.
  - Postprostate massage urine sample culture.
- **Management**
  - Antibiotic treatment third-generation cephalosporin or carbapenem and aminoglycoside if systemically unwell.
  - FLQ in mild illness.
  - Duration 2–4 weeks.
  - Avoid urethral catheterization as it impedes drainage of infected prostatic secretions.
- **Complications** include abscess formation, chronic infection, subsequent granulomatous inflammation that can mimic malignancy.

Chronic Bacterial Prostatitis

Often a cause of recurrent urinary tract infection in men **characterized by persistence of an infecting organism** (i.e., same organism in cultures over time). Patients can be asymptomatic in between exacerbations with bacteriuria. **Prostate examination is often normal**.

Pre- and postprostate massage samples can improve microbiologic yield. A 10-fold increase in bacterial count in postmassage urine samples supports the diagnosis.

- **Treatment failure** associated with:
  - Poor drug penetration.
  - Prostatic fluid pH change that occurs during infection.
  - Poor antibiotic compliance.
  - Infected stones.
- **Treatment duration**: 4–6 weeks with a fluoroquinolone. Consideration of chronic suppression of bacteriuria to minimize symptomatic episodes associated with bacteriuria.

Chronic Prostatitis/Chronic Pelvic Pain Syndrome

This is a **diagnosis of exclusion** with an **absence of bacteriuria,** but with significant perineal and pelvic pain impacting quality of life. There may or may not be leucocytes in mid-stream urine, postprostate massage urine, and semen. Current management strategies include antiinflammatory agents, empiric antibiotics, and analgesia, but outcomes are generally suboptimal.

Asymptomatic Inflammatory Prostatitis

These patients have evidence of prostatic inflammation or bacteriuria either on mid-stream urine, postprostate massage urine samples, or prostatic biopsy but are asymptomatic. Some advocate a course of antibiotics, but treatment goals are unclear.

Granulomatous Prostatitis

Typical histopathologic diagnosis in patient being worked up for prostatic malignancy after presentation with abnormal prostate examination.

Differential

- *Mycobacterium tuberculosis*: usually secondary to TB elsewhere in the urogenital tract.
- *Mycobacterium bovis* infection: iatrogenic infection post-intravesical BCG therapy.
- Nontuberculous mycobacteria.
- Less commonly
  - Deep seated endemic mycoses: blastomycosis, coccidioidomycosis, histoplasmosis.
  - Cryptococcosis (context of AIDS).

Prostatic Abscess

- Rare.
- **Ascending** infection caused by **usual organisms that cause urinary tract infection.**
- *S. aureus* can be implicated in context of prior *S. aureus* bacteremia.
- Other less common organisms to consider:
  - *Nocardia.*

- *Burkholderia pseudomallei* (melioidosis).
- Blastomycosis.
- Cryptococcosis.
- **Risk factors**
  - Diabetes mellitus.
  - Immunocompromise.
  - Inadequate treatment of acute bacterial prostatitis.
- **Presentation**
  - Similar to acute bacterial prostatitis, including abnormal prostatic exam with tenderness and fluctuant swelling.
- **Management**
  - Includes drainage (perineal or transurethral).
  - 4–6 weeks antibiotic duration.

Further Reading

1. Infectious Diseases Society of America guidelines for the diagnosis and treatment of asymptomatic bacteriuria in adults. *Clin Infect Dis.* 2005;40:653–654.
2. International clinical practice guidelines for the treatment of acute uncomplicated cystitis and pyelonephritis in women: a 2010 update by the Infectious Diseases Society of America and the European Society for Microbiology and Infectious Diseases. *Clin Infect Dis.* 2011;52(5):e103–e120.
3. Diagnosis, prevention, and treatment of catheter-associated urinary tract infection in adults: 2009 international clinical practice guidelines from the Infectious Diseases Society of America. *Clin Infect Dis.* 2010;50:625–663.
4. Lipsky BA, Byren I, Hoey CT. Treatment of bacterial prostatitis. *Clin Infect Dis.* 2010;50(12):1641–1652.
5. Bichler KH, Eipper E, Naber K, Braun V, Zimmerman R, Lahme S. Urinary infection stones. *Int J Antimicrob Agents.* 2002;19:488–498.

20

Infections of Pregnancy

RACHEL C. MOORES

Complications of Infection in Pregnancy: Overview

Some infections are associated with significant maternal and fetal complications during pregnancy (Table 20.1). This chapter focuses on the fetal complications. See Chapter 18 for further discussion on maternal complications of infection in pregnancy.

Key principles

- Predisposing factors:
  - Humoral immune responses in pregnancy are similar to the nonpregnant woman:
    - Cell-mediated immunity (CMI) is diminished.
    - The physiologic changes associated with pregnancy (altered smooth muscle and sphincter tone, increased oxygen consumption along with pressure effects of the enlarging gravid uterus) may also contribute to infection.
- The outcome of exposure to a pathogen during pregnancy is affected by:
  - Pre-existing maternal immunity/vaccination.
  - Gestation of pregnancy.
  - Ability of pathogen to cross the placenta.
- Infections in pregnancy can result in a number of different adverse outcomes:
  - Fetal loss/miscarriage/stillbirth (e.g., rubella).
  - Prematurity (e.g., herpes simplex virus [HSV], cytomegalovirus [CMV], *Toxoplasma*).

- Intrauterine growth restriction (IUGR) (e.g., rubella, CMV, *Toxoplasma*).
- Teratogenic effects (e.g., varicella-zoster virus [VZV]).
- Congenital disease (e.g., CMV).
- Perinatal acquisition of infection (e.g., HSV).
- Persistent infection (e.g., human immunodeficiency virus [HIV], hepatitis B [HBV]).
- Possible interventions include:
  - Antenatal screening: currently for syphilis, HBV, and HIV in the UK.
  - Risk reduction: advice about behavior change to avoid exposure to particular pathogens.
  - Active immunization: either prepregnancy (e.g., MMR [measles, mumps, rubella], VZV) or promptly following exposure.
  - Passive immunization after exposure with pooled human immunoglobulin products.
  - Drug treatment: e.g., aciclovir (ACV) for recurrent genital HSV, antiretroviral therapy (ART) in HIV.
  - Targeted screening and treatment: e.g., when fetal abnormalities are identified antenatally.

Coxiella burnetii

- Small gram-negative bacterium. Obligate intracellular organism, resides in phagolysosome.

Epidemiology and Transmission

- Hardy, resistant to heat/drying and common disinfectants.
- Zoonotic disease acquired from ungulates (sheep, goats, cattle) or domestic animals (dogs and cats). Present in

TABLE 20.1	Infections During Pregnancy Associated With Significant Maternal and/or Fetal Complications			
Bacterial	**Protozoa**	**Viral Rash/Fever**	**Herpesviruses**	**Chronic Viral Infections**
Coxiella burnetii	Toxoplasmosis	Measles	Cytomegalovirus	Hepatitis B
Listeriosis	*Trypanosoma cruzi*	Parvovirus B19	Herpes simplex virus	Human
Streptococcus agalactiae	(Chagas)	Rubella	Varicella-zoster virus	immunodeficiency
(group B streptococcus)		Zika		virus
Syphilis				

high concentrations in **birth products**, also in **urine, feces**, and **milk.**

- Persists in environment therefore **acquisition via aerosols from soil/dust contaminated** with animal excreta possible.
- **Very low inoculum required** to cause disease.
- Rarely reported to be acquired from a tick bite or unpasteurized milk or by person-to-person contact.

Clinical Features

Infection in pregnancy appears to **increase severity of disease and risk of progression** to chronic Q fever. Associated with increased risk of miscarriage, IUGR, intrauterine fetal death (IUFD), and preterm delivery. Evidence of these associations is of limited quality (small numbers of case series). **An association with fetal malformations has not been reported**.

- Complications probably arise from placental insufficiency through inflammation and appear to be more common if infection occurs during the 1st trimester.
  - Symptoms: nonspecific, febrile illness with fatigue, myalgia, sometimes dry cough and gastrointestinal (GI) upset.
  - May be complicated by pneumonia or hepatitis.
  - Onset of symptoms is within 2–3 weeks of exposure.
  - Up to 50% of infections may be asymptomatic (reflected by estimates of 3% seroprevalence in some US surveys).
- Progression to chronic Q fever occurs in <5% outside pregnancy, but it is thought this risk is higher in pregnancy-associated infection.

Diagnosis

- Predominantly via serology.
  - **Paired serum samples** to demonstrate rising antibody titer.
  - Counterintuitively, response to phase II antigen is associated with acute disease, with a shift to phase I response in chronic disease.
  - Polymerase chain reaction (PCR) may be performed on whole blood or serum.

Treatment

- Gold-standard treatment of acute Q fever is doxycycline/hydroxychloroquine combination, **both of which are contraindicated in pregnancy.** Some experts recommend long-term **suppressive treatment with co-trimoxazole and folic acid** (which is not bactericidal against *C. burnetii*) until after pregnancy, when definitive treatment can be given.
- **Serologic monitoring for relapse** is recommended for at least 2 years after treatment. Monitoring during future pregnancies is also recommended as there is **a risk of recrudescent infection.**

Listeriosis

- *Listeria monocytogenes*, aerobic gram-positive bacillus.
- Relatively resistant to heat/cold/alcohol/acid and able to grow at low temperatures (<5 °C).
- Killed by pasteurization or thorough cooking.

- Readily identified on sterile site cultures (blood or CSF), although may be mistaken for diphtheroids.
- Not identified on routine stool culture and not normally tested, as high environmental burden means asymptomatic individuals can excrete viable *Listeria*.

Epidemiology and Transmission

- Usually acquired from ingestion of contaminated food (fruit, salad, and dairy produce); also possible from animal contact, particularly lambing ewes.
- Pregnant women and neonates are more susceptible to clinical disease following exposure.
- Risk of illness after consuming contaminated food is **increased 10–20-fold in pregnancy.**

Clinical Features

- Causes a spectrum of illness from mild febrile illness or gastroenteritis to fatal invasive infection and meningoencephalitis.
  - Gastroenteritis (incubation hours–days) follows ingestion of large numbers of viable organisms. Usually self-limiting within 48 hours.
  - Invasive disease often has a longer incubation period (median 11 days but up to 28 days).
  - Consequences: miscarriage, stillbirth, preterm labor, neonatal disease.
  - Fetal/neonatal death in around 25% of cases.
- Neonatal disease divided into early and late:
  - **Early (<6 days):** probably result of transplacental spread, usually presents as **sepsis.** Granulomatosis infantiseptica is a severe manifestation of disease with disseminated abscesses and skin lesions, which is usually fatal.
  - **Late (7–28 days):** more often presents as **meningitis/encephalitis.**

> ### CLINICAL PEARLS
> - Usually causes bacteremia without central nervous system (CNS) involvement in pregnancy.
> - Outcomes worst in 1st trimester (usually fatal to fetus) but listeriosis more commonly diagnosed in 3rd trimester.

Treatment

- Pregnant women are treated with high dose IV **amoxicillin** (synergistic gentamicin often used for CNS disease). **If penicillin allergy, consider trimethoprim–sulfamethoxazole** (not in 1st trimester as folate antagonist or in last 4 weeks of pregnancy as risk of hemolytic anemia) or **carbapenem.**
- Neonatal disease usually treated with amoxicillin/gentamicin combination.

Streptococcus agalactiae

- Also known as group B streptococcus (GBS).
- Originally identified as a cause of fatal puerperal sepsis, causes morbidity in pregnancy and neonatal disease, as well as manifestations in nonpregnant adults.

Epidemiology and Transmission

- Commensal of human genital and lower GI tract, prevalence 10%–40% depending on population screened.
- Colonization is a risk factor for neonatal GBS disease.
- Screening usually involves low vaginal and rectal swabs, but incidental isolation of GBS on urine culture indicates high genital bacterial burden and should be managed as per positive genital screen.
- Vertical transmission occurs during labor.

Clinical Features

- Maternal GBS causes asymptomatic bacteriuria, urinary tract infection (UTI), pneumonia, bacteremia without focus, chorioamnionitis, postpartum endometritis, and wound infection.
- Also a cause of IUFD and preterm delivery.
- Neonatal disease divided into **early and late onset** (<7 days vs >7 days).
  - Early onset usually at <24 hours: sepsis, meningitis, pneumonia. Mortality 5%–10%.
  - Late onset usually manifests as bacteremia, but meningitis present in approximately 1/3, and focal infections such as cellulitis, septic arthritis, adenitis, or empyema can occur. Low case fatality rate.

Risk Factors for GBS Neonatal Disease

- Fever in labor >38 °C.
- Preterm labor (<37/40 gestation).
- Prolonged rupture of membranes.
- Previous infant affected by GBS disease.
- GBS bacteriuria in this pregnancy.

A risk factor-based approach **predicts only 30%** of cases, therefore **in the United States** the approach is **routine genital screening at 35–37/40 and intrapartum antibiotics for all who screen positive** (unless elective cesarean section is performed prelabor with intact membranes).

Prophylaxis is recommended **without screening** if the woman has had a previous infant with GBS disease, or a positive urine culture for GBS during the current pregnancy.

In the UK, where the prevalence of GBS carriage and the incidence of neonatal GBS disease is lower, a **risk-factor-based** approach is used.

Intrapartum Prophylaxis

Prophylaxis has had a significant impact on the incidence of early neonatal disease (reduced from approx. 1.7 to 0.6 cases per 1000 live births), but no impact on the incidence of late-onset disease (approx. 0.5 per 1000 live births) in the United States between 1993 and 1998.

- IV benzylpenicillin at least 4 hours before delivery and repeat doses every 4 hours until delivery.
- IV ampicillin/amoxicillin are alternatives (broader-spectrum).

- Clindamycin or vancomycin are recommended for those with penicillin allergy.

Guidelines for the management of neonatal sepsis routinely cover early-onset GBS disease, usually with either amoxicillin or benzylpenicillin plus aminoglycoside (synergy *in vitro*).

Syphilis

- Spirochete bacterium *Treponema pallidum* subsp. *pallidum*. See also Chapter 21.

Epidemiology and Transmission

- Sexually transmitted via a mucocutaneous lesion.
- Mother-to-child transmission (MTCT) can be transplacental or at delivery.
- The risk of fetal infection is greatest with **primary maternal syphilis.** Timely treatment of the pregnant woman usually prevents fetal infection.

Clinical Features

- **Fetal consequences**: spontaneous abortion, polyhydramnios, IUGR, hydrops fetalis, preterm delivery, or IUFD.
- Two-thirds of infants with congenital syphilis are asymptomatic at birth, but signs of disease usually present by 6-week check.
  - **Early** (<2 years): common signs are rhinitis, desquamating rash, hepatosplenomegaly, lymphadenopathy, skeletal abnormalities.
    - Rarer signs include condylomata lata, vesicular or bullous skin lesions, periostitis, hydrops, thrombocytopenia, hepatitis, jaundice, glomerulonephritis.
    - CNS involvement in >20%.
    - Death results from liver failure, pneumonia, hypopituitarism, or pulmonary hemorrhage.
  - **Late**: sensorineural deafness, intellectual impairment, saddle nose deformity, frontal bossing, jaw/dental/palatal abnormalities, saber tibia, short stature, keratitis. (See Figs. 20.1 and 20.2.)

Diagnosis

- Dark ground microscopy ± PCR on bodily fluids (e.g., nasal discharge, CSF) or samples from suspicious lesions.
- Serology: perform a non-treponemal (e.g., rapid plasma reagin [RPR]) quantitative test on infant venous blood; avoid using cord blood and avoid specific treponemal tests; CDC recommend comparing with paired maternal RPR; UK recommend infant IgM. If treated, will require CSF analysis, HIV screen, skeletal survey, CXR, ophthalmology and audiology assessments and cranial ultrasound.

Management

Syphilis in pregnancy should be managed by a physician with expertise in this area. Referral should be made as early as possible, and referral to fetal medicine should also be considered. Contact tracing and assessment of mother's older children for signs of congenital syphilis may also be needed.

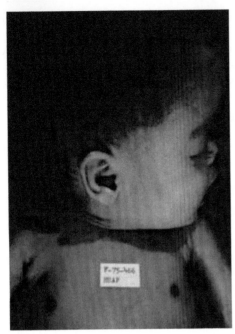

• **Fig. 20.1** Frontal bossing, interstitial keratitis, and saddle nose in congenital syphilis. (From James WD, Berger TG, Elson DM. *Andrews' Diseases of the Skin: Clinical Dermatology*. 12th ed. Elsevier; 2016.)

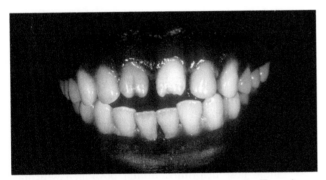

• **Fig. 20.2** Congenital syphilis with Hutchinson teeth. (From James WD, Elson DM, McMahon P. *Andrews' Diseases of the Skin: Clinical Atlas*. 1st ed. Elsevier; 2018.)

- **High-dose penicillin is the mainstay** of treatment for syphilis in pregnancy. The recommended regimen depends on the stage of syphilis in the mother, the presence of HIV co-infection, and the gestation of pregnancy.
- Corticosteroids may also be needed if there is evidence of cardiovascular or neurosyphilis.
- **Other regimes are inferior** and therefore desensitization should be undertaken to allow penicillin treatment if at all possible.
- Congenital syphilis in infants is treated with high-dose IV benzylpenicillin.

Prevention

- 1st trimester screening with either syphilis EIA or TPPA, followed by confirmation with an alternative treponemal

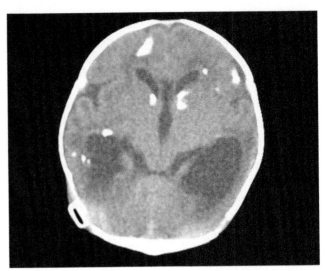

• **Fig. 20.3** Multiple calcified lesions in cerebral toxoplasmosis. (From Montoya JG, Boothroyd JC, Kovacs JA et al. Imaging studies of central nervous system toxoplasmosis in *Toxoplasma gondii*. In: Bennett JE, Dolin R, Blaser MJ, eds. *Mandell, Douglas, and Bennett's Principles and Practice of Infectious Diseases*. Updated 8th ed. Elsevier; 2015.)

test, allows antenatal treatment of undiagnosed syphilis and **largely prevents transmission to the fetus.**
- In the UK >95% of women are screened in pregnancy and <0.1% are found to have an active infection requiring treatment.
- High-risk women may be retested in the 3rd trimester.

Toxoplasmosis

- *Toxoplasma gondii*, ubiquitous protozoan parasite.
- Primary infection in children or adults causes a nonspecific febrile illness, sometimes accompanied by lymphadenopathy.

Epidemiology and Transmission

- Acquired from contact with feces of infected cat or consumption of undercooked meat (particularly beef).
- One-third of UK population seropositive; CDC estimates 11% US population ≥ 6 years old are seropositive.
- First trimester acquisition: 10%–15% risk of transmission. If transmission occurs, miscarriage or severe abnormalities are likely, e.g., hydrocephalus, cerebral calcifications, or chorioretinitis (Fig. 20.3).
- 2nd trimester acquisition: 25% risk of transmission. Miscarriage is less likely, but neurologic/ophthalmologic abnormalities as above.
- 3rd trimester acquisition: high risk of transmission (>80%) but consequences usually limited to chorioretinitis.

Clinical Features

- Congenital toxoplasmosis **rare:** affects approximately 1 in 10,000–30,000 live births in the UK. Occurs when *Toxoplasma* **acquired for the first time during or just before** pregnancy.

- Causes miscarriage, IUFD, and ophthalmologic abnormalities. Other neurologic abnormalities (hydrocephalus, cerebral palsy, epilepsy, deafness) as well as hepatosplenomegaly and jaundice may be noted after birth.
- **Diagnosis**: serology (*Toxoplasma*-specific IgM/IgG) ± amniocentesis/cordocentesis where appropriate.

Treatment and Prevention

- Spiramycin for maternal seroconversion (reduces the risk of transmission).
- Pyrimethamine/sulfadiazine if fetal infection confirmed.
- Routine advice to pregnant women to avoid pregnant/lambing ewes, avoid undercooked or cured meats, wear gloves for gardening/changing cat litter, and wash hands thoroughly.

Trypanosoma cruzi (Chagas Disease)

- **Transmission** may occur with both acute and chronic maternal infection. Most common during 2nd and 3rd trimester.
- **Risk factors** for congenital transmission:
  - Mother with detectable parasitemia.
  - Mother with reduced CMI.
  - Co-infection with HIV or malaria.
  - Sibling with congenital infection.
- **Effect on pregnancy**:
  - If no transmission, no effect on outcome of pregnancy.
  - If child infected:
    - Increased risk of premature delivery, low birth weight, preterm premature rupture of membranes (PPROM).
    - May be asymptomatic initially but develop symptoms day/weeks later.
    - If untreated, may develop chronic disease with GI and cardiac complications.

Clinical Manifestations

- Respiratory distress syndrome and low APGAR scores.
- Anemia, thrombocytopenia.
- Hepatomegaly, splenomegaly, jaundice.
- Meningoencephalitis ± microcephaly.
- Myocarditis with cardiomegaly and arrhythmias.
- Megaesophagus and megacolon: may be present at birth; high mortality rate associated.
- Ocular involvement: chorioretinitis and opacification of vitreous body.

Diagnosis

- All pregnant women who live or have lived in endemic areas should be tested for infection with *Trypanosoma cruzi*.
- All children born to seropositive mothers should be tested at birth, and again at 1 month and >9 months of age.
- Microscopy for blood parasites or PCR for DNA (birth, 1 month).
- Serology (>9 months).

Treatment

Benznidazole or nifurtimox for 60 days. Generally successful and well tolerated in first year of life (cure rate >90%).

Measles

- ssRNA, enveloped *Paramyxovirus*. (See Chapter 23.)

Effect on Pregnancy

- Rare in pregnant women in the UK and US due to vaccination and low levels of circulating virus, but causes:
  - Fetal loss (miscarriage, IUFD).
  - Preterm delivery.
  - Increased maternal morbidity (predominantly respiratory – direct pneumonitis and secondary bacterial pneumonia).
- **Measles is not a cause of congenital abnormalities.**

Management and Prevention

- Routine immunization with two doses of measles-containing vaccine (e.g., MMR) is 97% protective against clinical measles. However, MMR is a live vaccine and therefore **contraindicated during pregnancy.**
- **Passive immunization with HNIG** may be used:
  - In a susceptible pregnant woman in contact with a suspected/confirmed measles case, administration of HNIG **within 6 days of exposure attenuates illness.** However, there is no evidence it prevents IUFD or preterm delivery.
  - Infants born to a mother with active measles are passively immunized with HNIG (0.25 mL/kg IM) to prevent neonatal measles, which can be severe.

Parvovirus B19

- Small, nonenveloped ssDNA virus (genus *Erythrovirus*). (See Chapter 23.)
- Asymptomatic seroconversion is common.
- 50% seropositive by age 15. Seroprevalence in elderly >90%.
- Women of child-bearing age seroconvert 1.5% pa in the United States.

Clinical Features

- Infection in first 20 weeks of pregnancy can lead to IUFD and hydrops fetalis.
- Maternal infection before 20/40:
  - Transplacental transmission estimated at 33%.
  - **9% risk of infection overall.**
  - 3% risk of hydrops fetalis if infection from 9 to 20/40.
  - Risk of fetal anomalies less than 1%.
- Maternal infection after 20/40 not associated with any documented risk.

Diagnosis

- Pregnant women in contact with a proven parvovirus infection, or those with a nonspecific maculopapular rash in pregnancy, should have their immune status checked.

- Serology (IgM detectable in >90% by the onset of rash, IgG present by 7th day of illness) and molecular tests (**parvovirus DNA PCR on plasma**).
- Repeat serology 4 weeks after suspected exposure due to rates of asymptomatic infection.
- Fetal infection can be confirmed by PCR on amniotic fluid, fetal blood sampling, or postmortem tissue.

Management and Prevention

- Refer to fetal medicine for monitoring.
- **Intrauterine transfusion** improves fetal outcome in hydrops.
- No vaccine or passive immunization strategies are currently available.

Rubella

- +ssRNA *Togavirus*. (See Chapter 23.)

Epidemiology

In the prevaccine era, rubella was a common, usually mild infection of primary school-aged children. Now very rare due to high vaccine uptake, but imported cases occur. The **high rate of subclinical infection (20%–50%)** and **prolonged infectious period** mean that pregnant women **may not be aware** of exposure.

Congenital infection may be diagnosed by reverse transcription (RT) PCR on placental biopsy/cordocentesis or demonstration of a rising rubella antibody titer in the neonate's blood.

Clinical Features

- Rubella in the 1st trimester:
  - **1st trimester rubella** infection has major consequences for the fetus.
  - Up to 20% spontaneous abortion if infection before 8/40.
  - 90% incidence of fetal defects if infection before 10/40 (congenital rubella syndrome).
- Maternal rubella after the 1st trimester:
  - 13–18/40: hearing defects and retinopathy in 10%–20%.
  - **Maternal infection after 20 weeks carries no documented risk.**
- **Congenital rubella syndrome (CRS):** Multisystem. Major manifestations are:
  - Cardiovascular (pulmonary artery stenosis, patent ductus arteriosus).
  - Neurologic (including meningoencephalitis at birth, sensory and motor developmental delay, autism).
  - Ocular (including cataracts, glaucoma, and retinopathy) (Fig. 20.4).
  - **Nerve deafness (bilateral, sensorineural) = single most common finding.**
  - "**Blueberry muffin**" rash (Fig. 20.5) due to dermal extramedullary hematopoiesis.

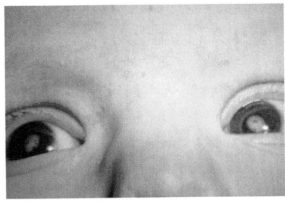

• Fig. 20.4 Bilateral cataracts in infant with congenital rubella syndrome. (From Mason WH. Rubella. In: Kliegman R, Stanton B, Behrman RE, et al., eds. *Nelson Textbook of Pediatrics.* 20th ed. Elsevier; 2016.)

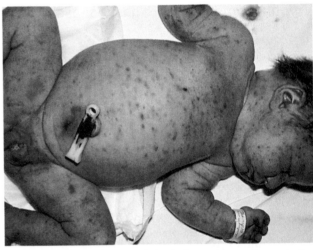

• Fig. 20.5 Infant with congenital rubella syndrome, demonstrating characteristic rash and jaundice (From Michaels MG, Williams JV. Infectious diseases. In: Zitelli BJ, McIntire S, Nowalk AJ. *Zitelli and Davis' Atlas of Pediatric Physical Diagnosis.* 7th ed. Elsevier; 2018.)

Management and Prevention

- **Isolation** precautions: infants with congenital rubella **shed high levels of virus for up to 1 year** after birth and therefore are infectious to others.
- **Prevention:** routine vaccination schedule: 2 doses of MMR >97% effective. If vaccination history unclear, check rubella IgG and vaccinate *before* pregnancy if possible. Otherwise, MMR may be given postpartum. **Routine antenatal care in the UK no longer includes screening for rubella immunity as exposure to the virus is considered unlikely for the majority of pregnant women.**

Zika

- Mosquito-borne flavivirus (female *Aedes* spp., most commonly *Aedes aegypti*). See also Chapter 23.
- An emerging infectious disease with outbreaks in the Pacific, Americas, and Caribbean. Sexual transmission also reported, and theoretical risk from blood transfusion/transplantation.

Prevention

- No vaccine available at present.
- **Pretravel advice** to women who are pregnant/considering pregnancy is the **main intervention** possible.
  - Current advice = **avoid travel to areas with evidence of current Zika transmission.**
  - **Barrier contraception** is recommended for 3 months following last possible Zika exposure for couples wishing to conceive, 2 months if only the female partner was potentially exposed.

Clinical Features

- **Effects on fetus**: miscarriage, still birth, and multiple birth defects, in particular microcephaly and severe brain abnormalities.
  - Effects of 1st trimester infection may include miscarriage.
  - In United States: birth defects reported in 8%–26% of fetuses with confirmed 1st trimester Zika infection; and approximately **10% of all Zika-infected pregnancies were affected** by Zika-associated defects.
  - In Brazil **>50% of 1st and 2nd trimester exposures resulted in adverse outcomes**, i.e., miscarriages or CNS abnormalities (42% of live-born infants).
  - 3rd trimester exposure: microcephaly, IUGR, cerebral calcifications, atrophy, hemorrhage, and ventricular enlargement were observed.
- **Congenital Zika syndrome** now described, including cognitive, motor, and sensory disabilities plus:
  - Severe microcephaly with partial collapse of skull (Fig. 20.6).
  - Decreased brain tissue with calcium deposition.
  - Retinal damage with pigmentation.
  - Hypertonia.
  - Joint abnormalities such as talipes.

Diagnosis and Management

- Serology and PCR (available through the UK Rare and Imported Pathogens Laboratory/CDC).
  - 1–7 days of illness: serum, EDTA blood, and urine.
  - 7–21 days after onset of symptoms: serum and urine.
  - Later than 21 days: serum only.
- If initial tests confirm Zika virus (positive PCR or seroconversion consistent with recent infection) refer to fetal medicine. Amniocentesis and USS-monitoring may be indicated. No specific treatment available.

Cytomegalovirus (CMV)

- Human herpesvirus: virus persists lifelong, reactivation results in further transmission.
- Commonest congenital infection, estimated to affect 0.3% of all infants born in the UK.
- Congenital CMV (cCMV) can result from **primary infection** during pregnancy (**risk of transmission 30%–40%**) or reactivation of latent infection (risk of transmission 1%).

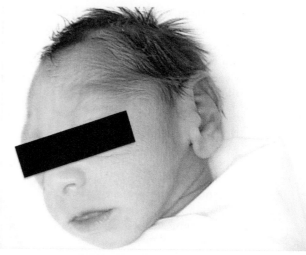

• **Fig. 20.6** Neonate with severe microcephaly (From Miranda HA, Costa MC. Expanded spectrum of congenital ocular findings in microcephaly with presumed Zika infection. *Ophthalmology.* 2016;123(8):1788–1794.)

- Disease only occurs in a minority:
  - Approx. 10% have evidence of disease at birth.
  - 5% mortality in "symptomatic" disease.
  - Long-term neurologic impairment in 10%.
- Features in fetus/neonate
  - IUGR.
  - Jaundice.
  - Hepatosplenomegaly.
  - Chorioretinitis.
  - Thrombocytopenia.
  - Encephalitis.
- Microcephaly/ventriculomegaly/calcifications.

> **CLINICAL PEARLS**
>
> - Approximately 15% of infected, asymptomatic neonates will later develop problems, principally sensorineural hearing loss and learning difficulties.

Diagnosis

- If cCMV is suspected antenatally, first look for evidence of maternal seroconversion (CMV IgG and IgM ± avidity assay) and then consider referral for detailed fetal USS ± amniocentesis.
- Where cCMV is suspected in the neonate, diagnosis is confirmed by positive CMV DNA PCR on **at least 2 independent samples** (urine and saliva commonly submitted for initial screening) within the **first 21 days of life.**

Treatment and Prevention

- If cCMV *infection* is confirmed, need to make an assessment of whether there is CMV *disease.* Current recommendations are for **6 months' treatment with ganciclovir** if there is neurologic or significant organ involvement. A pediatric infectious diseases specialist should be consulted.

- **Prevention**: Pregnant women concerned about CMV acquisition (in particular healthcare workers, child carers, and parents of older children) can be advised that **regular hand hygiene**, especially after nappy-changing, may reduce exposure. No vaccine/prophylaxis is licensed for prevention of MTCT.

Herpes Simplex Virus (HSV)

- Human herpesvirus: virus persists lifelong, reactivation results in further transmission.
- Routes of infection to fetus/neonate:
  - Fetal acquisition in utero by transplacental infection is rare, but can cause microcephaly, hepatosplenomegaly, and IUGR.
  - Ascending infection if premature rupture of membranes.
  - Direct contact with infected maternal genital secretions during delivery.
  - Oral herpes in mother postdelivery (kissing baby).
  - Contact with relatives or hospital staff in babies born to susceptible mothers.

Prevention

- Primary genital infection in the 3rd trimester poses the greatest risk of transmission to infant (occurs in 30%–50%).
  - Elective cesarean section recommended for primary HSV infection in final 6 weeks of pregnancy.
  - Prolonged rupture of membranes and invasive fetal monitoring in labor should be avoided if vaginal delivery is chosen.
- Type-specific HSV Ab testing and PCR from lesions should be performed if possible.
- In recurrent genital outbreaks maternal antibody offers some protection to infants in postnatal period, but may not prevent transmission (risk 2%–5% if lesions present at time of vaginal delivery). **Prophylactic/ suppressive aciclovir may be given from 36/40 of pregnancy**.
- Vaginal delivery in recurrent HSV, even in the presence of anogenital lesions, is not associated with an increased risk of neonatal HSV disease.

Clinical Features

- Neonatal herpes disease occurs 3 days to 6 weeks post delivery.
  - Lesions of skin, eye, mouth (SEM) 7–12 days (Fig. 20.7).
  - Neurologic symptoms ± SEM 2–6 weeks.
  - Disseminated disease with/without vesicles 4–11 days.
  - Mortality in untreated cases of disseminated disease exceeds 80%.
- **Diagnosis**: neonatal swabs (lesion, oral, rectal, mucosal, umbilical) ± EDTA blood ± CSF for HSV PCR.

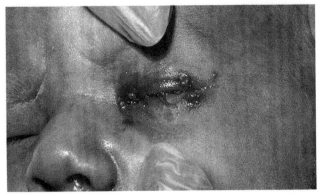

- **Fig. 20.7** Neonatal herpes simplex infection. (From Paller AS, Mancini AJ. Cutaneous disorders of the newborn. In: *Hurwitz Clinical Pediatric Dermatology*. 5th ed. Elsevier; 2016.)

Treatment

- Commence high-dose IV aciclovir immediately.

Varicella-Zoster Virus (VZV)

- Varicella-zoster virus (human herpesvirus 3) (see Chapter 23).
- Primary infection (chickenpox) in pregnancy can cause serious morbidity and even maternal mortality, but it is rare (affecting 3 in 1000 pregnancies). Also causes fetal varicella syndrome (FVS) and congenital/neonatal varicella.

Prevention

- In the UK and the US, over 90% of adults are seropositive for VZV IgG. Women born overseas (particularly in tropical or subtropical areas) are much more likely to be seronegative for VZV.
- Women seeking prepregnancy advice should be asked about history of clinical chickenpox. In the absence of a previous clinical illness consistent with chickenpox, VZV IgG can be checked, and vaccination considered PRIOR to conception. (Avoid pregnancy for at least 4 weeks after second dose of vaccine.)
- Vaccination can be offered postpartum for women who have been identified as seronegative during pregnancy. It is safe to breastfeed after VZV vaccination.
- Women who have not had chickenpox should be advised to avoid contact with chickenpox and shingles during pregnancy and to seek medical advice as soon as possible if an exposure occurs (defined as being in the same room for >15 minutes for chickenpox, or direct contact with active lesions of shingles, particularly if the person with shingles is significantly immunocompromised).
- If **exposure** occurs, and woman is **seronegative, VZIG** is advised (effective **up to 10 days** after exposure). Even if chickenpox does occur, the illness is likely to be less severe and FVS is less likely.

Clinical Features

- Complications including pneumonia (5%), hepatitis, and encephalitis are more common in pregnancy.

- The risk of severe chickenpox is increased in smokers, pre-existing lung disease, immunosuppression, and in the second half of pregnancy.
- A dense or hemorrhagic rash and mucosal involvement also predict potentially severe disease.

Fetal Consequences of Primary VZV Infection

- 1st trimester
  - No increased risk of miscarriage.
  - Congenital varicella syndrome (CVS): limb hypoplasia, eye defects (cataracts, chorioretinitis, microphthalmia), neurologic defects (microcephaly, cortical atrophy), intrauterine growth retardation (IUGR), and dermatomal skin scarring.
  - **Highest risk** if infection acquired **<20 weeks' gestation.**
  - Occurs in only 1%–2% of cases.
- 2nd trimester: undetected fetal chickenpox with no discernible sequelae.
- Neonatal varicella: severe or fatal chickenpox in neonates in whom primary varicella was acquired in mother **7 days before to 7 days after delivery** (mortality 30% untreated).

Management

Postexposure Prophylaxis

- Varicella immunoglobulin (VZIG) recommended for all pregnant women without evidence of immunity following a significant exposure. Neonates with significant exposure to chickenpox or shingles should receive VZIG for any of the following:
  1. A VZV-antibody negative neonate during the 1st 7 days of life.
  2. A premature infant still requiring intensive care.
  3. An infant born at >28/40 with no maternal immunity.
  4. An infant born at <28/40 or birthweight <1500g.
  5. If their mother develops chickenpox in the period 7 days before or after delivery.
- VZIG should be administered **as soon as possible** in neonates (ideally within 7 days), and **no later than 10 days** postexposure in pregnant women. Chickenpox may still occur. Cases should be monitored and treated with ACV should infection manifest.
- Prophylaxis with oral ACV/valACV may be considered in the absence of VZIG. Treatment should be commenced 7–10 days postexposure for 7 days.

Treatment

- Treat with **oral ACV if gestation >20 weeks,** particularly if rash <24 hours old.
- Consider treatment with oral ACV if <20 weeks gestation. It is not licensed for use in pregnancy (although it appears to be safe). Benefits may outweigh risk.
- Any respiratory or neurologic symptoms should prompt urgent assessment and consideration of admission.
- **Intravenous ACV is indicated in severe varicella in pregnancy at any gestation.**

If primary VZV infection occurs in the last weeks of pregnancy, where possible **delivery should be delayed** until at least 7 days after the appearance of the rash to allow transplacental antibody transfer, and to avoid maternal complications, e.g., coagulopathy and hemorrhage. Multiple specialists may need to be involved in management, including ITU and neonatology.

Monitoring

Women who have had chickenpox in the first 28 weeks of pregnancy should be referred to a fetal medicine unit for additional ultrasound examination at least 5 weeks after the illness and further discussion. Prenatal diagnosis of FVS by ultrasound is possible if characteristic abnormalities are detected. Amniocentesis may also be performed: amniotic fluid VZV DNA PCR has a high sensitivity but low specificity for FVS.

Hepatitis B (HBV)

- Routine antenatal care in UK includes screening for hepatitis B surface antigen (HBsAg) at booking appointment. If HBsAg-positive, refer to hepatology/gastroenterology/infectious diseases depending on local protocols, to be seen within 6 weeks to allow assessment and institution of treatment if needed by the 3rd trimester.

> **CLINICAL PEARLS**
>
> - Transmission largely occurs at the time of delivery, and risk is related to maternal viremia, hence the recommendation to treat maternal viral load >10^7 IU/mL with antivirals prepartum to reduce the 10% residual risk of perinatal transmission in this high-risk group despite active and passive immunization of the neonate.

Management

- **Offer tenofovir to women with HBV DNA >10^7 IU/ml** in the 3rd trimester to reduce the risk of transmission of HBV to the infant.
- Monitor quantitative HBV DNA 2 months after starting tenofovir and ALT monthly after the birth to detect postnatal HBV flares in the woman.
- Stop tenofovir 4–12 weeks after the birth unless the mother meets criteria for long-term treatment.
- **Offer active and passive hepatitis B immunization to infants.**
- Advise women that breastfeeding is safe, providing guidance on hepatitis B immunization of the infant is followed.
- Consider the need to test/immunize older children and other household members.

Vaccination

- Give hepatitis B vaccine at birth, 1, 2, and 12 months to all infants born to HBsAg positive mothers.
- Give hepatitis B immune globulin (HBIG) by deep intramuscular injection within 48 hours of birth to all high-risk infants.

TABLE 20.2	Other Infections Adversely Affecting Maternal Outcome	
	Maternal Complications	**Interventions**
Coccidioidomycosis	Risk of severe disease in pregnancy, especially in 3rd trimester or peripartum	Consider antifungals if evidence of active infection: New positive serology Increasing titers despite previous treatment Clinical evidence of disease First-line = amphotericin B (AmB) Avoid triazoles in 1st trimester, risk–benefit analysis for 2nd and 3rd May use intrathecal AmB
Hepatitis E	Mortality rate in 3rd trimester is 20%–25%, compared with overall case fatality rates of 1% during HEV outbreaks	Consider hospitalization for supportive management
Influenza	Increased risk of severe illness and death (4–5×); highest risk probably in 3rd trimester and first 4 postpartum weeks	Prevent with vaccination; treat suspected or proven infection promptly with antivirals (severe illness with admission to ITU and death more frequent with delay of antivirals)
Malaria	Severe disease more likely in pregnant women (particularly primigravida) Severe anemia Increased risk of hypoglycemia Maternal mortality	Choice of malarial drugs for both treatment and prophylaxis is affected by stage of pregnancy

- Follow-up by pediatric or primary care team according to local arrangements.

The **following infants are considered "high-risk" and should receive both vaccine and HBIG**

- Mother has acute hepatitis B in pregnancy.
- There is detectable maternal HBsAg and:
  - HBeAg is positive
  - HBeAg and anti-HBe are negative
  - e markers are not available
  - infant is born weighing <1500g
  - maternal HBV DNA known to be >200,000 IU/mL or >1 ×10^6 copies/mL

Human Immunodeficiency Virus (HIV)

- Universal opt-out screening in 1st trimester of pregnancy in UK; CDC recommend all pregnant women are screened. Aim is to identify all positive women in order to achieve undetectable viral load by 3rd trimester, allow normal labor and delivery, and prevent MTCT.
- **Scenarios**
  - Living with HIV prepregnancy.
  - New diagnosis: requiring ART for mother's health.
  - ART during pregnancy in asymptomatic mother for prevention of MTCT only.
  - Late presenter not on treatment.
- **Principles**
  - Make the diagnosis early, refer to expert care in order to start ART during 2nd trimester.
  - Viral load testing at 36/40 informs decision-making as to mode of delivery.

- **MTCT rates now <1%** with management according to current guidelines.

Best practice in this area is constantly changing, and all patients should be managed by a specialist multidisciplinary team. The British HIV Association guidelines for the management of HIV in pregnant women are regularly updated and a useful reference for information.

Other Infections in Pregnancy with Adverse Maternal Outcome

Table 20.2 summarizes the maternal complications and management of coccidioidomycosis, hepatitis E, influenza, and malaria in pregnancy.

Further Reading and Resources

1. British HIV Association. BHIVA Guidelines on the Management of HIV in Pregnancy and Postpartum; 2018. https://www.bhiva.org/pregnancy-guidelines.
2. Royal College of Obstetricians and Gynecologists. Chickenpox in Pregnancy. Green-Top Guideline No. 13; 2015. https://www.rcog.org.uk/globalassets/documents/guidelines/gtg13.pdf.
3. Public Health England (PHE). The Green Book; 2018. Chapter 34, Varicella https://www.gov.uk/government/collections/immunisation-against-infectious-disease-the-green-book#the-green-book.
4. Public Health England (PHE). Zika Virus (ZIKV): Clinical and Travel Guidance; 2019 (updated regularly) https://www.gov.uk/government/collections/zika-virus-zikv-clinical-and-travel-guidance.
5. Kingston M, et al. BASHH UK National Guidelines on the Management of Syphilis; 2015. https://www.bashh.org/documents/UK%20syphilis%20guidelines%202015.pdf.

21

Sexually Transmitted Infections

NICHOLAS VAN WAGONER, WESLEY WILLEFORD

Definitions

Syndromes caused by sexually transmitted infections (STIs) can be broadly categorized as:

Urethritis: inflammation of the urethra characterized by symptoms of dysuria, urethral pruritus, and/or urethral discharge. Signs may include mucoid, mucopurulent, or purulent discharge. (Table 21.1.)

Vaginitis: inflammation of the vagina characterized by symptoms of discharge, itching, discomfort, or odor. Signs include vulvovaginal inflammation characterized by erythema (diffuse or localized), edema, abnormal vaginal pH, and/or discharge. (Table 21.2.)

Cervicitis: inflammation of the cervix characterized by symptoms of vaginal discharge, unusual vaginal bleeding, vaginal irritation/pain, dyspareunia, or pelvic pressure/pain. Signs include purulent or mucopurulent endocervical exudate in the endocervical canal or on an endocervical swab specimen, endocervical friability, and edematous cervical ectopy. (Table 21.3.)

Pelvic inflammatory disease (PID): infection of the upper female reproductive tract characterized by abnormal vaginal discharge, pelvic pain, bleeding between periods, and dyspareunia. Signs include cervical motion tenderness with or without pain with palpation of the adnexa or uterus. Caused by extension of lower genital tract infection. Signs of cervicitis may or may not be present.

Proctitis: inflammation of the rectum characterized by symptoms of pus/blood on stools or when wiping, anorectal pain, tenesmus, and/or constipation. Signs on anoscopic exam include erythema of rectal tissue, purulent discharge, and erosions/ulcers.

Proctocolitis: inflammation of the colonic mucosa extending to 12 cm above the anus. Symptoms and signs include those observed with proctitis plus abdominal cramping and diarrhea.

Enteritis: inflammation of the small intestine characterized by diarrhea and abdominal cramping without signs of proctitis or proctocolitis. Signs may include fecal leukocytes and/or positive ova and parasites.

Epididymitis/orchitis: epididymitis and orchitis are inflammation of the epididymis and testicle(s), respectively. Characterized by swelling and pain of the scrotum, epididymis and/or testicle(s). Signs include edema, and/or tenderness to palpation of the scrotum, epididymis, and/or testicle(s).

Genital ulcer: skin defect characterized by ulceration (deep) or erosion (superficial) predominantly confined to the genitals, perineum, anus, and perianal skin. Lesions may be painful or pruritic (genital herpes) or painless (primary syphilis). Symptoms and signs may also include inguinal lymphadenopathy. Systemic symptoms may be observed at the time of genital herpes primary infection.

Approach to the Sexual History

- An effective sexual history is fundamental to determining STI risk.
- Sexual history-taking guidance is available from the National Coalition for Sexual Health, the Centers for Disease Control and Prevention, and the National LGBT Health and Education Center.
- Sexual behavior can vary between individuals and across an individual's life span. Routinely take a sexual history to determine current sexual health needs. When taking a sexual history, use inclusive and neutral terms, avoid assumptions, and avoid use of judgmental terms.
- Use information learned from the sexual history to guide counselling (i.e., STI risk reduction, sexual function, and sexual satisfaction).
- The sexual history can be an effective place to assess gender identity and sexual orientation.

INFLAMMATORY INFECTIONS

Chlamydia trachomatis

Microbiology

- *C. trachomatis* is a gram-negative obligate intracellular bacterium.

TABLE 21.1 **Summary Table of Common Urethral Infections**

	Urethritis		
	Neisseria gonorrhoeae	*Chlamydia trachomatis*	*Mycoplasma genitalium*
Symptoms	Dysuria, discharge	Dysuria, discharge	Dysuria, discharge
Quality of discharge	Cloudy, purulent	Often clear	Often clear
Diagnosis	Urine NAAT	Urine NAAT	Can do NAAT testing, but no FDA approved test. Usually sent to large centers
Treatment	Ceftriaxone 250 mg IM + azithromycin 1 g	Azithromycin 1 g stat *or* doxycycline 100 mg BD for 7 days	Azithromycin 1 g (resistance approximate 50% in some settings), may require moxifloxacin 400 mg daily for 14 days

TABLE 21.2 **Summary Table of Common Vaginal Infections**

	Vaginal Discharge (see also Chapter 18)		
	Bacterial Vaginosis	*Trichomoniasis*	*Candidiasis*
Symptoms	Discharge without pain or pruritus	May have pain with intercourse, dysuria, vaginal soreness	Vaginal dryness, pain with intercourse
Quality of discharge	Malodorous, homogenous discharge which may be clear, white, or gray. Fishy odor often present	Green-yellow, frothy discharge	White, thick, without odor
Diagnosis	3/4 of Amsel criteria	NAAT from vaginal, endocervical, or urine specimens. May also use wet mount	Wet prep demonstrating budding yeast, hyphae, or pseudohyphae with 10% KOH solution
Treatment	Metronidazole 500 mg twice daily for 7 days	Metronidazole 2 g orally as a single dose	OTC regimens including clotrimazole; but can use fluconazole 150 mg in a single dose

TABLE 21.3 **Summary Table of Common Cervical Infections**

	Cervicitis		
	Neisseria gonorrhoeae	*Chlamydia trachomatis*	*Mycoplasma genitalium*
Symptoms	Vaginal discharge, unusual vaginal bleeding, vaginal irritation/pain, dyspareunia, or pelvic pressure/pain	Vaginal discharge, unusual vaginal bleeding, vaginal irritation/pain, dyspareunia, or pelvic pressure/pain	Vaginal discharge, unusual vaginal bleeding, vaginal irritation/pain, dyspareunia, or pelvic pressure/pain
Diagnosis	Cervical discharge NAAT	Cervical discharge NAAT	Can do NAAT. Usually sent to large centers
Treatment	Ceftriaxone 250 mg IM + azithromycin 1 g stat	Azithromycin 1 g stat *or* doxycycline 100 mg BD for 7 days	Azithromycin 1 g stat (resistance approximate 50% in some settings), may require moxifloxacin 400 mg OD for 14 days

- Strains are divided into three biovars, then subtyped by serovar.
  - Trachoma biovar: serovars A–C cause infection of the eyes.
  - Genital tract biovar: serovars D–K are sexually transmitted and cause urogenital and anorectal infections.
  - Lymphogranuloma venereum (LGV) biovar: serovars L1–3 are sexually transmitted and cause invasive urogenital and anorectal infection.
- *C. trachomatis* has a biphasic life cycle.
  - Extracellular: infectious elementary body.
  - Intracellular: noninfectious reticulate body.
  - Elementary bodies enter mucosal cells, then differentiate into reticulate bodies in a membrane-bound compartment known as an inclusion. After several rounds of replication, reticulate bodies differentiate into elementary bodies, are released from the cell, and infect neighboring cells.
  - *C. trachomatis* cannot be grown on conventional bacteriologic medium.
  - The innate and adaptive branches of the immune system respond to *C. trachomatis* infection, yet **reinfection is common.**

Epidemiology of Genital Tract Serovars

- Most frequently reported infectious disease in the United States.
  - Highest rates observed in women 15–24 years of age.
  - Prevalence of *C. trachomatis* is increasing.
  - Rates are higher among racial/ethnic minorities compared to whites.

Clinical Manifestations of Genital Tract Serovars

The majority of people infected are asymptomatic.
- Cervicitis (Table 21.3)
  - 85% have no signs or symptoms.
  - Incubation period 7–14 days for symptomatic disease.
  - Duration of asymptomatic infection unknown.
  - May experience vaginal discharge, intermenstrual bleeding, or postcoital bleeding.
  - Signs include pelvic tenderness and cervical motion tenderness.
  - Complications include pelvic inflammatory disease, ectopic pregnancy, infertility, perihepatitis.
- Urethritis (Fig. 21.1A, Table 21.1).
  - Roughly 50% asymptomatic.
  - Incubation period 5–10 days.
  - When present, discharge is most often characterized as mucoid.
  - Complications: epididymitis, prostatitis, reactive arthritis (more commonly observed in men).
- Proctitis
  - *C. trachomatis* infection is often asymptomatic, in contrast to the LGV serovars.

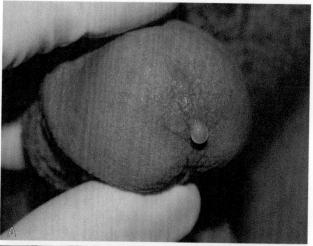

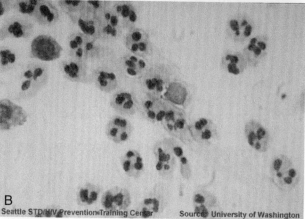

- **Fig. 21.1** (A) Mucoid to cloudy discharge of urethritis. (B) Urethral specimen gram stain consistent with nongonococcal urethritis for which *C. trachomatis* is a cause (i.e., presence of polymorphonuclear cells without intracellular diplococci. (From Geisler WM. Diseases caused by chlamydiae. In: Goldman L, Schafer AI, eds. *Goldman–Cecil Medicine.* 23rd ed. Elsevier; 2007.)

Diagnosis of Genital Tract Serovars

- Cervicitis
  - Leukorrhea with >10 WBC per high power field examination of vaginal fluid is associated with chlamydia (nonspecific).
  - Perform **nucleic acid amplification testing (NAAT)** for *C. trachomatis* on all persons with cervicitis from vaginal, cervical, or urine specimens.
- Urethritis
  - Point-of-care tests do not distinguish between infectious and noninfectious causes of nongonococcal urethritis (NGU). As a well-established cause of NGU, *C. trachomatis* should always be considered when symptoms of urethritis are present and supported by point-of-care evidence.
  - Mucoid, mucopurulent, or purulent discharge on examination.
  - Gram stain of urethral specimen with **≥2 white blood cells (WBC)** per oil immersion field (Fig. 21.1B).

- Positive leukocyte esterase from first-void urine or ≥10 WBC per high power field on sediment from spun first-void urine.
- Perform NAAT for *C. trachomatis* on all persons with urethritis from urethral or first-void urine specimens.
- First void urine = first catch urine. Instruct patients to hold their urine for ≥1 hour before testing. Capture the first 20 mL of urine as contains the highest organism load.
- Urethral swab: insert 2–4 cm inside urethra and rotate once before removal.
- Proctitis
  - Patients with symptoms of proctitis should undergo anoscopy to look for **mucosal edema, easy bleeding, and/or ulcerations** and to evaluate patency of the rectal lumen. Gram stain of anorectal exudate may show polymorphonuclear leukocytes (PMN).
  - Perform NAAT for *C. trachomatis* on all person with proctitis from rectal specimens. NAAT recently approved for extragenital use.

Screening

- **Women**
  - All sexually active women <25 years old and sexually active women ≥25 years old with risk factors (i.e., a new sex partner, more than one sex partner, a sex partner with concurrent partners, or a sex partner with a sexually transmitted infection). **Rescreen 3 months after treatment** of *C. trachomatis.*
  - All pregnant women <25 years old and pregnant women ≥25 years old with risk factors.
  - Retest pregnant women in the 3rd trimester if <25 years old or ≥25 years old with risk factors.
  - Pregnant women with chlamydia infection **need a test-of-cure 3–4 weeks after treatment.** Rescreen 3 months after treatment.

- **Men**
  - Consider screening young men in high prevalence clinical settings such as **adolescent clinics, correctional facilities, and STD clinics.**
  - In men who have sex with men (MSM), screen at least **annually** at sites of exposure (urethra and rectum) **independent of condom use.** Screen MSM every 3 to 6 months at increased risk, including those with human immunodeficiency virus (HIV).

Treatment of Genital Tract Serovars

- Primary regimens for infections of the cervix, urethra, and rectum.
  - Azithromycin 1 gram orally in a single dose (preferred in pregnancy).
  - Doxycycline 100 mg twice daily for 7 days (contraindicated in the 2nd and 3rd trimesters of pregnancy).
- Alternative agents include erythromycin, levofloxacin, and ofloxacin.
- Partner notification and treatment recommended.

Epidemiology of LGV Serovars

- Uncommon STI.
- LGV is endemic in certain areas of Africa, Southeast Asia, India, the Caribbean, and South America.
- In developed countries, LGV is predominantly associated with rectal infections. LGV is increasingly recognized as a cause of proctitis and proctocolitis among MSM.

Clinical Manifestations of LGV Serovars

- Genital tract infection is characterized by **transient genital ulcer(s) or papule(s)**, followed by the appearance of tender inguinal and/or femoral **lymphadenopathy** (typically unilateral) and **bubo** formation (Fig. 21.2A).

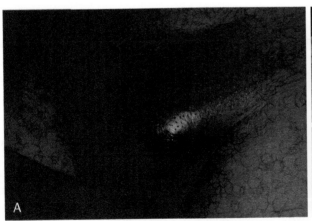
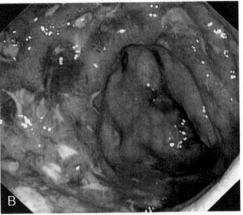

- **Fig. 21.2** (A) LGV with inguinal lymphadenopathy. (B) LGV proctitis. (Panel A from Pereira FA. Lymphogranuloma venereum. In: *Treatment of Skin Disease: Comprehensive Therapeutic Strategies.* 5th ed. Elsevier; 2017. Panel B from Felt-Bersma RJF, Bartelsman JF, et al. Hemorrhoids, rectal prolapse, anal fissure, perianal fistulae and sexually transmitted diseases. *Best Pract Res Clin Gastroenterol.* 2009;23(4):575–592. © 2009.)

- **Groove sign**, formed by swollen matted lymph nodes developing along the course of the inguinal ligament may be present.
- **Proctitis** (Fig. 21.2B) and **proctocolitis** characterized by rectal ulcerations, bleeding, tenesmus, mucoid discharge, and lower abdominal cramping and pain.
- LGV proctitis and proctocolitis can mimic inflammatory bowel disease.
- Complications: perirectal abscess(es), fissures, fever, malaise, weight loss, fatigue.

Diagnosis of LGV Serovars

- Diagnosis is usually based on epidemiologic and clinical findings, confirmation of *C. trachomatis* infection by NAAT, and exclusion of other potential etiologies of proctocolitis, lymphadenopathy, or genital ulcers. Gram stain of anorectal exudate may show PMNs.
- When available, persons with positive *C. trachomatis* NAAT and findings concerning for LGV should undergo molecular testing on the outer membrane protein A (*omp*A).
- Available NAATs for *C. trachomatis* do not distinguish between non-LGV and LGV serovars.

Treatment of LGV Serovars

- Primary regimen for genital and rectal infections
  - Doxycycline 100 mg twice daily for 21 days.
- Alternative regimen
  - Erythromycin 500 mg 4 times daily for 21 days.
- Partner notification and treatment recommended.
- When buboes are present, **aspiration** or incision and drainage should be considered to prevent development of ulcerations or fistulous tracts.

Neisseria gonorrhoeae

Microbiology

- *N. gonorrhoeae* is a gram-negative diplococcus with demanding nutritional and environmental *in vitro* growth requirements.
- **Thayer-Martin agar** is used to isolate *N. gonorrhoeae* from nonsterile sites.
- Chocolate agar is used to culture from sterile sites.
- *In vitro* culture requires **CO_2 enrichment.**
- It infects mucosal surfaces including the endocervix, urethra, rectum, pharynx, and conjunctiva.
- Type IV pili is an important virulence factor that allows *N. gonorrhoeae* to attach to mucosal epithelial cells and to polymorphonuclear leukocytes.
- The organism does not elicit a protective immune response and individuals can become repeatedly infected.
- *N. gonorrhoeae* has the capacity for antigenic variation whereby it can express different surface antigens which help the organism evade antibody response.

Epidemiology

- Rates of gonorrhea have increased annually since 2009 in the United States.
- Although rates increased in both sexes, higher rates are observed among men.
  - Rates of gonorrhoea are highest in men 20–29 years of age.
- Rates are higher among racial/ethnic minorities compared to whites.
- Antimicrobial resistance remains a persistent concern with *N. gonorrhoeae*.

Clinical Manifestations

- Cervicitis (Fig. 21.3A, Table 21.3).

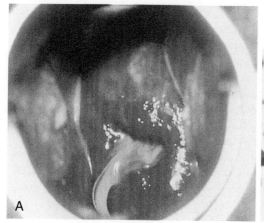
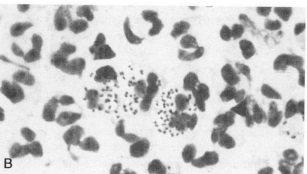

• **Fig. 21.3** (A) Mucopurulent discharge associated with cervicitis. (B) Gram stain consistent with gonococcal urethritis. (Panel A from Ison CA, Lewis DA. Gonorrhoea. In: Morse SA, et al. *Atlas of Sexually Transmitted Diseases and AIDS*. 4th ed. Elsevier; 2010. Panel B from Braverman PK. Urethritis, vulvovaginitis, and cervicitis. In: Long SS, Prober CG, Fischer M, eds. *Principles and Practice of Pediatric Infectious Diseases*. 5th ed. Elsevier; 2018.)

- Complications: pelvic inflammatory disease, ectopic pregnancy, infertility, disseminated gonococcal infection (DGI) (i.e., petechial or pustular acral skin lesions, asymmetric polyarthralgia, tenosynovitis, or oligoarticular septic arthritis).
- Urethritis (when present, discharge may be mucoid, mucopurulent, or purulent) (Table 21.1).
  - Complications: epididymitis, prostatitis, and DGI.
- Proctitis.
- Pharyngitis.
- *N. gonorrhoeae* infection is often asymptomatic.

Diagnosis

- Cervicitis
  - Leukorrhea with >10 WBC per high power field examination of vaginal fluid is associated with *N. gonorrhoeae* (nonspecific).
  - Perform nucleic acid amplification testing (NAAT) for *N. gonorrhoeae* on all persons with cervicitis from vaginal, cervical, or urine specimens.

Urethritis

- Mucoid, mucopurulent, or purulent discharge on examination.
- Gram stain of urethral specimen with ≥2 white blood cells (WBC) per oil immersion field with WBC containing gram-negative intracellular diplococci (Fig. 21.3B).
- Positive leukocyte esterase from first-void urine or ≥10 WBC per high power field on sediment from spun first-void urine.
- Perform NAAT for *N. gonorrhoeae* on all persons with urethritis from urethral or first-void urine specimens.
- Proctitis
  - Patients with symptoms of proctitis should undergo anoscopy to look for mucosal edema, easy bleeding, and/or ulcerations and to evaluate patency of the rectal lumen. Gram stain of anorectal exudate may show PMNs with or without gram-negative intracellular diplococci.
  - Perform NAAT for *N. gonorrhoeae* on all person with proctitis from rectal specimens.
- Pharyngitis
  - In most cases, **pharyngeal gonorrhea is asymptomatic.** When pharyngitis and risk for exposure are present, perform NAAT on pharyngeal specimens.

Screening

- **Women**
  - All sexually active women <25 years old and sexually active women ≥25 years old with risk factors (i.e., a new sex partner, more than one sex partner, a sex partner with concurrent partners, or a sex partner with a sexually transmitted infection). Rescreen 3 months after treatment of *N. gonorrhoeae*.
  - All pregnant women <25 years old and pregnant women ≥25 years old with risk factors. Rescreen 3 months after treatment.

- **MSM**
  - Screen at least annually at sites of exposure (pharynx, urethra, rectum) independent of condom use. Screen MSM every 3–6 months at increased risk including those with HIV.

Treatment

- Primary regimen for infections of the cervix, urethra, and rectum
  - **Ceftriaxone** 250 mg IM in a single dose *plus* azithromycin 1 g orally in a single dose.
- Alternative regimens cervix, urethra, and rectum
  - Cefixime 400 mg orally in a single dose *plus* azithromycin 1 gram orally in a single dose.
- Primary regimen for infections of the pharynx
  - Ceftriaxone 250 mg IM in a single dose *plus* azithromycin 1 g orally in a single dose.
- Partner notification and treatment recommended.
- Other treatment considerations
  - When cephalosporin treatment failure is suspected (symptoms do not resolve within 3–5 days of appropriate treatment and no sexual exposure; or positive cultures 72 hours post-treatment; or positive NAAT 7 days after appropriate treatment with no new exposure), perform culture with antimicrobial susceptibility testing and report case to CDC.
  - Gonococcal infections of the pharynx are more difficult to eradicate.

Mycoplasma genitalium

Microbiology

- *M. genitalium* is among the smallest known bacteria.
- It has a flask-like shape and lacks a cell wall.
- It is a facultative anaerobe.
- Culture requires cocultivation with Vero cells and may take up to several months to show growth.

Epidemiology

- The prevalence of *M. genitalium* from general population samples ranges from 1% to 3%.
- In persons presenting to STI clinics and with syndromes consistent with STI, the prevalence of *M. genitalium* is higher.
- Accounts for 15%–20% of nongonococcal urethritis (NGU) in men. Its role in other male anogenital tract syndromes is less well characterized.
- The pathogenic role for *M. genitalium* in women is less well understood. The organism is more often found in women with cervicitis than without cervicitis.

Clinical Manifestations

- Cervicitis: potential role (Table 21.3).
  - Complications may include PID.
- Urethritis (Table 21.1).

- Acute NGU similar in character to NGU that is caused by *C. trachomatis*.
- Thought to account for a large proportion of persistent and/or recurrent NGU.

Diagnosis

- NAAT testing of urine, urethral, vaginal, and cervical swabs is offered at some large centers and by some commercial laboratories.
- Consider *M. genitalium* in persistent or recurrent cases of urethritis and possibly in cases of persistent or recurrent cervicitis and PID.

Treatment

- **Agents targeting the bacterial cell wall are ineffective.**
- **Resistance to doxycycline and azithromycin is common.**
- Therapy is less well characterized than for other STI.
- Urethritis and cervicitis
  - Initial: azithromycin 1 g (resistance approximate 50% in some settings).
  - Treatment failures: moxifloxacin 400 mg daily for 7, 10, or 14 days.
- PID
  - Consider *M. genitalium* in cases that do not respond to standard therapy.
  - Consider moxifloxacin 400 mg for 14 days in these settings.
- Partner notification and treatment recommended.

Trichomonas vaginalis

Microbiology

- *Trichomonas vaginalis* is an **anaerobic**, single-cell, motile, **flagellated protozoan.**
- Varies in size and shape with a mean length and width of 10 μm × 7 μm.
  - It contains 5 flagella. Four are located at its anterior portion and 1 is embedded within its membrane.
  - It infects the **squamous epithelium** of the urogenital tract including the vagina, urethra, and paraurethral glands.
- *T. vaginalis* grows in broth culture (Diamond's TYI).

Epidemiology

- **Most prevalent nonviral STI** in the United States and worldwide.
- Found in 3%–5% of women in North America.
- Rates are higher among racial/ethnic minorities compared to whites.
- Unlike *C. trachomatis* and *N. gonorrhoeae*, *T. vaginalis* is not uncommonly found in women over 40 years of age.
- Associated with increased risk for HIV acquisition.
- Infection is linked to adverse pregnancy outcomes.
- Infection **may persist** for months to years if untreated.

Clinical Manifestations

- Most (70%–85%) infections are asymptomatic or present with minimal symptoms.
- Vaginitis may be characterized by (Fig. 21.4, Table 21.2)
  - Malodorous, green-yellow, frothy vaginal discharge.
  - Vulvar erythema and pruritus.
  - Vaginal inflammation.
  - Strawberry cervix.
  - Dyspareunia.
- Urethritis, epididymitis, prostatitis, in pregnancy, may cause
  - Premature rupture of membranes.
  - Preterm delivery.
  - Postpartum sepsis.
  - Low birth weight.

Diagnosis: Vaginitis and Urethritis

- **NAAT** from vaginal, endocervical, or urine specimens is recommended (FDA approved). NAAT may be used to detect *T. vaginalis* from urethral specimens in men if CLIA certified.
- **Wet mount** of vaginal specimens is highly specific but has low sensitivity.
  - Mobile flagellated protozoa may be seen.
  - Advantage of point-of-care testing.
  - Sample the posterior fornix.
- Culture was the reference standard prior to the development of molecular detection tests.
  - In women, culture of vaginal specimens is preferred over urine.
  - In men, culture of urethral swab, urine sediment, or semen is recommended.
- Other FDA point-of-care assays are available.

Screening

- Consider screening women in high prevalence settings, including STI clinics and correctional facilities.
- Consider screening women with risk for infection, including multiple sex partners, history of STI, substance use, and commercial sex work.
- Screen women with HIV at entry to care and then annually. More frequent screening may be indicated by risk.

Treatment

- Recommended treatment for women and men
  - Metronidazole 2 g orally as a single dose, *or*
  - Tinidazole 2 g orally as a single dose.
- Alternate treatment (use if treatment failure with above regimen and reinfection is not believed to be the cause)
  - Metronidazole 500 mg orally twice daily for 7 days.
- Recommended treatment in women with HIV
  - Metronidazole 500 mg orally twice daily for 7 days
- **Disulfiram-like reaction** is possible with nitroimidazoles. Caution patients about alcohol consumption when taking metronidazole or tinidazole.

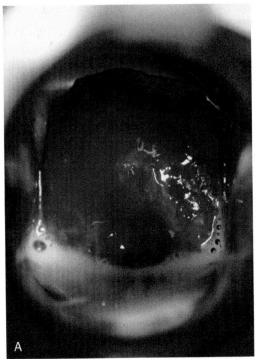

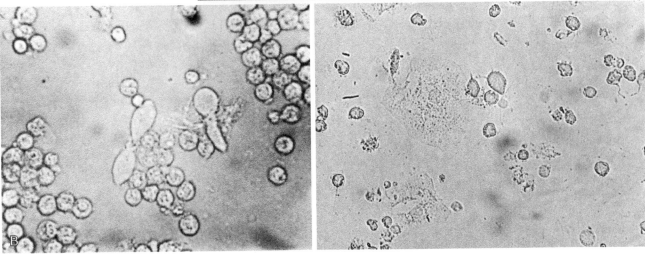

• **Fig. 21.4** (A) Frothy discharge of vaginal trichomoniasis with strawberry cervix. (B) Microscopic view of wet preparation with *T. vaginalis*. (Panel A from Lewis D. *Medicine.* 2014;42(7):369–371. Panel B(i) from Faro S. Trichomoniasis. In: Kaufman RH, Faro S, eds. *Benign Diseases of the Vulva and Vagina.* 4th ed. Mosby–Year Book; 1994. B(ii) from Friedrich EG. *Vulvar Disease.* 2nd ed. WB Saunders; 1983.)

- **Tinidazole reaches higher levels in the genital tract, has a longer half-life, and few side effects but is more expensive than metronidazole.**

Bacterial Vaginosis

- Bacterial vaginosis (Table 21.2) is a polymicrobial clinical syndrome resulting in the replacement of *Lactobacillus* spp. by organisms such as *Prevotella* spp., *Mobiluncus* spp., *Gardnerella vaginalis*, *Mycoplasma*, and *Ureaplasma*.
- Cause of alteration of vaginal microbes is incompletely understood.
- It is unclear whether bacterial vaginosis involves the sexual transmission of an instigating pathogen.
- See also Chapter 18.

Other Causes of Vaginitis

- Vulvovaginal candidiasis (Table 21.2) (see also Chapter 18).
- Consider irritant or allergic contact dermatitis, atrophic vaginitis and erosive lichen planus in women presenting with vaginitis.

GENITAL ULCERS

Treponema pallidum

Microbiology

- *T. pallidum* has a helicallycoiled corkscrew shape (6–15 μm × 0.1–0.2 μm).

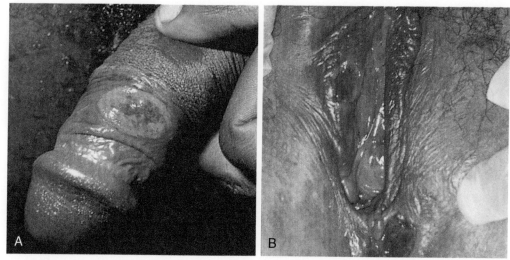

• **Fig. 21.5** (A and B) Primary syphilis. (From Cox D, Ballard RC. Syphilis. In: Morse SA, Ballard AC, Holmes KK, Moreland AA. *Atlas of Sexually Transmitted Diseases and AIDS*. 4th ed. Elsevier; 2010.)

- It grows slowly with a division time of 30 hours.
- *T. pallidum* cannot be cultured *in vitro*.
- The organism is too slender for visualization by conventional light microscopy. It can be visualized by dark-field microscopy.
- Epidemiology
- In low-income countries approximately 5 million cases are diagnosed yearly with **heterosexual transmission common and congenital infection not uncommon.**
- In the United States and other industrialized countries, rates of reported primary and secondary syphilis are increasing.
  - **MSM** account for most cases of primary and secondary syphilis.
  - Rates are higher among racial/ethnic minorities compared to whites.
  - There are high rates of syphilis and HIV co-infection.

Clinical Manifestations

- Direct lesion contact during sex is responsible for most cases of transmission.
- Time from exposure to first symptoms (primary syphilis) is approximately 3 weeks.
- Left untreated, *T. pallidum* will disseminate widely through the bloodstream and produce varying clinical manifestations (secondary syphilis), typically within 2–3 years of infection. Some infected persons will develop symptoms after a long period of latency (tertiary syphilis).

Stages of Disease

Primary Syphilis (Figs. 21.5A and B)
- **Localized, nontender, clean-based, indurated ulcer** at site of inoculation (i.e., chancre).
- The chancre can be located at nearly any location exposed (i.e., genitalia, oropharynx, rectum).

- The primary chancre may be accompanied by tender or nontender regional lymphadenopathy.
- Without treatment, the primary lesion(s) will usually resolve in 3–6 weeks.

Secondary Syphilis (Figs. 21.6A and 21.B)
- Typically characterized by **painless, macular rash** of 1–2 cm, reddish or copper lesions, and is often located on the **palms** of the hands or the **soles** of the feet. However, the rash of secondary syphilis can be widely variable and involve mucous membranes which are highly infectious (i.e., condyloma lata).
- Some other manifestations of secondary syphilis include diffuse lymphadenopathy, hepatosplenomegaly, hepatitis, nephrotic syndrome.

Latent Syphilis
- The **asymptomatic period** that occurs after resolution of manifestations of secondary syphilis.
  - Early latent infection is defined as infection <1 year.
  - Late latent infection is defined as infection >1 year.

Tertiary Syphilis
- About **one-third** of those with **untreated syphilis** will develop manifestations of neurosyphilis, cardiovascular syphilis, or gummatous syphilis.
- Cardiovascular manifestations most often include aneurysm of the ascending aorta, aortic valve insufficiency, or coronary artery disease.
- Gumma are reactive, granulomatous processes that lead to symptoms secondary to locally exerted **mass effect.**
- Neurologic manifestations include **general paresis** (dementia, seizures, or psychiatric syndrome) and **tabes dorsalis** from posterior column and spinal nerve root involvement (abrupt and severe radicular pain, ataxia from loss of proprioception, Argyll–Robinson pupil, loss of reflexes, and impaired vibratory sense).

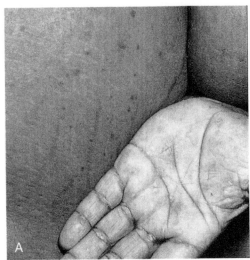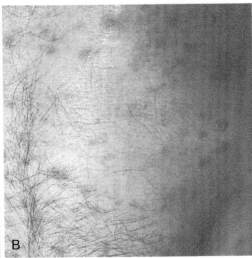

• **Fig. 21.6** (A and B) Dermatologic manifestations of secondary syphilis. (From Cox D, Ballard RC. Syphilis. In: Morse SA, Ballard AC, Holmes KK, Moreland AA. *Atlas of Sexually Transmitted Diseases and AIDS*. 4th ed. Elsevier; 2010.)

• Note that neurologic manifestation of syphilis can occur at any stage and include **uveitis, cranial nerve palsies, aseptic meningitis,** and **stroke-like meningovascular syphilis.**

Diagnosis

• Dark field microscopy is infrequently used due to decreased availability of equipment, requirement for specimen collection from active lesions, and improvement in serologic testing.
• **Nontreponemal tests** are based on antigens synthesized from lecithin, cholesterol, and cardiolipin that react with antibodies produced in response to *T. pallidum* infection.
  • The rapid plasma reagin (**RPR**) and Venereal Disease Research Laboratory (**VDRL**) tests detect IgG and IgM.
  • These are **quantitative tests** used to detect *T. pallidum* infection and to track response to therapy.
• **Treponemal** tests detect antibodies to treponemal antigens.
  • Examples include fluorescent treponemal antibody adsorbed (**FTA-ABS**) and *Treponema pallidum* particle agglutination (**TPPA**) assays.
  • Once infected, treponemal tests typically **remain positive.**
  • A treponemal test should be performed in persons with a positive nontreponemal test to **confirm** infection.
• When patients with syphilis exhibit signs of cranial nerve dysfunction, auditory or ophthalmic abnormalities, meningitis, stroke, acute or chronic altered mental status, or loss of vibration sense, further testing is warranted to evaluate for **neurosyphilis.**
  • The diagnosis of neurosyphilis depends upon multiple factors including **cerebrospinal fluid (CSF) cell count, protein,** and **CSF-VDRL** in the presence of reactive serologies.
  • CSF-VDRL is highly specific but insensitive.

Treatment

Stage of Disease	First-Line Treatment
Primary and secondary syphilis	Benzathine penicillin G 2.4 million units in a single IM dose
Early latent syphilis	Benzathine penicillin G 2.4 million units in a single IM dose
Late latent syphilis	Benzathine penicillin G 7.2 million units IM in 3 doses at 1-week intervals
Tertiary syphilis	Benzathine penicillin G 7.2 million units IM in 3 doses at 1-week intervals
Neurosyphilis	Aqueous crystalline penicillin 18–24 million units per day administered as 3–4 million units IV every 4 hours or continuous infusion for 10–14 days

Other Diagnostic and Treatment Considerations

• To confirm serologic response to therapy, repeat the same nontreponemal test used for initial diagnosis at **6 and 12 months post-treatment.** An appropriate serologic response is indicated by a **4-fold reduction in titer.**
• **Penicillin G is the preferred agent for syphilis treatment.** In cases of primary and secondary syphilis in penicillin-allergic individuals, doxycycline, tetracycline, azithromycin, and ceftriaxone can be used. When alternate treatment is used, close clinical and serologic follow-up is needed.
• Treat all pregnant women with syphilis with parenteral penicillin G. Desensitize in cases of penicillin allergy.
• The Jarisch–Herxheimer reaction is an acute, febrile reaction characterized by headache, fever, and myalgias. It typically occurs within 24 hours of treatment. It is seen more often in early syphilis.

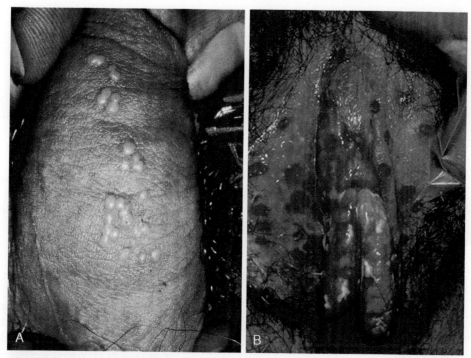

• **Fig. 21.7** (A and B). Clinical manifestations of genital herpes at initial infection. (From Patel R. Genital herpes. *Medicine*. 2014;42(7):354–358.)

- The **prozone phenomenon** is a **false-negative** serologic result from high antibody titers that interfere with antigen-antibody complex formation.
- **Partner treatment**
  - In cases of primary and secondary syphilis, treat partner(s) if exposed within 90 days regardless of serologic status.
  - In cases of primary and secondary syphilis in which exposure was >90 days, treat based upon serologic test results. If testing is unavailable or loss to follow up is likely, presumptively treat.
- All persons diagnosed with primary or secondary syphilis should be tested for HIV.

Herpes Simplex Virus Type 2 (and Type 1)

Virology

- Herpes simplex viruses Type 1 and Type 2 (HSV-2) are large, double-stranded DNA viruses in the *Herpesviridae* family.
- **Pathogenesis**
  - Virus is transmitted through **close contact** with the skin and genital secretions of an infected person who is shedding virus. Viral shedding occurs both in the **presence and absence of symptoms.**
  - HSV initially infects **epithelial or mucosal cells** at the site of entry. The virus then infects sensory nerve endings in the dermis and is transported to the cell's nucleus in the sensory root ganglion.
  - Periodic viral reactivation leads to anterograde transport down the sensory root ganglion and replication in epithelial or mucosal cells. Replication can cause symptoms or be asymptomatic.
- Virus can be grown in cell culture.

Epidemiology

- HSV-2 is the most common cause of genital ulcer disease worldwide.
- While HSV-1 is typically acquired in childhood and causes orolabial infection, it is becoming an important cause of genital herpes.
- **Most persons with genital herpes are unaware of their infection.**
- Rates of genital herpes are higher among women compared to men.
- Rates are higher among racial/ethnic minorities compared to whites.

Clinical Manifestations

Initial Infection

- Symptoms may or may not develop at the time of infection.
- When present, anogenital ulcers are typically **multiple, bilateral**, and last 10–14 days (i.e., more severe than genital ulcers observed in recurrences). Ulcers typically cause **pain or itching.** Associated symptoms may include **dysuria**, vaginal or urethral discharge, and **tender inguinal adenopathy.** Initial infection can cause cervicitis or urethritis (Figs. 21.7A and B).
- **Systemic symptoms**, including fever, headache, malaise, and myalgias, may also be present.

Symptomatic Recurrence (Fig. 21.8)

- Number and severity of recurrences is variable.
- Anogenital ulcers typically last 5–10 days and are **typically less severe** than observed after initial infection.

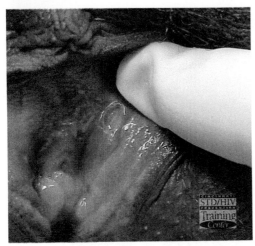

• **Fig. 21.8** Clinical manifestation of genital herpes recurrence. (Courtesy Cincinnati STD/HIV Prevention Training Center, Cincinnati, OH; with permission.)

• Less common manifestations of recurrent include urethritis, cervicitis, fissures.
• Systemic symptoms are absent.
• Often preceded by a **prodrome.**

Asymptomatic Reactivation (Shedding)

• Viral replication in the absence of symptoms. This can occur between clinical recurrences or in persons with no history of clinical symptoms.
• Shedding rates are highest in the first 3 months after infection.

Diagnosis

• **Virologic** tests: require presence of a lesion.
  • Cell culture: sensitivity is low, especially for recurrent lesions. Sensitivity wanes as lesions begin to heal.
  • **NAAT/PCR** is available for diagnosis in some laboratories and is more sensitive than culture.
• **Serologic** tests
  • Type-specific serologic assays are available.
  • In the absence of symptoms, a positive HSV-2 antibody implies genital infection whereas a positive HSV-1 antibody does not distinguish between orolabial and genital infection.
• When lesions are present, virologic and serologic tests are used concurrently to determine acute (cell/culture or NAAT-positive and serologically negative) or recurrent (cell/culture or NAAT-positive and serologically positive).

Screening

• Consider type-specific HSV serologic testing in women and men.
• Pregnant women: HSV-2 serologic screening is not recommended in pregnancy but may be useful in identifying and counseling women at risk for HSV genital infection.

Treatment

• First clinical episode
  • Aciclovir, valaciclovir, or famciclovir. Multiple dosing regimens are approved.
  • Treat for 7–10 days.
• Episodic therapy for recurrent genital herpes
  • Aciclovir, valaciclovir, or famciclovir. Multiple dosing regimens are approved.
  • Treat for 1–5 days depending upon regimen.
• Suppressive therapy
  • Used to reduce frequency of recurrences and rates of transmission.
  • Aciclovir, valaciclovir, and famciclovir are approved for suppressive therapy.
• **Other treatment considerations**
  • In patients living with HIV:
    • Length of therapy for recurrent genital herpes is longer.
    • Suppressive therapy dosing differs.
    • Although suppressive therapy reduces clinical manifestations, it does not reduce risk for transmission of HSV-2 or HIV to susceptible sex partners.
  • Consider resistance when lesions persist in the presence of appropriate therapy.
    • Foscarnet, cidofovir, and imiquimod may be used to treat aciclovir-, valaciclovir-, and famciclovir-resistant HSV.
  • In pregnant women with known genital herpes, suppressive aciclovir or valaciclovir reduces the frequency of recurrences and thus the need for cesarean delivery.

Haemophilus ducreyi (Chancroid)

• Small fastidious gram-negative coccobacillus; requires enriched media, high humidity, and high CO_2.

Epidemiology

• Rare in United States and other developed countries; incidence has dropped markedly elsewhere.
• Incubation period 4–7 days.

Clinical Manifestations

• Classically painful purulent ulcers with ragged undermined edge, which easily bleed.
• May develop inguinal lymphadenopathy, which can develop into painful buboes.
• Aspiration is recommended rather than incision and drainage. These may rupture spontaneously, which delays healing.
• Complications: phimosis, tissue loss, increased risk of HIV transmission.

Diagnosis and Treatment

• Gram stain = "school of fish," but sensitivity is poor.
• PCR more sensitive than culture if available.
• **Treatment**

- Azithromycin 1 g single dose.
- HIV infection: ciprofloxacin 500 mg BD for 3 days.
- Partner treatment recommended if contact within 10 days before symptom onset.

Donovanosis (granuloma inguinale)

- Caused by *Klebsiella granulomatis*, intracellular, encapsulated gram-negative bacteria.
  - Unusual infection, and limited geographically (tropical including India, Australia, Papua New Guinea, the Caribbean, and southern Africa).
  - Primarily a sexually transmitted infection of low infectivity.
  - Causes chronic progressive painless ulceration.
  - Classically: rolled edges, easily bleeds.
  - Ulcers may coalesce or spread subcutaneously and form pseudobuboes.
  - Heal by scarring; may cause lymphedema of the external genitalia.

Lipschutz Ulcer

- Nonsexually acquired acute genital ulceration.
  - Thought to be an immune response to distant infection such as EBV or CMV.
  - Single or multiple, large, bilateral, painful vulvar ulcers in young women and adolescent girls. Usually not sexually active.
  - Usually associated with prodrome of fever, malaise, lymphadenopathy, tonsillitis, and hepatitis.
  - Intense pain and dysuria usually reported.
  - Heal within 6 weeks.

Human Papillomavirus (HPV)

Virology

- Human papillomaviruses are small nonenveloped viruses with a small, circular double-stranded DNA genome belonging to the family *Papillomaviridae.*
- Over 100 types of HPV are defined, of which approximately 40 are sexually transmitted.
- HPV infects cells in the **basal layer of the skin and mucous membranes.** Once infected, differentiating epithelial cells that normally stop dividing continue to divide.
- The early genes *E6* and *E7* from high-risk types are the primary oncoproteins. They manipulate cell cycle regulators, induce chromosomal abnormalities, and block apoptosis.
- Because the infection is nonlytic and restricted to the epithelium, HPV is protected from the host's immune response.

Epidemiology

- HPV is the **most common STI** in the United States.

- Rates of exposure and infection are high shortly after sexual debut.
- HPV types **16 and 18** account for **most cases of cervical cancer** and half of high-grade cervical intraepithelial lesions, or dysplasia. These types also cause most penile, vulvar, vaginal, anal, and oropharyngeal cancers and dysplasia.
- 90% of *Condylomata acuminata* are caused by HPV types 6 and 11.

Clinical Manifestations

- Clinical presentation of HPV infection depends on which type of HPV is causing infection.
- **Most HPV infections are transient** and clear within 8 months to 2 years. However, high-grade HPV types are more likely to persist.
- Condylomata acuminata (anogenital warts) with 90% caused by low risk types 6 or 11.
- Anogenital and oropharyngeal dysplasia and malignancy.

Diagnosis

- **Anogenital warts** (Fig. 21.9)
  - Visual inspection.
  - Biopsy with confirmation should be considered in atypical presentations. Other HPV testing is not recommended.
- **HPV-associated cancers and precancerous lesions**
  - Cervical screening
    - Begin at age 21 through age 65.
    - Perform Pap testing every 3 years on women aged 21–29.
    - Perform Pap testing every 3 years or Pap testing plus HPV testing (detect viral DNA or RNA) every 5 years on women aged 30–65.
    - Perform Pap screening regardless of vaccination status.
    - Women with abnormal Pap screening should undergo HPV testing.
  - Anal cancer screening
    - There is insufficient data to recommend screening.
    - Some centers screen for anal cancer among high-risk populations. These include people with HIV, MSM, and others with a history of receptive anal sex. Anal cytology is initially performed. High-resolution anoscopy is performed when abnormal cytologic results are found.

Treatment and Prevention

- Anogenital wart removal
  - Patient applied: Imiquimod, Podofilox or Sinecatechins 15% ointment.
  - Provider administered: cryotherapy, surgical removal, trichloroacetic acid, or bichloroacetic acid.
  - If a high-grade squamous intraepithelial lesion or cancer is identified when screening for HPV-associated cancer (or from pathology on an excised lesion), refer to a specialist for treatment.

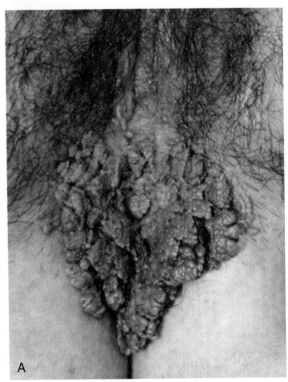
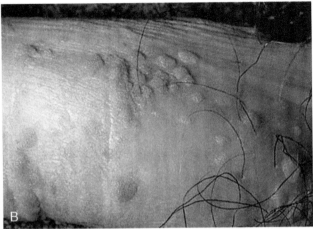

• **Fig. 21.9** (A and B) Anogenital warts. (Panel A reprinted with permission from the American College of Obstetricians and Gynecologists. From Gagné H. Colposcopy of the vagina and vulva. *Obstet Gynecol Clin North Am*. 2008;35:659–669. With permission from the Foreign Policy Research Institute. Panel B from Habit TP, ed. *Clinical Dermatology*. 4th ed. Mosby; 2004.)

• Vaccination
  • Vaccines are highly effective. See Chapter 45.

OTHER PATHOGENS WHICH MAY BE SEXUALLY TRANSMITTED

Hepatitis A

• Hepatitis A virus is shed in high rates in feces. Sexual transmission results from fecal–oral contact. MSM are at higher risk.
• MSM should be vaccinated against hepatitis A.
• See also Chapters 22 and 45

Hepatitis B

• Hepatitis B virus is found at highest concentrations in the blood. It is also found in semen, vaginal secretions, and saliva.
• Hepatitis B is efficiently transmitted by percutaneous or mucous membrane exposure to infected blood or body fluids. Risk factors include unprotected sex with an infected partner, MSM, history of an STI, and IVDU.
• Screening is recommended for men and women with risk factors, pregnant women, all MSM, and persons with HIV.
• See also Chapters 22 and 45.

Hepatitis C

• Hepatitis C virus is primarily considered a blood borne pathogen transmitted through exposure to infected blood. However, among MSM with HIV, increasing rates of hepatitis C infection have been observed and are believed to represent sexual transmission.
• Screen MSM born between 1945 and 1965 and other MSM with risk factors.
• Screen persons with HIV for hepatitis C at their initial evaluation for HIV.
• Annual screening is recommended for MSM with HIV.

Enteric Pathogens

• May include other organisms transmitted through oral–anal exposure.
• STI pathogens commonly associated with enteritis in MSM include
  • *Campylobacter* spp.
  • *Entamoeba histolytica.*
  • *Giardia lamblia.*
  • *Salmonella* spp.
  • *Shigella* spp.
• Diagnosis includes thorough history, stool culture, and ova, cysts, and parasite analysis.
• *Entamoeba histolytica* may also present as painful perianal/perineal ulceration.

Further Reading and Resources

1. CDC (Centers for Disease Prevention and Control). A Guide to Taking a Sexual History. CDC Stacks; 2005. Publication 99–8445 https://stacks.cdc.gov/view/cdc/12303.
2. Manhart LE. *Mycoplasma genitalium. Infect Dis Clin North Am.* 2013;l27:779–792.
3. Hook EW. Syphilis. *Lancet.* 2017;389:1550–1557.
4. Bachmann L. *Sexually Transmitted Infections in HIV-Infected Adults and Special Populations: A Clinical Guide.* Cham: Springer International Publishing; 2017.
5. BASHH (British Association for Sexual Health and HIV) guidelines. https://www.bashh.org/guidelines.
6. CDC (Centers for Disease Prevention and Control). Diseases characterized by vaginal discharge: 2010 STD treatment guidelines. https://www.cdc.gov/std/treatment/2010/vaginal-discharge.htm. CDC (Centers for Disease Prevention and Control) STD treatment guidelines. https://www.cdc.gov/std/tg2015/default.htm.
7. CDC (Centers for Disease Prevention and Control). *STD Treatment Guidelines: Screening Recommendations*; 2015. https://www.cdc.gov/std/tg2015/screening-recommendations.htm.

22

Hepatitis Viruses

RACHEL PRESTI

Clinical Presentation of Hepatitis

Acute Infection

- Acute inflammation of the liver.
- Early symptoms: fatigue, nausea, anorexia, right upper quadrant abdominal pain.
- Early labs: leukopenia, lymphocytosis, elevation of transaminases (ALT, AST).
- Late: jaundice (elevated bilirubin), weight loss, pruritus, hepatosplenomegaly.
- Hepatic failure: transaminases >10× upper limit of normal (ULN), elevated bilirubin, change in personality/hepatic encephalopathy, coma, elevation of prothrombin time and diffuse hemorrhage. Can ultimately lead to death or liver transplantation.
- Differential diagnosis: usually infectious, i.e., herpesvirus infections (herpes simplex virus [HSV], cytomegalovirus [CMV], Epstein–Barr virus [EBV]), leptospirosis, dengue, yellow fever. Potentially toxic exposures (acetaminophen/paracetamol, mushroom).

Chronic Infection

- Persistent infection 6 months after transmission.
- Early: asymptomatic.
- Early labs: usually ALT > AST, usually 2–5× ULN.
- Late (cirrhosis): weakness, abdominal swelling, peritonitis, edema, bruising, GI bleeding, hepatic encephalopathy.
  - Cirrhotic patients require screening every 6–12 months for hepatocellular cancer.
- Differential diagnosis: Wilson's disease, autoimmune hepatitis, nonalcoholic steatohepatitis (NASH), drug-induced, cryptogenic cirrhosis.

Summary of the Hepatitis Viruses

Table 22.1 provides a summary overview of the hepatitis viruses.

Hepatitis A (HAV)

Epidemiology

- Worldwide distribution.
- Humans are the only known reservoir.
- Fecal–oral transmission (person-to-person or via contaminated food/water).
- No maternal–fetal transmission.
- Sporadic or epidemic outbreaks, often associated with daycare, institutionalization, and foodborne outbreaks.
- Infection usually confers lifelong immunity.
- Infective from 2–3 weeks before symptoms to 1 week after onset.

Acute Infection (Fig. 22.1)

- >70% adults and 10% children <6 years old develop symptomatic illness.
- Acute infection may require hospitalization in ~10%.
- **Fulminant hepatic failure** with encephalopathy and deranged synthetic function occurs in **<1%.**
- Outcomes worse in older patients, or co-infection with HIV or HBV.
- Diagnosis: HAV IgM. HAV RNA can be detected in blood and stool.
- **Treatment = supportive.** Liver transplant may be required for fulminant infection.
- Most improve within 2 months with no long-term sequelae.
- 1 in 7 will experience **relapsing hepatitis** during 6 months after acute infection.
- **Prolonged cholestatic hepatitis** lasting >12 weeks occurs in <5%; usually resolves spontaneously.
- Chronic HAV infection does not develop.

Prevention

- Vaccination: 2 doses of vaccine. Safe and well-tolerated. See Chapter 45.
- Recommended childhood vaccination at age 1 year in the United States, but not in the UK.

TABLE 22.1 **Hepatitis Viruses**

	HAV	HBV	HCV	HDV	HEV
Pathogen (genus, genome structure)	*Picornavirus*, +RNA	*Hepadnavirus*, dsDNA	*Flavivirus*, +RNA	HBV satellite, –RNA circle	*Hepevirus*, +RNA
Epidemiology	1.4 million new incidence cases annually	350 million worldwide prevalence	170 million worldwide prevalence	15–20 million worldwide prevalence	20 million new incidence cases annually
Transmission	Fecal–oral	Blood, perinatal, sexual	Blood, perinatal, rarely sexual	Blood	Fecal–oral, zoonotic
Incubation	15–45 days	30–150 days	15–120 days	14–160 days	24–72 days
Acute infection/ mortality	Hospitalization in 13%; mortality 0.3%–2.1%	Jaundice in 30%, fulminant in 0.1%	Jaundice in 20%–30%, fulminant rare	Co-infection: severe acute disease	Up to 10% in elderly, pregnant
Chronic/latent infection	Never	>90% children; <10% adults	50%–80%	2% HBV co-infection; 90% HBV superinfection	Rare
Diagnosis	HAV IgM	HBsAg, HBcAb total and IgM	HCV Ab, RNA if HIV, acute	HDV Ab, IgM, RNA	HEV IgM
Treatment	Supportive	Supportive, treat chronic	Treat with DAA; monitor acute	Treat HBV	Supportive, ribavirin
Prevention	Vaccine; post-exposure prophylaxis: HAV vaccine ± Ig	Vaccine; perinatal: HBIg, vaccine	Standard precautions	HBV vaccination	Vaccine in China
Unique clinical features	Daycare, institutions; 10% develop relapsing cholestatic hepatitis	Highly infectious. Reactivates with immuno-suppression, treatment of HCV	Extrahepatic manifestations (rash, renal failure, autoimmune); no immunity	Requires HBV infection	Severe disease in pregnancy, associated with Guillain–Barré

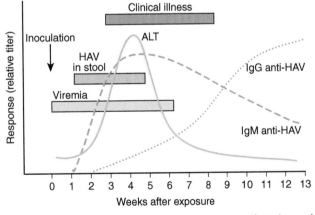

• **Fig. 22.1** Timeline of clinical and laboratory manifestations of acute hepatitis A. *ALT,* alanine aminotransferase; *HAV,* hepatitis A virus; *IgG,* immunoglobulin G; *IgM,* immunoglobulin M. (From Margolis HS, et al. Appearance of immune complexes during experimental hepatitis A infection in chimpanzees. *J Med Virol.* 1988;26:315–326.)

Hepatitis B (HBV)

Epidemiology

• 10 genotypes (A–J); prevalence varies geographically; genotype may influence outcomes.
• WHO have categorized countries based on prevalence of HBsAg into high (>8%), intermediate (2%–8%), and low (<2%) endemicity countries.
  • Both United States and UK are low prevalence areas (carriage rate 0.1%–0.5%).
  • **Rates may vary between individual communities.**
• Transmission: blood (intravenous drug use [IVDU], transfusion, highly infectious), sexual contact, perinatal.
  • Acquisition varies geographically with endemicity.
    • Transmission in highly endemic areas is predominantly vertical (perinatal); or horizontally acquired from another child in the first 5 years of life.

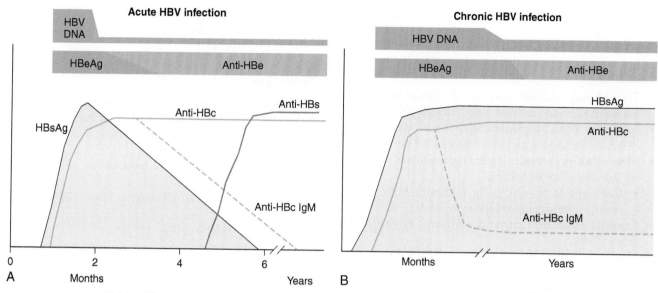

• **Fig. 22.2** Timeline of laboratory manifestations of acute and chronic hepatitis B infection. *HBV,* hepatitis B virus; *DNA,* deoxyribonucleic acid; *Ag,* antigen; *IgM,* immunoglobulin M. (From Konerman MA, Lok AS. Epidemiology, diagnosis and natural history of hepatitis B. In: Sanyal AJ, et al. *Zakim and Boyer's Hepatology.* 7th ed. Elsevier; 2018.)

- Sexual or percutaneous transmission more common routes in North America and Western Europe.
- 100X more infectious by needlestick than HIV, 10X more infectious than HCV.
- The virus can survive outside the body for at least **7 days.**
- 1% of persons living with HBV also have HIV.

Acute Infection (Fig. 22.2A)

- 70% subclinical.
- Rare cause of fulminant hepatitis.
- Treatment during acute infection is *supportive.*
  - Exceptions: fulminant disease, HIV co-infection.

Chronic Infection (Fig. 22.2B)

- Develops in ≥90% of infected neonates, 25% of 1–5-year-olds, but <5% of adults.
  - Inversely proportional to age at time of infection.
- 20%–30% of adults with chronic infection have progressive liver disease.
- Extrahepatic manifestations include polyarteritis nodosa and renal disease.
- Chronic hepatitis B has a number of different stages according to the level of HBV replication, the immune response, and associated liver disease. ALT, HBV DNA, eAg, and eAb levels are key determinants. (See Table 22.2.)
- Precore and core promoter mutants.
  - High error rate in reverse transcription of HBV.
  - **HBeAg production is reduced or prevented, but infectious virions are still produced.**
  - Prevalence may vary with genotype.

TABLE 22.2	Phases of Chronic HBV Infection
Immune tolerant	High levels of HBV replication, but no evidence of active liver damage May last 10–30 years, with very low rate of spontaneous HBeAg clearance during this phase
Immune clearance (immune active)	Increased rate of spontaneous HBeAg clearance with HBeAb seroconversion Associated with exacerbations of active hepatitis, with raised ALT
Inactive carrier state	Also known as latent/nonreplicative phase HBV DNA may be undetectable and liver disease in remission Predominantly important in the setting of anticipated immune compromise • Need to pre-emptively treat or screen for reactivated infection • Consider if HBV cAb positive
Reactivation HBeAg negative	Active HBV replication with active liver disease but undetectable HBeAg. This may be due to HBV virus that cannot produce HBeAg due to genetic variation (precore or core promoter mutants)

Diagnostics

- See Table 22.3 for interpretation of HBV serology.
- HBsAg: a marker of HBV infection, protein on the surface of HBV.
- Anti-HBs (HBV sAb): immunity (recovery vs. immunization).
- Anti-HBc (HBV cAb): previous or current HBV infection (lifelong).

- Anti-HBc IgM (HBV cAb IgM): recent infection (≤6 months).
- HBeAg: an indicator of viral replication.

Treatment

- Treat during chronic infection if transaminases are increased (immune active or reactivating HBV).
- Treatment slows progression of cirrhosis, reduces incidence of liver cancer, and improves survival rates.
- **Most effective therapies: entecavir, tenofovir.**
  - Tenofovir also treats HIV.
  - Case reports of reactivating fulminant HBV when tenofovir treatment for HIV is stopped.
- Lamivudine has high rate of development of viral resistance (30%).
- Clearance is rare, but suppression of HBV DNA and ALT normalization in 75%; most people therefore continue treatment for life.
- Interferon can be used for therapy but poorly tolerated.
- Treatment of HCV has been reported to result in HBV reactivation and flares of hepatitis with elevated transaminases, occasionally resulting in death or liver transplant.

Prognosis

- Risk of progression to cirrhosis, hepatic decompensation, and hepatocellular carcinoma (HCC).
- **Cirrhosis** develops with an incidence of ~300 per 100,000 person years.
  - The risk is increased with older age, male gender, HBeAg seropositivity, elevated ALT, elevated HBV DNA, elevated HBsAg, and HBV genotype C.
- Screening for HCC is recommended in all patients with cirrhosis, Asian males ≥40 years, Asian females ≥50 years, sub-Saharan Africans ≥20 years, and those with a family history of HCC.

- Screening is by 6-monthly liver ultrasound scan (USS) (± AFP) as the doubling time of HCC is estimated to be 4–6 months.

Prevention

- Mainstay is **vaccine.** See Chapters 20 and 45.
- Vaccination at birth has reduced incidence in the United States. Most cases are imported. Now also part of UK childhood schedule as of 2017.
- Protective antibody levels induced in >95% young adults/children/infants.
- Immunity lasts at least 20 years, and probably **lifelong.**

Hepatitis C (HCV) (Fig. 22.3)

Epidemiology

- Areas with high prevalence (>3.5%) include central and east Asia, North Africa, and the Middle East.
- Transmission: **blood exposure** (IVDU, transfusion), perinatal, can be transmitted sexually especially via **receptive anal intercourse.**
- Highest-risk populations are the **birth cohort from 1945–1965,** IVDU, receipt of blood products before 1990.
- HCV genotypes 1–6.
  - Geographic variation in expression of genotypes (Genotype 1 is most common in the United States and Europe).

Acute Infection

- **Usually asymptomatic.** Very rare cause of fulminant hepatitis.
- No indication for treatment during acute infection. Should monitor for spontaneous recovery. More likely to clear if acute infection is symptomatic or if infection is acquired at birth.

TABLE 22.3 Interpretation of Serologic Results for HBV

sAg	sAb	cAb IgM	cAb	eAg	eAb	HBV DNA	ALT	Clinical Scenario
–	–	–	–	–	–	–	Normal	Susceptible to infection
+	–	++	–	+	–	High	High	Acute infection
–	+	–	+	–	±	–	Normal	Immunity due to natural infection
–	+	–	–	–	–	–	Normal	Immunity due to vaccination
+	–	–	+	+	±	High	Low/normal	Chronic infection, immune tolerant
+	–	–	+	±	±	Var	High	Chronic infection, immune active. Consider treatment
+	–	–	+	+	+	Low	High	Chronic infection, seroconverting
+	–	–	+	–	+	Low	Low	Chronic infection, inactive carrier
+	–	–	+	–	+	Var	High	Chronic infection, reactivating. Consider treatment
–	–	–	+	–	–	–	Normal	Most likely resolved infection, at risk for reactivation

Chronic Infection

- 50%–80% of adults develop chronic infection.
- Normal or mildly elevated transaminases in chronic infection. Gammopathy (elevated protein–albumin ratio).
- Risk of cirrhosis is 15%–30% within 20 years. It is increased in patients with diabetes, co-infection with HIV or HBV, and with alcohol use.

- Patients with chronic HCV and cirrhosis have a 7%–14% 5-year risk of developing HCC.
- Risk higher with high alcohol intake.
- Prognosis once HCC diagnosed is poor (5-year survival 10%–15%).
- **Frequent extrahepatic manifestations:**
  - Systemic: autoimmune thyroiditis, B-cell non-Hodgkin lymphoma.
  - Skin: lichen planus, porphyria cutanea tarda, vasculitis (cryoglobulinemia).
  - Glomerulonephritis (cryoglobulinemia).

Treatment (Fig. 22.4)

Difficult to test in exams as rapidly moving field.
- Assessment for treatment
  - HCV RNA to confirm active infection.
  - HCV genotype.
- The first direct antivirals targeted only genotype 1, but now many are pangenotypic.
- Fibrosis staging: liver biopsy (gold standard, but used less commonly due to risk), FibroScan (ultrasound based), FibroSURE (blood test).
- Antivirals: all directly acting antivirals
  - Protease inhibitors: tela**previr**, boce**previr**, asuna**previr**, sime**previr**, grazo**previr**.
  - NS5A inhibitors: daclat**asvir**, ledip**asvir**, elb**asvir**.
  - NS5B polymerase inhibitors, nucleoside polymerase inhibitors: sofos**buvir**, mericitabine.

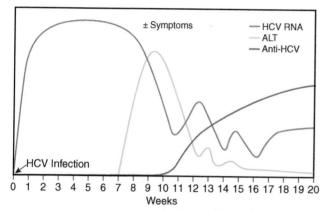

- **Fig. 22.3** Timeline of clinical and laboratory manifestations of acute and chronic hepatitis C infection. *HCV,* hepatitis C virus; *ALT,* alanine aminotransferase; *RNA,* ribonucleic acid. (From Ward JW, Holtzman D. Epidemiology, natural history and diagnosis of hepatitis C. In: Sanyal AJ, et al. *Zakim and Boyer's Hepatology.* 7th ed. Elsevier; 2018.)

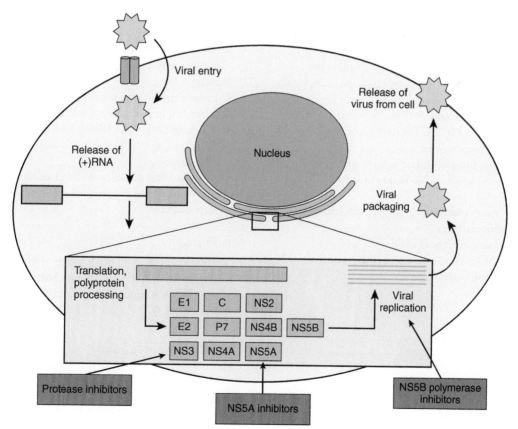

- **Fig. 22.4** Life cycle of hepatitis C virus and mechanism of action of directly acting antivirals. (From Muir AJ. Treatment of hepatitis C. In: Sanyal AJ, et al. *Zakim and Boyer's Hepatology.* 7th ed. Elsevier; 2018.)

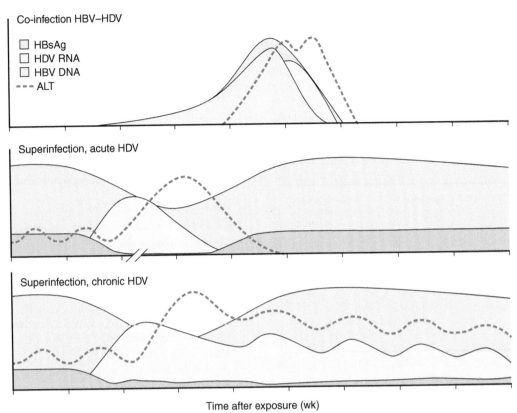

• **Fig. 22.5** Timeline of clinical and laboratory manifestations of hepatitis D infection. *HBV,* hepatitis B virus; *HDV,* hepatitis D virus; *HBsAg,* hepatitis B surface antigen; *RNA,* ribonucleic acid; *DNA,* deoxyribonucleic acid. (From Haller T. Hepatitis D. In: Sanyal AJ, et al. *Zakim and Boyer's Hepatology.* 7th ed. Elsevier; 2018.)

- NS5B polymerase inhibitors, nonnucleoside polymerase antivirals inhibitors: deleo**buvir**, fili**buvir**, tego**buvir.**
- Used in combination, sometimes with ribavirin.
- Usually 12-week therapy, can be extended to 24 weeks for cirrhotics or prior treatment failures.
- **High rates of success >95%.** Sustained virologic response (SVR) = HCV RNA undetectable >12 weeks after treatment completed.
- SVR is a cure, there is no latent form of HCV.
- Reinfection is possible. **No immunity to HCV with cure.**
- May still need monitoring for hepatocellular carcinoma if prior cirrhosis.
- Pediatric treatment not available.
- Treatment of HCV can result in reactivation of HBV with worsening hepatitis.

Prevention

- No vaccine available.
- No sterilizing immunity.
- Avoid blood exposures, use safe sexual practices.

Hepatitis D

Clinical Course (Fig. 22.5)

- Satellite of HBV.
- Requires infection with HBV.

- Can occur simultaneously with HBV or as a result of superinfection.
- Usually IVDU/transfusion, less likely transmitted sexually. No cases of perinatal transmission in the United States.
- Clinical course varies and can range from self-limited to acceleration of liver disease and liver failure.
  - Co-infection with HBV can cause a more severe acute infection syndrome, but usually clears with HBV clearance.
  - Superinfection can cause flares of hepatitis in chronically HBV-infected persons and can accelerate disease due to HBV.

Prevention

- Prevention is same as HBV prevention.
- There is no specific treatment. **Interferon is the only drug effective against HDV.** HBV antivirals have no effect on HDV.

Hepatitis E (Fig. 22.6)

Acute Infection

- Fecal–oral, zoonotic.
  - Genotype 1,2: Asia and North Africa. No animal reservoir. Fecal–oral transmission.
  - Genotype 3,4: Endemic in swine. Zoonotic transmission especially in butchers and farmers.

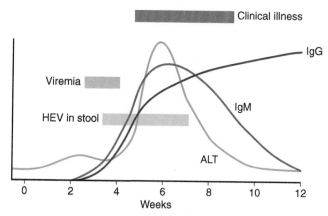

• **Fig. 22.6** Timeline of clinical and laboratory manifestations of hepatitis E infection. *ALT,* alanine aminotransferase; *HEV,* hepatitis E virus; *IgG,* immunoglobulin G; *IgM,* immunoglobulin M. (From Dalton HR, Izopet J, Bendall R. Hepatitis E. In: Sanyal AJ, et al. *Zakim and Boyer's Hepatology.* 7th ed. Elsevier; 2018.)

- Endemic in most developing world. Most common cause of acute viral hepatitis worldwide.
- Mild symptoms in general.
- Severe, fulminant disease: especially in **pregnant women** and patients with underlying liver disease.

Chronic Infection

- Not common, but immune suppression can lead to chronic carrier state.
- Extrahepatic manifestations described in chronic carriers (**cryoglobulinemia**, glomerulonephritis, **Guillain–Barré**).

Prevention

- Vaccine approved in China.

Other Infection-related Hepatic Conditions

Hepatitis G and Transfusion-Transmitted Virus (TTV)

- Isolated from patients with post-transfusion hepatitis.
- Viremia seen in 1% of blood donors without hepatitis.
- **No known disease.**

HIV and Viral Hepatitis Co-infections

- 10% of people with HIV in the United States are co-infected with HBV.

- 25% of people with HIV in the United States are co-infected with HCV; 75% of IVDU with HIV also have HCV. Co-infection with HIV and HCV triples risk for liver disease over HCV monoinfection.
- Tenofovir is antiviral for both HBV and HIV.
- HCV antiviral drugs may have drug interactions with antiretrovirals for HIV.
- MSM account for 20% of new HBV infections and 10% of new HAV infections in the United States.

Other Infectious Causes of Hepatic Parenchymal Disease

- *Mycobacterium avium*
- *Cryptococcus neoformans*
- *Microsporidium spp.*
- *Pneumocystic jirovecii*
- *Bartonella spp.*
- *Histoplasma capsulatum*
- Herpesviruses

Other Infection-related Causes of Hepatic Parenchymal Disease

- Antiretroviral therapy (ART) toxicity.
  - Abacavir, nevirapine classically, although have been seen with almost all ART.
  - Stopping HBV active therapy if HBV co-infected (look for history of HBV cAb+ or sAg+).
- Malignancy.
  - Kaposi sarcoma.
  - Hepatocellular carcinoma.
- Biliary disease.
  - AIDS cholangiopathy.

Likely Mimics for Viral Hepatitis

Infections that mimic viral hepatitis are covered in detail elsewhere (see Table 22.4).

Further Resources

1. CDC (Centers for Disease Control and Prevention): Viral Hepatitis. https://www.cdc.gov/hepatitis/resources/.
2. American Association for the Study of Liver Diseases: Practice Guidelines. https://www.aasld.org/publications/practice-guidelines-0.
3. AASLD and Infectious Diseases Society of America: HCV Guidance. http://www.hcvguidelines.org.

TABLE 22.4   **Hepatitis Mimics**

	Common Clinical Scenarios	Key Information
Acute Hepatitis Mimics		
Herpesvirus infection	Pregnant woman and HSV infection (genital or oral ulcer) Person with HIV Transplant patient and CMV HHV6 and syncytial giant-cell hepatitis	See Chapter 3
Adenovirus	Immune suppression, especially transplant Children, especially <5 years old Often presents as fulminant hepatic failure	Treatment is reduction of immunosuppression, potentially immunoglobulin or cidofovir. Often requires transplantation See Chapter 3
Parvovirus B19	Hepatitis in children Worsened liver failure with chronic HBV or HCV	See Chapter 23
Leptospirosis	Exposure to contaminated water, jaundice, and abdominal pain, also with fever, headache, and muscle aches Second phase: Weil's disease and liver failure	See Chapter 31
Yellow fever	Illness ranges from mild febrile disease to fulminant liver failure and bleeding Travel history, usually to South America or Africa	See Chapter 30
Dengue	Travel to endemic area and exposure to mosquitoes Retro-orbital headache, fever, rash	See Chapter 30
Toxic exposure/drug induced liver injury	Look for medication ingestions Acetaminophen, isoniazid, statins, methotrexate, amoxicillin–clavulanate, anesthetics, antiepileptics Toxic exposure • Alcoholic hepatitis, often associated with elevated AST • Herbal remedies • Recreational drug use (ecstasy and cocaine) • Ingestion of foraged mushrooms	
Chronic Hepatitis Mimics		
NASH	Look for other signs of metabolic syndrome	
Autoimmune hepatitis	ANA, ASMA, LKM-1 positive	
Wilson's disease	Under age 40, Kayser–Fleischer rings, neuropsychiatric disease	
Hemochromatosis	Cirrhosis with skin color change, congestive heart failure	

23
Viral Exanthems and Vaccine-Preventable Diseases

RACHEOL SIERRA

Introduction

Many viruses exhibit a classical exanthem or cutaneous skin rash as a feature of their clinical syndrome. The original six exanthematous illnesses of childhood were measles, scarlet fever (group A *streptococcus*), rubella, "Dukes' disease," exanthem infectiosum (parvovirus B19), and exanthem subitum (human herpesvirus 6). Exanthems may be particularly characteristic of their underlying viral etiology while many rashes are nonspecific. Distinct exanthems such as that described in the Gianotti–Crosti syndrome (Fig. 23.1) may be attributed to a number of viral pathogens.

Parvovirus B19

- Single-stranded DNA virus; small, nonenveloped, icosahedral.
- Genus *Erythrovirus*.

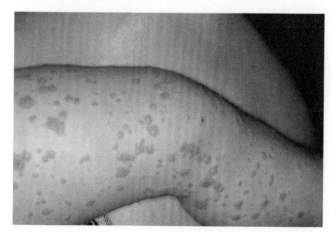

- **Fig. 23.1** Gianotti–Crosti syndrome. Flat-top red papules. Reported in association with hepatitis B, EBV, CMV, and enterovirus infections. (From Diseases of the epidermis. In: Kliegman R, Stanton B, Behrman RE, et al., eds. *Nelson Textbook of Pediatrics*. 20th ed. Elsevier; 2016.)

- Family *Parvoviridae*.
- Virus replicates in erythroid precursor cells.

Exanthems Caused by Human Parvovirus B19

Erythema Infectiosum (Fifth Disease)

- Principally a **self-limiting** childhood infection with a **worldwide** distribution. Peak age 5–18 years. Approximately 50% of children seropositive by 15 years.
- **Transmission via respiratory droplets.** Virus can be transmitted **vertically** from mother to fetus and has been acquired through transfusions of **blood** and blood-derived products.
- Viral entry via the upper respiratory tract. Short period of viremia occurs 7–10 days postexposure, lasting around one week. The latter stages represent the infectious period and precede the appearance of rash.

Clinical Features

- Prodrome of mild fever, malaise, and coryzal symptoms common before rash. Other symptoms: nausea, headache, diarrhea, and myalgia.
- **Biphasic rash**
  - **Slapped cheek** syndrome. Intense erythema over malar areas. Resolves once antibody production has occurred. At this stage the immunocompetent individual is no longer infectious (Fig. 23.2A).
  - Subsequent widespread **fine lacy maculopapular** rash of trunk and limbs (Fig. 23.2B).
- Arthralgia: usually in adults, women > men.
- Predominately **symmetrical small joint arthritis** of hands or fingers; may last several weeks to months.

Investigations

- Diagnosis confirmed with **serology**: IgM positivity from 7 to 10 days of exposure.
- IgG antibodies appear from 15 days after exposure.

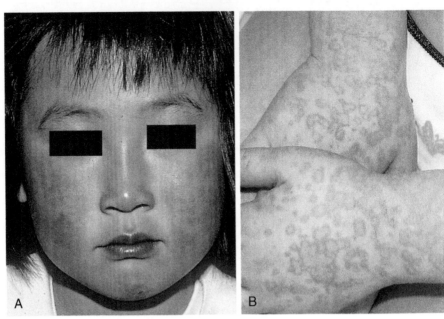

• **Fig. 23.2** Parvovirus B19. (A) Malar erythema, classic "slapped cheek." (B) Erythematous lacy rash. (Panel A courtesy Robert Hickey, MD, Children's Hospital of Pittsburgh, Pittsburgh, PA. Panel B from Cohen BA, Lehman V, eds. Dermatlas.org – Dermatology Image Atlas. Johns Hopkins University [website].)

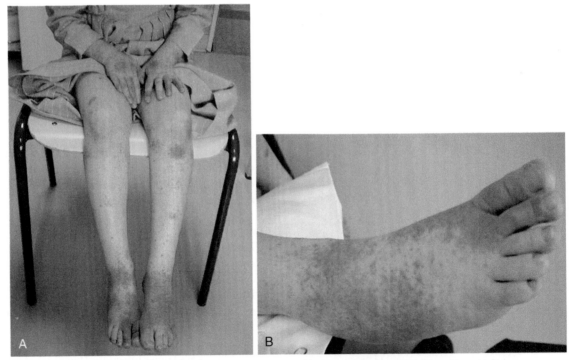

• **Fig. 23.3** PPGSS. Petechial exanthem of distal limbs with demarcation at ankles. (From Parez N, Dehee A, Michel Y, et al. Papular-purpuric gloves and socks syndrome associated with B19V infection in a 6-year-old child. *J Clin Virol.* 2009;44:167–169.)

- Serum parvovirus **DNA detection** by polymerase chain reaction (PCR) used in **immunocompromised** individuals when IgM less reliable. Molecular tests also used for diagnosis of fetal infection (see below).

Papular-Purpuric "Glove-and-Socks" Syndrome (PPGSS)

- Usually young adults, also children.

- Pruritic erythema and edema of distal extremities becoming petechial or purpuric = so-called "glove and socks" distribution. **Sharp demarcation** at level of wrists and ankles may occur (Fig. 23.3).
- Mucosal involvement with oral lesions, ulceration, and pharyngeal erythema.
- May be associated with fever and lymphadenopathy.
- Self-limiting; may take several weeks to resolve fully.

Other Manifestations of Parvovirus Infection

Aplastic Crisis in Patients with Hemolytic Anemia

- Parvovirus may be **fatal** in individuals with hematologic conditions such as sickle cell anemia or thalassemia. Transient but abrupt disruption to erythropoiesis triggers an **aplastic crisis.**
- **Supportive** measures, such as blood transfusions, are required until infection resolves.

Chronic Parvovirus Infection in the Immunosuppressed

- An **immunocompromised** host who fails to eradicate the virus may develop **severe chronic anemia.**
- Patients with chronic bone marrow suppression due to parvovirus infection **may remain infectious** for months or years.

Intrauterine Infection

- See Chapter 20
- Infection in **first 20 weeks** of pregnancy can lead to **intrauterine death and hydrops fetalis.**

Asymptomatic Infection

- 25% are asymptomatic.
- Approximately **50% will have nonspecific** flu-like symptoms alone – clinical suspicion of parvovirus infection in such cases will be low.

Treatment and Prevention

- There is **no specific antiviral treatment, prophylaxis, or licensed vaccine for parvovirus.**

Enterovirus

- Single-stranded RNA virus; nonenveloped, icosahedral.
- Family *Picornaviridae.*
- Viral replication occurs in the intestinal tract.
- Over 100 serotypes
  - Human enteroviruses include polioviruses (PV), Coxsackievirus (CV) groups A and B, enteric cytopathic human orphan (ECHO) viruses and "new" enterovirus types (numbered EV 68–71, 73–91, and 100–101).
  - Enteroviruses also classified as four species, human enterovirus A, B, C, and D. Polioviruses, part of enterovirus C group, will be discussed later in the chapter.

Clinical Features

- Wide spectrum of clinical disease from a mild febrile illness through to fatal and severe morbidity in presentations affecting the central nervous system (see Table 23.1).

TABLE 23.1   Clinical Disease Due to Enterovirus Serotypes

Syndrome	Serotypes Most Often Implicated
Aseptic meningitis	Coxsackieviruses A2, 4, 7, 9, and others and B2–5 Poliovirus types 1–3 Echoviruses 4, 6, 7, 9, 11, 30, and others Human parechoviruses 1–4
Aseptic meningitis with rash	Coxsackieviruses A9 and B4 Echoviruses 4 and 16 Enterovirus 71
Conjunctivitis (hemorrhagic)	Enterovirus 70 Coxsackievirus A24
Epidemic pleurodynia (Bornholm disease)	Coxsackieviruses B1–6
Hand, foot, and mouth disease	Coxsackieviruses A6, 9, 16, and others Coxsackieviruses B2–5 Enterovirus 71
Herpangina	Coxsackieviruses A2, 4–6, 8, and 10 Probably Coxsackieviruses B3 and others
Myopericarditis	Coxsackieviruses A4 and 16 and B1–5 Echoviruses 9 and human parechovirus 1
Paralysis	Polioviruses 1–3 Coxsackieviruses A7 and others Echoviruses 4, 6, 9, and others Enterovirus 71
Rash	Coxsackieviruses A9 and B1, 3, 4, and 5 (also implicated: A4–6 and 16) Echoviruses 9 and 16 (also 2, 4, 11, 14, 19, and 25)
Respiratory disease	Echoviruses 4, 8, 9, 11, 20, and others Coxsackieviruses A21 and 24 and B1 and 3–5 Enterovirus D68

- **Majority** of infections, especially in children, are **asymptomatic.**

Exanthems Caused by Enteroviruses

Hand, Foot, and Mouth Disease (HFMD)

- Also known as vesicular stomatitis with exanthem.
- Predominantly attributed to **Coxsackie A** but also Coxsackie B and enterovirus EV71 (Table 23.1).
- Usually considered a **common** self-limiting febrile illness in children, under the age of 10.

Epidemiology and Transmission

- Found worldwide, sporadic or epidemic. Outbreaks tend to occur in **warm temperatures**, summer or early autumn.

- Feco-oral transmission, or from respiratory secretions. **Highly infectious** with outbreaks seen in nursery or similar childcare settings.
- Outbreaks of EV71 causing HFMD, largely in Asia–Pacific region have also been associated with severe complications such as aseptic meningitis, meningoencephalitis and acute flaccid paralysis as well as effects on the cardiopulmonary system.
- Individuals may shed virus in stool for several weeks.

Clinical Features

- **Painful ulcerative lesions** in the oral cavity. Predominate on **hard palate, tongue, and buccal mucosa.**
- Vesicular eruptions arise on soles of feet and palms of the hands, usually following mouth lesions.
- Peripheral vesicles may be painful or asymptomatic.
- Maculopapular rashes may also occur on buttocks or genitals.
- Lesions usually resolve between 5–10 days without scarring.

Atypical HFMD

- Usually a more widespread vesiculobullous rash.
- May be multiple erythematous crusted papules, similar to Gianotti–Crosti rash.
- **Predilection** of lesions at sites of **atopic eczema** (eczema coxsackium).
- **Skin peeling or nail shedding** during the convalescent period.

Treatment and Prevention

- **No antiviral agents effective against enteroviruses.**
- Vaccines for EV71 under development; include inactivated whole-virus, live attenuated strains, virus-like particles (VLP), and DNA vaccines. Two EV71 vaccines have been granted Chinese FDA approval and are commercially available in China.

Measles

- One serotype.
- Single-stranded, negative-sense RNA virus; enveloped, helical.
- Genus *Morbillivirus.*
- Family *Paramyxoviridae.*

Epidemiology and transmission

- Humans are the **only reservoir.**
- **Worldwide** prevalence. It remains a significant cause of morbidity and mortality in children in low income countries.
- Airborne and contact transmission through **respiratory droplets.** The virus initially infects epithelial cells of the upper respiratory tract and conjunctiva, then spreads to regional lymph nodes. Primary viremia disseminates to reticuloendothelial system.

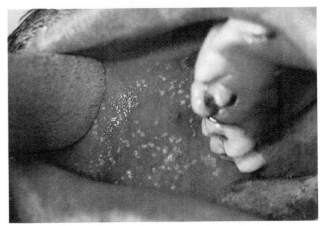

• **Fig. 23.4** Koplik's spots. Pathognomonic of measles. (From Emond RT, Welsby PD, Rowland HA, eds. *Color Atlas of Infectious Diseases.* 4th ed. Mosby; 2003.)

- **Secondary viremia results in viral dissemination** to other epithelial sites: skin, gastrointestinal tract, kidney, and central nervous system.
- **Infectious droplets may remain airborne for up to 2 hours.**
- Measles is **highly contagious**: >90% secondary attack rates in susceptible contacts (i.e., *9 out of 10 susceptible people exposed to an infected person will develop infection*).

Clinical Features

- Incubation period around 10 days, up to 3 weeks in adults.
- Usually 2–4 day prodrome of malaise, **high fever.** Typically 3Cs = "**cough, coryza, and conjunctivitis.**"
- Individuals are considered to be infectious during this prodrome and **until 4 days after the onset of rash.**
- **Koplik's spots,** pathognomonic white papules on an erythematous base affecting the buccal mucosa, may be seen during this phase. Appearance is brief (Fig. 23.4).
- The **measles exanthem** results from a **cell-mediated immune response** to the virus.
  - While the typical measles rash is clinically distinctive, the presentation of this disease in patients with impaired **immunity** or those who have had **prior vaccination** or **received immunoglobulin** may be quite different.
  - Appears around day 3–4 of illness, usually accompanied with high fever.
  - Usually **starts behind ears**, spreading over the face, then trunk, and finally to limbs. Palms of hands and soles of feet may be involved.
- Erythematous and maculopapular, becoming confluent as disease progresses (Fig. 23.5).

Complications

- People at high risk for complications and severe illness include children <5 years, adults >20 years, pregnant women, and those with cell-mediated immunodeficiencies.

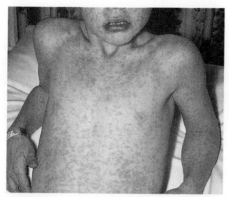

• **Fig. 23.5** Morbilliform rash of measles. (From Hobson RP. Infectious disease. In: Walker BR, Colledge NR, Ralston SH, Penman ID, eds. *Davidson's Principles and Practice of Medicine.* 22nd ed. Elsevier; 2014.)

• Respiratory: secondary bacterial infections, including pneumonia, otitis media or croup.
• Central nervous system:
    • **ADEM** (acute disseminated encephalomyelitis) occurs soon after the initial illness. Approximately **1 in 1000 children with natural infection**; $1–2 / 1 \times 10^6$ following vaccination with live attenuated virus.
    • MIBE (measles inclusion body encephalitis), progressive and fatal occurring in children with impaired cellular immunity.
    • SSPE (subacute sclerosing panencephalitis), rare but again **fatal degenerative** neurologic condition presenting **5–10 years after** infection. Cases largely in children who had measles **under** the age of **2 years**, with a preponderance in boys. **Measles vaccination reduces the incidence of SSPE.**

Other Manifestations of Measles Infection

Atypical Measles

• Syndrome described in individuals who had early measles vaccination with inactivated (killed) virus and were subsequently exposed to wild-type virus.
• Response thought to be due to hypersensitivity to measles virus in a partially immune host.
• Severe illness characterized by high fever, atypical rash (varies from urticarial, vesicular, maculopapular, or hemorrhagic), and associated with peripheral or pulmonary edema.
• Vaccination with killed measles virus ceased in 1967, therefore this clinical manifestation is rare.

Modified Measles

• Milder illness with less dramatic rash: patients who have **received normal immunoglobulin** as postexposure prophylaxis, babies with **residual maternal antibody**, and in some cases individuals who have received **standard vaccination.**

Measles in Certain Groups

• Immunosuppressed: Patients with an **abnormality in cell-mediated immunity** may have **severe** disease with absence of rash. They are at **higher risk** of CNS involvement and less common disease presentations such as primary measles or giant cell pneumonitis.
• Malnourished children: particularly those with **vitamin A deficiency.** Disease is **more severe with augmented complications**, e.g., severe corneal lesions, blindness, life-threatening pneumonia, severe otitis media, diarrhea, and delayed recovery. In vulnerable populations, measles remains a significant cause of death in childhood.
• **Measles in pregnancy** can be associated with **severe maternal morbidity**, as well as higher risk of spontaneous abortion, premature labor, and low-birthweight infants.

Treatment and Prevention

A safe and effective vaccine for measles has been available since the 1960s. Despite this, in 2016 nearly 90,000 deaths occurred from measles, the majority in children under the age of 5. Increasing routine childhood vaccination globally is a key strategy to reduce deaths attributed to measles.

• Available measles vaccines contain **live attenuated** strains.
• Vaccine usually given combined with measles, mumps, and rubella (MMR) or a measles, mumps, rubella, and varicella (MMRV) vaccine.
• Standard MMR immunization is a **two-dose** program (approx. 97% effective).
• Initial dose 12–15 months followed by second dose usually at school entry (4–6 years).
• Single dose MMR provides adequate immunity in 93% of individuals.
• In outbreaks, age for initial dose may be lowered to 6–12 months. As vaccine response is unreliable in this age group, a further 2 doses are still recommended at 12–15 months and preschool.
• High vaccine coverage (**at least 90%**) central to maintaining **high population immunity.**
• **Postexposure prophylaxis with MMR** given **within 72 hours** of exposure may prevent disease and is indicated in susceptible measles contacts.
• **Normal immunoglobulin** given as postexposure prophylaxis in cases known, or likely to be **antibody-negative** to measles. May prevent or modify disease if given **within 6 days** of exposure.

Rubella

• Single-stranded, positive-sense RNA virus; enveloped, icosahedral.
• Genus *Rubivirus.*
• Family *Togaviridae.*

Key Facts
- Rubella is predominately a mild febrile illness of childhood.
- Infection acquired during pregnancy poses a major risk to the developing fetus, resulting in significant congenital morbidity and mortality.
- Person-to-person transmission is through droplet spread.
- Incubation period 16–23 days.

The Rubella Exanthem

- Prodrome of **mild,** generalized malaise; occasionally mild conjunctivitis or tender **posterior auricular lymphadenopathy.**
- Maculopapular rash appears concurrently, or 1–5 days after onset of symptoms and resolves within 3–4 days.
- Rash first appears on forehead, then face, spreading rapidly to trunk and limbs. Pinpoint lesions.
- Infectious period is variable: **from 7 days before to 7 days after** the appearance of rash. Viral shedding maximal when rash is erupting.
- **A significant proportion** (at least 50%) of rubella infections are **asymptomatic** or do not manifest with rash. **These patients are still able to transmit virus.**

Complications

- Post-infectious **thrombocytopenia:** usually self-limiting but can cause epistaxis, gastrointestinal bleeding, or hematuria during the convalescent period (1:3000 cases have bleeding complications).
- **Arthritis:** more common in adults, women > men. Usually hands and wrists. **May take several weeks** to resolve.
- Encephalitis (1:6000 cases). Usually good prognosis.
- Progressive rubella panencephalitis (PRP): rare, similar to SSPE in measles. Death occurs 2–5 years after onset.

Congenital Rubella Syndrome

- First trimester rubella infection has major consequences for the fetus: 90% risk of adverse fetal outcome including miscarriage, still birth, premature labor, and severe birth defects. See Chapter 20 for more detail.

Treatment and Prevention

Rubella is vaccine-preventable. Targeted by the World Health Organization (WHO) within the Measles and Rubella initiative with the aim of elimination of both in five WHO regions by 2020. Rubella infections in the UK and United States are at levels defined as eliminated by the WHO.
- Live attenuated vaccine given as combined MMR or MMRV (see measles vaccination).
- Single dose of rubella-containing vaccine confers 95%–100% protection.
- Susceptible women of childbearing age should be offered MMR.
- The vaccine is contraindicated in pregnancy although there is no evidence that rubella-containing vaccines are teratogenic. Women should be counselled in appropriate contraceptive advice for 1 month postvaccination.

Varicella-Zoster Virus (VZV)

- Double-stranded DNA virus; enveloped.
- Family *Herpesviridae.*
- Humans are the only reservoir.
- Primary infection with VZV causes varicella (chickenpox); reactivation causes herpes zoster (shingles).

Varicella

Varicella is **endemic worldwide**.
- Primary varicella infection is considered a mild childhood infection in Europe and North America. 90% of cases occur in children younger than 13 years of age.
- In tropical climates, it is more common in young adults.
- Groups at risk of severe disease include infants; immunosuppressed patients; adults, particularly smokers or persons with chronic lung disease; and pregnant women.
- Virus transmitted in respiratory secretions or spread by virus released from fluid filled vesicles, through **direct contact or aerosolized.**
- Chickenpox is contagious with an attack rate of 90% in susceptible contacts.
- Incubation period 10–21 days.
- VZV becomes **latent** in the sensory dorsal root ganglia.
- Infection leads to **lifetime immunity.**

The Varicella Exanthem

- Nonspecific prodrome of fever and malaise precedes rash by 1–2 days.
- Lesions often first appear on the scalp, face, or trunk, starting as crops of red flat macules which quickly morph into **fluid-filled vesicles.** Rash **intensely pruritic.**
- Any epithelial surface can be affected. Lesions can be found on the conjunctiva of the eyes or epithelia of the genital tract.
- Lesions tend to appear in **clusters** over a 48 hour period from first onset, with vesicles sometimes becoming pustular before drying out and crusting over.
- Infectious period **48 hours before onset of rash until all lesions have dried completely.**

Breakthrough Varicella

- Individuals vaccinated can still succumb to wild-type varicella virus. Usually mild illness with atypical maculopapular rather than vesicular rash but in 25%–30% cases will present as classic chickenpox.

- Approximately **1 in 5 children** who have been vaccinated may get **breakthrough** varicella infection.

Complications

- More common in at-risk groups.
- Predominant complication is **secondary bacterial infection**: *Staphylococcus aureus* or *Streptococcus pyogenes*, particularly in children.
- **Varicella pneumonia** occurs in **1 in 400 adult cases**: increased severity in smokers and patients with chronic lung disease.
- Complications include hepatitis, thrombocytopenia, severe purpuric hemorrhagic rash, arthritis and myocarditis, pericarditis, nephritis, and acute retinal necrosis.
- Acute cerebellar ataxia, encephalitis, and meningitis are rare but can occur in otherwise healthy individuals.
- Progressive varicella, with involvement of the visceral organs and the development of hemorrhagic varicella is life-threatening; more commonly in immunosuppressed.
- **All immunosuppressed individuals presenting with primary varicella should have an urgent clinical assessment and commence high-dose intravenous aciclovir.**
- Consider treatment in **all at-risk groups**. Adults: treat with oral aciclovir. **Proven benefit only if given within the first 24 hours.**

Varicella and Pregnancy

- Increased severity and risk of maternal and fetal complications, particularly maternal **pneumonitis** and **congenital varicella syndrome.**
- See Chapter 20.

Treatment and Prevention

- Varicella vaccines have been available since the mid-1980s. Both varicella and herpes zoster vaccine are based on the Oka strain and are **live attenuated vaccines.**
- Licensed vaccines available as a single-antigen vaccine or in combination (MMRV).
- Two-dose schedule confers greatest degree of immunity in children (>98%) compared to approximately 75% in adults.
- Routine varicella vaccination has been implemented by certain countries including Australia, Canada, and European countries such as Greece and Germany. In the United States vaccination was introduced in 1995 with a two-dose schedule universally adopted in 2006.
- In the UK the aim of varicella vaccination is to **protect those individuals most at risk of serious disease.** As such recommended for nonimmune healthcare workers and susceptible close household contacts of immunocompromised patients.
- The **epidemiology of varicella infections is likely to change** with the implementation of childhood vaccination programs. Falling rates of disease in children will be evident but the impact on other aspects of the disease,

such as **adult incidence** or **epidemiology of herpes zoster**, are yet unquantified.

Postexposure Prophylaxis

- Varicella immunoglobulin (VZIG) recommended in individuals **without evidence of immunity** who are at **high risk of severe varicella** following a **significant exposure.** This includes immunocompromised patients, pregnant women, neonates, and premature infants. See Chapter 20.
- VZIG should be administered **as soon as possible** in immunocompromised hosts. Chickenpox may still occur. Cases should be monitored and treated with aciclovir should infection manifest.
- Prophylaxis with oral aciclovir may be considered in the absence of VZIG. Treatment should be commenced 7–10 days postexposure for 7 days.

Herpes Zoster (HZ)

When cell-mediated immunity declines, reactivation of virus occurs. Most common in elderly (risk increases with age) or **immunocompromised** host. Neonates who developed intrauterine chickenpox or were infected during the postnatal period or those acquiring infection as young infants, can present with shingles in childhood.

- Shingles may occur in varicella acquired naturally or following vaccination.
- Increased morbidity in immunocompromised patients. Evolution of lesions continues for **longer** with definitive resolution taking several weeks. Patients at **higher risk of disseminated zoster**; widespread cutaneous rash and progression to severe disease if not treated.
- Other manifestations: CNS disease such as encephalitis, myelitis, cranial and peripheral nerve palsies, and stroke syndrome; pneumonitis; hepatitis.
- **Postherpetic neuralgia:** a debilitating dermatomal pain persisting beyond resolution of rash.
  - Occurs in **20%** of individuals with herpes zoster.
  - More common with increasing age; adults over 70 have a four times greater risk than those age 60.

The Herpes Zoster Exanthem

- Pain may be the first symptom of HZ, occurring in the dermatome where lesions subsequently arise.
- Uncomplicated HZ, distribution limited to single dermatome, without crossing the midline. Reactivation in thoracic and lumbar dermatomes occurs most frequently.
- Ramsay Hunt syndrome; peripheral facial (VII) nerve palsy with vesicles in ear (Fig. 23.8) or mouth. May be associated with auditory (VIII) nerve symptoms; tinnitus, vertigo, nystagmus, and nausea.
- Ophthalmic zoster: reactivation in the trigeminal nerve and other ocular manifestations such as zoster keratitis, corneal ulceration, or optic neuritis, are sight-threatening.

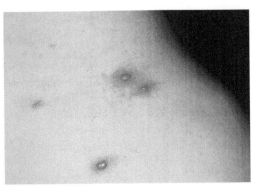

• **Fig. 23.6** Fluid-filled vesicles characteristic of chickenpox, in varying stages of development. (From Paller AS, Mancini AJ. *Hurwitz Clinical Pediatric Dermatology*. 5th ed. Elsevier; 2016.)

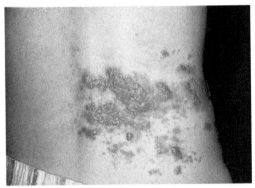

• **Fig. 23.7** Herpes zoster involving the lumbar dermatome. (From Whitley RJ. Chickenpox and herpes zoster. In: Bennett JE, Dolin R, Blaser MJ, eds. *Mandell, Douglas, and Bennett's Principles and Practice of Infectious Diseases*. Updated 8th ed. Elsevier; 2015.)

• Acute retinal necrosis, a rare but also potentially blinding process associated with zoster or varicella, is attributed to viral dissemination rather than dermatomal reactivation.

Treatment and Prevention

• **Treatment** with oral antivirals (Table 23.2) is recommended in:
  • Immunocompetent hosts if lesions <72 hours old; should be considered if new lesions appearing beyond this time.
  • All immunocompromised patients presenting with shingles.
  • Any suspicion of disseminated or progressive disease warrants urgent clinical assessment and initiation of high dose IV aciclovir, 10 mg/kg (adults).

Prevention
• Herpes zoster vaccine has been shown to reduce the incidence of shingles in older people. Current licensed preparations contain live attenuated varicella virus (i.e., Zostavax).
• Zostavax **reduces incidence of shingles** by 51% in adults between 60 and 70 years of age. **Reduces risk of postherpetic neuralgia** by 66% in persons over age 60.

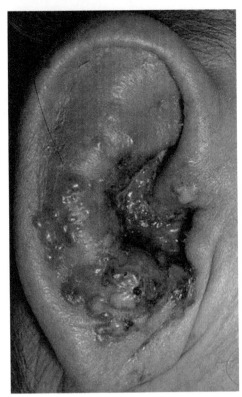

• **Fig. 23.8** Typical skin lesions associated with Ramsey–Hunt syndrome. (From Steven D. Waldman. *Pain Review*. 2nd ed. Elsevier; 2017.)

TABLE 23.2	Oral Antiviral Agents Used for Uncomplicated Herpes Zoster (Adults)	
Aciclovir		800 mg five times a day 7 days
Valaciclovir	Prodrug of aciclovir	1 g tds 7 days
Famciclovir	Prodrug of penciclovir	500 g tds 7 days

From the MSD Manual [Merck Manual] Professional Version, edited by Robert Porter. Copyright 2018 by Merck Sharp & Dohme Corp., a subsidiary of Merck & Co., Inc., Kenilworth, NJ. Available at http://www.msd manuals.com/professional.

• Shingles vaccine advocated in certain middle to high income countries where programs are deemed beneficial and cost-effective. Targeted age recommendations may vary (Sweden >50; United States and Canada ≥60; Australia 60–79; UK 70–79).
• Duration of protection not known.

Human Herpes Virus 6 and 7

• Double-stranded DNA viruses; enveloped.
• Beta herpesviruses; family *Herpesviridae*.
• Two HHV-6 species: HHV 6A and HHV 6B. HHV 6B causes the majority of recognized clinical disease.
• HHV-7 infections are in the majority asymptomatic.

- Following primary infection, both HHV-6 and HHV-7 establish viral latency.

Exanthem Subitum

Also known as sixth disease or roseola infantum, caused predominantly by HHV-6B.

- Usually self-limiting febrile illness in infants (4 months to 2 years) following loss of maternal antibody. Small proportion caused by HHV-7, but present later in childhood, usually from age 3.
- Transmission is likely via **respiratory** secretions.
- Clinical presentation of **acute high-grade fever**, lasting 3 days. Other symptoms: irritability, coryzal symptoms, and gastrointestinal upset.
- Resolution of fever is heralded by appearance of rash: rose-pink papules or maculopapular blanching non-pruritic rash. Usually trunk and face.
- Encephalopathy can occur. HHV-6B infection is the most common cause of **febrile convulsions.**
- HHV-6 infections in immunocompetent adults rare. An infectious mononucleosis-type syndrome, hepatitis and myocarditis have been described with primary disease.
- Encephalitis with HHV-6 is likely secondary to re-activation and has been described in both immuno-competent and immunocompromised individuals.
- HHV-6 is frequently detected post-transplant in both solid organ and hematopoietic stem cell transplant recipients (HSCT), but the clinical consequences of this re-activation are not fully understood.

Other Viral Exanthems

Smallpox

Smallpox at one time was the most feared of all infectious diseases, famed for influencing the course of history from as far back as the Roman Empire. Virus was most effective in naïve populations. Large epidemics occurred every 5–15 years in the presence of adequate numbers of susceptible individuals.

Smallpox was eradicated worldwide in 1980 following an international vaccination program. Virus stock is still maintained in two facilities, within the United States and Russia.

- Double-stranded DNA virus, from the *Orthopoxvirus* genus, family *Poxviridae*.
- Humans were the only reservoir.
- Disease transmission via **respiratory droplets**; or occasionally by **contact** with infectious lesions.
- Two forms of smallpox – different virus strains – variola major and variola minor with **mortality rates of 20%–30% and 1%** respectively.
- Incubation period of 10–12 days. Symptoms of fever, backache, headache, or vomiting before appearance of rash.
- Lesions progressed from macules to papules, eventually vesicular, and finally pustular. Lesions would scab and fall off leaving characteristic pockmarks.

- Distribution was predominately face, oral mucosa, and limbs. Individuals were **most infectious during the exanthem phase.**
- **Mortality proportional to extent of rash and nature of lesions.** Flat smallpox and hemorrhagic smallpox were invariably fatal.
- There was, and still is, **no effective antiviral for smallpox.** Concerns regarding its use as a potential bioterrorist weapon remain.

Primary Human Immunodeficiency Virus (HIV)

See also Chapter 36, Natural history of HIV.

- An acute HIV seroconversion illness estimated to occur in 40%–90% of individuals newly infected with HIV.
- Symptoms usually 2–4 weeks after viral transmission. Often nonspecific generalized malaise, fever, lymphadenopathy, hepatitis, fatigue, and arthralgia. Lymphadenopathy may persist for several weeks.
- **Viral exanthem in approximately 70% of cases.**
  - Erythematous macules or maculopapular; may develop hemorrhagic or necrotic lesions.
  - Distribution typically trunk, calves, palms of hands, and soles of feet.
  - Develops 2–3 days after onset of fever.
  - Shallow, painful mucocutaneous ulcers may occur in the oral cavity or genitals.

Epstein–Barr Virus

- Epstein–Barr virus (EBV), one of the herpesviruses; enveloped double-stranded DNA viruses.
- Virus enters via epithelial cells in the pharynx or upper respiratory tract and targets B-lymphocytes. Infection of B-lymphocytes results in viral latency.
- Primary EBV causes the majority (80%) of cases of **infectious mononucleosis** (IM).
  - IM largely a disease of children and young adults. Principal signs: lymphadenopathy, fever, and sore throat, followed by hepatitis. Generalized malaise and fatigue are common. Occurs in up to 50% of primary infections.
- **Rash develops in 3%–15 % of patients with IM.**
  - Usually maculopapular, may be urticarial or petechial.
  - Erythema multiforme and Gianotti–Crosti syndrome are associated with EBV.
  - Ampicillin/**amoxicillin rash** associated with EBV occurs in 95%–100% of individuals given these antibiotics. Rash is maculopapular, pruritic, and **usually develops 5 days into treatment.**

Cytomegalovirus

Primary CMV accounts for remaining **20% of IM.** Most cases are asymptomatic. Severe, and life-threatening disease

TABLE 23.3	Principal Viruses Causing Viral Hemorrhagic Fevers		
Family	**Virus/Disease**	**Vector or Animal Host**	**Endemic Countries**
Filoviridae	Ebola	Unknown	Africa
	Marburg	Unknown	Africa
Arenaviridae	Lassa	Rodent	West Africa
	Junin	Rodent	Argentina
	Machupo	Rodent	Bolivia
	Guanarito	Rodent	Venezuela
	Sabia	Rodent	Brazil
Bunyaviruses	Crimean-Congo	Tickborne Infected livestock	Africa Middle East Eastern Europe Central Asia
	Hantavirus	Rodent	Asia Europe South America
	Rift Valley fever	Mosquitoborne	Sub-Saharan Africa Middle East
Flaviviridae	Yellow fever	Mosquitoborne	South America Africa
	Dengue hemorrhagic fever	Mosquitoborne	Africa, Asia, South America
	Kyasanur Forest	Tickborne, monkey	India
	Omsk	Tickborne	Central Asia

in immunocompromised individuals occurs by both primary CMV infection, for example in solid organ transplants or as a consequence of CMV reactivation.

- CMV, like other herpesviruses, establishes latency following primary infection.
- Transmission horizontally through close contact or sexual contact.
  - Virus secreted in saliva, urine, cervical or vaginal secretions, and semen.
  - Vertical transmission occurs in utero, resulting in congenital CMV disease.
  - Blood transfusion and organ donations have also been a source of transmission.

Cutaneous Manifestations of CMV Infection

- Maculopapular or urticarial rash as part of an infectious mononucleosis syndrome
- Antibiotic (ampicillin/amoxicillin)-induced rash, characteristic of EBV infection, also occurs in CMV.
- **Cutaneous CMV with vesicular lesions or ulceration.** Seen rarely in advanced HIV, solid or bone marrow transplants, i.e., patients with significant cell-mediated immunodeficiencies. Presentation can mimic HSV or VZV, particularly as **reactivation** of latent disease. CMV can be isolated from vesicular fluid or tissue biopsy of ulcers. Histology may

demonstrate classic **nuclear inclusion "owl's eye"** morphology.
- Nonspecific manifestations of CMV, particularly in disease reactivation, include macules, papules, hyperpigmented plaques, or generalized erythematous morbilliform exanthems.
- **Valganciclovir** has a role in treatment of specific skin manifestations of CMV in the immunocompromised host.

Viral Hemorrhagic Fever (VHF)

Hemorrhagic rashes represent the severe and invariably fatal spectrum of diseases caused by VHF viruses. VHFs caused by several families of enveloped RNA viruses (Table 23.3).
- VHFs associated with specific animal hosts or vectors, hence **restricted geographical spread.**
  - Countries or specific regions within countries may be endemic for a named viral species.
  - **Humans are incidental hosts.**
  - Person-to-person spread may occur, resulting in local outbreaks or transmission beyond areas of endemicity.

Clinical Features

- Early clinical presentation often nonspecific.
  - Usually fever, myalgia, headache, diarrhea, vomiting, or sore throat.

- The spectrum of disease varies from mild or asymptomatic infections to case fatality rates of up to 70% (Marburg) and 90% (Ebola).
- Maculopapular rash may occur.
- Conjunctival injection, petechiae, spontaneous bruising, or mucosal hemorrhages can develop.
- Vascular endothelial damage in severe disease results in circulatory collapse and multiorgan failure.

Prevention

There are few widely available vaccines for VHF.
- Yellow fever; live attenuated vaccine. Single-dose confers immunity in >95% of individuals. The objectives of yellow fever immunization are twofold. To protect individual travelers visiting areas where there is risk of transmission and prevent international spread of yellow fever into susceptible regions where the mosquito vector and potential nonhuman primate hosts co-exist. As such, evidence of yellow fever vaccine may be required for entry into certain countries.
- Kyasanur Forest; formalin-inactivated tissue-culture vaccine. Mass vaccination has been used to control outbreaks and spread of disease in local populations. Vaccine is short-lived.

Dengue

Dengue is a flavivirus with four serotypes. Transmitted by species of *Aedes* mosquito.
- Endemic in countries of Southeast Asia, the Americas, the Western Pacific, Africa, and the Middle East, in climates and geographical locations where vector survives.
- Primary infection with one serotype results in lifelong immunity to this serotype only, and transient (<6 months) cross-protection to the others.
- Dengue virus causes a wide spectrum of disease including asymptomatic infections. In the majority an acute self-limiting illness: dengue fever. Small proportion progress to severe disease: dengue hemorrhagic fever or dengue shock syndrome.
- Incubation period 4–7 days (range 3–14 days).

Clinical Features

- Dengue fever classically consists of **sudden onset fever**, **retro-orbital pain**, myalgia, arthralgia, lymphadenopathy, and **rash.**
- Diffuse macular or maculopapular rash appears usually **2–5 days from onset of fever.**
  - Characteristically markedly erythematous, blanching, resembling sunburn (Fig. 23.10).
  - Rash may coalesce with resultant widespread generalized erythema with white areas of sparing.
  - Mucosal involvement may be mild and include conjunctival or scleral infection, vesicles or erythema of the soft palate, mild bleeding of gums or epistaxis.

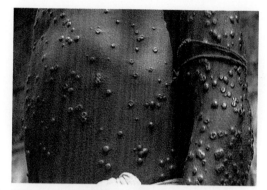

● **Fig. 23.9** Smallpox: semiconfluent umbilicated pustular lesions. (Courtesy Centers for Disease Control and Prevention Public Health Image Library. Image #10661.)

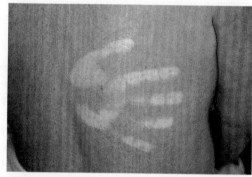

● **Fig. 23.10** Widespread macular erythematous blanching rash of early stage dengue fever. (From Morris-Jones R, Morris-Jones S. Travel-associated skin disease. *Infect Dis Clin North Am.* 2012;26(3):675–689.)

- **No specific antiviral or currently licensed dengue vaccine** in the UK or United States.

Chikungunya

- An arbovirus infection transmitted by *Aedes aegypti* and *Aedes albopictus.*
- Genus *Alphavirus:* enveloped positive-stranded RNA virus from the *Togaviridae* family.

Chikungunya fever has been associated with outbreaks in the many tropical and subtropical regions in Asia, the Indian subcontinent, Pacific islands, and sub-Saharan Africa. However, since chikungunya first emerged in the Caribbean in 2013, it has caused widespread disease in North, Central, and South America.

Clinical Features

- **Hallmark features are fever, arthralgia, and rash.** The name "chikungunya" is a Makonde word in Tanzania, the country where the illness was first characterized, and means "to walk bent over."
- Other symptoms: generalized malaise, headache, gastrointestinal symptoms, and myalgia. Majority (85%) of patients present with symptoms. Incubation period 3–7 days.

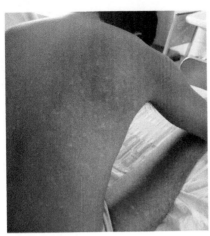

• **Fig. 23.11** White areas of sparing. (From Freedman DO. Infections in returning travelers. In: Bennett JE, Dolin R, Blaser MJ, eds. *Mandell, Douglas, and Bennett's Principles and Practice of Infectious Diseases.* Updated 8th ed. Elsevier; 2015.)

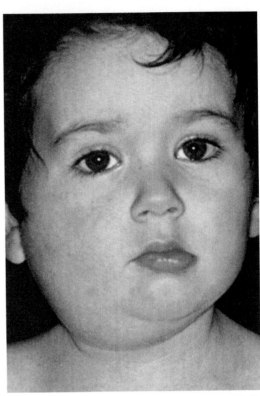

• **Fig. 23.12** Mumps in childhood. (From Emond RT, Welsby PD, Rowland HA, eds. *Colour Atlas of Infectious Diseases.* 4th ed. Mosby; 2003.)

- Arthralgia: usually 3–5 days after onset of fever but may present much earlier. Symmetrical oligo- but usually polyarthralgia. Any joint may be affected, usually distal joints (wrists, hand, ankles). In the majority arthralgia resolves in up to 4 weeks, but a significant proportion of patients continue to have chronic or relapsing joint disease for many months or even years.
- **Rash: skin manifestations reported in 40%–75%** of cases. Predominately **nonspecific** morbilliform or maculopapular eruption. Less commonly generalized urticarial lesions or, in infants, a vesiculobullous rash.
- Other skin changes following initial exanthem include **hypermelanosis of skin** and **desquamation of the palms of hands.**
- Disease is usually self-limiting but can be fatal in a small proportion of cases. **There is no vaccine.**

Zika

- Zika is a single-stranded RNA virus from the genus *Flavivirus.*
- Transmission, like chikungunya and dengue, by the bite of infected *Aedes* species mosquito.

  Until recently infections have occurred largely in Africa, where it was first identified, and Asia. In 2015, Zika was recognized in Brazil with a reported increase in one of the most significant associations of the disease, microencephaly in neonates, born to mothers who had acquired infection during pregnancy (see Chapter 20). This outbreak of Zika virus has now spread across South and Central America and the Caribbean, Southeast Asia, and the Indian subcontinent, sub-Saharan Africa, and the Pacific islands.
- Incubation period 3–14 days.

Clinical Features

- In contrast to chikungunya, a reported **80% of infections are asymptomatic.** Illness is usually mild and self-limiting.

- **Predominant features are fever, rash, arthralgia, and conjunctivitis.** Post-infectious Guillain-Barré syndrome, as well as other neurologic complications, such as transverse myelitis and meningoencephalitis have been associated with the disease.
- Exanthem reportedly more common in symptomatic patients than in dengue or chikungunya, composed of:
  - Pruritic maculopapular rash.
  - Malar erythema.

Prevention and Management

- Prevention is through bite avoidance.
- Where possible, pregnant women or couples planning pregnancy are advised to avoid regions where outbreaks are ongoing.
- Zika infection has been reported via sexual transmission and can be detected in semen for some time post-infection.
- There is **no vaccine** for Zika.

Mumps

Worldwide mumps is an infection of childhood recognized by its characteristic parotid gland swelling.
- Single-stranded RNA virus, member of the *Paramyxovirus* genus.
- Transmitted by **droplet spread.**
- Initial infection via the upper respiratory or eye spreads to lymph nodes followed by primary viremia. Virus disseminates to salivary and other glands and sites such as testes and pancreas.

- Incubation period 14–24 days.

Clinical Features

- **Parotitis**, the consequence of viral replication in the parotid glands and ensuing inflammation and interstitial edema, occurs in **95% of symptomatic cases** of mumps.
- Subclinical infection occurs in up to a third of patients.
- Orchitis or epididymoorchitis in up to 30% of symptomatic cases. More common in adults than children and may occur in isolation or following presentation with parotitis. Oophoritis occasionally occurs in females.
- CNS involvement. Primary mumps meningitis (1%–10%) and encephalitis (0.1%) most frequently, with around 50% of presentation occurring without parotitis. Long-term morbidity is uncommon.
- Sensorineural deafness well-known complication of mumps but permanent hearing loss is rare.
- Other manifestations include pancreatitis, myocarditis, thyroiditis, interstitial nephritis, mastitis, hepatitis, and a migratory polyarthritis.

Laboratory Diagnosis

- Serologic, with detection or mumps IgM antibodies.
- Detection of viral nucleic acid (**PCR**). **Saliva or buccal or throat swabs most reliable specimens.** Virus can be isolated from CSF, urine, and semen.
- Serum IgM should be taken as soon as mumps suspected clinically but, in some cases, may not be detectable until 5 days after onset of illness.

Prevention and Treatment

- Vaccines contain **live attenuated** strain of mumps virus.
- Usually administered in combination with measles and rubella (MMR) within childhood immunization schedule.
- Single dose confers around 60%–90% immunity and therefore **second dose is required.**
- **Vaccine protection wanes** while natural infection confers lifelong immunity.
- Response to vaccine is not sufficiently rapid to confer protection in an outbreak.
- **No antiviral treatment.** Management is supportive.

Polio

Poliovirus, one of the enteroviruses, is infamous for its devastating effects on the central nervous system of young children. Epidemic poliomyelitis appeared at the turn of the 20th century in Europe and the United States, becoming an illness of school-age children and young adults. The introduction of vaccine was dramatic.

The Global Polio Eradication Initiative has seen cases drop from an estimated 350,000 cases in 1988 to 37 reported cases in 2016. Endemic transmission remains only in Pakistan, Nigeria, and Afghanistan, but risks of re-introduction to countries in Africa and Asia is a concern.

- Three serotypes, 1, 2, and 3 exist, all of which cause motor neurone disease.
- Polio now mainly affects **children under 5 years** of age.
- Transmission is universally feco-oral but oral–oral transmission also occurs.
- Virus replicates in the gastrointestinal tract and adjacent lymphoid tissue. If disease progresses, neurones are infected, principally **motor and autonomic neurones.**
- Incubation period 9–12 days for onset of viral prodrome, 11–17 days for onset of paralysis.

Clinical Features

- **95% cases are asymptomatic.**
- Abortive poliomyelitis (4%–8% cases); prodrome of fever with nonspecific symptoms of fatigue, loss of appetite, headache, or gastrointestinal symptoms.
- Nonparalytic poliomyelitis; clinical signs of viral meningitis.
- Spinal paralytic poliomyelitis (0.1%); asymmetrical flaccid paralysis, with absent reflexes, proximal muscles groups with legs affected more than arms. Bulbar paralytic poliomyelitis occurs in 5%–35% of paralytic cases.

Prevention

- Inactivated polio vaccine (IPV): Salk vaccine, contains all three serotypes.
  - A primary time-determined three-dose schedule provides >95% coverage.
  - Lifelong protection is reliably achieved through two further booster vaccinations.
  - Compared to oral polio vaccine (OPV), IPV induces low levels of immunity in the intestine. When an individual immunized with IPV is challenged with wild-type polio, virus is able to replicate in the intestine resulting in prolonged viral shedding in stool, a risk to unimmunized contacts.
  - IPV, however, has been shown to boost both humoral and intestinal immunity in children who have received OPV.
- OPV: Sabin vaccine is a live attenuated oral vaccine. Vaccines now in use have only serotype 1 and serotype 3; type 2 was removed following wild-type elimination.
  - Postvaccination, OPV virus is shed from oropharynx for up to 14 days and in the stool for up to 8 weeks.
  - This is considered beneficial for boosting community immunity. OPV-related poliomyelitis, however, can occur through two rare, but key processes.
    - Vaccine-associated paralytic poliomyelitis (VAPP). Vaccinated individuals (usually infants) or their contacts. Increased risk also reported in individuals with B-cell deficiency.
    - Circulating vaccine-derived polioviruses (cVDPV) derived from OPV.
- IPV vaccine is recommended in countries free of polio. Usually in combination with diphtheria, tetanus, and/or pertussis as part of childhood immunization.
- Widespread use of OPV remains in endemic countries. For lasting elimination of polio, however, it is recognized that OPV vaccination must cease, an objective central in the Polio Eradication and Endgame Strategy Plan.

Further Reading and Resources

1. Public Health England (PHE). The Green Book. https://www.gov.uk/government/collections/immunisation-against-infectious-disease-the-green-book#the-green-book.
2. CDC Centers for Disease Control and Prevention. https://www.cdc.gov.
3. World Health Organization. Global Measles and Rubella Strategic Plan 2012–2020. http://www.who.int/immunization/documents/control/ISBN_978_92_4_150339_6/en/.
4. Kliegman R, Stanton B, Behrman RE, et al., eds. *Nelson Textbook of Pediatrics*. 20th ed. Elsevier; 2016.
5. Kuesia G, Wreghitt T. *Clinical and Diagnostic Virology*. Cambridge: Cambridge University Press; 2009.

24

Disease Due to Spirochetes, Excluding Syphilis

GILL JONES, ALBERTO SAN FRANCISCO RAMOS

Spirochetes

Spirochetes are spiral-shaped bacteria. This chapter will look at the endemic treponematoses; relapsing fevers, leptospirosis; and Lyme disease.

Syphilis is not included here; it is covered in detail in Chapter 21, Sexually Transmitted Infections. Rat bite fever is covered in Chapter 31, Infections Associated with Animal Exposure. There is further discussion of Lyme disease in Chapter 30, Arthropod-Borne Diseases.

Endemic Treponematoses

The endemic or nonvenereal treponematoses are a group of chronic, primarily cutaneous diseases caused by **spirochetes** which are morphologically and serologically indistinguishable from *Treponema pallidum*, causative agent of venereal syphilis:

- **Yaws** (*Treponema pallidum* subsp. *pertenue*).
- **Endemic syphilis** or **bejel** (*Treponema pallidum* subsp. *endemicum*).
- **Pinta** (*Treponema carateum*).

As with venereal syphilis, the clinical course can be divided in clinical stages:

- Primary stage: characterized mainly by **cutaneous lesions.**
- Secondary stage: **recurrence of skin manifestations** and even cartilage/bone involvement months or years after primary illness.
- Latency stage: **regression** of symptoms following the host immune response.
- Tertiary stage: occurs late in the clinical history, often many years after the primary infection and is characterized by **bone and soft tissue destruction.**

Despite all these similarities, the endemic treponematoses have some **key differences from venereal syphilis** in their epidemiologic distribution, transmission, and clinical manifestations (Table 24.1).

Epidemiology

- Historic overview:
  - Before the antibiotic era, endemic treponematoses were widely spread in areas of South America, Africa, Southeast Asia, and the Pacific.
  - Mass treatment campaigns led by the World Health Organization (WHO) and United Nations Children's Fund (UNICEF) in the 1950s and 1960s led to worldwide reduction in incidence and prevalence.
  - After the 1970s, they slowly re-emerged. In 1978, a World Health Assembly Resolution renewed efforts to eradicate yaws.
- Geographic distribution:
  - Yaws, pinta, and endemic syphilis (bejel) are **endemic in rural areas** among communities living **in overcrowded conditions and poor hygiene.**
  - Varied geographic distribution, **rarely found above or below the 30th parallel** (Fig. 24.1):
    - Yaws: humid and tropical forests of Africa, Asia, Latin America, and the Pacific.
    - Pinta: low-altitude areas and river basins of Central and South America, and the Caribbean.
    - Endemic syphilis (bejel): found in seminomadic tribes in isolated, dry areas of the Sahel (southern border of the Sahara desert) and the Arabian Peninsula.

Microbiology

The causative agents of the endemic treponematoses belong to the order Spirochaetales, family Spirochaetaceae, genus *Treponema*. Four species are human pathogens: *T. pallidum* subsp. *pallidum* (venereal syphilis), *T. pallidum* subsp. *pertenue* (yaws), *T. pallidum* subsp. *endemicum* (endemic syphilis), and *T. carateum* (pinta).

- Long and thin (8–13 ×0.15 μm) Gram-negative, **spiral-shaped bacteria.**
- Invisible to light microscopy, can be observed under dark field illumination or fluorescent antibody techniques, demonstrating characteristic **corkscrew motility.**

TABLE 24.1	Key Differences Between Endemic Treponematoses and Venereal Syphilis	
	Endemic Treponematoses	**Venereal Syphilis**
Who?	Childhood diseases	Adolescents and young adults
Where?	Confined to deprived, rural, tropical communities	Global distribution
What route?	Transmitted by **direct contact**	Primarily transmitted by **sexual contact**
Complications?	**Congenital infection** in endemic treponematoses and **systemic manifestations** outside the musculoskeletal system are **rare**	Congenital and tertiary syphilis are well-recognized complications of untreated venereal syphilis

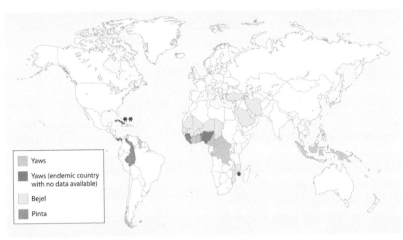

• **Fig. 24.1** Geographic distribution of the endemic treponematoses. (From Giacani L, Lukehart SA. The endemic treponematoses. *Clin Microbiol Rev.* 2014;27(1):89–115.)

• **Cannot be cultured *in vitro*,** diagnosis is based on clinical and serologic findings and visualization of spirochetes on microscopy from clinical specimens.
• Each species is morphologically and immunologically **indistinguishable** from each other.
• Whole genome sequencing analysis reveals over 99% similarity within the different *Treponema pallidum* subspecies and *T. carateum*.
• Easily killed by drying, heating, and oxygen exposure, they replicate slowly (every 30 hours) and cannot survive outside the mammalian host.

Pathogenesis

Understanding of the disease mechanisms in treponemic diseases is limited by the inability to grow spirochetes *in vitro*, their fragile cellular structure, and inability to survive outside the host.
• Treponemes infect the human host by **penetrating through the skin.**
• They move through tight junctions between epithelial cells and attach to fibronectin-coated surfaces on the extracellular matrix of host cells.
• Organisms reach the lymphatic nodes and then disseminate through the body within hours.

• Main virulence factor is their **corkscrew motility**, allowing them to move within the connective tissue.
• *T. pallidum* might stimulate trafficking on T-cells, also surface protein antigen variation may play a role in immune evasion and establishment of chronic infection.

Yaws (Frambesia, Pian, Buda, Bouba)

Yaws is a chronic, disfiguring, and debilitating childhood infectious disease caused by *Treponema pallidum* subsp. *pertenue*.
• **Most prevalent** of all endemic treponematoses, with over 250,000 cases reported in 13 countries between 2010 and 2013.
• Yaws is on the WHO list of Neglected Tropical Diseases.
• Usually seen in **children <15 years**, especially in poor communities in warm, humid, and tropical forest areas of Africa, Asia, Latin America, and the Pacific.
• Male to female ratio is 1:1, **humans are the only reservoir.**
• Transmission is by close contact with the infected lesions of another individual through a break in the skin, commonly the lower legs, head, face, and mouth.
• There is no sexual or vertical transmission.

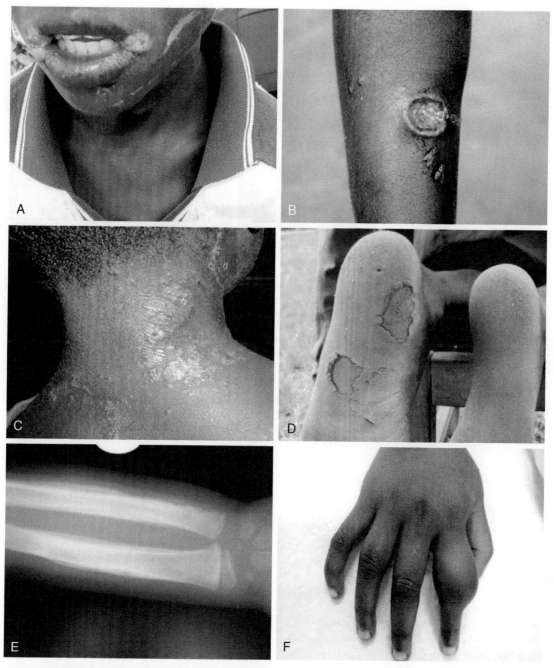

• **Fig. 24.2** Primary and secondary yaws. (A) Papilloma with yellow crust in the peribuccal area of a patient with primary yaws. (B) Early stage ulcer, round in shape with raised margins and a reddish, friable bed. (C) Scaly patches on the skin of a patient with secondary yaws. (D) Cracks and discoloration of the soles of the feet of a patient with secondary yaws. (E) Loss of clarity of the cortex of the distal radius and ulna and organized periosteal reaction (widespread onion layering) in a patient with osteoperiostitis. (F) Fusiform swelling of the second digit of a patient with dactylitis. (Images copyright © Oriol Mitja and Kingsley Asiedu. From Oriol M, Asiedu K. Yaws. *The Lancet.* 2013;381(9868):763–773.)

• Incubation period is between 9 days and 3 months, usually around 3 weeks.

Clinical Manifestations

Primarily a cutaneous infection but can subsequently extend into deeper tissues. Infection can be divided into stages:

• **Primary lesion:** "*mother yaw*" or "*frambesioma.*"
  • Raised, papular lesion appears at the inoculation site (Fig. 24.2A and B).

• Highly contagious and pruritic, facilitating **autoinoculation by scratching.**
• Enlarges into nodules 2–5 cm long which subsequently ulcerate.
• Ulcers have raised dark margins and erythematous center, **resembling raspberries** (hence the name frambesia, from "framboise" in French).
• Regional lymphadenopathy can occur.

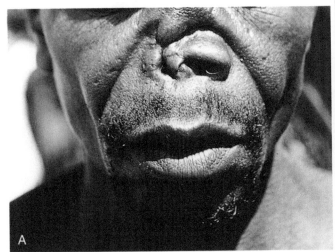
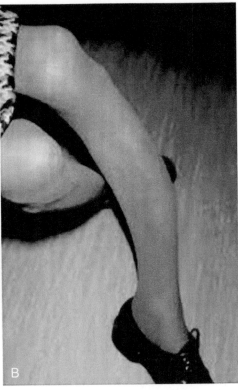

• **Fig. 24.3** (A) Gangosa in late stage of yaws (rhinopharyngitis mutilans; occurs also in endemic syphilis). (B) Clinical photograph showing tibial "saber shins." (Panel A courtesy WHO. Panel B from Agrawal A. Musculoskeletal colloquialisms based on weapons. *J Clin Orthop Trauma.* 2017;8(1):1–10.)

- Heals after several months into a hypopigmented area of skin with hyperpigmented borders.
- **Secondary** manifestations (Fig. 24.2C–F): due to systemic dissemination of treponemes, they usually appear at the time the primary lesion is healing. If untreated, they heal without scarring within weeks/months.
  - Fever + malaise common at this stage.
  - **Skin lesions**
    - Secondary papules or "daughter yaws."
    - Plantar/palmar hyperkeratosis, causing "crab yaws" (painful crab-like gait in children).
    - Condyloma lata in moist crevices and mucous membranes.
    - Secondary bacterial infection of cutaneous lesions can occur.
  - **Periostitis** and **osteitis**: in long bones and phalanges (causes **digital swelling**).
- **Clinical latency**: asymptomatic stage, recognized only by serologic tests. Recurrences of secondary lesions can occur, usually within 5 years.
- **Tertiary stage:** occurs in 10% of untreated yaws patients, characterized by destructive lesions in bone (periostitis and osteomyelitis) and cartilage.
  - "Gangosa" (Fig. 24.3A): disfiguring chronic destruction of nasal and facial bone, cartilage, and soft tissue; also termed *rhinopharyngitis mutilans.*
  - "Goundou": hypertrophic periostitis causing exostosis of the paranasal maxillae (last reported in 1989).

- "Saber shins" (Fig. 24.3B): bowing of the tibia due to chronic periostitis.
- Gummatous subcutaneous nodules and destructive lesions of cartilage and bone.
- Central nervous system (CNS) and cardiovascular complications have been reported in yaws, as in syphilis.

Endemic Syphilis (Bejel, Njovera, Siti, Dichuchwa)

Endemic syphilis or bejel is caused by *T. pallidum* subsp. *endemicum.* This treponemic disease occurs primarily in nomadic rural communities living in arid areas of North Africa and the Arabian Peninsula.
- Commonest in **children** aged 2–15 with equal sex distribution.
- Transmitted through **direct contact** or **fomites** such as drinking or food preparation utensils.
- Incubation period is approximately 3 weeks.
- **Primary lesion**: painless papula or ulcer inside the oropharynx which can often be absent or go unnoticed. Can last for months to years.
- **Secondary lesions** appear after 3–6 months and resemble those of venereal syphilis.
  - Lesions of **mucous membranes** of oropharynx, tongue, nasopharynx, tonsils (Fig. 24.4, bejel).

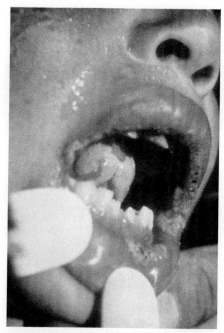

• **Fig. 24.4** Secondary lesions of bejel. (From Syphilis, yaws, bejel, and pinta. In: James WD, Elston DM. *Andrews' Diseases of the Skin: Clinical Atlas.* Elsevier; 2018.)

- Skin manifestations include maculopapular lesions, condylomata in intertriginous areas, angular stomatitis, and a generalized nonpruritic rash.
- Laryngitis.
- Cervical lymphadenopathy can also occur.
- Long bone and hand osteitis and periostitis (similar to yaws, causing nocturnal bone pain).
- **Latency:** secondary manifestations heal within 6–9 months, and disease enters a quiescent state.
- **Tertiary disease** is relatively common, affects 25%–50% of patients, usually in late teenage years or early adulthood.
  - Resembles tertiary yaws or syphilis.
  - **Gummatous** lesions in skin and mucosal areas which can progress to destructive ulcers.
  - Destruction of palate and nasal septum (= "gangosa," as in yaws)
  - **Periostitis of long bones:** "saber tibia" is the commonest bone manifestation.
  - Neurologic and cardiac involvement, as well as congenital transmission, has been reported but is rare and milder than in venereal syphilis.

Pinta (Mal del Pinto, Carate, Enfermedad Azul)

Pinta is a treponemic disease caused by *Treponema carateum*. It is the mildest of the endemic treponematoses, with **only cutaneous manifestations and no evidence of systemic involvement.**

- Distribution is limited to tropical countries of Central and South America and the Caribbean, predominately among those living in poverty.

- Can occur at any age but commonest in children and young adults; no sex predilection.
- Transmission by **direct contact** through breaks in the skin; no congenital transmission.
- Incubation period is 2–3 weeks.
- **Primary lesions** are small erythematous papules on exposed areas of the body which gradually enlarge and then coalesce. The lesions become hyperpigmented over the next few months.
  - Regional lymphadenopathy may occur.
  - In contrast with other treponematoses, lesions do not usually disappear if untreated.
- **Secondary lesions** or "pintids" appear after several months on any area of the skin, following treponemic dissemination. They are small scaly erythematous papules which get darker over time.
- **Tertiary stage** is characterized by slow depigmentation of preexisting lesions, similar to vitiligo.

Diagnosis of Endemic Treponematoses

The endemic treponematoses can be diagnosed by:
- **Recognition** of **clinical signs and symptoms** in patients with a relevant epidemiologic background.
- **Direct visualization of treponemes** in clinical specimens (not readily available in some endemic areas) by dark field microscopy or immunofluorescence.
- **Rapid point-of-care testing** by immunochromatographic strips.
- **Treponemal serology:** the serologic tests used to diagnose endemic treponematoses are the same as those used for venereal syphilis. Antibody response to all treponematous diseases is identical, therefore serology alone cannot differentiate between them. Serologic tests are divided into "nontreponemal" and "treponemal" tests:
  - **Nontreponemal tests:** based on cross-reactivity between cardiolipin-cholesterol-lecithin antigens with antibodies to *T. pallidum.*
    - Rapid plasma reagin (RPR) and Venereal Disease Research Laboratory (VDRL).
    - Become **positive 2–4 weeks** after the appearance of the primary lesion.
    - **Quantitative** tests: can be used for screening and to monitor treatment response. **Four-fold reduction in antibody titers** indicates successful treatment.
    - False-positive results occur in malaria, leprosy, or autoimmune conditions.
  - **Treponemal tests:** based on antibody reactivity to native or recombinant *T. pallidum* subsp. *pallidum* antigens:
    - Examples include fluorescent treponemal antibody adsorbed (FTA-ABS) and *Treponema pallidum* particle agglutination (TPPA) assays.
    - Help **confirm** a positive nontreponemal test.
    - Remain **positive for life,** therefore cannot be used to monitor treatment.

Treatment

- **Intramuscular benzathine penicillin G** has traditionally been the treatment of choice for endemic treponematoses.
  - Adults: 1.2 million units single dose.
  - Children <10 years: 600,000 units.
  - Highly effective and long acting.
- More recently, oral **azithromycin 30 mg/kg** (up to 2 g once daily) has been demonstrated to be noninferior to benzathine penicillin G for treatment of yaws.
- WHO has adopted mass treatment with oral azithromycin as part of its global strategy for yaws eradication by 2020.

Leptospirosis

Leptospirosis is a zoonosis caused by pathogenic spirochetes from the genus *Leptospira*. It was first described by Weil as a multisystemic illness with jaundice and renal dysfunction in 1886.

Epidemiology and Transmission

- Leptospirosis is **endemic worldwide**, with higher incidence in the tropics during the rainy season and late summer in temperate areas.
- In developing countries, outbreaks occur after heavy rainfall and flooding in areas with poor housing standards.
- WHO's Leptospirosis Burden Epidemiology Group estimates approximately 873,000 cases worldwide annually with 48,600 deaths.
- Leptospirosis is maintained in nature by **chronic renal infection of carrier animals.**
  - Mammal hosts: **rodents**, cattle, swine, dogs, sheep, goats.
  - Infected animals shed *Leptospira* in their **urine** contaminating the environment, especially **water.**
- Humans are infected incidentally after **animal or environmental exposure.**
  - Contact with animal urine or tissue, contaminated water or soil.
  - *Spirochetes* enter through cuts, abraded skin, mucous membranes, or conjunctiva.
  - Transplacental transmission can occur.
- **Risk factors** for infection:
  - **Recreational exposure:** fresh water swimming (linked with outbreaks in sporting events), canoeing, kayaking, etc.
  - **Occupational** exposure: farmers, veterinarians, abattoir (slaughterhouse) workers, laboratory staff, sewer workers, pet traders.
  - **Rodent infestation**, walking barefoot in water, contaminated rainwater catchment systems.

Microbiology

Leptospira derives from the Greek *lepto* (thin) and Latin *spira* (coiled).
- Leptospires measure 0.1 μm in diameter by 6–20 μm in length (Fig. 24.5).

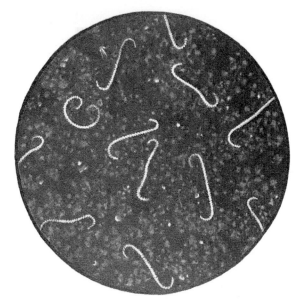

- **Fig. 24.5** Leptospira microscopy. Appearance of living leptospires as seen by dark field microscopy. Note the very fine coils and characteristic hooked ends. (From Picardeau M. Leptospirosis; Weil's disease. In: Murray PR, et al. *Medical Microbiology*. 7th ed. Elsevier; 2012. From an original painting by Dr. Cranston Low. In: Low RC, Dodds TC *Atlas of Bacteriology*. Livingstone; 1947.)

- They are highly motile spirochetes, with approx. 18 coils per cell.
- Can be visualized by dark field, fluorescence, or silver stain microscopy.
- Characteristic terminal **"question mark" hook.**
- Genus *Leptospira* contains 21 species, 9 of which are pathogenic (*L. interrogans, L. kirschneri, L. noguchii, L. alexanderi, L. weilii, L. alstonii, L. borgpetersenii, L. santarosai,* and *L. kmetyi*).
- Can be grown in special media in the laboratory within 1–2 weeks.

Pathogenesis

- *Leptospira* infection leads to rapid hematogenous dissemination, allowing organisms to penetrate different tissues, including the CNS.
- Transendothelial migration of spirochetes is facilitated by **systemic vasculitis.**
- **Vascular injury** is responsive for some of multiorgan manifestations of leptospirosis:
  - Pulmonary hemorrhage.
  - Renal cortical and tubulo-epithelial necrosis.
  - Disruption of hepatic architecture and liver cell injury.
- Virulence factors.
  - Leptospiral lipopolysaccharide (LPS) (is not bound by TLR-4 unlike other gram-negative LPS).

Clinical Manifestations

Leptospirosis has a variety of clinical manifestations and disease severity.
- Incubation period is 2–20 days (average 10 days).
- Some patients have a mild or subclinical presentation.

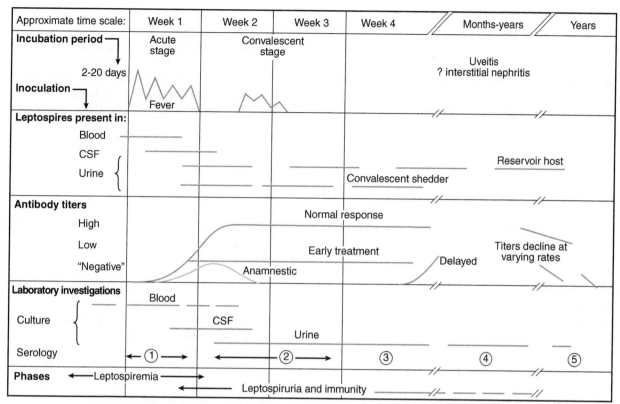

• **Fig. 24.6** Biphasic nature of leptospirosis and relevant investigations at different stages of disease. Specimens 1 and 2 for serology are acute-phase specimens; 3 is a convalescent-phase sample; and 4 and 5 are follow-up samples. (From Haake DA, Levett PN. *Leptospira* species (leptospirosis). In: Bennett JE, Dolin R, Blaser MJ, eds. *Mandell, Douglas, and Bennett's Principles and Practice of Infectious Diseases.* Updated 8th ed. Elsevier; 2015.)

- **90% of patients have a self-limited, systemic disease.**
- Others present with **severe multisystemic** disease with a combination of renal failure, liver failure, pneumonitis, and hemorrhagic diathesis.
  - **Weil's disease:** eponym for severe presentation of leptospirosis with **hepatic dysfunction** (jaundice) and **renal failure.**

Leptospirosis has been described in some patients as a **biphasic disease** (Fig. 24.6). However, in many cases both phases **may merge**, particularly in severe disease.

- **Acute, septicemic stage:** characterized by high, remittent fevers (38–40°C), headache, rigors, myalgia, anorexia, nausea and vomiting, and sore throat.
  - **Conjunctival suffusion** (55% of patients) and **muscle tenderness** (calf and lumbar spine) are the most characteristic features.
  - Less common features: nonproductive cough, hepatomegaly, splenomegaly, skin rash, abdominal pain, cholecystitis, and pancreatitis.
  - Lasts for 5–7 days.
  - Leptospires can be found in blood and cerebrospinal fluid (CSF).
- **Immune, leptospiuric phase:** lasts 4–30 days, leptospires are cleared from blood and CSF while IgM antibody response develops.
  - Organisms can be detected in urine and other organs.

- In addition to acute phase symptoms, the immune phase can present with:
  - **Jaundice** as a result of acute liver failure.
  - **Renal failure:** usually nonoliguric hypokalemic renal insufficiency with impaired sodium reabsorption and potassium wasting.
    - Renal biopsy demonstrates acute interstitial or immune complex glomerulonephritis.
  - Aseptic meningitis: occurs in up to 80% of cases.
    - Intense fronto-temporal headache.
    - Lymphocytic CSF pleocytosis with counts <500/mm^3.
    - Mildly raised CSF protein with normal glucose.
  - Rarer neurologic complications include encephalitis, transverse myelitis, and Guillain–Barré syndrome.
  - **Pulmonary symptoms**: severe pulmonary hemorrhage syndrome (SPHS) is the most serious manifestation, presenting with diffuse lung injury, ARDS picture with impaired gas exchange ± hemoptysis.
- **Severe leptospirosis cases** can progress directly from the acute phase to fulminant illness, with hyperpyrexia (>40°C) and rapid onset of liver and renal failure, hemorrhagic pneumonitis, cardiac arrhythmias, and circulatory collapse. Mortality rates can be up to 40%.

Diagnosis

- Leptospirosis diagnosis requires high clinical suspicion on the basis of epidemiologic exposure and clinical symptoms.
- Biochemistry and hematology laboratory findings are nonspecific:
  - WBC 3,000–26,000/μL. Thrombocytopenia and pancytopenia reported.
  - **Hyponatremia** and **renal failure** occur in severe leptospirosis.
  - 40% of patients have **elevated transaminases** (usually <200 IU/L) and **bilirubin.**
  - Urinalysis often shows proteinuria, leucocytes, casts, and microscopic hematuria.
- Direct visualization of leptospires in blood or urine by dark field microscopy can be used for diagnosis but has low sensitivity and specificity.
- **Polymerase chain reaction (PCR)** may be used in the acute stage – within 5 days of symptom onset.
- **Serology** is the most used diagnostic method. Microscopic agglutination test (MAT) is the reference assay.
  - Detects agglutinating antibodies, may be present from 5 days after onset.
  - Single titer of >1:800 is strongly suggestive of recent *Leptospira* infection.
  - Ideally compare two samples, at least 1 week apart.
  - **Serologically confirmed case: four-fold rise in MAT titer between acute-phase and convalescent serum.**
  - Cross-reaction occurs with syphilis, relapsing fever, Lyme, viral hepatitis, HIV, etc.
- Leptospires can be cultured from blood, CSF, peritoneal fluid (first 10 days), and urine (after 10 days).
  - Special media required, growth can take several weeks.

Treatment

Antibiotic therapy for leptospirosis should be started as soon as possible for symptomatic patients.
- **Mild disease:** oral therapy (adults).
  - Doxycycline 100 mg twice daily for 7 days.
  - Azithromycin 500 mg once daily for 3 days.
- **Severe leptospirosis:** in addition to **supportive care** with renal replacement therapy, ventilatory support, or blood products, **intravenous antibiotics** are recommended (adults).
  - Penicillin 1.5 million units every 6 hours.
  - Ceftriaxone 2 g once daily.
  - Doxycycline 100 mg twice daily.
- Jarisch–Herxheimer reactions occur in up to 20% of patients following antimicrobial therapy.

Relapsing Fevers

Relapsing fevers are arthropod-borne infections characterized by recurrent pyrexial episodes with concomitant spirochetemia:
- Caused by spirochetes from the *Borrelia* genus.

- Divided in two groups depending on the arthropod vector
  - **Epidemic tickborne relapsing fever** (TBRF): zoonosis caused by >20 different *Borrelia* species, transmitted mainly by soft ticks of the family Argasidae.
  - **Endemic louseborne relapsing fever** (LBRF): caused by *B. recurrentis* and transmitted by *Pediculus humanus* (body louse).

Microbiology

The spirochetes belonging to the family Borreliaceae are now recognized to be divided into two distinct genera on the basis of their genotypic and phenotypic groupings:
- Species causing Lyme disease, e.g., *Borrelia burgdorferi*.
- Species causing relapsing fevers:
  - Louseborne (LBRF): *Borrelia recurrentis*.
  - Tickborne (TBRG): *B. hermsii*, *B. mazzottii*, etc.
- 8–30 μm long and 0.2–0.5 μm wide, they have a helical shape.
- Cannot be seen by light microscopy but can be **visualized by dark field microscopy.**
- Microaerophilic organisms with complex nutritional requirements, grow on specific media.
- *Borrelia* spirochetes undergo **spontaneous antigenic variation** of membrane proteins, variable major proteins (***vmp***). *Vmp*s are responsible for the different serotypes and play a role in the pathogenesis of the recurrent febrile episodes.

Epidemiology

Tickborne Relapsing Fever

- TBRF is a **zoonosis**, with **rodents** acting as the main reservoir.
- Occurs on every continent except Antarctica and Australia, given the global distribution of the vector ticks.
- *Borrelia* spp. causing TBRF and their corresponding tick vectors vary on different geographic areas (Table 24.2).
- Cases are usually **sporadic** (e.g., returning travelers) or appear in **small outbreaks** within certain geographic areas, more common in the summer months.
- Transmission
  - **Ticks:** obligate blood feeders, live close to vertebrates (rodents, chipmunks, squirrels, rabbits, etc.), which act as reservoirs for *Borrelia* spp.
  - Spirochetes survive in the salivary glands of the ticks.
  - When ticks take a blood meal, spirochetes are released and penetrate through the skin, reaching the bloodstream.
  - **Risk factors for exposure:** cave dwelling, living in rodent-infected houses, and sleeping in log wood cabins.
  - **50% risk of disease transmission after infected tick bite.**
  - Transplacental and transfusion related transmission has been reported.

Louseborne Relapsing Fever

- *B. recurrentis* is transmitted by *Pediculus humanus corporis*, the **human body louse.**

TABLE 24.2   *Borrelia* Species Causing Relapsing Fever

Borrelia spp.	Disease	Arthropod Vector	Reservoir	Geographic Distribution
B. hermsii	TBRF	Ornithodoros hermsi	Rodents	Western United States, Canada
B. turicatae	TBRF	O. turicata	Rodents	Southwestern United States
B. parkeri	TBRF	O. parkeri	Rodents	Western United States and Baja California
B. mazzottii	TBRF	O. talaje	Rodents	Mexico and Central America
B. venezuelensis	TBRF	O. rudis	Rodents	South America
B. crocidurae	TBRF	O. erraticus		Middle East
B. hispanica	TBRF	O. marocanus		Iberian Peninsula and North Africa
B. miyamotoi	TBRF	Ixodes spp.	Rodents	United States and Japan
B. recurrentis	LBRF	Pediculus humanus	Humans	Eastern Africa, previously worldwide

Modified from Horton JM. Relapsing fever caused by *Borrelia* species. In: Bennett JE, Dolin R, Blaser MJ, eds. *Mandell, Douglas, and Bennett's Principles and Practice of Infectious Diseases.* Updated 8th ed. Elsevier; 2015.

- Endemic in the **Horn of Africa** (Ethiopia, Somalia, and Sudan), commonest in the rainy season.
- Overcrowding, refugee concentration, poor hygiene, famine, and wars predispose to **epidemics of LBRF**, as lice move from one person to another, spreading the disease.
- Large epidemics occurred during the First and Second World Wars.
- Reported on homeless people in Europe in the context of crowded shelters.
- Body lice live on clothing (not on the skin) and feed only from **humans, who are the only reservoir for LBRF.**
- Transmission: lice are crushed by humans following blood meals, releasing the spirochetes close to the bite side where they enter the bloodstream. Conjunctival infection also occurs through eye rubbing.

Pathogenesis

- Relapsing fever is primarily an extracellular bloodstream infection.
- Spirochetes migrate from the bloodstream to invade body organs (brain, eye, liver, spleen, etc.).
- Febrile episodes coincide with rapid *Borrelia* replication, where spirochetes are visible on blood smears.
- *Vmp* antigenic variation is responsible for fever relapse.
  - Specific humoral immune response to the predominating *vmp* serotype clears the spirochetes from the blood, resulting in an afebrile period.
  - Clones expressing a different *vmp* through antigenic variation will predominate, eventually causing a febrile relapse by escaping immunologic control.
  - Cyclic process of antigenic variation followed by specific antibody production is responsible for the relapsing course of the illness.

Clinical Manifestations

- Median incubation period is 7 days (range 2–18).

- Relapsing fever is characterized by recurrent febrile episodes.
  - Sudden onset of fever, usually >39 °C.
    - **TBRF: multiple** recurrent episodes if untreated, lasting 1–3 days.
    - **LBRF:** unremitting first febrile episode (3–6 days) with usually **one recurrence**.
- **Crisis phase:** occurs at the end of the first febrile episode:
  - Hyperpyrexia, hypertension, and tachycardia followed by profuse diaphoresis, falling temperature, and hypotension.
  - Lasts 15–30 min, period of highest mortality in untreated relapsing fever.
- Each febrile relapse is usually less severe than the previous.
- **Systemic symptoms:** headache, myalgias, arthralgias, rigors, dizziness, and vomiting.
- Hepatosplenomegaly, lymphadenopathy, and rash may occur in 30% of patients.
- **Neurologic** complications:
  - Confusion, apathy, delirium, and coma are secondary to spirochetemia.
  - Neurologic symptoms such as meningitis, paralysis, seizures, cranial nerve palsies, and radiculopathies are a consequence of CNS invasion by spirochetes.
- **Ophthalmologic** complications: uveitis and endophthalmitis.
- **Cardiopulmonary** complications: myocarditis, arrhythmias, acute respiratory distress syndrome (more common in TBRF).

Diagnosis

- General laboratory findings
  - Normocytic anemia, leukocytosis or leukopenia, and thrombocytopenia.

- Elevated ESR and CRP.
- Hepatitis with elevated transaminases and bilirubin.
- Hypoalbuminemia.
- Diagnosis of relapsing fever is made by a combination of:
  - Relapsing fever symptoms + epidemiologic history of tick/lice exposure in endemic geographic areas.
  - Direct visualization of spirochetes on blood smear on Giemsa or Wright blood smear.
    - Blood smear sensitivity during a febrile period is approx. 70%.
    - Negative blood smears do not exclude relapsing fever.
  - Acute and convalescent **serologic assays** can confirm diagnosis in patients with negative blood smears.
  - **PCR** testing is available in some centers.

Management

- If untreated, mortality rates are up to 10% for TBRF and 70% for LBRF.
- **TBRF** (adults)
  - Doxycycline 100 mg twice daily orally for 10 days.
  - Tetracycline 500 mg every 6 hours orally for 10 days.
  - Erythromycin 500 mg every 6 hours orally for 10 days.
  - In patients with CNS involvement.
    - IV penicillin G 3 million units every 4 hours for 14 days.
    - IV Ceftriaxone 2 g once daily for 14 days.
- **LBRF** (adults)
  - Tetracycline 500 mg single dose orally/IV.
  - Doxycycline 200 mg single dose orally.
  - Procaine penicillin G 400,000–800,000 units IM.
  - Erythromycin 500 mg single dose orally/IV.
- All patients should be monitored for **Jarisch–Herxheimer** reactions.
  - Occur in 50% of patients within the first 2–3 hours after first antibiotic dose.
  - Rigors, fever, and leukopenia; can be complicated by hypotension, ARDS, and death.
- **Postexposure prophylaxis** with doxycycline (200 mg OD, then 100 mg OD for 4 days) is effective for **TBRF** prevention.

Lyme Borreliosis (Lyme Disease)

- Most common tickborne infection in Europe and North America.
- First described in 1975 in Old Lyme, Connecticut, USA.
- Lyme disease diagnosis and management is controversial.
- Public perception of Lyme disease is that it is highly pathogenic and difficult to treat and diagnose.
- Other syndromes may be wrongly labeled as Lyme disease.
- Many activist groups exist.
- Nonstandard diagnostic techniques and treatment approaches are employed. These can be detrimental to vulnerable patients.

- New guidelines from both the IDSA and BIA are awaited after extensive consultation with many stakeholders, including patient representative groups.

Epidemiology

- Genus *Borrelia*, previously known as *Borrelia burgdorferi* sensu lato group. Six species are able to cause Lyme disease.
- *Borrelia burgdorferi* (previously *B. burgdorferi* sensu stricto) (associated with arthritic and neurologic presentations).
- *Borrelia garinii* (associated with neurologic presentations).
- *Borrelia afzelii* (associated with *Acrodermatitis chronica atrophicans*).
- *Borrelia bavariensis*.
- *Borrelia mayonii*.
- *Borrelia spielmanii*.
  United States
- *Borrelia burgdorferi* = **only pathogenic species in North America.**
- Approximately 300,000 cases per year.
- 95% of Lyme cases are from 14 states.
- High infection rates (>20% of ticks with *B. burgdorferi*) are documented in:
  - New England.
  - Parts of the mid-Atlantic states.
  - Parts of Minnesota and Wisconsin.
  Europe
- *B. garinii* and *B. afzelii* more common than *B. burgdorferi*.
- *B. garinii* most frequently found in the UK.
- Highest incidence is in central Europe, e.g., Slovenia 155/100,000.
- UK incidence 0.7/100,000.

Vector
- Lyme disease is transmitted by the bite of the hard-bodied ixodid ticks (*Ixodes ricinus* complex) (Fig. 24.7).
  - See Fig. 24.7 for the 2-year life cycle of the *Ixodes* vector.
- Birds and mammals are the usual feeding hosts.
- Humans are incidental hosts (usually nymphal stage).

Clinical Presentation

Traditionally subdivided into early and late Lyme disease – see Table 24.3.
- Initial infection is cutaneous (typically erythema migrans) but can disseminate to other tissues and organs.
- Clinical manifestations include:
  - Mild "flu-like" illness including arthralgia (which can be misdiagnosed as arthritis); and cutaneous, articular, neurologic, and cardiac manifestations.

Early Lyme Disease
  Erythema Migrans
- Cutaneous infection.

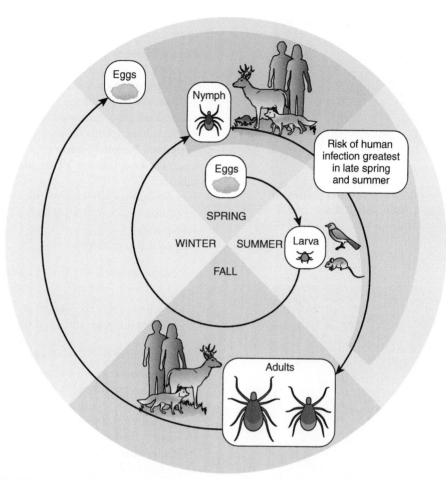

• **Fig. 24.7** Life cycle of the *Ixodes* tick. (From Schoen RT. Management of Lyme disease. In: Weisman MH, et al. *Targeted Treatment of the Rheumatic Diseases.* Elsevier; 2010. Adapted from http://www.cdc.gov/ncidod/dvbid/lyme/ld_transmission.htm.)

TABLE 24.3	**Traditional Classification of Early and Late Lyme Disease**		
	Cutaneous	**Neurologic**	**Other**
Early	Erythema migrans, borrelial lymphocytoma	Lyme meningitis, VIIth cranial nerve palsy	Lyme carditis
Late	Acrodermatitis chronica atrophicans	Encephalitis, encephalomyelitis, peripheral neuropathy	Lyme arthritis

- Most common manifestation of Lyme disease (~ 90% of cases).
- Distinctive target-like lesion with central clearing (Fig. 24.8).
- Usually appears within **7–14 days of the bite** but can be up to 30 days.
- >5cm diameter
- **Tick hypersensitivity reactions appear in first 48 hours** and usually less than 5 cm.
- Primary erythema migrans occurs at the site of a tick bite.
- Multiple lesions suggest early disseminated disease.

- **Clinical diagnosis sufficient, as serologic tests may be negative in early disease.**
- **Prompt antibiotic therapy may abrogate antibody response.**
  Borrelial Lymphocytoma
- Solitary red–blue lesion (Fig. 24.9).
- Painless.
- Few centimeters in diameter.
- Often found on ear, nipple, or scrotum.
- Polyclonal B cell infiltrate histologically.
- Rare in North America, more common with the Eurasian strain *B. afzelii.*

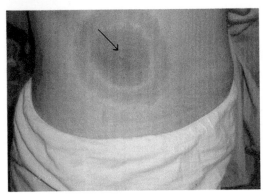

• **Fig. 24.8** Erythema migrans lesion with punctum (*arrow*). (From Nadelman RB. Erythema nigrans. *Infect Dis Clin North Am.* 2015;29(2):211–239.)

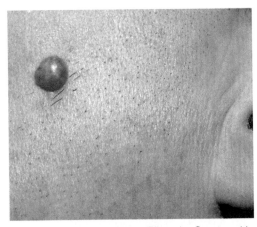

• **Fig. 24.9** Borrelial lymphocytoma. (Photo by Spectrum11 – Own work. Licensed under Creative Commons Zero, Public Domain Dedication via Wikimedia Commons – http://commons.wikimedia.org/wiki/File:Borrelial_lymphocytoma.jpg#mediaviewer/File:Borrelial_lymphocytoma.jpg.)

- Emerges later than erythema migrans lesions and can last a year or longer.
- Treatment as per erythema migrans.
  Cardiac Disease
- Rare **atrioventricular block;** myopericarditis even less common.
- Usually occurs **within 2 months** of infection.
- Requires serologic confirmation (usually positive at presentation).
- **Resolves within 6 weeks, but antibiotic therapy advised to prevent sequelae.**
- Criteria for admission to hospital for monitoring:
  - 1st-degree with prolonged PR interval (>300 milliseconds).
  - 2nd- or 3rd-degree block.
  - Symptomatic.
  - Dyspnea.
  - Chest pain.
  - Syncope.

Clinical Presentation: Early Neurologic Lyme Disease

Central Nervous System
- Subacute lymphocytic meningitis.
  - Longer onset than viral meningitis, median 7 days.
  - Cranial nerve palsies.
  - Papilledema common in children.
  - Encephalomyelitis (rare).

Peripheral Nervous System
- Cranial nerve lesions: **VIIth most common,** may be bilateral.
- Usually resolves without treatment but treatment advocated to avoid complications, e.g., Lyme arthritis.
- Radiculopathy.
- Mononeuritis multiplex.

Clinical Presentation: Ocular Lyme Disease

- Rare.
- Usually presents as conjunctivitis.
- Uveitis, papillitis, keratitis, and episcleritis also described.

Clinical Presentation: Late Lyme Disease

- Less common in era of recognition and treatment of erythema migrans lesions.
- **Arthritis**
  - Typically involves **knee.**
  - **Large effusions common.**
  - Other large joints and temporomandibular joint can be involved.
  - Characterized by **intermittent episodes** lasting weeks to months.
  - Granulocytic infiltrate of synovial fluid.
  - Synovial fluid PCR recommended.
  - Oral regimens usually effective if neurologic involvement excluded.
  - Treatment failures with oral regimens may require further course (consider parenterals).
  - NSAIDs effective.
  - Antibiotic refractory arthritis may be an autoimmune reaction to OspA.
- **Encephalopathy**
  - Mild memory and cognitive disturbance.
  - CSF findings may be normal.
  - Seropositivity expected.
  - Response to antibiotic therapy slow (months after treatment).
- **Encephalomyelitis**
  - Rare.
  - Progresses slowly.
  - Can resemble multiple sclerosis but MRI findings not present.
  - Seropositivity.
  - **Intrathecal antibody production.**
  - **CSF lymphocytic pleocytosis.**
  - **Elevated CSF protein.**
  - **Normal CSF glucose.**

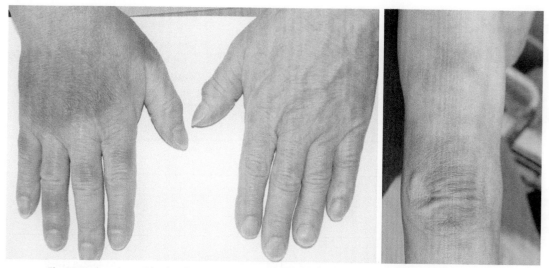

• **Fig. 24.10** Acrodermatitis chronica atrophicans. (With permission from Elsevier. The Lancet. From Joanna Zajkowska, et al. Acrodermatitis chronica atrophicans. *Lancet Infect Dis*. 2011;11(10):800.)

- CSF PCR: low yield.
- **Peripheral neuropathy**
  - Intermittent paresthesia.
  - Typically glove and stocking.
- **Acrodermatitis chronica atrophicans** (Fig. 24.10)
  - Rare in North America, commoner in Europe.
  - Late skin manifestation (years post infection).
  - More common in women.
  - 20% patients have history of erythema migrans.
  - Most commonly associated with *B. afzelii*.
  - **Early: blue–red discoloration of skin.**
  - **Late: cutaneous atrophy "tissue paper skin."**
  - Two-thirds have associated peripheral neuropathy.
  - May develop nodules over bony prominences.

Investigations

Note: IDSA and BIA guidelines are both under revision.

Erythema Migrans
- Clinical diagnosis of cutaneous Lyme disease with the typical erythema migrans rash sufficient

Extracutaneous Lyme Disease
- A history of plausible tick exposure must be obtained.
- Supporting diagnostics required.
- Culture of spirochetes from patient specimens (gold standard, rarely performed as sensitivity low and difficult/slow to perform).
- Histology: may see spirochetes or typical morphology, e.g., acrodermatitis chronica atrophicans
- **Serology: acute and convalescent** (>2 weeks after onset of symptoms).
- CSF can also be tested for intrathecal antibody production.
- **PCR**
  - Higher yield from tissue than fluid.
  - Tissue, e.g., skin, synovium, endomyocardium.

- Fluid, e.g., CSF, synovial, and ocular fluid.

Serology
- Should be performed in accredited laboratories.
- If testing has been performed in nonaccredited laboratories, it should be repeated by the clinician.
- Paired serum specimens to assess for seroconversion usually advocated if symptoms develop. Not recommended simply following a bite.
- Early treatment may prevent antibody production.
- **2-Tier testing algorithm**
  - Tier 1 = polyvalent ELISA
    - False-positives reported with:
      - Autoimmune conditions.
      - Cross-reacting antibodies, e.g., EBV.
      - Other spirochete infections, e.g., syphilis.
      - Inappropriate cut-off values/interpretation.
  - Proceed to tier 2 testing if tier 1 positive = separate IgM and IgG immunoblot (Western blot).
    - False-positives more common with IgM.
    - Appropriate history regarding timing of tick exposure required for interpretation.
    - Antibody response can take weeks to develop so repeat testing advocated in early disease.
    - IgG can persist for months or years despite therapy.
- Clinicians are advised to be cautious of other testing offered by "Lyme specialty" laboratories with poor specificity including:
  - Microscopic examination blood/body fluids for spirochetes.
  - CD-57+/CD3- lymphocyte subpopulation typing.
  - Lymphocyte transformation tests.

Treatment Options

Treatment options vary depending on the stage of infection at diagnosis. See Table 24 4.
- *B. burgdorferi* antibiotic susceptibilities:

TABLE 24.4	Treatment Recommendations for Lyme Disease	
Clinical Presentation	Antibiotic(s) Recommended	Duration of Therapy
Early		
Erythema migrans	PO regimen[a]	14 days (14–21 days)
Acute disseminated nonneurologic Lyme	Doxycycline 100 mg BD or ceftriaxone 2 g OD	21 days 14 days
Cardiac disease	In hospital: ceftriaxone 2 g OD[b] Ambulatory: PO regimen[a]	14 days (14–21 days)
Neurologic Meningitis Radiculopathy VIIth nerve palsy	Ceftriaxone 2 g OD[b] Ceftriaxone 2 g OD[b] PO regimen[a]	14 days (10–28 days) 14 days (10–28 days) 14 days (14–21 days)
Late Neurologic Central nervous system Peripheral nervous system	Ceftriaxone 2 g OD[b] Ceftriaxone 2 g OD[b]	14 days (14–28 days) 14 days (14–28 days)
Arthritis (no neurologic involvement)	PO regimen[a]	28 days
Acrodermatitis chronica atrophicans	PO regimen[a]	21 days (14–28 days)

[a]PO regimen = Amoxicillin 500 mg TDS PO or doxycycline 100 mg BD PO (first line) or cefuroxime axetil, 500 mg BD PO (second line). Azithromycin (third line).
[b]Alternative regimens = cefotaxime or penicillin G.

- Tetracyclines.
- Most penicillins.
- Second- (e.g., cefuroxime) and third-generation (e.g., ceftriaxone) cephalosporins.
- Macrolides less effective.
- Mild Jarisch–Herxheimer type intensification of symptoms reported in approximately 15% of patients in first 24 hours of therapy.

Prevention

Prevention of Lyme disease centers upon tick bite avoidance. Protective clothing, e.g., long sleeves and trousers, combined with tick repellent and vigilance for, and quick removal of, attached ticks.

Vaccination with OspA Lyme Disease vaccine does not confer long-lasting protection.

Prophylaxis

- Chemoprophylaxis is not recommended in Europe.
- United States: single-dose chemoprophylaxis with doxycycline can be considered if *all* of the following criteria are fulfilled:
  - Reliable identification of *I. scapularis* tick estimated to have been attached for a minimum of 36 hours.
    - *I. pacificus* infection rates rarely reach 20%, therefore prophylaxis generally not necessary.
  - Prophylaxis can be started within 72 hours of tick removal.
  - Estimation of local infection rates of ticks estimated to be at least 20%.
  - Treatment with doxycycline is not contraindicated.

Post Lyme Disease Syndrome

- Controversial,
- Symptoms despite appropriate therapy for Lyme disease.
- Symptoms usually reported usually involve
  - Fatigue.
  - Widespread musculoskeletal pain.
  - Cognitive disturbance.
  - Reduced activity levels.
- IDSA suggest "must have objective evidence of prior Lyme Disease."
- Testing should be in accredited laboratories using validated methods.
- No convincing evidence for repeating the initial appropriate antibiotic treatment course.
- Long-term antibiotic therapy not advocated.
- May be related to other conditions, e.g., chronic fatigue syndrome and fibromyalgia.
- Patients may seek unorthodox or non-evidence-based therapies.

Further Reading and Resources

1. Giacani L, Lukehart SA. The endemic treponematoses. *Clin Microbiol Rev.* 2014;27(1):89–115.
2. Wormser G, Dattwyler RJ, Shapiro ED. The clinical assessment, treatment, and prevention of Lyme disease, human granulocytic anaplasmosis, and babesiosis: Clinical Practice Guidelines by the Infectious Diseases Society of America. *Clin Infect Dis.* 2006;43:1089–1134.
3. British Infection Association. The epidemiology, prevention, investigation and treatment of Lyme borreliosis in United Kingdom patients: a position statement by the British Infection Association. *J Infect.* 2011;62:329–338.

4. Stanek G, Fingerle V, Hunfeld KP, et al. Lyme borreliosis: clinical case definitions for diagnosis and management in Europe. *Clin Microbiol Infect.* 2011;17(1).

5. WHO resources: http://www.who.int/mediacentre/factsheets/fs31 6/en/; http://www.who.int/yaws/disease/en/.

6. Centers for Disease Prevention and Control (CDC). Lyme webpage. https://www.cdc.gov/lyme/stats/index.html.

25

Skin and Soft Tissue Infections and Toxin-Mediated Diseases

STEPHEN Y. LIANG

General Principles

- Skin and soft tissue infections (SSTI) rank high among infectious disease syndromes frequently encountered in clinical medicine.
- Gram-positive bacteria are responsible for the majority of SSTIs, with *Staphylococcus aureus* and beta-hemolytic streptococcus (particularly group A streptococcus) implicated in most cases. Community-acquired methicillin-resistant *S. aureus* (MRSA) is strongly associated with SSTI and should be considered when selecting empiric antibiotic therapy in high prevalence populations and geographic areas.
- A rational approach to SSTI begins with a review of major infections progressing from superficial to deep skin and soft tissue structures affected. Next, unique clinical situations associated with SSTIs will be addressed, followed by a discussion of several organism-specific SSTIs and toxin-mediated diseases.

MAJOR SKIN AND SOFT TISSUE INFECTIONS

Impetigo

- Superficial, intraepidermal infection caused by group A streptococcus and/or *S. aureus*.
- Vesicles and pustules rupture yielding honey-yellow crusted lesions (*nonbullous impetigo*), frequently involving the face and extremities (Fig. 25.1). Bacterial superinfection can also occur at sites of minor skin trauma or viral infection (e.g., varicella-zoster virus, herpes simplex virus).
- *Bullous impetigo* accounts for 10% of all impetigo cases and is caused by toxin-producing *S. aureus*. Superficial flaccid bullae rupture and give rise to crusted lesions, resembling *Toxicodendron* dermatitis (e.g., poison ivy).

- Commonly encountered in children and during hot, humid weather. Other risk factors include low socioeconomic status, living in close quarters, and poor hygiene.
- Streptococcal impetigo has been associated with epidemics, particularly in tropical regions, and can be complicated by post-streptococcal glomerulonephritis.
- Systemic therapy with an oral penicillin (e.g., amoxicillin–clavulanate, dicloxacillin) or cephalosporin (e.g., cephalexin) is effective. Empiric coverage for MRSA can be achieved with trimethoprim/sulfamethoxazole (TMP–SMX), doxycycline, or clindamycin depending on local antibiotic susceptibility patterns. Topical bacitracin or mupirocin can be used in mild, limited infections.

Folliculitis

- Infection of the hair follicle caused primarily by *S. aureus*.
- Small, raised, erythematous lesions, with or without a visible pustule at the base of the hair follicle, commonly involving the scalp, face (including nares), trunk, buttocks, and lower extremities (Fig. 25.2). Infection can progress deeper to form furuncles and carbuncles.
- Risk factors include skin trauma (e.g., repetitive shaving), hyperhidrosis, occlusion of hair follicles, and nasal *S. aureus* carriage.
- Infection is usually self-limited. Treatment with topical mupirocin is appropriate for mild infections. When folliculitis is severe or widespread, an antistaphylococcal oral antibiotic (e.g., dicloxacillin or cephalexin for methicillin-susceptible *S. aureus*, MSSA; TMP–SMX, doxycycline, or clindamycin for MRSA) is recommended.
- Folliculitis has also been associated with other organisms in certain contexts:

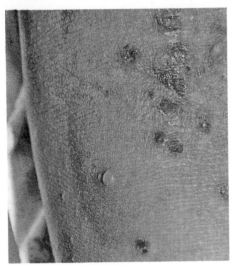

• **Fig. 25.1** Nonbullous impetigo, with initial vesicles giving way to crusted lesions. (From Stevens DL. Cellulitis, pyoderma, abscesses, and other skin and subcutaneous infections. In: Cohen J, Powderly W, Opal S, eds. *Infectious Diseases*. 4th ed. Elsevier; 2017.)

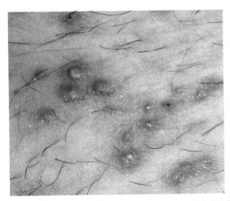

• **Fig. 25.2** Methicillin-resistant *Staphylococcus aureus* folliculitis. (From Habif TP. *Clinical Dermatology*. 6th ed. Elsevier; 2016.)

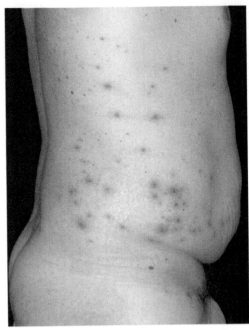

• **Fig. 25.3** *Pseudomonas aeruginosa* folliculitis (hot tub folliculitis). (From Habif TP. *Clinical Dermatology*. 6th ed. Elsevier; 2016.)

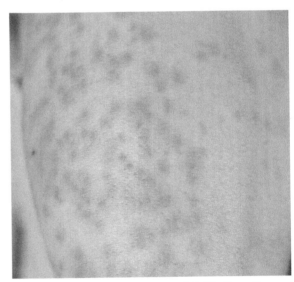

• **Fig. 25.4** Cercarial dermatitis ("swimmer's itch"). (From Stevens DL. Cellulitis, pyoderma, abscesses, and other skin and subcutaneous infections. In: Cohen J, Powderly W, Opal S, eds. *Infectious Diseases*. 4th ed. Elsevier; 2017.)

- *Pseudomonas aeruginosa*: after contact with contaminated or incompletely chlorinated water (hot tub folliculitis) (Fig. 25.3). While self-limited in most instances, severe infections can be treated with oral ciprofloxacin.
- Fungi (including *Malassezia*, dermatophytes, and *Candida*): more often encountered in patients who have received broad-spectrum antibiotics or corticosteroids (topical or oral), or who are immunocompromised. Topical clotrimazole or systemic antifungal therapy (e.g., fluconazole, itraconazole) is effective.
- Avian schistosomes (cercarial dermatitis or "swimmer's itch"): molluscan intermediate hosts release cercaria that trigger an allergic reaction within human hair follicles and pores after freshwater exposure, resulting in intense pruritus (Fig. 25.4). The reaction is self-limited and may be treated with antipruritics and topical corticosteroids. Antibiotic therapy is not necessary.

Furuncles and Carbuncles

- Abscess formation within the dermis or subcutaneous tissues most commonly due to *S. aureus*.
- A furuncle (boil) is a deep infection of a hair follicle (Fig. 25.5). Several furuncles merge to form a carbuncle, a more extensive skin infection associated with purulent fluid collection.
- Painful, tender, fluctuant, and/or erythematous lesions that like folliculitis involve hair-bearing surfaces, particularly on the face, neck, axillae, and buttocks. Lesions

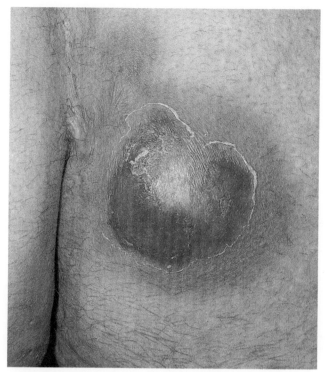

• **Fig. 25.5** Furuncle (boil). (From Habif TP. *Clinical Dermatology*. 6th ed. Elsevier; 2016.)

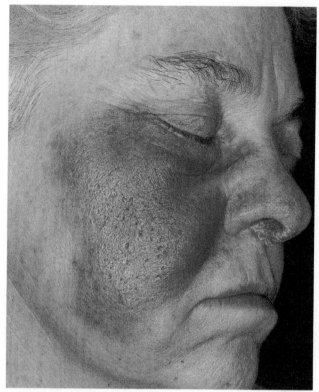

• **Fig. 25.6** Erysipelas. (From Habif TP. *Clinical Dermatology*. 6th ed. Elsevier; 2016.)

may spontaneously drain along the course of a hair follicle. Systemic signs and symptoms including fever and lymphadenopathy may be present, more commonly with carbuncles.

• Risk factors include skin trauma, obesity, immunosuppression, and nasal *S. aureus* carriage.

• While empiric antibiotic therapy alone may be effective in treating a furuncle, incision and drainage of an abscess is the mainstay of treatment for a carbuncle.

• Abscess culture obtained during incision and drainage can help tailor appropriate antibiotic therapy.

• For uncomplicated infections, empiric antibiotic therapy with an oral antistaphylococcal antibiotic (e.g., dicloxacillin or cephalexin for MSSA; TMP–SMX, doxycycline, or clindamycin for MRSA) is appropriate. If the patient has extensive infection requiring hospitalization, intravenous antibiotic therapy with nafcillin, oxacillin, or cefazolin is appropriate for treating MSSA. Vancomycin, linezolid, daptomycin, or ceftaroline may be used to treat MRSA infection.

• Furuncles and carbuncles involving the nares and/or medial third of the face can be complicated by septic cavernous sinus thrombosis. Headache, fever, periorbital edema, ptosis, proptosis, chemosis, and cranial nerve deficits (involving III, IV, V, VI) should prompt concern for this infectious disease emergency.

• Apart from *S. aureus*, other organisms can also cause abscess formation:
  • Gram-negative bacteria and anaerobes are associated with perioral, perirectal, and vulvovaginal abscesses.

• *Mycobacterium fortuitum* has been associated with infectious outbreaks involving nail salons and footbaths.

Erysipelas

• Infection of the upper dermis and superficial lymphatics classically associated with group A streptococcus and other beta-hemolytic *Streptococci*.

• Raised, well-demarcated, intensely erythematous and indurated lesion involving the face (butterfly distribution) or lower extremities (Fig. 25.6). Onset is acute in nature and accompanied by pain and systemic symptoms, including fever and chills.

• More common in young children and older adults.

• Risk factors include obesity, diabetes mellitus, venous insufficiency, lymphedema, tinea pedis, prior regional surgery (e.g., lymph node dissection, saphenous vein graft), and skin trauma.

• Treatment of mild infections consists of an oral penicillin (e.g., penicillin V, amoxicillin), cephalexin, or clindamycin. For moderate to severe infections warranting hospitalization, intravenous aqueous penicillin G is recommended. Erysipelas can be challenging to differentiate from cellulitis, which can be caused by streptococcus or *S. aureus*. In such instances, nafcillin, oxacillin, or cefazolin are appropriate options.

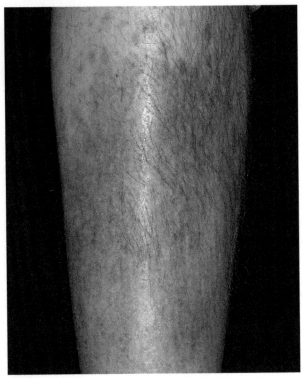

• **Fig. 25.7** Cellulitis. (From Habif TP. *Clinical Dermatology.* 6th ed. Elsevier; 2016.)

Cellulitis

- Infection of the deeper dermis and subcutaneous tissue commonly caused by *S. aureus,* group A streptococcus, or other *Streptococcus* species
- Skin erythema, edema, and warmth, with or without purulent drainage or exudate, most frequently involves the lower extremities with associated tenderness and lymphadenopathy (Fig. 25.7). Systemic symptoms including fever and chills, particularly with cellulitis due to group A streptococcus. In contrast to erysipelas, the borders of cellulitis are not well-demarcated due to the depth of infection.
- Risk factors include obesity, venous insufficiency, lymphedema, tinea pedis, prior regional surgery, and skin trauma. Underlying infections (e.g., furuncle, carbuncle, deep soft tissue abscess, osteomyelitis) can manifest with cellulitis. Chronic decubitus ulcers and wounds can become infected and develop surrounding cellulitis.
- Blood cultures are rarely positive.
- Empiric antibiotic therapy should be guided by clinical suspicion for infection with *S. aureus* vs. *Streptococcus* species.
  - Oral antibiotic options to cover MSSA and *Streptococcus* include dicloxacillin, amoxicillin/clavulanate, or cephalexin. If MRSA is strongly suspected or confirmed, TMP–SMX, doxycycline, or clindamycin are reasonable choices.

- Intravenous antibiotic options to cover MSSA and *Streptococcus* include nafcillin, oxacillin, cefazolin, or clindamycin. If MRSA is suspected, vancomycin, daptomycin, ceftaroline, or linezolid is recommended.
- Thrombophlebitis can complicate lower extremity cellulitis. Orbital cellulitis can progress to orbital abscess, subperiosteal abscess, brain abscess, and/or septic cavernous sinus thrombosis.
- While *Streptococcus* spp. and *S. aureus* are responsible for most cases of cellulitis, infection due to a wide range of other organisms including *Enterococcus*, gram-negative bacteria (e.g., *Pseudomonas aeruginosa, Enterobacteriaceae*), anaerobes, and fungi are also possible depending on the anatomic location of the infection, host immune status, and environmental exposures (e.g., water, soil, vegetation).

Necrotizing Soft Tissue Infection

- Fulminant infection of the muscle, fascia, and fat, typically classified by microbiologic etiology.
  - Type I: mixed aerobic (e.g., Enterobacteriaceae) and anaerobic bacteria (e.g., *Fusobacterium, Peptostreptococcus, Bacteroides, Clostridium*).
  - Type II: monomicrobial infection with group A streptococcus, *S. aureus* (including MRSA), *Aeromonas hydrophilia,* or *Vibrio vulnificus.*
- Infection may initially spare overlying skin, manifesting as pain out of proportion to physical findings, rapidly progressing to skin crepitus, discoloration (red to purple), blisters, bullae, and tissue necrosis with systemic toxicity (fever, hemodynamic instability, sepsis) (Fig. 25.8). The extremities are most commonly affected, although infection can also involve the neck (cervical necrotizing fasciitis), abdominal wall, perineum (Fournier's gangrene), or surgical wounds.
- Risk factors include diabetes mellitus, peripheral vascular disease, immunosuppression, recent surgery or trauma, and injection drug use (IDU).
- As early clinical presentations may overlap with cellulitis and other SSTIs, a high index of suspicion is necessary to establish the diagnosis.
  - Laboratory values, even when used as part of a prediction tool such as the Laboratory Risk Indicator for Necrotizing Fasciitis (LRINEC) score (Table 25.1), are of limited utility.
  - Blood cultures are more frequently positive than in cellulitis (25%).
  - Imaging, including plain radiography and computed tomography (CT), can demonstrate gas and edema along fascial planes and in subcutaneous tissue. Magnetic resonance imaging (MRI) is overly sensitive and may unnecessarily delay timely surgical intervention.
  - In cases where imaging is equivocal, diagnosis is clinical and surgical exploration may serve both diagnostic and therapeutic purposes.

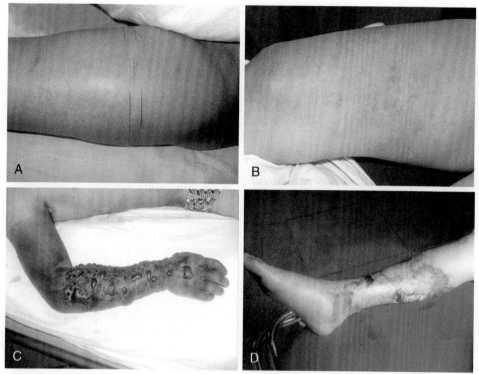

• **Fig. 25.8** Progressive stages of necrotizing soft tissue infection due to *Vibrio* species. (A) Left thigh infection, early presentation of skin damage with rapid swelling and pain. (B) Right thigh, late presentation of skin damage with swelling, ecchymoses, and evolving necrosis. (C) Right arm, late presentation with swelling, hemorrhagic bullae. (D) Right leg, late presentation with subcutaneous tissue necrosis and bullae. (From Hong GL, Lu CJ, Lu ZQ, et al. Surgical treatment of 19 cases with *Vibrio* necrotising fasciitis. *Burns.* 2012;38(2):290–295.)

TABLE 25.1	Laboratory Risk Indicator for Necrotizing Fasciitis (LRINEC)[a]	
Variable		**Points**
CRP >150 mg/L		4
Leukocytosis		1
WBC count between 15,000 and 25,000/mm³		2
WBC count >25,000/mm³		
Anemia		1
Hgb between 11 and 13.5 g/dL		2
Hgb <11 g/dL		
Hyponatremia		2
Na <135 mmol/L		
Renal insufficiency		2
Cr >1.6 mg/dL		
Serum glucose >180 mg/dL		1

Cr, creatinine; CRP, C-reactive protein; Hgb, hemoglobin; WBC, white blood cell.

[a]LRINEC score <6 points is considered low risk for necrotizing soft tissue infection but does not rule out the diagnosis. High clinical suspicion for necrotizing soft tissue infection warrants surgical debridement, irrespective of LRINEC score.

- Emergent and aggressive surgical debridement is imperative to achieve source control and prevent further progression of infection.
    - Operative cultures should be obtained to help guide antibiotic therapy.
- Empiric antibiotic therapy should consist of a combination of broad-spectrum agents such as vancomycin or linezolid to cover gram-positive bacteria (including MRSA) and piperacillin–tazobactam or meropenem to cover gram-negative and anaerobic bacteria.
- Clindamycin may be added to suppress bacterial protein synthesis and toxin production, but should not be relied upon solely for gram-positive coverage.
- Mortality may be as high as 35%.

Pyomyositis

- Primary skeletal muscle abscess predominantly due to *S. aureus.*
- Fever accompanied by localized skeletal muscle swelling tenderness, swelling, and fluctuance progress in severity over time. Overlying skin erythema and warmth develop followed by hemodynamic instability and sepsis.

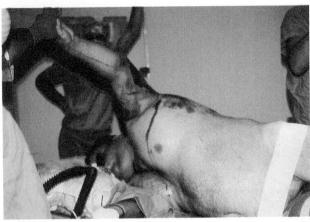

• **Fig. 25.9** Clostridial myonecrosis with characteristic bronze discoloration of the skin over the shoulder. (From Pasternack MS, Swartz MN. Myositis and myonecrosis. In: Bennett JE, Dolin R, Blaser MJ, eds. *Mandell, Douglas, and Bennett's Principles and Practice of Infectious Diseases*. 8th ed. Elsevier; 2015. Fig. 96.2.)

• More common in tropical regions.
• Risk factors include IDU, trauma (due to penetrating injury, blunt injury, or vigorous exercise), human immunodeficiency virus infection, diabetes mellitus, chronic corticosteroid therapy, liver disease, malnutrition, and hematologic malignancy. Toxocariasis has also been associated with the development of pyomyositis.
• Plain radiography may demonstrate soft tissue gas and edema. Ultrasound and CT are well-suited to identifying significant abscess formation. MRI is highly sensitive in identifying focal muscle edema (myositis) prior to abscess formation and mapping the extent of the infection in greater detail.
• Treatment is composed first of surgical or percutaneous drainage of the abscess with culture to guide antibiotic therapy.
• Empiric antibiotic therapy should include coverage of MSSA and MRSA, usually with vancomycin. Broader coverage to include gram-negative and anaerobic bacteria should be considered in severe infection and immunocompromised patients.
• Compartment syndrome is a potential complication, particularly when pyomyositis involves the anterior tibial compartment.

Clostridial Myonecrosis

• Rapidly progressive infection of skeletal muscle, due to *Clostridia* (primarily *Clostridium perfringens*), also known as gas gangrene.
• Initial muscle pain out of proportion to physical findings progresses to tense muscle swelling, crepitation, overlying skin discoloration (red to purple) and bullae, and subsequent systemic toxicity (Fig. 25.9).
• Often seen in the setting of a contaminated open fracture, penetrating wound, surgical wound (particularly, bowel or biliary tract surgery), septic abortion, or limb-threatening

peripheral vascular disease. Intramuscular and subcutaneous injections as well as skin popping with black tar heroin have also been associated with infection. Other risk factors include diabetes mellitus, hematologic malignancy, and gastrointestinal disease.
• Myonecrosis due to *C. septicum* can be seen in the setting of bacteremia due to occult gastrointestinal malignancy or neutropenic colitis.
• Plain radiography and CT demonstrate gas and edema along fascial planes and in soft tissue. CT and MRI are particularly helpful in diagnosing early infection.
• Emergent and aggressive surgical debridement of infected muscle and fasciotomy to decompress muscle compartments are tantamount. Operative cultures should be obtained to guide antibiotic therapy.
• Initial empiric antibiotic therapy should broadly cover for necrotizing infection using a combination of vancomycin or linezolid, piperacillin–tazobactam or meropenem, and clindamycin. Targeted therapy for clostridial myonecrosis is best achieved through a combination of penicillin G and clindamycin, both of which are highly active against *C. perfringens*, with the latter also capable of suppressing toxin production.

SKIN AND SOFT TISSUE INFECTIONS ENCOUNTERED IN UNIQUE CLINICAL SITUATIONS (TABLE 25.2)

Infections Associated with Aquatic Exposures

• Skin trauma followed by environmental water exposure has been associated with SSTI due to several aquatic bacteria.

Aeromonas species

• Associated with freshwater (lakes, rivers, streams), estuarine (brackish) water, and floodwater exposures as well as medicinal leech therapy.
• Cellulitis and traumatic wound infections are the most common SSTIs associated with *A. hydrophila*, but myonecrosis and necrotizing soft tissue infection are also possible.
• Antibiotic therapy utilizing a third-generation cephalosporin, fluoroquinolone, or TMP–SMX is recommended pending antibiotic susceptibility testing from a positive wound culture.
• Patients undergoing medicinal leech therapy should receive prophylactic ciprofloxacin.

Vibrio vulnificus

• Associated with exposure to salt water or estuarine water (e.g., Gulf of Mexico), or from handling and/or ingesting raw or undercooked shellfish (e.g., oysters).
• Cellulitis complicating a traumatic wound directly exposed to contaminated water or shellfish (e.g., while

TABLE 25.2	Differential Diagnosis for Skin and Soft Tissue Infections Associated With Unique Clinical Situations	
Clinical Situation	**Unique Organisms**
Aquatic exposure	
Estuarine (brackish) water, floodwater	*Aeromonas* spp., *Vibrio vulnificus*
Handling raw seafood	*Vibrio vulnificus* (shellfish) *Erysipelothrix rhusiopathiae* (shrimp, crab, fish)
Aquarium or swimming pool water	*Mycobacterium marinum*
Foot baths, nail salons	*Mycobacterium fortuitum*
Contact with animal products (e.g., hides, wool)	*Bacillus anthracis*
Animal bite	
Dog	*Pasteurella canis* *Capnocytophaga canimorsus* (asplenia, underlying liver disease)
Cat	*Pasteurella multocida* *Bartonella henselae* (cat scratch disease)
Human bite	*Eikenella corrodens*
Macaque monkey	B virus
Leech therapy	*Aeromonas* spp.
Traumatic injury	
Puncture through tennis shoe	*Pseudomonas aeruginosa*
Inoculation with soil or vegetation	*Mucorales, Aspergillus, Fusarium, Sporothrix schenckii*
Burn	*Staphylococcus aureus, Pseudomonas aeruginosa*

opening oysters) can rapidly progress to hemorrhagic bullae, tissue necrosis, and potentially necrotizing soft tissue infection.

- Primary septicemia secondary to ingestion of contaminated shellfish, particularly in those with underlying liver disease or hemochromatosis, can manifest hemorrhagic bullae and develop systemic toxicity leading to septic shock.
- Wound and blood cultures have significant utility in confirming diagnosis.
- Antibiotic therapy consists of doxycycline in combination with ceftriaxone or cefotaxime.

Mycobacterium marinum

- Associated with exposure to aquarium, swimming pool, and some natural bodies of water.
- Minor skin trauma followed by aquatic exposure leads to small, violet papules that ulcerate superficially and scar over the course of several weeks (Fig. 25.10).
- Presentation is similar, and the differential diagnosis includes *Sporothrix schenckii.*
- Antibiotic therapy may consist of a combination of clarithromycin with either ethambutol or rifampin, for typically three to four months, and should be guided by antibiotic susceptibility testing.

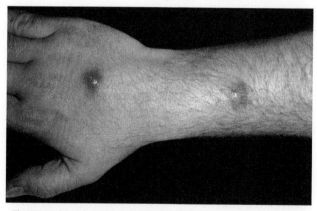

• **Fig. 25.10** *Mycobacterium marinum* infection. (From Habif TP. *Clinical Dermatology.* 6th ed. Elsevier; 2016.)

Animal Bite Infections

- Soft tissue infections associated with animal bites typically derive from either the normal oral flora of the biting animal or the skin flora of the human patient (*Staphylococcus, Streptococcus*).
- Erythema, edema, tenderness, and purulent drainage at the bite wound are common with infection. Fever and lymphangitis may be present. Tenosynovitis,

septic arthritis, and osteomyelitis are also possible depending on the anatomic location and depth of the bite.

Dog and Cat Bites

- Canine and feline oral flora include *Pasteurella* spp., *Capnocytophaga canimorsus*, and anaerobes, as well as *Streptococcus* and *Staphylococcus*. *Bartonella henselae* is also present in the saliva of cats.
- While dog bites comprise ≥80% of all animal bites, only 5% become infected as most bites involve relatively shallow skin tears and lacerations. In contrast, more than 80% of cat bites become infected as most involve deep puncture wounds.
- Antibiotic prophylaxis after a dog or cat bite should include coverage for *P. multocida*.
  - Amoxicillin–clavulanate is recommended, usually for 3–5 days. Ciprofloxacin, TMP–SMX, or doxycycline in combination with clindamycin are acceptable alternative regimens.
  - Rabies postexposure prophylaxis may be indicated.
- Treatment of soft tissue infection after dog or cat bite consists of the same antibiotics used for prophylaxis. In severe infections requiring hospitalization, ampicillin–sulbactam provides appropriate broad-spectrum coverage. Empiric MRSA coverage should also be considered depending on local prevalence.
- Other infections associated with dog and cat bites:
  - *C. canimorsus* infection can progress to bacteremia and sepsis, particularly in patients with asplenia or underlying liver disease.
  - *B. henselae* is the etiologic agent for cat scratch disease.

Human Bites

- Human oral flora includes *Streptococcus*, *Staphylococcus*, and anaerobes, including most notably, *Eikenella corrodens*.
- Amoxicillin–clavulanate is active against *E. corrodens* and is appropriate for prophylaxis and treatment of infection. In severe infections requiring hospitalization, ampicillin–sulbactam is recommended with or without the addition of MRSA coverage.

Wild Animal Bites:

- Amoxicillin–clavulanate is a reasonable choice for antibiotic prophylaxis and empiric treatment of soft tissue infection in most cases.
  - Unusual organisms may be associated with bites involving certain wild animals and antibiotic therapy should be guided by wound culture. *Aeromonas* spp. have been associated with bites from leeches, alligators, and snakes sustained in fresh or brackish water. *Vibrio* spp. have been described in infections involving shark bites and *Serratia marcescens* with iguana bites.
- Postexposure rabies prophylaxis may be indicated.

- Macaque monkey bites carry a risk of transmitting B virus, a herpesvirus.
  - Postexposure prophylaxis with valaciclovir or aciclovir is recommended.
  - B-virus infections in humans can present with vesicles or ulcers localized at the site of the bite, influenza-like illness, or fatal encephalomyelitis. Treatment with intravenous aciclovir is recommended.

Infections After Traumatic Injury

- *Staphylococcus* and *Streptococcus* remain the most common organisms associated with SSTI after penetrating trauma.
- Punctures to the foot through a rubber-soled shoe have classically been associated with wound infection, septic arthritis, and osteomyelitis due to *P. aeruginosa*.
- Penetrating wounds contaminated with soil, vegetation, or feces may be encountered in agricultural, livestock/farmyard, and industrial injuries leading to uncommon infections involving animal bowel flora as well as mycobacteria and fungi found in the natural environment.
- Invasive fungal infections (IFI) involving *Mucorales*, *Aspergillus*, and *Fusarium* species as well as other fungi have been associated with traumatic wounds sustained after motor vehicle crashes (particularly motorcyclists and unrestrained passengers), natural disasters (e.g., tornado), and military blast injury involving improvised explosive devices).
- Surgical debridement may be necessary in the setting of severe infections, particularly IFI. Operative bacterial and fungal cultures and histopathology are paramount to tailoring appropriate antibiotic and/or antifungal therapy and establishing a diagnosis of IFI.

Infections Associated With Burn Injury

- *S. aureus* and *P. aeruginosa* are the most common organisms associated with burn wound infection (impetigo, cellulitis, or surgical site infection) and burn wound sepsis (invasive infection).
  - The microbiology of infection shifts from gram-positive skin flora (*Staphylococcus*, *Streptococcus*) during the initial days following injury to gram-negative bacteria (e.g., *P. aeruginosa*, *Acinetobacter baumannii*, *Enterobacteriaceae*).
  - Multidrug-resistant organisms (including MRSA) and fungi (e.g., *Candida*, *Mucorales*, *Aspergillus*, and *Fusarium* species) emerge with prolonged hospitalization and use of broad-spectrum antibiotics.
- Risk factors for burn wound sepsis include a total body surface area (TBSA) burn >20%, delayed burn wound excision (which can increase bacterial colonization of the burn eschar), extremes of age, and immunosuppression.

- Diagnosis of burn wound sepsis requires the presence of clinical features consistent with wound infection and systemic signs and burn wound biopsy demonstrating bacterial count $>10^5$ bacteria per gram of tissue obtained with evidence of microbial invasion into unburned tissue on histopathology.
- While antibiotic therapy alone is adequate to treat a burn wound infection, both aggressive surgical wound debridement and antibiotic therapy guided by operative culture are necessary to effectively treat burn wound sepsis.

Surgical Site Infections

- *S. aureus* (including MRSA), coagulase-negative *Staphylococcus*, *Enterococcus* species, *P. aeruginosa*, and other enteric gram-negative bacteria are all organisms commonly associated with SSI.
  - Group A streptococcus and *Clostridium* species should be considered in SSIs that develop rapidly within the first 48 hours of surgery.
- Superficial surgical site infections (SSI) encompass the epidermis, dermis, and subcutaneous tissue, while deep infections involve the muscle, fascia, and other tissue. Erythema, edema, tenderness, and purulent drainage from the surgical site are common signs.
- SSIs are generally attributed to a surgical procedure if they develop within the ensuing 30 days; this window may be extended when prosthetic implants or other devices are involved.
- Risk factors include diabetes mellitus, obesity, old age, immunosuppression, malnutrition, tobacco dependence, preexisting infection, colonization with *S. aureus*, and prolonged hospitalization.
- Empiric broad-spectrum antibiotics and early surgical debridement when indicated are key to optimizing clinical outcomes. Operative cultures should be obtained to help tailor antibiotic therapy.

OTHER ORGANISM-SPECIFIC SKIN AND SOFT TISSUE INFECTIONS

Cutaneous Anthrax

- Inoculation and infection of the subcutaneous tissue with the spores of *Bacillus anthracis*.
- Pruritic papules evolve into vesicles and bullae that ulcerate, leaving behind a painless black eschar with surrounding induration (Fig. 25.11). Fever may be present.
- Spore exposure usually results from direct contact with infected animals or contaminated animal products (e.g., hides, wool).
- Antibiotic therapy entails ciprofloxacin or doxycycline for 60 days.

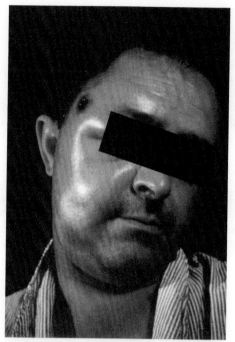

- **Fig. 25.11** Cutaneous anthrax with prominent surrounding soft tissue edema. (From Rao GR, Walker DH. Anthrax. In: Guerrant R, Walker D, Weller P, eds. *Tropical Infectious Diseases*. 3rd ed. Elsevier; 2011.)

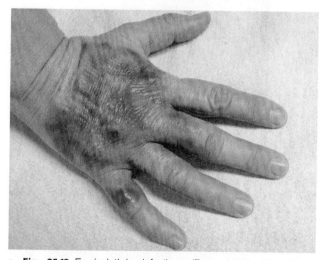

- **Fig. 25.12** *Erysipelothrix* infection. (From Habif TP. *Clinical Dermatology*. 6th ed. Elsevier; 2016.)

Erysipelothrix Infection

- Indolent infection of cutaneous tissue due to *Erysipelothrix rhusiopathiae*.
- Cellulitis leads to painful, violaceous lesions with associated lymphangitis, often stemming from an abrasion to the hand (Fig. 25.12).
- Associated with occupational exposures involving persons who handle contaminated shrimp, crab, fish, and animal meat and hides.

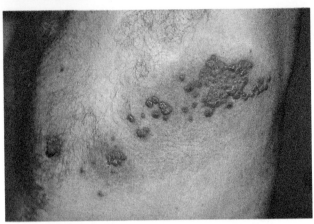

• **Fig. 25.13** Herpes zoster. (From James WD, Berger TG, Elson DM. *Andrews' Diseases of the Skin: Clinical Dermatology*. 12th ed. Elsevier; 2016.)

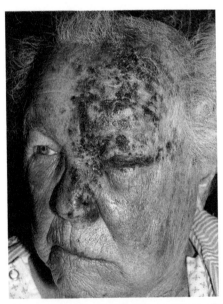

• **Fig. 25.14** Herpes zoster involving the V1 dermatome. (From James WD, Berger TG, Elson DM. *Andrews' Diseases of the Skin: Clinical Dermatology*. 12th ed. Elsevier; 2016.)

• Antibiotic therapy usually consists of penicillin V, cephalexin, or ciprofloxacin for localized infections. More extensive infections can be treated with intravenous penicillin G, ceftriaxone, or imipenem.

Herpes Zoster

• Reactivation of latent varicella-zoster virus (VZV) with cutaneous manifestations, also known as "shingles."
• Prodromal pain followed by a vesicular eruption along a dermatomal distribution (typically thoracic or lumbar) is typical in the immunocompetent host. Vesicles evolve into pustules that finally crust over (Fig. 25.13). A single dermatome is usually involved, although neighboring dermatomes may be affected.

• Vesicular eruption along a dermatome of cranial nerve V (trigeminal nerve, usually V1), particularly involving the nose (Hutchinson's sign), with associated eye pain and conjunctivitis should raise the concern for herpes zoster ophthalmicus, which can lead to keratitis, iritis, and vision loss (Fig. 25.14).
• Vesicular eruption within the auricle and auditory canal with ear pain and unilateral facial paralysis should raise the concern for herpes zoster oticus (Ramsay Hunt syndrome).
• Treatment with aciclovir or valaciclovir within 72 hours reduces duration and severity of pain, speeds healing of lesions, and may decrease the likelihood of postherpetic neuralgia.

Dermatophytosis

• A constellation of superficial fungal infections involving the skin, hair, and nails due to dermatophytes which comprise the genera *Epidermophyton*, *Microsporum*, and *Trichophyton*.
• Common dermatophyte infections include:
  • Tinea corporis ("ringworm"): pruritic, annular, serpiginous rash with central clearing and raised borders involving any part of the body, excluding the face, hands, feet, or inguinal region (Fig. 25.15).
  • Tinea cruris ("jock itch"): pruritic, erythematous patches with central clearing involving the inguinal region.
  • Tinea pedis ("athlete's foot"): pruritic, erythematous erosions or scaly patches often favoring the interdigital spaces.
  • Tinea capitis: scaly patches involving the scalp with destruction of hair cuticles leading to alopecia.
• With the exception of hair (tinea capitis) or nail (tinea unguium) infections, initial antifungal therapy usually consists of a topical azole; topical nystatin is not effective against dermatophytes. Oral azoles (itraconazole, fluconazole), terbinafine, or griseofulvin may be used in refractory or extensive infections. Tinea capitis and tinea unguium are typically treated with terbinafine or griseofulvin.

Sporotrichosis

• Indolent infection of the cutaneous and subcutaneous tissue due to the dimorphic fungus *S. schenckii*.
• Minimally painful papules or nodules develop at the site of injury over days to weeks, with or without ulceration. Subsequent lesions may follow a lymphatic distribution proximally along an extremity (sporotrichoid spread) (Fig. 25.16).
• Classically associated with traumatic inoculation of an extremity with soil or vegetation (e.g., rose gardener pricked by a rose thorn).
• The antifungal agent of choice is itraconazole.

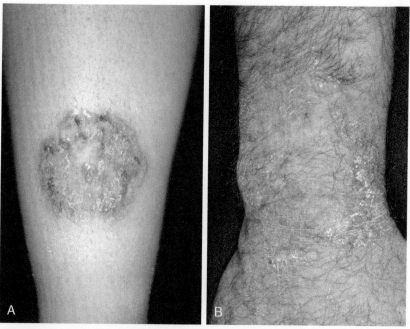

• **Fig. 25.15** Tinea corporis. (A) Classic round annular lesion; (B) extensive lesions with diffuse scale. (From Habif TP. *Clinical Dermatology*. 6th ed. Elsevier; 2016.)

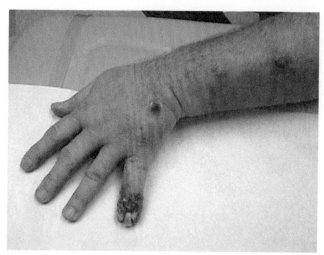

• **Fig. 25.16** Sporotrichosis. (From Rex JH, Okhuysen PC. *Sporothrix schenckii*. In: Bennett JE, Dolin R, Blaser MJ, eds. *Mandell, Douglas, and Bennett's Principles and Practice of Infectious Diseases*. Updated 8th ed. Elsevier; 2015.)

DIFFERENTIAL DIAGNOSES FOR ORGANISM-SPECIFIC SSTI BASED ON SKIN LESION CHARACTERISTICS (TABLE 25.3)

Toxin-Mediated Diseases

Toxic Shock Syndrome (TSS)

- Superantigen-mediated disease due to toxic shock syndrome toxin-1 (TSST-1) and enterotoxins produced by toxigenic *S. aureus*.

- The US Centers for Disease Control and Prevention case definition describes TSS in its severest form (Table 25.4). Clinical disease can span from a nonspecific febrile illness to hemodynamic instability, multiorgan dysfunction, and diffuse erythroderma (a painless, sunburn-like rash that gives way to desquamation) (Fig. 25.17).
- Risk factors include colonization with *S. aureus*, presence of a foreign body (e.g., nasal packing material, highly absorbent tampon), and the absence of TSST-1 host antibodies.
- Blood cultures are rarely positive.
- Antibiotic therapy typically consists of nafcillin, oxacillin, or vancomycin (depending on the concern for MRSA) in combination with clindamycin (to inhibit toxin production). Linezolid can also be used to treat MRSA and may suppress TSST-1 production.
- Aggressive fluid resuscitation and removal of any retained foreign body that can serve as a reservoir for toxigenic *S. aureus* should be undertaken promptly.
- Mortality is low (<5%).

Streptococcal Toxic Shock Syndrome (STSS)

- Superantigen-mediated disease due to exotoxins produced by group A streptococcus.
- The CDC case definition describes fulminant STSS (Table 25.5). Clinical disease can be variable. Rash is less pronounced in STSS than TSS.
- Risk factors include recent surgery, vaginal or cesarean delivery, traumatic injury, and viral infection (e.g., varicella, influenza).

TABLE 25.3 | **Differential Diagnoses for Specific Skin and Soft Tissue Infections by Skin Lesion Characteristics**

Clinical Condition	Organisms
Bullous Lesions	
Bullous impetigo	*Staphylococcus aureus*
Staphylococcal scalded skin syndrome	*Staphylococcus aureus*
Necrotizing soft tissue infection	Type I: mixed aerobic and anaerobic bacteria Type II: group A streptococcus, *Staphylococcus aureus*, *Vibrio vulnificus*
Clostridial myonecrosis	*Clostridium perfringens*, *Clostridium septicum*
Crusted Lesions	
Impetigo	*Staphylococcus aureus*, group A streptococcus
Nocardiosis	*Nocardia asteroides*
Tinea corporis	Dermatophytes
Systemic fungal infection	*Histoplasma capsulatum* *Coccidioides immitis* *Blastomyces dermatitidis*
Cutaneous mycobacterial infection	*Mycobacterium marinum* *Mycobacterium tuberculosis*
Cutaneous leishmaniasis	*Leishmania tropica*
Ulcerative Lesions	
Cutaneous anthrax	*Bacillus anthracis*
Cutaneous diphtheria	*Corynebacterium diphtheriae*
Ecthyma gangrenosum	*Pseudomonas aeruginosa*
Ulceroglandular tularemia	*Francisella tularensis*
Bacillary angiomatosis	*Bartonella henselae*, *Bartonella quintana*
Bubonic plague	*Yersinia pestis*
Buruli ulcer	*Mycobacterium ulcerans*
Cutaneous leishmaniasis	*Leishmania tropica*
Sexually transmitted infections (genital ulcerative disease)	*Treponema pallidum* (primary syphilis) *Haemophilus ducreyi* (chancroid) *Chlamydia trachomatis* (lymphogranuloma venereum) Herpes simplex virus

Adapted from: Stevens DL. Cellulitis, pyoderma, abscesses, and other skin and subcutaneous infections. In: Cohen J, Powderly W, Opal S, eds. *Infectious Diseases*. 4th ed. Philadelphia: Elsevier; 2017. p. 84–94.

- Blood cultures may be positive in up to 60% of cases.
- Antibiotic therapy narrowly targeting group A *Streptococcus* is achieved with penicillin in combination with clindamycin. Broader coverage with piperacillin–tazobactam or meropenem in combination with clindamycin, with or without additional MRSA coverage, may be warranted until streptococcal infection has been confirmed, as fulminant STSS may be indistinguishable from septic shock.
- Aggressive fluid resuscitation, vasopressor/inotropic support, mechanical ventilation, and prompt surgical debridement of infected wounds (surgical or traumatic) are crucial to improving survival.
- Mortality can range from 20% to 45%.

TABLE 25.4   Case Definition for Toxic Shock Syndrome (TSS)ᵃ

Clinical Criteria

- Fever: temperature ≥38.9°C or 102.0°F
- Rash: diffuse macular erythroderma
- Desquamation: 1–2 weeks after onset of rash
- Hypotension: systolic blood pressure ≤90 mmHg (adult) or <5th percentile by age (children <16 years of age)
- Multiorgan involvement (≥3 organ systems):
  - Gastrointestinal: vomiting and/or diarrhea at onset of illness
  - Muscular: severe myalgia or CPK ≥2 times the upper limit of normal
  - Mucous membrane: vaginal, oropharyngeal, or conjunctival hyperemia
  - Renal: BUN or serum Cr ≥2 times the upper limit of normal for laboratory or urinary sediment with pyuria (≥5 leukocytes per high-power field) in the absence of urinary tract infection
  - Hepatic: total bilirubin, ALT, or AST ≥2 times the upper limit of normal
  - Hematologic: platelet count <100,000 per mm³
  - Central nervous system: disorientation or alterations in consciousness without focal neurologic signs when fever and hypotension are absent

Laboratory Criteria

Negative results on the following tests, if obtained:
- Blood or cerebrospinal fluid cultures (blood culture may be positive for *Staphylococcus aureus*)
- Serologies for Rocky Mountain Spotted Fever, leptospirosis, or measles

Case Classification

- Probable: ≥4 clinical criteria + laboratory criteria met
- Confirmed: 5 clinical criteria + laboratory criteria met, including desquamation (unless death occurs prior to desquamation)

ALT, alanine aminotransferase; AST, aspartate aminotransferase; BUN, blood urea nitrogen; CPK, creatine phosphokinase; Cr, creatinine.
ᵃCase definitions are updated periodically and can be found at http://wwwn.cdc.gov/nndss.

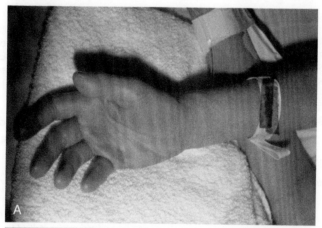

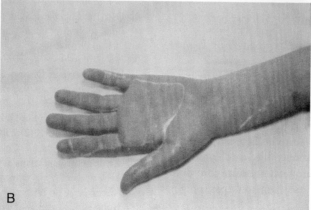

• **Fig. 25.17** Toxic shock syndrome. (A) Sunburn-like rash and subcutaneous edema. (B) Desquamation in late disease. (From CDC Public Health Image Library. Panel A, Image #5114; panel B, Image #5113. Photo credit: CDC. http://phil.cdc.gov.)

TABLE 25.5	Case Definition for Streptococcal Toxic Shock Syndrome (STSS)[a]

Clinical Criteria

- Hypotension: systolic blood pressure ≤90 mmHg (adult) or <5th percentile by age (children <6 years of age)
- Multiorgan involvement (≥2 organ systems):
  - Renal: serum Cr ≥2 mg/dL (≥177 μmol/L) for adults or ≥2 times the upper limit of normal for age. In patients with preexisting renal disease, >2-fold elevation above baseline
  - Coagulopathy: platelet count ≤100,000 per mm³ (≤100 ×10⁶/L) or disseminated intravascular coagulation, defined by prolonged clotting times, low fibrinogen level, and presence of fibrin degradation products
  - Hepatic: total bilirubin, ALT, or AST ≥2 times the upper limit of normal for the patient's age. In patients with preexisting liver disease, >2-fold elevation above baseline
  - Acute respiratory distress syndrome: acute onset of diffuse pulmonary infiltrates and hypoxemia in the absence of cardiac failure or by evidence of diffuse capillary leak manifested by acute onset of generalized edema, or pleural or peritoneal effusions with hypoalbuminemia
  - Skin: generalized erythematous macular rash that may desquamate
  - Soft tissue necrosis, including necrotizing fasciitis or myositis, or gangrene

Laboratory Criteria

- Isolation of group A *Streptococcus*

Case Classification

- Probable: All clinical criteria met + absence of other identified etiology for illness + isolation of group A streptococcus from a nonsterile site
- Confirmed: All clinical criteria met + isolation of group A streptococcus from a sterile site (e.g., blood, cerebrospinal fluid, synovial fluid, pleural fluid, or pericardial fluid)

ALT, alanine aminotransferase; AST, aspartate aminotransferase; Cr, creatinine.

[a]Case definitions are updated periodically and can be found at http://wwwn.cdc.gov/nndss.

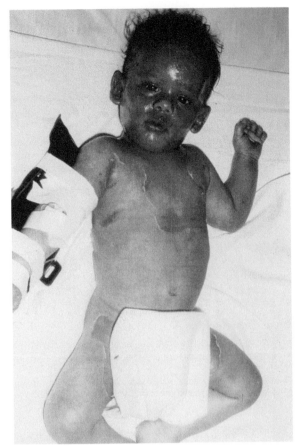

• **Fig. 25.18** Staphylococcal scalded skin syndrome. (From Pasternack MS, Swartz MN. Cellulitis, necrotizing fasciitis, and subcutaneous tissue infections. In: Bennett JE, Dolin R, Blaser MJ, eds. *Mandell, Douglas, and Bennett's Principles and Practice of Infectious Diseases*. Updated 8th ed. Elsevier; 2015.)

- Mortality is low in children (<3%) despite severity and extent of disease, but higher in adults.

Staphylococcal Scalded Skin Syndrome

- Blistering disease due to exfoliative toxin A or B produced by toxigenic *S. aureus*.
- Superficial scarlatiniform rash rapidly progresses to large flaccid bullae that rupture easily, giving way to widespread exfoliation exposing bright red areas of skin (Fig. 25.18). A positive Nikolsky sign (easy rupturing of bullae with gentle traction applied to the surrounding skin) is present, and clinical findings may resemble toxic epidermal necrolysis (TEN). Fever and skin tenderness are common.
- More common in children and neonates (pemphigus neonatorum).
- Antistaphylococcal antibiotic therapy should consist of nafcillin, cefazolin, or vancomycin. Fluid resuscitation is paramount.

Further Reading

1. Abrahamian FM, Goldstein EJ. Microbiology of animal bite wound infections. *Clin Microbiol Rev*. 2011;24(2):231–246.
2. Diaz JH, Lopez FA. Skin, soft tissue and systemic bacterial infections following aquatic injuries and exposures. *Am J Med Sci*. 2015;349(3):269–275.
3. Liu C, Bayer A, Cosgrove SE, et al. Clinical practice guidelines by the Infectious Diseases Society of America for the treatment of methicillin-resistant *Staphylococcus aureus* infections in adults and children. *Clin Infect Dis*. 2011;52(3):e18–e55.
4. Norbury W, Herndon DN, Tanksley J, et al. Infections in burns. *Surg Infect*. 2016;17(2):250–255.
5. Stevens DL, Bisno AL, Chambers HF, et al. Practice guidelines for the diagnosis and management of skin and soft tissue infections: 2014 update by the Infectious Diseases Society of America. *Clin Infect Dis*. 2014;59(2):e10–e52.
6. Wong CH, Khin LW, Heng KS, et al. The LRINEC (Laboratory Risk Indicator for Necrotizing Fasciitis) score: a tool for distinguishing necrotizing fasciitis from other soft tissue infections. *Crit Care Med*. 2004;32(7):1535–1541.

26

Bone and Joint Infections

SHADI PARSAEI

Diabetic Foot Infections and Associated Osteomyelitis

Definition: inflammation of bone due to infecting microorganism(s).

Epidemiology

- **Mechanism of infection**: **contiguous** as a result of direct extension from the diabetic foot ulcer to tissue and bone.
- **Risk factors**: poor blood glucose control, **peripheral neuropathy**, **peripheral vascular disease (PVD)**, antecedent trauma, chronic ulceration, history of recurrent ulcer, wound with palpable bone.
- **Causative organisms**: diabetic foot infections (DFI) are frequently polymicrobial and may consist of gram-positive, gram-negative, and/or anaerobic organisms. The choice of an empiric regimen should be based upon the severity of infection, suspected organism(s), and their prevalence in the community.
  - **Gram-positive** organisms, (*Staphylococcus* spp. *Streptococcus* spp.) comprise the majority of DFI. Methicillin-resistant *Staphylococcus aureus* (MRSA) has emerged as an important pathogen and can be present in up to a third of infections.
    - Empiric therapy for gram-positive organisms only can be considered for mild to moderate infections; coverage for MRSA should be considered if the patient has a history of previous MRSA infection, evidence of MRSA colonization, presence of severe infection, or in the setting of high community prevalence of MRSA.
  - **Gram-negative** organisms such as *Enterobacteriaceae* can be present in moderate to severe infections; empiric coverage for these organisms should be considered.
  - While often buzzed about, *Pseudomonas aeruginosa* has been implicated in a small percentage of DFI. Empiric coverage can be considered if certain risk factors are present (e.g., history of water exposure or

clinical failure while receiving nonpseudomonal antibiotic therapy).
  - **Anaerobes** such as *Bacteroides* spp. can be involved, especially if tissue necrosis or ischemia is present; empiric coverage should be considered in moderate to severe infections.

Diagnosis (see Fig. 26.1)

- **Laboratories**
  - Complete blood count (CBC), comprehensive metabolic panel (CMP), hemoglobin A1c (Hgb A1c), erythrocyte sedimentation rate (ESR), and C-reactive protein (CRP).
- **Imaging**
  - An X-ray can demonstrate bony erosion but may take **2–4 weeks** to demonstrate radiographic changes. A negative X-ray does not rule out osteomyelitis.
  - Magnetic resonance imaging (MRI) is sensitive and is useful in suspected **early (<2 weeks)** osteomyelitis (OM) and for evaluating for concomitant deep tissue infection or soft tissue abscess.
  - MRI can be limited in detecting Charcot changes.
  - Computed tomography (CT) scans or nuclear imaging can be helpful in cases when MRI is not feasible (e.g., pacemaker placement).
- **Culture data**
  - Blood cultures (preferably two sets) especially if systemic symptoms of infection are present.
  - If the patient is clinically stable, empiric antibiotic therapy should be withheld until culture data can be obtained.
  - Ideally, cultures should be obtained after the area has been debrided or by sampling deep tissue and/or bone.
  - Care must be taken in utilizing superficial swabs as it may reflect surface colonization but may not be indicative of the underlying causative organism(s).
    - However, recovery of MSSA or MRSA on superficial cultures may correlate with the presence of deep tissue infection.

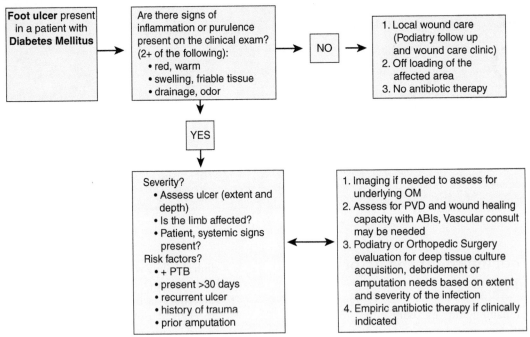

• **Fig. 26.1** Evaluation of the diabetic foot ulcer. PTB, probe-to-bone; OM, osteomyelitis; PVD, peripheral vascular disease; ABI, ankle–brachial index. (Lipsky BA, Berendt AR, Cornia PB, Pile JC et al., 2012 Infectious Disease Society of America Clinical Practice Guideline for the Diagnosis and Treatment of Diabetic Foot Infections, *Clinical Infectious Diseases,* Volume 54, Issue 12, 15 June 2012, pp. e132-e173.)

Treatment

- Often requires a **multidisciplinary team** (Podiatry, Vascular, Wound Care, Infectious Diseases, Primary Care).
- Obtain appropriate culture data.
- Imaging to further elicit the depth and involvement of the infection.
- Assess for presence of PVD (e.g., ankle–brachial index [ABI]), as poor blood flow can impact wound healing and hamper antibiotic delivery to the site of infection. Revascularization may be required for some patients.
- In systemically ill patients, empiric antibiotic therapy with de-escalation to definitive therapy based on culture data. In stable patients, it is reasonable to await culture data.
- Medical management only (e.g., antibiotics) can be considered if there is **no associated abscess or gangrene** present.
- Length of antibiotic therapy ranges from 4 to 6 weeks but can be shortened based on the surgical debridement completed, and if proximal surgical margins do not exhibits signs of inflammation on histopathologic review.

Septic Arthritis

Definition: infection of a native joint.

Epidemiology

- **Mechanism of infection:** joints can become infected **hematogenously** from a distant foci of infection (e.g., endovascular infection, odontogenic source, etc.) or **contiguously** through direct inoculation (e.g., corticosteroid injection, trauma) or extension from osteomyelitis of the long bones.
- The **knee is the most commonly involved** joint (50% of cases) followed (in order of frequency) by the hip, shoulder, elbow, and ankle.
- **Sternoclavicular** joint or **sacroiliac** joint involvement should prompt concern for **intravenous drug use (IVDU).**
- **Risk factors:** older age, bacteremia or endovascular infection, recent history of or active IVDU, history of corticosteroid injections, comorbid conditions such as diabetes mellitus, rheumatoid arthritis, or history of recent joint surgery.
- **Clinical presentation**
  - Pain, warmth, and swelling in the affected joint.
  - Inability to ambulate or bear weight on the joint.
  - Systemic symptoms such as fever may be present.
- Certain **conditions can mimic septic arthritis.** This includes cellulitis, bursitis, inflammatory arthritis such as **crystal arthropathy** (gout and pseudogout), rheumatoid arthritis, and reactive arthritis.
- The presence of crystals in the joint fluid does not rule out the presence of septic arthritis; while less frequently encountered, more than one inflammatory process can be present.

Diagnosis

- **Laboratories**
  - CBC, CMP, ESR, and CRP.
  - Blood cultures (preferably two sets); cultures can be positive in up to 50% of cases.

TABLE 26.1   Categorization of Arthrocentesis Synovial Fluid Findings

Variable	Normal	Non-inflammatory[a]	Inflammatory[b*]	Septic Arthritis	Hemarthrosis
Synovial fluid	Transparent	Transparent	Mildly opaque	Opaque/cloudy	Bloody
WBC (mm³)	<200	<200	>2,000	>50,000[c, d]	Can appear falsely elevated due to RBCs
PMN (%)	<25	<25	≥50	≥75[c, d]	>50 to <75
Synovial fluid culture	Negative	Negative	Negative	Positive[d]	Negative

[a]E.g., osteoarthritis.
[b]E.g., gout, pseudogout, rheumatoid arthritis.
[c]Of note, septic arthritis secondary to *Neisseria gonorrhoeae* may present with a lesser cell count in comparison to nongonoccal arthritis.
[d]Of note, antibiotic pre-treatment may blunt cell count, differential, and culture-yield.
Shoulter DE and Russell AS. (2019). Synovial fluid analysis. In M. R. Curtis (Ed.), *UptoDate.*

- **Arthrocentesis** remains the **gold standard** in the diagnosis of septic arthritis. Provided that the patient is clinically stable, antibiotic therapy should ideally be withheld until joint aspiration can be completed. The fluid should be sent for the following:
  - Cell count and differential.
  - Gram stain and culture (aerobic/anaerobic, fungal, acid-fast bacilli [AFB]).
  - Crystal analysis to evaluate for gout and pseudogout.
  - Refer to Table 26.1 for etiologies based on synovial fluid results.
- **Imaging**
  - X-rays can demonstrate joint space widening, which can be suggestive of joint space effusion.
  - An MRI can detect an associated contiguous osteomyelitis and joint space effusion.
  - A CT can be obtained when an MRI is not feasible (e.g., in cases of pacemaker placement or other noncompatible hardware).
  - Echocardiogram can be obtained in cases where an endovascular infection such as endocarditis is suspected (e.g., *S. aureus, Streptococcus* spp., *Candida* spp., etc.).

Causative Organisms (see Table 26.2)

Bacterial. Can be divided into gonococcal and nongonococcal etiologies.

- **Gonococcal arthritis** is due to infection by *Neisseria gonorrhoeae* and is an important cause of pyogenic arthritis in sexually active adults up to 40 years of age.
- A small percentage of mucosal infections disseminate as a result of bacteremic spread of the organism. Disseminated gonococcal infection (DGI) typically manifests as arthralgias, tenosynovitis, and rash (**arthritis-dermatitis syndrome**), but a purulent distal mono- or oligoarthritis can be seen (e.g., knees, wrists, and ankles) in up to a third of untreated cases.

TABLE 26.2   Causative Organisms and Common Clinical Associations

Organism(s)	Clinical Scenario
Staphylococcus aureus (MSSA or MRSA)	Healthy and immunocompromised, rheumatoid arthritis, IVDU
Group B streptococci	Poorly controlled DM, malignancy
Streptococcus pneumoniae	Splenic dysfunction
Enteric gram-negatives (e.g., *Klebsiella* spp., *Escherichia coli*)	GI tract infection, immunocompromised, trauma, IVDU
Pseudomonas spp.	DM, immunocompromised, water exposure/contamination, trauma
Aeromonas spp.	Brackish water, water exposure/contamination
Salmonella spp.	Sickle cell disease, HIV
Eikenella corrodens *Peptostreptococcus* spp.	Inoculation by oral flora, (e.g., fight bite, oral flora, contamination of needle in setting of IVDU)
Pasteurella multocida	Cat bite
Capnocytophaga spp.	Dog bite
Mycoplasma hominis	Postpartum septic arthritis, recent history of GU tract manipulation, immunocompromised

DM, diabetes mellitus; GI, gastrointestinal; GU, genitourinary; HIV, human immunodeficiency virus; IVDU, intravenous drug use.

- Cutaneous findings can range from a maculopapular rash to a pustular dermatosis of the palms or soles (on average 10–15 lesions).

- Lab testing for suspected DGI should include indirect evaluation with testing of urogenital and/or extragenital mucosal sites (oropharyngeal and rectal) by nucleic acid amplification (**NAAT**).
- This organism can be extremely difficult to culture on routine media, requiring **chocolate agar or Thayer-Martin medium** instead.
- Blood cultures typically have low diagnostic yield with the exception of the early stages of dissemination.
- While not FDA-approved, NAAT of the synovial fluid can be performed but may not be readily available in all laboratories.
- It is important to highlight that synovial fluid cell counts in septic arthritis due to *Neisseria gonorrhoeae* are less pronounced than other routine bacterial etiologies.
- Involved joints may require recurrent aspirations of the joint effusions. Involved joints tend to respond quickly to antibiotic therapy. Once improved, the patient can be transitioned to step-down therapy.
- **Therapy**
  - Initial therapy: ceftriaxone 1 g IV Q24h + azithromycin 1 g PO ×1.
  - Step-down therapy: doxycycline. Cefixime is associated with increasing rates of resistance and is no longer recommended as first-line therapy.
  - 7–14 total days of antibiotic therapy may be required.
  - If recurrent infections are noted, screen for late complement deficiency.
- **Nongonococcal** arthritis: see Table 26.2 for common associations.
  - **Lyme** arthritis (see Chapter 30)
    - *Borrelia burgdorferi* infection transmitted by *Ixodes scapularis* ticks in the spring–summer months.
    - Arthritis is the most common late-stage manifestation of the disease. It commonly presents as a monoarthritis with the **knee** most commonly involved. Systemic manifestations of disease may be absent.
    - Synovial fluid can be sent for PCR testing in order to confirm the diagnosis.
    - Oral antibiotic therapy (e.g., doxycycline, amoxicillin, or cefuroxime) with a 30-day duration of therapy is recommended. If an inadequate response is observed, then intravenous therapy with ceftriaxone can be utilized.
  - *Mycobacterium* arthritis (see Chapters 32–33)
    - *M. tuberculosis*, septic arthritis is the second most common manifestation of osteoarticular disease after the spine (Pott's disease). While any joint can be involved, **commonly large joints are affected** (hips, knees).
    - *M. chelonae* and *M. fortuitum* are the most common species of nontuberculous mycobacteria which can cause infection in immunocompetent hosts. Infection occurs through direct inoculation during trauma or as a direct extension to bone from skin and soft tissue infections. Surgical management is often required.

- **Fungal (see Chapters 27–28)**
- Comprises a small percentage of septic arthritis, but when encountered, is most commonly due to *Candida* species.
- Other etiologies include blastomycosis, *Cryptococcus*, coccidiomycosis, and sporotrichosis. Infection occurs as a result of direct inoculation or disseminated disease (more commonly in immunocompromised hosts).
- **Viral**
- Important etiologies include human immunodeficiency virus (HIV), hepatitis B, hepatitis C, parvovirus B19, and alphaviruses (such as chikungunya virus).
- Viral arthritis often presents acutely in a symmetric polyarticular pattern and as part of a constellation of symptoms which commonly include fever and rash.
- **Pathogenesis**: this may occur as result of direct infection of the synovium versus immune-complex formation due to viral infection.
- **Laboratories**
  - CBC, CMP, creatine kinase, ESR, CRP, and viral serologies (based on clinical suspicion).
  - Rheumatoid factor (RF), anticyclic citrullinated peptide (CCP), and antinuclear antibodies (ANA) can help for rheumatic disease.
    - Low titer autoantibodies (e.g., ANA or RF) can be present in the setting of viral arthritis (false-positive due to antibody cross-reactivity).
- Most cases of viral arthritis are self-limited and require only supportive care with nonsteroidal antiinflammatory agents (NSAIDs).
- Joint involvement secondary to **parvovirus** can be observed in up to 60% of infected adults, with women more commonly affected. The pattern of joint involvement is **rheumatoid arthritis (RA)-like** given symmetric involvement of wrists, metacarpophalangeal, and proximal interphalangeal joints.
- Arthralgia due to **hepatitis B** can be seen in the **prodromal stage** (RA-like) or in the setting of **chronic infection.** It is thought to occur due to immune-complex formation.
- Arthralgia due to **hepatitis C** is thought to occur due to immune-complex formation and can present in an RA-like pattern (more common) or as oligoarthritis with involvement of larger joints; this presentation is more typically associated with mixed essential cryoglobulinemia.
- **Rubella** is less commonly encountered given immunization (more commonly seen in the developing world, involves the small joints of the hand).
- **Chikungunya** is vectorborne and transmitted by the *Aedes aegypti* and *Aedes albopictus* mosquitoes. It is encountered in Asia, Africa, Europe, and more recently, the Caribbean. It can affect both small and large joints with typically **>10 joints** affected. The prominent joint symptoms are associated with a rash and high fevers. Up to a third of patients can develop chronic symptoms with relapsing-remitting or unremitting patterns

of joint involvement. Diagnosis can be made with RT-PCR testing for chikungunya virus RNA (up to a week after symptom onset); if symptoms have been present greater than a week, then serologic testing can be utilized (IgM can be present up to 3 months from symptom onset).

- **Reactive arthritis** is **sterile inflammation** of the joints hypothesized to be secondary to a dysregulatory immune response from an antecedent infection. There is a weak association with **HLA-B27.**
- Mainly occurs in young adults, with **men and women equally affected.** Presents as an **asymmetric oligoarthritis** of large joints with extraarticular manifestations such as urethritis, uveitis, or conjunctivitis (classic triad).
  - Reminder: "Can't see, can't pee, can't climb a tree."
- Antecedent infections associated with reactive arthritis include *Chlamydia trachomatis* (organism may be identified by NAAT testing of the urine), *Shigella*, *Salmonella*, *Campylobacter*, and *Yersinia*.
- This is often a diagnosis of exclusion.
- With the exception of *C. trachomatis* (which should be treated), supportive care is recommended for all other etiologies.

Treatment

- Aspiration and surgical drainage, in combination with antibiotics are the mainstay of therapy. Suspicion of septic arthritis constitutes a surgical evaluation for diagnosis and treatment in order to preserve joint function.
- In cases of pyogenic (nongonococcal) arthritis, up to 4 weeks of pathogen-directed antibiotic therapy is recommended. Intravenous antibiotics or highly bioavailable oral antibiotic therapy (e.g., fluoroquinolones) may be utilized. Gonococcal arthritis can be treated for shorter durations (7–14 days).
- Atypical infections such as fungal and mycobacterial arthritis will require a combined surgical and medical approach, with a prolonged course of therapy, at minimum of 6 months.

Vertebral Osteomyelitis

Definition: infection of the vertebral bodies and adjacent disk spaces.

Epidemiology

- There has been an increase in incidence in the United States which has been attributed to:
  - Increasing rates of IVDU.
  - Use of indwelling vascular catheters.
  - Increase in immunosuppressed individuals.
- Approximately 50% of cases involve individuals >60 years of age with males more commonly affected.
- **Mechanism of infection**: infection usually occurs **hematogenously**, due to seeding from a distant focus of infection (e.g., endovascular infection, dental source,

etc.) versus **contiguously** through direct inoculation (e.g., corticosteroid injection, trauma) or extension (e.g., esophageal perforation, skin and soft tissue infection [SSTI], gastrointestinal tract in inflammatory bowel disease [IBD] patients) with involvement of disk with extension to the neighboring vertebral bodies.

- The lumbar spine is the site of most frequent involvement followed by thoracic and then cervical spine.
- **Risk factors** for infection include comorbid conditions such as diabetes mellitus, IVDU, corticosteroid injections, and history of previous spinal surgery.
  - Commonly **monomicrobial** with 70% due to gram-positive organisms.
  - Gram-negative infections are more common in the lumbar spine.
  - Up to 30% of patients may experience neurologic complications.
  - **Clinical presentation**: back pain that does not respond to conservative management, plus or minus the presence of fever.

Diagnosis

- **Laboratories**
  - CBC, CMP, ESR, and CRP.
  - Blood cultures (preferably two sets), which can be positive in up to 75% of cases, given the hematogenous nature of the infection.
- **Imaging**
  - MRI is the gold standard for diagnosis.
  - CT can be an alternative when use of MRI is contraindicated (e.g., pacemaker).
  - Radionuclide imaging, while sensitive, lacks specificity.
  - X-ray may not demonstrate erosive changes until late in the disease course.
- **Bone/tissue biopsy** for culture (aerobic/anaerobic, AFB, and fungal if index of suspicion present) and histopathology is recommended in order to attain a microbiologic diagnosis. 16sPCR testing is not routinely recommended as it may have low sensitivity and may not be readily available, but can be employed in a case-by-case basis.
  - If the patient is clinically stable and without neurologic compromise, antibiotics can be held prior to culture acquisition in order to not diminish culture yield.

Causative Organisms

- *S. aureus* (MSSA and MRSA) constitute greater than 50% of cases.
- Enteric gram-negative bacilli comprise up to 30% cases (more predominant in the lumbar spine).
- Group B streptococcus is associated with poorly controlled diabetes.
- Coagulase-negative *Staphylococcus* species (CoNS) commonly *S. epidermidis* is associated with hardware-associated infections.
- *Pseudomonas* is associated with immunocompromise and IVDU.
- *Salmonella* is associated with sickle cell disease patients.

- *Candida* is associated with IVDU and indwelling vascular catheters.
- **Atypical etiologies**
  - *M. tuberculosis* vertebral osteomyelitis (**Pott's disease**) represents the **most common** form of osteoarticular tuberculosis.
    - Comprises 50%–60% of cases and often **thoracolumbar** in location.
    - Initially involves contiguous vertebrae with **extension to the disc later in the disease course** (anterior superior or inferior end plates, posterior aspect is spared) in contrast to pyogenic vertebral osteomyelitis.
  - Brucellosis is endemic to the Middle East and the Mediterranean. It is associated with the consumption of unpasteurized cheeses and milks.
    - Commonly presents as sacroiliitis or spondylodiscitis in the **lumbosacral** region.

Treatment

- At minimum requires 6–8 weeks of pathogen-directed therapy often with an intravenous or highly bioavailable oral antibiotic.
- Atypical organisms will require a combination of surgical and medical management with extended courses of antibiotic therapy. *Brucella* may require a minimum of 12 weeks. Fungal and infections due to AFB can require up to 24 weeks of therapy.

Prosthetic Joint Infections (PJI)

Definition: infection involving a joint endoprosthesis. Diagnosis can be challenging as there is no standardized definition or diagnostic criteria.

Epidemiology

- PJI complicates 1.5% of primary total hip arthroplasties (THA) and 2.5% of primary total knee arthroplasties (TKA).
- Revisions are associated **with greater risk** of infection.
  - Classification
  - **Early** PJI: onset <3 months from surgery, contiguous, acquired during joint implantation.
  - Delayed PJI: onset between 3 and 24 months from surgery, contiguous, acquired during joint implantation.
  - Late PJI: onset >24 months from surgery, hematogenous spread with joint involvement (distant site involvement).
- **Risk factors**
  - **Preoperative**: prior surgery of joint in question, prior infection of the bone, tobacco abuse, diabetes mellitus, obesity, rheumatoid arthritis, immunosuppression.
  - **Postoperative**: presence of a surgical site infection, hematoma, *S. aureus* bacteremia.

Clinical Presentation

- Can be challenging as symptoms are often protean in nature, but symptoms of PJI may include:
  - Sudden onset of pain in prosthetic joint.
  - Chronically painful prosthesis.
  - Erythematous joint.
  - Draining sinus tract or wound drainage.
  - Presence of purulence involving the prosthesis without another identified etiology.
- Conditions that can **mimic** PJI: metallosis (metal-on-metal wear of the endoprosthesis leading to a local hypersensitivity reaction), aseptic loosening (loss of fixation not due to an underlying infectious etiology such as osteolysis or wear), crystalline arthropathy (gout, pseudogout).
- **Common causative organisms**
  - CoNS, commonly *S. epidermidis*.
  - *S. aureus* (MSSA or MRSA).
  - *Streptococcus* spp.
  - *Cutibacterium acnes* (formerly *Propionibacterium acnes*), associated with shoulder PJI, but a rare cause of PJI of the hips or knees.
  - Enteric gram-negatives.
  - Atypical organisms such as *Brucella*, *Coxiella*, fungi (most common, *Candida* spp.), and mycobacteria such as *M. tuberculosis*.
  - Culture-negative (can be due to antibiotic pretreatment or atypical organisms such *Brucella* or *Coxiella*, which are diagnosed through high index of suspicion and serologic testing).

Diagnosis

- **Laboratories**
  - CBC, CMP, ESR, and CRP.
  - Blood cultures (preferably two sets) if there is a concern for bacteremia.
- **Imaging**
  - Echocardiogram can be obtained if endovascular infection is suspected.
  - X-ray can demonstrate loosening of the endoprosthesis or associated osteomyelitis.
  - MRI and CT can be limited by hardware artifact.
- **Arthrocentesis** remains the **gold standard** in diagnosing PJI; if the patient is clinically stable, recommend holding antibiotic therapy until aspiration can be completed. The fluid should be sent for the following:
  - Cell count and differential.
  - Gram stain and culture (aerobic/anaerobic, fungal, AFB).
  - Crystal analysis to evaluate for gout and pseudogout.
  - Molecular biomarkers such as **alpha-defensin** are being increasingly utilized in the diagnosis of PJI and do not appear to be affected by antecedent antibiotic therapy. However, they may not be readily available at all institutions.
  - **Cultures** (aerobic/anaerobic, fungal, AFB) should be attained by CT-guided aspiration or intraoperatively;

sonication/vortexing of prosthesis (if biofilm-producing organism is suspected) can be utilized operatively to increase the culture yield; however, this can be subject to contamination or false-positive results and may not be available at all institutions.
- Specimen should be sent for histopathology review.
  - 16sPCR is not routinely recommended as it can demonstrate low sensitivity, but can be utilized on a case-by-case basis.

Treatment

- Proven infection often requires a combination of surgical and medical management.
  - Debridement, antibiotics, and implant retention (DAIR) followed by chronic oral antibiotic suppression.
    - This technique may be considered in early PJI infections with <3 weeks of symptoms with a well-fixed prosthesis, with no sinus tract on presentation; may be associated with increased risk of failure, especially when an organism such as *S. aureus* is involved.
  - Late infections are optimally treated by a two-stage exchange; however, in certain scenarios, a one-stage exchange may be utilized by the orthopedic surgeon.
  - In cases of retained hardware in infections due to *Staphylococcus* spp. (e.g., *S. epidermidis*, MSSA, MRSA), adjunctive oral rifampin can be added given its activity against biofilms.

27

Infections Caused by Yeasts and Yeast-Like Fungi

ILAN S. SCHWARTZ

Cryptococcosis

Microbiology

- Two main species complexes: *Cryptococcus neoformans* and *C. gattii*.
  - Now recognized to be at least 7 pathogenic cryptic species within these. However, formal classification has not been modified.
- Large polysaccharide **capsule** is a defining feature of these fungi. It is required for the virulence, and strains without a capsule rarely cause disease.

Epidemiology

- Cryptococcosis is usually associated with immunocompromise (IC).
  - Advanced human immunodeficiency virus (HIV), transplantation, long-term corticosteroids, cirrhosis are some of the biggest risk factors.
  - Cryptococcosis in HIV is associated with CD4 <100 cells/μL.
  - In United States, HIV-associated cases now comprise a minority; HIV remains the dominant comorbidity in resource-poor settings.
  - 15%–25% of all cases are in otherwise immunocompetent patients.
- *C. neoformans* is classically associated with **pigeon** guano, rotting trees, and has a global distribution.
- *C. gattii* is classically associated with **eucalyptus** trees in endemic areas (Vancouver Island in British Columbia, Canada; **Pacific Northwest** in United States, Australia). More detailed studies are suggesting that the range may be larger and even growing.

Clinical Presentation

Cryptococcal Meningitis (CM)

- Although called meningitis, this syndrome is really a meningoencephalitis.
- A high index of suspicion is frequently needed to make the diagnosis because clinical signs are unreliable.
- Classic meningeal signs like meningismus and photophobia are present in a minority of patients (~1/4 to 1/3).
- Fever is also an unreliable finding and may be absent in half of patients.
- Encephalopathic symptoms like lethargy, altered mentation may result from increased intracranial pressure (ICP) as well as direct neuroinvasion.
- Cranial nerve palsies occur late in the disease, and are most common with increased ICP. They may appear during treatment, most often as a result of a paradoxical immune reconstitution inflammatory syndrome (**IRIS**). The optical nerves are frequently involved.
- Space-occupying lesions (cryptococcomas) may also occur in a minority of patients.

Lung

- Disease can be asymptomatic or can mimic subacute or chronic pneumonias.
- Abnormalities on chest imaging include pulmonary nodule(s), lymphadenopathy, infiltrates, and cavitation.

Skin

- Cutaneous disease can take any appearance, but the classic lesions are widespread papules with central umbilication, resembling molluscum contagiosum (Fig. 27.1).
- Direct inoculation into the skin has been described, but in the vast majority of cases skin lesions are due to dissemination.

Other

- Ocular and ocular nerve involvement are common in CNS disease.
  - Ocular palsies, papilledema, and/or retinal exudates are the most common findings.
  - Papilledema is usually a sign of increased ICP.
- Chronic prostatitis
  - Prostatic cryptococcosis is usually subclinical but may serve as a reservoir leading to relapse in inadequately treated patients with disseminated cryptococcosis.
- Bone and soft tissue
  - Osteoarticular lesions occur in fewer than 10% of patients with disseminated cryptococcosis.

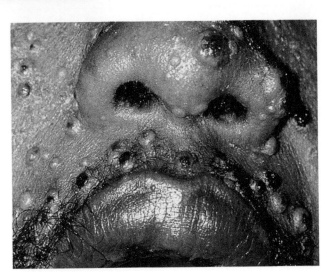

• **Fig. 27.1** Molluscum-like lesions of cryptococcosis. (From James WD, Berger TG, Elston DM. Diseases resulting from fungi and yeasts. In: *Andrews' Diseases of the Skin: Clinical Dermatology*. 12th ed. Elsevier; 2016.)

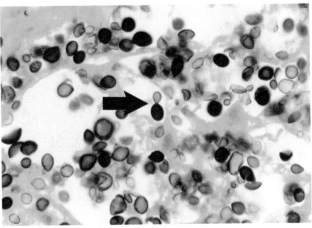

• **Fig. 27.2** Grocott's methenamine stain showing narrow-based budding and variable yeast size of *Cryptococcus neoformans*. ×1000. (From Wojewoda C, Procop GW. Infections with yeasts and yeastlike fungi. *Pathol Infect Dis.* 2015;26:531–572.)

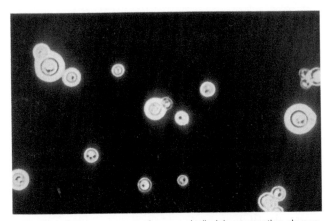

• **Fig. 27.3** *Cryptococcus neoformans*. India ink preparation demonstrating the large capsule surrounding budding yeast cells. ×1000. (From Pfaller MA, McGinnis MR. The laboratory and clinical mycology. In: Anaissie EJ, McGinnis MR, Pfaller MA, eds. *Clinical Mycology*. 2nd ed. Elsevier; 2009.)

- Vertebral osteomyelitis is the most common presentation.
- Well-circumscribed, osteolytic lesions may be seen on radiography.
- Septic arthritis is uncommon but reported, usually involving the knee.
- Peritonitis can occur, especially in patients with cirrhosis and those receiving peritoneal dialysis. Although sometimes described as spontaneous fungal peritonitis in the literature, this should be treated as disseminated disease. Mortality is very high (~80%).

Diagnosis

- Cerebrospinal fluid (CSF) analysis
  - Typical profile includes mildly elevated protein, low to normal glucose, lymphocytic pleocytosis.
  - Lumbar opening pressure elevated in many cases of CM. If the opening pressure is negative on the first lumbar puncture (LP), clinical increase in headache, confusion, or any clinical deterioration might be related to elevations in pressure that have developed during the treatment.
  - Testing for CM should include cryptococcal antigen (CrAg), India Ink (where available, although not largely used since advent of CrAg), and fungal culture.
- Culture
  - *Cryptococcus* spp. can be cultured from blood, CSF, and tissue, usually within a few days.
  - Will grow on most aerobic and fungal media.
  - Isolation from blood is enhanced by use of lysis centrifugation.
  - Concanavalin-glycine-thymol agar turns blue for *C. gattii* but *not C. neoformans*. However, speciation is more commonly determined by matrix-assisted laser desorption/ionization-time of flight (MALDI-TOF).
- Cytopathology/histopathology
  - Hematoxylin and eosin stain demonstrates 4–10 μm yeasts which appear to have a large clearing around them because the large polysaccharide capsule does not stain.
  - Fungal stains, i.e., Grocott's methenamine silver (GMS) or periodic acid–Schiff (PAS) stains, show narrow-based budding and variable sizes (Fig. 27.2).
  - India Ink is useful for visualization in CSF, but this test is no longer widely available in the United States (Fig. 27.3).
  - **Mucicarmine** stains the polysaccharide capsule pink or red (Fig. 27.4), and **Alcian blue** stains the capsule blue; these can help in the differentiation from other fungi of similar size and morphology, which lack capsules.
- **CrAg** detection
  - CrAg is detectable in serum and CSF months before the appearance of any signs/symptoms of CM.
  - Lateral flow assay now preferred over older methods (latex agglutination, enzyme immunoassays), as it appears to have higher sensitivity, specificity, is less expensive, and requires less training and technologist time.

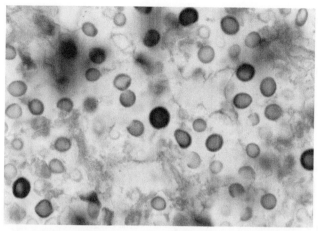

• **Fig. 27.4** The capsule of a metabolically active *Cryptococcus* may be highlighted with the mucicarmine stain. ×1000. (From: Wojewoda C, Procop GW. Infections with yeasts and yeastlike fungi. *Pathol Infect Dis.* 2015;26:531–572.)

• Serum should be routinely tested for CrAg in people with HIV with CD4 ≤100 cells/μL in countries with high incidences of cryptococcal meningitis. If screening serum CrAg is positive, then CSF examination is necessary to rule out CM. If active CM ruled out, pre-emptive fluconazole 400 mg PO daily × ≥12 months. If findings suggest CM, treat as CM (see below).
• CrAg titers correlate poorly with total fungal burden.
• There is no role for serial monitoring to assess response to treatment. Patients can stay positive for years after the infection, and changes in titer are not associated with clinical course.
• CrAg testing has low sensitivity for diagnosing isolated pulmonary cryptococcosis.
• **All** patients diagnosed with cryptococcosis (including diagnoses of extra-CNS disease or asymptomatic antigenemia) need CSF examination to rule out CM.

Management

Management of CM involves three phases: induction, consolidation, and maintenance (see Fig. 27.5).
• **Induction phase** consists of 2 drugs for ≥2 weeks
  • Amphotericin B (AMB)
    • IV liposomal 3–4 mg/kg daily (preferred) *or* deoxycholate 0.7 mg/kg daily (alternative).
  • Flucytosine 100 mg/kg daily PO
    • Also known as 5-fluorocytosine (5-FC).
    • Its addition to AMB is shown in trials to result in faster CSF sterilization and improved survival.
    • Adverse effects include cytopenias, hepatotoxicity, and gastrointestinal (GI) toxicity.
    • Where flucytosine is not available, AMB + fluconazole 800 mg PO/IV daily is superior to AMB alone (but inferior to AMB + flucytosine).
  • If after ≥2 weeks, there is clinical improvement and a repeated CSF culture is negative, then de-escalate to consolidation phase.
• **Consolidation phase**
  • Fluconazole 400 mg PO daily for ≥8 weeks.

• **Maintenance phase**
  • Fluconazole 200 mg PO daily for at least 1 year of azole therapy.
    • Non-CNS, extrapulmonary cryptococcosis, or diffuse/severe pulmonary disease should be treated the same as CM. Limited pulmonary disease (or asymptomatic CrAg+ with CM excluded) can be treated with fluconazole 400 mg PO/IV daily for ≥1 year.
  • The timing of antiretroviral therapy (ART) initiation is important.
  • Increased mortality has been demonstrated in a trial of patients starting ART within 2 weeks of initiating antifungal therapy for CM.
    Thus it is prudent to wait *at least* until after completion of induction therapy (≥2 weeks, although some experts recommend waiting ≥10 weeks).

Other Considerations in Management
• Management of **increased cranial pressure** (ICP) is critical.
  • Patients may clinically deteriorate, even with effective therapy, due to ICP.
  • Lumbar opening pressure should be measured in all patients at the time of diagnosis.
  • If lumbar pressure is elevated, CSF should be drained (via serial LPs or insertion of lumbar drain/ventriculostomy).
  • In rare cases, the chronically elevated pressure will require a ventriculoperitoneal drain, as the pressure may never return to normal.
• Management of **IRIS**
  • ~30% of people with HIV and CM who are newly started/re-started on ART develop a paradoxical IRIS.
  • Usually absent or minimal inflammation observed in CSF pre-ART initiation.
  • Presents as CNS deterioration despite microbiological efficacy (**sterilized CSF** vs. treatment failure in which CSF cultures remain positive).
  • Management is generally supportive; **continue antifungals and ART** (and ensure ICP managed); role of corticosteroids uncertain.
• Corticosteroids
  • Routine administration of corticosteroids in the treatment of CM results in increased disability and mortality.
  • A role for corticosteroids in patients with IRIS and edema from stroke and/or cryptococcoma may still be of benefit but should be of limited duration.

Pneumocystis

Microbiology

• *Pneumocystis jirovecii* is the cause of *Pneumocystis* pneumonia (PCP).
• Thought initially to be protozoan, *P. jirovecii* is now proven by genetic analyses to be a fungus.
• Life cycle of *P. jirovecii* includes trophic forms and cysts.

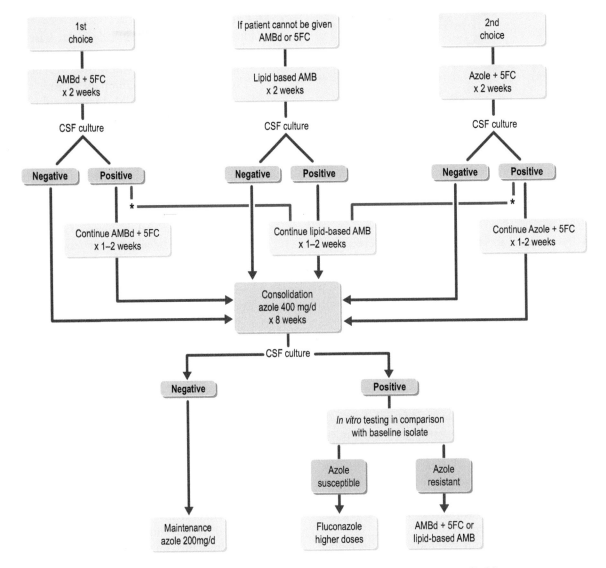

* if yeast burden is unchanged or increased compared to baseline, or AMBd or 5FC had to be discontinued because of toxicity.
AMBd = amphotericin B deoxycholate; 5FC = flucytosine

• **Fig. 27.5** Treatment algorithm for cryptococcal meningitis. (From Viviani MA, Tortorano AM. Cryptococcus. In: Anaissie EJ, McGinnis MR, Pfaller MA, eds. *Clinical Mycology.* 2nd ed. Elsevier; 2009.)

Epidemiology of Infection and Disease

- Inoculation is presumably respiratory, with primary infection occurring in first 2 years of life in the majority of individuals.
- Disease occurs almost exclusively in IC hosts. Most commonly affected are patients with the following conditions:
  - Advanced HIV (CD4 <200 cells/μL, but especially <100 cells/μL).
  - Prolonged use of corticosteroids or other immunosuppressants for chronic autoimmune diseases, post-transplantation, etc.
  - Chemotherapy for malignancies (especially lymphoma).
  - Congenital immunodeficiencies.

Clinical Features of PCP

- Patients typically present with fever, dyspnea, **nonproductive cough** and weight loss.

- **Hypoxia** is a *sine qua non* of PCP.
- Clinical deterioration is generally gradual in patients with HIV and more rapid in non-HIV-associated disease.
- Radiographs usually demonstrate bilateral interstitial disease (Fig. 27.6).

Diagnosis

- Pathology is the standard diagnostic for PCP.
  - The characteristic pathologic findings of lung tissue are acellular, foamy, **eosinophilic**, intraalveolar exudates seen on H&E (Fig. 27.7).
  - Fungal stains (like PAS or GMS) demonstrate cysts (Fig. 27.8), allowing differentiation from alveolar proteinosis.
  - Immunofluorescent antibodies can be used to highlight the organism and significantly improve the sensitivity of pathologic examination.
- Molecular diagnostic tools are not yet widely employed

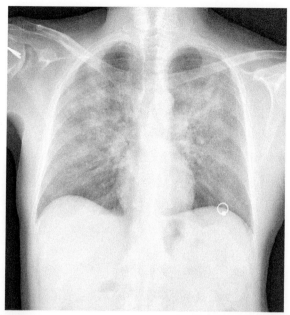

• **Fig. 27.6** Chest radiograph showing bilateral infiltrates. (From Walzer PD, Smulian AG, Miller RF. *Pneumocystis* species. In: Bennett JE, Dolin R, Blaser MJ, eds. *Mandell, Douglas, and Bennett's Principles and Practice of Infectious Diseases*. 8th ed. Elsevier; 2015.)

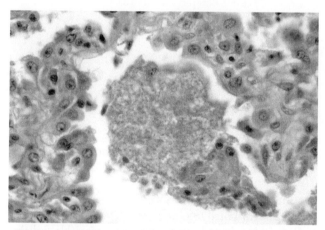

• **Fig. 27.7** An alveolar eosinophilic cast seen in pneumocystosis. H&E stain, 500× magnification. (From Wojewoda C, Procop GW. Infections with yeasts and yeastlike fungi. *Pathol Infect Dis*. 2015;26:531–572.)

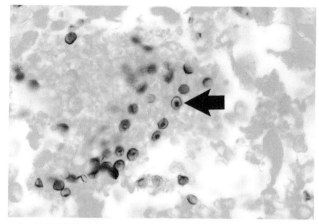

• **Fig. 27.8** GMS stain demonstrates the cyst forms of *Pneumocystis* in lung tissue. These do not bud. Some demonstrate the distinctive intracystic bodies (*arrow*). 1000×. (From Wojewoda C, Procop GW. Infections with yeasts and yeastlike fungi. *Pathol Infect Dis*. 2015;26:531–572.)

for the diagnosis of PCP. In-house PCR assays are sensitive and specific but not commercially available.
• There is no role for culture in the diagnosis of PCP because *P. jirovecii* will not grow on artificial media.
• Nonspecific biomarkers that can be elevated in PCP include serum lactate dehydrogenase and 1,3-beta-D-glucan.

Treatment

Treatment recommendations for PCP are shown in Table 27.1.

Prevention

Secondary prophylaxis is indicated in patients with prior PCP. Additionally, primary prophylaxis is recommended for people with HIV with CD4 ≤200 cells/μL or comprising <14% of total lymphocyte count, or in situations where CD4 count ≤250 cells/μL, but ART cannot be initiated and q3monthly CD4 monitoring is not possible.

The preferred regimen is trimethoprim–sulfamethoxazole (TMP–SMX) 1 DS PO daily. An advantage of this regimen is that it also protects against toxoplasmosis.

Alternative regimens include the following:
• TMP–SMX 1 DS PO 3 times per week (preferred), *or*
• Dapsone 100 mg PO daily or 50 mg PO BID (second-line, check G6PD), *or*
• (Dapsone 50 mg + pyrimethamine 75 mg + leucovorin 25 mg) PO weekly, *or*
• Aerosolized pentamidine 300 mg monthly (associated with breakthrough infections in the upper lobes where the medication does not reach well), *or*
• Atovaquone 1500 mg PO daily (with food), *or*
• (Atovaquone 1500 mg + pyrimethamine 25 mg + leucovorin 10 mg) PO daily.

Candidiasis

Microbiology

• *Candida* spp. are common colonizers of GI tract, skin.
• *Candida albicans* is by far the most common cause of clinical disease; the next most common is usually *C. glabrata*, although this may depend in part on geography and prior antifungal exposure.
• *C. glabrata* is an important species because it is the second most frequently encountered species, causing invasive disease in many settings and exhibits reduced susceptibility to azoles (and rarely echinocandins).
• *C. krusei* is important because of resistance to fluconazole and reduced susceptibility to other antifungals.
• *C. parapsilosis* is susceptible to fluconazole but increased minimum effective concentration (MIC) to echinocandins. Strong biofilm former leading to association with central lines and implantable devices.

TABLE 27.1 **Treatment of PCP**

Indication	Regimen	Drug	Route	Dose	Comments
Moderate to severe PCP Severe PCP:	Preferred	TMP–SMX	IV	15 mg/kg per day TMP, 75 mg/kg per day SMX in 3 divided doses	Switch to PO upon clinical improvement
PaO_2 <70 mmHg or A–a O_2 gradient >35 mmHg Moderate PCP:	Alternative	Pentamidine	IV	3–4 mg/kg QD	Infuse >60 min; watch ↑/↓ glycemia, renal function, torsades de pointe
A–a O_2 gradient 35–45 mmHg; (can use PO)	Alternative	Clindamycin plus	IV	600 mg Q6H or 900 mg Q8H	Switch to PO upon improvement
		Primaquine	PO	30 mg (base) QD	Test for G6PD
	Preferred	Prednisone	PO	40 mg BID ×5 days; 40 mg QD ×5 days; 20 mg QD ×11 days	Begin ASAP and within 72 hours
Mild PCP PaO_2 ≥70 mmHg *and* A–a O_2 gradient ≤35 mmHg	Preferred	TMP–SMX	PO	2 DS (160 TMP+ 800 SMX) tablets TID	
	Alternative	TMP plus	PO	5 mg/kg TID (15 mg/kg/d)	Test for G6PD deficiency
		Dapsone	PO	100 mg QD	
	Alternative	Clindamycin plus	PO	450 mg QID or 600 mg TID	Test for G6PD deficiency
		Primaquine	PO	30 mg (base) QD	
	Alternative	Atovaquone	PO	750 mg BID	Take with food

Notes: Patients with HIV should receive 21 days of therapy; non-HIV patients should receive at least 14 days of therapy depending on severity of immunocompromise.
A-a, alveolar:arterial; *TMP*, trimethoprim; *SMX*, sulfamethoxazole; *DS*, double-strength; *G6PD*, glucose-6-phosphate dehydrogenase; *QD*, daily.
Adapted from Kovacs JA. Pneumocystis pneumonia. In: Goldman L, Schafer AI, eds. *Goldman–Cecil Medicine*, 25th ed. 2091–2099.e3.

- *C. lusitaniae:* Resistant to AMB but remains susceptible to fluconazole and echinocandins. Very rare species.
- *C. auris* is emerging as a cause of nosocomial infection. The convergence of several factors make this fungus difficult to identify, eradicate from environmental surfaces, and to treat.
- *C. auris* is capable of effective horizontal spread. Most cases of disease are due to exogenous strains, unlike other *Candida* spp., which usually emerge from endogenous microbiota already colonizing a person when they enter a hospital.
- *C. auris* can cause invasive disease such as candidemia or deep-seated infection. It also causes otomycosis (ear infections) and mastoiditis.
- Identification can be challenging because *C. auris* is typically misidentified by commercial identification systems. *C. auris* may be misidentified by VITEK-2 as *C. haemulonii* or *C. famata,* or by API-20C as *Rhodotorula glutinis, C. sake,* or *Saccharomyces cerevisiae.* The correct identification can be made by MALDI-TOF or DNA sequencing.
- *C. auris* strains are typically resistant to one or more classes of antifungals. Almost all strains are fluconazole resistant, and 50% of all isolates are resistant to two or more classes of antifungals. Rarely, panresistance is encountered making these infections untreatable.

Mucosal Candidiasis

Cutaneous Candidiasis Syndromes
- Include intertrigo, paronychia, onychomycosis, balanitis, folliculitis, generalized cutaneous candidiasis.

Oropharyngeal Candidiasis (OPC)
- Usually attributed to *C. albicans* (80%–90%).
- Risk factors include immunocompromise (HIV, diabetes, corticosteroid use, cancer), antibiotic exposure, and use of dentures.
- Clinical
  - Thrush causes mouth pain, dysgeusia (altered taste), and dysphagia.
  - Examination reveals diffuse erythema with white patches (Fig. 27.9); these can be scraped off, revealing bleeding/irritated mucosa.
- Treatment
  - Mild disease can be treated with topical clotrimazole, miconazole, or nystatin for 7–14 days. However, these treatments have high failure rates and can be difficult to tolerate due to poor taste, making fluconazole the preferred treatment in most cases.
  - Moderate to severe disease should be treated with fluconazole 100–200 mg PO daily ×7–14 days.

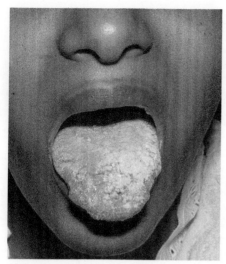

• **Fig. 27.9** Thrush. (From James WD, Berger TG, Elston DM. *Diseases resulting from fungi and yeasts.* In: *Andrews' Diseases of the Skin: Clinical Dermatology.* 12th ed. Elsevier; 2016.)

Alternatives are itraconazole solution 200 mg PO once daily or posaconazole suspension 500 mg PO BID for 3 days, then 400 mg daily for up to 4 weeks.

• When oral therapy is not tolerated, parenteral therapy with fluconazole can be considered; an echinocandin or AMB are alternatives. AMB is very rarely necessary.

Esophageal Candidiasis

• Risk factors include IC conditions such as advanced HIV infection, as well as inhaled corticosteroids, antibiotic use, and radiation therapy to the head and neck.
• Esophageal candidiasis occurs in the absence of OPC in 2/3 of cases.
• Symptoms include dysphagia, odynophagia, and retrosternal pain.
• Diagnosis is often made by response to empiric antifungal therapy. When performed, esophagoscopy may show yellow or white plaques on an erythematous background with some degree of ulceration.
  • Definitive diagnosis requires biopsy for histopathology, but in practice this is rarely done.
• **Management**
  • Fluconazole 200–400 mg PO daily ×14-–21 days is first-line treatment.
  • If unable to tolerate oral therapy, IV fluconazole or an echinocandin is recommended with de-escalation to PO fluconazole when able.
  • If disease is recurrent or recalcitrant to therapy, samples may need to be obtained by esophagoscopy and submitted for culture and antifungal susceptibility testing.

Vulvovaginal Candidiasis (VVC) (See Chapter 18)

• **Microbiology**
  • VVC is caused by *C. albicans* in the vast majority of cases.
• **Epidemiology**
  • VVC is extremely common in women of reproductive age (75% of women will experience ≥1 episode).

• Risk factors include postmenarche and premenopause (or in postmenopausal women taking hormone replacement therapy), pregnancy, corticosteroids, diabetes, and antibiotic use.
• Recurrent VVC occurs in a small subset of women; often these are caused by non-*albicans Candida* spp.

• **Presentation**
  • The most common symptoms encountered are pruritus; vaginal discharge which can range from watery to like "cottage cheese" and which is *not* malodorous; vulvar irritation; dyspareunia; external dysuria.
• **Examination**
  • Erythema, swelling of external genitalia, often pustulopapular lesions peripherally; erythema of vaginal mucosa; normal cervix.
• **Diagnosis**
  • VVC must be differentiated from bacterial vaginosis and trichomoniasis (see Chapter 18).
    • **Normal pH** (4–4.5), in contrast to bacterial vaginosis, trichomoniasis, which characteristically have pH >4.5.
    • Fungal elements are seen on KOH wet mount.
  • Culture not routinely indicated.
• **Management**
  • For uncomplicated VVC, topical antifungals recommended.
  • Alternatively: fluconazole 150 mg PO ×1.
  • Severe acute VVC, fluconazole 150 mg PO q3d ×2–3 doses
    • For VVC with fluconazole-resistant isolates, alternatives include topical intravaginal boric acid, nystatin, or flucytosine ± 3% AMB cream.
    • Recurrent VVC: induction therapy with fluconazole or topical therapy for 10–14 days, followed by fluconazole 150 mg PO weekly ×6 months.

Chronic Mucocutaneous Candidiasis

• **Epidemiology**
  • Associated with several specific defects of innate immunity.
  • These include, among others, mutations involving the following:
    • Autoimmune regulator (*AIRE*) gene.
    • Signal transducer and activation of transcription 1 (*STAT1*).
    • Interleukin-17 (IL-17) receptor.
    • *Dectin-1* deficiency.
    • Toll-like receptor 3 defect.
• **Clinical presentation**
  • Chronic noninvasive candidiasis of skin, nails, and mucus membranes.
  • Disfiguring hyperkeratotic lesions.
  • Severe esophageal candidiasis can lead to structuring.
  • Sometimes associated with autoimmune polyendocrine syndrome type 1 (also known as autoimmune polyendocrinopathy-candidiasis-ectodermal

dystrophy/dysplasia [APECED]). This autosomal recessive syndrome is characterized by CMC, hypoparathyroidism, and adrenal insufficiency, a triad present in <90% of affected patients. Additional findings may include hypogonadism, vitiligo, alopecia, malabsorption, anemia, and/or cataracts.

- Usually present from infancy but depends on subtype.
- **Diagnosis**
  - Definitive diagnosis is only by genetic analysis of *AIRE* gene for associated mutations.
  - Look for endocrinopathies such as hypothyroidism (check thyroid stimulating hormone ±free T4 and T3 levels); hypogonadism (in males, follicle-stimulating hormone [FSH] and luteinizing hormone [LH] and additionally in postmenarchal women with irregular or absent menses, measure estradiol and prolactin); hyperadrenalism (check adrenocorticotropic hormone [ACTH] and cosyntropin stimulation test); hypoparathyroidism (check calcium, phosphorus, magnesium). Pernicious anemia (characterized by macrocytic anemia and low vitamin B12 levels) may also be noted.
  - Consider an endocrine autoantibody screen (although negative results do not exclude the diagnosis).
  - Rule out other primary and secondary immunodeficiencies (check immunoglobulins, complete blood count for leukopenia, HIV test, etc).
- **Treatment**
  - Systemic fluconazole, itraconazole, or ketoconazole with unknown duration, to be guided by symptoms.

Otomycosis

- *Candida auris* is increasingly reported as a cause of community or healthcare-acquired otomastoiditis.
- This syndrome can be diagnosed by swab of discharge for fungal culture.
- The optimal therapy for *C. auris* otomycosis is not established.
- In severe cases of mastoiditis, debridement may be necessary.

Invasive Candidiasis

Candidemia

- Microbiology
  - *C. albicans* is the species most commonly implicated in invasive disease; the next most common cause is *C. glabrata* in most centers although *C. tropicalis* is more common in some regions outside North America. *C. krusei* and *C. parapsilosis* are also common causes of invasive candidiasis.
- **Epidemiology**
  - Risk factors fall into three categories: those that break down the mucocutaneous border, those that interfere with neutrophil function and count, and those that shift the microbiome in the favor of *Candida* spp.

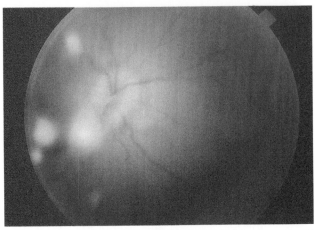

- **Fig. 27.10** *Candida* endophthalmitis. All candidemic patients should be examined for such well-demarcated, white chorioretinal lesions. (From Bicanic TA, Harrison TS. Systemic fungal infections. *Medicine*. 2014;42(1):26–30.)

These include: central venous catheter (CVC), broad-spectrum antibiotic use, recent gastrointestinal surgery, total parenteral nutrition, neutropenia.
- *C. auris* infection should be considered in patients hospitalized in areas where cases have been reported.
- **Clinical Presentation**
  - Fever and hemodynamic instability may be present, as with bacterial sepsis.
  - Complications notably include the following conditions:
    - Chorioretinitis (Fig. 27.10), which should be considered in all patients with candidemia.
    - Endocarditis is uncommon but should be considered in patients with prosthetic valves, injection drug users, and patients with persistently positive cultures.
- **Diagnosis**
  - Blood cultures are the hallmark of diagnosis; however, these are limited by slow growth of *Candida* species (2–5 days usually). In addition, blood cultures will miss ~50% of cases of invasive candidiasis (i.e., hepatosplenic disease).
  - Clinical microbiology labs usually identify species by commercial ID systems, MALDI-TOF.
    - ***Candida auris* will be misidentified** by commercial ID systems. Specifically, it will be misidentified by Vitek-2 as *C. haemulonii* most commonly, and less commonly as *C. famata*, and by API-20C as *Rhodotorula glutinis*, *Candida sake*, or *Saccharomyces cerevisiae*.
    - The correct identification can be made by DNA sequencing or MALDI-TOF.
  - Non-culture-based diagnostic assays are also commercially available (see Table 27.2).
- **Management**
  - First-line therapy for invasive candidiasis should be an **echinocandin** until speciation +/- antifungal susceptibility testing confirms fluconazole susceptible strain.

TABLE 27.2   Operating Characteristics of Non-Culture-Based Diagnostic Tests for Invasive Candidiasis

Test	Sensitivity	Specificity	Notes
1,3-β-D-glucan	75%–80%	80%	False-positives with colonization, blood products, some β-lactam antibiotics, dialysis
Combined Mannan/ anti-Mannan IG	83%	86%	↓ sensitivity in IC hosts Time needed to mount detectable response Positive results unable to distinguish acute vs. past infection
T2 magnetic resonance (T2Candida)	89%–91%	98%	Can detect 5 most common *Candida* spp., provides identification to 1 of 3 groups: *C. albicans/C. tropicalis*, *C. glabrata/C. krusei*, and *C. parapsilosis* Other species will be missed

- Alternative (in selected patients who are not critically ill and unlikely to have fluconazole-resistant strain): Fluconazole (800 mg IV/PO loading, followed by 400 mg IV/PO daily)
- Transition from echinocandin to fluconazole is recommended in patients who are stable, are infected by fluconazole-sensitive *Candida* isolates, and who have negative repeat blood cultures.
- Lipid formulation AMB is an alternative (if intolerance to, unavailability of, or isolates resistant to other antifungals).
- Dilated **ophthalmologic exam** for all cases of candidemia; this should occur within a week of diagnosis (except in neutropenic patients, who should be examined within a week of neutrophil recovery).
- **Repeat blood cultures** daily to document date of clearance of fungemia to determine duration of treatment.
- Continue treatment 2 weeks from clearance of fungemia and resolution of attributable symptoms in the absence of deep-seated infection.
- In cases of central line-associated candidemia, the CVC should be removed as early as can be safely achieved.
- Patients with *C. auris* infection or colonization need contact isolation precautions; patient rooms should be cleaned daily and terminally with a sporicidal detergent.

Chronic Disseminated Candidiasis (Hepatosplenic Candidiasis)
- **Epidemiology**
  - The most common risk factor for this syndrome is neutropenia.
- **Clinical presentation**
  - This syndrome usually affects liver and spleen. Although involvement of other organs is common, disease in these sites may be less evident on imaging.
  - Chronic disseminated candidiasis often presents as fever that does not respond to antibiotics; abdominal pain and/or elevated liver enzymes (especially alkaline phosphatase) after recovery from neutropenia.

- **Diagnosis**
  - Abdominal imaging shows hepatic and/or splenic infiltration or abscesses (Fig. 27.11).
  - Blood and biopsy cultures are often negative.
  - Biopsies will show inflammation with yeasts and – unless *C. glabrata* is implicated – pseudohyphae.
- **Management**
  - Lipid formulation AMB OR an echinocandin should be prescribed for several weeks, followed by fluconazole (so long as fluconazole-resistant isolate not suspected).
  - Treatment duration is until radiographic resolution (median treatment is 9 months).

Urinary Tract Candidiasis
- **Microbiology**
  - *Candida* spp. cause ~25% of urinary tract infections (UTIs) in patients with indwelling urinary catheters.
  - Majority of positive urine cultures can be cleared by removal or exchange of the catheter.
- **Clinical presentation**
  - *Candida* spp. can cause lower and occasionally upper UTI.
  - Renal candidiasis may be a complication of systemic candidemia.
  - UTI can be complicated by fungal balls (both in the renal pelvis and the bladder), leading to obstruction.
- **Diagnosis**
  - Asymptomatic candiduria unlikely to be clinically important.
  - Disseminated candidiasis should be *considered* in a septic patient with candiduria.
  - To make the diagnosis, consider blood cultures and renal imaging.
- **Management**
  - Asymptomatic candiduria can be managed by removal of the indwelling catheter; no treatment is required unless there is high risk for dissemination (such as in patients with neutropenia, very low birth weight infants, or undergoing a urologic procedure).

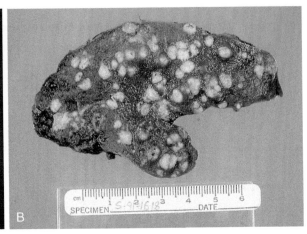

• **Fig. 27.11** Radiologic and pathologic findings in chronic disseminated candidiasis. (A) Computed tomography and (B) gross specimen showing multiple granulomatous lesions of *Candida albicans* in the liver and spleen in a 5-year-old boy with acute lymphoblastic leukemia, prolonged granulocytopenia, and fever despite amphotericin B therapy. (From Smith PB, Steinbach WJ. *Candida* species. In: Long SS, Prober CG, Fischer M, eds. *Principles and Practice of Pediatric Infectious Diseases.* 5th ed. Elsevier; 2018.)

- Symptomatic cystitis: fluconazole (if susceptible) 200 mg PO daily × 2 weeks.
- Pyelonephritis: fluconazole (if susceptible) 200–400 mg PO daily × 2 weeks.
- Management of fungal balls should include surgical intervention, plus antifungals as for pyelonephritis. If nephrostomy tubes are *in situ*, irrigation with AMB deoxycholate can be considered.

Other Yeasts

Trichosporon spp.

- **Microbiology**
  - These yeasts cause superficial and (rarely) deep infections.
  - *Trichosporon asahii* is the most common species implicated in invasive disease.
  - Other species implicated in disease:
    - *T. asteroides, T. cutaneum* cause superficial infections.
    - *T. ovoides* causes white piedra (hair shaft infection) of the scalp.
    - *T. inkin* causes white piedra of pubic hair.
    - *T. mucoides* and *T. inkin* are also rarely implicated in systemic disease.
  - Uniquely, these fungi produce septate hyphae, arthroconidia, and budding yeasts.
- **Epidemiology**
  - Risk factors for disease include medically and surgically complex patients in hospitals, including patients with malignancies or neutropenia, those taking corticosteroids, patients with prosthetic heart valves, transplantation recipients, and injection drug users.
  - The portal of entry is usually via gastrointestinal or respiratory tracts; occasionally the portal of entry is a CVC.

- **Clinical presentation**
  - Superficial fungal diseases caused by these species include white piedra, onychomycosis, and otomycosis.
  - Invasive syndromes caused by *Trichosporon* spp. include pneumonia as well as acute and chronic disseminated diseases.
    - Acute disease clinically resembles invasive candidiasis.
    - Chronic dissemination disease similar to chronic hepatosplenic candidiasis: a chronic infection of liver, spleen, other tissues after recovery from neutropenia.
- **Diagnosis**
  - Definitive diagnosis of infection is achieved through biopsy of affected tissue for histopathology and fungal culture.
  - Blood culture can sometimes be helpful for diagnosing systemic disease.
  - For chronic disseminated abdominal disease, alkaline phosphatase is usually elevated. Abdominal imaging shows hepatosplenic infiltration or abscesses.
  - *Trichosporon* spp. can cross-react with **CrAg.**
- **Treatment**
  - Minimum inhibitory concentrations are high for AMB and echinocandins and lower for triazoles.
  - Treatment of systemic disease is generally with triazoles.

Rhodotorula

- **Microbiology**
  - Usually this fungus recovered from a clinical specimen represents a contaminant, although occasionally it is a pathogen of IC hosts.
  - *Rhodotorula mucilaginosa* (formerly *R. rubra*) is the species most frequently implicated in disease.
- **Clinical presentation**
  - Syndromes include central-line associated fungemia, fever of unknown origin, and rarely meningitis.

- **Diagnosis**
  - Isolation from bloodstream should be considered diagnostic of invasive disease in the right clinical setting. Isolation from other sites may or may not represent true pathogenicity.
- **Management**
  - Removal of CVC and treatment with antifungals are appropriate in sick patients, although the evidence for either intervention is very weak.
  - AMB/flucytosine can be considered as these are generally active. *Rhodotorula* spp. are generally less sensitive to triazoles and resistant to echinocandins.

Malassezia spp.

- **Microbiology**
  - These are **lipophilic** dimorphic fungi.
  - *Malassezia furfur* species complex are most commonly implicated in causing human disease.
  - *M. pachydermatis* can be involved in invasive (but not cutaneous) disease.
  - *M. furfur* cannot synthesize medium- or long-chain **fatty acids**, growth requires exogenous supply. Knowing this can help understanding the epidemiology and improve diagnosis of infections.
    - These fungi tend to colonize oily areas of skin (scalp, shoulders, chest, back); highest colonization rate in teenagers.
    - They can contaminate parenteral lipids.
    - They are difficult to recover unless the microbiology lab is notified of the suspicion, since isolation requires use of media **enriched with fatty acid supplements** (e.g., Dixon's media, or Sabouraud dextrose agar supplemented with olive oil or tween).
  - Clinical syndromes
- Colonization is extremely common.
  - These fungi commonly colonize human skin.
  - This is most commonly noted in teenagers (>90% prevalence of colonization).
  - Colonization is extremely common among neonates in neonatal intensive care units.
  - Skin infections are the most common clinical syndrome caused by *Malassezia* spp.
- **Pityriasis (tinea) versicolor** (Fig. 27.12)
  - Clinical
    - Hypo- or hyperpigmented macules that coalesce into scaling plaques (Fig. 27.12A).
    - Usually the trunk or proximal limbs are affected.
  - Diagnosis
    - Biopsy may show yeasts and hyphae with "basket weave" splaying of the stratum corneum (Fig 27.12B).
    - Skin scrapings examined microscopically with KOH may show yeasts and hyphal forms with the classic appearance of **"spaghetti and meatballs"** (Fig. 27.12C). Calcofluor staining can also help highlight fungal elements (Fig. 27.12D).

- Treatment
  - Topical azole or terbinafine cream is usually the first-line therapy.
  - Systemic itraconazole may be needed in severe cases.
  - Patients should be aware that pigmentary changes can take many months to resolve.
- Folliculitis can also be caused by *Malassezia* spp.
- Most often, *Malassezia* spp. cause seborrheic dermatitis and dandruff.
- Systemic disease is rare.
- **Epidemiology**
  - Systemic disease occurs most commonly in **preterm neonates.**
  - Risk factors include prematurity, CVC, **parenteral lipids**, IC states.
  - Clinical findings include fever unresponsive to broad-spectrum antibiotics, bradycardia, respiratory distress, hepatosplenomegaly, lethargy.
  - The diagnosis of invasive disease can be difficult.
    - Common, nonspecific findings include leukocytosis and thrombocytopenia.
    - Bilateral pulmonary infiltrates are observed on chest X-ray in >50%.
    - Fungemia can occasionally be diagnosed by Gram stain of the buffy coat.
    - Blood cultures are usually negative in the absence of lipid-enriched media (hence the importance of communicating the clinical suspicion with the microbiology laboratory).
    - Lysis centrifugation improves recovery from blood.
- **Management**
  - Removal of CVC and discontinuation of IV lipids is usually all that is needed unless deep-seated infection is present.
  - If fungemia persists, systemic therapy (e.g., AMB or fluconazole) should be started.

Blastoschizomyces capitatus

- A yeast species formerly described as *Geotrichum capitatum* or *Trichosporon capitatum*.
- An uncommon cause of clinical infection.
- Risk factors for infection appear similar to those for *Trichosporon*: IC conditions, including neutropenia and hematologic malignancy.
- Systemic infection, including fungemia, or localized disease involving various organ sites can occur.
- Most common clinical syndrome is fever without localizing findings and which does not respond to antimicrobials.
- Diagnosis of systemic disease is usually made by blood culture.
- Optimal treatment is not established, but isolates are usually susceptible *in vitro* to AMB. Newer triazoles like itraconazole, voriconazole, and posaconazole can also be considered.

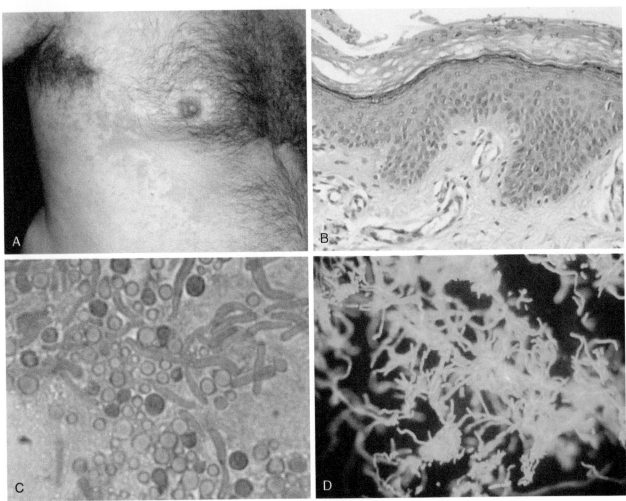

• **Fig. 27.12** Clinical, histologic, and direct microscopy findings in pityriasis versicolor. (A) Typical lesion of pityriasis versicolor on the trunk of 54-year-old man. (B) Histology of pityriasis versicolor, with evident absence of inflammatory infiltrate in the dermis and the abundant yeasts and hyphae in the entire stratum corneum (H&E stain; original magnification ×200). (C) "Spaghetti and meatballs" appearance of the hyphae and yeast cells of *Malassezia* on the direct microscopy of pityriasis versicolor skin scales stained with Parker's ink (original magnification ×1000). (D) Pityriasis versicolor skin scales after Calcofluor staining. (From Gaitanis G, Velegraki A, Mayser P., Bassukas ID. Skin diseases associated with *Malassezia* yeasts: facts and controversies. *Clin Dermatol.* 2013;31(4):455–463.)

Saccharomyces spp.

- *Saccharomyces cerevisiae* is commonly known as "baker's yeast" or "brewer's yeast."
- Occasionally, *Saccharomyces* spp. are implicated in causing human disease.
- Risk factors include immunocompromising conditions, chemotherapy, presence of a CVC, GI surgery, and antimicrobial exposure.
- Rare cases of vaginitis have been linked to commercial *S. cerevisiae* strains used in baking.
- Clinical disease includes fungemia in the majority of reports, although this is presumably distorted by the difficulty in attributing pathogenicity when isolates from other sites. Urinary tract infection, including symptomatic vaginitis, is also convincingly reported. Pneumonia and empyema have been reported, as have peritonitis, cholecystitis, and prosthetic-valve endocarditis.
- Isolation from blood culture can establish the diagnosis; isolation from other sites requires careful review of before attributing pathogenicity.
- Management should include removal of CVCs (where applicable) with or without systemic antifungals.

Further Reading

1. Pappas PG, Kauffman CA, Andes DR, et al. Clinical practice guideline for the management of candidiasis: 2016 update by the Infectious Diseases Society of America. *Clin Infect Dis.* 2016;62(4):e1–e50.
2. Kullberg BJ, Arendrup MC. Invasive candidiasis. *N Engl J Med.* 2015;373(15):1445–1456.

3. Chowdhary A, Sharma C, Meis JF. *Candida auris*: A rapidly emerging cause of hospital-acquired multidrug-resistant fungal infections globally. *PLoS Pathog*. 2017;13(5):e1006290.

4. Panel on Opportunistic Infections in HIV-Infected Adults and Adolescents. Guidelines for the prevention and treatment of opportunistic infections in HIV-infected adults and adolescents: recommendations from the Centers for Disease Control and Prevention, the National Institutes of Health, and the HIV Medicine Association of the Infectious Diseases Society of America. Available at: http://aidsinfo.nih.gov/contentfiles/lvguidelines/adult_oi.pdf.

5. Perfect JR. Cryptococcosis (*Cryptococcus neoformans* and *Cryptococcus gattii*). In: Bennett JE, Dolin R, Blaser MJ, eds. *Mandell, Douglas, and Bennett's Principles and Practice of Infectious Diseases*. Updated 8th ed. Philadelphia: Elsevier; 2015. pp. 2934–2948.

28

The Dimorphic Mycoses

LAURIE PROIA

Definitions

Thermal dimorphism: Fungi that exhibit thermal dimorphism grow in mycelial (mold) form in the environment (21–25 °C) and convert to yeast form at body temperature (37 °C) through a complex process of gene upregulation called phase transition.

Dimorphic fungi
- *Histoplasma capsulatum, H. duboisii.*
- *Blastomyces dermatitidis.*
- *Coccidioides immitis, C. posadasii.*
- *Paracoccidioides brasiliensis.*
- *Talaromyces (Penicillium) marneffei.*
- *Sporothrix schenckii.*
- *Emmonsia* spp.

Histoplasma capsulatum, H. duboisii

Epidemiology

- Histoplasmosis is the most common endemic mycosis.
- Found worldwide (every continent except Antarctica) but endemic to North America, notably the central United States and Ohio–Mississippi River valley, Central and South America, Caribbean (Figs. 28.1A and B).
- US states with highest infection rates are southern Illinois, Indiana, western Ohio, Missouri, Kentucky, Tennessee, Mississippi, and Arkansas.
- Exposure to bird or bat guano: *spelunking* (cave exploration), exposure to bird roosts, chicken coops, prison yards/school yards, or any soil exposure.
- Infection occurs with inhalation of aerosolized microconidia (spores) into the lungs.
- African histoplasmosis, caused by *Histoplasma capsulatum* var. *duboisii*, is mainly seen in West Africa and Madagascar, noted to have a "triple tropism" with infection of lymph nodes, skin (cold abscesses), and bones/joints, rarely the lungs.

Clinical Features

- 50%–90% of infections may be asymptomatic or subclinical and nonprogressive, especially in a healthy host with low-titer exposure to spores.

- Prior infection may be the incidental finding of splenic calcifications on CT scans done on persons residing in endemic regions.

Acute Pulmonary Histoplasmosis

- Influenza-like symptoms (fever, cough, chest pain) develops after ~14 day incubation; imaging may show patchy pneumonitis ± mediastinal or hilar adenopathy (which may be a clue!).
- Severity of symptoms may correlate with higher burden of spore exposure.
- Rheumatologic manifestations occur in 5%–10% and may include arthralgias, erythema nodosum or erythema multiforme, pericarditis; usually self-limited.
- Persistent mediastinal adenitis occurs in <10% with enlarged, inflamed lymph nodes compressing local structures such as the airways, pulmonary vessels, or esophagus; symptoms (e.g., cough, dyspnea, chest pain, dysphagia) may last for months and antifungal therapy is generally of no benefit.

Chronic Pulmonary Histoplasmosis

- Symptoms >6 weeks' duration with progressive pulmonary infiltrates or lung cavities (Fig. 28.2).
- More common in older men with chronic obstructive pulmonary disease (COPD); resembles pulmonary TB or lung cancer with fever, sweats, cough, hemoptysis, and weight loss with upper lobe predominance.
- Bronchopleural fistula formation rarely seen.

Disseminated Histoplasmosis

- Hematogenous spread of *Histoplasma* outside the lungs occurs in a large proportion of individuals but is limited by development of cellular immunity in healthy hosts.
- Progressive disseminated histoplasmosis more common in the elderly or those who are immunocompromised, such as persons with HIV/AIDS (CD4 <100 cells/μL),

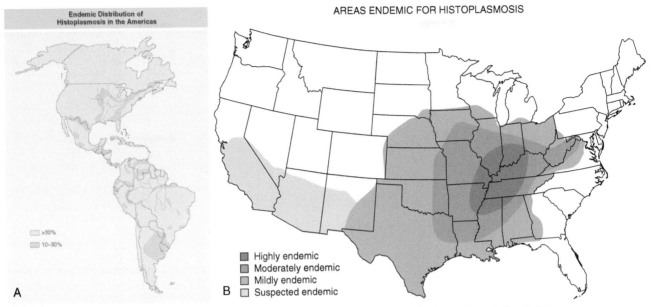

• **Fig. 28.1** Endemic distribution of histoplasmosis in the Americas. (Panel A from Cohen J, Powderly W, Opal S, eds. *Infectious Diseases*. 2nd ed. Mosby; 2004. Panel B from Miller AS, Wilmott RW. The pulmonary mycoses. In: Wilmott RW, et al., eds. *Kendig's Disorders of the Respiratory Tract in Children*. 9th ed. Elsevier; 2019.)

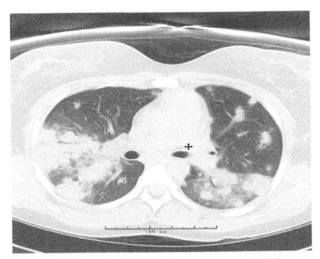

• **Fig. 28.2** CT chest showing bilateral consolidative and nodular pneumonia of pulmonary histoplasmosis in a renal transplant recipient.

solid organ transplant recipients, patients on tumor necrosis factor (TNF) antagonists, and rarely in the setting of gamma-interferon deficiency.

• Symptoms may be acute and fulminant or a more subacute "febrile wasting illness."

• Fevers, sweats, respiratory symptoms, and weight loss are common; spread through the reticuloendothelial system with lymphadenopathy, hepatomegaly, and bone marrow infiltration; adrenal insufficiency may be present.

• Other sites of involvement include GI mucosa with oral ulcers, colonic mass lesions or colitis with ulcerations; cutaneous dissemination usually characterized by a diffuse papular rash but can also manifest as a focal necrotizing cellulitis (Figs. 28.3A and B).

• Lab evaluation shows pancytopenia and transaminitis (possible clue: AST > ALT) with elevated alkaline phosphatase; diffuse reticulonodular (miliary) infiltrates on imaging.

• Histoplasma can be transmitted via organ transplant, usually manifests 2 weeks post-transplant involving allograft with secondary dissemination; usually severe and often fatal.

• May be associated with hemophagocytic lymphohistiocytosis (HLH).

Fibrosing Mediastinitis

• Thought to be a sequela of pulmonary histoplasmosis (though other causes include TB, sarcoid, lymphoma, idiopathic/autoimmune).

• An abnormal and robust host inflammatory response to *Histoplasma* antigens leads to necrotizing lymphadenitis; calcification and fibrosis occur late with airway compromise, compression of the great vessels, and entrapment of mediastinal structures.

• Histopathologic exam of tissues reveals granulomas and fibrosis with an absence of yeast (if yeast forms present, they are usually nonviable and cultures are negative).

• No effective treatment (antifungals and steroids not beneficial); stent placement may relieve airway or vessel obstruction.

Diagnosis of Histoplasmosis

• Culture is gold standard for diagnosis of chronic pulmonary and disseminated infection. Histoplasma may take up to 2 weeks to grow on fungal media.

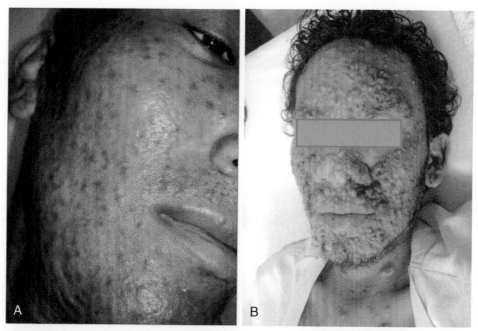

• **Fig. 28.3** Skin lesions of disseminated histoplasmosis. (Panel A from Chang P, Rodas C. Skin lesions in histoplasmosis. *Clin Dermatol.* 2012;30 (6):592–598. Panel B courtesy Andrej Spec MD.)

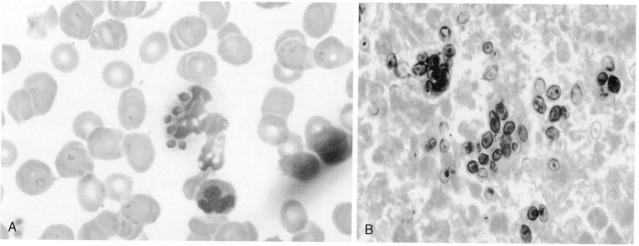

• **Fig. 28.4** Histoplasmosis. (A) Blood smear showing small intracellular yeast cells of *Histoplasma* within a neutrophil. GMS (silver) stain showing small yeast forms of *Histoplasma* (cell walls stain black). (B) *Histoplasma capsulatum* yeast forms fill phagocytes in the lung of a patient with disseminated histoplasmosis; inset shows high power of pear-shaped thin-based budding yeasts (silver stain). (Panel A from Deepe GS. *Histoplasma capsulatum* (Histoplasmosis). In: Bennett JE, Dolin R, Blaser MJ, eds. *Mandell, Douglas, and Bennett's Principles and Practice of Infectious Diseases*. 8th ed. Elsevier; 2015. Panel B from Husain A. The lung. In: Kumar V, Abbas AK, eds. *Robbins & Cottran Pathologic Basis of Disease*. 9th ed. Elsevier; 2015.)

- Small (2–4 μm) intracellular and extracellular yeast forms may be seen on direct exam of sputum/lavage fluid in patients with chronic pneumonia.
- Blood, bone marrow, or other tissue may demonstrate the characteristic yeast forms in cases of disseminated disease (Wright's stain for blood, Gomori–Methenamine–Silver (GMS) stain or periodic acid–Schiff (PAS) for tissue) (Figs. 28.4A and B).
- The *Histoplasma* antigen enzyme immunoassay (EIA) measures cell wall galactomannan in serum or urine,

can also be measured in bronchoscopic lavage fluid or cerebral spinal fluid (CSF); highest sensitivity seen with disseminated infection in immunocompromised host (>90%); may sometimes be detected in cases of severe acute pulmonary pneumonia. Cross-reactivity seen with *Blastomyces*, *Paracoccidioides*, *Talaromyces*, less common with *Coccidioides* and rarely with *Aspergillus*. A negative urine antigen does not exclude infection. Clearance of antigenuria can be indicative of treatment response.

- Antibodies to *Histoplasma* can be measured by immunodiffusion or complement fixation. Immunodiffusion detects H and M precipitin bands (M bands more commonly detected, may persist for years). Complement fixation antibody titers of >1:8 are useful for diagnosis of chronic pulmonary/mediastinal histoplasmosis; can remain positive for years, thus may be less specific for active infection.

Treatment of Histoplasmosis

Indications for Antifungal Therapy (adapted from IDSA Guidelines, 2007)

- **Definite indication**, proven or probable efficacy
  - Acute diffuse pulmonary infection, moderately severe or severe symptoms.
  - Chronic cavitary pulmonary infection.
  - Disseminated or central nervous system (CNS) infection.
- **Uncertain indication**, unknown efficacy
  - Acute focal pulmonary infection, asymptomatic, or mild symptoms that persist.
  - Mediastinal lymphadenitis.
  - Mediastinal granuloma, inflammatory syndromes treated with corticosteroids.
- **Not recommended**, unknown efficacy or ineffective
  - Mediastinal fibrosis.
  - Pulmonary nodule, isolated, asymptomatic.

Treatment

Pulmonary Histoplasmosis

Acute, self-limited, healthy host	None, observation
Mild to moderate	Itraconazole
Moderate to severe	Lipid formulation of amphotericin B (L-AMB, 3–5 mg/kg per day) for 1–2 weeks until clinical improvement, then stepdown to oral itraconazole

Disseminated Histoplasmosis

Mild to moderate	Itraconazole
Moderate to severe	L-AMB for 1–2 weeks until improvement, then stepdown to itraconazole
CNS infection	L-AMB for up to 4–6 weeks as tolerated and until improvement, then stepdown to oral itraconazole (could consider voriconazole due to better CNS/CSF penetration)

- Avoid fluconazole, echinocandins due to poor *in vitro* activity.
- Avoid azoles in first trimester pregnancy due to potential teratogenicity.
- Itraconazole capsules require gastric acid for enhanced bioavailability (take with food, acidic beverage), concomitant use of antacids, H2 blocker, or proton pump inhibitor (PPI) may be cause for treatment failure.

- Negative inotropy and congestive heart failure (CHF) exacerbation may be seen with itraconazole use.
- No comparative data on use of newer azoles (voriconazole, posaconazole, isavuconazole), although *in vitro* activity and some clinical efficacy reported.

Blastomyces dermatitidis

Epidemiology

- Blastomyces thrives in moist, acidic soil rich in organic debris along rivers and waterways.
- Ohio and Mississippi River basin, upper midwestern United States (blastomycosis was formerly known as Chicago's Disease), down through the south central US and regions bordering the Great Lakes (northern New York and Canadian provinces) (Fig. 28.5).
- Historically affected men with outdoor occupations or hobbies, e.g., forestry workers or hunters and their dogs (dogs may be harbingers for community outbreaks).
- Primary infection acquired through inhalation of airborne conidia (spores) from soil; cutaneous inoculation rarely reported with laboratory accidents or farming injuries.

Clinical Features

- ~50% of infected individuals will have asymptomatic or subclinical infection.
- Incubation period typically 4–6 weeks.
- More severe infection has been linked to a newly described strain of *Blastomyces dermatitidis*, renamed *Blastomyces gilchristii*.

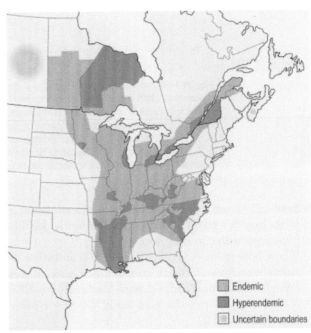

- **Fig. 28.5** Endemic regions for blastomycosis in North America. (From Amstead GM, et al. Histoplasmosis, blastomycosis, coccidioidomycosis and cryptococcosis. In: Guerrant RL, Walker DH, Weller PF, eds. *Tropical Infectious Diseases: Principles, Pathogens and Practice.* 3rd ed. Elsevier; 2011.)

Acute Pulmonary Blastomycosis

- Influenza-like illness with fever, fatigue, productive cough.
- Some spontaneous cures of infection reported.
- May progress to adult respiratory distress syndrome (ARDS).

Chronic Pulmonary Blastomycosis

- Respiratory symptoms lasting generally 2–6 months or more.
- Lobar infiltrate or mass-like consolidation on imaging may be mistaken for TB or lung cancer; often misdiagnosed or diagnosis delayed (Fig. 28.6).

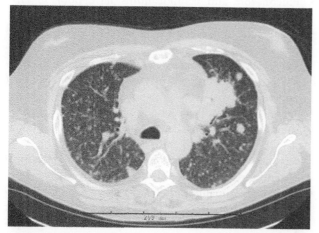

• **Fig. 28.6** CT scan of a liver transplant recipient with severe pulmonary blastomycosis; note the large left upper lobe cavitary mass lesion, numerous smaller nodules and diffuse reticulonodular infiltrates.

- Typical patient is treated for community-acquired pneumonia with numerous courses of antibacterials without response, eventual diagnosis made by bronchoscopy or lung biopsy.
- May spread contiguously through tissue planes like *Actinomyces* or tuberculosis (TB); pneumonia may be complicated by empyema, adjacent rib or vertebral osteomyelitis, or a draining sinus tract through the chest wall.

Disseminated Blastomycosis

- Extrapulmonary dissemination more common with *Blastomyces* than with *Histoplasma* or *Coccidioides*, seen in 25%–75% of patients.
- Extrapulmonary disease occurs in both immunocompetent and immunocompromised although individuals with impaired cell-mediated immunity (e.g., HIV, diabetes, solid organ transplant, chronic steroid or TNF antagonist use) are more likely to disseminate.
- Patients may present with signs of dissemination without active pulmonary infection (although may see an area of parenchymal scar on chest X-ray or computed tomography).
- Common sites of extrapulmonary spread include: skin, bone/joint, genitourinary (GU) tract, and CNS.
- Skin is most common site for dissemination; lesions may be single or multiple, papular or pustular. Chronic skin lesions are ulcerative or verrucous (resembles basal cell carcinoma with raised pearly border). Skin lesions may occur anywhere on body but predilection for face, especially along nasolabial folds (Figs. 28.7A and B).

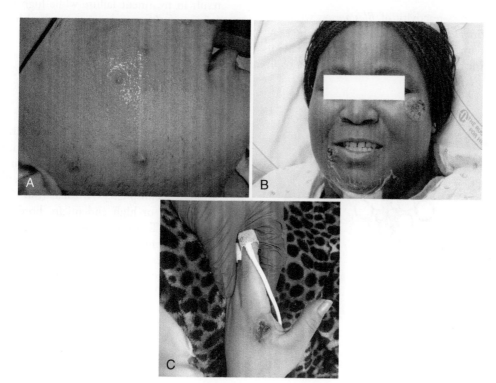

• **Fig. 28.7** Skin lesions of disseminated blastomycosis. (A) Papulopustular rash. (B and C) Large, raised, verrucous lesions.

- Osteoarticular blastomycosis results in chronic osteomyelitis, usually of long bones or axial skeleton, or septic arthritis; spinal infection may present as epidural abscess, paravertebral, or psoas abscess with adjacent vertebral osteomyelitis.
- GU tract infection usually manifests as epididymoorchitis or chronic prostatitis in men (sterile pyuria); GU tract infection in women is rare.
- CNS blastomycosis develops in 5%–10% of cases of disseminated infection, more common in diabetics; usually with chronic headache and/or focal neurologic deficit associated with a single mass lesion, sometimes concomitant meningitis is present.

Diagnosis of Blastomycosis

- Gold standard is culture with growth usually observed in 5–10 days on fungal media (Sabaroad's dextrose agar), but a presumptive diagnosis may be made by direct visualization of the characteristic yeast form in body fluids or tissue.
- Yeast cells are large (8–15 μm), have a refractile cell wall, and produce a single bud with a broad base of attachment between mother and daughter cell (broad-based budding) (Fig. 28.8).
- Sputum or BAL fluid may be treated with 10% KOH or Calcofluor white; GMS or PAS stains may aid in identification of yeast forms in tissue.
- Inflammatory response to *Blastomyces* is both neutrophilic and cell-mediated; on histopathologic exam of tissue can see both microabscesses and granulomas.
- *Blastomyces* antibody testing is available commercially, but historically serologies have lacked sensitivity and specificity.
- High degree of cross-reactivity of *Blastomyces* with the serum/urine *Histoplasma* antigen enzyme immunoassay (EIA); a *Blastomyces*-specific EIA for measurement of galactomannan in serum or urine is available (may still cross-react with *Histoplasma*).

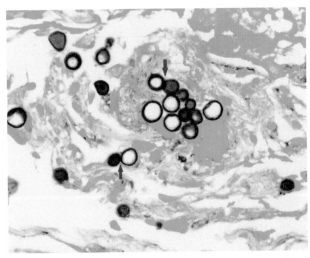

• **Fig. 28.8** GMS stain of lung biopsy with a cluster of yeast cells and two examples of broad-based budding (*arrows*).

Treatment of Blastomycosis

- Treatment generally recommended for all patients, even those with mild infection due to the potential for untreated pulmonary blastomycosis to progress or disseminate.
- Most patients with pulmonary blastomycosis present with prolonged or chronic symptoms that would warrant treatment.
- Itraconazole may be given first-line to those with mild to moderate, non-CNS, infection.
- A lipid formulation of AMB should be given first-line to patients with moderate to severe pulmonary blastomycosis, CNS infection, or women in early pregnancy; later may stepdown to oral azole such as itraconazole (could consider voriconazole for CNS blastomycosis).
- Fluconazole and echinocandins have poor *in vitro* activity.
- Therapeutic drug monitoring is recommended for all patients taking either formulation of itraconazole (capsule or suspension) owing to the drug's variable bioavailability (low serum levels may be a reason for treatment failure).
- All azoles inhibit the hepatic cytochrome P450 system to some degree; in transplant recipients itraconazole inhibits CYP3A4 and will raise calcineurin inhibitor (e.g., tacrolimus) and cyclosporine levels leading to toxicity of coadministered drug (renal, CNS side-effects).
- Voriconazole mainly inhibits the isoenzyme CYP2C19 and to a lesser degree CYP2C9 and CYP3A4; genetic polymorphisms in CYP2C19 may also lead to interpatient variability in voriconazole metabolism; thus therapeutic drug monitoring required (low serum vori levels (<1 μg/mL) may be seen with rapid metabolizers and result in treatment failure while high serum vori levels (>5.5 μg/mL) may be associated with toxicity such as encephalopathy).

Coccidioides immitis, C. posadasii

Epidemiology

- *C. immitis* causes infection in southern California, *C. posadasii* causes infection outside of southern California; the two species are indistinguishable clinically.
- Thrives in soil found in the arid, desert regions of the Western hemisphere: Arizona (the "Cocci corridor" is a region of high endemicity bordered by Phoenix, Scottsdale, Tucson), New Mexico, southern California, west Texas, northern Mexico, and parts of Central and South America; some isolated foci of infection found in Washington state, Dinosaur National Monument in Utah (Fig. 28.9).
- Cases often occur outside of endemic areas, usually in persons with recent travel to or residence in the southwestern United States; spores may be carried on fomites that cover the surfaces of automobiles or produce that is harvested in endemic regions and spread remotely.

- Increased infection rates after rainy seasons, dust storms, earthquakes.
- Exists as a single-celled arthroconidia (spore) in the environment; primary portal of entry is the lungs and one inhaled spore may produce infection.

- Inhaled arthroconidia revert from their characteristic barrel shape to a yeast phase consisting of an enlarged spherule (up to 70 μm); endospores pinch off the inner cell membrane and, once mature, rupture from the spherule and are released into surrounding tissue (they in turn become spherules and the process continues).

Acute Pulmonary Coccidioidomycosis

- Incubation period usually 1–3 weeks; approximately 60% of infections are subclinical.
- May mimic community-acquired pneumonia with fever, fatigue, cough, pleurisy, dyspnea (aka "San Joaquin Valley Fever"); high erythrocyte sedimentation rate (ESR) and peripheral eosinophilia in 10%–15%.
- More severe symptoms can develop with higher inoculum exposures.
- Associated dermatologic and rheumatologic syndromes ("Desert Rheumatism") more common in women than men, consist of polyarthralgias, erythema nodosum, or erythema multiforme, may be a clue for primary *Coccidioides* infection.
- Infection may resolve without sequelae although 5% will develop a residual lung nodule or thin-walled cavity; these lesions usually resolve in 1–2 years but can enlarge or rupture into adjacent pleura; may require surgical resection (Fig. 28.10).

Chronic Pulmonary Coccidioidomycosis

- May develop in diabetics, immunocompromised hosts.
- Productive cough, chest pain, dyspnea, and hemoptysis with constitutional symptoms of night sweats, fatigue, and weight loss.
- Chest imaging shows consolidation and cavitation; hilar adenopathy may be present.

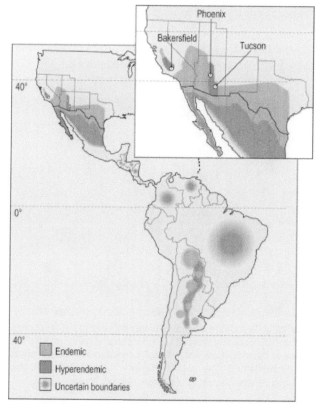

• **Fig. 28.9** Map showing regions of southwestern United States, Central and South America endemic for *Coccidioides*. (From Amstead GM, et al. Histoplasmosis, blastomycosis, coccidioidomycosis and cryptococcosis. In: Guerrant RL, Walker DH, Weller PF, eds. *Tropical Infectious Diseases: Principles, Pathogens and Practice*. 3rd ed. Elsevier; 2011.)

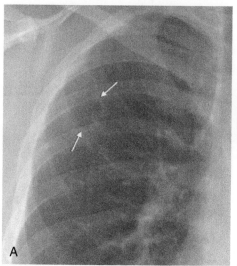
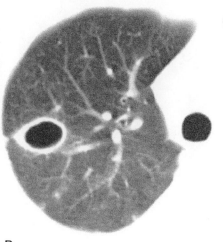

• **Fig. 28.10** Thin-walled cavity of *Coccidioides* in the right upper lung on chest X-ray and chest CT. (Courtesy of Drs. Rebecca M. Lindell and Thomas E. Hartman, Mayo Clinic, Rochester, MN.)

Disseminated Coccidioidomycosis

- Extrapulmonary, hematogenous dissemination is rare, usually seen in <1%, and typically occurs during the first year of infection.
- More common in persons with cell-mediated immunodeficiencies but can develop in otherwise normal hosts.
- High-risk groups for dissemination include male gender, pregnancy, persons of African or Filipino ancestry, and immunosuppression due to HIV, organ transplant, TNF antagonist use.
- Most common site for dissemination is the meninges, can also spread to skin, bone/joints (especially knees or vertebral column sometimes with adjacent paraspinal abscess) (Fig. 28.11).
- Most common symptom of *Coccidioides* meningitis is chronic progressive headache; patients may present with a febrile stroke due to vasculitis or concomitant back pain from spinal arachnoiditis. CSF shows lymphocytic pleocytosis, low glucose, and high protein; CSF eosinophils may be elevated; CSF culture usually negative.
- Donor organ transmission of *Coccidioides* reported; usually occurs within 2 weeks post-transplant; severe and often fatal.

Diagnosis of Coccidioidomycosis

- Culture is gold standard for diagnosis, but histopathologic exam of body fluids or tissue may reveal the characteristic large spherule with endospores (Figs. 28.12 and 28.13).
- Mature colonies are highly infectious, alert lab personnel when *Coccidioides* suspected.
- Serologic testing is useful; *Coccidioides* antibodies may take a few weeks to develop with an initial IgM response within 1–2 weeks, IgG detected later and may last for months.

- Anticocci antibodies may be measured by immunodiffusion, EIA or complement fixation; IgM and IgG measured by EIA more sensitive at detection of early infection and useful for initial screening but can lack specificity (especially if IgM alone is positive); immunodiffusion is more specific than EIA.
- *Coccidioides* antibodies measured quantitatively by complement fixation can be detected in serum or CSF; often useful for diagnosing meningeal disease as CSF culture is usually negative. High or rising IgG titers may be associated with progressive or disseminated disease.

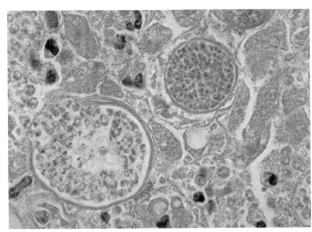

• **Fig. 28.12** Yeast form of *Coccidioides* showing the large spherule (mother cell) containing intracellular endospores; spherule on left shows rupture of the mother cell with release of endospores into adjacent tissue. (From Klatt EC. The lung. In: Kumar V, Abbas AK, eds. *Robbins and Cotran Pathologic Basis of Disease.* 9th ed. Elsevier; 2015.)

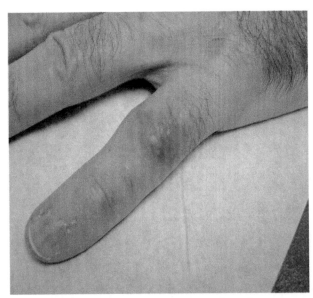

• **Fig. 28.11** Skin lesion of disseminated *Coccidioides.*

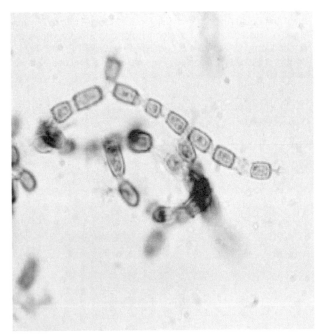

• **Fig. 28.13** Barrel-shaped arthroconidia of the mycelial (mold) form of *Coccidioides.* (From Shehab KW, Shehab ZM. Coccidioidomycosis. In: Cherry JD, Harrison GJ, Kaplan SJ, Steinbach WJ, Hotez PJ, eds. *Feigin and Cherry's Textbook of Pediatric Infectious Diseases.* 8th ed. Elsevier; 2019.)

- Similar to the *Histoplasma* antigen assay, there is a *Coccidioides* antigen assay for detection of galactomannan in urine, serum or CSF; sensitivity higher in immunocompromised hosts with disseminated infection

Treatment of Coccidioidomycosis

- In general, antifungal therapy is **not** indicated for healthy hosts with early uncomplicated infection since most will resolve their illness without treatment.
- Treat high-risk individuals (patients at risk for more severe disease or dissemination), patients with severe or prolonged pneumonia or disseminated infection.
- Fluconazole or itraconazole are effective.
- A lipid formulation of amphotericin B should be used as initial therapy for severe infection or in pregnant women in the first trimester (azoles teratogenic).
- Meningeal *Coccidioides* is fatal if untreated and requires lifelong therapy due to high risk for relapse; initial therapy is with high-dose fluconazole (400–1200 mg daily), which has excellent CNS/CSF penetration. For severe or refractory CNS infection, intrathecal amphotericin B administered via lumbar or ventricular instillation has been used.
- Echinocandins poorly active.

Paracoccidioides brasiliensis, P. lutzii

Epidemiology

- Paracoccidioidomycosis is a common systemic mycosis found in South America (was formerly referred to as South American blastomycosis).
- Majority of cases occur in Brazil, followed by Venezuela, Colombia, Ecuador, Argentina (Fig. 28.14).
- Traditionally affected persons living in rural, agricultural regions of Brazil, though increasing incidence in urban areas paralleling the HIV epidemic.
- Acquired through inhalation of soil-residing spores, but symptomatic infection is uncommon (<5%) and determined by underlying host immune responses.
- Primary mucocutaneous infection from direct inoculation is rare but possible.
- Infection may manifest many years after an individual has left an endemic region, average latency period may be >10–15 years.
- There are two patterns of infection: acute/subacute (juvenile) form and chronic form.

Acute/Subacute Paracoccidioidomycosis

- Represents <10% of all cases and is more common in children and young adults.
- Acute form of disease may also be seen in people with HIV.
- Manifested by disseminated infection with spread through the reticuloendothelial system.

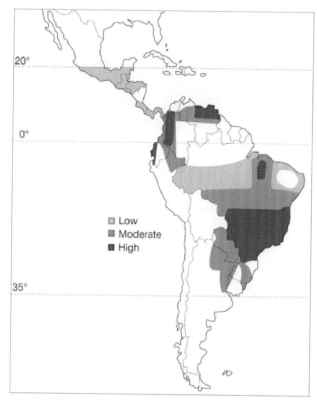

• **Fig. 28.14** Endemic regions for *Paracoccidioides* with highest incidence in Brazil. (From Negroni R, Anstead GM, Graybill JR. Paracoccidioidomycosis. In: Guerrant RL, Walker DH, Weller PF, eds. *Tropical Infectious Diseases: Principles, Pathogens and Practice.* 3rd ed. Elsevier; 2011.)

- Symptoms include fever, weight loss, peripheral and central adenopathy, hepatosplenomegaly, pancytopenia from bone marrow infiltration; pneumonia uncommon.
- Disease mimics disseminated TB, *Histoplasma,* or lymphoma; persons with acute paracoccidioidomycosis and risk factors should be tested for HIV infection.

Chronic Paracoccidioidomycosis

- 90% of cases of paracoccidioidomycosis present as the chronic form, symptoms may develop months or years following primary infection.
- Usually seen in men, 30–60 years old, who work in farming or agriculture.
- Manifests clinically as pneumonia with mucous membrane involvement in >50%. Oral mucosa most frequently affected, usually presents as painful ulcers (Figs. 28.15A and B).
- Can disseminate from lungs to other sites, including skin, lymph nodes, adrenal glands, CNS similar to TB or *Histoplasma.*

Diagnosis of Paracoccidioidomycosis

- Diagnosis can be made by culture of sputum, blood, skin, and other tissue; may take 3–4 weeks to grow.
- **Direct exam of body fluids or tissue reveals the characteristic yeast form**: a large, round mother cell with multiple, narrow-based budding daughter cells

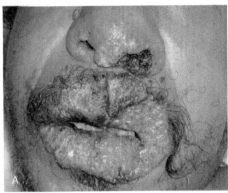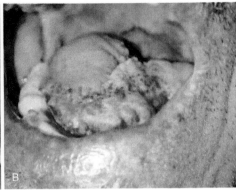

• **Fig. 28.15** Mucocutaneous lesions of *Paracoccidioides*. (Panel A from Restrepo A, Tobón AM, Cano LE. Paracoccidioidomycosis. In: Bennett JE, Dolin R, Blaser MJ, eds. *Mandell, Douglas, and Bennett's Principles and Practice of Infectious Diseases*. Updated 8th ed. Elsevier; 2015. Panel B from Negroni R, Anstead GM, Graybill JR. Paracoccidioidomycosis. In: Guerrant RL, Walker DH, Weller PF, eds. *Tropical Infectious Diseases: Principles, Pathogens and Practice*. 3rd ed. Elsevier; 2011.)

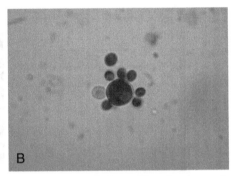

• **Fig. 28.16** Yeast phase of *Paracoccidioides* showing characteristic multiple budding daughter cells resembling Mickey Mouse ears (A lower left) or pilot wheel (B). (Panel A from Restrepo A, Tobón AM, Cano LE. Paracoccidioidomycosis. In: Bennett JE, Dolin R, Blaser MJ, eds. *Mandell, Douglas, and Bennett's Principles and Practice of Infectious Diseases*. 8th ed. Elsevier; 2015. Fig. 269.1. Panel B from Negroni R, Anstead GM, Graybill JR. Paracoccidioidomycosis. In: Guerrant RL, Walker DH, Weller PF, eds. *Tropical Infectious Diseases: Principles, Pathogens and Practice*. 3rd ed. Elsevier; 2011.)

attached to it resembling a "pilot's wheel" on a ship or, if there are only two daughter buds, "Mickey Mouse" ears (Figs. 28.16A and B).
• Serologic assays are available but may be less sensitive in immunocompromised individuals.

Treatment of Paracoccidioidomycosis

• Most azoles, amphotericin B, and trimethoprim–sulfamethoxazole (TMP–SMX) are active.
• Itraconazole recommended for mild to moderate disease; lipid formulation of amphotericin B or high-dose TMP–SMX for severe infection; high-dose TMP–SMX or voriconazole may also be used for CNS infection.
• Use of TMP–SMX may require longer course of treatment to prevent relapse.

Talaromyces (Penicillium) marneffei

Epidemiology

• Major opportunistic pathogen in people with HIV living in Southeast Asia or in immunocompromised individuals with extensive travel to endemic regions.

• Endemic to Southeast Asia, especially northern Thailand and Vietnam, northeast India, southern China (Guangxi Province), Hong Kong, and Taiwan (Fig. 28.17).
• The exact ecologic niche of *Talaromyces* is unknown, but infection is presumed to result from inhalation of spores from the environment; rarely infection acquired through cutaneous inoculation has been described.

Clinical Features of Talaromycosis

• Majority of affected patients are men with underlying cell-mediated immunodeficiency due to HIV infection (CD4 <100 cells/μL), organ transplant, chronic steroid use, or gamma-interferon deficiency; older age and malnutrition may also increase risk.
• Most infections are asymptomatic or subclinical; symptomatic disease results from reactivation of latent infection with subsequent dissemination particularly to organs of the reticuloendothelial system (lymph nodes, liver, spleen, bone marrow).
• Talaromycosis may be mistaken for disseminated TB, histoplasmosis or melioidosis; common symptoms include fever, weight loss, cough, diarrhea, lymphadenopathy, hepatosplenomegaly, and pancytopenia.

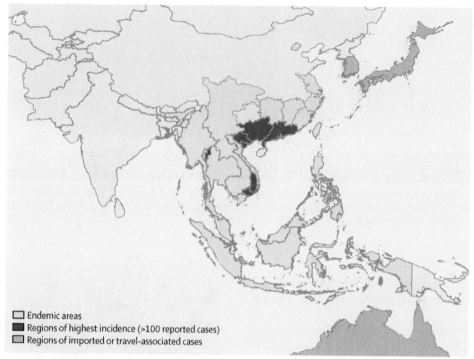

• **Fig. 28.17** Endemic regions for talaromycosis. (Reprinted with permission from Elsevier. The Lancet. From Limper AH, Adenis A, Le T, Harrison TS. Fungal infections in HIV/AIDS. *Lancet Infect Dis*. 2017;17: 334–343.)

• Diffuse papular skin rash seen in 60%–70%; papules may develop central umbilication resembling disseminated cutaneous cryptococcosis or molluscum contagiosum.
• Positive blood cultures (fungemia) present in 50% of patients.
• Lung imaging reveals diffuse reticulonodular (miliary) infiltrates but may see mass-like consolidation or cavitary lesions.

Diagnosis of Talaromycosis

• Grows readily in culture of sputum, blood, skin scrapings, lymph node tissue, and bone marrow, usually within 2–7 days.
• A unique feature of the mold form is production of a soluble red pigment that diffuses into the agar.
• Intracellular and extracellular yeast cells are oval-shaped and divide by fission, not budding, thus have a characteristic central or transverse septum.
• Can see cross-reactivity of *Talaromyces* with galactomannan antigen assays used to diagnose *Histoplasma* or *Aspergillus* infection.
• Serologic assays not yet proven useful.

Treatment of Talaromycosis

• Itraconazole given for mild to moderate infection, lipid formulation of amphotericin B for moderate to severe infection, including CNS disease.
• Voriconazole may be given as an alternative to itraconazole; fluconazole has poor activity and echinocandins not recommended.
• In general, initiation of antiretroviral therapy (ART) should be delayed for 2 weeks after start of antifungal treatment in people with HIV with CD4 >50 cells/μL to lessen risk for immune reconstitution inflammatory syndrome (IRIS); no delay in ART recommended if CD4 <50 cells/μL.
• Secondary prophylaxis with a maintenance dose of itraconazole (200 mg once daily) is recommended for people with HIV until there is immune reconstitution with ART, usually CD4 >100 cells/μL for at least 6 months.

Sporothrix spp.

Epidemiology

• Found worldwide though most cases reported from North and South America, particularly Mexico, Colombia, Brazil, and Uruguay; a region of hyperendemicity has been observed in children and adults living in the rural central highlands of Peru.
• *Sporothrix schenckii* is the primary pathogenic species although other less common species have been identified around the world (e.g., *Sporothrix brasiliensis* in Brazil).
• Infection results from traumatic inoculation of soil or other vegetative matter containing the fungus into skin and subcutaneous tissue.
• Historically referred to as "rose handler's disease" with infection resulting from the prick of a rose thorn.
• *Sporothrix* found in soil, straw, hay, wood, and sphagnum moss; risk groups include gardeners, landscapers, florists, forestry workers, or construction workers.
• Zoonotic transmission is common; cutaneous inoculation may result from a bite or scratch from a digging animal, especially cats, dogs, even armadillos (sporotrichosis described in armadillo hunters in South America).
• Inhalation of aerosolized *Sporothrix* may result in pulmonary infection.

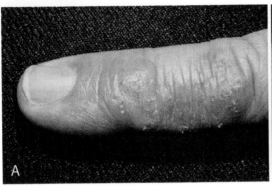
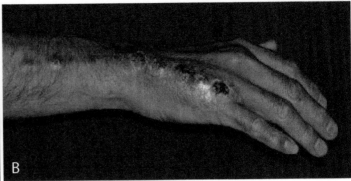

• **Fig. 28.18** Sporotrichosis. (A) Chronic indurated plaque on digit. (B) Characteristic lymphocutaneous pattern of spread. (Panel A from Cohen BA. *Pediatric Dermatology*, 4th ed. Elsevier; 2013. Panel B courtesy Adrina Motta MD, Universidad El Bosque, Bogota, Colombia.)

Clinical Features of Sporotrichosis

- Patterns of infection include lymphocutaneous form, pneumonia, bone/joint infection, and disseminated disease.
- Disseminated infection occurs in individuals with underlying immune defects including malnutrition, alcoholism, diabetes, and HIV infection.
- **Lymphocutaneous sporotrichosis**
  - Initial site of inoculation usually involves finger or hand but may be anywhere on body depending on site of trauma.
  - Within a few weeks a painless papule develops at the site of inoculation. This lesion may remain as a fixed papule or plaque; in some cases the papule will ulcerate followed by secondary spread along regional lymphatics, local adenopathy may be absent (Figs. 28.18A, 28.18B).
  - Differential diagnosis for a sporotrichoid lesion (nodular lymphangitis) includes *Nocardia, Mycobacterium marinum* (or other atypical mycobacteria), and *Leishmania.*
- **Pulmonary sporotrichosis**
  - Seen more commonly in middle-aged men with alcoholism or chronic obstructive pulmonary disease.
  - Can present as a fibrocavitary pneumonia resembling TB, outcomes usually poor.
- **Osteoarticular sporotrichosis**
  - May cause septic arthritis or osteomyelitis and results from direct inoculation of the fungus through skin into the underlying joint space or bone.
  - Alternatively hematogenous dissemination from the lungs to a single joint or multiple joints may occur.
- **Disseminated sporotrichosis**
  - Disseminated infection is rare and most often described in individuals with underlying advanced HIV infection.
  - Can disseminate from the lungs or a site of lymphocutaneous infection.
  - May spread to any organ such as eye, meninges, liver, spleen, bone marrow, and lymph nodes; may also be associated with diffuse cutaneous involvement.

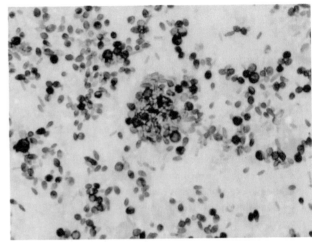

• **Fig. 28.19** GMS stain of small oval-shaped yeast forms of *Sporothrix.* (Courtesy Dr. Rene Gerhard, São Paulo, Brazil.)

Diagnosis

- Culture of skin, sputum, or other tissue remains the gold standard for diagnosis; *Sporothrix* grows readily on fungal media (Sabaroad's dextrose agar), usually within 1–2 weeks.
- Yeast cells are small and oval, sometimes referred to as cigar-shaped (Fig. 28.19).
- Histopathologic exam of tissue may demonstrate a mixed neutrophilic and granulomatous inflammatory response, similar to that seen with *Blastomyces.*
- Serologic assays not useful.

Treatment

- Infection does not resolve without treatment, even in healthy hosts or those with the fixed cutaneous form.
- Itraconazole considered the treatment of choice for mild to moderate infection, including lymphocutaneous and osteoarticular disease or uncomplicated pneumonia.
- Amphotericin B, preferably a lipid formulation, preferred for moderate to severe sporotrichosis with step down to oral itraconazole for a prolonged course.
- Fluconazole is less effective than itraconazole and considered second-line therapy; terbinafine appears effective but clinical data limited.

- Oral saturated solution of potassium iodide (SSKI) has been used to treat sporotrichosis, particularly before the availability of azoles; treatment now replaced by itraconazole but SSKI may still be prescribed in developing countries due to low cost. Side-effects such as metallic taste, emesis, and salivary gland enlargement may limit its use.

- Local hyperthermia may be effective treatment for fixed cutaneous sporotrichosis, especially in pregnant women in whom azoles are contraindicated.

Emmonsia spp.

- Soil-dwelling dimorphic fungi found worldwide.
- Some species associated with granulomatous lung infection in rodents.
- Rare cause of human disease but disseminated infection observed in individuals with advanced HIV infection and in solid organ transplant recipients.
- May be misdiagnosed as disseminated histoplasmosis.
- Largest series of emmonsiasis described in 13 people with HIV in South Africa, median CD4 16 cells/μL.
- Associated with fever, fungemia, pneumonia (imaging may mimic pulmonary TB), and diffuse skin lesions including papules, crusted plaques, and ulcers
- Grows readily on fungal media; yeast colonies are small and oval-shaped with single or multiple narrow-based buds.

- Recommended treatment with amphotericin B followed by step down to itraconazole.

Further Reading

1. Wheat LJ, Freifeld AG, Kleiman MB, Baddley JW, et al. Clinical practice guidelines for the management of patients with histoplasmosis: 2007 update by the Infectious Diseases Society of America. *Clin Infect Dis.* 2007;45:807–825.
2. Chapman SW, Dismukes WE, Proia LA, et al. Clinical practice guidelines for the management of blastomycosis: 2008 update by the Infectious Diseases Society of America. *Clin Infect Dis.* 2008;46:1801–1812.
3. Galgiani JN, Ampel NM, Blair JE, et al. 2016 Infectious Diseases Society of America (IDSA) Clinical practice guideline for the treatment of coccidioidomycosis. *Clin Infect Dis.* 2016;63:717–722.
4. Kauffman CA, Bustamante B, Chapman SW, et al. Clinical practice guidelines for the management of sporotrichosis: 2007 update by the Infectious Diseases Society of America. *Clin Infect Dis.* 2007;45:1255–1265.
5. Shikanai-Yasuda MA, Mendes RP, Colombo AL, et al. Brazilian guidelines for the clinical management of paracoccidioidomycosis. *Rev Soc Bras Med Trop.* 2017;50:715–740.
6. Supparatpinyo K, Khamwan C, Baosoung V. Disseminated *Penicillium marneffei* infection in Southeast Asia. *Lancet.* 1994;344:110–113.
7. Nelson KE, Sirisanthana T. Disseminated *Penicillium marneffei* infection in a patient with AIDS. *N Engl J Med.* 2001;344:1763.
8. Kawila R, Chaiwarith R, Supparatpinyo K. Clinical and laboratory characteristics of *Penicilliosis marneffei* among patients with and without HIV infection in Northern Thailand. *BMC Infect Dis.* 2013;13:464.
9. Kenyon C, Bonorchis K, Corcoran C, et al. *Emmonsia*: a dimorphic fungus causing disseminated infection in South Africa. *N Engl J Med.* 2013;369:1416–1424.

29
Monomorphic Mold Infections

PASCHALIS VERGIDIS

Microbiology

Hyaline hyphomyces are molds that have colorless, septate hyphae and produce arthroconidia. They include *Aspergillus*, *Fusarium*, and *Penicillium*.

Aspergillus

- Members of the genus *Aspergillus* grow rapidly. They mature within 3 days. On histology *Aspergillus* forms septate hyphae (3–12 μm in diameter) that demonstrate dichotomous branching at approximately 45° angles (Fig. 29.1). Hyphae are nearly parallel to one another.
  - *A. fumigatus* is the most common species.
  - *A. terreus* is resistant to amphotericin B.
  - *A. flavus* can cause sinusitis without tissue invasion in the immunocompetent host.
  - *A. niger* is usually colonizing the airways but can sometimes be associated with invasive disease. *A. niger* can cause otomycosis, which is a noninvasive disease.
- *Aspergillus* is ubiquitously found in solid, water, air, and decaying vegetation.
- Dispersed spores have caused disease outbreaks after hospital construction or renovation.

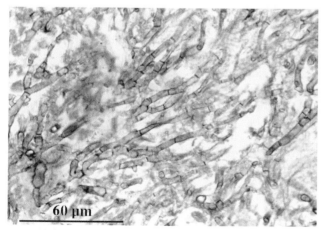

• **Fig. 29.1** Septate hyphae of *Aspergillus* with dichotomous branching at approximately 45° angles. (From Kaminski's Slide Atlas, University of Adelaide. https://mycology.adelaide.edu.au/.)

Fusarium

- *F. solani* and *F. oxysporum* are the most common species associated with human disease.
- *Fusarium* produces characteristic fusoid macroconidia (banana or canoe-shaped macroconidia) (Fig. 29.2). On histology *Fusarium* forms septate hyphae (3–8 μm in diameter) that branch at acute angles.

Penicillium

- *Penicillium* spp. are commonly colonizing the airways without causing disease.
- See also *Talaromyces marneffei* (formerly *Penicillium marneffei*) in Chapter 28 (Dimorphic Fungi).

Zygomycetes

- Zygomycetes are a class of fungi that form broad, ribbon-like hyphae (3–25 μm in diameter) that have no or very few septa (Fig. 29.3). Branching is irregular, nondichotomous, sometimes at right angles.
- The Zygomycetes include *Rhizopus*, *Mucor*, *Rhizomucor*, *Cunninghamella*, *Lichtheimia* (formerly *Absidia*), and other species.
- *Rhizopus* and *Rhizomucor* produce rootlike hyphae (rhizoids).
- Disease risk factors include poorly controlled diabetes mellitus with hyperglycemia and ketoacidosis, hematologic malignancy/HSCT/SOT, corticosteroid use, skin and soft tissue infection in severe trauma (combat injury, tornados, post-tsunami).

Scedosporium

- Produces a pale to yellow-brown diffusible pigment. Produces septate hyphae (2–4 μm in diameter). Resembles *Aspergillus* but demonstrates dichotomous branching at 60° to 70° angles.
- *Scedosporium apiospermum* (asexual form of *Pseudallescheria boydii*).
- *Lomentospora prolificans* (no asexual form).

Dematiaceous Fungi

- This is a diverse group of fungi found in the soil and air. They grow on plants and in organic debris. They produce dark colonies due to melanin pigment in their cell walls.
- Many infections are caused by traumatic implantation from the environment into the cutaneous or subcutaneous tissue.

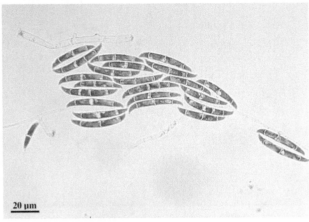

• **Fig. 29.2** Banana-shaped macroconidia typical of *Fusarium* spp. (From Kaminski's Slide Atlas, University of Adelaide. https://mycology.adelaide.edu.au/.)

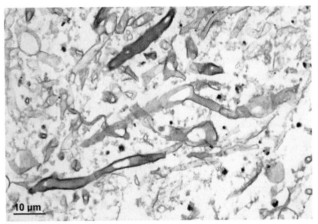

• **Fig. 29.3** Ribbon-like aseptate hyphae of Mucor. (From Kaminski's Slide Atlas, University of Adelaide. https://mycology.adelaide.edu.au/.)

- Pulmonary infection can occur by inhalation. The disease can disseminate.
- Most important human pathogens: *Alternaria, Bipolaris, Curvularia,* and *Exserohilum.*
- Eumycetoma and chromoblastomycosis are distinct entities caused by dark-walled fungi.
  Dermatophytes
- Dermatophytes are filamentous fungi that can digest and obtain nutrients from the keratin.
- Most commonly dermatophytosis is caused by *Microsporum canis, Trichophyton rubrum,* and *Epidermophyton floccosum.*

Invasive Pulmonary Mycoses

Clinical Syndromes

- The most common cause of invasive pulmonary mycoses is *Aspergillus.*
- Risk factors for invasive aspergillosis include severe and prolonged neutropenia, hematopoietic stem cell transplant (HSCT), graft-versus-host disease, solid organ transplant (SOT), tumor necrosis TNF-α antagonists, chronic corticosteroid treatment, AIDS, chronic

granulomatous disease. Among SOT recipients the risk is highest in lung transplant recipients.
- Other pulmonary mold infections typically occur in patients with severe neutropenia and HSCT/SOT recipients. These include the zygomycetes, other hyaline hyphomycetes like *Fusarium,* and dematiaceous molds such as *Alternaria, Bipolaris,* and *Curvularia.*
- Lung infections are usually the primary site of entry. The infection may disseminate to other tissues (including the central nervous system).

Pathogenesis

- Inhaled conidia germinate and transform into hyphae upon entry into the lungs.
- Vascular invasion causes thrombosis and tissue infarction. Vessel disruption can cause hemoptysis.
- Angioinvasion leading to necrosis is the hallmark of mucormycosis. If the spores are swallowed by immunocompromised patients during periods of malnutrition, gastrointestinal mucormycosis may develop. This rare syndrome mainly affects the stomach and may lead to rupture of the hollow organs with secondary bacterial infections in addition to the mold infection.
- Mucormycosis may present as breakthrough infection on antifungal prophylaxis effective against *Aspergillus* but not *Mucor* (such as voriconazole or echinocandin prophylaxis).
- Scedosporiosis results from inhalation but has also been reported after near-drowning in dirty fresh water. Pneumonia with dissemination to the central nervous system can occur in this setting.

Clinical Presentation

- Cough, dyspnea, pleuritic chest pain, and hemoptysis are common in invasive pulmonary aspergillosis. The diagnosis should be considered in high-risk patients having persistent fever despite the use of broad-spectrum antibiotic treatment. Other clinical features include pleural effusion and pneumothorax. Symptoms may be blunted due to impaired host defenses in the immunocompromised host.
- Ulcerative *Aspergillus* tracheobronchitis occurs typically among lung transplant recipients and is characterized by the presence of extensive pseudomembranous or ulcerative lesions.
- Fungemia is uncommon except for *Fusarium* infections. Disseminated disease can rapidly progress to death.
- Pulmonary mucormycosis may present as a necrotic mass. The disease can manifest with hemoptysis and may extend to the mediastinum or pericardium through angioinvasion.

Diagnosis

- **Invasive aspergillosis**
  - Diagnosis is typically made by recovery of *Aspergillus* in respiratory samples of high-risk patients with consistent radiographic findings.

- Serum *Aspergillus* galactomannan: sensitivity 82% in patients with neutropenia. Sensitivity is lower in SOT recipients. Bronchoalveolar lavage (BAL) fluid galactomannan has increased sensitivity compared to serum. Note that galactomannan can be positive in other mycoses (such as histoplasmosis, fusariosis).
- Serum beta-D-glucan is associated with low sensitivity and low specificity for the diagnosis of aspergillosis.
- Imaging: pulmonary nodular infiltrates are found in aspergillosis and other mold infections. The halo sign presents as ground glass opacity surrounding a nodule and reflects hemorrhage in the setting of angioinvasion. Cavitation occurs late in the course of disease.
- **Fusariosis**
  - Beta-D-glucan is released by *Fusarium* spp. The assay is not specific.
  - *Aspergillus* galactomannan may cross-react and give positive result.
  - Radiographic findings are similar to other invasive mold infections (pulmonary nodules, halo sign, cavitation).
  - High rates of fungemia occur in invasive disease (unlike other mold infections).
- **Pulmonary mucormycosis**
  - The diagnosis is typically established by histopathology.
  - Tissue cultures have low sensitivity due to the friability of the nonseptate hyphae. The yield may be improved by mincing (and not homogenizing) the tissue sample.
  - *Aspergillus* galactomannan and beta-D-glucan assays are negative in mucormycosis.
  - Cavitation occurs in pulmonary disease. Tissue thrombosis can result in wedge-shaped infarcts.
- **Scedoporiosis**
  - The diagnosis is usually established by culture. Histopathology may show angioinvasion and thrombosis.

Treatment

- **Invasive aspergillosis**
  - Primary regimen: voriconazole is associated with improved survival and fewer side-effects compared to amphotericin B. In a randomized controlled trial, isavuconazole was found to be noninferior compared to voriconazole for the treatment of invasive mold disease.
  - A lipid formulation of amphotericin B or posaconazole can be used alternatively. Better serum concentrations are achieved with the use of delayed-release posaconazole tablets compared to the oral suspension.
  - Amphotericin B, posaconazole, and isavuconazole have activity against *Mucorales* and other non-*Aspergillus* molds and are useful for empiric treatment.
  - Combination treatment is not routinely recommended. In a randomized controlled study among patients with hematologic malignancies and HSCT recipients, combination with anidulafungin failed to demonstrate superiority compared to voriconazole monotherapy. However, mortality was lower with combination therapy in the galactomannan-positive group. Combination treatment may be considered in patients with severe, prolonged neutropenia or those with elevated serum/BAL galactomannan.
- **Invasive fusariosis**
  - It is generally recommended to use an amphotericin B lipid formulation in combination with voriconazole until antifungal susceptibilities are available. Of note, *Fusarium* spp. are intrinsically resistant to the echinocandins.
  - Adjunctive treatments include granulocyte colony-stimulating factor (CSF), granulocyte-macrophage CSF and granulocyte infusions but their efficacy is largely unproven.
- **Mucormycosis**
  - A lipid formulation of amphotericin B (such as liposomal amphotericin B 5–10 mg/kg) is used for primary treatment.
  - Combination treatment with an echinocandin may be beneficial.
  - Adjunctive treatment with deferasirox failed to demonstrate benefit and may actually cause harm.
  - Posaconazole or isavuconazole can be used as salvage or step-down therapy once the disease is controlled.
  - Other measures include: (i) surgical debridement of affected tissue; (ii) correction of hyperglycemia, ketoacidosis; (iii) reduction of immunosuppression (if possible); (iv) granulocyte CSF, granulocyte-macrophage CSF, granulocyte infusions.
  - Mucormycosis is associated with high mortality rates among HSCT and SOT recipients.
- **Scedosporiosis**
  - *Scedosporium apiospermum* is typically resistant to amphotericin B. Voriconazole should be used for treatment.
  - *Lomentospora* (formerly *Scedosporium*) *prolificans* is usually resistant to all antifungal agents. Surgical debridement should be undertaken. Reduction in immunosuppression should be considered. Combination antifungal treatment may be beneficial. Synergy with terbinafine and echinocandins has been reported *in vitro*.

Chronic Pulmonary Aspergillosis

Clinical Syndromes

- Chronic pulmonary aspergillosis (CPA) is typically encountered in patients with underlying structural lung disease (pre-existing lung cavity due to tuberculosis or non-tuberculous mycobacterial infection, prior thoracic surgery, etc.).
- Chronic pulmonary aspergillosis typically affects middle-aged patients, predominantly male.

Disease Forms

- Aspergillus nodules: One or more nodules that are typically measuring <3cm and do not cavitate.

- Chronic cavitary pulmonary aspergillosis is the most common form. It is characterized by the presence of multiple cavities that may or may not contain an aspergilloma. If left untreated, cavitary disease may progress to chronic fibrosing pulmonary aspergillosis. Extensive fibrotic destruction can lead to loss of lung function.
- Subacute invasive aspergillosis occurs in mildly immunocompromised or very debilitated patients. The disease has similar features with chronic cavitary pulmonary aspergillosis but progresses more rapidly.
- Aspergilloma is a fungal ball within a pulmonary or pleural cavity or an ectatic bronchus (Fig. 29.4). This can be a complication of chronic cavitary pulmonary aspergillosis or subacute invasive aspergillosis.

Clinical Presentation

- The disease presents with dyspnea, chronic productive cough, and constitutional symptoms such as weight loss, malaise, and anorexia.
- Aspergillomas may be asymptomatic.
- Hemoptysis is a serious, potentially life-threatening complication.

Diagnosis

- Elevated *Aspergillus* IgG.
- Growth of *Aspergillus* from sputum/BAL cultures, strongly positive BAL *Aspergillus* galactomannan.
- Histopathology demonstrating fungal hyphae consistent with *Aspergillus*.
- Imaging: chronic cavitary pulmonary aspergillosis is characterized by areas of consolidation associated with one or more thick-walled lung cavities that may contain aspergillomas. Aspergillomas present as solid, round, or oval intracavitary masses. They do not enhance on contrast CT imaging.

Treatment

- Azole therapy provides benefit in progressive/symptomatic disease and may be useful in preventing or treating

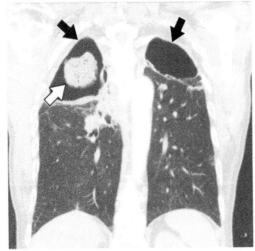

- **Fig. 29.4** Aspergilloma (fungus ball) within a right upper lobe lung cavity.

hemoptysis. Response to therapy is generally slow and duration of treatment may be prolonged (6–12 months or longer).
- Voriconazole is the primary antifungal used in the treatment of CPA. Alternative antifungals are itraconazole, posaconazole, and isavuconazole.
- Tranexamic acid can be used to control mild to moderate hemoptysis. Severe hemoptysis is managed by bronchial artery embolization.
- Single aspergillomas can be resected surgically.

Allergic Bronchopulmonary Aspergillosis

- **Clinical syndrome**
  - Allergic bronchopulmonary aspergillosis (ABPA) is a hypersensitivity reaction in response to airway colonization with *Aspergillus* among patients with asthma or cystic fibrosis.
- **Pathogenesis**
  - ABPA is caused by an aberrant inflammatory host response to *Aspergillus*.
- **Clinical presentation**
  - ABPA is characterized by bronchial mucoid impaction. During exacerbations of the disease patients present with transient pulmonary infiltrates. Central bronchiectasis occurs after years of disease. ABPA can progress to pulmonary fibrosis or chronic pulmonary aspergillosis.
- **Diagnostic criteria**
  - Predisposing condition (one must be present): asthma, cystic fibrosis.
  - Obligatory criteria (both must be present): elevated *Aspergillus* IgE. Elevated total IgE (typically >1000 IU/mL).
  - Other criteria (at least two must be present): precipitating serum antibodies or elevated *Aspergillus* IgG, radiographic pulmonary opacities consistent with ABPA, eosinophilia (>500 cells/µL) in glucocorticoid-naïve patients.
  - Patients with severe asthma, not fulfilling criteria for ABPA, may have severe asthma with fungal sensitization.
- **Treatment**
  - Treatment is aimed at controlling the allergic response and reducing fungal burden.
  - Corticosteroid treatment is recommended for exacerbations of the disease.
  - In a randomized trial, itraconazole given for 16 weeks significantly reduced corticosteroid use, reduced IgE levels, and improved exercise tolerance and pulmonary function. Itraconazole is usually used because of the history of studies performed. There is no reason to believe that other *Aspergillus*-active azoles would not be efficacious.
  - Interaction between itraconazole and some inhaled corticosteroids may lead to Cushing's syndrome.
  - Relapse after discontinuing antifungal therapy is common. Long-term antifungal therapy may be necessary.

- Avoidance of fungal exposure (house renovation, composting, farming) may prevent exacerbations.

Ocular Disease

- **Clinical syndromes**
  - Keratitis results from traumatic introduction or poor hygiene practices of contact lens wearers. An outbreak due to *Fusarium* spp. linked to contaminated contact lens solution occurred in 2004–2006. *Aspergillus* keratitis can result from trauma or corneal surgery. Swimming in natural bodies of freshwater with contacts is a risk factor.
  - *Aspergillus* is the most common cause of mold endophthalmitis. The disease is usually exogenous. Endogenous endophthalmitis typically occurs in intravenous drug users and immunocompromised patients with disseminated disease.
  - Sinus mucormycosis may extend to the orbital space causing periorbital edema, proptosis, chemosis, and preseptal edema. Involvement is usually unilateral.
- **Diagnosis**
  - Diagnosis of keratitis is established by obtaining corneal scrapings for Calcofluor stain and fungal culture.
  - The diagnosis of mold endophthalmitis is established by culture of the vitreous or aqueous fluid.
- **Treatment**
  - Keratitis is treated with natamycin eye drops. Alternatively, amphotericin B eye drops can be used.
  - Endophthalmitis is treated by intravitreal injection of amphotericin B or voriconazole in combination with systemic voriconazole (voriconazole has good penetration into the vitreous fluid). Antifungal therapy should be combined with vitrectomy.

Invasive Fungal Sinusitis

- **Clinical syndrome**
  - Invasive fungal sinusitis occurs in patients with uncontrolled diabetes, neutropenia, HSCT/SOT recipients, and those receiving corticosteroid treatment. The infection can cause local invasion and dissemination.
  - Agents of invasive fungal sinusitis include *Aspergillus*, *Mucor*, *Rhizopus*, *Fusarium*, *Pseudallescheria boydii*, and the dematiaceous fungi (such as *Alternaria*, *Bipolaris* and *Curvularia* spp.).
- **Clinical presentation**
  - Invasive fungal sinusitis presents with fever, epistaxis, sinus discharge, and headache.
  - A black necrotic eschar in the nasal mucosa is a characteristic finding but is not always present. The disease may progress to perforation of the nasal septum.
  - Complications include periorbital edema, visual loss, diplopia, ptosis, ophthalmoplegia, proptosis, cavernous sinus thrombosis, and cerebral abscess.
  - Mucormycosis can extend into the orbit or brain in patients with diabetic ketoacidosis or profound neutropenia.

- **Diagnosis**
  - Culture of sinus aspirates is helpful in diagnosing the disease.
  - The diagnosis is established by histopathology demonstrating tissue invasion.
  - Consider invasive fungal sinusitis if radiographic evidence of pansinusitis in severely immunocompromised individuals.
- **Treatment**
  - A lipid formulation of amphotericin B should be used for empiric treatment.
  - If mucormycosis has been ruled out, the infection can be treated with voriconazole.
  - Surgical debridement may be required.
  - After clinical improvement, treatment can be stepped down to an oral agent (posaconazole and isavuconazole are active against *Mucor*).

Allergic Fungal Rhinosinusitis

- **Clinical syndrome**
  - Allergic fungal rhinosinusitis (AFRS) is an allergic fungal reaction that results in the accumulation of eosinophilic mucin among immunocompetent patients.
  - The disease is mainly caused by dematiaceous fungi (*Alternaria*, *Bipolaris*, *Curvularia*) and *Aspergillus* spp.
- **Pathogenesis**
  - AFRS is caused by an aberrant inflammatory host response to dematiaceous fungi and *Aspergillus*.
- **Clinical presentation**
  - AFRS is a form of chronic rhinosinusitis often associated with nasal polyposis and sometimes ABPA. Exacerbations can follow a bacterial or viral infection.
- **Diagnostic criteria**
  - AFRS is characterized by chronic rhinosinusitis in the presence of nasal polyposis and eosinophilic mucin with fungal hyphae in the paranasal sinuses. Histopathology does not demonstrate evidence of tissue invasion. Fungus-specific IgE is elevated.
- **Treatment**
  - Corticosteroid treatment can control the inflammatory response and result in shrinking of the polyps. Relapse is common after short courses of corticosteroid treatment.
  - Endoscopic sinus surgery with polyp removal is indicated if medical management fails. Surgical treatment should be followed by systemic glucocorticoid therapy.
  - Itraconazole may be beneficial in patients with refractory disease or in patients with frequent exacerbations.

Central Nervous System Infection

Clinical Syndromes

- Cerebral aspergillosis is usually accompanied by pulmonary infection in the immunocompromised host. Isolated cerebral disease can affect intravenous drug users.

- Central nervous system (CNS) mucormycosis usually results from extension of rhinosinusitis. Isolated CNS disease can again be encountered in intravenous drug users.
- Brain abscess by dematiaceous fungi is most commonly caused by *Cladophialophora bantiana* and typically occurs in the immunocompromised host.
- A multistate outbreak of fungal meningitis among patients who received epidural methylprednisolone injections contaminated with *Exserohilum* spp., a dematiaceous mold, occurred in 2012.
- Disseminated *Scedosporium* infection in the immunocompromised host has a predilection for the CNS.

Clinical presentation

- Cerebral fungal infection may present with mental status changes, headaches, or focal neurologic deficits. CNS infection is associated with high mortality.

Diagnosis

- The diagnosis is established by histopathology or culture.
- The cell wall melanin of dematiaceous fungi may appear yellowish-brown on hematoxylin and eosin stain. Use of Fontana–Masson stain may allow easier identification of these dark-walled fungi.
- The imaging findings are nonspecific. Abscesses present as ring-enhancing lesions.

Treatment

- Treatment for brain abscess involves surgical drainage/ excision in combination with antifungal treatment.
- Voriconazole is the drug of choice for *Aspergillus* brain abscess.
- Mucormycosis is treated with liposomal amphotericin B. Posaconazole or isavuconazole can be considered for step-down therapy after clinical improvement.
- CNS infection due to dematiaceous fungi should probably be treated with liposomal amphotericin B followed by voriconazole (or another triazole).
- *Scedosporium apiospermum* is resistant to amphotericin B. Voriconazole is the treatment of choice.

Dermatophytosis

Clinical Syndromes

- Tinea corporis.
- Tinea pedis (athlete's foot).
- Tinea cruris (crural fold of groin).
- Tinea capitis (scalp).
- Tinea barbae (beard hair).
- Onychomycosis.

Clinical Presentation

- Tinea corporis presents as a pruritic annular scaling patch or plaque that spreads centrifugally followed by central clearing. This gives the impression of a ring (hence the term ringworm infection) (Fig. 29.5). The condition can be misdiagnosed as eczema or psoriasis.
- Tinea pedis can present in one of the three following forms: interdigital (pruritic, erythematous erosions or scales), hyperkeratotic (hyperkeratotic eruption of the soles and medial/lateral foot surface) or inflammatory (vesicular or bullous lesions). The main symptom is pruritus. The skin usually cracks and may become macerated. Main complications are bacterial cellulitis and onychomycosis.
- Tinea cruris (jock itch) presents with scaling of the groin area. The rash may spread to the perineal or perianal area.
- Tinea capitis typically occurs in young children. The disease presents with scaling of the scalp associated with a variable degree of erythema, inflammation, and alopecia. Pruritus is common. The infection may resemble seborrheic dermatitis.
- Onychomycosis typically occurs in the presence of infection of the toe or palmar skin. Most commonly presents with distal and subungual involvement.

Diagnosis

- Skin scrapings of affected areas demonstrate segmented hyphae with potassium hydroxide (KOH) preparation.
- The infecting organism can be recovered by culture of skin scrapings or nail clippings.

Treatment

- Dermatophytosis is usually managed by topical agents such as azole antifungals (miconazole, clotrimazole, or other).

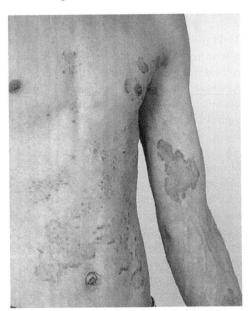

• **Fig. 29.5** Multiple ringworm lesions in a pediatric patient with tinea corporis.

- Systemic antifungals are reserved for extensive disease or for patients who failed topical therapy. The main oral antifungal used to treat dermatophytosis is terbinafine. Alternatively, itraconazole or fluconazole can be used.
- Hepatic failure is a rare but severe side-effect of terbinafine use.
- Topical treatment is usually ineffective for onychomycosis. Systemic treatment (with terbinafine or itraconazole) is given for several weeks. Urea paste can be added to remove residual areas of infection.

Other Cutaneous Mold Infection

Clinical Syndromes

- Fusariosis can present as localized cutaneous disease (cellulitis) or disseminated disease with multiple erythematous lesions (papules, nodules, or necrotic skin lesions). The most classic presentation is **toe cellulitis surrounding onychomycosis** in a neutropenic patient, which then turns into a disseminated necrotic rash (Fig. 29.6).
- *Scedosporium* can cause skin infection from direct inoculation (typically traumatic).
- Minor trauma typically results in inoculation of agents of phaeohyphomycosis (dematiaceous fungi). The infection is more prevalant in males and has been associated with outdoor activities such as farming and woodcutting, usually while barefoot.
- Eumycetoma and chromoblastomycosis are distinct entities caused by dark-walled fungi. Infection typically occurs after traumatic inoculation of the organism, most commonly in tropical and subtropical areas.
- Healthcare-associated outbreaks due to *Mucorales* have been associated with adhesive bandages, hospital linens, and construction. These usually present as necrotic lesions resembling ecthyma gangrenosum at the contact site.

Clinical Presentation

- Invasive fusariosis may present as refractory fever in a neutropenic patient with metastatic skin lesions at different stages. The necrotic lesions may resemble ecthyma gangrenosum. In a study of HSCT recipients, metastatic skin lesions were encountered in 75% (see Fig. 29.6).
- Cutaneous mucormycosis can present in the form of plaques, vesicles, nodules, or ulcerations. Deeper involvement may present with necrotizing fasciitis, myositis, or osteomyelitis.
- *Scedosporium* infection can cause papular skin lesions that progress to necrosis. Another presentation is chronic subcutaneous infection (mycetoma).
- Subcutaneous phaeohyphomycosis typically presents as a single erythematous nodule, usually on the extremities. In rare cases the infection may disseminate in immunocompromised patients.
- Eumycetoma (Madura foot) is a chronic subcutaneous skin and soft tissue infection usually affecting

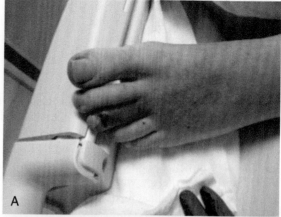
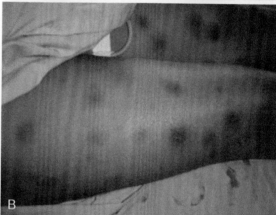

• **Fig. 29.6** (A) *Fusarium*-associated toe infection resembling cellulitis surrounding onychomycosis. (B) Disseminated *Fusarium* rash, resembling multiple ecthyma gangrenosum. (Panel A from Biesbroeck LK, Shinohara MM. Inpatient Consultative Dermatology. *Med Clin North Am.* 2015;99(6):1349–1364. © 2015. Panel B from Narayanan G, et al. Disseminated *Fusarium* fungemia in a patient with acute myeloid leukemia. *Mayo Clin Proc.* 2016;91(4):542–543. © 2016.)

the lower extremity (typically single foot). It is most commonly caused by *Madurella mycetomatis*. It typically affects healthy adults who work in rural areas and have frequent exposure to soil (such as farmers). The disease presents with nodular lesions and sinus tracts draining macroscopic grains. The infection may extend to the bone. The lesions may evolve over months to years.

- Chromoblastomycosis is a chronic, localized fungal infection of the skin and subcutaneous tissue usually involving the lower extremities. Most commonly it is caused by *Fonsecaea pedrosoi*. Frequently the lesions are warty or cauliflower-like. The lesions may persist for many years. Many cases have been reported in Madagascar.

Diagnosis

- Madura foot can be diagnosed by the microscopic examination of the grains. Culture of the grains will establish a microbiologic diagnosis. Imaging can be used to determine the extent of the disease (such as bone involvement).

- The diagnosis is confirmed by the identification of muriform organisms on KOH preparation. The infecting fungal organism can be recovered by culture of skin biopsy specimens.

Treatment

- Eumycetoma caused by *M. mycetomatis* is treated with itraconazole for 6–24 months. Typical surgical debulking is employed after weeks of antifungal therapy. Relapse rates after debulking of large lesions remain high.
- Chromoblastomycosis is difficult to cure even with prolonged antifungal therapy with itraconazole or terbinafine. Treatment modalities include surgical removal and topical treatments such as cryotherapy.
- Madura foot and chromoblastomycosis are prevented by avoiding skin trauma in endemic areas (wearing of shoes and protective clothing covering the extremities).

Further Reading

1. Leeflang MM, Debets-Ossenkopp YJ, Visser CE, et al. Galactomannan detection for invasive aspergillosis in immunocompromised patients. *Cochrane Database Syst Rev.* 2015;(12):CD007394.
2. Maertens JA, Raad II , Marr KA, et al. Isavuconazole versus voriconazole for primary treatment of invasive mould disease caused by *Aspergillus* and other filamentous fungi (SECURE): a phase 3, randomised-controlled, non-inferiority trial. *Lancet.* 2016;387(10020):760. Epub 2015 Dec 10.
3. Marr KA, Schlamm HT, Herbrecht R, et al. Combination antifungal therapy for invasive aspergillosis: a randomized trial. *Ann Intern Med.* 2015;162(2):81–89.
4. Stevens DA, Schwartz HJ, Lee JY, et al. A randomized trial of itraconazole in allergic bronchopulmonary aspergillosis. *N Engl J Med.* 2000;342(11):756.
5. Nucci M, Marr KA, Queiroz-Telles F, et al. *Fusarium* infection in hematopoietic stem cell transplant recipients. *Clin Infect Dis.* 2004;38(9):1237–1242.

30
Arthropod-Borne Diseases

ALFREDO J. MENA LORA

Arthropod-borne diseases are of growing importance in the United States and around the world. These diseases are transmitted through vectors and are among the most common causes of infectious diseases morbidity and mortality worldwide. Over the past century, a dramatic change in our ability to travel among regions of the world has caused a shift in the distribution of these diseases. In the mid-20th century, dengue became endemic in tropical and subtropical regions in the Americas. In recent years, Zika virus transitioned from a handful of cases in a distant part of Africa, to a major public health threat affecting millions of people in tropical and subtropical regions worldwide. Changing temperatures and climate patterns may cause the geographic distribution of these diseases to shift. Arthropod-borne diseases will remain high yield for clinical practice and for review boards.

MAJOR ARTHROPOD-BORNE DISEASES IN THE UNITED STATES

Lyme Disease

- Lyme disease is a tickborne multi-stage condition caused by *Borrelia burgdorferi*. It is the most common tickborne disease in the United States. In Europe, other strains may cause Lyme disease, such as *Borrelia garinii* and *Borrelia afzelii*.
- Vectors: *Ixodes scapularis* (deer tick), *Ixodes pacificus*.
- Reservoirs depend by region. In the northeastern United States, the principal reservoir hosts of *B. burgdorferi* are the white-footed mouse, chipmunks, short-tailed and masked shrews, and eastern gray squirrels. In California, *B. burgdorferi* has been isolated from several host species including western gray squirrels, dusky-footed wood rats, and California kangaroo rats.
- Geography: New England, Mid-Atlantic states, Wisconsin, Minnesota, Pacific Northwest (Table 30.1).
- Season: spring, summer, or fall, when the weather is warm.

- Clinical presentation: multiple stages.
  - Early Lyme: typically occurs within 30 days of a tick bite.
    - Early localized: target lesion at bite site (erythema migrans). Flu-like symptoms may occur (Fig. 30.1). Erythema migrans may appear one week after tick bite. History of tick exposure may not be elicited, as >25% of patients do not recall a tick bite. Thus obtaining epidemiologic history with geographic exposure is key.
    - Early disseminated: spread of infection to skin and other organs. Multiple smaller lesions of erythema migrans, carditis with varying degrees of AV block, myocarditis, and neurologic complications. Third-degree heart block can occur and may be life-threatening. Neurologic manifestations of Lyme disease can include cranial nerve palsies, radiculitis, or aseptic meningitis.
  - Late Lyme: has an onset of months to years after tick bite.
    - Manifestations can include arthritis, encephalitis, peripheral neuropathy, lymphocytoma, or acrodermatitis chronica.
    - Lyme arthritis typically involves joint swelling and pain in weight-bearing joints. Most patients have knee involvement. Effusion may have neutrophilic pleocytosis and may be confused as bacterial septic arthritis.
    - Cranial nerve palsies can occur with CN VII, the most commonly affected cranial nerve. Radiculitis with pain, paresthesia, or weakness may occur as well.
    - Aseptic meningitis with lymphocytic pleocytosis may occur. Lyme CSF index, a ratio of CSF Lyme Ab to serum Lyme Ab, normalized for protein amount, can assist in the diagnosis of neuroborreliosis. A suggestive ratio is greater than 1–1.2.
    - Bannwarth syndrome is a manifestation of early neuroborreliosis characterized by painful radiculoneuritis and lymphocytic pleocytosis. It is often associated with cranial nerve involvement and peripheral paresis.

TABLE 30.1 **Diseases, Ticks, and Geography**

Disease	Vector	Geography
RMSF, tularemia	American dog tick *Dermacentor variabilis*	American dog tick (*Dermacentor variabilis*)
RMSF, tularemia	Rocky Mountain wood tick *Dermacentor andersoni*	Rocky Mountain wood tick (*Dermacentor andersoni*)
Ehrlichiosis, tularemia, and STARI	Lone Star tick *Amblyomma americanum*	Lone Star tick (*Amblyomma americanum*)
Anaplasmosis, babesiosis, and Lyme disease.	Blacklegged tick or deer tick *Ixodes scapularis*	Blacklegged tick (*Ixodes scapularis*)

TABLE 30.1	Diseases, Ticks, and Geography—cont'd	
Disease	**Vector**	**Geography**
Anaplasmosis, Lyme disease	 Western blacklegged tick *Ixodes pacificus*	 **Western blacklegged tick** *(Ixodes pacificus)*
RMSF (*R. rickettsia*)	 Brown dog tick *Rhipicephalus sanguineus*	 **Brown dog tick** *(Rhipicephalus sanguineus)*
Spotted fever (*R. parkeri*)	 Gulf Coast tick *Amblyomma maculatum*	 **Gulf Coast tick** *(Amblyomma maculatum)*

RMSF, Rocky Mountain spotted fever; STARI, southern tick-associated rash illness.

- Acrodermatitis is a blue–red discoloration on distal extremities with swelling over months to years. Skin becomes thin and atrophic, and sclerotic plaques may develop.
- Lyme arthritis is usually monoarticular and involves major joints such as the knee.
- Post-Lyme syndrome: Post-Lyme syndrome, or post-treatment Lyme disease syndrome, is a nonspecific fatigue syndrome that may occur after Lyme disease. It is considered a postinfectious fatigue syndrome. Long-term antibiotics do not improve symptoms.

- Diagnosis: testing will depend on stage.
  - Early Lyme with erythema migrans or disseminated erythema migrans is a clinical diagnosis. Serologies may be falsely negative in early infections. Serology is only sent for atypical or difficult cases.
  - All other manifestations of Lyme disease require a combination of risk factors, manifestations, and serologic diagnosis. EIA plus western blot is performed and should be combined with end-organ disease.

- For central nervous system (CNS) disease, cerebrospinal fluid (CSF) studies, serologies, and Lyme CSF index (ratio of Lyme antibody in CSF to serum).
- Treatment: will depend on stage and severity of disease (Fig. 30.2).
  - Early disease can be treated with amoxicillin or doxycycline for 10 days.
  - CNS manifestations require IV ceftriaxone or cefotaxime for 14–28 days.
  - Lyme arthritis may require longer duration of therapy, typically 28 days.
  - Prophylaxis after a tick bite: removal of tick and treatment with doxycycline within 72 hours post tick bite is 87% effective in highly endemic regions (>10% of ticks positive for Lyme).

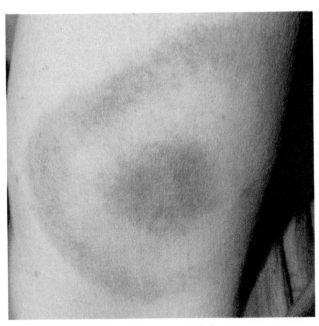

• **Fig. 30.1** Lyme target lesion.

HIGH YIELD POINTS

Lyme can be localized or disseminated. Remember the co-infections that can occur with Lyme disease: babesiosis and anaplasmosis. A phrase to help you remember: "**Ana** gives **lime** juice to her **babies**" (anaplasmosis, Lyme, babesiosis). All these co-infections except babesiosis can be treated with doxycycline. Thus if a patient is not responding while on doxycycline, consider babesiosis.

Human Granulocytic Anaplasmosis (HGA)

- HGA is caused by *Anaplasma phagocytophilum*, an intracellular pathogen that infects granulocytes.
- Vectors: *Ixodes scapularis* and *Ixodes pacificus*.
- Geography: primarily in the upper East Coast, mid-Atlantic, and West Coast.
- Season: spring, summer, or fall, when the weather is warm.
- Clinical presentation: febrile illness with malaise, myalgia, nausea, vomiting, and headache. A maculopapular rash is present in 10% of patients. It is generally milder than human monocytic ehrlichiosis (HME) or Rocky Mountain spotted fever. CNS involvement is rare. Transaminitis, leukopenia, and thrombocytopenia are common.
- Diagnosis: serologies and PCR can be helpful. Morulae within neutrophils can be seen on blood smear and is much more likely to be seen with HGA than HME (Fig. 30.3).
- Treatment: doxycycline.

HIGH YIELD POINTS

Remember how to differentiate HGA from HME, and remember the co-infections that can occur: babesiosis and Lyme disease. A phrase to help you remember: "**Ana** gives **lime** juice to her **babies**" (anaplasmosis, Lyme, babesiosis) (Table 30.2).

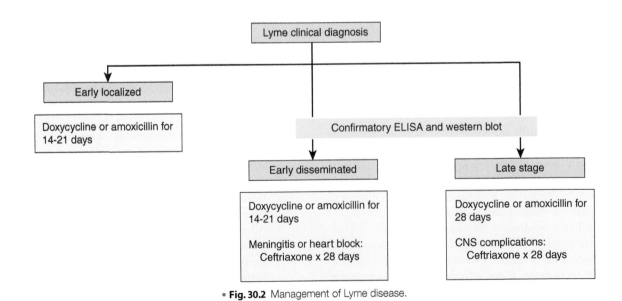

• **Fig. 30.2** Management of Lyme disease.

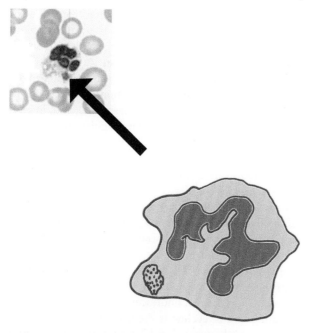

• **Fig. 30.3** Morula within a neutrophil.

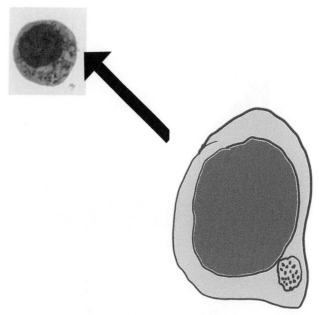

• **Fig. 30.4** Morula within a monocyte.

TABLE 30.2	Key Features of Human Monocytic Ehrlichiosis (HME) and Human Granulocytic Anaplasmosis (HGA)	
	HME	**HGA**
Tick	*Amblyomma*	*Ixodes*
Geography	Southeast, mid-Atlantic, South Central	New England, mid-Atlantic, Upper Midwest
Differentiating symptoms	CNS involvement Rash in 40% Abnormal smear in 20%	CNS involvement and rash are rare Abnormal smear is present in >50%
Peripheral smear	Monocyte	Polymorphonuclear leukocytes

Human Monocytic Ehrlichiosis (HME)

- HME, or ehrlichiosis, is caused by *Ehrlichia chaffeensis*, an intracellular pathogen that infects monocytes.
- Vectors: *Amblyomma americanum* (Lone Star tick).
- Geography: primarily in the East Coast, mid-Atlantic, and Midwest.
- Season: spring, summer, or fall, when the weather is warm.
- Clinical presentation: febrile illness with malaise, myalgia, nausea, vomiting, diarrhea, and headache. Leukopenia and transaminitis are common and a clue to the diagnosis. A maculopapular rash is present in 30%–50% of patients. It is generally more severe than HGA and can be more severe in children. CNS involvement can occur along with progression to multiorgan dysfunction syndrome and acute respiratory distress syndrome.

- Diagnosis: serologies and PCR can be helpful. Morulae within monocytes can be seen on blood smear and are less likely to be seen with HME than HGA (Fig. 30.4).
- Treatment: doxycycline.

> **HIGH YIELD POINTS**
>
> Remember how to differentiate HGA from HME (Table 30.2). Remember the co-infections that can occur: tularemia and STARI (see below).

Babesiosis

- Babesiosis is a malaria-like illness caused by *Babesia microti*, a tickborne protozoan organism that infects red blood cells and causes hemolysis. Think of this infection if you see a malaria-like presentation without travel to an area endemic for malaria.
- Vectors: *Ixodes* spp.
- Geography: primarily in Northeast and upper Midwestern states.
- Season: spring, summer, or fall, when the weather is warm.
- Incubation period can range from 1 to 6 weeks.
- Clinical presentation: ranges from subclinical to severe. Mild disease is common, with recurrent fevers, myalgias, and hemolysis. Illness can progress and cause organ dysfunction, renal failure, and respiratory distress. Laboratory findings typically include hemolytic anemia, elevated LDH, transaminitis, thrombocytopenia, and elevated creatinine.
- Diagnosis: blood smear or PCR. Thick/thin smear will show intra-erythrocytic ring forms and Maltese crosses (Fig. 30.5). If parasitemia is >5%, that constitutes high burden and thus severe disease. Patients with asplenia, malignancy, immunocompromise (use of tumor necrosis

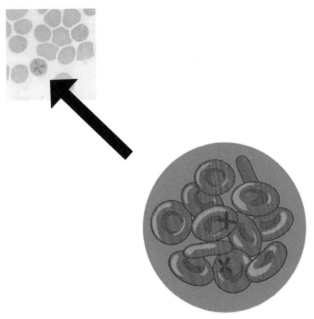

• **Fig. 30.5** Maltese crosses in red blood cells.

factor [TNF] antagonists, human immunodeficiency virus [HIV]) heart failure, liver disease, or hemoglobinopathies are at high risk for severe babesiosis.
• Treatment: asymptomatic disease does not require treatment. For mild disease, atovaquone plus azithromycin for 7–10 days. Severe disease requires clindamycin plus quinine in parenteral forms.

> **HIGH YIELD POINTS**
>
> *Babesia* infection has many similarities to malaria, and this may help you remember both. Key similarities include its hemolysis, overall clinical presentation, and the importance of the level of parasitemia to risk stratify. Remember the common tickborne co-infections that can occur. A phrase to help you remember: "**Ana** gives **lime** juice to her **babies**" (anaplasmosis, Lyme, babesiosis).

Rocky Mountain Spotted Fever

• Rocky Mountain spotted fever (RMSF) is caused by *Rickettsia rickettsii* and can be transmitted by a variety of ticks. The geography of these individual ticks can vary, but the presence of different ticks in different geographic areas makes RMSF a disease that can occur anywhere in the continental United States.
• Vectors: *Dermacentor variabilis* (dog tick), *Dermacentor andersoni* (wood tick), *Rhipicephalus* (dog tick), *Amblyomma americanum* (Lone Star tick).
• Geography: continental United States.
• Season: most cases occur in summer, between May and September.
• Clinical presentation: RMSF can be rapidly progressive and lethal. The usual triad involves rash, headache, and fever. A rash is present in 90% of cases. Half of patients present with a rash, thus 50% may also present without a rash, and clinicians should have a high index of

suspicion. Constitutional symptoms that resemble a viral illness are also present (Fig. 30.6). The rash is typically faint, pink macules that starts peripherally and spreads from limbs to the thorax. The rash usually spares the face. Lab findings can include leukocytosis or leukopenia, thrombocytopenia, anemia, abnormal liver function tests (LFTs), elevated creatine kinase (CK), and, in severe cases, disseminated intravascular coagulation (DIC), and coagulopathy. However, unlike ehrlichiosis and anaplasmosis, low white blood cell counts and transaminitis are not common findings. Lymphocytic pleocytosis can be present on CSF studies.
• Diagnosis: a clinical diagnosis is usually made. It is not advised to delay treatment to pursue advanced diagnostic modalities due to high mortality with lack of treatment. Organ failure and mortality can occur within 5–7 days without treatment. Diagnostic options include serologies, skin biopsy with *Rickettsia* polymerase chain reaction (PCR), or direct fluorescent antibody (DFA).
• Treatment: doxycycline is the drug of choice. Duration of therapy is between 3 and 7 days. Due to high mortality, treatment should be initiated immediately for cases with high index of suspicion.

> **HIGH YIELD POINTS**
>
> Remember RMSF can present anywhere in the United States. The key feature is the rash (Table 30.3). Also remember the co-infections that can occur: tularemia.

Rickettsialpox

• Rickettsialpox is a spotted fever syndrome caused by *Rickettsia akari*.
• Vectors: house mites.
• Geography: northeastern United States, think of large cities like New York with possible house mites.
• Season: present all year.
• Clinical presentation: fever, malaise, disseminated vesicular rash, and a black eschar at the site of the bite. Geography and exposure to house mites are the differentiating features.
• Diagnosis: mostly clinical. Serologies, biopsy, and PCR techniques can be pursued when diagnosis is unclear.
• Treatment: doxycycline.

> **HIGH YIELD POINTS**
>
> • Think of rickettsialpox in a patient from the northeastern United States, usually in major cities, and exposure to house mites.

Spotted Fever Associated with *R. parkeri*

• *R. parkeri* causes a spotted fever syndrome in the Gulf Coast and mid-Atlantic region of the United States.
• Vectors: *Amblyomma maculatum* (Gulf Coast tick).
• Geography: Gulf Coast.
• Season: present all year.

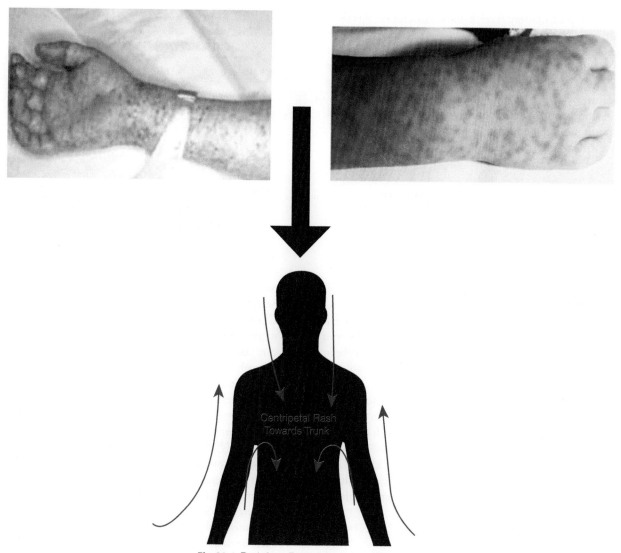

• **Fig. 30.6** Rash from Rocky Mountain spotted fever.

TABLE 30.3 **Key Features of *Rickettsia* spp.**

Organism	Disease	Geography	Vector	Presentation
Rickettsia rickettsii	RMSF	Continental United States	*Dermacentor*, *Rhipicephalus*, and *Amblyomma* ticks (dog, wood, and Lone Star tick)	Headache, fever, centripetal rash involving palms and soles
Rickettsia akari	Rickettsialpox	Northeastern United States	House mites	Mild rash
Rickettsia parkeri	Spotted fever	Mid-Atlantic region	*Amblyomma maculatum* (Gulf Coast tick)	Mild rash similar to RMSF, dark eschar ("tache noire")
Rickettsia prowazekii	Epidemic typhus	Worldwide	Human body louse	Fever, centripetal rash
Rickettsia typhi	Murine typhus	Worldwide	Fleaborne	Fever, myalgia, leukocyte adhesion deficiency, confusion, black eschar

- Clinical presentation: fever, malaise, disseminated vesicular rash, and a black eschar at the site of the bite. Overall presentation and rash is very similar to RMSF but milder and with a black eschar at the bite site, known as a "tache noire." Geography and exposures are the differentiating features.
- Diagnosis: mostly clinical. Serologies, biopsy, and PCR techniques can be pursued when diagnosis is unclear.
- Treatment: doxycycline.

HIGH YIELD POINTS

- Think of *R. parkeri in* a patient from the southeastern United States with a mild version of RMSF plus a tache noir.

STARI (Southern Tick-Associated Rash Illness)

- A mild febrile illness with a rash similar to erythema migrans and Lyme disease that may appear one week after the tick bite. The causative organism may be *Borrelia lonestari* based on a single case report that has not been reproduced. The true cause is still uncertain. It is a relatively new disease, first described in the 1980s.
- Vectors: *Amblyomma americanum* (Lone Star tick).
- Geography: Mississippi, Missouri, Southern Illinois, Maryland, Georgia, South Carolina, and North Carolina.
- Season: mainly in the summer.
- Clinical presentation: mild febrile illness with malaise, headache, and skin lesions that may be single or multiple but is not associated with systemic multiorgan manifestations as Lyme disease.
- Diagnosis: usually a diagnosis of exclusion, in areas where STARI is present and Lyme disease is not.
- Treatment: self-resolving without treatment on most patients.

HIGH YIELD POINTS

Think of STARI when you see a vignette or case similar to Lyme disease with erythema migrans, in an area where Lyme disease is not prevalent.

Tick Paralysis

- Tick paralysis is caused by neurotoxins within the salivary glands of ticks. *Dermacentor andersoni* (the Rocky Mountain wood tick) and *Dermacentor variabilis* (the American dog tick) are the most commonly associated ticks. *Amblyomma americanum* can cause tick paralysis as well.
- Geography: Pacific northwest.
- Season: more common during the summer.
- Clinical presentation: ascending paralysis, respiratory failure, and death.
- Diagnosis: clinical diagnosis, with paralysis and embedded tick usually found in scalp or other areas not immediately obvious.
- Treatment: supportive care and removal of tick.

HIGH YIELD POINTS

Remember tick paralysis disease for any patient with unexplained neurologic weakness after hiking. Look for ticks in places that are not obvious, such as the scalp (Table 30.1).

Tickborne Relapsing Fever

- Tickborne relapsing fever can be caused by a variety of organisms. In the United States, *Borrelia recurrentis*, *Borrelia hermsii*, and *Borrelia parkeri* are the most important.
- Key clinical findings are fever, headache, flu-like syndromic presentations in the setting of poor hygiene.
- Vectors: *Ornithodoros* soft ticks. Patients may not remember tick bite.
- Geography: Southwestern regions of the United States, particularly in areas of high elevation.
- Season: all year round.
- Clinical presentation: fevers, chills, headache, myalgia, nausea, recurring every week or every 10 days. Illness can last for several months. Hepatosplenomegaly, thrombocytopenia, and even DIC can occur. Altered mental status and neurologic deficits can occur with CNS disease.
  - Epidemic louseborne relapsing fever is also caused by *B. recurrentis* and is transmitted by the human body louse (*Pediculus humanus*). It usually occurs in poor socioeconomic settings and poor hygiene, increasing in incidence during war, famine, and in refugees.
- Diagnosis: Giemsa staining of blood smear can reveal spirochetemia. Serology and PCR testing can be performed.
- Treatment: doxycycline or tetracycline for 5–10 days. Ceftriaxone if CNS manifestations.

HIGH YIELD POINTS

Think of tickborne relapsing fevers (*B. recurrentis*, *B. hermsii*, and *B. parkeri*) in patients with recurrent fevers in the southwestern United States.

Trench Fever

- Trench fever is a louseborne relapsing fever which can be caused by a *Bartonella quintana*.
- Key clinical findings are fever, headache, flu-like syndromic. Constellation of symptoms last 4–5 days, recurring over a period of 5–6 weeks. The name *quintana* refers to this timing. Think of this organism in patients with homelessness or poor hygiene.
- Vectors: human body louse (*Pediculus humanus*).
- Geography: worldwide.
- Season: all year round.
- Clinical presentation: fevers, chills, headache, myalgia, nausea, malaise, dizziness, splenomegaly, and occasionally a macular truncal rash. Fever persists for weeks, recurring in 4–5-day episodes.
- Diagnosis: Fastidious organism that is difficult to culture. Longer incubation at lower temperatures may yield

positive blood cultures. Indirect fluorescence assay (IFA) and enzyme-linked immunosorbent assay (ELISA) may be used in the right clinical setting as well. New PCR tests are available and will likely play a wider role in the diagnosis.
- Treatment: doxycycline or aminoglycosides can be used for treatment.

> **HIGH YIELD POINTS**
>
> Think of this illness in patients with recurrent fevers who are homeless or have poor hygiene.

Typhus Fevers

Scrub Typhus

- Scrub typhus is an illness caused by *Orientia tsutsugamushi*. Scrub typhus is also known as bush typhus.
- Vectors: chigger.
- Geography: Southeast Asia.
- Clinical presentation: inoculation eschar followed by a febrile illness and rash.
- Diagnosis: serologic testing, direct immunofluorescent testing or PCR from skin biopsy.
- Treatment: doxycycline.

> **HIGH YIELD POINTS**
>
> Remember the inoculation eschar in patients with exposure to Southeast Asia.

Epidemic Typhus

- Epidemic typhus is an illness caused by *Rickettsia prowazekii*, present worldwide. It is associated with poor sanitation.
- Vectors: lice, human body louse, or *Pediculus humanus.*
- Geography: worldwide
- Clinical presentation: fever, maculopapular rash starting in the trunk and spreading outward. It can also cause a recurrent febrile illness (Brill–Zinsser disease). Disease can progress to coma and death.
- Diagnosis: serologic testing, direct immunofluorescent testing, or PCR from skin biopsy.
- Treatment: doxycycline.

> **HIGH YIELD POINTS**
>
> Think of this disease in febrile patients that are homeless, unkept, or in refugee camps. Also associated with flying squirrel fleas.

Murine/Endemic Typhus

- Murine typhus or endemic typhus is a fleaborne febrile illness caused by *Rickettsia typhi*. Murine typhus is spread to people through contact with infected fleas.
- Geography: worldwide. Present in California, Hawaii, and Texas.

- Clinical presentation: fevers, chills, myalgias, nausea, vomiting, occasional rash and lymphadenopathy. The disease can progress to altered mental status and confusion. A necrotic eschar can develop at the bite site.
- Diagnosis: serologies, immunofluorescent testing, and biopsy.
- Treatment: doxycycline.

> **HIGH YIELD POINTS**
>
> Endemic typhus has global reach. In the United States, typically in Hawaii and southeastern United States in border with Mexico.

MAJOR ARTHROPOD-BORNE DISEASES IN THE UNITED STATES TRANSMITTED BY MOSQUITOES (Table 30.4)

Mosquito-Borne Illnesses

Dengue Fever

- Dengue fever (DENF) is caused by the dengue virus (DENV). It is the most common mosquito-borne viral disease worldwide. The disease spectrum can range from a mild febrile illness to severe disease with plasma leakage, shock, and death. It is the most common cause of hemorrhagic fever worldwide. It is a significant cause of morbidity and mortality worldwide, with 50–100 million infections and 22,000 deaths per year.
- Pathogen: DENV is a flavivirus with five known DENV serotypes (DENV 1–5). These are antigenically distinct serotypes, each generating a unique host immune response to the infection. Antibody-dependent enhancement may occur, causing patients to develop higher immune responses on subsequent exposures to DENV. This promotes higher immune response, plasma leakage, and progression to severe forms of dengue
- Vectors: transmitted by *Aedes aegypti* and *Aedes albopictus.*
- Geography: tropical and subtropical regions worldwide, with cyclical outbreaks affecting large urban areas (Fig. 30.7).
- Season: year-round in tropical and subtropical regions. Outbreaks occur more commonly in rainy seasons when water accumulates and mosquito reservoirs develop.
- Clinical presentation: WHO classification includes dengue with or without warning signs and severe dengue for those with capillary leak and shock (Fig. 30.8).
  - Dengue has an incubation period of 4–10 days and should be considered as a cause of fever in a traveler returning from endemic regions.
  - Dengue without warning signs (mild–moderate): viral illness with fever, nausea, vomiting, faint maculopapular rash, myalgia.
  - Dengue with warning signs occurs as patients develop endothelial damage and plasma leakage, causing symptoms such as abdominal pain, thrombocytopenia, hemoconcentration, edema, effusions, hepatomegaly, bleeding, and persistent vomiting.

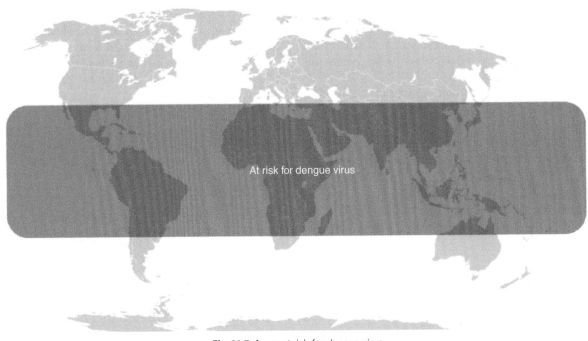

• **Fig. 30.7** Areas at risk for dengue virus.

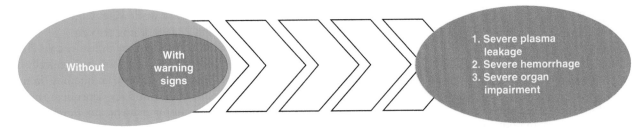

Dengue with or without warning signs	Severe dengue

1. Severe plasma leakage
2. Severe hemorrhage
3. Severe organ impairment

Without · With warning signs

CRITERIA FOR DENGUE ± WARNING SIGNS

Probable dengue
live in /travel to dengue endemic area.
Fever and 2 of the following criteria:
• Nausea, vomiting
• Rash
• Aches and pains
• Tourniquet test positive
• Leukopenia
• Any warning sign

Laboratory-confirmed dengue
(important when no sign of
plasma leakage)

Warning signs*
• Abdominal pain or tenderness
• Persistent vomiting
• Clinical fluid accumulation
• Mucosal bleed
• Lethargy, restlessness
• Liver enlargement >2 cm
• Laboratory: increase in HCT
  concurrent with rapid decrease
  in platelet count

*(requiring strict observation
and medical intervention)

CRITERIA FOR SEVERE DENGUE

Severe plasma leakage
leading to:
• Shock (DSS)
• Fluid accumulation with respiratory
  distress

Severe bleeding
as evaluated by clinician

Severe organ involvement
• Liver: AST or ALT >=1000
• CNS: Impaired consciousness
• Heart and other organs

• **Fig. 30.8** World Health Organization classification of dengue.

• Severe dengue corresponds to continuation of plasma leakage with significant edema, third-spacing, effusions, bleeding, and hypotension.
• Diagnosis: often a clinical diagnosis in areas of high prevalence. Dengue IgM via ELISA is usually positive by day 6. Serum dengue nonstructural protein-1 (NS-1)

antigen testing can be positive starting day 1. Blood viral culture or PCR may also detect in viremia on day 1 of disease.
• Treatment: supportive care with oral or intravenous hydration and frequent monitoring of hemodynamic status, platelets, and hemoglobin. Hospitalization is

TABLE 30.4 Other Arthropod-Borne Illnesses in the United States

Organism	Disease	Geography	Vector	Presentation
Heartland virus	Heartland virus disease	Midwest	*Amblyomma americanum* (Lone Star tick)	Fever, fatigue, diarrhea, leukopenia, thrombocytopenia
Powassan virus	Tickborne encephalitis	Upper Midwest, Canada	*Ixodes* and *Dermacentor* ticks	Fevers, chills, confusion, acute disseminated encephalomyelitis
Bourbon virus	Bourbon fever	Midwest and mid-Atlantic region	*Dermacentor* or *Amblyomma* ticks	Fever, headache, malaise, maculopapular rash. Severe disease can progress to bone marrow suppression and acute respiratory distress syndrome
Coltivirus	Colorado tick fever, Mountain tick fever	Rocky Mountain region, usually at high altitude	*Dermacentor andersoni* (wood tick)	Fever, chills, malaise, maculopapular rash. Severe disease can progress to hemorrhagic fever and meningitis

TABLE 30.5 Differences Between Dengue, Chikungunya, Yellow Fever, and Leptospirosis

	Dengue	Chikungunya	Yellow Fever	Leptospirosis
Key features	Febrile illness, mosquito exposure Thrombocytopenia Shock	Febrile illness, mosquito exposure Joint pains Milder disease than dengue	Febrile illness, mosquito exposure Transaminitis, jaundice, no vaccine prior to travel	Febrile illness, water exposure Hyperbilirubinemia out of proportion to transaminitis Conjunctival suffusion

recommended for patients with warning signs, to monitor, hydrate, and prevent progression to severe dengue. There is no antiviral treatment. Steroids or platelet transfusions are not recommended.

HIGH YIELD POINTS

Think of dengue in any febrile traveler returning from endemic regions. Remember key differences between yellow fever (more transaminitis and jaundice, lack of immunization prior to travel), chikungunya (more joint disease, less plasma leakage), and leptospirosis (water exposure, conjunctival suffusion) (Table 30.5).

Chikungunya Fever

- Chikungunya fever (CHIKF) is caused by the chikungunya virus (CHIKV). The name is taken from the Mozambique Makonde language and means "that which bends up," in reference to the severe joint disease it can cause. CHIKF can cause a mild febrile illness with polyarthralgia. A subset of patients can have prolonged residual joint pain that may be neuropathic in nature, although there is evidence for ongoing replication of virus in the affected joints.
- Vectors: transmitted by *Aedes aegypti* and *Aedes albopictus*.
- Geography: tropical and subtropical regions. CHIKV is now present worldwide, after the emergence of CHIKV in the Americas in 2014. Locally acquired cases in Florida and Puerto Rico have been documented as well (Fig. 30.9).

- Season: year-round in tropical and subtropical regions. Outbreaks occur more commonly in rainy seasons when water accumulates and mosquito reservoirs develop.
- Clinical presentation: fever, chills, fatigue, headache, maculopapular rash, nausea, vomiting, back pain, myalgias, polyarthralgia, lymphadenopathy, and conjunctivitis. Fever abates usually by day 3 of illness. Polyarthralgia and fatigue can persist for months after illness. Rare cases of encephalitis have been reported. Labs can reveal mild thrombocytopenia, leukopenia, and elevated CK.
- Diagnosis: often a clinical diagnosis in areas of high prevalence. Serum PCR can be diagnostic during illness. Serum IGM can be detected by day 2 and persists for 3 months. Serum IgG remains positive for years. Serologies can be helpful for travelers, as patients from endemic regions may have prior asymptomatic exposure.
- Treatment: no specific treatments. Supportive care with hydration and rest. NSAIDs and acetaminophen can abate fevers and lessen joint pain.

HIGH YIELD POINTS

Remember how to differentiate from similar travel-related diseases (Table 30.5).

Zika Virus Disease

- Zika virus disease is caused by the Zika virus (ZIKV), a flavivirus closely related to dengue and yellow fever. It was first discovered in Uganda in 1947. Only 13 cases

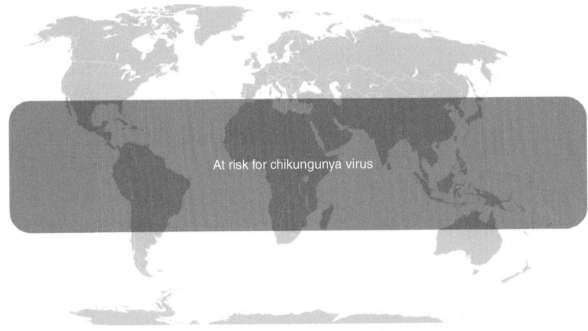

• **Fig. 30.9** Areas at risk for chikungunya virus.

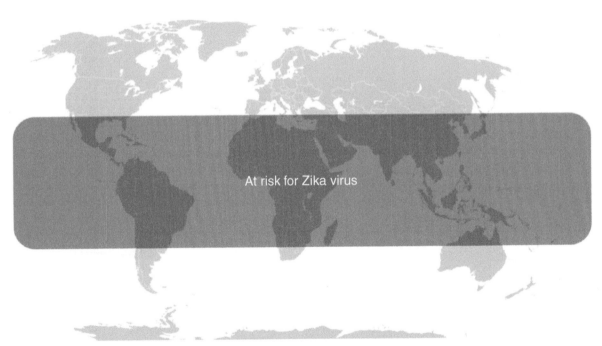

• **Fig. 30.10** Areas at risk for Zika virus.

were described until an outbreak occurred in Micronesia (2007), with 5000 infected. A larger outbreak occurred in the French Polynesian islands (2013) before ZIKV emerged in the Americas. It is now endemic in Asia, Africa, and the Americas.

- Vectors: transmitted by *Aedes aegypti* and *Aedes africanus*. Maternal transmission vertically and via breast milk. Sexually transmitted via semen.
- Geography: tropical and subtropical regions. ZIKV is now present worldwide. Locally acquired cases in Florida and Puerto Rico have been documented as well (Fig. 30.10).

- Season: year-round in tropical and subtropical regions. Outbreaks occur more commonly in rainy seasons when water accumulates and mosquito reservoirs develop.
- Clinical presentation: most infections are asymptomatic. Clinical symptoms may occur and are usually mild. These include low-grade fever, arthralgia, nonpurulent conjunctivitis, and a diffuse maculopapular rash. Post-infectious complications include Guillain–Barré syndrome. Maternal–fetal transmission can cause abortion, ophthalmologic complications, and microcephaly.

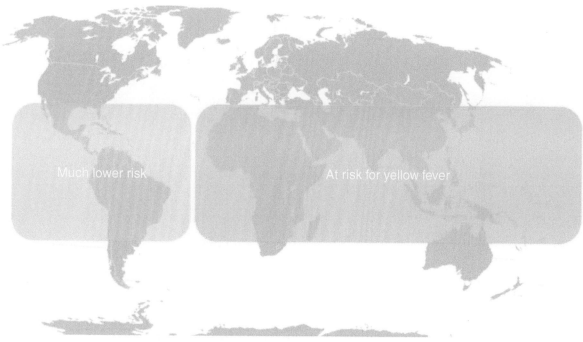

• **Fig. 30.11** Areas at risk for yellow fever virus.

- Diagnosis: testing via ELISA and PCR techniques is available. Indications for testing have evolved and are likely not testable in review boards at time of writing.
- Treatment: no specific treatments. Supportive care with hydration and rest. NSAIDs and acetaminophen can lessen acute symptoms.

> ### HIGH YIELD POINTS
>
> Remember the high association with fetal malformations and Guillain–Barré. Remember that Zika is the **only vectorborne illness that can also be transmitted sexually.** Travel advisories and abstinence may be needed for patients who are currently pregnant or are planning to become pregnant.

Yellow Fever

- Yellow fever is caused by the yellow fever virus (YFV). It is a flavivirus closely related to dengue and Zika viruses. The disease spectrum ranges from an asymptomatic infection to a potentially lethal multiorgan viral hemorrhagic fever.
- Vectors: transmitted by *Aedes aegypti* and *Haemagogus* spp.
- Geography: endemic in Africa and the Americas, occurring both in high density urban areas and jungles/forests (Fig. 30.11).
- Season: year-round in tropical and subtropical regions. Outbreaks occur more commonly in rainy seasons when water accumulates and mosquito reservoirs develop.
- Clinical presentation: usually a mild febrile illness and self-resolving febrile disease. There are three stages of infection:
  - Stage 1: Infection: fever, headache, photophobia, myalgia, nausea, vomiting. Minimal increase in transaminases.
  - Stage 2: Remission: afebrile and resolution of symptoms. Patients typically fully recover and do not progress to further stages.
  - Stage 3: Intoxication: Progression to most severe forms of disease, with return of fevers, nausea, vomiting, and jaundice. Multiorgan dysfunction occurs, with oliguric renal failure, azotemia, transaminitis (AST > ALT), and hyperbilirubinemia. Hemorrhagic complications can occur, with hematuria, melena, hematemesis, mucosal bleeding, and ecchymoses. Patients who progress to neurologic findings such as convulsions, stupor, or coma can have a mortality as high as 70%.
- Diagnosis: PCR and ELISA testing can be performed.
- Treatment: supportive care.
- Prevention: yellow fever vaccine is recommended for patients above the age of 9 months who will travel to certain parts of the Americas and sub-Saharan Africa where the disease is endemic. This live attenuated vaccine is not recommended for immunocompromised patients. Booster doses after 10 years are recommended if new exposure may occur.
  - Yellow fever vaccine can cause a vaccine-associated neurotropic disease (YEL-AND) and vaccine-associated viscerotropic disease (YEL-AVD). YEL-AND causes fever and headache that can progress to encephalitis or demyelinating disease with peripheral or central nervous involvement at 3–50 days after the vaccine. Most patients will completely recover. YEL-AVD causes fever, malaise, headache, and myalgia that can progress to hepatitis, hypotension, multiorgan failure, and death.

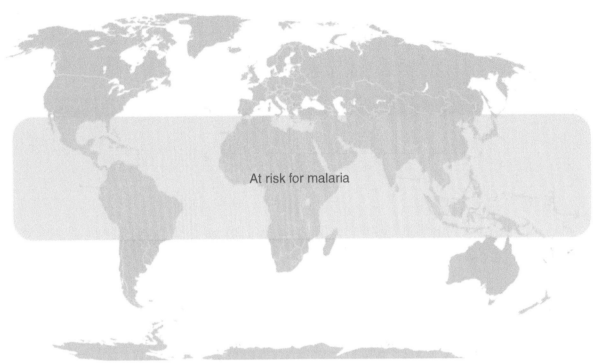

• **Fig. 30.12** Areas at risk for malaria.

HIGH YIELD POINTS

Think of yellow fever in patients who did not receive pretravel vaccinations. Remember how to differentiate from similar travel-related diseases (Table 30.5).

Malaria (see also Chapter 34)

- Malaria is caused by *Plasmodium falciparum*, *P malariae*, *P vivax*, *P ovale*, and *P knowlesi*. It is a major cause of morbidity and mortality worldwide and should always remain on the differential in febrile travelers.
- Malaria's life cycle is complex but rarely tested in depth on review boards.
  - *P. falciparum* invades RBCs of all ages, and thus can causes the most severe disease via microvascular end-organ damage. *P. falciparum* is the most common species reported in the United States and is the most common cause of severe malaria. Severe malaria is characterized by sequestering of red blood cells and endothelial damage, leading to organ failure.
  - *P. vivax* invades reticulocytes and can persist in hepatocytes as hypnozoites for months to years.
  - *P. ovale* can also persist in hepatocytes for months to years. This can be a cause of relapsing fevers long after a return from a trip.
  - *P. malariae* causes low-level parasitemia and is typically a mild disease.
  - *P knowlesi* morphologically resembles *P. malariae* but causes severe disease like *P. falciparum* and is only found in Southeast Asia, including Malaysia.

- Vectors: *Anopheles* mosquito. Prefers night-time or pre-dawn biting and transmission.
- Geography: tropical and subtropical regions worldwide. Burden of disease and resistance can vary geographically (Fig. 30.12).
- Season: year-round in tropical and subtropical regions.
- Clinical presentation: the cardinal symptom of malaria is fever, that may follow typical fever cycles known as paroxysms. Attacks also known as the malarial paroxysms. The paroxysms are dependant on antibody release as erythrocytes rupture and release merozoites. These paroxysms will exhibit patterns of 48 hours for *P. vivax*, *P. ovale*, and *P. falciparum*, and a 72-hour pattern for *P. malariae*. Initially fevers may be irregular. *P. falciparum* may exhibit distinct paroxysms, a continuous fever, or irregular cycles of fever.
  - Beyond fever, in clinical practice (and review boards), differentiation between uncomplicated or severe malaria is of utmost importance, as it changes the management:
  - Uncomplicated malaria: jaundice, cyclical fevers, chills, sweats. No signs of end-organ damage.
  - Complicated malaria: same symptoms as uncomplicated, but with end-organ damage such as renal failure, metabolic acidosis, encephalopathy, or pulmonary edema. Hyperparasitemia >5% is also diagnostic for severe malaria.
- Diagnosis: Giemsa-stained thick and thin smears are used to diagnose, determine the species, and the degree of parasitemia. Rapid diagnostic tests are available and can give a prompt diagnosis but cannot confirm degree of

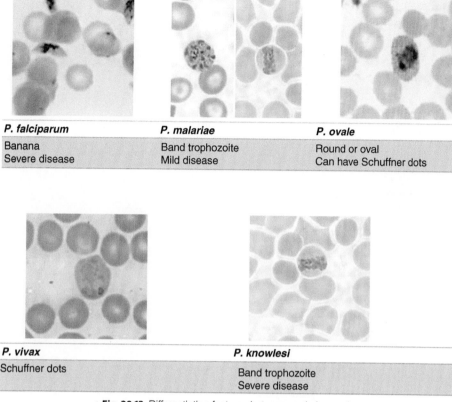

P. falciparum	P. malariae	P. ovale
Banana Severe disease	Band trophozoite Mild disease	Round or oval Can have Schuffner dots

P. vivax	P. knowlesi
Schuffner dots	Band trophozoite Severe disease

• **Fig. 30.13** Differentiating features between malaria species.

parasitemia. Rapid antigen tests may miss low-level parasitemia, so a thick smear should always be performed.

- Fig. 30.13 illustrates differentiation between species on malaria slides.
- Treatment: chloroquine-susceptible *Plasmodium* is only present in a handful of countries, and management will depend on resistance trends, clinical presentation, and severity. The CDC provides a free hotline for the treatment of malaria that is a great resource for this rarely encountered disease (Fig. 30.14).
  - Uncomplicated: atovaquone–proguanil ×3 days, artemether–lumefantrine ×2 days, quinine sulfate plus doxycycline or clindamycin ×7 days, or mefloquine. If from chloroquine susceptible region, chloroquine phosphate ×2 days or hydroxychloroquine ×2 days.
  - Severe malaria: intravenous quinine plus doxycycline, tetracycline, or clindamycin. Intravenous treatment should continue until parasitemia is <1% and patient can tolerate oral medications. Intravenous artesunate can be used as well. Once parasitemia is <1%, transition to any of the oral therapies above.
  - For severe malaria, admission to the hospital and telemetry is needed to monitor QTc and QRS widening from intravenous medications.
  - There is no role for exchange transfusion.
  - Pregnancy: preferred agents are quinine or chloroquine. Avoid primaquine.
  - For *P. malaria* and *P. ovale*, must also clear hypnozoites with primaquine for 14 days.
- Prophylaxis: atovaquone–proguanil for most places. Chloroquine can be used only in susceptible areas (see map, Fig. 30.14). Mefloquine is the drug of choice for prophylaxis in the setting of pregnancy. Mefloquine may cause vivid dreams, insomnia, and dizziness.
  - Terminal prophylaxis: most malarious regions have at least 1 species of relapsing malaria. Travelers to those areas, particularly those with prolonged exposure, should be offered terminal prophylaxis with primaquine for 2 weeks.

HIGH YIELD POINTS

Remember key differences between malaria species. Assessing severity is key and understanding the need for telemetry, QTc monitoring, and electrolyte monitoring while on IV antimalarials for severe disease.

ARTHROPOD-BORNE ILLNESSES ACQUIRED ABROAD

Visceral and Cutaneous Leishmaniasis

- Leishmaniasis involves multiple clinical syndromes caused by several different pathogens. The syndromes involve cutaneous, mucosal, and visceral forms. The infection

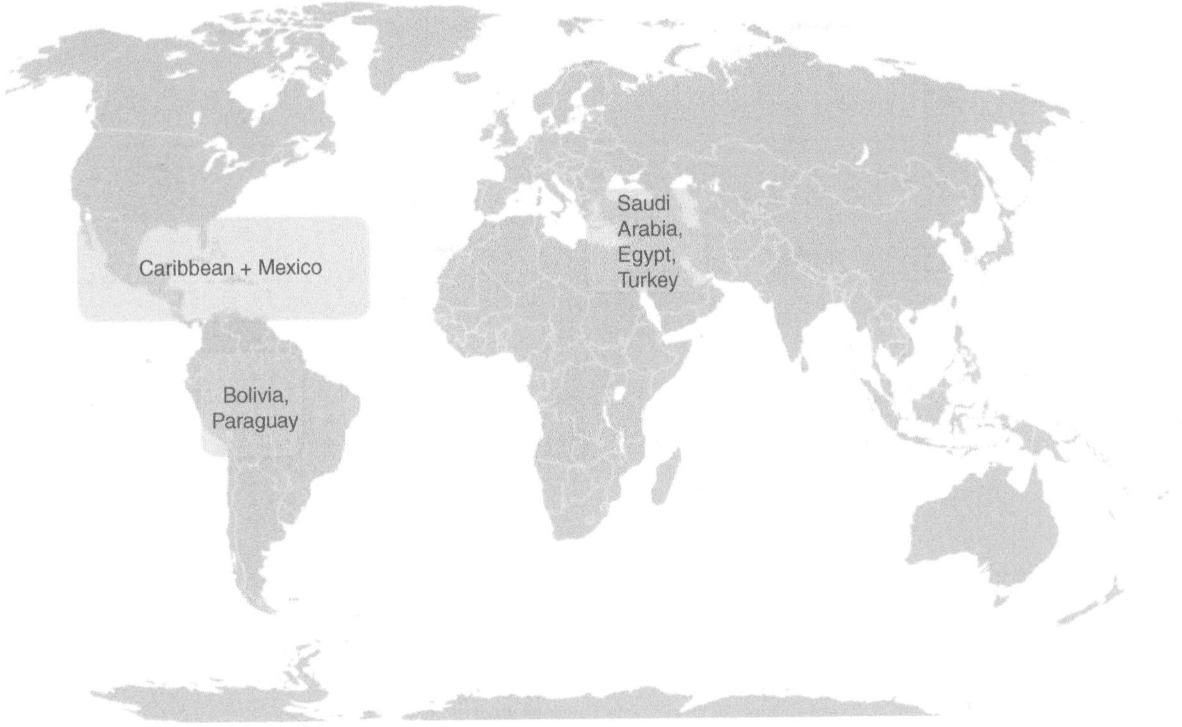

Caribbean + Mexico

Bolivia, Paraguay

Saudi Arabia, Egypt, Turkey

• **Fig. 30.14** Areas with chloroquine-susceptible malaria.

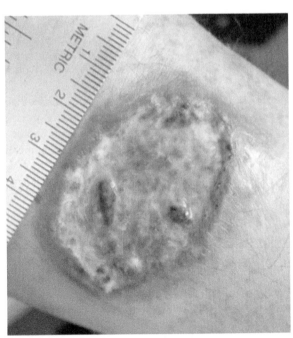

• **Fig. 30.15** Leishmania ulcer.

can range from asymptomatic to severe. Cutaneous and mucosal leishmaniasis can cause substantial morbidity while visceral disease can be life-threatening. Visceral leishmaniasis is caused by a protozoa, *L. donovani* and *L. chagasi*. Cutaneous leishmaniasis is caused by *L. major*, *L. tropica*, *L. mexicana*, *L. amazonensis*, *L. peruviana*, and *L. braziliensis*. Disease can be classified as Old World leishmaniasis vs. New World leishmaniasis depending

on the organism and geographic region where it was acquired. Both can cause systemic or cutaneous disease.
• Vectors: transmitted by various species of sandfly.
• Geography: visceral leishmaniasis is more common in India, Bangladesh, Nepal, Sudan, and Brazil. Cutaneous leishmaniasis is more common in Afghanistan, Algeria, Iran, Brazil, Colombia, and Peru.
• Clinical presentation
  • Old World leishmaniasis: cutaneous or mucocutaneous disease can be transient and may leave a scar. Visceral disease (Dumdum fever, kala-azar, meaning black fever) presents with fever, weight loss, hepatosplenomegaly, and marrow involvement (Fig. 30.15).
  • New World leishmaniasis: cutaneous and mucosal involvement is common in Chile and Uruguay. Visceral involvement similar to Old World disease can occur.
• Diagnosis: biopsy, histologic exam, culture, serologic studies, and PCR techniques. Bone marrow biopsy may be needed. It may mimic histoplasmosis on biopsy.
• Treatment: localized disease can be treated with topical paromomycin and methylbenzethonium ointment or intralesional antimonials. Surgical excision or local cryotherapy can be used as well. Systemic therapy with fluconazole, pentavalent antimonials, or amphotericin is recommended for severe systemic disease.

HIGH YIELD POINTS

Look for pizza-like borders on cutaneous lesions.

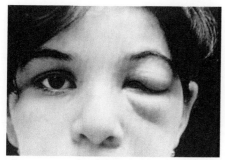

• **Fig. 30.16** Romaña sign. (From Ryan ET, Durand M. Ocular disease. In: Guerrant RL, Walker DH, Weller PF. *Tropical Infectious Diseases: Principles, Pathogens and Practice.* 3rd ed. Elsevier; 2011.)

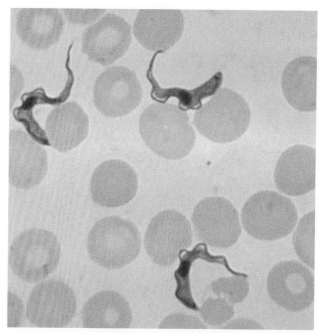

• **Fig. 30.17** *Trypanosoma cruzi.*

Chagas Disease

- Chagas disease is caused by a protozoan, *Trypanosoma cruzi*, that is transmitted in rural areas of Latin America by the "kissing" bug. Chagas can also be transmitted vertically and through transfusions.
- Vectors: *Rhodnius*/reduviid "kissing" bug. The infection is not introduced through the bite, but rather through feces that the reduviid bug leaves behind during feeding. Those feces are then scratched and rubbed into the wound by the patient. Similar species of reduviid bugs are also present in North America, but they do not defecate at the time of feeding and are not able to complete the life cycle.
- Geography: endemic in the Americas.
- Clinical presentation: disease can present in both acute and chronic forms:
  - Acute disease: may start 1–2 weeks after initial infection. Presentation can include a red lesion at the site of inoculation (Chagoma) and progress to periorbital edema (Romaña sign). This is accompanied by fever and malaise. Lymphadenopathy and HSM can occur (Fig. 30.16).
  - Chronic disease: usually involves end-organ damage. Cardiac problems are most common, with biventricular dilation. GI disease can occur as well, including mega-colon or mega-esophagus. CNS disease can occur in the setting of AIDS, with re-activation, meningoencephalitis, and brain abscess.
- Diagnosis: serologies, Giemsa-stain of blood. PCR technology available (Fig. 30.17).
- Treatment: nifurtimox or benznidazole. May need pacemaker if cardiac involvement is severe. End-organ damage may progress, and solid organ transplant needed.

HIGH YIELD POINTS

Remember the Romaña sign and the chronic complications such as enlarged heart, esophagus, or GI tract.

African Sleeping Sickness

- A zoonotic infection caused by a protozoa, *Trypanosoma brucei*. This disease is a zoonotic infection of cattle transmitted via the tsetse fly. Vertical or sexual transmission can also occur.
- Vectors: tsetse fly.
- Geography: *T. brucei gambiense* occurs in western Africa, while *T. brucei rhodesiense* occurs in eastern parts of Africa.
- Clinical presentation: there are three stages associated with this disease: ulceration, systemic symptoms, and CNS phase.
  - Ulcerative phase: usually a chancre at the site of the tsetse fly bite.
  - Systemic phase: occurs with dissemination via venous and lymphatic system. Fever, malaise, and lymphadenopathy occur.
  - CNS phase: invasion of the CNS causes meningoencephalitis with headache, somnolence, and behavioral changes.
- Diagnosis: direct observation of trypanosomes via Giemsa-stained thick blood smears or smears of chancres or lymph node aspirates (Fig. 30.18). Serologic testing can be helpful as well. CSF analysis and staining if CNS infection is a concern.
- Treatment: pentamidine, melarsoprol, or eflornithine.

HIGH YIELD POINTS

Remember, tsetse fly for "tsleeping" sickness.

Oroya Fever

- Also known as Carrion's disease, Oroya fever is a disease caused by *Bartonella bacilliformis* and is transmitted by sandflies. It typically presents as a febrile disease in returning travelers from South America.
- Vectors: sandfly of the genus *Lutzomyia*.
- Geography: Peru, Ecuador, and Colombia. Typically occurs at high elevations.

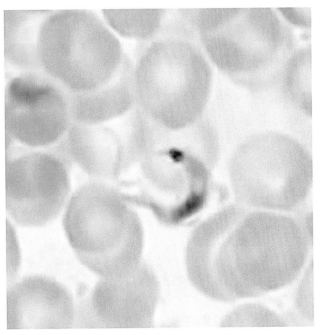

• **Fig. 30.18** *Trypanosoma brucei.*

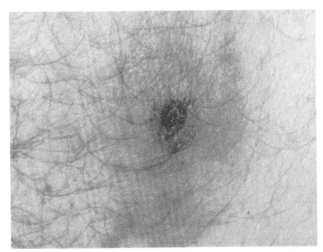

• **Fig. 30.19** Tache noire. (From Faccini-Martínez AA, García-Álvarez L, Hidalgo M, Oteo JA. Syndromic classification of rickettsioses: An approach for clinical practice. *Int J Infect Dis*. 2014;28:126–139.)

- Clinical presentation: can present as an acute febrile illness with lymphadenopathy, splenomegaly, and hemolytic anemia. In its chronic form, it can present with small nodular lesions known as Peruvian warts, along with malaise, weight loss, and fever.
- Diagnosis: histopathology using Warthin–Starry stain can yield multiple bacilli in lymph nodes or skin lesions. Serologies can be helpful but can cross-react with other *Bartonella* species.
- Treatment: ciprofloxacin.

> **HIGH YIELD POINTS**
>
> Think of Oroya fever in patients from endemic regions, such as Peru.

African Tick Bite Fever

- Febrile illness caused by *Rickettsia africae.* This disease should always be considered in returning travelers with a history of a skin lesion or eschar.

- Vectors: *Amblyomma* species.
- Geography: sub-Saharan Africa.
- Season: present all year round.
- Clinical presentation: febrile illness with headache and vesicular rash. Hallmark of the condition is to find a black eschar (tache noire) at the site of tick bite (Fig. 30.19).
- Diagnosis: The diagnosis is mostly clinical. Serologies, biopsy, and PCR techniques can be pursued when diagnosis is unclear.
- Treatment: doxycycline.

> **HIGH YIELD POINTS**
>
> Think of this disease in a febrile patient, with travel to Africa, possible tick exposure, and a tache noire.

Other Travel-Related Vectorborne Spotted Fevers

Table 30.6 illustrates features of other travel-related fever syndromes that are vectorborne.

TABLE 30.6   Key Features of Travel-Related Vectorborne Fever Syndromes

Organism	Disease	Geography	Vector	Presentation
Rickettsia slovaca	TIBOLA	Europe and Asia	*Dermacentor*, *Rhipicephalus*, and *Amblyomma* ticks (dog, wood, and Lone Star tick)	Lymphadenopathy, fever, and malaise
R. slovaca or *D. marginatus*	DEBONEL	Europe and Asia	House mites	*Dermacentor*-borne necrosis and lymphadenopathy, fever, and malaise
R. slovaca, *R. raoultii* or *R. rioja*	SENLAT	Europe and Asia	*Dermacentor*	Scalp eschar, neck lymphadenopathy, fever, and malaise
Rickettsia conorii	Mediterranean spotted fever, boutonneuse fever	Mediterranean, Southeast Asia	*Rhipicephalus* (dog tick)	Fever and papular skin rash Boutonneuse is a French description of this appearance
Rickettsia japonica	Oriental spotted fever, Japanese spotted fever	Japan and northern Asia	*Haemaphysalis flava*	Fever, macular rash, and petechiae
Rickettsia sibirica	Siberian spotted fever	Russia, China, Mongolia	*Dermacentor*	Fever, black eschar, headache, myalgia, lymphadenopathy
Rickettsia felis	Fleaborne spotted fever	Worldwide except Antarctica	Cat fleas	Fever, thrombocytopenia
Rickettsia africae	African tick bite fever	Africa	*Amblyomma*	Fever, black eschar (tache noire)
Rickettsia australis	Queensland tick fever	Australia	*Ixodes*	Fever, headache, myalgia, rash

TIBOLA, tickborne lymphadenopathy; DEBONEL, *Dermacentor*-borne-necrosis-erythemalymphadenopathy; SENLAT, scalp eschar and neck lymph adenopathy after a tick bite.

Further Reading

1. Wormser GP, Dattwyler RJ, Shapiro ED, et al. The clinical assessment, treatment, and prevention of Lyme disease, human granulocytic anaplasmosis, and babesiosis: clinical practice guidelines by the Infectious Diseases Society of America. *Clin Infect Dis.* 2006;43:1089–1134.
2. Biggs HM, Behravesh CB, Bradley KK, et al. Diagnosis and management of tickborne rickettsial diseases: Rocky Mountain spotted fever and other spotted fever group rickettsioses, Ehrlichioses, and anaplasmosis -- United States. *MMWR Recomm Rep.* 2016;65:1–44.
3. Sanchez E, Vannier E, Wormser GP, et al. Diagnosis, treatment, and prevention of Lyme disease, human granulocytic anaplasmosis, and babesiosis: a review. *JAMA.* 2016;315:1767–1777.
4. Talagrand-Reboul E, Boyer PH, Bergström S, et al. Relapsing fevers: neglected tick-borne diseases. *Front Cell Infect Microbiol.* Epub ahead of print 4 April 2018. http://doi.org/10.3389/fcimb.2018.00098.
5. Marcondes CB, Contigiani M, Gleiser RM. Emergent and re-emergent arboviruses in South America and the Caribbean: why so many and why now? *J Med Entomol.* Epub ahead of print 2 March 2017. http://doi.org/10.1093/jme/tjw209.
6. Ashley EA, Pyae Phyo A, Woodrow CJ. Malaria. *Lancet.* 2018;391:1608–1621.
7. Aronson N, Herwaldt BL, Libman M, et al. Diagnosis and treatment of leishmaniasis: clinical practice guidelines by the Infectious Diseases Society of America (IDSA) and the American Society of Tropical Medicine and Hygiene (ASTMH). *Clin Infect Dis.* 2016;63:1539–1557.
8. Bern C. Antitrypanosomal therapy for chronic Chagas' disease. *N Engl J Med.* 2011;364:2527–2534.

31

Infections Associated with Animal Exposure

GEROME ESCOTA

This chapter will highlight important bacterial and viral infections associated with animal exposure. Zoonotic parasitic infections are discussed in Chapters 34, 35, and 46.

Leptospirosis

Leptospirosis is a zoonotic infection acquired from **rodent exposure**. Rodents act as the main reservoir of *Leptospira* spp., which excrete the bacteria in their urine. Human infection occurs with exposure to damp soil or water contaminated by rodent urine. Risk factors are summarized in Box 31.1.

Microbiology and Pathogenesis

- *Leptospira* is a spirochete (helical and coiled bacteria).
- Medically important spirochete infections can be remembered by "**SwiRLL**" (see Box 31.2).
- Best visualized by dark field microscopy, these bacteria are highly motile. *Leptospira interrogans* is the most important species that causes human disease.
- With exposure to contaminated water, humans acquire the bacteria through skin breaks, mucous membranes, or conjunctivae (with no associated focal lesion at the inoculation site).
- Hematogenous dissemination and penetration of tissue barriers follow next.
- Widespread vasculitis ensues, mainly involving the kidneys (acute tubular necrosis, interstitial nephritis), lungs (pulmonary hemorrhage), liver (cholestasis, hepatocyte degeneration; **frank hepatic necrosis is often absent**).

Epidemiology

- Infection is widespread and endemic in all regions of the world. Surveillance studies suggest that it may be the most common zoonotic infection.
- Outbreaks occur in late summer or early fall in temperate countries and during rainy seasons in tropical regions.
- The highest incidence of leptospirosis in the United States is in Hawaii.

Clinical Presentation

- Leptospirosis has a broad clinical spectrum. The infection is most commonly self-limited (2–20 days incubation period). Some patients develop a **biphasic illness**, as shown in Fig. 31.1.
- Some patients do not progress to severe disease while others develop severe disease without a brief improvement in symptoms. In fulminant cases, patients can present with symptoms that rapidly progress to severe disease.
- **Calf and/or lumbar muscle tenderness** is a characteristic physical exam finding.
- **Conjunctival suffusion** (redness without exudate) is also a characteristic finding (Fig. 31.2).
- **Weil's disease** is a syndrome of severe renal and hepatic dysfunction (Box 31.3).

Diagnosis

- During the first 10 days of the illness, leptospires can be isolated from the blood and cerebrospinal fluid (CSF). The organism can be seen in the urine after the first week of the illness.
- Direct examination of the leptospires under dark field microscopy is not routinely done because of its low sensitivity and specificity (artifacts can be mistaken for leptospires).
- The organism can be cultured in appropriate media; however, positive cultures are uncommon.
- Detection of the organism by polymerase chain reaction (PCR) is a promising tool that needs further clinical validation.
- The **microscopic agglutination test (MAT)** is the most common method of diagnosing leptospirosis. It consists of exposing serum samples with *Leptospira* spp. antigens and detection of agglutination under dark field microscopy. It relies on the rise of Ig M antibodies against *Leptospira* spp. that begins after the first week of illness. A diagnosis is made by demonstrating:
  - A four-fold rise between acute-phase and convalescent MAT titers.

- A single MAT titer of **≥1:800** in the presence of compatible symptoms.
- A single MAT titer of **≥1:200** suggests recent or current infection.

Treatment

- Intravenous **penicillin** G is the treatment of choice for severe disease. Ceftriaxone has equivalent efficacy as penicillin G. Mild disease is treated with oral antibiotics (doxycycline, amoxicillin, ampicillin).
- Treatment can be complicated by Jarisch-Herxheimer reaction (Box 31.4).

Prevention

- Doxycycline once-weekly for prophylaxis may be indicated during high-risk exposure (e.g., frequent flooding in highly endemic areas).

Bartonellosis

Microbiology and Pathogenesis

- *Bartonella* spp. are fastidious and intracellular gram-negative bacilli. There are three species that cause human disease: *Bartonella henselae*, *Bartonella quintana*, and *Bartonella bacilliformis*.
- ***Bartonella henselae*** infection is associated with **exposure to cats** (i.e., cat scratch, cat bite).

> **• BOX 31.1** **Risk Factors for Leptospirosis: Buzzwords**
>
> - Recreational activities: freshwater swimming, canoeing, kayaking, trail biking, triathlons.
> - Natural calamities: flooding, increased rainfall.
> - Occupational or household exposure to rodents.

> **• BOX 31.2** **Medically Important Spirochete Infections: SwiRLL**
>
> - Syphilis (*Treponema pallidum*)
> - Relapsing fever (*Borrelia recurrentis*)
> - Leptospirosis (*Leptospira*)
> - Lyme disease (*Borrelia burgdorferi*)

- ***Bartonella quintana*** (causative agent for **trench fever**) and ***Bartonella bacilliformis*** (causative agent for **Oroya fever** and **verruga peruana**) are associated with arthropod exposure and hence will be discussed in Chapter 30, Arthropod-Borne Diseases.
- *Bartonella henselae* is transmitted to humans through cat scratch or bite that permits the inoculation of the infected feces of cat fleas (*Ctenocephalides felis*). Direct exposure to cat fleas has also been linked to human infection.
- Note that cats can be bacteremic with *Bartonella* without causing symptoms for years (usually kittens).
- Inoculation of the organism into humans is followed by a localized inflammatory reaction (i.e., regional lymphadenopathy) that leads to systemic dissemination by endothelial invasion.

Epidemiology

- *Bartonella henselae* infection has worldwide distribution. Although it usually affects children and adolescents, infection occurs in all age groups and among immunocompetent and immunocompromised hosts.

Clinical Presentation

- **Cat-scratch disease** is the major clinical syndrome associated with *Bartonella henselae* infection.
  - Papules and/or pustules appear at the inoculation site (e.g., extremities, scalp, eyes) within 1 week after a cat bite or scratch (these must be sought out as they are often missed). This is followed by regional lymphadenopathy (usually in the axilla, epitrochlear, neck, inguinal; at the same side of inoculation) that appears 1–7 weeks after the bite or scratch.
  - Patients may complain of fever, malaise, headache, arthralgia, and myalgia for several days.
  - The lymph nodes can last for many months and is usually the main complaint of patients seeking medical attention. It can cause a lot of pain and may suppurate in some patients. The lymph nodes resolve with or without antibiotic treatment.
- Atypical manifestations that can precede or occur with the development of lymphadenopathy (or even in the absence of it) are seen in 10% of patients:
  - **Parinaud's oculoglandular syndrome** (Fig. 31.3): granulomatous conjunctivitis with concurrent ipsilateral periauricular (rarely submandibular) lymphadenopathy.

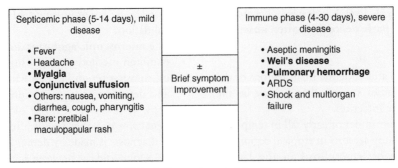

• Fig. 31.1 Biphasic illness characteristic of leptospirosis

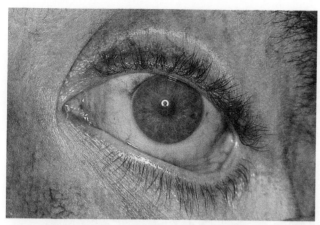

Fig. 31.2 Conjunctivitis in a patient with Weil's disease. (From Cohen J, Powderly WG, eds. *Infectious Diseases*. 2nd ed. Mosby; 2004.)

BOX 31.3   Hepatic Dysfunction in Leptospirosis: Buzzword

Hepatic dysfunction is characterized by:
- Total bilirubin elevation (often extremely elevated) **out of proportion** to the mildly elevated AST and ALT (rarely >200 U/L).

BOX 31.4   Jarisch–Herxheimer Reaction

- Characterized by fever, chills, rash, myalgia, or headache that occur within a few hours after the receipt of antibiotics (cytokine release from the rapid killing of organisms).
- Usually seen in patients with spirochete infection (see Box 31.1).
- Treatment: most are self-limited; antipyretics, supportive care.

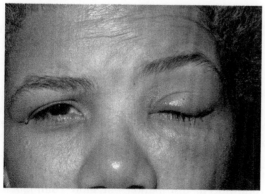

Fig. 31.3 Parinaud's oculoglandular syndrome (conjunctivitis with swollen eyelid and unilateral regional lymphadenopathy, not shown). (From Kaiser PK, Friedman NJ. Conjunctiva and sclera. In: *The Massachusetts Eye and Ear Infirmary Illustrated Manual of Ophthalmology*. 4th ed. Elsevier; 2014.)

- Encephalopathy/encephalitis
  - Headache is a common complaint; patients can be afebrile.
  - Other symptoms: restlessness, confusion, cranial nerve palsy, focal neurologic deficits, seizure, coma.
  - CSF exam usually shows lymphocytic predominant, mild pleocytosis, and normal glucose.
  - Magnetic resonance imaging of the brain is often normal.
- Neuroretinitis
  - Sudden loss of visual acuity (usually involving one eye) is the most common scenario.
  - Papilledema with **stellate exudates (star formation)** on ophthalmologic exam is pathognomonic.
  - Spontaneous resolution with excellent prognosis is the rule.
- Fever of unknown origin (even in the absence of localizing signs).
- Granulomatous hepatitis or splenitis: manifesting as prolonged fever and abdominal pain; abdominal CT scan usually shows enlarged liver or spleen with hypodense lesions (Fig. 31.4).
- Others: atypical pneumonitis, disabling musculoskeletal manifestations (arthritis, osteitis, myalgia), transverse myelitis, hypercalcemia (related to overproduction of vitamin D associated with granuloma formation).

The other clinical syndromes associated with *Bartonella henselae* infection are **bacillary angiomatosis** and **bacillary peliosis**. They are mostly seen among **people living with HIV (PLWH) with CD4 count <200 cells/μL** and other immunosuppressed patients. Of note, *Bartonella quintana* can also cause bacillary angiomatosis/peliosis.

- Bacillary angiomatosis
  - Neovascular proliferation that manifests as cutaneous nodules/masses (usually red/purple) that bleed profusely when incised.
  - Nodules/masses can also involve the liver, spleen, lungs, bone, brain, gastrointestinal tract.
  - Fever and other constitutional symptoms frequently occur.
  - **Can look like Kaposi sarcoma among HIV-infected patients.**
- Bacillary peliosis
  - Commonly involves the **liver and spleen**; manifests as numerous cysts filled with blood.
  - Fever and constitutional symptoms often occur.
  - Abdominal CT scan usually shows enlarged **liver or spleen with hypodense lesions.**
- *Bartonella henselae* and *Bartonella quintana* are also important causes of **culture-negative endocarditis** (see Chapter 15).

Diagnosis

When patients present with any of the syndromes mentioned above and cat exposure (**even in the absence of a bite or a scratch**) is elicited on history, a diagnosis of bartonellosis is

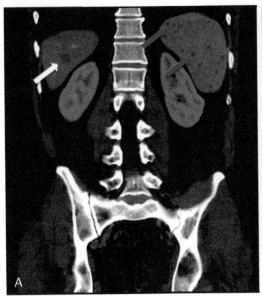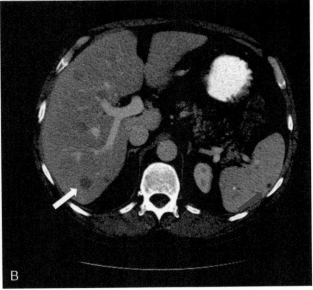

• **Fig. 31.4** Hepatosplenic bartonellosis. Computed tomography scan of the abdomen and pelvis. (A) Coronal view; (B) transverse view. Hypodense lesions shown by *red arrows*. (From Bieraugel K, Oehler D, NeSmith M, Chiovaro J. Cat got your spleen? Hepatosplenic *Bartonella* infection. 2015; *Am J Med.* 128(3):246–249.)

often made when a serologic test is positive, or characteristic histopathologic findings are seen, or molecular evidence of *Bartonella* is present.

- Serologic test
  - Ig G titer <1:64: low likelihood of disease but does not rule it out.
  - Ig G titer 1:65 to 1:256: possible infection; repeat testing should be done in 2 weeks.
  - Ig titer **>1:256**: strongly suggests recent or active disease.
- Necrotizing granuloma (often stellate) with demonstration of bacilli on Warthin–Starry staining is the pathologic hallmark of bartonellosis.
- Bartonella PCR testing can be done on tissue specimen to further confirm the diagnosis.

Treatment

- Antibiotic treatment as detailed in Table 31.1 typically accelerates resolution of symptoms.

Brucellosis

Microbiology and Pathogenesis

Brucella spp. are small, gram-negative, intracellular coccobacilli. Brucellosis is a zoonosis of **wild and domestic animals** (e.g., **cattle, sheep, goats, swine**). It is also an occupational disease since it is most common among farmers, veterinarians, and laboratory technicians.

- Multiple routes of transmission:
  - Ingestion of infected and **unpasteurized milk.**
  - Direct contact with infected animals or their secretions though any break in the skin (during hunting).
  - Inhalation of aerosols from infected animals.
  - Others: blood transfusion, organ transplantation.

TABLE 31.1 Treatment of Bartonellosis

Cat-scratch disease	Usually self-limited Consider antibiotics for severe manifestation: macrolide × 5 days
Encephalitis	Doxycycline + rifampin × 4–6 weeks
Neuroretinitis	Doxycycline + rifampin × 4–6 weeks
Bacillary angiomatosis	Macrolide or doxycycline × 3 months
Bacillary peliosis	Macrolide or doxycycline × 4 months
Endocarditis	Proven case: Doxycycline × 6 weeks (to 3 months if no surgical intervention) + gentamicin × 14 days Suspected case: Ceftriaxone + doxycycline × 6 weeks plus gentamicin × 14 days

- Three species that cause the majority of human infection:
  - *Brucella melitensis*: sheep, goats, camels
  - *Brucella abortus*: cattle
  - *Brucella suis*: domestic/feral swine.

Brucella, after gaining entrance into the body, migrates to the lymph nodes and spreads systemically through the reticuloendothelial system. It causes formation of granuloma in tissues.

Epidemiology

- Worldwide in distribution but more common in the Mediterranean countries, the Persian Gulf, parts of Mexico, Central and South America, the Indian subcontinent, the Balkan Peninsula, and the former Soviet Union.

- Brucella has long been successfully eradicated from the herds in the United States, and all cases are associated with travel, migration, or exposure to imported unpasteurized milk.

Clinical Presentation

Due to its wide spectrum of disease manifestations, like tuberculosis, it is often called a "**great mimic**."

- It is an important cause of **fever of unknown origin (FUO)**, especially in patients with known exposure to domestic animals.
  - After the typical incubation period of 1–4 weeks, it manifests as acute or insidious onset of fever associated with **malodorous perspiration (moldy odor)**, pronounced myalgia and arthralgia, fatigue, malaise, abdominal pain, anorexia, and depression. Hepatomegaly, splenomegaly, and lymphadenopathy maybe apparent on examination or imaging.
  - These symptoms can persist or relapse for days, weeks, or years ("**undulant fever**").
- Brucellosis is a disseminated illness that can involve virtually any organ system (similar to tuberculosis although respiratory involvement in brucellosis is not as common as in tuberculosis).
- Osteoarticular involvement (sacroiliitis in young patients; spondylodiskitis and peripheral arthritis in older patients) is the most common localized infection seen in more than half of patients.
- **Pedro-Pons sign** is said to be pathognomonic of brucellar spondylitis. On plain radiograph, it is the characteristic **anterosuperior step-like erosion** of the involved vertebra, usually the lumbar spine.
- Neurologic involvement is often a serious complication. **Neurobrucellosis** manifests as acute or chronic meningoencephalitis, myelitis, cranial nerve palsies, and radiculoneuropathy. The symptoms can evolve gradually and the manifestations often subtle as to elude diagnosis for a long period of time. CSF usually shows lymphocyte-predominant pleocytosis, high protein, and hypoglycorrhachia (similar to tuberculosis).
- Epididymoorchitis is another common complication; manifests as testicular swelling. In the right epidemiologic setting, any patient who complains of testicular pain/swelling and joint pains should be ruled out for brucellosis.
- Endocarditis, pericarditis, myocarditis.
- Others: hepatosplenic abscesses, colitis, peritonitis, pneumonia, hematologic manifestations (anemia, thrombocytopenia, leucopenia, disseminated intravascular coagulation), skin and ocular lesions.

Diagnosis

- **Culture of the bone marrow** is the gold standard for diagnosis. It is more sensitive than blood culture, remains positive even with prior antibiotic use, and most useful in patients with chronic brucellosis. It should be obtained if the index of suspicion is high, even in the absence of a positive serologic test.

TABLE 31.2 Treatment of Brucellosis

Uncomplicated, nonfocal disease	Doxycycline + streptomycin (or gentamicin) × 6 weeks Alternative: doxycycline + rifampin × 6 weeks
Osteoarticular disease	Doxycycline + streptomycin (or gentamicin) × 3 months
Neurobrucellosis	(Ceftriaxone × 1 month) + (doxycycline + rifampin × 4–5 months); oral antibiotics must be continued generally until CSF parameters normalize
Endocarditis	Lacks data: combination of an aminoglycoside, doxycycline, and rifampin × 6 weeks to 6 months

- Serologic test
- Ig G titer **>1:80** is considered positive in nonendemic regions.
- Ig titer **>1:160** is considered positive in endemic regions.
- Of note, serologic tests become harder to interpret in the setting of chronic infection, reinfection, and relapse as titers remain elevated after an acute infection.
- False-positive results: **antibodies can cross-react with Francisella tularensis** and other bacteria.
- PCR-based molecular testing is a promising tool.

Treatment

- Antibiotic treatment is as detailed in Table 31.2.
- Despite antibiotic treatment, relapses can occur in 5%–15% of cases.
- Even if antibody titers decline with antibiotic treatment, it is an unreliable marker to monitor after a course of antibiotics. Interpretation of serologic tests requires correlation with clinical examination during follow-up.

Q Fever

Microbiology and Pathogenesis

Like brucellosis, Q fever is a zoonosis associated with **domestic animal exposure** (e.g., **cattle**, **sheep**, **goats**). Other animals such as horses, dogs, swine, and camels can harbor the organism and transmit to humans. Unlike brucellosis, it is still present in domestic herds in the United States.

- *Coxiella burnetii*, a gram-negative coccobacilli and the causative agent of Q fever, gets shed in the feces, urine, milk, and most especially in placental products of infected animals. Humans get infected by inhalation of aerosolized organisms.
- Close contact to infected animals, although the most common kind of exposure, is not required for human infection. Outbreaks of Q fever have occurred in communities adjacent to roads on which vehicles carrying infected animals pass through.

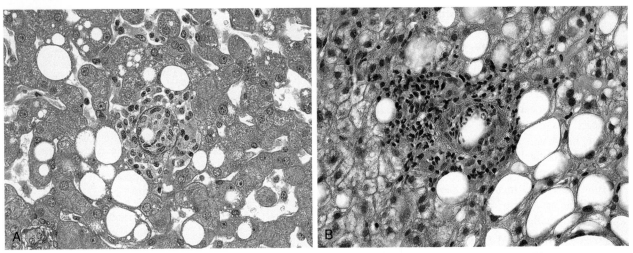

• **Fig. 31.5** Donut granuloma, with a clear center surrounded by an eosinophilic ring. (From Kanel GC, Korula J. Infectious disorders, non-viral. In: *Atlas of Liver Pathology*. Elsevier; 2011.)

• The most dangerous time for infection is during the birthing process of the animal.
• An inoculum of as little as one bacterium is enough to establish disease in humans.

Epidemiology

• Worldwide in distribution, except New Zealand.
• Urbanization of sheep and cattle farming contributed to recent large outbreaks in Europe.

Clinical Presentation

• The most common presenting illness is mild and self-limiting fever that lasts from a few days to 2 weeks. Some infections are also asymptomatic.
• **Pneumonia**
    • Q fever is one of the causes of **atypical pneumonia** (i.e., subacute illness, dry cough, predominance of nonrespiratory manifestations such as diarrhea, hepatitis, and headache).
    • Cough is seen in less than one-third of patients but fever and headache predominate. Headache is sometimes so severe that it may be the chief complaint of a patient seeking medical attention.
    • Although not unique to Q fever, the appearance of **round pneumonia** (coin-sized pulmonary infiltrate) should raise suspicion for *Coxiella burnetii* infection in the right epidemiologic setting.
• **Endocarditis**
    • The most well-recognized form of chronic Q fever; occurs as a complication of acute Q fever (some have had asymptomatic acute infection).
    • Occurs predominantly in older adults (>40 years), those with prior valvular disease/surgery, immunocompromised patients, and pregnant women.
    • Patients present with mild, prolonged, and intermittent fever, fatigue, and malaise.
• Other common manifestations: hepatomegaly, splenomegaly, digital clubbing, purpuric skin eruption, immune-complex glomerulonephritis.

• Patients can also have **hypergammaglobulinemia and elevated levels of autoantibodies** (e.g., rheumatoid factor, antismooth muscle antibodies, antimitochondrial antibodies, antiphospholipid antibodies, positive Coombs test).
• **Hepatitis**
    • Can be the presenting symptom of acute Q fever in some patients.
    • Often occurs in patients with fever of unknown origin related to chronic Q fever infection.
    • Can persist despite antibiotic treatment; in these patients, autoimmune hepatitis may be contributing, and a short course of corticosteroids is sometimes beneficial.
• **Fever of unknown origin**
    • Can have concurrent pneumonia, hepatitis, or hematologic manifestations.
• **Lipoid or donut or fibrin ring granuloma** seen on tissue biopsy (Fig. 31.5) suggests Q fever infection (although this finding is also seen in Hodgkin lymphoma, EBV infection, and drug hypersensitivity reactions).
• Others: osteoarticular infection, hemolytic anemia, reactive thrombocytosis, erythema nodosum, postinfective fatigue syndrome.

Diagnosis

Serologic tests has been the mainstay of diagnosing Q fever. The test relies on antibody responses to antigenic phase variation that is characteristic of *Coxiella burnetii* (phase I and II; morphologically similar but antigenically and biochemically different).

• Acute Q fever (acute pneumonia, hepatitis)
    • During acute infection, *Coxiella burnetii* is phase II-dominant. As the infection becomes chronic, it switches to phase I-dominant.
    • Acute infection: phase II (Ig G, Ig M) >> phase I antibodies (Ig G, Ig M).
    • A four-fold rise in phase II Ig G antibodies after 2–4 weeks also makes the diagnosis of acute Q fever.

- Chronic Q fever (endocarditis, prolonged fever of unknown origin, etc.)
  - Chronic infection: phase I (Ig G, Ig M usually negative) >> phase II antibodies (Ig G, Ig M usually negative).
  - **A single phase I Ig G titer >1:800 makes a diagnosis of chronic Q fever.**

Treatment

- **Acute Q fever**: doxycycline × 14 days.
  - Alternative agents include a macrolide, trimethoprim–sulfamethoxazole (TMP–SMX), or fluoroquinolone.
  - For pregnant women, TMP–SMX is recommended.
- **Chronic Q fever** (including endocarditis): doxycycline + hydroxychloroquine × 18 months (24 months for prosthetic valve endocarditis).
  - Alternative regimen, include doxycycline + rifampin, doxycycline + fluoroquinolone.
  - For pregnant women, TMP–SMX is recommended.
  - Serologic tests should be performed every 3 months during and up to 2 years after stopping antibiotic treatment. In general, cure is achieved when phase I Ig G falls below 1:800, anemia and hypergammaglobulinemia improve, and the erythrocyte sedimentation rate declines.

Tularemia

Microbiology and Pathogenesis

Francisella tularensis, the causative agent of tularemia, is a gram-negative coccobacillus. *Francisella tularensis* subsp. *tularensis* and *Francisella tularensis* subsp. *holarctica* cause the majority of human illness.

- Tularemia is mostly associated with exposure to rabbits, squirrels, voles, muskrats, and beavers. Dogs, cats, and other carnivorous animals that prey on them can transmit the disease by carrying the organism in their claws or mouths.
- Tularemia has multiple routes of transmission:
  - **Arthropod bite** (ticks in most cases, flies in California and Nevada, mosquitoes in some European countries; can transmit the organism via the saliva or feces) and **contact with contaminated animal products** (e.g., skinning, dressing infected animals) are the most common routes.
  - Others: **inhalation** via aerosolized droplets, **ingestion** of contaminated water or mud (or even meat), animal bites.
  - Inhalation of contaminated materials (e.g., dust, hay, water) during activities such as **lawn mowing** (outbreak of infection in Martha's Vineyard in 2000).
  - **There is no risk of human-to-human spread.**
- After cutaneous entry, it incites a localized inflammatory reaction characterized by tissue necrosis. The bacteria then spread to regional lymph nodes and spread via the blood (most are bacteremic) and the lymphatic system. Tissue specimens can sometimes reveal caseating granuloma.
- Because of its high attack rate, it is a potential agent of bioterrorism (see Chapter 47). Laboratory personnel handling a specimen from a patient suspected of having tularemia need to be notified.

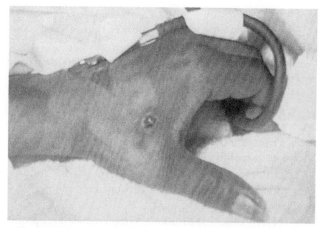

- **Fig. 31.6** Tularemic eschar. (From Beard CB, Dennis DT. Tularemia. In: Cohen J, Opal S, Powderly W, eds. *Infectious Diseases*. 3rd ed. Elsevier; 2010.)

Epidemiology

- Confined mostly to the Northern hemisphere; most notably absent in the United Kingdom, Africa, South America, and Australia.
- More than half of cases in the United States are reported from Arkansas, Missouri, Kansas, South Dakota, California, and Oklahoma during the summer months.

Clinical Presentation

The incubation period is typically 3–5 days. The most common symptoms are abrupt onset of fever, chills, fatigue, headache, myalgia, cough, abdominal pain, and diarrhea.

There are six classic presentations of tularemia **that often overlap** with one another.

- **Ulceroglandular**
  - Skin ulcer + regional lymphadenopathy (inguinal > cervical).
  - The skin ulcer may become an eschar (Fig. 31.6) over time and can precede, coincide with, or come after the appearance of the lymph node; the ulcers can sometimes appear sporotrichoid in distribution.
- **Glandular**
  - Together with ulceroglandular tularemia, represents the most common presentation.
  - No skin ulcer (or have resolved already).
  - Lymph nodes are painful and often persist for weeks; fever and other constitutional symptoms may have already resolved on presentation.
  - Differential diagnoses: pyogenic infection, cat-scratch disease, sexually transmitted diseases (syphilis, chancroid, lymphogranuloma venereum), sporotrichosis, tuberculosis.
- **Oculoglandula**r
  - Usually affects only one eye.
  - Occurs after the organism gains entry via the conjunctiva through contaminated fingers, splashes of water, or aerosol.
  - **Similar in presentation with cat-scratch disease** (Parinaud's oculoglandular syndrome).

- **Pharyngeal**
  - Occurs via oropharyngeal route of transmission (contaminated food or water).
  - Often with concurrent cervical lymphadenopathy.
- **Pneumonic**
  - Occurs via inhalational route of transmission or via hematogenous spread from other forms of tularemia (typhoidal > ulceroglandular).
  - Presents as community-acquired pneumonia that does not respond to conventional antibiotics; pneumonic symptoms and infiltrates can even last for months mimicking other causes of chronic pneumonia.
- **Typhoidal**
  - Fever + other constitutional symptoms without prominent skin lesions or lymphadenopathy.
  - The most difficult to diagnose and hence presents usually as **fever of unknown origin**; severe cases can present acutely with rapid deterioration.
  - Prominent manifestations: abdominal pain, diarrhea, nausea, vomiting, headache, hepatitis (with splenomegaly and hepatomegaly in chronic cases).
  - Rarely, may be complicated by meningitis.

Diagnosis

- Serologic tests remain the most common method of diagnosing tularemia.
  - A single titer **>1:128** (microagglutination) or **>1:160** (tube agglutination), with compatible symptoms, suggest active disease.
  - Note that antibodies against *Francisella tularensis* tend to persist for several years after an acute infection.
  - A fourfold rise in antibody titer repeated after 10–14 days is the definitive serologic diagnosis for tularemia.
- The organism can be isolated in culture using special media from the blood, lymph node, wound drainage/biopsy, sputum, or pleural fluid.

Treatment

- Moderate to serious illness: streptomycin or gentamicin × 7–10 days.
- Mild disease: ciprofloxacin or doxycycline × 14 days.
- Meningitis: streptomycin or gentamicin + doxycycline or chloramphenicol × 2–3 weeks.

Other Important Infections

Anthrax

Anthrax is caused by *Bacillus anthracis*, one of several medically important gram-positive bacilli (Box 31.5).

Actinomyces and *Nocardia* are also gram-positive bacilli but usually described as "**branching filamentous organisms**" (BFO).

- Associated with exposure to **infected grazing herbivores** (e.g., cattle) and **contaminated animal products** (e.g., hide, wool, hair, horn) by either **inhalation** or

---

> • **BOX 31.5** **Medically Important Gram-Positive Bacilli**
>
> "*CARE*er in *P*roblem-*B*ased *L*earning"
> - C, *Corynebacterium*, *Clostridium*
> - A, *Arcanobacterium hemolyticum*
> - R, *Rhodococcus equi*
> - E, *Erysipelothrix rhusiopathiae*
> - P, *Propionibacterium* (or *Cutibacterium*) *acnes*
> - B, *Bacillus*
> - L, *Listeria*, *Lactobacillus*

ingestion, or **contact** (even with trivial trauma) with bacterial spores that can remain in the environment for long periods of time.
- Sporadic cases occur most commonly in Africa, the Middle East, and Latin America; anthrax has been used in bioterrorism (refer to Chapter 47).

The infection manifests in different ways depending on the route of transmission.

- **Cutaneous anthrax**
  - Painless, nonpurulent papule that develops, within days, into a vesicle and then to a black eschar surrounded by a significant amount of induration or nonpitting edema that is out of proportion to the size of the wound (the entire extremity may become edematous); the edema is secondary to bacterial production of edema factor (Fig. 31.7).
  - Cutaneous anthrax acquired through injection drug use presents atypically (no eschar, presents with extensive skin infection; relatively painless and with pronounced edema and systemic symptoms).
- **Inhalational anthrax**
  - Almost always raises suspicion for bioterrorism.
  - Serious infection with very high mortality rate despite use of appropriate antibiotics and intensive care.
  - Starts with flu-like illness (prodromal phase) that progresses into an intermediate phase characterized by high fever, dyspnea, pleuritic chest pain, and confusion (chest X-ray typically shows widened mediastinum and hemorrhagic pleural effusion); progresses (even with antibiotic use) to a fulminant phase with multiorgan failure.
  - Regarded as a disease of the mediastinum rather than a lung parenchymal disease.
- **Gastrointestinal anthrax**
  - Usually through ingestion of undercooked meat.
  - Oropharyngeal anthrax: marked inflammation of the pharynges with ulcer and pseudomembrane formation (similar to diphtheria); marked edema of the face and neck.
  - Intestinal anthrax: diarrhea, severe abdominal pain, nausea, vomiting, massive ascites (can be bloody), bloody diarrhea.
- **Anthrax meningitis** (Box 31.6)
  - Arises as a complication of bacteremia (usually from inhalational and gastrointestinal anthrax) in 50% of cases.

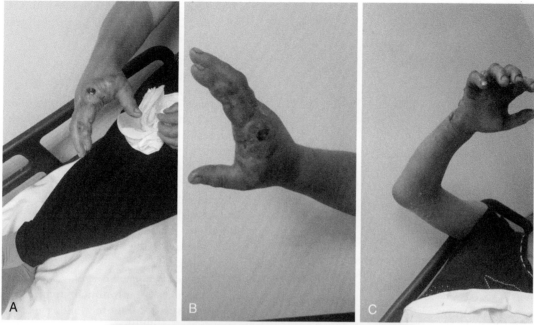

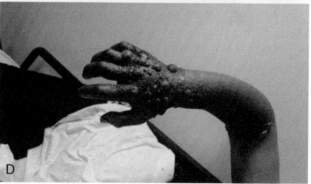

• **Fig. 31.7** Cutaneous anthrax. Note the prominent eschar surrounded by a significant amount of edema which is pathognomonic of the infection. Hemorrhagic blisters can sometimes develop. (From Emet M, Tortum F, Karagoz S, Calbay A. Cutaneous anthrax. *J Emerg Med.* 2017;52(2):240–241.)

• BOX 31.6 Anthrax Meningitis

Maintain high index of suspicion in all cases of inhalational, gastrointestinal, or cutaneous anthrax with severe and systemic manifestations. **Lumbar puncture should be performed** in these patients to rule out meningitis, unless contraindicated.
- **Harbinger of death** (usually a day after onset).
- Manifests as acute onset headache and rapidly progressing mental status deterioration.
- Characterized by subarachnoid hemorrhage, widespread parenchymal bleed, and cerebral edema.

Treatment

- Cutaneous anthrax (naturally acquired): fluoroquinolone or doxycycline x 7-10 days.
- Cutaneous anthrax (suspected bioterrorism): fluoroquinolone or doxycycline × 60 days.
- Systemic anthrax (inhalational, gastrointestinal, severe cutaneous anthrax) **and meningitis ruled out**: ciprofloxacin + clindamycin/linezolid × 2–3 weeks (followed by postexposure prophylaxis to prevent recurrence → single agent therapy to complete 60 days of treatment).

- Systemic anthrax (inhalational, gastrointestinal, severe cutaneous anthrax) **with meningitis (or in cases where meningitis cannot be ruled out with a lumbar puncture)**: ciprofloxacin + meropenem + linezolid × 2–3 weeks (followed by postexposure prophylaxis to prevent recurrence → single agent therapy to complete 60 days of treatment).
- All patients with systemic anthrax should also receive **antitoxin therapy (raxibacumab, obiltoxaximab)**.
- In addition, all patients with inhalational anthrax should receive **anthrax immunoglobulin.**
- Glucocorticoid therapy should be considered in patients with meningitis, cutaneous anthrax with extensive edema, or septic shock.

Plague

- Caused by *Yersinia pestis*, a gram-negative bacilli.
- Associated with close contact with **infected rodents and their predators** (usually dogs and cats).
- Human transmission occurs via flea bite (most common), direct inoculation (e.g., handling of carcasses of

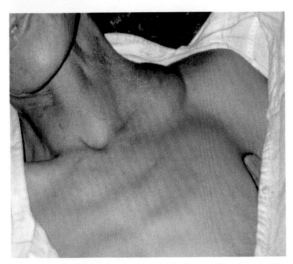

• **Fig. 31.8** Cervical bubo in a patient with plague. (Reprinted with permission from Elsevier. The Lancet. From Prof. Michael B Prentice PhD, et al. Plague. *Lancet Infect Dis.* 2007;369(9568):1196–1207.)

infected animals during hunting), or inhalation of aerosols (pneumonic plague).
• Most cases reported in sub-Saharan Africa, particularly **Madagascar**, Tanzania, and Democratic Republic of the Congo; in the United States, most cases are reported from **New Mexico**, **Arizona**, **Colorado**, and **California.**
• Clinical manifestation
  • **Bubonic plague**
    • Usually arises after a flea bite to an extremity.
    • Characterized by the acute and sudden appearance of a **bubo** (exquisitely painful and tender lymphadenopathy in the groin, axilla, or head and neck region) (Fig. 31.8) associated with high fever and chills.
    • The bubo lacks signs of ascending lymphangitis that is characteristic of other causes of infectious lymphadenitis.
  • **Septicemic plague**
    • Abrupt onset of high fever, chills, and other constitutional symptoms in the absence of lymphadenopathy.
    • Rapidly progressive disease; death can ensue in a few days.
  • **Pneumonic plague**
    • Primary pneumonia occurs after inhalation of infectious aerosols (e.g., close contact with a person with pneumonic plague, dogs or cats with pharyngeal bacterial contamination, exposure related to laboratory work or **bioterrorism**).
    • Secondary pneumonia occurs as a complication of septicemic or bubonic plague.
    • Heralded by high fever, chills, cough (often with blood-tinged sputum) that rapidly progress to respiratory compromise within a few days; chest imaging shows bilateral alveolar infiltrates and consolidation.

• Treatment: streptomycin or gentamicin is the treatment of choice. Doxycycline is an alternative agent. Treatment is continued for 7–14 days.

Rat-Bite Fever

• Caused by *Streptobacillus moniliformis* (North America, Europe) and *Spirillum minus* (Asia) which are part of rodent nasopharyngeal flora.
• Associated with **rodent exposure** (e.g., bites, **even from pet rats**, are the most common route of transmission but patients can develop infection without recalling an actual bite); bites from carnivores that prey on rodents have also transmitted the infection.
• Infections caused by *Streptobacillus moniliformis* and *Spirillum minus* differ but both are characterized by the abrupt onset of fever, chills, and headache.
  • *Streptobacillus moniliformis*: characterized by the development of **prominent migratory arthralgia/arthritis** and diffuse morbilliform or petechial rash that can involve the palms and soles.
  • *Spirillum minus*: characterized by the development of an ulcer at the inoculation site associated with regional lymphadenopathy; the ulcer forms into an **eschar** over time; **arthritis/arthralgia is absent.**
• Both can be visualized on peripheral blood smear but only *Streptobacillus moniliformis* grows on culture; *Spirillum minus* is mainly diagnosed by direct visualization of the organism on smear.
• Treatment: penicillin G is the treatment of choice.

Hantavirus

• Caused by viruses in the *Bunyaviridae* group; human transmission occurs through exposure (e.g., inhalation, contact) to aerosols or from **contamination with rat urine, feces, or saliva.**
• Usually infects otherwise healthy individuals; cleaning a room infested with mice/rats is a common risk factor.
• Causes two syndromes of medical importance:
  • Hemorrhagic fever and renal syndrome (HFRS)
    • Hantaan virus (Korea, China, eastern Russia) and Dobrava virus (Balkan peninsula) cause severe HFRS.
    • Recent epidemic of Seoul virus causing HFRS in the United States December 2016 to January 2017.
    • Puumala virus (Scandinavian region) causes *nephropathia epidemica* (a milder form of HFRS).
  • Hantavirus pulmonary syndrome (HPS)
    • **Sin Nombre virus**, found in the western part of the United States (highest cases in Utah, Colorado, Arizona, and New Mexico).
• Clinical manifestation: see Box 31.7.
• Diagnosis: detection of IgM in the serum, PCR testing of blood or tissue samples.
• Treatment is supportive; excessive fluid hydration should be avoided and use of cardiotonic drugs is recommended.

• BOX 31.7 **Hallmark of Hantavirus Infection (HFRS and HPS)**

- Fever, thrombocytopenia (more severe in HFRS), leukocytosis with left shift (immature myeloid cells in the smear), atypical lymphocytosis, elevated hematocrit (from increased capillary permeability).
- HFRS is characterized by fever, severe thrombocytopenia (leading to hemorrhagic petechiae and bleeding), and acute renal failure (acute interstitial nephritis); hemodynamic instability leading to shock and multiorgan failure is secondary to the development of acute and profound capillary leak syndrome.
- HPS manifests similarly as HFRS but without the early development of acute renal failure and hemorrhagic diathesis; characterized by the rapid development of respiratory failure secondary to pulmonary edema from increased capillary leakage.

Monkeypox and Cowpox

- Monkeypox virus is so named because it was first isolated from monkeys, but since then it has been found to infect a wide variety of small mammals.
  - Infections are confined to Africa, however in 2003, an outbreak in the United States (Illinois, Indiana, Kansas, Missouri) occurred, linked to exposure to **prairie dogs and South American rodents**; outbreak investigation demonstrated that the guinea pigs were infected by monkeypox virus from small animals imported from Ghana.
  - Characterized by fever and **vesicular rash**; the vesicles appear in the **same stage of development (unlike the varicella or chickenpox rash); rash is indistinguishable from smallpox** but monkeypox is distinguished from the latter by the prominent development of submandibular/cervical **lymphadenopathy** in monkeypox infection.
- **Cowpox** is a related virus associated with exposure to infected **cows**; characterized by the appearance of localized vesicles (usually the hands and face) in association with mild fever and malaise.

Orf

- Orf virus infection is associated with exposure to sheep, goats, cattle, camels.
- Characterized by the appearance of a solitary nodule at the inoculation site (usually the finger); the nodule first appears as a papule and slowly develops into a vesicle and a granulomatous nodule over 4–6 weeks (Fig. 31.9).
- Usually self-limited but the use of topical cidofovir and imiquimod has anecdotally been reported to be effective.

Herpes B Virus

- Herpes virus B (also called B virus) infection is associated with exposure to **Old World macaques.**

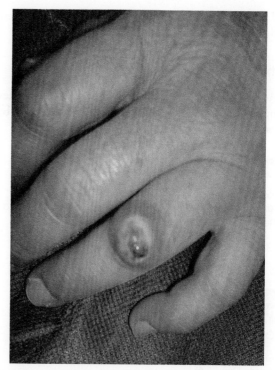

• **Fig. 31.9** Orf. Solitary lesion at the site of inoculation. (From Saçar H, Uyar B, Saçar T, Duran A. Investigation of the complications and incidences of orf disease during and after the Feast of the Sacrifice period. *Dermatologica Sinica.* 2015;33(4):191–195.)

- Routes of acquisition: bites, scratches, nonintact skin exposure to mucosal secretions.
- The most common and dreaded manifestation in humans is **encephalitis** that mimics herpes simplex virus encephalitis; other patients complain of a localized vesicular rash around the inoculation site accompanied by paresthesias.
- Patients with potential herpes B virus exposure should receive postexposure prophylaxis with aciclovir/valaciclovir for 14 days.
- Patients with herpes B virus infection should be treated with intravenous ganciclovir/aciclovir and receive oral aciclovir/valganciclovir for long periods of time after an infection.

Psittacosis

- Caused by *Chlamydia psittaci.*
- Associated with contact with infected birds (asymptomatic or sick); human infection mostly comes from parakeets, cockatoos, and parrots, but many bird species can transmit the disease.
- Humans acquire the disease when bacteria from dried bird feces become aerosolized and inhaled.
- Outbreaks associated with exposure to pet shops or poultry farms.
- Causes symptoms characteristic of atypical pneumonia (i.e., dry cough, predominance of nonrespiratory symptoms, including headache, myalgia, diarrhea, liver enzyme abnormalities).
- Diagnosis is mainly through serologic testing.

- Treatment is with the use of doxycycline, macrolides, or fluoroquinolones.

Rabies

- Associated with exposure to **rabid dogs** (mostly in developing countries) and **wild animals**, **particularly bats**, **raccoons**, **skunks**, and **foxes** (in the Unites States).

• BOX 31.8   Risk of Person-to-Person Transmission

Of the zoonoses that have been presented here, only the pneumonic form of plague (*Yersinia pestis*) can be transmitted from person to person.

- Transmitted by exposure to the saliva of infected animals (rarely via aerosolized virus in bat caves or organ transplantation).
- Characterized by a fatal form of central nervous system infection.
- See Chapter 12 (Central Nervous System Infections) for more information.

For risk of person-person transmission see Box 31.8.

Other Animal-Associated Infections

A miscellany of other infections arising from animal exposure is presented in Table 31.3.

TABLE 31.3   Other Infections

Organism/Infection	Animal Exposure	Clinical Pearls
Rhodococcus equi (see Box 31.5)	Horses	• Subacute pneumonia (often cavitary), extrapulmonary (brain and skin abscess) • Think of *R. equi* in a patient with pulmonary **malakoplakia** (chronic granulomatous infection) + epidemiologic exposure
Pasteurella multocida	Cats	• Wide spectrum of infections
Capnocytophaga canimorsus	Dogs	• Severe sepsis and shock in asplenic/immunocompromised patients
Mycobacterium marinum	Fish, fish tank	• Lymphangitic (or sporotrichoid), nodular cellulitis, deep infections (e.g., tenosynovitis)
Salmonella (non-typhi)	Pet reptiles and amphibians (snake, turtle, frogs)	• Bacteremia, gastroenteritis
Lymphocytic choriomeningitis virus	Rodents	• Common during winter months • Aseptic meningitis (but can also look bacterial) • Case of infection derived from organ transplantation
Toxoplasma gondii	Cats	• Important in pregnant and immunocompromised patients • Mononucleosis-like illness; pneumonia and brain abscess in immunocompromised patients
Erysipelothrix rhusiopathiae (see Box 31.5)	Swine, sheep, horses, fish	• Commonly infects slaughterhouse workers, butchers, fishermen, aquarium workers • Causes a well-demarcated **violaceous rash (erysipeloid of Rosenbach)** with minimal swelling (usually in the hands, site of inoculation)
Mycobacterium bovis	Cattle (unpasteurized milk)	• Clinically and radiographically indistinguishable from tuberculosis
Listeria monocytogenes (see Box 31.5)	Foodborne (unpasteurized dairy products)	• Elderly (>60 years), immunocompromised hosts • Causes a distinctive form of central nervous system infection, **rhombencephalitis** that predominantly affects the brain stem in patients who are immunocompetent
Ebola and Marburg virus	Primates (bats are possible reservoir hosts, but bat-to-human transmission has not been shown)	• Exclusively found in Africa • Contact with infected animals (e.g., butchering, hunting) • Viral hemorrhagic fever • High mortality and person-to-person transmission rates

32

Tuberculosis

CARLOS R. MEJIA-CHEW, THOMAS CHARLES BAILEY

Etiology

Tuberculosis (TB) is caused by any of the species from the *Mycobacterium tuberculosis* complex (MTB):
- *M. tuberculosis.*
- *M. africanum.*
- *M. bovis* (commonly associated with intestinal tract TB via consumption of unpasteurized dairy products).
- *M. canetti* (cases seen in the Horn of Africa).
- *M. pinnipedii* (exposure to seals).
- *M. microti* (a rodent pathogen).
- Bacillus Calmette–Guérin (BCG).

Epidemiology

- MTB has a worldwide distribution, and one-third of the world's population is infected.
- There are 10 million new cases of TB disease yearly, but only 6.4 million get access to TB care.
- TB is the top infectious disease killer in the world (1.6 million deaths in 2017) and the leading killer among people living with human immunodeficiency virus HIV (one in three AIDS-related deaths), the majority of whom live in sub-Saharan Africa.
- There is a worldwide increase of drug-resistant TB, especially in India, China, Russia, and Eastern Europe.
  - Multidrug-resistant (MDR) TB: resistance to both isoniazid (INH) and rifampin (RIF).
  - Extensively drug-resistant (XDR) TB: MDR, plus resistance to any fluoroquinolone (FLQ), and at least one of the three injectable agents (amikacin, capreomycin, or kanamycin).

Natural History

- Risk of acquiring TB infection is higher in close contacts of patients with acid-fact bacilli (AFB) smear-positive pulmonary TB (~30%) than smear-negative (~10%).
- Latent TB infection (LTBI) is a misnomer since mycobacteria bacilli are not truly in a dormant phase; however, this term is still commonly used (Fig. 32.1) (Table 32.1).

TB Infection

- Asymptomatic infection is diagnosed through a positive **Mantoux** tuberculin skin test (TST) (see Table 32.2) or an interferon gamma release assay (IGRA).
- Chest imaging can either have no abnormalities, show granulomas, and/or pleural/parenchymal scarring.
- TST conversion occurs 3–6 weeks after exposure.
- There are two types of IGRA tests available (see Fig. 32.2):
  - QuantiFERON®-TB Gold Plus (**QFT-Plus**).
  - T-SPOT® *TB* test (**T-Spot**).
- IGRAs have excellent specificity (>90%) and are unaffected by previous BCG vaccination.
- In people living with HIV, both IGRA and TST may be negative (>10%). In the setting of advanced disease (i.e., CD4 count <50) and if there has been recent exposure to a person with infectious TB, LTBI treatment should be considered despite negative screening tests.

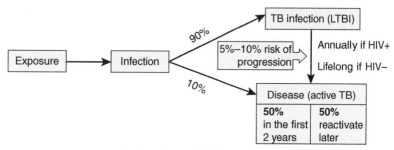

• **Fig. 32.1** Latent TB infection diagram.

465

TABLE 32.1	Risk Factors for TB	
Risk Factors for INFECTION	**Risk Factors for PROGRESSION**	
Homelessness	Diabetes	
Work-related exposure (Healthcare/ Penitentiary)	Intravenous drug use	
Immigrants from an endemic area	Intestinal bypass	
	TNF-α inhibitors	
Exposure to someone with active pulmonary TB	CXR abnormalities c/w prior inadequately treated infection	
	HIV or other immunosuppression	
Incarceration	End-stage renal disease	
Intravenous drug use	Recent TB infection	
	Silicosis	
At **Home** or **Work** I'm Exposed to **Infection.**	**DITCHERS**	

TABLE 32.2	Tuberculosis Skin Testing Interpretation
TST Induration (not erythema)	**Population in Which Is Considered POSITIVE**
≥5 mm	HIV, close contact with active TB case, CXR consistent with TB, immunosuppressed (patients with transplant or on prednisone ≥15 mg/day for >3 weeks), receiving anti-tumor necrosis factor (TNF) agents
≥10 mm	Dialysis, diabetes, IV drug users, lymphoma/leukemia, head/neck cancer, children ≤4-year-old, foreign born from countries of higher incidence, high-risk patients (i.e., healthcare workers, incarcerated, homeless, nursing home or long-term care facility residents, microbiology lab personnel)
≥15 mm	Healthy persons without risk factors for TB
False negative	Live virus vaccinations, hypoproteinemia, lymphoproliferative disorders, old age, use of immunosuppressants (corticosteroids), improper administration, interpretation, or storage

- During pregnancy, there is an increased risk of hepatotoxicity due to INH, extending up to 3 months postpartum. Therefore LTBI treatment in pregnancy is usually reserved for those recently exposed, those living with HIV or those who have other significant immunosuppression.

Treatment of TB Infection

- The single most important thing before treating TB infection is to rule out active TB disease (symptom review, physical exam, and baseline chest X-ray–CXR).

- Effective treatment of LTBI reduces the risk of progression to TB disease by 60%–90% (Table 32.3).
- <60% of patients complete the 9-month INH monotherapy regimen.
- The short course (3 months) of once-weekly (12 doses) combined INH + rifapentine (RPT) enhances adherence.
- For those exposed to MDR-TB, treatment of LTBI is based upon drug susceptibilities. Twelve months of a FLQ-based regimen, alone or in combination with a second drug (ethambutol [EMB] favored if susceptible) is recommended.
- Baseline alanine aminotransferase (ALT), aspartate aminotransferase (AST), alkaline phosphatase (ALP), and total bilirubin can help distinguish preexisting abnormalities from TB-drug induced hepatotoxicity. However, they are only routinely recommended with:
  - Underlying liver disease.
  - Active alcohol consumption.
  - Concomitant hepatotoxic drugs.
  - Pregnancy, up to 3 months postpartum.
  - People living with HIV.
- Monitor monthly for clinical symptoms of hepatitis.

TB Disease: Clinical Syndromes

- TB disease most commonly involves the lungs, but it can affect any organ.
- The characteristic histopathologic feature of TB is the presence of caseating ("cheese-like") granulomatous inflammation.
- TB is divided into primary and reactivation disease (postprimary), and by pulmonary vs. extrapulmonary disease, based on timing and organ involved, respectively.
- Extrapulmonary TB is more common in people living with HIV and may present without systemic symptoms.
- Subacute/chronic symptoms are typical and commonly include fever, chills, night sweats, weight loss, cough, and hemoptysis.
- If there is parenchymal lung involvement (not exclusively pleural) the patient is potentially contagious and should be placed in a negative-pressure isolation room.
- The most common extrapulmonary site of involvement is the lymphatic system (Table 32.4).

Pulmonary TB

Primary TB
- Remains undiagnosed in the majority of cases, as symptoms are absent or mild and usually self-resolving (fever and nonproductive cough). Chest pain can be seen but is less common, and there may be bulky intrathoracic adenopathy that may cause bronchial compression in children.

Reactivation TB
- Is generally progressive and has upper lobe predilection with cavitation but not bulky adenopathy.
- Fever and night sweats are seen in 50% of cases.

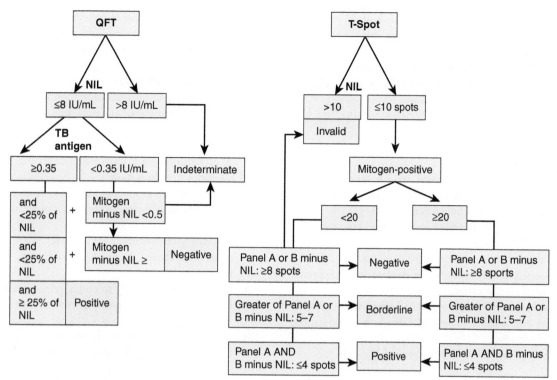

• **Fig. 32.2** Indeterminate (QFT) or invalid (T-spot) results may be caused by either a failed positive (mitogen) or negative (NIL) control. When the controls are valid, results are interpreted after subtraction of the NIL result from the patient result.

TABLE 32.3   Treatment of Latent Tuberculosis Infection

Regimen	Duration	Doses
INH + RPT once a week	3 months	12
RIF daily	4 months	120
INH daily	6 months	180
INH daily	9 months	270
INH twice weekly	6–9 months	52–76

INH isoniazid; RPT rifapentine; RIF rifampin

TABLE 32.4   Typical Patterns of TB Disease: Primary vs. Reactivation

Primary TB	Reactivation TB
Usually a child or immunocompromised (endemic areas or close contacts of infectious persons with TB)	Usually an adult
	Upper-lobe disease
	Pulmonary cavitation and nodules
Mid-lower lobe disease in >80% of patients	Extrapulmonary more common
Hilar adenopathy in 2/3 of patients (R>L)	
Pleural effusion in 1/3 of patients	

• Hemoptysis is seen in 25% of the cases and is uncommonly due to Rasmussen's aneurysm (aneurysm in the setting of a cavitation).
• Typically affects apical-posterior segments of the upper lobes > superior segments of the lower lobes > apical anterior segment of the upper lobes.
• Cavitation is more common (20%–40%) than in primary TB.
• Other typical chest CT findings: hilar adenopathy, centrilobular nodules, and branching linear lesions (tree-in-bud-sign).
• Lower lung field TB → TB disease occurring below the hila.

TB pleuritis
• Pleural effusion is seen in up to 25% of cases of primary TB.
• Although it can resolve spontaneously in 2–4 months, it may leave pleural thickening/calcifications.
• If not treated it can cause rapidly progressive disease in infants and immunosuppressed patients and carries a high risk of reactivation in immunocompetent patients.
• A presumptive diagnosis is based on the presence of a lymphocytic predominant exudative effusion with an adenosine deaminase (ADA) >40 IU/L, or the presence of caseating granulomas on pleural biopsy (>70% of cases).
• AFB smear sensitivity in the pleural effusion is very low (<10%). Nucleic acid amplification tests (NAAT) also have low sensitivity (~45%).

- Definitive diagnosis is based on isolation of *M. tuberculosis* on pleural fluid culture (<30% sensitivity) or pleural biopsy culture (40%–80% sensitive).
- >95% of patients with granulomatous pleuritis have tuberculosis. Other causes: rheumatoid arthritis, fungal infection, tularemia, and sarcoidosis.
- With therapy, most patients defervesce within 2 weeks, and pleural fluid is resorbed within 6 weeks.

Endobronchial TB
- Infection of the tracheobronchial tree is more commonly seen in extensive TB disease (cavitation), caused by extension from a parenchymal focus.
- Causes barking productive cough, wheezing, rhonchi and, rarely, lithoptysis.
- Bronchial stenosis is present in 90% of cases and bronchial ulceration (hemoptysis) or perforations (fistulas) are potential complications.
- CXR can be normal in up to 20% of cases. Although CT can show endobronchial lesions. Diagnosis established by bronchoscopy.
- Bronchoscopy brushing and lavage are high yield for cultures (>90%).

Miliary TB

- Represents disseminated disease (hematogenous), usually seen in the first 6 months after the TB exposure, although it also occurs in reactivation disease.
- Acute miliary TB may be fulminant (multiorgan system failure/septic shock/acute respiratory distress syndrome).
- Most commonly affects elderly, infants, and immunosuppressed patients (including people living with HIV).
- Lung involvement is almost always present, and chest imaging typically shows diffuse micronodules (≤3 mm), predominantly in the lower lobes ("millet seeds" in the lungs).
- Clinical evaluation should include funduscopy.
- Anemia is the most common laboratory abnormality, but other cytopenias are not uncommon, and leukemoid reactions have been described.
- High-yield biopsy sites for culture: bone marrow, liver, lymph nodes, pleura/bronchi.

Extrapulmonary TB

TB Lymphadenitis
- After the lung, it is the second most common site of involvement and is usually due to reactivation disease.
- More common in people living with HIV, women, and children.
- Involvement of the cervical region is called scrofula.
- Most often presents as chronic nontender lymphadenopathy with or without fever; but can also present as a bulky mass due to conglomeration of lymph nodes.
- Incision and drainage of a fluctuant mass can lead to fistula formation.

- Diagnosis requires tissue samples for AFB smear, culture, and histologic evaluation. Fine needle aspiration first, followed by biopsy if needed is a reasonable approach.

Central Nervous System TB
- Presents as three clinical entities: meningitis, intracranial tuberculoma, and spinal arachnoiditis.
- **TB meningitis**
  - Occurs in primary (usually high incidence settings) or reactivation (usually low incidence settings) via hematogenous dissemination.
  - Specific risk factors include HIV, immunosuppression, advanced age, alcoholism, malnutrition, and cancer.
  - Presents as subacute/chronic basilar meningitis (i.e., general malaise, headache, confusion, low-grade fever).
  - It can progress quickly to coma, seizures, and paresis.
  - Untreated, the outcome is typically death within weeks.
  - 50% of patients have CXR abnormalities.
  - CSF findings: very low glucose, elevated proteins, and moderate lymphocytic pleocytosis.
  - Recently, a new molecular test, the Xpert MTB/RIF Ultra (Xpert Ultra) showed above 90% sensitivity and specificity for tuberculous meningitis.

TB Endophthalmitis
- Can involve any part of the eye but usually presents as uveitis (anterior or posterior) due to hematogenous spread.
- A clinical diagnosis based on risk exposure and known TB disease elsewhere or positive test for TB infection and typical findings of choroidal granulomas.
- Other causes of choroidal granulomas include syphilis, sarcoidosis, and fungal infection.
- Definitive diagnosis is established by ocular tissues smear/cultures, but is rarely done. Rapid molecular tests can help if samples are obtained, but yield is low.

Bone and Joint TB
- Caused by hematogenous, not contiguous, dissemination and can affect any bone.
- Two histopathologic types: exudative (caseous) and granular. Exudative is associated with bone/joint destruction/inflammation and abscess formation, whereas granular is more insidious and less destructive (more common in adults).
- TB vertebral discitis/osteomyelitis (Pott's disease) most commonly affects the lower thoracic and upper lumbar region. It may be associated with a "cold" psoas abscess.
- Poncet's disease is an acute, symmetrical, immune-mediated polyarthritis that may be seen in patients with active TB.
- Half of patients have evident pulmonary disease.
- Diagnosis requires tissue samples for microscopy, culture, and histologic evaluation (needle aspiration and/or biopsy).

TB Pericarditis

- Occurs in 1% of pulmonary TB cases.
- Symptoms are nonspecific (fever, weight loss, night sweats), but commonly presents as insidious pericarditis (chest pain, orthopnea, cough).
- Four progressive stages: Fibrinous exudation → Serosanguineous → Granulomatous caseation → Constrictive scarring.
- Constrictive pericarditis will occur in ~50% of patients despite prompt antituberculous therapy.
- Diagnosis requires pericardiocentesis or biopsy.
  - Presumptive diagnosis can be made if pericarditis develops in someone with known TB disease elsewhere, lymphocytic pericardial exudate with ADA level (>30 IU/L), or clinical response to antituberculous therapy.
  - Steroids are indicated only if there is high risk of developing constrictive pericarditis: large effusions, high levels of inflammatory cells, or early signs of constriction.
  - Pericardiectomy is sometimes required for constrictive pericarditis.

BCG disease

- BCG is a live-attenuated strain of *M. bovis* designed as vaccine to protect infants from miliary TB and TB meningitis.
- BCG has no impact in preventing TB in adults.
- Disseminated BCG infection can occur in immunosuppressed patients.
- Has been used as adjuvant immunotherapy in bladder cancer through direct bladder instillation since the 1970s.
- Granulomatous BCG-disease (prostatitis, diskitis/osteomyelitis, pneumonitis, hepatitis, miliary disease/sepsis) can occur in those receiving intravesicular BCG instillations.
- BCG (*M. bovis*) is inherently resistant to pyrazinamide (PZA), thus it is treated with a three-drug regimen of RIF, INH, and EMB.

TB Diagnosis

- All patients diagnosed with TB should get an HIV test, and all persons living with HIV should be screened for TB.
- Neither TST nor IGRA tests distinguish TB infection from TB disease (supports, but neither rules in or out disease).
- Patients with risk of TB exposure, or progression to active disease if infected, should be screened for LTBI.
- In all ≥2 years of age IGRA tests are preferred for screening for LTBI (some experts advocate for ≥1 year of age). Otherwise, TST is preferred.
- Typical chest abnormalities (upper lobe infiltrate or cavitation) and/or histopathology findings (granulomas) can be suggestive of TB infection but are not specific.

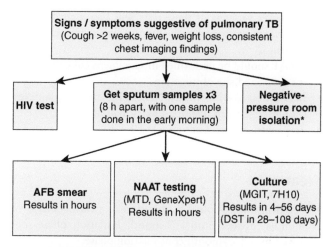

Possible results of rapid tests	Interpretation
Smear + / NAAT +	TB
Smear + / NAAT −	Consider NTMs
Smear − / NAAT +	TB
Smear − / NAAT −	Consider alternate diagnosis

- **Fig. 32.3** Diagnostic testing in suspected cases of pulmonary tuberculosis. Abbreviations: TB, tuberculosis; HIV, human immunodeficiency virus; AFB, acid-fast bacilli; NAAT, nucleic acid amplification test; MTD, Hologic Amplified Mycobacterium Tuberculosis Direct Test; GeneXpert, Xpert MTB/RIF® test; MGIT, Becton Dickinson BACTEC MGIT; 7H10, Middlebrook 7H10/sel7H11 agar; DST, drug susceptibility testing; NTM, nontuberculous mycobacteria. *In the hospital setting.

- Mycobacterial culture is the gold standard for diagnosing TB: >90% sensitive for pulmonary TB (most sensitive diagnostic method) but less sensitive for extrapulmonary TB.
- Mycobacterial cultures.
  - Solid media (e.g., Löwenstein–Jensen): growth is slow (4–8 weeks), colonies look "rough and buff" and are nonchromogens (not pigmented).
  - Liquid broth media allows more rapid growth (6–10 days).
- Three initial sputum cultures should be obtained within 24 hours (Fig. 32.3).
- Cultures should be obtained monthly until negative on 2 consecutive months, to determine total duration of therapy.
- Noninfectiousness is determined by three consecutive negative smears over at least 2 separate days after 2 weeks of therapy with clinical response.

AFB smear is 50%–60% sensitive (30%–50% in people living with advanced HIV), but other organisms can also be AFB-positive on smear (Box 32.1).

- Nucleic acid amplification tests (NAAT) that detect MTB DNA are highly specific, but sensitivity varies among different types of samples.
- Appropriate NAAT include:
  - Hologic Amplified Mycobacterium Tuberculosis Direct (MTD) Test.
  - Xpert MTB/RIF® test, that also detects RIF resistance (*rpoB* gene mutations), which predicts MDR-TB.

- Newer versions of these tests will also identify resistance mutations for the second-line antituberculous drugs.
- NAAT should be performed in specimens collected from the suspected site of infection.
- In addition to AFB smears, NAAT, and cultures, samples should be sent for histologic examination.
- Test sensitivities: Culture (1–10 CFU/mL) > NAAT (100 CFU/mL) > AFB smear (10,000 CFU/mL).

Treatment

- For drug-susceptible TB, duration of treatment is 6–9 months, divided into a 2-month initiation phase followed by a 4–7-month continuation phase.
- In culture-negative TB (multiple, adequate cultures obtained) continuation phase can be shortened to 2 months.
- Longer duration of therapy is indicated in:
  - CNS TB → 9–12 months.
  - Pulmonary disease with cavitation and persistent positive cultures after 2 months of therapy → 9 months.
  - People living with HIV not on ART → 9 months.
  - Bone and joint TB → 9–12 months, with 12 months favored in setting of hardware.
- Corticosteroids are indicated for TB meningitis but not routinely for TB pericarditis.

• BOX 32.1 Other AFB-Positive Organisms

NTM (all *Mycobacterium* spp. – from respiratory samples suspect MAC, *M. kansasii*, and *M. abscessus* group)
Rhodococcus equi
Nocardia spp. (partially acid-fast, gram-positive, branching filamentous organisms)
Legionella micdadei
Isospora, *Cyclospora*, and *Cryptosporidium* (modified stool AFB)
NTM, nontuberculous mycobacteria; MAC, *Mycobacterium avium* complex.

- Daily therapy has demonstrated superior efficacy. Intermittent therapy is often adopted for directly observed therapy but is not recommended for people living with HIV because of decreased efficacy and increased emergence of RIF resistance.
- First-line drugs include RIF, INH, PZA, EMB (RIPE). For detailed information about antimycobacterial drugs, including dosing, common side effects, and drug interactions, see Chapter 6, Antimycobacterial Agents.
- In children EMB can be omitted if they are HIV-negative, smear-negative, and do not have cavitary disease or if the source case is known and has pansensitive TB.
- Follow-up:
  - Baseline liver function test, creatinine, and complete blood counts.
  - After 2 weeks of therapy, obtain weekly sputum smears until smear-negative. Once a negative sputum smear is first documented, obtain two additional sputa on separate days to confirm the patient is noninfectious.
  - Monthly sputum culture until two consecutive cultures are negative.
  - Monthly clinical (including Ishihara color discrimination test while/if on EMB) evaluation until completion of therapy.
- TB treatment failure = positive cultures after 4 months of therapy.
  - Often associated with lack of weight gain and/or persistent night sweats during treatment.
  - Lack of adherence, drug resistance, malabsorption, extensive disease (bilateral pulmonary, cavitary, or extrapulmonary disease).
- TB relapse = recurrent TB after completion of treatment and apparent cure (Table 32.5).

People with HIV

- The treatment of tuberculosis in people living with HIV is not different from those without HIV, except:
  - Drug–drug interactions, especially with RIF, are more common. Rifabutin can be used instead of RIF if the ART regimen includes a protease inhibitor.

TABLE 32.5 Effective Treatment Regimens for Tuberculosis

| Regimen | Intensive Phase (8 weeks) | | Continuation Phase (18 weeks) | |
	Drugs	Interval and Dosage	Drugs	Interval and Dosage
1	RIF INH PZA EMB	7 doses/week for 56 doses *or* 5 doses/week for 40 doses	INH RIF	7 doses/week for 126 doses *or* 5 doses/week for 90 doses
2	RIF INH PZA EMB	7 doses/week for 56 doses *or* 5 doses/week for 40 doses	INH RIF	3 doses/week for 54 doses

Modified from the 2016 ATS/CDC/IDSA Treatment of Drug-Susceptible Tuberculosis guidelines. Regimen 1 is preferred and is the most effective regimen.

- HIV increases the risk of progression from TB infection to disease, and CD4 counts influence the severity/clinical manifestations of TB disease.
- TB accelerates HIV progression (can increase HIV viral load).
- In people living with advanced HIV and TB, Immune Reconstitution Syndrome (IRIS) can occur after starting ART:
  - Paradoxical worsening of TB symptoms.
  - Unmasking of unknown (clinically not recognized) TB disease.
  - IRIS usually appears 2–3 weeks after starting ART and may require treatment with corticosteroids. Both TB treatment and ART should be continued.
- For timing on antiretroviral initiation in people with HIV/TB co-infection see Chapter 38, Antiretroviral Therapy, section on HIV-TB co-infection.

MDR-TB

- Treatment regimen is based on multiple drugs to which the isolate is susceptible (see Table 32.6).
- Never add a single drug to a failing regimen.
- Classical treatment regimens are continued for >18 months after sputum culture becomes negative. Intensive phase with five active drugs for 6 months and continuation phase with four active drugs.
- The World Health Organization endorsed the use of a standardized 9–12-month treatment regimen as first line for MDR-TB (conditional recommendation; low level of evidence):
  - The following seven drugs for 4–6 months: high dose INH + PZA + EMB + kanamycin (KAN) + moxifloxacin (MXF) + clofazimine (CFZ) + prothionamide (PTO).

TABLE 32.6   Second-Line TB Drugs

Injectables	Kanamycin (KAN) Amikacin (AMK) Capreomycin (CM) Streptomycin (STM)
Fluoroquinolones	Levofloxacin (LFX) Moxifloxacin (MFX)
Oral bacteriostatics	Ethionamide Cycloserine (DCS) Linezolid (LZD)
Unclear role	Clofazimine (CFZ) Amoxicillin–clavulanate (AMX/ClV) Imipenem (IPM) High-dose isoniazid (INH) Clarithromycin (CLR) Para-aminosalicylic acid (PAS)
New TB drugs (third-line)	*Bedaquiline* *Delamanid*

- Followed by 5 months PZA + ETB + MXF + CFZ.
- In 2012 bedaquiline, an *M. tuberculosis* ATP synthase inhibitor, was the first new TB drug approved by the FDA in 40 years.
- Delamanid is another new nitroimidazole drug used for MDR and XDR-TB but is not approved in the United States.

33

Nontuberculous Mycobacterial Infections

YASIR HAMAD

Introduction

Nontuberculous mycobacteria (NTM) are a group of ubiquitous acid-fast bacilli (AFB) positive organisms other than *Mycobacterium tuberculosis* complex (MTBC). There are more than 150 species that have been characterized so far, with about half of them thought capable of causing human or animal disease.

Microbiology and Classification

Previously, morphology and rate of growth were used for species identification (Fig. 33.1). Biochemical methods and, more recently, molecular methods have been adopted which have led to more accurate identification of NTM species. Molecular methods have also led to identification of many new species.

The **rate of growth** alone can give a clue to the identity of the NTM while molecular testing is being conducted. Practically, NTMs can be classified into two large groups: rapidly growing mycobacteria (RGM) and slowly growing mycobacteria. RGM usually grow within 7 days while slowly growing mycobacteria take longer. This is specifically when referencing the growth on solid media after subculture. Growth in liquid media is heavily influenced by the quantity of inoculum and often violates these rules.

Runyon Classification
- Developed to help with phenotypic identification of NTMs.
- In addition to rate of growth, the organism's ability to produce yellow pigment with or without exposure to light is assessed.
  - **Photochromogens** are slow growing and produce a yellow–orange pigment only in the presence of light exposure.
  - **Scotochromogens** can produce pigment with or without light exposure.
  - **Nonchromogens** produce no pigment.
    - All of the RGMs are nonchromogens.

See Table 33.1 for examples of rapidly and slowly growing mycobacteria and their characteristics.

Most NTM will grow between 28°C and 37°C within 2–3 weeks. The Infectious Diseases Society of America (IDSA) recommends that all NTM cultures should include both liquid and solid media cultures. Some NTM require special media supplementation, different incubation temperatures, or longer incubation periods. These mycobacteria are summarized in Table 33.2.

Epidemiology

- Nontuberculous mycobacteria (NTM) are **ubiquitous environmental** organisms worldwide.
- Organisms can be found in **soil** and **water** (natural and treated).
  - They are generally resistant to chlorination of water.
  - *M. kansasii*, *M. xenopi*, and *M. simiae* are recovered almost exclusively from municipal water sources.
- There are higher rates of isolation and clinical disease in the southeastern United States, particularly for *M. kansasii*, *M. avium* complex (MAC), and *M. abscessus*.

Risk Factors for NTM Disease
- Pulmonary NTM disease: bronchiectasis, cystic fibrosis, cigarette smoking, and chronic obstructive pulmonary disease (COPD).
- Disseminated disease: **cell-mediated immunodeficiency** (e.g., AIDS and steroids use); genetic syndromes with **interferon (IFN)-γ** or **interleukin (IL)-12 pathway defects**.
- Risks of tumor necrosis factor (TNF)-α blockers in NTM infection as yet unclear.

Routes of Transmission
- **Inhalation** of infected **aerosols from environment** (e.g., shower head, hot tub).
- Ingestion of the organism (the presumed route for *M. avium* disseminated disease).

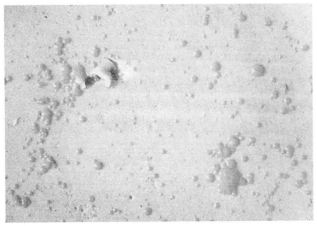

• **Fig. 33.1** *Mycobacterium kansasii* colonies on Middlebrook agar; yellow pigment develops after brief exposure to light. (From Murray PR, Rosenthal K, Pfaller M. *Medical Microbiology.* 8th ed. Elsevier; 2016.)

TABLE 33.2	NTM Species Requiring Special Culture Techniques	
Special Culture Requirement		**NTM Species**
Lower incubation temperature 28–30°C (consider for all skin, joint fluid, and bone specimens)		*M. conspicuum* *M. genavense* *M. haemophilum* *M. marinum*
Supplementation with iron		*M. haemophilum*
Supplementation with mycobactin		*M. avium* subsp. *paratuberculosis* *M. genavense*
Supplementation with egg yolk		*M. ulcerans*
Longer incubation (8–12 weeks)		*M. genavense* *M. ulcerans*
In vivo growth only		*M. leprae*

TABLE 33.1	Runyon Classification of Nontuberculous Mycobacteria
Rapidly Growing Mycobacteria (RGM)	**Slowly Growing Mycobacteria**
M. abscessus *M. abscessus* subsp. abscessus *M. abscessus* subsp. bolletii *M. abscessus* subsp. massiliense *M. chelonae* *M. fortuitum complex* *M. fortuitum* *M. peregrinum* *M. porcinum* *M. immunogenum* *M. mucogenicum* *M. smegmatis*	Photochromogens *M. kansasii* *M. marinum* Scotochromogens *M. gordonae* *M. scrofulaceum* Nonchromogens *M. avium* complex (MAC) *M. avium* *M. intracellulare* *M. chimaera* *M. haemophilum* *M. malmoense* *M. simiae* *M. terrae complex* *M. ulcerans* *M. xenopi* *M. szulgai*

TABLE 33.3	Common Clinical Syndromes Caused by NTM Species
Syndrome	**Most Common Cause**
Pulmonary infection	MAC *M. kansasii* *M. abscessus*
Lymphadenitis	MAC
Skin, soft tissue, and bone disease	*M. fortuitum* group *M. chelonae* *M. abscessus* *M. marinum* *M. ulcerans* (rare in United States)
Disseminated infection	With HIV: *M. avium*, *M. kansasii* Without HIV: *M. abscessus*, *M. chelonae*
Hypersensitivity pneumonitis	Metal workers: *M. immunogenum* Hot tub: *M. avium*

MAC, M. avium complex; HIV, human immunodeficiency virus.

• Direct inoculation through skin breaks or trauma (e.g., skin and soft tissue infection in RGM).
• **No evidence of human-human or animal-human transmission.**
  • Not communicable, so not reportable/notifiable.

Clinical Presentation

Invasive infection can be classified into four major clinical syndromes:
1. Pulmonary disease (commonest manifestation).
2. Lymphadenitis.
3. Skin, soft tissue, and bone disease.
4. Disseminated disease.

The most common causes of each of the syndromes are summarized in Table 33.3.

Diagnosis

Since NTM are ubiquitous organisms, their isolation in culture by itself is not sufficient to make the diagnosis of clinical disease. The diagnosis of NTM disease requires **compatible clinical presentation in addition to the organism recovery.** The diagnosis of pulmonary disease, in particular, has well-developed criteria that are summarized below.

Pulmonary Disease
• MAC is the most common cause of pulmonary disease, followed by *M. kansasii* and *M. abscessus*

> ### ▪ BOX 33.1 Minimum Evaluation for Suspected NTM Lung Disease
>
> - Chest X-ray, if negative high-resolution computed tomography (HRCT) scan.
> - 3 or more sputa for acid-fast bacilli (AFB) stains.
> - Exclusion of other disorders, e.g., TB.

> ### ▪ BOX 33.2 Clinical and Microbiological Criteria for Diagnosing NTM Lung Disease
>
> #### Clinical (both required)
>
> 1. Pulmonary symptoms, nodular or cavitary opacities on chest radiograph, or an HRCT scan that shows multifocal bronchiectasis with multiple small nodules AND
> 2. Appropriate exclusion of other diagnoses.
>
> #### Microbiologic
>
> 1. Positive culture results from at least two separate expectorated sputum samples
>   OR
> 2. Positive culture result from at least one bronchial wash or lavage
>   OR
> 3. Transbronchial or other lung biopsy with mycobacterial histopathologic features (granulomatous inflammation or AFB) and positive culture for NTM or biopsy showing mycobacterial histopathologic features (granulomatous inflammation or AFB) and one or more sputum or bronchial washings that are culture positive for NTM.

- Diagnosis of NTM pulmonary disease requires clinical, microbiological, and radiological evaluation (Boxes 33.1 and 33.2).
- If diagnosis is not confirmed based on these criteria, the patient should be followed until the diagnosis is either confirmed or excluded.

CLINICALLY IMPORTANT NONTUBERCULOUS MYCOBACTERIA

M. avium Complex (MAC)

- Slowly growing, nonpigmented mycobacteria.
- The **most common cause of NTM disease** in the United States.
- Includes two major species: *M. avium* and *M. intracellulare*.
- *M. intracellulare* is the most common cause of NTM lung disease.
- *M. avium* infection is the most common cause of disseminated NTM disease in acquired immunodeficiency syndrome (AIDS) patients.

MAC Lung Disease

There are two types of clinical and radiologic presentation:

1. Apical fibrocavitary lung disease
   - This is an aggressive form of disease that usually affects **males in their 40s–50s** with history of **cigarette smoking ± excessive alcohol use.**
   - Untreated, progresses in 1–2 years to extensive lung cavitation with respiratory failure.
2. Nodular bronchiectatic disease
   - "Lady Windermere Syndrome": slowly progressive form.
   - Usually affects **postmenopausal, nonsmoking, white females.**
   - Frequently right middle lobe or lingula affected.

Treatment

- Only macrolide sensitivity testing is recommended.
- Use of **combination therapy** is the basis of therapy.
- Standard regimen = **rifampin + ethambutol + macrolide** (azithromycin or clarithromycin).
- Daily dosing is used for fibrocavitary disease while three-times-weekly can be used in nodular bronchiectatic form.
- Continue treatment for **12 months after achieving culture-negativity.**
- IV aminoglycosides and surgical resection can be used in refractory cases.

MAC Disseminated Disease

- Fever is the main symptom, occurs in >80% of cases.
- Other less common symptoms are night sweats and weight loss.
- Physical signs include abdominal tenderness, hepatosplenomegaly, and lymphadenopathy.
- Most commonly occurs in **AIDS patients with CD4 count <50** cells/μL.
- Diagnosis is by **culture of MAC from a sterile site.**
  - Mycobacterial **blood cultures are positive in 90%** of cases (increased to 98% by taking a second sample).
  - Others might be diagnosed by bone marrow, lymph node, or liver biopsy.

Treatment

- Treatment with MAC therapy and antiretroviral therapy (ART) usually results in a good response (Box 33.3).
  - Clarithromycin has more rapid clearance of MAC.
  - Azithromycin is better tolerated and has fewer drug interactions.
- Watch out for interactions between rifamycins, protease inhibitors, and nonnucleoside reverse transcriptase inhibitors.
- Rifabutin used in patients with high risk of short-term mortality and those with significant drug–drug interactions.
- Monitor for development of immune reconstitution inflammatory syndrome (**IRIS**) as the immune system recovers with ART treatment.
- Continue MAC treatment until:
  - Clinical response for at least 3 months.

• BOX 33.3 Disseminated MAC Treatment and Prevention

- Treatment: Macrolide (clarithromycin or azithromycin) + ethambutol ± Rifabutin
- Prevention: if CD4 count <50 cells/μL azithromycin 1200 mg weekly or clarithromycin 500 mg twice daily

---

- Good viral load response to ART (<50 copies/mL on two consecutive occasions).
- Good CD4 count response to ART (>100 cells/μL on two occasions at least 3 months apart).

MAC Lymphadenitis

- MAC is the most common cause of mycobacterial lymphadenitis in the United States.
- Children affected >>>> adults
  - Majority <3 years of age.
  - Immunocompetent adults rarely affected.
- Usually **cervical glands** are involved.
- **Surgical resection** alone results in **cure in 95%** of cases.
- TB has to be excluded.
- Avoid use of TB drugs without a macrolide and incisional biopsy without excision, as high rates of persistent disease with sinus tract formation and chronic drainage may occur.

MAC Hypersensitivity Pneumonitis

- Also known as "hot tub lung."
- **Hypersensitivity lung disease** associated with MAC exposure caused by exposure related to undrained **pool or spa** with overgrowth of MAC (resistant to disinfectants).
- Similar syndrome associated with metalworking fluid has been linked to *M. immunogenum.*
- Diagnosis is made using clinical, radiologic, and microbiologic studies (Box 33.4).
- Treatment is controversial but usually consists of removal of the source (e.g., hot tub), ± steroids, and a short course antimicrobial therapy (3—6 months) depending on clinical response and disease severity.

M. chimaera

- *M. chimaera* is also a member of the *Mycobacterium avium* complex.
- Caused a recent outbreak in **cardiac surgery patients** (risk factors – see Box 33.5).
- Infection was linked to **contaminated heater-cooler devices** that are used in cardiac surgeries or ECMO (extracorporeal membrane oxygenation).
- Common features of infection include fever, malaise, weight loss, lymphopenia, and elevated alkaline phosphatase.
- Infections include endocarditis, severe disseminated infection, and chronic sternal wound infection.

• BOX 33.4 Diagnosis of MAC Hypersensitivity Pneumonitis

Clinical Criteria

1. Subacute respiratory symptoms (dyspnea, cough, and fever) AND
2. Hot tub exposure

Radiologic

1. Diffuse infiltrate with nodularity
   ±
2. Ground glass opacity and mosaic pattern

Microbiologic

MAC isolate in sputum, bronchoalveolar lavage, tissue, and hot-tub water

---

• BOX 33.5 Risk Factors for *M. chimaera* Infection

- Cardiothoracic operations since January 2013.
- Heart valve surgery (replacement or repair) >>> CABG or transplant surgery.
- Other reported infection-related procedures were heart–lung transplant, left ventricular assist device (LVAD) implantation, and vascular grafts.

- Disseminated infection can involve liver, bone marrow, lung, skin, brain, lymph nodes, and bone (spine).
- Incubation period can be long, with a median of 19 months (range: 3 months to 5 years).
- Antibiotic treatment is similar to that of *Mycobacterium avium* complex.
- Surgical treatment might be needed in cases of prosthetic valve endocarditis.
- Mortality rate is high and can reach up to 50%.

M. kansasii

Epidemiology

- *M. kansasii* is the second most common cause of NTM disease in the United States after MAC.
- More prevalent in central and southern US states.
- SE England and Wales also have higher rates of infection with *M. kansasii.*
- **Tap water** is the major reservoir.
- Disease mostly affects **middle-aged white men.**
- Risk factors for acquiring the infection are summarized in Box 33.6.

Clinical Presentation

Pulmonary Disease

- Very similar presentation to pulmonary tuberculosis.
- **Upper lobe** predilection and **cavitary disease** are common.
- Nodular bronchiectatic lung disease similar to MAC has been reported.
- Without treatment the disease is usually progressive in nature.

BOX 33.6 Risk Factors for *M. kansasii* Infection

- Pneumoconiosis
- Chronic obstructive pulmonary disease
- Previous mycobacterial disease
- Malignancy
- Alcoholism
- HIV

Disseminated Disease

- *M. kansasii* is the second most common cause of disseminated NTM disease in AIDS patients.
- Unlike MAC disseminated disease, 50% of cases also have pulmonary disease.
- Blood cultures are only positive in 25% of patients.
- Treatment is the same as pulmonary disease treatment.
- Watch out for interactions between rifamycins, protease inhibitors, and nonnucleoside reverse transcriptase inhibitors.

Treatment

- Typical regimen used for treatment is **rifampin, isoniazid,** and **ethambutol.**
- Treatment duration is 12 months from culture negativity.
- Sensitivity testing to rifampin is recommended.
- Rifampin is critical for treatment success.
- Response is usually good, and there is no role for surgical intervention.

M. abscessus (RGM)

Microbiology and Epidemiology

M. abscessus is a **rapidly growing** mycobacterium (RGM) that consists of three subspecies:
- *M. abscessus* subsp. *abscessus.*
- *M. abscessus* subsp. *massiliense.*
- *M. abscessus* subsp. *bolletii.*

M. abscessus disease is more prevalent in southeastern US states (Florida to Texas).

Clinical Presentation

Skin, soft tissue, and bone disease
- Can present as ulcerations, abscesses, draining sinuses, or nodules (Fig. 33.2).
- Usually resulting from **trauma or surgery** (e.g., cosmetic surgeries).
- Resolves spontaneously or requires surgical debridement.
- Can show good results to medical treatment chosen on the basis of susceptibility testing.

Pulmonary Disease

- Third most common cause of NTM lung disease.
- Responsible for about 80% of pulmonary disease caused by RGM.
- Mostly affects white female nonsmokers in their 60s.

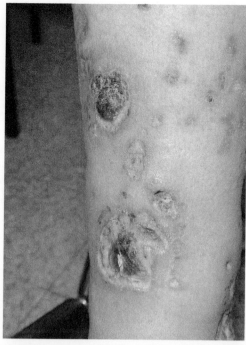

Fig. 33.2 Nodules and ulcers on lower leg in patient with *Mycobacterium abscessus* skin infection. (Courtesy Roni Dodiuk-Gad.)

BOX 33.7 Risk Factors for *M. abscessus* Infection

- Bronchiectasis
- Prior mycobacterial disease
- Cystic fibrosis
- Alpha-1-antitrypsin deficiency
- Lipoid pneumonia
- Chronic vomiting

- Risk factors for pulmonary disease in younger adults are listed in Box 33.7.
- Clinical presentation is usually similar to that of MAC lung disease, though only 15% develop cavitary lesions.

Treatment

Treatment should be guided by antimicrobial susceptibilities.
- Typically resistant to standard antituberculous agents.
- *M. abscessus* is usually susceptible to **clarithromycin** (esp. *M. massiliense*) and **amikacin.**
- Low MICs to cefoxitin, imipenem, tigecycline, and linezolid.
- MICs to clofazimine are generally low but there is no established cutoff.
- Treatment duration:
  - Severe skin, soft tissue 4 months.
  - Bone disease treat 6 months.
  - Pulmonary disease 12 months from negative culture.
- **Source control** is important: **drainage** of all abscesses and removal of any infected foreign bodies.
- Treatment is very **challenging** due to medication toxicities and lack of a reliable empiric antibiotic regimen.

• BOX 33.8 Duration of Treatment for *M. chelonae* Infection

- Skin and soft tissue infection 4 months.
- Bone infection 6 months.
- Pulmonary infection 12 months from negative culture.

- *M. abscessus* subsp. *massiliense* has better prognosis than *M. abscessus* subsp. *abscessus* due to the lack of functional erythromycin resistance methylase (*erm*) gene, which causes inducible resistance to macrolides.

M. chelonae (RGM)

Clinical Presentation

- Previously used to be reported as part of *M. chelonae/abscessus* group.
- Treatment is usually easier than that of *M. abscessus*.
- Skin, soft tissue, and bone disease are the most important clinical manifestations.
- Disseminated skin infection is seen in immunocompromised patients.
- Cases of keratitis have been associated with contact lenses and ocular surgeries (e.g., Lasik).
- Pulmonary disease has been reported but is not common.

Treatment

- Isolates are usually susceptible to macrolides, tobramycin, linezolid, and imipenem.
- Regimen usually consists of a macrolide and a companion drug, based on susceptibility testing.
- Duration of therapy varies by clinical presentation (Box 33.8).

M. fortuitum group (RGM)

Clinical Presentation

- Responsible for 60% of localized cutaneous NTM infections in previously healthy individuals.
- Has no predilection for immunocompromised patients.
- Skin, bone, and soft tissue infections can occur in sporadic or clustered cases.
- Whirlpool footbaths during pedicure procedures in nail salons have been identified as a source of some outbreaks.
- Pulmonary disease is rare but can occur in patients with chronic vomiting and acid reflux.

Treatment

- Usually susceptible to macrolides, quinolones, doxycycline, minocycline, aminoglycosides, and sulfamethoxazole–trimethoprim.
- Carries the *erm* gene with risks of inducible macrolide resistance.
- Treatment duration is the same as *M. chelonae* (see Box 33.8).

• BOX 33.9 Epidemiology of Leprosy

- The World Health Organization (WHO) reported 211,009 new cases in 2017.
- 81% of new cases in 2013 were from India (59%), Brazil, and Indonesia.
- Adolescents and those older than 30 years seem to be more susceptible to the disease, with predilection to males.

- Source control is important, and should include drainage of all abscesses and removal of infected foreign bodies.

M. leprae

Microbiology and Epidemiology

- The causative agent of leprosy (see Box 33.9).
- **Cannot be cultured *in vitro*.**
- Can be cultured in the footpad of immunodeficient mice.
- Transmission is thought to occur through **nasal secretions and respiratory droplets**, **transplacental**, **breast-feeding**, **skin contact**, and through zoonotic transmission from contact with armadillos.

Clinical Presentation

- Key features are hypopigmented skin lesions with hypoesthesia.
- Lesions can also be erythematous and infiltrative.
- Other neurologic manifestation include weakness, autonomic dysfunction, and peripheral nerve thickening.
- **Subtypes:**
  - Spectrum of manifestations range from tuberculoid (paucibacillary) to lepromatous (multibacillary) leprosy (see Table 33.4).
  - These two forms represent the extremes of presentations based on the immune system response to the infection.
  - In-between these two polar forms exist three borderline forms: borderline tuberculoid, borderline intermediate, and borderline lepromatous leprosy.
- Manifests as tissue damage with bone resorption.
- Long-term complications result mostly from neuropathy as well as systemic manifestations of the disease.
- Eye is frequently involved as a consequence of facial nerve palsy (dryness) or iridocyclitis.

Immune-Mediated Reactions

- Reversal reaction
  - Manifests as increased warmth, erythema, and edema of preexisting lesions.
  - Results from the development of exuberant local T-cell-mediated immune response directed at living or dead bacilli.
  - Can occur with any form of leprosy except tuberculoid form.
  - If left untreated can lead to permanent nerve damage.
- Erythema nodosum leprosum (ENL)

TABLE 33.4	Clinical Spectrum of Leprosy	
Type	**Tuberculoid Leprosy**	**Lepromatous Leprosy**
Number of skin lesions	<5	Innumerable
Type of skin lesions	Macules or plaques	Nodules, papules, macules, or infiltrative dermopathy
Sensation in the skin lesion	Hypoesthetic	Intact
Systemic involvement	Limited to skin and nerves	Can affect eye, nasal mucosa, nerves, kidney, and bone
Pathological Findings		
Granuloma formation	Well formed	Absent
Acid-fast bacilli	Absent to rare	Abundant
Lymphocytes	Abundant	Few
Image	See Fig. 33.3	See Fig. 33.4

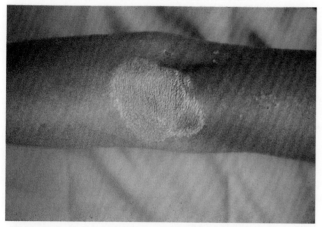

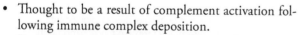

• **Fig. 33.3** Tuberculoid leprosy. Early tuberculoid lesions are characterized by anesthetic macules with hypopigmentation. (From Britton WJ. Leprosy. In: Cohen J, Powderly WG, Opal SM. *Infectious Diseases*, 3rd ed. Philadelphia: Mosby; 2010.)

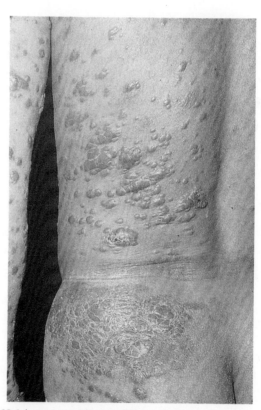

• **Fig. 33.4** Lepromatous leprosy. Diffuse infiltration of the skin by multiple nodules of varying size, each with many bacteria. (From Britton WJ. Leprosy. In: Cohen J, Powderly WG, Opal SM. *Infectious Diseases*, 3rd ed. Philadelphia: Mosby; 2010.)

- Thought to be a result of complement activation following immune complex deposition.
- Presents as acute development of **new subcutaneous nodules** that are red, painful, and tender (Fig. 33.5).
- Most commonly affects the extensor surface of the skin of the legs and the face.
- Occasionally affects other organs including the eye, nasal mucosa, joints, kidneys, and testes.

Diagnosis

- Clinical exam and slit-skin testing is used to make the diagnosis in endemic countries.
- Histopathological examination of skin biopsy is the gold standard.
- Serologic and PCR testing are of limited use and are not available commercially.

Treatment

- Use of multiple drug treatment is recommended.
- Dapsone, rifampin and clofazimine are first-line agents.
- Prolonged courses of therapy: 12–24 months.
- **Baseline G6PD deficiency screen**, periodic complete blood count, and complete metabolic panel are recommended while on therapy.
- Alternative agents include fluoroquinolones, minocycline, and clarithromycin.

- WHO recommendations and the US National Hansen's Disease Program differ with respect to:
  - The number of agents for tuberculoid disease.
  - Monthly vs. daily rifampin.
  - Treatment duration.
- **Reactions are treated with courses of corticosteroids, along with continuation of multidrug antibiotic regimens.**
- Clofazimine has been used for reversal reactions.

- Thalidomide can be used as a steroid-sparing agent in ENL.

Other Clinically Relevant Nontuberculous Mycobacteria Species

Other less commonly encountered NTM species are summarized in Table 33.5. These are organisms that are known to be clinically significant.

TABLE 33.5 Clinical Presentation of Less Commonly Encountered NTM Species

NTM Species	Clinical Presentation	Comment
M. genavense	• Disseminated infection in AIDS patients	Consider when disseminated infection is suspected but cultures are negative Needs special conditions for optimal growth (Table 33.2)
M. gordonae	• Mostly considered a contaminant • Can rarely cause pulmonary disease	• Avoid drinking or rinsing with tap water prior to respiratory specimen collection
M. haemophilum	• Skin, soft tissue, and joint disease • Disseminated infection in immunocompromised hosts	• Needs special conditions for optimal growth (Table 33.2)
M. immunogenum (RGM)	• Central venous catheter-related bacteremia • Skin infection • Hypersensitivity pneumonitis due to metalworking fluid contamination	• Has been implicated in pseudo-outbreaks due to contaminated scopes
M. malmoense	• Lymphadenitis • Pulmonary disease	• Mostly a disease of children in Europe and Asia
M. marinum	• Skin and soft tissue infection due to exposure to a wound to contaminated water • Mostly affecting upper extremities (See Fig. 33.6)	• The cause of "fish tank granuloma" • Needs special conditions for optimal growth (Table 33.2)
M. mucogenicum (RGM)	• Central venous catheter-related bacteremia • Peritoneal catheter-related peritonitis	• Usually considered a contaminant when isolated from a pulmonary specimen
M. scrofulaceum	• Lymphadenitis in children • Pulmonary disease in gold miners	• Fading disease, likely due water treatment
M. simiae	• Rare cause of clinical disease	• Pseudo-outbreaks due to water contamination have been reported
M. smegmatis (RGM)	• Rare cause of skin, soft tissue, and bone disease • Pulmonary disease in patients with lipoid pneumonia	• Considered resistant to macrolides
M. szulgai	• Pulmonary disease similar to TB and M. kansasii	• Isolation in culture is usually significant (not commonly found in the environment)
M. terrae complex	• M. nonchromogenicum is associated with hand tenosynovitis	• Otherwise considered a nonpathogen
M. ulcerans	• Chronic necrotic progressive ulcer of skin and soft tissues (Buruli ulcer) (See Fig. 33.7)	• 3rd most common cause of mycobacterial disease worldwide (after TB and M. leprae) • Rare in the United States • Needs special conditions for optimal growth (Table 33.2)
M. xenopi	• Pulmonary disease with apical cavitation • Chronic obstructive pulmonary disease is a risk factor	• 2nd most common NTM in Canada (after MAC) • Thermophilic bacteria, colonizes hot water systems

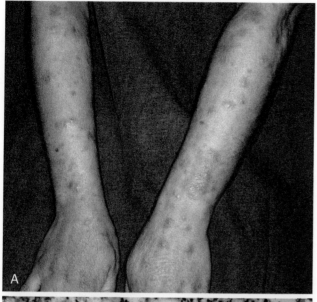

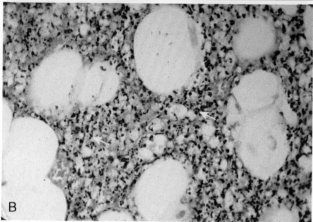

• **Fig. 33.5** Erythema nodosum leprosum (ENL). (A) Patient with lepromatous leprosy undergoing ENL reaction with bright-pink papules, plaques, and nodules occurring on bilateral upper extremities. (B) High-power view of the lobular panniculitis and characteristic polymorphonuclear cell infiltrate (*yellow arrows*) seen in ENL biopsy specimens. (H&E; original magnification ×400. Courtesy Sonia Kamath.)

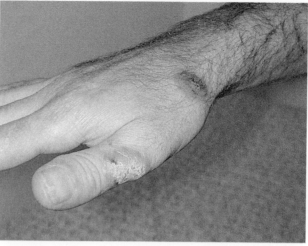

• **Fig. 33.6** Plaques on thumb and back of hand in patient with *Mycobacterium marinum* skin infection. (Courtesy Roni Dodiuk-Gad.)

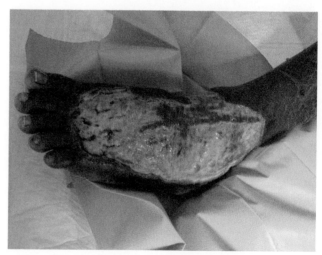

• **Fig. 33.7** Large ulceration of the left foot before treatment of *Mycobacterium ulcerans*. (Courtesy Nicolas Vignier.)

Further Reading and Resources

1. Griffith DE, et al. An official ATS/IDSA statement: diagnosis, treatment, and prevention of nontuberculous mycobacterial diseases. *Am J Respir Crit Care Med.* 2007;175(4). https://doi.org/10.1164/rccm.200604–571ST.

2. Haworth CS, et al. British Thoracic Society guidelines for the management of non-tuberculous mycobacterial pulmonary disease (NTM-PD). *Thorax.* 2017;72(suppl 2).

3. World Health Organization. *Guidelines for the Diagnosis, Treatment and Prevention of Leprosy.* Geneva: WHO; 2018. https://apps.who.int/iris/handle/10665/274127.

34

Protozoa

FRANCESCA LEE, NICOLAS BARROS, DOMINICK CAVUOTI

Introduction

Only a small number of the protozoa species identified are known to cause human disease. Microbiological identification has traditionally depended on morphology, but technological advances are leading to the increased use of alternate techniques, including antigen detection and nucleic acid amplification tests (NAAT). Clinically, these organisms are often categorized by their primary sites of infection (although several species can disseminate). As with many infections, epidemiology is key to assessing the likelihood of a particular pathogen being the cause of a patient's symptoms. Treatment is well-studied and validated for some of the infectious conditions caused by protozoa, but in other cases only limited evidence exists to support recommendations.

BLOOD AND TISSUE PROTOZOA

Malaria

Malaria symptoms have been described in Chinese writings from 2700 BC, as well as by the ancient Egyptians in 1550 BC, and the ancient Greeks around 413 BC. It was originally thought to be a disease transmitted by bad air (mala aria). It was not until the late 1800s that French and British physicians identified the parasite and demonstrated the life cycle.

Microbiology and Pathogenesis

- This disease is caused by five species of the genus *Plasmodium*. They include *Plasmodium falciparum*, *Plasmodium vivax*, *Plasmodium ovale*, *Plasmodium malariae*, and the more recently recognized *Plasmodium knowlesi* (Box 34.1).
- The life cycle (Fig. 34.1) is complex, involving two hosts. The vector is the female *Anopheles* mosquito, which generally feeds at night (Fig. 34.2). Human infection begins when a malaria-infected female *Anopheles* mosquito inoculates sporozoites into the human host. These sporozoites

infect hepatocytes, where they mature into schizonts. The schizonts then rupture and release merozoites. The merozoites next infect red blood cells, initially visible as a ring, or trophozoite, stage. These mature into schizonts, which again rupture and release more merozoites. A portion of the merozoites will undergo sexual differentiation into gametocytes (rather than form schizonts). It is these gametocytes which are ingested by the next *Anopheles* mosquito. Inside the mosquito gut, the sporogonic cycle takes place.

Epidemiology

- World Health Organization statistics indicate that in 2016 there were 216 million cases in 91 countries, with 445,000 deaths.
- Disease burden and species prevalence vary by geography and also by seasonality. Ninety percent of disease and death occur in Africa. Other areas with high incidence include Central America, South America, Southeast Asia, the Indian subcontinent, and the Middle East. The parasite requires temperatures above 60°F (15.5°C) for growth; below this, it cannot be transmitted (Table 34.1).
- Risk factors for acquisition are environmental and human. Environments that are conducive to the *Anopheles* mosquito include warm rainy seasons, shallow water collections, and a lack of mosquito netting or other protective measures in the home. Humans living in these environments are often at risk for mosquito bites. In areas of low transmission, partial immunity explains why adults generally have less severe disease than children. Rates of severe illness and death are highest for children under age 5.

> **• BOX 34.1 It's not OVer!**
>
> *P. ovale* and *P. vivax* are notable for a dormant (hypnozoite) stage which can persist in the liver for years, leading to future relapses. **"It's not OVer!"**

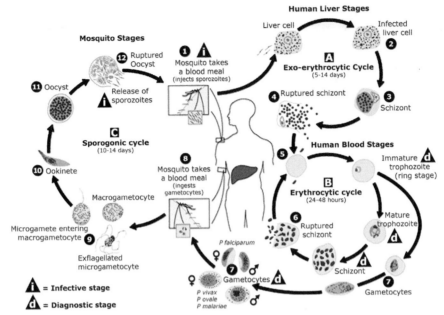

• **Fig. 34.1** Blood stage parasites are the cause of symptoms. (Courtesy Centers for Disease Control and Prevention. About malaria. http://www.cdc.gov/malaria/about/biology/.)

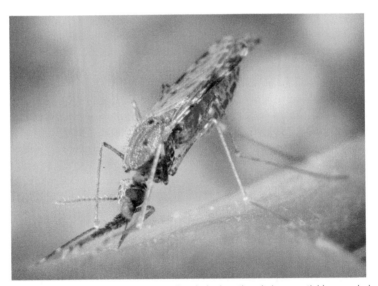

• **Fig. 34.2** The *Anopheles* mosquito, the vector of malaria, has the abdomen sticking up during feeding. (From Feder HM, Mansilla-Rivera K. Fever in returning travelers: a case-based approach. *Am Fam Phys*. 88(8):524–530. Courtesy Centers for Disease Control and Prevention.)

TABLE 34.1	**Geographic Distribution of *Plasmodium* Species**				
	P. falciparum	*P. vivax*	*P. ovale*	*P. malariae*	*P. knowlesi*
Geographic distribution	Tropical and subtropical Central and South America, Africa, Southeast Asia	Tropical and subtropical Central and South America, India, Southeast Asia; key areas Korea and the former Soviet Union	Sub-Saharan Africa	Tropical and subtropical Central and South America, Africa, Southeast Asia	Southeast Asia (especially Myanmar, Thailand, and Cambodia)

Clinical Features

- For all species, fever is the most common symptom. This is often accompanied by, or preceded by, vague complaints such as fatigue, headache, myalgias, arthralgias, abdominal pain, cough.
  - Physical exam may be normal, or may reveal pallor, splenomegaly, jaundice.
  - Laboratory findings may include anemia, elevated bilirubin, thrombocytopenia, acute renal failure, transaminitis.
- *P. falciparum*
  - Can cause severe malaria, manifested by acidosis, coma, seizure, shock, renal failure, profound anemia, and jaundice (Box 34.2).
  - Severity is often correlated to parasitemia (proportion of RBCs infected with parasites), although this is not absolutely predictable.

> ### • BOX 34.2 Malaria Complications (You need a CHAPLIN)
>
> - **C**erebral malaria/Coma/Convulsions
> - **H**ypoglycemia/Hemorrhage/Hemoglobinuria (blackwater fever)
> - **A**nemia
> - **P**ulmonary edema
> - **L**actic acidosis
> - **I**cterus
> - **N**ecrosis of renal tubules (ATN)

- The other species are much less likely to have severe disease, although *P. knowlesi* case reports are increasing.
- Fever pattern is sometimes used to differentiate species. Fever is caused by the rupture of mature schizonts. Fever patterns are not reliable in early infection (Table 34.2).

Diagnosis

- Diagnosis has depended upon microscopy for years – the thick and thin blood smears. There are certain features which increase the likelihood of a particular organism (thin delicate rings in normal-sized RBCs point toward *P. falciparum*), but there is often overlap (Table 34.3). **In particular, early *P. knowlesi* infections look just like *P. falciparum*, but as the infection progresses, the morphology changes to resemble *P. malariae* (Box 34.3 and Fig. 34.3).** Treatment also impacts microscopy, as the morphology of dying parasites becomes altered. For this reason, it is challenging for a laboratory to make an initial diagnosis once therapy has been started.
- Given these challenges, both rapid diagnostic tests and molecular assays have been developed. The rapid diagnostic tests are run directly on a blood sample and usually have a panmalaria target and a specific *P. falciparum* target (histidine-rich protein 2/HRP-2). Molecular assays are promising but not readily available outside of reference laboratories. Rapid tests have low sensitivity for non-*falciparum* malaria, low parasite burden disease, and cannot quantify parasite burden. Hence, malaria cannot be ruled out based on a rapid test. For that reason, rapid tests should always be followed by microscopy.

TABLE 34.2 Fever Pattern in Malaria

	P. falciparum	P. vivax	P. ovale	P. malariae	P. knowlesi
Erythrocytic cycle duration	48 hours	48 hours	48 hours	72 hours	24 hours
Fever pattern	Irregular tertian fever	Tertian fever	Tertian fever	Quartan fever	Quotidian fever
Memory trick	Sounds "false" – no clear pattern			Malariae is "meh" about fever	Every day you "knowlesi" it's coming

TABLE 34.3 Erythrocyte and Parasite Morphology

	P. falciparum	P. vivax	P. ovale	P. malariae	P. knowlesi
Multiple infected RBC	Common	Maybe	Maybe	No	Yes
Schuffner's dots	No	Yes, fine	Yes, large	No	No
Size of infected cells	Normal	Enlarged	Enlarged	Small to normal	Small to normal
No. of merozoites in schizont	8–24 (rarely seen)	12–24	6–14	6–12, rosettes	6–16
Gametocyte	Crescent	Ameboid	Round/elongated with fimbriation	Round	Variable

• BOX 34.3 **"Know About Knowlesi!"**

Don't be fooled by *P. knowlesi*: if a patient presents with severe malaria but the slides look like *P. malariae*, it could be *P. knowlesi* as *P. malariae* is usually benign. **"Know about knowlesi!"**

Treatment

Prophylaxis

In persons living in endemic areas, prevention is far more important than treatment. This means eliminating standing water, using mosquito nets, avoiding being outside during peak hours, and possible use of insecticide to reduce the

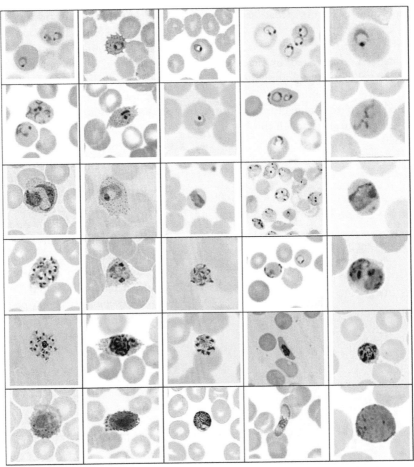

• **Fig. 34.3** Morphology of malaria parasites. (*Left to right*) Column 1: *Plasmodium vivax* (note enlarged infected RBCs). (*Top to bottom*) (1) Early trophozoite (ring form) (note one RBC contains 2 rings – not that uncommon); (2) older ring, note ameboid nature of rings; (3) late trophozoite with Schüffner dots (note enlarged RBC); (4) developing schizont; (5) mature schizont with 18 merozoites and clumped pigment; (6) microgametocyte with dispersed chromatin. Column 2: *Plasmodium ovale* (note enlarged infected RBCs). (1) Early trophozoite (ring form) with Schüffner dots (RBC has fimbriated edges); (2) early trophozoite (note enlarged RBC, Schüffner dots, and RBC oval in shape); (3) late trophozoite in RBC with fimbriated edges; (4) developing schizont with irregular-shaped RBC; (5) mature schizont with 8 merozoites arranged irregularly; (6) microgametocyte with dispersed chromatin. Column 3: *Plasmodium malariae* (note normal or smaller than normal infected RBCs). (1) Early trophozoite (ring form); (2) early trophozoite with thick cytoplasm; (3) late trophozoite (band form); (4) developing schizont; (5) mature schizont with 9 merozoites arranged in a rosette; (6) macrogametocyte with compact chromatin. Column 4: *Plasmodium falciparum*. (1) Early trophozoites (the rings are in the headphone configuration with double chromatin dots); (2) early trophozoite (accolé or appliqué form); (3) early trophozoites (note the multiple rings/cell); (4) late trophozoite with larger ring (accolé or appliqué form); (5) crescent-shaped gametocyte; (6) crescent-shaped gametocyte. Column 5: *Plasmodium knowlesi* – with the exception of image 5, these were photographed at a higher magnification (note normal or smaller than normal infected RBCs). (1) Early trophozoite (ring form); (2) early trophozoite with slim band form; (3) late trophozoite (band form); (4) developing schizont; (5) mature schizont with merozoites arranged in a rosette; (6) microgametocyte with dispersed chromatin. Note: Without the appliqué form, Schüffner dots, multiple rings per cell, and other developing stages, differentiation among the species can be very difficult. It is obvious that the early rings of all 4 species can mimic one another very easily. Remember: One set of negative blood films cannot rule out a malaria infection. (Columns 1–4 from Garcia LS. Malaria. *Clin Lab Med.* 2010;30(1):93–129. Column 5 courtesy Centers for Disease Control and Prevention.)

• **BOX 34.4** **Malaria Prophylaxis in Pregnant Women**

Available agents for malaria prophylaxis in pregnant women: **mefloquine, chloroquine, hydroxychloroquine.**

• **BOX 34.5** **Warning**

Mefloquine can induce neuropsychiatric adverse reactions that can persist even after discontinuation of therapy. Agranulocytosis and aplastic anemia have been described. Quinine can lead to serious cardiac conduction abnormalities including QT prolongation and torsades de pointes. Its use with other QT prolonging agents is not recommended.

mosquito population. For travelers, the most important consideration (besides use of repellant, bed nets, and adequate clothing), is prophylaxis. The risk of malaria transmission and appropriate prophylaxis should be reviewed prior to travel.

- *P. falciparum* chloroquine resistance: extensive. Limit to areas with low chloroquine resistance, such as the Caribbean, Central America west of the Panama Canal, and some areas of Middle East.
- *P. falciparum* mefloquine resistance: increasing. Myanmar/Thai border, Cambodia, southern Vietnam.
- *P. vivax* chloroquine resistance: Papua New Guinea, Indonesia.
- When in doubt:
  - Atovaquone–proguanil: starting 1–2 days prior to travel, continuing 7 days after leaving malarious area.
    - Contraindicated if creatinine clearance <30 mL/min; pregnant women; young children (Box 34.4).
  - Doxycycline: starting 1–2 days prior to travel, continuing 4 weeks after leaving malarious area.
    - Contraindicated if pregnant, young child.
  - Mefloquine: in areas with mefloquine-sensitive malaria. Begin >2 weeks prior to travel. Dose weekly. Continue 4 weeks after leaving malarious area.
    - Contraindicated in patients with psychiatric disorders, cardiac conduction abnormalities.
  - Primaquine: Primarily for *P. vivax/P. ovale* prophylaxis. Start 1–2 days prior to travel, continuing 7 days after leaving malarious area.
    - Terminal prophylaxis (or presumptive antirelapse prophylaxis) is the practice of taking primaquine for 14 days after leaving the malarious area, to prevent relapse or delayed onset of *P. vivax/P. ovale* infection. This is generally reserved for people with prolonged exposure to endemic areas.
    - Contraindicated if G6PD deficiency, pregnancy/lactation.

Treatment

- The first step to treat malaria is to determine the severity of disease.
- Complicated malaria is defined by:
  - Cerebral malaria/coma/convulsions.
  - Hypoglycemia/hemorrhage/hemoglobinuria (black-water fever).
  - Severe anemia (<5g/dL in children less than 12 or <7 g/dL in children older than 12 or adults).
  - Pulmonary edema.
  - Lactic acidosis (plasma bicarbonate <15 mmol/L or lactic acid >5 mmol/L).

- Icterus (serum bilirubin >3 mg/mL).
- Necrosis of renal tubules (ATN).
- Shock.
- Hyperparasitemia (*P. falciparum* parasitemia >10%).
- Management of complicated malaria
  - The treatment of choice is intravenous artesunate. However, if artesunate is not available, quinine or chloroquine can be used. Parenteral therapy should be continued for a minimum of 24 hours and then transitioned to an oral regimen once the patient is able to tolerate oral medications (to complete a full course).
- Management of uncomplicated malaria
  - The management of uncomplicated malaria depends on the species and drug resistance.
  - In areas with chloroquine-resistant *P. falciparum*, the preferred regimens include:
    - Artemether–lumefantrine (Coartem) for 3 days.
    - Atovaquone–proguanil for 3 days total.
  - Alternative regimens:
    - Quinine sulfate plus doxycycline or tetracycline or clindamycin ×7 days (Box 34.5).
    - Mefloquine ×2 doses (Box 34.5).
- If a patient presents with *P. falciparum* from an area with no known resistance, uncomplicated *P. malariae* or *P. knowlesi*:
  - Chloroquine or hydroxychloroquine for 48 hours.
- If a patient presents with *P. vivax* from an area with no known resistance or *P. ovale*
  - Chloroquine or hydroxychloroquine plus primaquine phosphate for 14 days.
- If a patient presents with *P. vivax* from an area with known chloroquine resistance:
  - Quinine sulfate plus doxycycline/tetracycline plus primaquine phosphate ×7 days.
  - Atovaquone–proguanil plus primaquine phosphate ×3 days.
  - Mefloquine plus primaquine phosphate.

American Trypanosomiasis: Chagas Disease

Microbiology and Pathogenesis

- *Trypanosoma cruzi* is a protozoan parasite. The main form of transmission is via the triatomine insect (kissing bug). This insect takes a blood meal, followed by

• BOX 34.6   Bottom of the Pile

To get this infection, one is literally at the bottom of the (insect's) crap pile.

defecation near the bite wound (Box 34.6). The feces contain trypomastigotes, which enter via the bite wound or via mucosal membranes (for example, scratching the wound then rubbing eyes). Transmission has been also been documented vertically from mother to child, via blood transfusion, organ transplantation, consumption of contaminated food, or laboratory inoculation.

- Vector: Triatomine insects (kissing bugs) (Fig. 34.4).

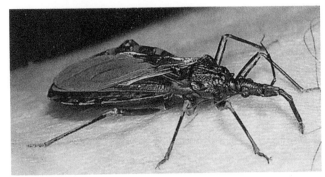

• Fig. 34.4 *Triatoma infestans*, a vector of *Trypanosoma cruzi*. (From Wallace P, Pasvol G. 2007. *Atlas of Tropical Medicine and Parasitology.* 6th ed. Elsevier; 2007. Image #1TF231.)

Epidemiology

- Endemic to the Americas, from southern United States to the north of Argentina and Chile, but the highest prevalence is found in Bolivia, Argentina, Paraguay, Ecuador, El Salvador, and Guatemala. Despite being confined to the Americas; vertical transmission allows for transmission in nonendemic areas. Triatomine insects are found in many parts of the United States, and they have been found to harbor *T. cruzi*.
- The main protection against this infection is housing with plastered walls and sealed entryways, which limits the ability of these nocturnal insects to feed on humans.

Clinical Features

- Most patients are asymptomatic.
- The **acute phase** may be characterized by fever, inflammation at the inoculation site (if occurs in the conjunctival site leads to unilateral palpebral edema: Romaña sign) (Fig. 34.5), lymphadenopathy, and hepatosplenomegaly. Myocarditis, generally subclinical, may also be present during the acute phase.
- The **chronic phase** will come to medical attention due to disease of the heart and GI tract. Chronic Chagas cardiomyopathy can present with biventricular heart failure, a wide range of electrical abnormalities/arrhythmias, thromboembolic disease, including stroke. Of note, **apical aneurysm** is a unique structural change associated with this infection. Less commonly, chronic infection can manifest as motility dysfunction of the esophagus or colon, from mild transit delay to megaesophagus or megacolon.
- An **indeterminate** form of Chagas diseases is commonly encountered, in which patients have laboratory evidence of infection (usually serology) but no apparent signs or symptoms.
- **Reactivation** of chronic Chagas disease has been seen in immunosuppressed patients, either secondary to HIV, or in the setting of solid organ transplantation. In these patients, presentations have included meningoencephalitis, brain abscess, acute myocarditis, skin nodules, panniculitis, and organ rejection.
- **Congenital Chagas** via vertical transmission has been diagnosed in up to 10% of infants born to infected

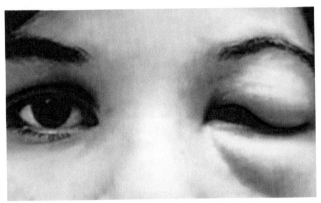

• Fig. 34.5 Romaña sign: unilateral palpebral edema at site of inoculation. (From Miles MA. Chagas disease (American trypanosomiasis). In: Cohen J, Powderly W, Opal S, eds. *Infectious Diseases*. 4th ed. Elsevier; 2017.)

mothers. Manifestations of infection include low birthweight, anemia, hepatosplenomegaly, and in some cases severe CNS disease and respiratory failure.

Diagnosis

- Acute phase: Microscopic visualization of trypomastigotes in blood or buffy coat; PCR if available.
- Chronic phase: Based on serology, generally using either ELISA or IFA technology. If positive, the results should be confirmed by a recognized reference lab (in the United States this is the Centers for Disease Control and Prevention [CDC]). This can also be diagnosed by tissue biopsy showing amastigotes (Fig. 34.6).
- Reactivation: Microscopic visualization of trypomastigotes in blood or buffy coat; PCR if available. If diagnosis of reactivation in transplant is confirmed, then a monitoring protocol should be implemented of weekly specimens for 2 months, then every other week for a month, then monthly until 6 months (or longer, if parasitemia persists or if the patient is treated for organ rejection).
- Congenital: diagnosis should be confirmed in the mother. The infant is acutely infected, so parasites should be visualized in blood, and PCR may be helpful. Serology is of limited use in this population as antibodies reflect the maternal population.

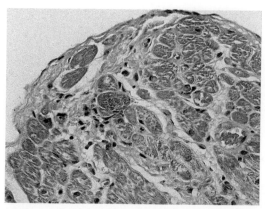

• **Fig. 34.6** Myocardial amastigote nest in a heart transplant patient with Chagas disease. (H&E, original magnification ×40). (Courtesy Dr Paula Carmo, MD, Belo Horizonte, Minas Gerais, Brazil.)

Treatment

- Patients with acute or congenital *T. cruzi* infection or those with reactivation disease should be treated. Patients under 19 with chronic infection should also be treated. Recommendations are less clear for those with chronic or indeterminate disease up to age 50. Patients with advanced cardiomyopathy or severe GI disease, those who are pregnant, or who have severe renal or hepatic dysfunction should not be treated (Table 34.4).
- The two agents used are benznidazole or nifurtimox. Dosing is dependent on age and weight. Duration of therapy can range from 60 to 120 days, depending on agent chosen and patient age.

African Trypanosomiasis: Sleeping Sickness

Microbiology and Pathogenesis

- *Trypanosoma brucei gambiense* and *Trypanosoma brucei rhodesiense*.
- Vector: tsetse fly. *Glossina palpalis* for *T. b. gambiense*. *Glossina morsitans* for *T. b. rhodesiense*.
- When a human is bitten by an infected fly, trypomastigotes are injected into the skin, forming a painful chancre at the site. The parasites then disseminate via the regional lymphatics and spread throughout the bloodstream. They are able to pass through vessel walls and enter the cerebrospinal fluid (CSF).
- Transmission: via the bite of the tsetse fly (Fig. 34.7). Other reported methods of transmission include blood transfusion, congenital infection, laboratory inoculation.

Epidemiology

- Both parasites are endemic to Africa but the geographical distribution is dependent on the species.
  - *T. b. gambiense* is found in West and Central Africa (mainly in the Democratic Republic of Congo, Central African Republic, and Chad), in humid habitats.
  - *T. b. rhodesiense* in found in East Africa (mainly Malawi and Uganda), in drier habitats.

TABLE 34.4	When to Treat American Trypanosomiasis	
Presentation		**Should I Treat?**
Acute *Trypanosoma cruzi* infection		Yes
Early congenital *T. cruzi* infection		Yes
Children <18 years with chronic *T. cruzi* infection		Yes
Reactivation of *T. cruzi* in immunocompromised host		Yes
Adults (19–50 years) with no or mild cardiomyopathy		Yes
Adults >50 years without advanced cardiomyopathy		Maybe
Gastrointestinal diseases without advanced cardiomyopathy		Maybe
Advanced cardiomyopathy with congestive heart failure		No
Megaesophagus with impaired swallowing		No
During pregnancy		Absolutely not
Severe renal or hepatic failure		Absolutely not

Clinical Features

Both parasites have two stages: early or hemolymphatic, or stage I, during which the parasites circulate in the blood/lymphatics, and the late stage/stage II, notable for central nervous system (CNS) manifestations (Box 34.7). If untreated, stage II mortality is 100%.
- Stage I
  - *T. b. gambiense* has a prolonged early stage, characterized by intervals of fever, headache, lymphadenopathy, hepatosplenomegaly, and endocrine disorders that may last several years.
  - *T. b. rhodesiense* stage I is characterized by a trypanosomal chancre at the site of inoculation, fever, lymphadenopathies, hepatosplenomegaly, and myocarditis. Duration is much shorter, weeks to months.
- Stage II
  - Severe neuropsychiatric and sleep disorders followed by coma and death within weeks if untreated. This may occur more slowly in *T. b. gambiense*.

Diagnosis

- Direct microscopic visualization of the trypomastigotes in blood smear, tissue aspirates, or CSF (Fig. 34.8). Antibodies are only commercially available for the diagnosis of *T. b. gambiense*.
- Staging is mandatory for all patients suspected of having human African trypanosomiasis. If the cerebrospinal fluid collected by a lumbar puncture reveals more than five white blood cells per μL or parasites the patient is categorized as having stage II disease.

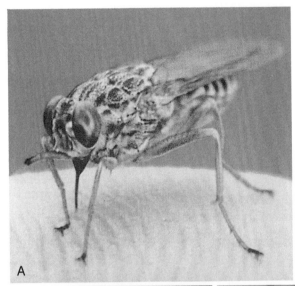

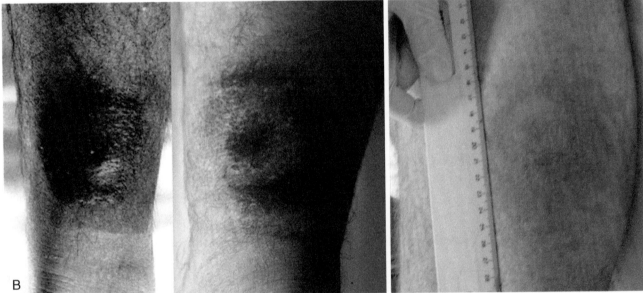

• **Fig. 34.7** (A) Tsetse fly. (B) Chancres of African trypanosomiasis. (Panel A courtesy Wellcome Foundation, Berkhamsted, England. Panel B courtesy Prof. Denis Malvy, Bordeaux, France [*left*, *middle*] and Prof. Joachim Richter, Düsseldorf, Germany [*right*].)

• **BOX 34.7** **East and West**

Just like time zone changes, African sleeping sickness is worse in the east than in the west. So **"East is least, West is best"** – at least in reference to a slower, less aggressive disease presentation.

Treatment

- *Trypanosoma brucei gambiense*
  - First-stage: pentamidine for 7 days.
  - Second-stage: nifurtimox for 10 days + eflornithine for 7 days.
- *Trypanosoma brucei rhodesiense*
  - First-stage: suramin ×5 weeks.
  - Second-stage: melarsoprol for 10 days.

Babesiosis

Microbiology and Pathogenesis

- *Babesia* species are intracellular protozoan parasites of erythrocytes. *B. microti* is the most common species seen in the United States. *B. duncani* and *B. duncani*-like are less common. *B. divergens* is the predominant species in Europe.
- Vector: *Ixodes scapularis* (black-legged tick or deer tick); *I. pacificus* is the likely vector on the west coast. The main animal host is the white-footed mouse (*Peromyscus leucopus)* and the white-tailed deer (*Odocoileus virgianianus*) (Box 34.8).
- Transmission is primarily via tick bite from the nymphal form (although adult ticks can also transmit). Infections have been acquired via blood transfusion, organ transplantation, and transplacental transmission. As these are

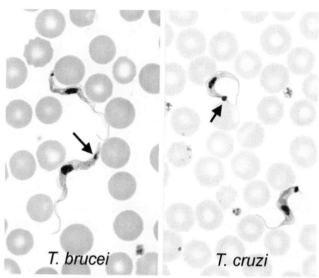

Fig. 34.8 *T. brucei*: small kinetoplast (*arrow*); *T. cruzi*: large kinetoplast (*arrow*) Also, classically, *T. cruzi* are described as "C" shaped, but you can tell from this image that this is not always the case. (From Schmitt BH, Rosenblatt JE, Pritt BS. Laboratory diagnosis of tropical infections. *Infect Dis Clin North Am.* 2012;26(2):513–554.)

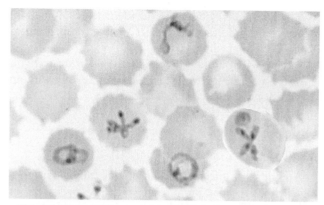

Fig. 34.9 Maltese Cross. (From McAdam A, Milner DA, Sharpe AH. Infectious diseases. In Kumar V, Abbas AK, Aster JC. *Robbins & Cotran Pathologic Basis of Disease.* 9th ed. Elsevier; 2015.)

BOX 34.8 A Colorful Disease

It's a colorful disease: **Black**-legged ticks bite **White**-footed mice and infect **Red** cells.

BOX 34.9 Good to Know

Remove the tick in <36 hours, and infection risk drops significantly.

---

mainly vectorborne, the majority of patients present during summer months. Humans are inadvertent, dead-end hosts. When the ticks feed, they release sporozoites into the dermis during prolonged attachment (Box 34.9). These sporozoites then enter the bloodstream and invade erythrocytes, where they become merozoites. Most clinical symptoms are due to the release of merozoites from the RBCs causing a host inflammatory response, as well as hemolysis and anemia.

Epidemiology

- The infection is most common in the northeastern United States, including Nantucket, Martha's Vineyard, and Long Island. The parasites have rarely been reported in Wisconsin, Washington, Oregon, and California.

Clinical Features

- The clinical features range from subclinical to life-threatening. Fever and flu-like symptoms are common but unlike malaria there is no periodicity to the fever cycle.

Severe cases can appear similar to malaria with high fever, chills, night sweats, myalgia, hemolytic anemia, hematuria, hepatosplenomegaly, and jaundice.

- Unlike other tickborne illnesses, the incubation period is long and ranges from 1 to 4 weeks. However, in patients with transfusion-related infection the incubation period can extend to up to 9 weeks.
- Risk factors for severe disease include asplenia, advanced age, and immunosuppression (HIV, malignancy, corticosteroids).
- Given that *Babesia* is transmitted by *Ixodes scapularis*, co-infection with anaplasmosis and Lyme is common and should be considered if the patient continues to have fever despite appropriate therapy (see Chapter 30).

Diagnosis

- Travel history and recent antimicrobial use are important. The organism can look very similar to malaria, especially *P. falciparum*, so travel history is important for the laboratorian to know.
- Thick and thin blood smears should be prepared from blood collected with EDTA as the preservative. The smears can be stained with Wright or Giemsa stains.
- The morphologic features include:
  - Infected RBCs are normal size.
  - No intracellular pigment.
  - Delicate rings with varying morphologies (round, oval, spindled).
  - Multiply infected RBCs.
  - Extracellular forms common (not seen with malaria).
  - Maltese Cross: intracellular tetrad of merozoites that are rarely seen (Fig. 34.9).
- Molecular assays are available from reference labs for difficult cases.
- Serology does not have a role in the diagnosis of babesiosis.

Treatment

- The preferred regimen is a combination of atovaquone plus azithromycin for 7–10 days.

- Clindamycin and quinine are the alternative combination.
- Severity of infection determines whether dosing and to use IV vs. oral administration.
- Patients with immunosuppression should be treated with 6 weeks of therapy with at least the last 2 weeks with no evidence of *Babesia* sp. in the blood.

Leishmaniasis

Microbiology and Pathogenesis

- A number of infectious conditions are caused by single-celled intracellular protozoa of the genus *Leishmania*. At least 21 different species have been implicated in human disease. All share female sandfly vectors (Old World, genus *Phlebotomus*; New World, genus *Lutzomyia*). These are mostly nocturnal feeders.
- The infected vector carries promastigotes in her gut, which enter mammals when the fly feeds. The

promastigotes transform into amastigotes within the vertebrate phagolysosomes. Amastigotes continue to multiply both in tissue and in macrophages. At the next blood meal, the sandfly takes up infected macrophages, and the cycle continues. Most species have zoonotic reservoirs.

Epidemiology

- *Leishmania* species are endemic to tropical and subtropical areas around the world. They have classically been divided into two groups: Old World and New World.
- The Old World *Leishmania* species extend from southwestern Europe and northeastern Africa, across the Arabian Peninsula and through Asia, with sporadic cases across Africa.
- The New World *Leishmania* species are found in the western hemisphere, from Texas through Central and South America. No autochthonous infections have been described in Australia, Antarctica, or the Pacific Islands.

Clinical Features

The disease manifestations are differentiated into visceral leishmaniasis vs. disease limited to the skin and mucosal services. For this review we identify cutaneous leishmaniasis, mucocutaneous leishmaniasis, and visceral leishmaniasis (Box 34.10 and Fig. 34.10).

• BOX **34.10**	**Leishmania Leaps the Lands: Old and New World Presentations**

- Old World: **kala-azar** = visceral leishmaniasis
- New World: **espundia** = mucocutaneous leishmaniasis

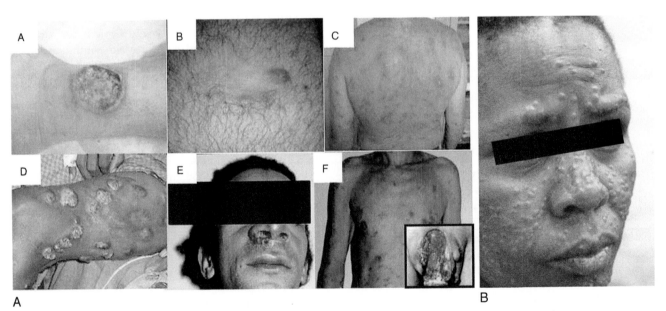

• **Fig. 34.10** (Panel A) (a) LCL presenting a single ulcer on the leg. (b) Leishmaniasis recidiva cutis presenting papules and vesicles around the healed lesion of cutaneous leishmaniasis on the leg. (c) Disseminated cutaneous leishmaniasis presenting numerous small ulcers on the back. (d) DCL presenting tumoral lesions and nodules associated with crusts and several scars from previous injuries on the left thigh. (e) Mucocutaneous leishmaniasis lesion in the nose and infiltration in nasal mucosa. (f) Atypical cutaneous leishmaniasis in a patient infected with human immunodeficiency virus presenting multiple macules on the chest and abdomen; (inset) extensive ulcer on the penis of a patient with acquired immune deficiency syndrome. (Panel B) Post kala azar dermal leishmaniasis. (Panel A: (a) courtesy Luiza K. Oyafuso, Instituto de Infectologia Emilio Ribas, São Paulo, Brazil; (b) courtesy Maria Edileuza Brito, Centro de Pesquisas Aggeu Magalhães, Fundação Oswaldo Cruz, Brazil; (c) courtesy Edgar M. Carvalho, Universidade Federal da Bahia, Brazil; (d) courtesy Jackson ML Costa, Centro de Pesquisas Gonçalo Muniz, Fundação Oswaldo Cruz, Brazil. (e and f) From Goto H, Lauletta Lindoso JA. *Infect Dis Clin North Am.* 2012;26(2):293–307. Panel B: From Magill AJ, Ryan ET, Hill DR, Solomon T. *Hunter's Tropical Medicine and Emerging Infectious Diseases.* 9th ed. Elsevier; 2013.)

- **Cutaneous leishmaniasis (CL)**, the most common presentation, is characterized by one or multiple ulcers that develop in exposed areas of the body (where the sandflies bite) (Box 34.11). Lesions develop weeks to months following the inoculation of the parasite. The ulcers have raised indurated borders, with some undermining. These lesions are typically **painless** and can persist for long periods of time. The appearance is quite varied and has been described as a single ulcer to sporotrichoid pattern to eczematous lesions, among other patterns.
  - **Diffuse cutaneous leishmaniasis (DCL)** is a rare condition resulting from dissemination of the parasite to macrophages distal from the inoculation site, with minimal lymphocytic reaction. This is usually seen in patients with a defect in cell-mediated immunity. Due to its appearance, it is sometimes known as lepromatous leishmaniasis.

> **BOX 34.11 Question: What Species Cause Cutaneous Leishmaniasis?**
>
> Answer:
> - Old World: *L. major, L. tropica, L. aethiopica*
> - New World (the species names help): *L. mexicana, L. venezuelensis, L. amazonensis, L. braziliensis, L. peruviana, L. guyanensis, L. panamensis*
> - Anything beyond Nicaragua (species other than *L. mexicana*) should be treated, due to higher risk of mucosal disease.

> **BOX 34.12 Question: What Species Cause Visceral Leishmaniasis?**
>
> Answer:
> - *L. donovani, L. infantum chagasi*

- **Leishmaniasis recidivans (LR)**: *L. tropica*. Persistent papule formation around healed primary lesion; organisms present along with notable granulomatous immune response.
- **Mucocutaneous leishmaniasis (ML)**, or espundia, is a concurrent or late complication of cutaneous leishmaniasis. It is characterized by destructive lesions in the oral and nasal mucosa that can progress to destruction of the nose, palate, throat, and surrounding tissues. Genital mucosa involvement has also been described. This is primarily a New World condition, as Old World infections rarely progress into ML.
- **Visceral leishmaniasis (VL)**, or kala-azar, is the result of dissemination of amastigotes into the reticuloendothelial system (Box 34.12). It typically presents with splenomegaly (± liver enlargement), and evidence of cytopenias such as pallor, epistaxis. Laboratory testing reveals pancytopenia, elevated transaminases, and low albumin. This presentation has a high mortality when untreated. A rare late sequela of treated VL is **post-kala-azar dermal leishmaniasis**, which is characterized by diffuse hypopigmented macules.
  - **Viscerotropic disease**: milder version of visceral leishmaniasis, seen in US military veterans of the Gulf War in the early 1990s.

Diagnosis

- Direct visualization of the amastigotes using light microscopy is the preferred technique and can be performed on dermal scrapings, tissue biopsies, and touch preparations. Sensitivity varies depending on the clinical presentation and sample type. Bone marrow aspirate is the preferred sample for diagnosis of VL with a sensitivity of 60%–85%. In CL, DCL, and ML a smear, biopsy, or scraping of the edge of the ulcer should be submitted for microscopy. Specialized culture techniques also exist (Figs. 34.11 and 34.12).

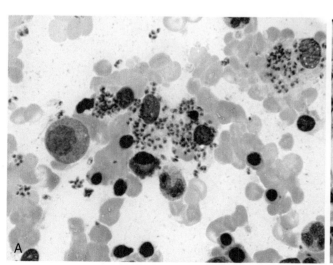
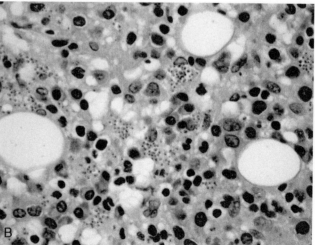

• **Fig. 34.11** Bone marrow leishmaniasis. (A) The *Leishmania* amastigotes in this aspirate smear are both extracellular and within histiocytes (Wright–Giemsa stain). (B) Intrahistiocytic amastigotes can also be visualized on a thin trephine biopsy section (H&E stain). (From Kradin RL. *Diagnostic Pathology of Infectious Disease*. 2nd ed. Elsevier; 2018.)

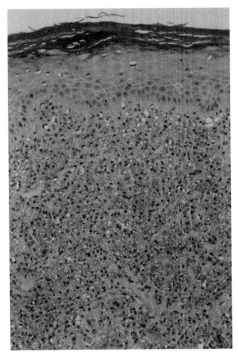

• **Fig. 34.12** Staining of a nodule on the forearm reveals numerous round, basophilic intracellular amastigotes with kinetoplasts, indicative of leishmaniasis. (H&E; original magnification ×40.) (From Handler MZ, Patel PA, Kapila R, Al-Qubati Y, Schwartz RA. Cutaneous and mucocutaneous leishmaniasis: differential diagnosis, diagnosis, histopathology, and management. *J Am Acad Dermatol.* 2015;73:911–926.)

- Tissue PCR has been developed and has a higher sensitivity for the diagnosis of all clinical presentations of *Leishmania.*
- Serological tests are most useful for VL. Otherwise, serology cannot discriminate between past or active infection and have limited availability.

Treatment

- The decision to treat CL is dependent on the risk of dissemination or local disfigurement, based either on knowing the species, or the host immune status, as well as patient preference. Observation may be sufficient, or local treatment only.
- Treatment options are limited, but include:
  - Pentavalent antimonials: generally first line for CL and ML. Can be administered systemically or intralesionally.
  - Amphotericin B (deoxycholate and liposomal formulations): most effective against CL.
  - Miltefosine: New World CL and ML; Old and New World VL. Teratogenic.
  - Azoles: mainly for CL.
  - Paromomycin has activity against certain strains causing cutaneous leishmaniasis, but it is rarely used.
- "Donovan destroys"
- "Infants invade"

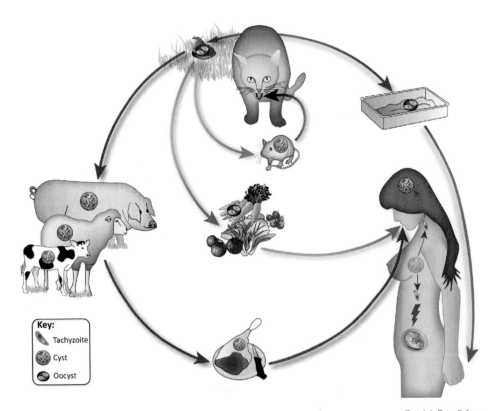

Key:
- Tachyzoite
- Cyst
- Oocyst

Trends in Parasitology

• **Fig. 34.13** Life cycle of *Toxoplasma gondii*. (From Rougier S, Montoya JG, Peyron F. Lifelong persistence of toxoplasma cysts: a questionable dogma? *Trends Parasitol.* 2017;33(2):93–101.)

Toxoplasmosis

Microbiology and Pathogenesis

- *Toxoplasma gondii* has a complex life cycle involving a definitive host (felines, including domestic cats) and intermediate hosts (many, from rodents to birds to farm animals) (see Fig. 34.13).
- The sexual cycle occurs within the intestinal epithelial cells of the definitive host. The oocysts are excreted with the cat feces and become infectious within 1–5 days.
- Intermediate hosts are infected by consuming the mature oocysts. Within the intermediate host, the oocysts rupture, releasing sporozoites which develop into tachyzoites. These travel via the lymphatic system and bloodstream, reaching neural and muscle tissue, where they isolate into cysts, becoming bradyzoites.
- Cats acquire the infection by eating infected tissue containing cysts or direct ingestion of sporulated oocysts in the environment.
- Humans (intermediate hosts) acquire infection by direct consumption of food or water that contains mature oocysts or by eating undercooked meat harboring tissue cysts, as well as via blood transfusion or transplantation (Box 34.13).
- *T. gondii* can be transmitted transplacentally from mother to the fetus, when the tachyzoite stage crosses the placenta. Notably, increased gestational age increases the risk of acquiring congenital toxoplasmosis if the pregnant mother becomes acutely infected but paradoxically is associated with a decreased disease severity.

Epidemiology

- Toxoplasmosis is a worldwide zoonosis. Seropositivity rates vary from 10% to over 90% and are highest in populations living in humid, warm climates and having extensive exposure to contaminated soil (kids playing in the dirt) (Box 34.14). In the United States seroprevalence is around 11%, with higher numbers found in those born outside the US, and lower numbers in US-born patients. Congenital toxoplasmosis rates are notably elevated in South America, parts of the Middle East, and some areas of Africa. In the United States incidence is estimated at 1 per 10,000 live births.

• BOX 34.13   Food for Thought

While humans are technically intermediate hosts (like mice), we are also dead-end hosts, since our pets don't generally eat us. But in theory, perhaps a lion could become infected by eating a toxoplasma-filled human?

• BOX 34.14   Cat vs. Human Diagnosis of Toxoplasmosis

Remember, *Toxoplasma* is shed in cat stool, not human stool. So, the "stool O&P" (ova and parasite) is not a good diagnostic assay for your human patient.

In pregnancy, the diagnosis is crucial, and dependent on serology.

Clinical Features

- In immunocompetent persons, toxoplasmosis is usually asymptomatic. If symptoms develop, they most commonly present as a flu- or mononucleosis-like illness, often with lymphadenopathy. These symptoms resolve spontaneously over weeks to months. *T. gondii* can also cause chorioretinitis in otherwise healthy patients, manifesting as visual loss or floaters.
- Manifestations of transplacentally acquired infection vary dependent on the trimester during which the disease was acquired and also the genotype of the pathogen (with certain genotypes being associated with more severe disease). The congenital toxoplasmosis triad includes **chorioretinitis**, **hydrocephalus**, and **intracranial calcifications**, although this is rarely present outside of textbooks. Most babies will be subclinical on routine physical examination. If severe manifestations are noted, this usually reflects infection during the first trimester.
- Immunocompromised individuals are at increased risk of reactivation. Persons living with HIV with CD4 counts below 200 cells/µL are a well-recognized population, most commonly presenting with encephalitis, followed by pneumonitis (clinically similar to *Pneumocystis jirovecii*). Imaging of these patients will show multiple intracerebral mass lesions (Fig. 34.14). Solid organ transplant recipients have been diagnosed with reactivation disease. Lesions may vary according to the net state of immunosuppression and can include toxoplasmic encephalitis, pulmonary toxoplasmosis, or allograft failure, particularly in heart transplant recipients.

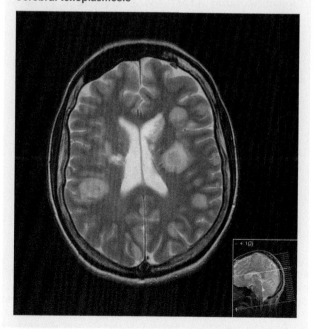

Cerebral toxoplasmosis

• Fig. 34.14 MRI showing multiple ring-enhancing lesions typical of cerebral toxoplasmosis. (From Croucher A, Winston A. Neurological complications of HIV. *Medicine*. 2013;41(8):450–455.)

Diagnosis

Diagnosis can be challenging, but the most commonly available tests are IgM and IgG via ELISA, PCR, and tissue biopsy (Fig. 34.15). In immunocompetent individuals the diagnosis is usually obtained by a combination of clinical signs and symptoms and serologic studies. If the *Toxoplasma gondii* IgM is negative and IgG is positive, acute infection can be ruled out with reasonable certainty. If only the IgM is positive, this likely indicates acute infection, but if both are positive, interpretation is complicated as *Toxoplasma* IgM antibodies can remain detectable for 12 months or more.

In people with HIV/AIDS, the diagnosis is based on a combination of a low CD4 T-cell count, encephalitis, positive *T. gondii* IgG, and multiple ring-enhancing masses in the brain parenchyma. In otherwise immunocompromised patients, serology is also challenging. It is helpful to have IgG results prior to transplantation, especially for bone marrow transplant patients. Often, the diagnosis relies on histopathology or molecular techniques (including PCR).

Treatment

- Acute infections in immunocompetent hosts are usually self-limiting and do not warrant treatment, unless the patient has severe or prolonged symptoms or has evidence of end-organ involvement. Oral pyrimethamine plus sulfadiazine plus leucovorin (folinic acid) for 2–4 weeks is the regimen of choice.
- Ocular disease should be treated for a minimum of 6 weeks.
- Immunocompromised patient (HIV/AIDS, solid and stem cell transplant patients) with suspected or confirmed infection should be treated for a minimum of 6 weeks. After completion of therapy immunocompromised patients should remain in prophylaxis with either trimethoprim–sulfamethoxazole (TMP–SMX), dapsone + pyrimethamine or atovaquone until immunologic reconstitution occurs or the overall net state of immunosuppression is low.

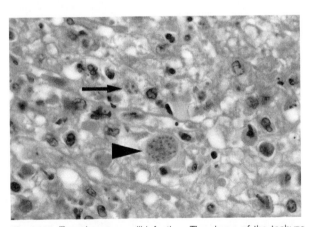

• **Fig. 34.15** *Toxoplasma gondii* infection. The shape of the tachyzoites is more difficult to appreciate in tissue sections than in impression smears, but cysts (*arrowhead*) can be more easily appreciated than tachyzoites (*arrow*). (Reproduced with permission from Pritt BS. Protozoal infections. In: Procop GW, Pritt BS, eds. *Pathology of Infectious Diseases: A Volume in the Series: Foundations in Diagnostic Pathology*. Philadelphia: Elsevier; 2015:610–43.)

- Treatment of pregnant women and infants is complicated. Pregnant women in whom infection is suspected or confirmed before 18 weeks' gestation, but in whom the fetus does not show infection, should receive spiramycin. If infection is acquired at or after 18 weeks' gestation, or in women with a positive amniotic fluid PCR or suspicious ultrasound, then a combination of pyrimethamine plus sulfadiazine plus folinic acid is indicated. These same agents are used in infants and older children with weight-based doses, along with prednisone in many cases.

INTESTINAL PROTOZOA

- While many protozoa can be found in stool, only a few species have been identified as human pathogens. Others generally indicate consumption of contaminated food or water and might trigger the clinician to keep testing for true pathogens.
- A common presenting symptom is diarrhea. While there may be key epidemiologic clues on exam questions, in reality, most patients either have multiple risk factors, or no clear risk factors to differentiate one pathogen from another. It is important to know what can be reliably diagnosed with the ova and parasite exam (O&P), and which pathogens require additional testing.

Neobalantidiasis

Microbiology and Pathogenesis

This infection is caused by *Neobalantidium coli* (formerly *Balantidium coli*), the only ciliated protozoan to infect humans. The life cycle is simple: cysts are ingested from contaminated food or water, or via the fecal–oral route. The organism undergoes excystation in the small intestine, while trophozoites colonize the large intestine. Cysts are then excreted in the stool.

Epidemiology

It is worldwide, mainly tropical and subtropical regions. Pigs are a common reservoir.

Clinical Features

- Asymptomatic infection.
- Acute colitis
  - Watery stool or blood stool (dysentery).
  - Nausea, vomiting, diarrhea, abdominal pain.
- Chronic infection: rare
  - Intermittent bloody diarrhea and pain.
- May lead to colonic perforation.

Diagnosis

- Stool microscopy (O&P exam).
  - Saline for trophozoites (40-200 µm) and cysts (50-70 µm) in fresh stool (rarely performed).
  - Polyvinyl alcohol (PVA) for permanent stain for cysts and trophozoites.
  - Formalin concentration for cysts.
- Can be found in the colonic mucosa (Fig. 34.16).
- NAAT (not commonly available).

• BOX 34.15 Beware the Swimming Pool!

Be suspicious if there are multiple cases in a community, especially during summer months.

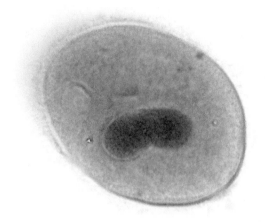

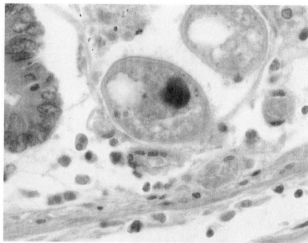

• **Fig. 34.16** *Neobalantidium coli* trophozoite, intestine (H&E, ×1000). (From Rifai N. *Neobalantidium coli*. In: Rifai N, et al., eds. *Tietz Textbook of Clinical Chemistry and Molecular Diagnostics*. 6th ed. Elsevier; 2018.)

Treatment

- Tetracycline.
- Metronidazole or paromomycin.

Cryptosporidiosis

Microbiology and Pathogenesis

Cryptosporidium parvum and *C. hominis* are the most common human pathogens. Multiple other species exist with particular vertebrate niches, although several have also been found in humans. These apicomplexan protozoa are acquired via ingestion of oocysts. Disease occurs primarily in proximal small bowel. Autoinfection can maintain disease persistence (in other words, eating one's own stool via poor hand hygiene).

Epidemiology

This pathogen has a global distribution and is often found in sources of drinking water or in **swimming locations**

(Box 34.15). Notably, the oocysts are resistant to chlorination and often not adequately filtered.

Clinical Features

- 3- to 28-day incubation, usually 7–10 days.
- Asymptomatic infection.
- Immunocompetent hosts
  - Symptoms range from acute to subacute to chronic, watery diarrhea, sometimes high-volume output.
  - May have associated gastrointestinal symptoms such as nausea, pain.
  - Generally self-resolving within 14 days.
- Immunocompromised hosts (especially HIV/AIDS)
  - Can have profound diarrhea and severe wasting.
  - Biliary tract involvement, including acalculous cholecystitis, cholangitis, pancreatitis.

Diagnosis

- Antigen detection assays (usually simultaneously detect *Giardia*)
  - Direct immunofluorescence assays (DFA).
  - Enzyme-linked immunosorbent assays (ELISA).
- NAAT
  - Usually as a part of a multiplex panel.
- Stool microscopy (Fig. 34.17)
  - Oocyst size 4.2-5.4 µm diameter.
  - Routine O&P exam rarely adequate.
  - Requires special stain, most commonly modified acid-fast stain.
- Small bowel or colonic biopsies demonstrate oocysts on luminal surface (intracellular but extracytoplasmic) (Fig. 34.18).

Treatment

- Supportive therapy, including fluid replacement and antidiarrheal agents.
- Immunocompetent patients generally self-resolve.
  - If profound disease or symptoms beyond 2 weeks, can consider nitazoxanide or paromomycin.
- Immunocompromised patients: no evidence that treatment helps.
  - HIV: antiviral therapy.
  - Non-HIV immunocompromised: reduction of immunosuppression, possibly nitazoxanide.

Cyclosporiasis

Microbiology and Pathogenesis

Caused by *Cyclospora cayetanensis,* a coccidian protozoan. Humans are the only known host. Transmission is via ingestion of contaminated water or food. Person-to-person

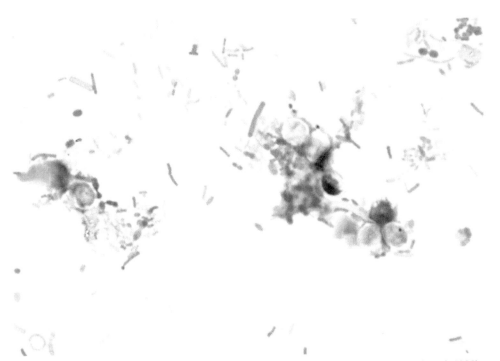

• **Fig. 34.17** *Cryptosporidium* spp. Modified acid-fast staining of oocysts in stool preparations (×1000). Note the variable intensity of staining. (From Pritt BS. Protozoal infections. In: Procop GW, Pritt BS, eds. *Pathology of Infectious Diseases*. Elsevier; 2015.)

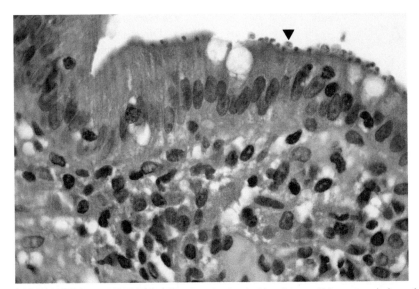

• **Fig. 34.18** The small, round, pale blue objects at the luminal border or within a vacuole in peripheral enterocyte cytoplasm are *Cryptosporidium parvum* organisms. The organisms rarely invade or disseminate. There is no inflammation, necrosis, or hemorrhage. (From Klatt EC. The gastrointestinal tract. In: Kumar V, Abbas AK, Aster JC. *Robbins & Cotran Pathologic Basis of Disease*. 9th ed. Elsevier; 2015.)

(fecal–oral) transmission seems unlikely as there is an environmental sporulation phase that takes several days. Unsporulated oocysts are the infectious forms, excreted in stool. Infection is primarily in the small bowel.

Epidemiology

There is a broad range of distribution. Most cases are reported from Mexico, Central and South America, the Indian subcontinent, Southeast Asia. In North America, most cases are associated with contaminated, imported fresh produce (peas, salad mix, cilantro, raspberries are some examples) (Box 34.16). In endemic areas, there may be seasonal patterns to infection, but these are not well established.

Clinical Features

- Incubation: 2–14 days, average 7 days.
- Asymptomatic infection, notably in endemic regions.
- Watery diarrhea.
  - Stools may be explosive.

- Weight loss, decreased appetite, abdominal cramping and bloating, flatus, nausea, fatigue.
- "Flu-like" symptoms: body aches, emesis, low-grade fever.
  - May be self-limited or have a prolonged course, lasting months.
- Severity highest in the young and the old.
- HIV infection may be complicated by acalculous cholecystitis.
- Postinfectious reactive arthritis has been reported.

Diagnosis

- Stool microscopy
  - Requires special stain, most commonly modified acid-fast stain. Oocysts (spherical; 7.5-10 μm) are larger than *Cryptosporidium* (Fig. 34.19). They will autofluoresce under UV microscopy.
- NAAT
  - Usually as a part of a multiplex panel.
- Small bowel biopsy for histology: cysts present in enterocytes.

Treatment

- TMP–SMX.
- Nitazoxanide in sulfa-allergic patients.

Cystoisosporiasis (formerly Isosporiasis)

Microbiology and Pathogenesis

Caused by *Cystoisospora belli* (previously *Isospora belli*), a coccidian protozoan. Humans appear to be the only host for this pathogen, while other members of the genus can infect other vertebrates. Transmission is via ingestion of contaminated water or food. Oocysts are the infectious forms (excreted in stool). Like *Cyclospora*, there is a

component of maturation in the environment, so person-to-person transmission is unlikely. Disease occurs primarily in the small intestine but also large intestine. It is rarely extraluminal.

Epidemiology

This organism has a worldwide distribution, usually tropical and subtropical regions.

Clinical Presentation

- Watery, nonbloody diarrhea.
  - May have malaise, anorexia, abdominal pain, emesis, fever, sometimes steatorrhea.
- Immunocompetent: self-limited.
- Immunocompromised: chronic, protracted, severe diarrhea with wasting.
  - HIV: acalculous cholecystitis.

Diagnosis

- Stool microscopy
  - Oocysts large, ellipsoidal, 25-30 μm.
  - Modified acid-fast stain.
- NAAT
- Small bowel biopsy for histology: oocysts in enterocytes (oval and larger than *Cyclospora*) (Fig. 34.20).

Therapy

- TMP–SMX (Box 34.17).
- Ciprofloxacin.

> **• BOX 34.16** **Think *Cyclospora***
>
> Think about this pathogen in a vegetarian with explosive diarrhea, bloating, and flatus.

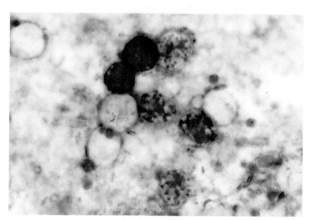

• **Fig. 34.19** *Cyclospora cayetanensis* oocysts. (From Babady E, Pritt BS. Parasitology. In: Rifai N, et al., eds. *Tietz Textbook of Clinical Chemistry and Molecular Diagnostics.* 6th ed. Elsevier; 2018.)

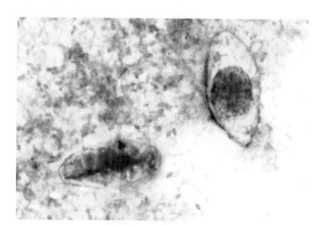

• **Fig. 34.20** *Cystoisospora belli* oocysts, each with a single sporoblast. (From Babady E, Pritt BS. Parasitology. In: Rifai N, et al., eds. *Tietz Textbook of Clinical Chemistry and Molecular Diagnostics.* 6th ed. Elsevier; 2018.)

> **• BOX 34.17** **TMP–SMX: Did You Know?**
>
> - Prophylaxis for *Pneumocystis jirovecii pneumonia* (PJP/PCP) with TMP–SMX (trimethoprim–sulfamethoxazole) reduces the risk of developing cystoisosporiasis and cyclosporiasis.

Amebiasis

Microbiology and Pathogenesis

- The etiologic agent is primarily *Entamoeba histolytica.* Multiple other species of intestinal amebae are recognized. *E. dispar* is not pathogenic. *E. moshkovskii* is being increasingly reported as associated with disease. *E. bangladeshi* pathogenicity is unclear.

- The mature cyst form of this organism is acquired via ingestion of contaminated food or water, as well as fecal–oral, sexually-associated transmission. It undergoes excystation in the small intestine, releasing trophozoites. These migrate to and invade the colonic mucosal barrier, multiply, and produce cysts. Both cyst and trophozoite forms are excreted in stool, but the latter are destroyed quickly outside the body (Fig. 34.21).

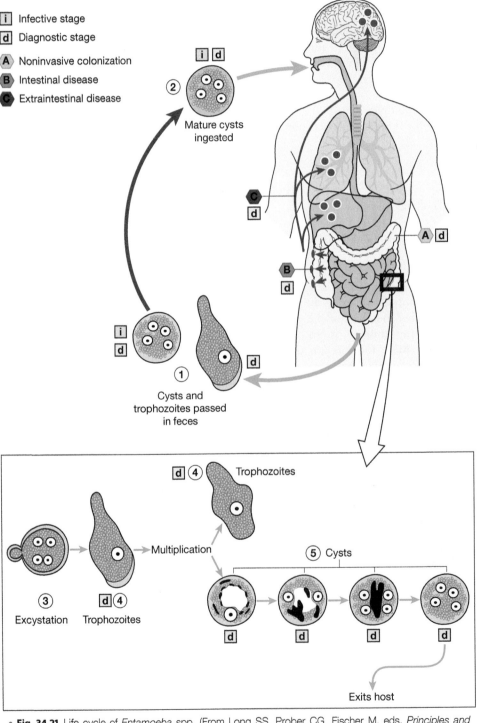

- **Fig. 34.21** Life cycle of *Entamoeba* spp. (From Long SS, Prober CG, Fischer M. eds. *Principles and Practice of Pediatric Infectious Diseases.* 5th ed. Elsevier; 2018.)

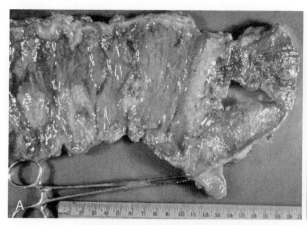
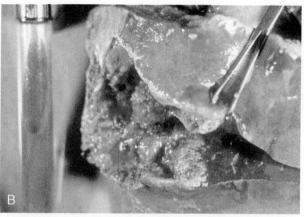

• **Fig. 34.22** *Entamoeba histolytica* infection demonstrating severe amebic colitis (A) and amebic liver abscess (B). The material aspirated from the amebic liver abscess (B, test tube) is said to resemble "anchovy paste." (Courtesy Centers for Disease Control and Prevention, Public Health Image Library.)

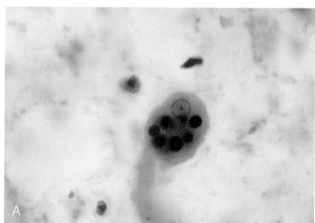
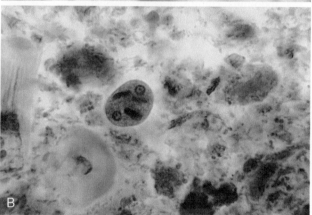

• **Fig. 34.23** *Entamoeba histolytica* trophozoite (A) and cyst (B). Trophozoites are motile and vary in size from 12 to 60 µm (average, 15–30 µm). The single nucleus in the cell is round with a central dot (karyosome) and an even distribution of chromatin granules around the nuclear membrane. Ingested erythrocytes may be in the cytoplasm. Cysts are smaller (10–20 µm [average, 15–20 µm]) and contain one to four nuclei (usually four). Round chromatoidal bars may be in the cytoplasm. (Courtesy Centers for Disease Control and Prevention, Public Health Image Library.)

Epidemiology

• This pathogen has a worldwide distribution but is particularly prevalent in India, Africa, Mexico, parts of Central and South America. It is more common in areas with poor sanitation and socioeconomic conditions. In the United States and other industrialized countries affected populations include travelers, recent immigrants from endemic areas, and men who have sex with men.

Clinical Features

• Incubation 2–4 weeks.
  • Clinical disease may not be apparent for years, especially extraintestinal forms.
• Intestinal infection
  • Asymptomatic colonization – 80%–90%.
  • Mild diarrhea, often bloody.
  • Abdominal pain.
  • Fever.
  • Fulminant colitis with bowel necrosis, perforation, peritonitis (rare, high mortality).
  • Persistent or chronic diarrhea (Fig. 34.22A).
• Ameboma: localized infection with surrounding granulation tissue. Uncommon.
• Extraintestinal disease
  • Amebic liver abscess: fever, right upper quadrant pain, appropriate epidemiology, and imaging (Fig. 34.22B).
    • Ten times more common in men.
    • Can occur even after short exposure in travelers.
    • Features include fever, right upper quadrant pain, hepatomegaly, diarrhea, cough, malaise, vomiting.
    • Jaundice is uncommon.
• Other rarely reported infections include pleuropulmonary, cardiac (usually from rupture of liver abscess), brain abscess, cutaneous infection.

Diagnosis

• Stool microscopy (O&P exam) (Fig. 34.23).
  • Saline preparation of fresh stool to detect motile trophozoites (not often performed).

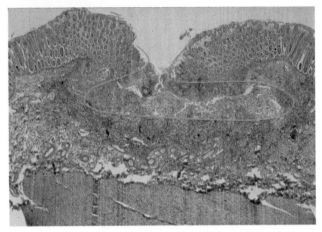

• **Fig. 34.24** *Entamoeba histolytica* trophozoite in stool sample showing ingested red blood cells. (From the collection of Herman Zaiman, "A Presentation of Pictorial Parasites.")

- Polyvinyl alcohol for permanent stain to detect trophozoites (single nucleus, 10-60 μm, usually 15-20 μm) and cysts (4 nuclei, 12-15 μm).
- Formalin fixation for concentration to detect cysts.
- Cannot differentiate species: classically the teaching was that an *Entamoeba* ingesting an RBC indicated *E. histolytica*, but this has been challenged recently.
- Stool antigen detection.
- Serum antigen detection.
- Serology
  - Most useful for exclusion of disease, as positive result cannot differentiate acute and previous infection.
- NAAT
  - Usually as a part of a multiplex panel, may cross-react with *E. dispar.*
- Endoscopy with biopsy in select cases.
  - Classic description is "flask-shaped ulcer" (Fig. 34.24).
  - Trophozoites will be at the margin of the ulcer.

Treatment

- Invasive colitis: metronidazole *plus* a luminal agent such as diiodohydroxyquin or paromomycin.
- Asymptomatic patients: intraluminal agent only.
- Amebic liver abscess: metronidazole or tinidazole *plus* a luminal agent (even if stool negative for parasites).

Giardiasis

Microbiology and Pathogenesis

- This infection is caused by the flagellated protozoan *Giardia duodenalis* (previously known as *G. lamblia*, or *G. intestinalis*). This is another pathogen ingested via contaminated water or food or via the fecal–oral route. Cysts are the infectious forms, secreted in stool. As few as 10 cysts can lead to infection. Trophozoites are the metabolically active form, found mainly in the small bowel.
- Other members of the genus *Giardia* infect nonhuman hosts, including cats and dogs. While *G. duodenalis* can also infect pets, it is less common than other *Giardia* species, which do not infect humans (Box 34.18).

• BOX 34.18 **Transmission From Pets**

- Can you get diarrhea from your giardiasis-infected dog? Yes, but it's unlikely.

Epidemiology

- This parasite is truly globally distributed and is often found in sources of water supplies (lakes, streams, ponds).
- Particularly common in areas with poor sanitation.
- Rates of infection are frequently highest in young children, and employment in a childcare setting is a recognized risk factor.
- Cysts are quite hardy and can survive cold water, meaning that water from mountain streams should be treated and filtered before drinking.

Clinical Features

- Asymptomatic infection/colonization.
- Acute giardiasis
  - 7- to 14-day incubation.
  - Symptoms may persist for 2–4 weeks
  - Diarrhea, often with foul-smelling stool and steatorrhea; malaise; abdominal cramping, bloating, and flatulence; nausea; weight loss. Less common symptoms include emesis, fever, constipation, itching.
- Chronic giardiasis
  - May develop after acute illness, or independently.
  - Loose stools without overt diarrhea; steatorrhea; weight loss and malabsorption; malaise/fatigue; abdominal cramps, bloating, flatulence.
- Common complications
  - Sequelae of malabsorption and weight loss, notably restricted growth in children.
  - Acquired lactose intolerance.
  - Irritable bowel syndrome symptoms.
  - Reactive arthritis.

Diagnosis

- Stool microscopy (O&P exam) (Fig. 34.25).
  - Saline preparation for trophozoites and cysts (not often performed).
  - Polyvinyl alcohol for permanent stain to detect trophozoites (pear-shaped, 2 nuclei, flagella, 10-20 μm) and cysts (10-14 μm, mature 4 nuclei, immature 2 nuclei).
  - Formalin concentration for cysts.
- Antigen detection assays (usually simultaneously detects *Cryptosporidium*).
  - Direct immunofluorescence assays (DFA).
  - Enzyme-linked immunosorbent assays (ELISA).
- NAAT
  - Usually as a part of a multiplex panel.
- Duodenal biopsy or aspirate for trophozoites (Fig. 34.26).

Treatment

- Tinidazole: for patients 3 years or older.
- Nitazoxanide: can be used for patients 1 year and older.

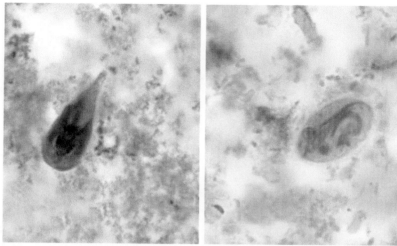

• **Fig. 34.25** Trophozoite (*left*) and cyst (*right*) of *Giardia duodenalis* (trichrome, original magnification ×1000). (Courtesy Centers for Disease Control and Prevention, DPDx Image Library.)

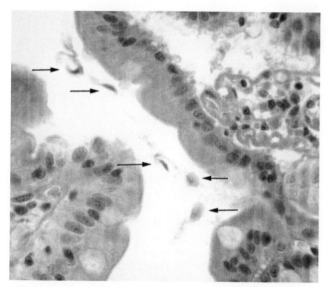

• **Fig. 34.26** *Giardia duodenalis*, intestinal biopsy, trophozoites (*arrows*) (H&E, ×500). (From Rifai N. *Giardia duodenalis* (a.k.a., *G. lamblia*, *G. intestinalis*). In: Rifai N, et al., eds. *Tietz Textbook of Clinical Chemistry and Molecular Diagnostics*. 6th ed. Elsevier; 2018.)

• Metronidazole.
• Paromomycin: in first trimester of pregnancy.

A Few More Notable Intestinal Organisms

Blastocystis species (previously *B. hominis*)

• The pathogenicity of this globally distributed organism is questionable. Many animal species also have these protozoa in stool, so it is likely a zoonotic organism (Fig. 34.27).
• It is generally found on O&P exam, in both cyst and trophozoite form.
• It is rarely pathogenic, and in most cases it only indicates consumption of contaminated food or water, and should spur the clinician to **continue searching** for other pathogens.

• Case reports exist of successfully treating patients with chronic gastrointestinal complaints, found to have *Blastocystis* in stool, with metronidazole or tinidazole.

Dientamoeba fragilis

• The pathogenicity of this globally distributed organism is controversial. It is likely underrecognized as many laboratories are unable to adequately identify it. It likely does cause diarrhea, colitis, and may have a more severe presentation in children.
• Transmission is thought to be fecal–oral, and possibly via attachment to helminth eggs.
• It is diagnosed on stool O&P exam, in the trophozoite stage (Fig. 34.28).
• Therapy is recommended only if it is the sole organism found in stool in patients with symptoms exceeding one week. Options include metronidazole, tinidazole, paromomycin.

Microsporidia

• Previously considered protozoa, now classified as obligate, intracellular, spore-forming fungi.
• There are at least 15 recognized pathogenic genera including *Encephalitozoon*, *Enterocytozoon*, *Pleistophora*, *Nosema*. Speciation is not routine.
• Distribution is worldwide. Infection is via inhalation of spores, contact with water containing spores, and may be zoonotically transmitted.
• Infection occurs mainly in immunocompromised patients, most commonly AIDS.
• These organisms can disseminate, or cause keratoconjunctivitis, skin and muscle infection, diarrhea, acalculous cholecystitis, pneumonitis, urinary tract infection, among other manifestations.
• They can be detected in any of the infected tissues, usually via chromotrope-based stains, immunofluorescence assays, hematoxylin and eosin (H&E), and tissue Gram stains (Fig. 34.29).

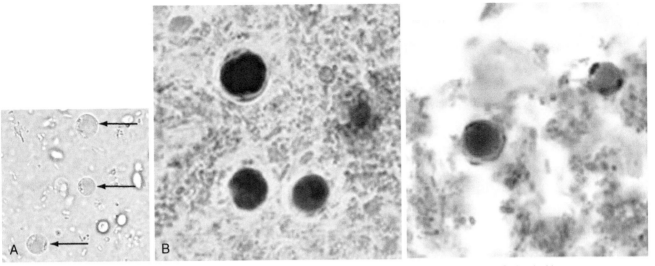

• **Fig. 34.27** *Blastocystis hominis* cysts. (A) Unstained wet mount. *Arrows* indicate cysts. (B) Stained with trichrome. Vacuoles vary from red to blue. (Courtesy Centers for Disease Control and Prevention, DPDx Image Library.)

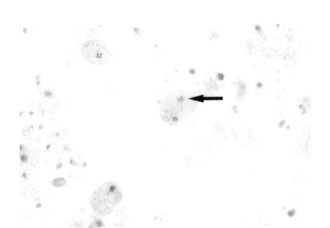

• **Fig. 34.28** *Dientamoeba fragilis* trophozoites showing the characteristic "fragmented" appearance (*arrow*). (From Pritt BS. *Parasitology Benchtop Reference Guide: An Illustrated Guide for Commonly Encountered Parasites.* Northfield, IL: College of American Pathologists; 2014.)

• **Fig. 34.29** Stool showing microsporidia using modified trichrome stain. (From Babady E, Pritt BS. Parasitology. In: Rifai N, et al., eds. *Tietz Textbook of Clinical Chemistry and Molecular Diagnostics.* 6th ed. Elsevier; 2018.)

- PCRs for stool have been developed for the most common species.
- Treatment options include albendazole (not effective against *Enterocytozoon*), fumagillin, fluoroquinolones.

Intestinal Pathogens: Summary

Table 34.1 summarizes risk factors and likely pathogens causing intestinal infection. Table 34.2 summarizes the diagnostic tests that will aid the differential diagnosis.

FREE-LIVING AMEBA

These organisms are called free-living because they do not require a host for survival. Instead, they exist quite happily in the environment and only cause human disease in limited circumstances. But when they cause disease, it

is often a deadly. *Balamuthia* and *Sappinia* cause granulomatous amebic encephalitis. *Acanthamoeba* causes this, as well as disease outside of the central nervous system (CNS). *Naegleria fowleri* is the etiology of primary amebic meningoencephalitis.

Naegleria

Microbiology and Pathogenesis

- **Agent:** *Naegleria fowleri.* This ameba is able to survive in adverse conditions in cyst form. When it reaches a conducive environment, it then exists in trophozoite form. It has a third, nonfeeding, flagellated form. The trophozoite form is infective. Humans acquire *Naegleria* when contaminated water is inhaled, allowing it to penetrate via the nasal mucosa, and migrate up the olfactory nerves to the brain.

TABLE 34.1 Risk Factors, Presenting Symptoms and Likely Pathogens

	Neobalantidium coli	Cryptosporidium	Cyclospora cayetanensis	Cystoisospora belli	Entamoeba histolytica	Giardia	Dientamoeba fragilis	Blastocystis
Foodborne outbreak	X	X	X					
Unpasteurized dairy		X						
Raw produce		X	X					
Swimming in or drinking untreated fresh water	X	X				X		
Swimming in recreational facility with fresh water		X						
Institutionalization		X				X		
Childcare center		X				X		
Travel to resource-limited areas	X	X	X	X	X	X	X	X
Exposure to pig feces	X	X						
Farm or petting zoo exposure		X						
AIDS		X	X	X				
Immunosuppressive medications		X	X	X				
Anal–genital/oral/digital contact		X			X	X		
Chronic diarrhea	X	X	X	X	X	X	?	?
Dysentery (blood in stool)	X				X			
Fever					X if high			

TABLE 34.2 Which Test to Order?[a]

	Neobalantidium coli	Cryptosporidium	Cyclospora cayetanensis	Cystoisospora belli	Entamoeba histolytica	Giardia
Stool O&P exam	X				X	X
Stool modified acid-fast stain		X	X	X		
Stool antigen detection		X			X	X
Stool NAAT (if available)		X	X	X	X	X
Stool immunoassay		X			X	X

[a]Why not *Dientamoeba* and *Blastocystis*? Because rarely would they be in the true differential diagnosis.
O&P, ova and parasite; NAAT, nucleic acid amplification test.

• BOX 34.19 *Naegleria* Memory Trick

- *Naegleria* needs nice warm water before it sprays your brain with PAM.

• BOX 34.20 Did You Know?

- *Balamuthia mandrillaris* was initially identified in the brain of a dead mandrill baboon, hence the name.

Epidemiology

- It has a worldwide distribution but needs warm freshwater, including: lakes, rivers, geothermal hot springs, warm water discharged from industrial plants, poorly maintained swimming pools, water heaters, and tap water. This organism's preferred temperature is up to 115°F (46°C). It has also been found in soil.
- The most common risk factor is recreational water activity in one of the above sources (Box 34.19).

Clinical Features

- Primary amebic meningoencephalitis (PAM).
  - Incubation period averages 5 days.
  - 99% mortality.
- Acute meningoencephalitis
  - Fever, headache, photophobia, nausea, vomiting, behavioral changes, altered mental status, seizure.
  - Meningeal signs, cranial nerve palsies, cranial hypertension leading to herniation and death.

Diagnosis

- CSF wet mount showing motile trophozoites (see Fig. 34.34A).
- Wright stain of cytospin cerebrospinal fluid (CSF).
- NAAT on CSF or brain biopsy (not commercially available).
- Antigen testing on CSF or biopsy.
- CSF has significant leukocytosis with polymorphonuclear cell predominance and often high numbers of RBCs. Glucose is low, protein is high. Opening pressure is elevated.

Treatment

- Regimen unclear.
- Miltefosine (amebicidal) in combination with other agents has been used successfully in several cases.
- Additional agents used have included conventional amphotericin B, rifampin, fluconazole, azithromycin.

Balamuthia

Microbiology and Pathogenesis

- **Agent:** *Balamuthia mandrillaris* (Box 34.20).
- Environmental forms include both cysts and trophozoites and can both be infective. Human disease occurs when the parasite enters via broken skin or is inhaled across the respiratory tract.

Epidemiology

- It has a worldwide distribution and has been found in soil and dust. It may also exist in water. Disease has been reported in immunocompetent and immunocompromised patients. In US cases there is a high proportion of patients of Hispanic ethnicity. Transmission has been reported via solid organ transplantation.

Clinical Presentation

- Incubation period unknown.
- Granulomatous amebic encephalitis (GAE)
  - Usually preceded by a granulomatous skin lesion in the midface/nose area (Fig. 34.30).

- Weeks to months of worsening headache, fever, visual changes, behavioral changes, focal neurologic deficits.
- Eventually will develop increased intracranial pressure, seizures, coma, death.
- CNS symptoms may be preceded by sinus or ear infections and often by skin lesions.
  - Skin lesions are often on the face.
- History of trauma and environmental exposure may be elicited.

Diagnosis
GAE
- Brain imaging (computed tomography [CT] or magnetic resonance imaging [MRI]) reveal abscesses (Fig. 34.31A and B).
- Lumbar puncture often contraindicated (focal lesions).
  - If CSF obtained, will usually have lymphocytic pleocytosis, low-normal glucose, very high protein. Trophozoites rarely seen.
- Brain tissue biopsy is needed.

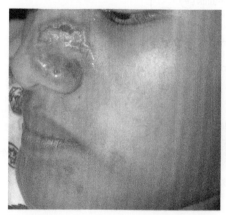

• **Fig. 34.30** Cutaneous free living amoebic infection. (Courtesy Francisco Bravo, MD.)

- H&E stain will show trophozoites and cysts (Fig. 34.31C).
- Culture of tissue.
- NAAT not widely available.

Cutaneous Lesions
- Biopsy with tissue stain. This will show primarily hemorrhagic necrosis (granulomatous inflammation can be seen in more immunocompetent hosts), cysts, trophozoites.
- Immunofluorescence or immunoperoxidase stain (at CDC).

Treatment
- Regimen unclear.
- Combination therapy has included pentamidine, sulfadiazine, flucytosine, fluconazole, macrolide, miltefosine.

Acanthamoeba

Microbiology and Pathogenesis
- **Agent:** *Acanthamoeba* spp.; at least nine species have been reported to cause human disease. Environmental forms include both cysts and trophozoites; trophozoites are infective (Fig. 34.32).
- When the organism enters the eye, it causes keratitis (Box 34.21).
- When entry is via respiratory tract or skin, can disseminate hematogenously to CNS or other sites.
- It can migrate along the olfactory nerves to the brain.

Epidemiology
- This ameba has a worldwide distribution. It has been identified in soil and dust; fresh water sources; brackish water; seawater; swimming pools, hot tubs; drinking water systems; HVAC (heating, ventilation, and air conditioning) systems.

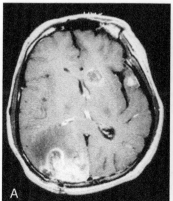
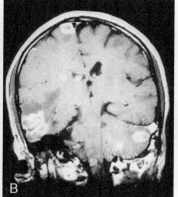
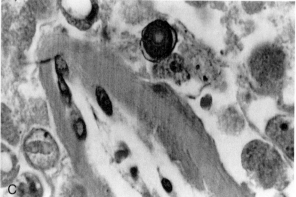

• **Fig. 34.31** (A and B) MRIs of the brain of a patient with *Balamuthia mandrillaris* granulomatous amebic encephalitis. Multiple enhancing lesions are seen in the right hemisphere, left cerebellum, midbrain, and brainstem. (C) Photomicrograph of the brain lesion from the same patient showing perivascular amebic trophozoites. A round amebic cyst with a characteristic double wall is seen in the top center (H&E, original magnification ×100). (From Deol I, Robledo L, Meza A, et al. Encephalitis due to a free-living amoeba [*Balamuthia mandrillaris*]: case report with literature review. *Surg Neurol.* 2000;53:611–616.)

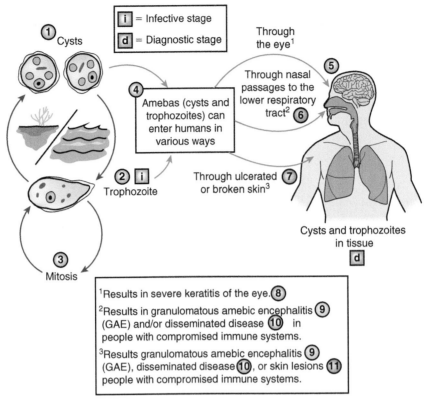

• **Fig. 34.32** Life cycle of *Acanthamoeba* spp. (From Nelson J, Singh U. *Acanthamoeba* species. In: Long SS, Prober CG, Fischer M. eds. *Principles and Practice of Pediatric Infectious Diseases.* 5th ed. Elsevier; 2018.)

• **BOX 34.21** **Keratitis Memory Trick**

- Which free-living ameba causes keratitis? *Acanthamoeba* – sounds like "canthus," part of the eye!

- Keratitis risk factors involve prolonged use of contact lenses and poor contact lens hygiene, especially with tap water exposure. Commercial contact lens solutions have also been contaminated.
- CNS and other infections are most often seen in immunocompromised patients (HIV, solid organ and stem cell transplant recipients, cirrhosis, etc.).

Clinical Features

- Incubation period unknown.
- Granulomatous amebic encephalitis (GAE)
  - Weeks to months of worsening headache, fever, visual changes, behavioral changes, focal neurologic deficits.
  - Eventually will have increased intracranial pressure, seizures, coma, death.
- Keratitis
  - Usually unilateral.
- Other
  - Cutaneous infection (Fig. 34.33)
    - Reported in both healthy and immunosuppressed patients.
    - Presentation includes papules or nodules which progress to necrotic ulcers; plaques; cellulitis. Can be painful or painless.

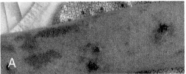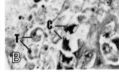

• **Fig. 34.33** (A) Patient with human immunodeficiency virus/acquired immunodeficiency syndrome with skin ulcers caused by *Acanthamoeba*. (B) A section through the ulcer showing *Acanthamoeba* trophozoites (T) and cysts (C). (H&E, ×1000.) (From Visvesvara GS, Roy SL, Maguire J, eds. Pathogenic and opportunistic free-living amebae. In: Guerrant RL, Walker DH, Weller PF, eds. *Tropical Infectious Diseases: Principles, Pathogens and Practice.* 3rd ed. Elsevier; 2011.)

- Nasopharyngeal infection
  - Severely immunocompromised patients.
  - Chronic nasal discharge and sinusitis, septal erosion.
- Disseminated infection
  - Severely immunocompromised patients.
  - Skin, lungs, ±CNS.

Diagnosis

GAE

- Lumbar puncture often contraindicated (focal lesions).
  - If CSF obtained, will usually have lymphocytic pleocytosis, low–normal glucose, high protein. Trophozoites rarely seen.
- Brain tissue biopsy is needed.
- H&E stain will show trophozoites and cysts with hemorrhagic necrosis.
- Culture of tissue.
- NAAT not widely available.

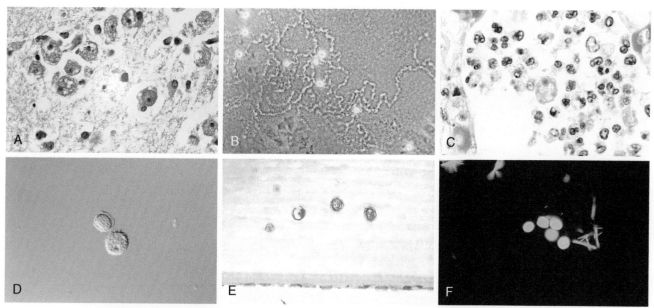

• **Fig. 34.34** (A) *Naegleria fowleri* trophozoites in primary amebic meningoencephalitis (H&E; ×100). (B) *Acanthamoeba* sp. culture showing trails left by motile trophozoites on a lawn of *Escherichia coli* (phase contrast microscopy; ×100). (C) *Acanthamoeba* sp. trophozoites within a cutaneous lesion in an individual infected with the human immunodeficiency virus (Giemsa stain; ×1000). (D) *Acanthamoeba* sp. trophozoite and cyst (differential interference contrast microscopy; ×400). (E) Double-walled cysts of *Acanthamoeba* sp. within corneal stroma (H&E; ×1000). (F) Cysts of *Acanthamoeba* sp. stained with Calcofluor white (epifluorescence microscopy; ×400). (From Fritsche TR, Pritt BS. Medical parasitology. In: McPherson RA, Pincus MR, eds. *Henry's Clinical Diagnosis and Management by Laboratory Methods.* 23rd ed. Elsevier; 2017.)

Keratitis

- Cornea scraping stained with Calcofluor, Giemsa, or Hemacolor to visualize trophozoites and/or cysts (Fig. 34.34D–F).
- Cornea scraping for culture and NAAT (Box 34.22).

Other

- Cutaneous: biopsy with tissue stain (Fig. 34.34C).
- Nasopharyngeal: biopsy with tissue stain.
- Disseminated: biopsy with tissue stain (usually diagnosed postmortem).

Treatment

GAE

- Regimen unclear.
- Miltefosine (amebicidal) in combination with other agents has been used successfully in several cases.
- Additional agents used have included pentamidine, fluconazole, TMP–SMX, metronidazole.

Keratitis

- Regimen unclear.
- Combination therapy recommended: polyhexamethylene biguanide or biguanide–chlorhexidine plus propamidine or hexamidine drops.

Other

- Cutaneous: various topical combinations plus systemic agents have been tried, including miltefosine.
- Nasopharyngeal: excision plus combination therapy.
- Disseminated: combination therapy.

• **BOX 34.22** Fun With Micro

Acanthamoeba and *Naegleria* culture can be performed by placing the tissue sample on a nonnutrient agar covered with a lawn of enteric bacteria (usually *E. coli*). This is because the parasite eats the bacteria and moves around the plate. Feeding tracks will be visible, and a wet mount can demonstrate the parasite (Fig. 34.34B).

Sappinia

Microbiology and Pathogenesis

- **Agent**: *Sappinia pedata* and *Sappinia diploidea*. Exists in cyst and trophozoite forms.

Epidemiology

- Widespread distribution, particularly in areas with elk and buffalo feces. Also near farm animals, soil with rotting plants, and possibly fresh water sources.

Clinical Features

There has been one case of granulomatous amebic encephalitis secondary to *Sappinia pedata*. The patient, a farmer with livestock, initially had symptoms of a sinus infection. This progressed to encephalitis. Resection of a focal lesion revealed trophozoites.

He recovered after treatment with azithromycin, pentamidine, itraconazole, and flucytosine.

35

Helminths

JENNIFER M. FITZPATRICK

SOIL-TRANSMITTED HELMINTHS

- Leading cause of helminth infections worldwide, with estimates of approximately 1.5 billion people infected.
- World Health Organization (WHO) suggests more than 880 million children require treatment today.
- **Geohelminths:** eggs or larvae mature on soil before becoming infective.
- Phylum Nematoda.
- Most common:
  - Roundworm (*Ascaris lumbricoides*).
  - Whipworm (*Trichuris trichiura*).
  - Hookworms (*Necator americanus* and *Ancylostoma duodenale*).
- Majority of infections are asymptomatic, yet contribute to poor nutritional status, growth retardation, impaired cognitive development, reduced school attendance and performance (and future economic potential).
  - Recognized as most common cause of iron deficiency anemia worldwide.
  - Individuals are often co-infected with other helminths and/or parasitic conditions; additive effect on nutrition, pathology, and morbidity.
  - Individual susceptibility to infection includes:
    - Behavior, epidemiology, host factors such as genetic predisposition and immunity.
  - Individual morbidity is related to degree of worm burden.
    - Heavy worm burden infections instigate majority of morbidity; highest risk of severe disease.

Remarkably, despite the vast array of niche adaptation to differing hosts, life cycle stages, reproduction, ecological environments, and pathological consequences, the human immune response differs little among helminth infections.

- Th$_2$-like production of significant quantities of interleukin-4 (IL-4), IL-5, IL-9, and IL-10.
- Development of strong immunoglobulin E (IgE), eosinophil, and mast cell responses.

Worldwide control programs are based around WHO resolutions to reduce Neglected Tropical Diseases (NTD):

- Periodic mass population de-worming (school-age children).
  - Financially subsidized, effective, and low toxicity chemotherapy.
- Health education and local community involvement.
- Improved sanitation to reduce soil contamination (infective transmission).

Ascaris Lumbricoides (Roundworm)

Pathogenesis

- Transmission typically through ingestion of eggs: contaminated hands, food, and/or water.
- Humans only known host.
- Eggs embryonate and require up to 3 weeks development on soil (in warm humid environments) prior to becoming infectious (transmission may therefore be seasonal).
- Early in infection, larvae invade across tissues resulting in hypersensitivity immune responses and inflammation.
- Adult worms survive free in small bowel lumen, primarily jejunum.
- Children develop only partial immunity.
- Large volume egg producers: 200,000 eggs/day.
- Asymptomatic egg-shedding facilitates transmission.
  - Eggs are particularly resilient, can remain viable up to six years in moist soil but may also survive freezing and/or periods of desiccation.
- Adult worms do not replicate in human host.
  - Tourists/travelers, visiting from areas of low endemicity, usually lose infection within 12–18 months as the adult worms die.
- *Ascaris suum* intestinal pig parasite; can also cause human infection (genotypically similar to *A. lumbricoides* but associated with pig husbandry and fertilizer usage).
- **Life cycle** (Fig. 35.1): adult worms (15–35 cm in length) live and mate in luminal jejunum and single-cell eggs are passed in the feces. Once ingested or inhaled, larvae hatch in the small intestine, penetrate the mucosa, and migrate via venous circulation through the liver to the heart and lungs (around 4 days postingestion).

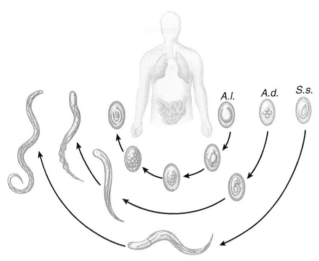

• **Fig. 35.1** Life cycle of intestinal nematodes with a migratory phase through the lungs. Eggs are passed with feces in *Ascaris lumbricoides* (A.l.) (roundworm), *Necator americanus*, or *Ancylostoma duodenale* (A.d.) (hookworms) infection or hatch in bowel lumen in *Strongyloides stercoralis* (S.s.). Ascaris eggs mature in soil, human infection following ingestion. Hookworm and strongyloidiasis; humans are infected via skin penetration. (From Maguire JH. Intestinal nematodes (roundworms). In: Bennett JE, Dolin R, Blaser MJ, eds. *Mandell, Douglas, and Bennett's Principles and Practice of Infectious Diseases*. Updated 8th ed. Elsevier; 2015.)

Maturing worms enter alveoli, ascend the tracheobronchial tree, where they can be swallowed and thus return to the intestine.

Clinical Manifestations

The majority of infections are asymptomatic; 15% result in significant morbidity.
- Early infection may develop pulmonary symptoms with larval transpulmonary migration.
  - Eosinophilia, fever, dry cough, shortness of breath (SOB), and chest pain
  - Severe: eosinophilic pneumonia (**Löffler-type syndrome**).
  - Self-limiting and resolves when worms reach maturity and travel to final location.
- Most pathology is adult worm-associated (developing after 6–8 weeks).
  - Malnutrition; nutritional deficiencies, including dietary protein, vitamins A and C, lactose, fatty-acids.
  - Pancreatic and hepatobiliary morbidity with adult worms obstructing biliary tree/pancreatic duct leading to biliary colic, acalculous cholecystitis, ascending cholangitis, luminal strictures, pancreatitis.
  - Rarely intestinal obstruction can develop due to very high worm burden.
  - Symptoms also relating to migrating worms at distant extragastrointestinal sites.

Management
- **Diagnosis** through stool microscopy identification of eggs (Fig. 35.2) or examination for adult worms.

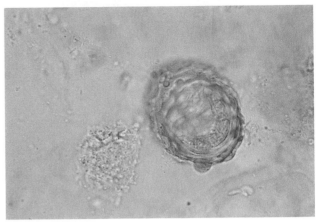

• **Fig. 35.2** *Ascaris lumbricoides* egg in feces. The elliptical ovum measures 50–70 × 40–50 μm. (From Curtis CM. Parasitic infections of the gastrointestinal tract. In: Cohen J, Powderly W, Opal S, eds. *Infectious Diseases*. 3rd ed. Elsevier; 2010.)

  - Fecal, urine, or sputum samples.
  - Larvae found in gastric aspirates or endoscopy specimens, or sputum during pulmonary migration.
  - Adult worms passed per rectum, or more rarely mouth/nose.
- Radiographic imaging as per clinical syndrome suggests; adult worms may be visible on plain radiograph, while ultrasound, computed tomography, and/or ERCP (endoscopic retrograde cholangiopancreatography) can also reveal worms and inflammatory pathology in the biliary tree.
- Molecular analysis including polymerase chain reaction (PCR) on blood and/or stool is not yet standard diagnostic tool, particularly in resource-poor countries.
- **Treatment:** albendazole single oral dose (can be extended to 3 days); alternatively mebendazole or ivermectin single dose.

Trichuris Trichiura (Whipworm)

- Epidemiology similar to *Ascaris*.
- Estimated 25% world population may be infected, mostly school-age children.
- Associated with poor hygiene, poor sanitation, and poverty.
- Ingestion via soil contaminated hands, food, and/or water.

Pathogenesis
- Life cycle (Fig. 35.3): eggs shed from feces embryonate within soil and become infective within 1–2 months.
- Larvae hatch within the small/large bowel, subsequently penetrate cecum mucosal crypts and embeds within the epithelial layer (after secretion of lipid bilayer pore-forming protein).
- Adults thus frequent the cecum and ascending colon after around 2–3 months; worms may also be seen in distal colon and rectum in heavy infections.

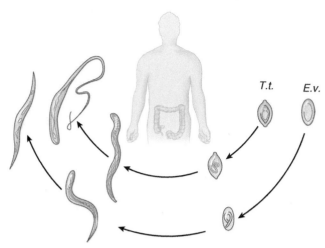

• **Fig. 35.3** Life cycle of nematodes without a migratory phase through the lungs. *Trichuris trichiura* (T.t.) eggs are passed with feces; those of *Enterobius vermicularis* (E.v.) are deposited at the perianal region. They embryonate within a short time, and infection is acquired by ingestion. Eggs hatch in the intestine, and larvae migrate to their final habitat in the colon (T.t.) or cecum (E.v.). (From Maguire JH. Intestinal nematodes (roundworms). In: Bennett JE, Dolin R, Blaser MJ, eds. *Mandell, Douglas, and Bennett's Principles and Practice of Infectious Diseases.* Updated 8th ed. Elsevier; 2015.)

- Pathologic changes will include an inflamed friable and edematous mucosa, macrophage and cytokine infiltrated lamina propria.
- Adult worms live 1–2 years (7000–20,000 eggs daily) and lay eggs around 12 weeks post-infection.
- No lung-stage.

Clinical Manifestations

- Majority asymptomatic infections with occasional high blood eosinophilia.
- Heavy worm burdens result in (~200 worms, commonly individuals harbor fewer than 20).
- Infection in childhood: long-term colitis.
  - Chronic abdominal pain, malabsorption, diarrhea, iron deficiency anemia, growth retardation, nail clubbing.
- *Trichuris* dysentery syndrome.
  - Loose stool with mucus/blood and tenesmus.
- Recurrent rectal prolapse.

Management

- **Diagnosis**
  - Stool microscopy for identification of eggs or examination of adult worms (Fig. 35.4).
  - Endoscopy: observe adult worms on mucosa/prolapsed rectum.
- **Treatment**
  - First-line treatment single dose mebendazole.
  - Alternatively, albendazole for 3 days, mebendazole for 3 days (mild–moderate infections), or ivermectin for 3 days.
  - Heavy infections: treat for at least 5 days and up to 7.

Interestingly, in recent years, experimental clinical trials have shown infection with some pathogenic

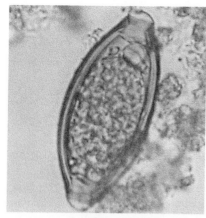

• **Fig. 35.4** Egg of *Trichuris trichiura*. Typically measure 50–55 μm × 22–24 μm; however, much larger (78 × 30 μm) eggs can occasionally be observed. (From Bogitsh B, Carter C, Oeltman T, eds. *Human Parasitology.* 5th ed. Elsevier; 2019.)

helminths can modify disease progress of some inflammatory conditions.

- *Trichuris* can secrete molecules that induce antiinflammatory cytokines.
- Studies have shown porcine *T. suis* may improve clinical progress in patients with inflammatory bowel disease, notably Crohn's disease.
- Helminth parasites are exquisitely adapted to evading, modulating host immune responses, and release many antiinflammatory molecules.
- Much further work is required to elucidate underlying mechanisms of worm immunomodulation and its direct effect on concomitant immune diseases, but it has ongoing clinical appeal.

Necator americanus and *Ancylostoma duodenale* (Hookworm)

- Approximately 10% of world's population may be infected.
- Leading worldwide cause of iron-deficiency anemia, particularly problematic in school-age children and women of child-bearing age.
- Endemic in tropical and subtropical areas of the world.

Pathogenesis

- Life cycle (see Fig. 35.1): eggs hatch in soil, releasing rhabditiform larvae that mature into filariform larvae (infective larval stage) that actively penetrate skin by releasing various proteases (infiltrate usually hair follicles/small fissures/trauma).
- Transmitted percutaneously from soil (larval invasion): barefoot walking on contaminated soil (oral transmission secondary).
- Larvae migrate through the lungs, travel via trachea and oesophagus, eventually mature and attach to small bowel mucosal wall (via buccal capsules, biting plates, or teeth).

- Chronic blood loss with parasitic feeding, exposure of mucosal capillaries with powerful enzymes, and production of anticoagulants/inhibitors of platelet activation.

Clinical Manifestations

- Majority asymptomatic although anemia may become symptomatic if severe.
- "Ground itch:" previously exposed/sensitized, pruritic maculopapular rash.
- Transient pneumonitis: larval migration through lungs, less frequent and less severe than *Ascaris*.
- Naïve patients more commonly develop epigastric pain, diarrhea, anorexia, peripheral blood eosinophilia (often around 1 month postexposure).
- Adult hookworms can generate chronic abdominal pain, persistent high peripheral blood eosinophilia; coupled with iron deficiency anemia and long-term malnutrition.

Management

- **Diagnosis**: Stool microscopy for eggs (note eggs are morphologically indistinguishable) or examination of adult worms (fecal larval culture) (Fig. 35.5).
- PCR analysis of fecal material/culture such as assays based on internal transcribed spacers (ITS-1 and 2) of the nuclear ribosomal DNA (rDNA) or real-time PCR methods (both commonly used for epidemiological surveillance).
- **Treatment**
  - Single dose albendazole.
  - Alternatively, mebendazole 3 days or albendazole for 3 days.
  - Pyrantel pamoate can be used but may require multiple dosing to achieve total elimination.
  - Ivermectin not as effective and therefore not recommended (although may be utilized within mass drug treatment programs as single dose).

Other Nematode Roundworms

Strongyloides Stercoralis

- Endemic in rural areas of tropical/subtropical regions, occurs only sporadically in temperate areas.
- *S. stercoralis* can complete its life cycle entirely within the human host (as well as soil) and thus generate a cycle of indefinite **autoinfection** – unique in the intestinal nematodes.

Pathogenesis

- Life cycle (see Fig. 35.1): infective filariform larvae found in soil or other materials contaminated with human feces penetrates human skin.
- As per hookworm infections, larvae migrate similarly through the lungs, travel via trachea and esophagus, eventually mature, and attach to small bowel mucosal wall.

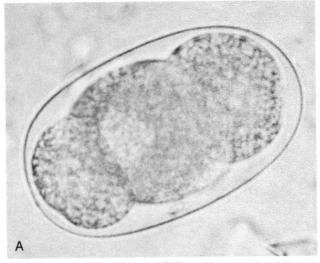
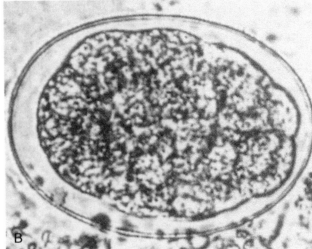

• **Fig. 35.5** Hookworm eggs. (A) Immature egg showing developing larva. (B) Mature egg. (From Brooker SJ. Soil-transmitted helminths (geohelminths). In: Farrar J, et al., eds. *Manson's Tropical Diseases*. 23rd ed. Elsevier; 2014.)

- Notably, small numbers of rhabditiform larvae mature into filariform larvae within the perineum or colon and re-enter the mucosa, enabling autoinfection and completion of full life cycle without leaving host.
- Eggs produced by parthenogenesis as no male adult form.
- On occasion direct person-to-person transmission observed.

Clinical Manifestations

- Most infections asymptomatic ± peripheral blood eosinophilia (neither diagnostic nor prognostic).
- "Ground itch" when larvae penetrate the skin.
- Mild intermittent gastrointestinal, cutaneous, or pulmonary symptoms that can persist for many years.
- Classic inflammatory edema, petechiae, serpiginous or urticarial tracts, and severe pruritus.
- Larva currens: **pathognomonic** of strongyloidiasis, migratory larvae within the dermis, evanescent (and fast

moving) pick/erythematous tracts, periumbilical purpura in disseminated infections, nonpalpable purpura, angioedema, and erythroderma (Fig. 35.6).

- Transpulmonary larval migration can produce mild pneumonitis (or, rarely, a Löeffler's-like syndrome) with cough, dyspnea, wheeze, and occasionally hemoptysis.
- Gastrointestinal manifestations include abdominal pain (duodenitis, enterocolitis, and malabsorption); anorexia, nausea, diarrhea, and vomiting.

Hyperinfection Syndrome
- Increased generation of filariform larvae: enhanced auto-infection.
- Immunosuppressed, high-risk individuals.
  - Congenital immune-deficiency, malignancy, immune-modulation therapy (including anti-TNF agents), corticosteroids, cytotoxic agents, neutropenia, hematopoietic stem cell transplant, solid organ transplants, splenectomy.
  - Underlying co-infections, e.g., HIV, especially HTLV-1 (T-lymphotropic virus type I).
  - Other conditions, such as excess alcohol intake and malnutrition.
  - Dysfunctional Th$_2$ activity with disseminated strongyloidiasis and treatment failure.
  - Increased numbers of worms seen in pulmonary/intestinal tracts but also unusual sites such as central nervous system (CNS), kidney, liver, and other organs.
- Clues to diagnosis in patients with risk factors:
  - Occult gram-negative or polymicrobial bacteremia; as the worm migrates out of the gut, it carries with it intestinal bacteria causing occult bacteremia.
  - Gram-negative meningitis in the absence of neurosurgical device or recent history of neurosurgical procedures.

Management
- Fecal sampling: identification rhabditiform larvae, 50% sensitivity (Fig. 35.7).
  - Fecal material inoculated on bacterial agar plates, 48 hours at room temperature.
  - Larvae crawl on the agar, spreading bacteria in their paths, creating bacterial growth patterns.
  - Macroscopic examination and formalin washing of agar plates confirms larvae.
  - Education to reduce infection (basic such as shoe-wearing) and community programs to improve sanitation.
- Larvae can also be identified from other nonfecal specimen in hyperinfection syndrome: sputum, bronchoalveolar lavage, pleural/peritoneal fluid.
- Serology – usually ELISA – assay IgG to filariform larvae.
  - Can be falsely negative in immunocompromised patients.
  - PCR assays in commercial development.
- **Treatment**
  - First-line treatment is ivermectin: 2 single doses on 2 consecutive days.

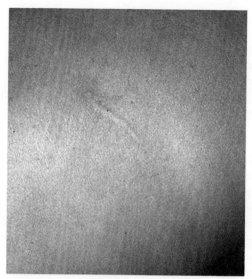

• **Fig. 35.6** Larva currens. Migratory urticarial rash of larva currens (*Strongyloides* infection). (Copyright Dr. Alison Grant, Hospital for Tropical Diseases, London, UK. Reproduced from Checkley AM. Eosinophilia in returning travellers and migrants from the tropics: UK recommendations for investigation and initial management. *J Infect.* 60(1):1–20.)

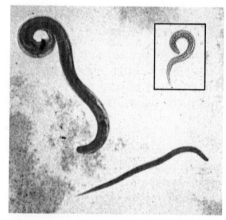

• **Fig. 35.7** Filariform larva (550 μm in length) and immature adult worm (1.3 mm) in feces following *Strongyloides stercoralis* infection. (From Siddiqui AA. Strongyloidiasis. In: Guerrant RL, Walker DH, Weller PF, eds. *Tropical Infectious Diseases: Principles, Pathogens and Practice.* 3rd ed. Elsevier; 2011.)

- Albendazole as alternative agent for 3 days, may be repeated after 3 weeks if required.
- **Hyperinfection syndrome**, optimal treatment regimen not fully elucidated:
  - Immune reconstitution.
  - Extended course of ivermectin ± addition of albendazole.
  - Treat with broad-spectrum antibiotics to cover enteric flora (often gram-negative bacteremia occurs).
  - Pretransplants, preinitiation of immunosuppression; serology if previous untreated infection or evidence of exposure.

Enterobius vermicularis (Pinworm)

- Most common nematode in Western world.
- Humans the only host.
- Temperate/tropical climes.
- *E. gregorii* second identified species, identical clinical features.

Pathogenesis

- School-age children (rare <2 years), close living conditions, especially common within families.
- Person-to-person transmission, auto-infection and infection through environmental contact.
- Life cycle (see Fig. 35.3): embryonated eggs are ingested, larvae hatch in the small intestine, subsequent adults establish themselves in the colon, cecum/appendix.
- Time from eggs to fecund adult worms usually around 4 weeks.
- Adults release around 10,000 eggs daily, adult lifespan is 2–3 months.
- Eggs can survive in different environments: up to 3 weeks (warm acrid areas just a few days) and become infective around 6 hours after exposure to oxygen (facilitating fecal–oral transmission).

Clinical Manifestations

- Most infections are asymptomatic and self-limiting.
- Gravid adult female (adult male rarely seen) migrates from intestine onto perianal region, usually at night; often intensely itchy (facilitating egg fecal–oral transmission).
- Eggs deposited on perianal skin folds (Fig. 35.8).
- Scratching/superficial skin irritation may lead to secondary bacterial infection.
- Female genital tract infection.
- Disturbed sleep.
- Significant psychological distress and anxiety.

Management

- Sellotape test: low power microscopy eggs, performed early morning prior to washing (to increase sensitivity).
- Inspect perianal area for adult worms during sleep: white, pin-shaped, and around 8–13 mm length.
- **Treatment**
  - Albendazole one dose initially, repeated in 2–3 weeks or mebendazole single dose, again repeated.
  - Pyrantel pamoate most frequently used in United States; single dose, repeated 2–3 weeks.
  - Chemotherapy to adult/developing worms, eggs not consistently destroyed; repeat treatment often required.
  - As re-infection and transmission common, **treat all members of shared household.**
  - Meticulous hygiene; hand-washing, keep fingernails short, wash bedding, and no shared towels/personal clothing, etc.

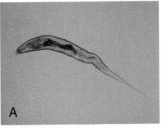
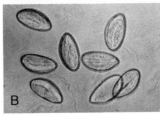

- **Fig. 35.8** (A) Adult female *Enterobius vermicularis* worm; small white roundworm, measuring 9–12 × 0.5 mm. (B) Characteristic eggs are ovoid in shape and measure 50 × 25 μm. The eggs are flattened on one side giving them the classic bean shape appearance. (From Moore TA. Enterobiasis. In: Guerrant RL, Walker DH, Weller PF, eds. *Tropical Infectious Diseases: Principles, Pathogens and Practice.* 3rd ed. Elsevier; 2011.)

TISSUE NEMATODES

Trichinella spp.

- 9 species and at least 12 genotypes.
- Most common: *Trichinella spiralis*, typically associated with the pig host.
- Other species include *T. brivoti, T. pseudospiralis,* and *T. murrelli*: often associated with consumption of wild game.
- While all species can potentially infect humans, seven have been implicated in human disease.
- Distinguished by those able to encapsulate in host muscle tissue of mammals only and those that do not encapsulate and infect mammals, birds (one species), or reptiles (two species).
- **Transmitted through ingestions of raw or undercooked contaminated meat (encysted larvae).**

Pathogenesis and Clinical Manifestations

Larvae are released from cysts (contaminated meat) following exposure to gastric acid and pepsin after ingestion. Parasite maturation and pathology then follow two distinct stages (Fig. 35.9).

- **Intestinal (2 to 7 days postingestion)**
  - Larvae invade the small bowel mucosa and develop into mature adult worms.
  - Fertilized female worms release newborn larvae; asymptomatic or may be accompanied by nonspecific symptoms, including:
    - Watery diarrhea, abdominal pain, nausea, and vomiting.
  - Local villous atrophy, mucosal, and submucosal infiltration (neutrophils/eosinophils/macrophages; mixed Th_1 and Th_2 response).

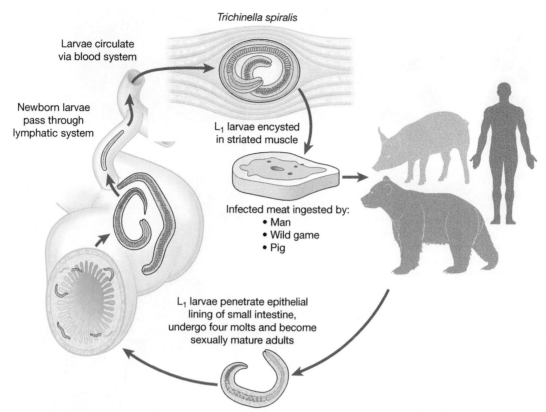

Trichinella spiralis

Larvae circulate via blood system

Newborn larvae pass through lymphatic system

L₁ larvae encysted in striated muscle

Infected meat ingested by:
• Man
• Wild game
• Pig

L₁ larvae penetrate epithelial lining of small intestine, undergo four molts and become sexually mature adults

• **Fig. 35.9** Life cycle of *Trichinella spiralis* showing stages and locations of development. (From Bruschi F. Trichinellosis. In: Magill AJ, Hill DR, Solomon T, Ryan E, eds. *Hunter's Tropical Medicine and Emerging Infectious Diseases*. 9th ed. Elsevier; 2013.)

- **Muscle (> 7 days postingestion)**
  - Muscle stage develops when the intestinal adult-derived larvae disseminate hematogenously (or via lymphatics) and invade striated muscle causing a constellation of distinctive symptoms:
    - Muscle pain, tenderness, swelling, and weakness, high fevers, macular or urticarial rash, headache, cough, dyspnea, dysphagia.
    - Subungual splinter hemorrhages, conjunctival and retinal hemorrhages, periorbital edema and chemosis, visual disturbance, ocular pain.
    - Symptoms peak 2–3 weeks postexposure.
  - Infection severity correlates directly with the number of original ingested larvae.
- **Other clinical pathology**
  - High peripheral blood eosinophilia is common; has no correlation with disease severity.
  - Elevated serum muscle enzymes (creatine kinase and lactate dehydrogenase) and hypergammaglobulinemia.
  - Cardiac involvement (larvae do not encyst in cardiac muscle: local inflammatory reactions and myocarditis); fatal acute trichinellosis myocarditis.
  - Multiorgan involvement
    - CNS (meningitis/encephalitis), renal, and/or pulmonary.

Management

- Serum serology (usually by ELISA, indirect immunofluorescence or latex agglutination); Western blot/immunoblot can be used for confirmation.
  - Seroconversion at least 3 weeks postinfection.
  - Co-infection, other helminths and autoimmune diseases all cause cross-reactivity and reduce specificity.
  - Antigen assay poor sensitivity.
- Demonstration of larvae on muscle biopsy: painful and not often required (Fig. 35.10).
- No commercially available PCR assay.
- **Treatment**
  - In mild self-limiting infection, anthelmintic treatment not necessarily required.
  - Albendazole for 10–14 days.
  - Alternatively, mebendazole for 3 days, then an increased dose for 10 days.
  - Prednisone may be administered concurrently in severe cases for 10–15 days.
  - Treatment after muscle invasion may fail to eliminate infective larvae from muscle.
  - Postexposure prophylaxis may be considered if given within 6 days of potential exposure; mebendazole for 5 days.

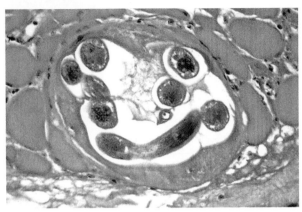

• **Fig. 35.10** Coiled *Trichinella spiralis* larvae within a skeletal muscle cell. (From Kazura JW. Tissue nematodes (trichinellosis, dracunculiasis, filariasis, loiasis, and onchocerciasis). In: Bennett JE, Dolin R, Blaser MJ, eds. *Mandell, Douglas, and Bennett's Principles and Practice of Infectious Diseases*. Updated 8th ed. Elsevier; 2015.)

Dracunculiasis: *Dracunculus medinensis* (Guinea Worm)

- Transmission by ingestion of unfiltered contaminated water containing copepods (small crustaceans) infected with *D. medinensis* larvae.
- Copepods die, release larvae that can penetrate gastric/intestinal mucosa wall; thereafter enter the abdominal cavity and retroperitoneal space.
- Migration through subcutaneous tissue and muscle planes.
- Mature female emerges through subcutaneous tissues (males die and encapsulate).

Clinical Manifestations

- Initial reaction can include fever, urticaria, pruritus, dizziness, nausea, vomiting, and diarrhea.
- Formation of local skin papule.
- High peripheral blood eosinophilia.

Management

- Treatment is based around slow percutaneous extraction of the adult worm (Fig. 35.11).
  - Wound around a stick, aiming to extract a few cm/day (can take weeks/months).
  - In the event worm is damaged/not fully extracted, an intense local painful inflammatory reaction may develop.
- Wound care, occlusive dressings, and good pain management.

Control and Prevention

In recent years exceptional progress has been made by WHO and international partners to treat and eradicate dracunculiasis worldwide:

- Community surveillance and education.
- Nylon filters for drinking water.
- Insecticides.

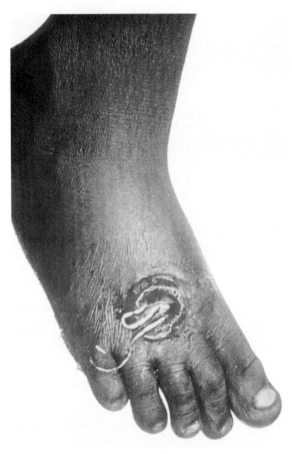

• **Fig. 35.11** *Dracunculus medinensis* emerging from the skin over the foot. (From Kazura JW. Tissue nematodes (trichinellosis, dracunculiasis, filariasis, loiasis, and onchocerciasis). In: Bennett JE, Dolin R, Blaser MJ, eds. *Mandell, Douglas, and Bennett's Principles and Practice of Infectious Diseases*. Updated 8th ed. Elsevier; 2015.)

- 1986: 3.5 million cases/year, around 20 African/Asian countries; now <25 cases/per year worldwide.
- In January 2016 the WHO certified 198 countries free from dracunculiasis, at present only 8 remaining to fully certify eradication (all in Africa).

Lymphatic Filariasis: *Wuchereria bancrofti* and *Brugia malayi*

- Nematodes of the lymphatics and subcutaneous tissues.
- Three major filarial species:
  - Most common worldwide: *Wuchereria bancrofti* (causes 90% lymphatic filariasis).
  - *Brugia malayi* and *B. timori*.
- Transmission by blood-feeding mosquito vectors; humans are definitive hosts.
- Humans only hosts for bancroftian filariasis; in contrast, brugian filariasis infects humans as well as domestic and wild animals.
- In Africa the most common vector is *Anopheles*, in the Americas, *Culex quinquefasciatus, Aedes,* and *Mansonia*.
- Major cause of disfigurement and disability; both urban and tropical areas.

- Filarial nematode parasites (and arthropods) are hosts for the bacterial endosymbiont *Wolbachia*.
  - Required for normal development and survival (target for drug discovery).

Clinical Manifestations

Most infections are asymptomatic or subclinical lymphatic dilation and dysfunction.
- Adult worm is responsible for pathology.
- Infection often first acquired in childhood.
- **Filarial lymphadenopathy**
  - Acute filarial lymphangitis; accompanied by headache or fever and other systemic symptoms (dying adult worms generate acute inflammatory response which progresses distally (retrograde) along the affected lymphatic vessel.
  - Postpubertal adolescent males; adult *W. bancrofti* found most commonly in intrascrotal lymphatic vessels; systemic symptoms may present as funiculitis, epididymitis, orchitis, or a tender granulomatous nodule.

Chronic manifestations will develop in approximately 30% of infected individuals.
- **Chyluria**
  - Rupture of dilated lymphatics into the renal pelvis (bancroftian filariasis).
  - Microscopic hematuria and proteinuria.
- **Lymphedema**
  - Most commonly legs, but can also occur in the arms, breasts, and genitalia.
  - Most people develop these symptoms years postinitial infection.
  - Recurrent secondary bacterial infections.
  - Advanced lymphedema also known as "elephantiasis" (Fig. 35.12).
- **Filarial hydrocele**
  - Lymphatic damage caused by adult worms (Fig. 35.13).
- **Tropical pulmonary eosinophilia (TPE) syndrome**
  - Cough, fever, marked eosinophilia, high serum IgE, and positive antifilarial antibodies.
  - Absent peripheral microfilaremia.
  - Most cases reported in long-term residents from Asia.
  - Men 20–40 years old are most commonly affected.
  - In contrast, Löeffler syndrome is an eosinophilic pneumonia caused by the parasites *A. lumbricoides*, *S. stercoralis*, and the hookworms *A. duodenale* and *N. americanus*.

Management

- Identification of microfilariae from blood, other fluids (peak intensity of microfilariae at night) (Fig. 35.14).
- Serology: ELISA *Wolbachia*: allows detection in absence of microfilariae.
- 1-day or 12-day treatment diethylcarbamazine citrate (DEC) (1-day treatment is often as effective as the 12-day regimen).

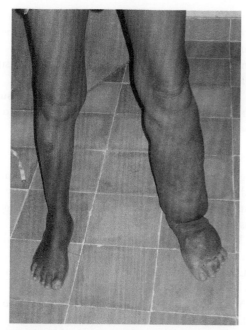

- **Fig. 35.12** Advanced lymphoedema of lower limb (elephantiasis). (Courtesy Thomas Fürst, PhD, Swiss Tropical and Public Health Institute, Basel, Switzerland.)

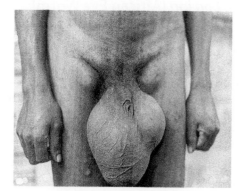

- **Fig. 35.13** Hydrocele and inguinal lymph node enlargement in bancroftian filariasis. (Nutman TB. Lymphatic filariasis. In: Guerrant RL, Walker DH, Weller PF, eds. *Tropical Infectious Diseases: Principles, Pathogens and Practice.* 3rd ed. Elsevier; 2011.)

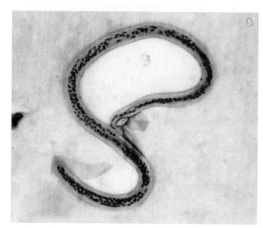

- **Fig. 35.14** Microfilaria of *Wuchereria bancrofti*. Microfilariae are differentiated by morphologic features, such as the presence of a sheath and placement of internal nuclei. (Giemsa, thick blood film, original magnification ×1000). (Schmitt BH. Laboratory diagnosis of tropical infections. *Infect Dis Clin North Am.* 2012;26(2):513–554.)

- Some studies have shown antimacrofilarial activity (adult worm killing) with doxycycline (4–6 weeks) and may reduce pathology in mild to moderate infections.
- Lymphedema therapist, basic principles of care such as hygiene, exercise, and treatment of wounds.

Note: definitive treatment for hydrocele is surgery (may be evidence of active infection but typically does not improve clinically following treatment with DEC).

Control

- Target disease by WHO and international partners for eradication.
- Aims: lymphatic filariasis elimination by reducing transmission through preventive chemotherapy.
- WHO recommended preventive mass drug administration (MDA)
  - Combination therapy given annually to an entire at-risk population.
  - Albendazole together with either ivermectin or with DEC.
  - Reduction of microfilariae in the bloodstream: preventing transmission to the insect vector.

Loiasis: *Loa loa* (African Eye Worm)

Loa loa is transmitted through repeated bites of the genus *Chrysops* (*C. silacea* and *C. dimidiata*): female tabanid redflies.
- Daylight blood-feeding, especially during rainy seasons.
- Most commonly found in Central and West Africa.
- An estimated 14.4 million people live in areas of high transmission.
- Another 15.2 million reside where 20%–40% of individuals report previous eye worm *L. loa* infective larvae.
- Long duration to maturation of adult worm (6 months to 1 year).
- *L. loa* do **not** harbor *Wolbachia* endosymbiotic bacteria.
- Infection usually requires prolonged, repeated exposure (or repeat intense exposure even in short residence).
- Microfilariae released from fecund adult female, migrate to blood with diurnal periodicity.
- Resident in subcutaneous tissues; often between tissue layers (ligaments/tendons) and/or between fascia, most often in lungs.
- Fertilized females can make thousands of microfilariae a day.
- 20-year survival in the human host (adult worms).

Clinical Manifestations

- Majority of infections asymptomatic; high peripheral blood eosinophilia.
- Transient itch/swelling, angioedematous response to adult worms (traveling through subcutaneous tissue), often on face and exposed extremities, termed **"Calabar" swelling** (Fig. 35.15).
- Myalgia, joint pains, and fatigue.

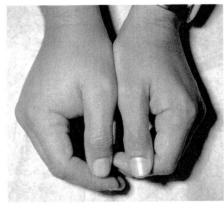

- **Fig. 35.15** Calabar swelling of the right hand. (From Klion AD. Loiasis and *Mansonella* infections. In Guerrant RL, Walker DH, Weller PF, eds. *Tropical Infectious Diseases: Principles, Pathogens and Practice.* 3rd ed. Elsevier; 2011.)

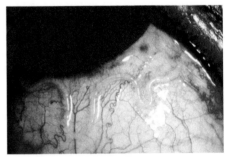

- **Fig. 35.16** Subconjunctival migration of an adult *Loa loa.* (From Armed Forces Institute of Pathology.)

- Migrate to conjunctiva and produce an **"eye worm"** (Fig. 35.16).
- Endomyocardial fibrosis causing myocarditis.
- Immune-complex nephropathy.
- Encephalitis: generally in association with DEC or ivermectin treatment; exact mechanism of posttreatment neurological complications unknown.

Management

- Standard diagnostic test is identification of microfilariae at daytime (10.00 h to 14.00 h); Giemsa-stained thin or thick blood smear.
- Concentration methods can be used; quantitative parasite counts for treatment guidance.
- Serology demonstrates high sensitivity/low specificity; *Wuchereria, Brugia, Onchocerca,* and *Mansonella* infections.
- One PCR assay for loiasis approved for diagnosis in the United States; RT-PCR developed at the Laboratory of Parasitic Diseases, National Institutes of Health, can detect and quantify *L. loa* microfilaremia (also adapted as a point-of-care test).
- First line treatment usually DEC; DEC (and ivermectin) is avoided, however, in patients with high microfilaremia as high risk of fatal encephalopathy from rapid killing of worms (**Mazzotti reaction**). These patients are often

pretreated with albendazole or apheresis (encephalopathy risk is **not** eliminated with corticosteroid treatment).

- **Mazzotti reaction post-DEC treatment**
  - Characterized by fever, urticaria, swollen and tender lymph nodes, tachycardia, hypotension, arthralgias, edema, and abdominal pain; can be life-threatening encephalitis and shock.
  - Usually occurs around 7 days posttreatment with DEC.
  - Associated with rapid killing of the microfilariae and acute severe inflammatory reactions.
  - Can be useful as diagnostic technique by skin patch testing.
  - Albendazole can be used as an alternative agent.
- **Note: DEC is contraindicated in individuals co-infected with onchocerciasis** due to risk of blindness and/or severe exacerbation of skin disease.
  - Treat onchocerciasis first then loiasis with DEC.
- There are no international programs to control or eliminate loiasis in affected endemic areas.
- No commercial vaccine available.
- Short-term travelers can use DEC chemoprophylaxis.

Onchocerciasis: *Onchocerca volvulus* (River Blindness)

- Humans only definitive host.
- Dioecious species: separate male and female reproductive organs in different individuals (not hermaphroditic).
- Transmission by blood-feeding *Simulium* spp., blackfly insect vector.
- Blackflies deposit infective third-stage larvae subcutaneously; these subsequently mature into adult parasites (macrofilariae) over 6–12 months.
- Females live in subcutaneous or deeper intramuscular tissues, surrounded by a fibrous capsule; males migrate to fertilize females (producing microfilariae).
- *O. volvulus* adults and microfilariae harbor endosymbiotic *Wolbachia* bacteria; essential for macrofilariae fertility and survival.

Clinical Manifestations

- Adult worms (macrofilariae) aggregate in subcutaneous tissue/intramuscular, encapsulated by fibrous tissue and form subcutaneous nodules (nonpainful, vascularized fibrous nodules).
- Microfilariae migrate through subcutaneous, dermal, ocular tissues, and lymph system.
- Generate minimal host immune response while alive.
- Dying/dead microfilariae generate a clinical inflammatory response.
- Unsheathed microfilaria migrate to dermis and eye; corneal inflammation appears to occur in response to both *Wolbachia* and *Onchocerca* antigens while dermal pathology *Onchocerca* only.

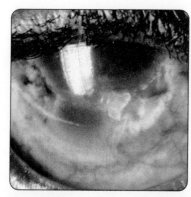

- **Fig. 35.17** Onchocerciasis: advanced sclerosing keratitis. (From Kanski J, Bowling B. *Synopsis of Clinical Ophthalmology*. 3rd ed. Saunders; 2013.)

- Onchocercal skin disease; pruritis, depigmentation (leopard skin), papular dermatitis, lichenified dermatitis, and atrophy (Fig. 35.17).
- Onchocercal skin disease (leopard skin); pruritus, papular dermatitis, lichenified dermatitis, atrophy, depigmentation (Fig. 35.18).
- Subcutaneous nodules, "onchocercomata"; usually contain one or two adult male and two or three adult female worms; do not cause significant symptoms, but often appear on bony prominences.
- Inguinal lymph node fibrosis and skin atrophy causing "hanging groin" (Fig. 35.18).

Management

- Identification of microfilariae in eye/skin:
  - Corneoscleral instrument – skin snips/biopsy; parasites emerge after 24 hours incubation in saline.
  - Ophthalmology slit-lamp examination.
- **Treatment**
  - Ivermectin single dose repeated every 3–6 months until asymptomatic.
  - Doxycycline has been shown to be effective for *Wolbachia* and therefore used as adjunctive therapy for 6 weeks.
  - No accepted alternative therapy; DEC is contraindicated due to risk of **Mazzotti reaction** (as *L. loa*: see above).

Control

- Sustainable community-directed treatment with ivermectin (CDTI) and vector control (environmentally safe methods).
- Goals of eliminating ocular morbidity and interruption of transmission.
- Expanded Special Project for the Elimination of Neglected Tropical Diseases in Africa (ESPEN) currently is supporting control programs, including onchocerciasis.
- WHO currently recommends treating onchocerciasis with MDA ivermectin at least once yearly for between 10 and 15 years.

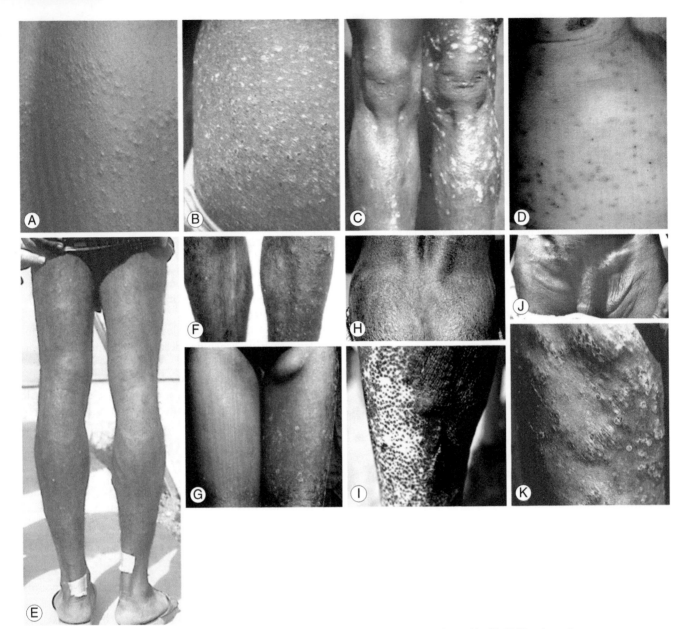

• **Fig. 35.18** Cutaneous lesions in onchocerciasis. (A) Acute pustular onchodermatitis. (B, C) Chronic onchodermatitis. (D) Dermatitis in Guatemala, erisipela de la costa. (E, F, G) Sowda with unilateral preference and dark skin as well as swollen femoral lymph node. (H) Skin atrophy in a 15-year-old boy. (I) Leopard skin. (J) Hanging groin. (K) Lichenified onchodermatitis. (Hoerauf AM. Onchocerciasis. In Tropical Infectious Diseases: Principles, Pathogens and Practice. 3rd ed. Elsevier; 2011.)

Other Important Tissue Nematodes

Angiostrongylus

- Cause of severe gastrointestinal or CNS disease in humans, depending on species.
- *Angiostrongylus cantonensis* (rat lungworm) causes **eosinophilic meningitis (>10% eosinophils in the CSF).**
- Risk factor: eating raw or undercooked snail.
- Predominant in Southeast Asia.

- Supportive management only, and no antiparasitic treatment is required (often contraindicated).

Baylisascaris

- Roundworm: host raccoons (humans acquire infection from ingestion of contaminated soil).
- Parasites invade the eye (ocular larva migrans), organs (visceral larva migrans), or the brain (neural larva migrans/**eosinophilic meningitis**).

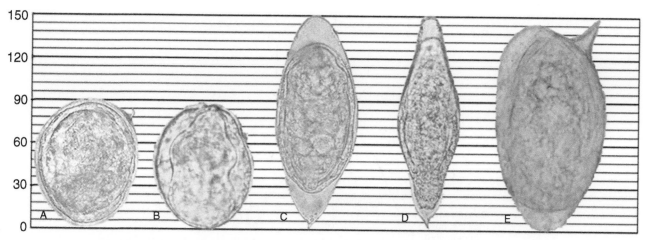

• **Fig. 35.19** Eggs from different *Schistosoma* parasites of humans. (A) *S. japonicum*; (B) *S. mekongi*; (C) *S. haematobium*; (D) *S. intercalatum*; (E) *S. mansoni*. Measurements expressed in μm. *S. haematobium* displays characteristic terminal spine whereas *S. mansoni* has a lateral spine. (From Bustinduy AL. Schistosomiasis. In: Farrar J, et al., eds. *Manson's Tropical Diseases*. 23rd ed. Elsevier; 2014.)

• Rare infection but found in United States (especially in children).
• No antiparasitic chemotherapy indicated.

Anisakis

• Parasitic nematode found in squid/fish and transmitted through ingestion of raw/undercooked seafood.
• Manifests acutely after eating raw fish (e.g., sushi); acute abdominal pain, nausea, vomiting, allergic reaction; often mistaken as acute abdomen.
• Antiparasitic agent rarely required (albendazole could be used but not FDA approved).
• **Treatment:** removal of worm (endoscopically or surgery).

Toxocara

• Dog (or cat) roundworm; transmission through ingestion contaminated soil/dirt.
• Self-limiting infection and antiparasitic agent not normally required.

SCHISTOSOMES AND OTHER FLUKES (TREMATODE FLATWORMS)

• Flatworms of the phylum Platyhelminths.
• Schistosomes create a heavy global disease burden, and schistosomiasis is devastating socioeconomically.
  • While mortality rate is low, the morbidity is high.
  • **Second most socioeconomically devastating parasitic disease after malaria.**
  • In resource-poor countries where endemic, symptoms of chronic illness can cause reduction in work productivity that ultimately leads to loss of income and a financial and emotional burden on an already impoverished society.

• Population at risk: 500–600 million people in 74 countries.
• Population infected: over 200 million at any one time and still growing.
• Global disease burden: est. 200,000 deaths/year and around 2 million DALYs (disability-adjusted life years) lost/year (up to 20 million).
• Over 23 species identified. Five main species of clinical importance; distinguished by molluscan vectors, location within host vasculature and egg morphology:
  • *S. mansoni* prevalence highest in sub-Saharan Africa but also endemic in South America.
  • *S. hematobium* sub-Saharan and Northern Africa, Middle East.
  • *S. japonicum* China and Southeast Asia.
  • *S. intercalatum* parts of western and central Africa.
  • *S. mekongi* found along the Mekong river basin region, from Cambodia to Laos.
• Species can usually be identified by egg morphology alone (Fig. 35.19).
The parasite rotates between three environmental niches (freshwater aquatic dwelling, intermediate molluscan, and definitive vertebrate hosts) and undergoes two distinct types of reproduction:
• Digenetic: alternate generations between sexually reproducing adult and asexually reproducing larval stages.
• Novel in platyhelminths: dioecious not hermaphroditic; separate male and female reproductive organs in different individuals.
• Adult worms absorb host proteins and coat themselves with host antigens, allowing prolonged residence in the bloodstream with evasion of immune attack.
• Life cycle (Fig. 35.20): fresh water, free-living motile miracidia hatch from the eggs to infect aquatic snails, here they undergo two rounds of asexual multiplication; released as infective cercariae into water.

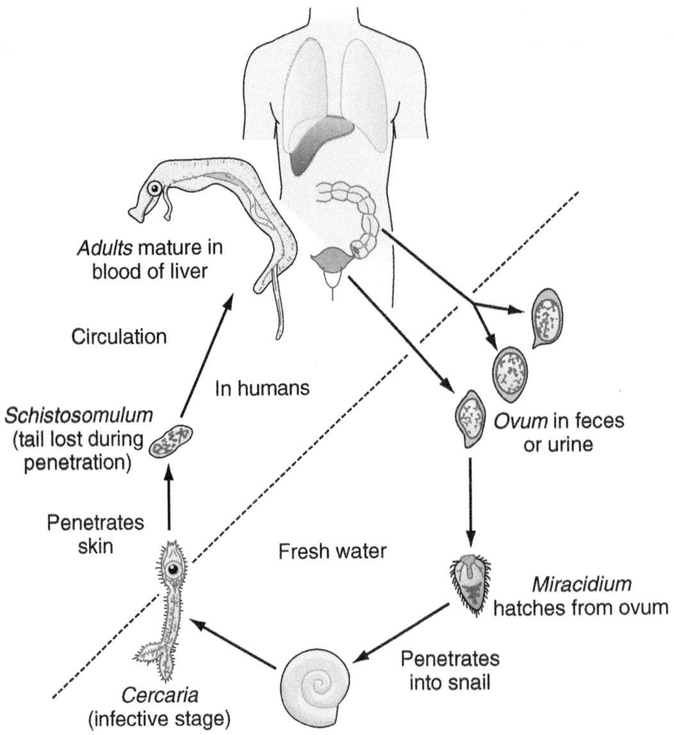

• **Fig. 35.20** Life cycle of *Schistosoma* and occurrence of schistosomiasis. Fresh water, free-living motile miracidia hatch from the eggs to infect aquatic snails and undergo two rounds of asexual multiplication – released as infective cercariae into water. Cercariae infect the human host, penetrating skin, and the cercarial head separates from its tail to become the parasitic schistosomules. After several days the parasites exit cutaneous tissue via blood (or lymphatic) vessels, travel first to the lungs through venous circulation and onward into the systemic vasculature. Worms feed on blood, mature, and pair up; female egg-laying begins around 5–6 weeks post-infection. Eggs are passed into snail-dwelling freshwater environments via urine or feces (depending on species). (From Montgomery SP. Blood trematodes: schistosomiasis. In: Long SS, Prober CG, Fischer M, eds. *Principles and Practice of Pediatric Infectious Diseases.* 5th ed. Elsevier; 2018.)

• Cercariae infect the human host, by penetrating unbroken skin. The cercarial head separates from its tail to become the parasitic schistosomula.
• After several days the parasites exit the cutaneous tissue via blood (or lymphatic) vessels, travel first to the lungs through venous circulation and onward into the systemic vasculature.
• Worms feed on blood, mature, and pair up, the whole process taking approximately 5 weeks. Egg laying begins around this time and completes the cycle.

Pathogenesis and Clinical Manifestations

• Endemic rural areas; urban sites usually lack the freshwater conditions for intermediate host to thrive.
• Infection through contaminated (cercarial larvae) freshwater ponds, lakes, and rivers.
• Clinical disease is caused by host immune response to migrating eggs; Th$_2$-type to eggs deposited in tissue leading to chronic inflammation and fibrosis.
• Egg production, host immune polarization, and pathology are all intimately associated.
• Natural course of the infection depends on age of primary exposure, intensity of ongoing exposure, development of immunity against repeat infection, and genetic susceptibility.

• In endemic areas, worm burden increases gradually, peaks during first two decades of life and subsequently declines to very low levels in adults.
• Infection associated with eosinophilia, IgE, IL-4, and IL-5.
• Tourism; single exposure, minimal worm burden: mild parasite load with limited morbidity.
• Adult male/female pairs exist in the body for around 5 years, yet can survive 20–30 years.
  • Interestingly, adult worms tend to stay together in partnership (egg-producing female lies within the gynecophoric canal of the larger male).
Many individuals can be asymptomatic and have subclinical disease during both acute and chronic stages of infection
• Cercariae manipulate host local immune response by releasing excretory/secretory products from their acetabular glands.
• Dermal penetration by cercariae usually asymptomatic.
• Hypersensitivity reaction with repeat exposure (not initial exposure); occasional localized inflammation with itchy rash ("swimmer's itch"); develops from within hours to up to one week post contaminated water exposures.
• **Avian schistosomiasis**: cercarial dermatitis caused by *Schistosoma* species where usual hosts are birds/mammals

and not humans. Cercariae penetrate through skin but do not mature into adult worms in the human body. Offending schistosomes include *Austrobilharzia variglandis* (normal host ducks), other common genera *Trichobilharzia*, and *Gigantobilharzia*.

Acute Schistosomiasis

- **Katayama fever**: acute onset constellation of symptoms may include fever, urticarial rash, angioedema, chills, myalgia, arthralgia, dry cough, diarrhea, abdominal pain, and headache.
  - Mild, self-limiting, and resolves over days, weeks, or months.
  - Liver, spleen, and lymph nodes often enlarged; often painful.
  - CNS involvement possible.
  - Hypersensitivity reaction to antigens and circulating immune complexes.
  - 2–8 weeks postinitial exposure.
  - Correlates with adult worm maturation, increasing antigen burden, and new egg production (usually 5-week adults).
  - Relatively common in nonimmune hosts such as travelers/tourists.
  - Elevated peripheral eosinophil count
- Schistosomule (larval) worms migrate through lung vascular system and may generate cough and/or dyspnea.
  - Respiratory symptoms and signs (in ~75% patients).
  - Transient pulmonary infiltrates.

Chronic Infection

Chronic infection can remain asymptomatic for years.
- Relies on repeated exposure, repeated reinfection posttreatment.
- Severity of disease correlates:
- Number of eggs trapped in tissues and anatomic distribution (organ tropism of infecting species).
- Duration and intensity.
- Human host immune response: as stated; Th$_2$ with high levels IL-4, IL-5, IL-9, and IL-10, and circulating IgE, eosinophils, and mast cell responses.
- While these Th$_2$ responses are clearly implicated in immunopathology, they can also permit host survival in the face of continuing infection.

Pathology Directly Related to Schistosome Species

Intestinal/Hepatosplenic Schistosomiasis: *S. mansoni* and *S. japonicum*
- Adult worms tropic for mesenteric venous plexus.
- Chronic inflammation can lead to bowel wall ulceration, hyperplasia, and polyposis and with heavy infections, to liver fibrosis and portal hypertension.
  - Nonfibrotic granulomatous inflammation around trapped eggs in the presinusoidal periportal spaces of the liver.
  - Egg deposition in the periportal spaces; causes periportal fibrosis (Symmers' pipestem fibrosis).

- Occlusion of the portal veins: portal hypertension with splenomegaly, portocaval shunting, and gastrointestinal varices.
- IL-13 may play a significant role in fibrosis development (certainly the case in murine infection model).
- Liver is firm and nodular.
- Childhood hepatosplenomegaly is not benign and is associated with both dilated portal system and stunting of growth.
- Colonic ulceration: intestinal bleeding and iron deficiency anemia (often exacerbated by hookworm co-infection).
- Chronic or intermittent abdominal pain, poor appetite, and diarrhea.
- Anemia, malnutrition, and developmental delay result from repeated infections in school-age children.
- Prompt treatment and re-treatment can lead to reversal/partial reversal of end-organ damage (6 months to 1 year posttreatment).
- See Fig. 35.21.

Urogenital Schistosomiasis: *S. haematobium*
- Adult worms generally reside in the venous plexus of the lower urinary tract.
- Eggs are excreted in the urine, and patients present with microscopic or macroscopic hematuria and/or pyuria (terminal hematuria, hematospermia).
- Eggs lodge in the urinary tract causing damage, dysuria, and hematuria.
- Contracted, fibrotic, thick-walled bladder with calcifications (calcified eggs/fibrosed bladder wall).
- Granulomatous inflammation, ulcerations, and development of pseudopolyps in the bladder and ureteral walls.
- Other long-term complications include bladder neck obstruction, hydroureter, and hydronephrosis.
- Immune complex glomerulopathy, leading to proteinuria and nephrotic syndrome.
- Increased risk of bladder cancer; usually squamous cell carcinoma.
- Female genital tract, causing female genital schistosomiasis that can affect the cervix, fallopian tubes, and vagina.
- Increased susceptibility to other infections (particularly *Salmonella*); may be an independent risk factor for HIV infection.
- Hypertrophic and ulcerative lesions of the vulva, vagina, and cervix.

Central Nervous System
- Neuro-schistosomiasis can involve the spinal cord (acute myelopathy) and/or the brain, myelopathy more common than cerebral disease.
- Extremely rare.
- Aberrant migration/embolization of adult worms to spinal cord or microcirculation.
- Egg production/ectopic deposition of eggs; intense inflammatory granulomatous reaction with local tissue destruction and scarring.
- Occasional embolic CNS egg granulomas; act as space-occupying lesions.

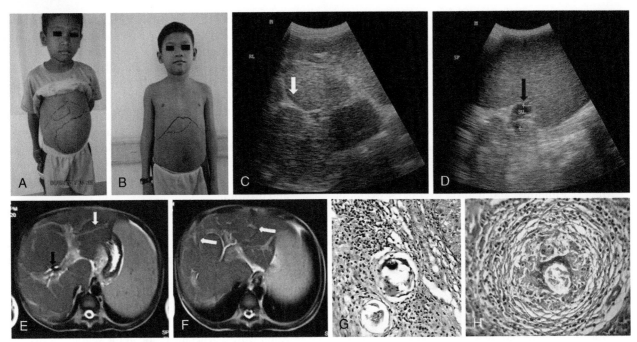

• **Fig. 35.21** The abdomen of a 12-year-old boy with severe schistosomiasis (A) before and (B) after sple-nectomy. Ultrasound of the patient showing (C) a markedly thickened branch of the main portal vein (*white arrow*), and (D) a markedly enlarged spleen with dilated splenic vein (*black arrow*). MRI depicting (E) a cav-ernous transformation of the right portal vein (*black arrow*) and periportal fibrosis running along the second branch of the portal vein (*white arrow*), and (F) curvilinear tracts scattered throughout the liver parenchyma consistent with periportal fibrosis (*arrows*). Histopathology sections showing (G) early *Schistosoma japoni-cum* egg granuloma and (H) late granuloma in the liver. (From Olveda DU. The chronic enteropathogenic disease schistosomiasis. *Int J Infect Dis.* 2014;28:193–203.)

Diagnosis

- Egg identification in fecal microscopy (Fig. 35.22).
- Eggs are shed intermittently and in low amounts in light-intensity infections (such as returning travelers).
- Increase the sensitivity of stool and urine; three samples collected on different days.
- Classification of intestinal schistosomiasis intensity:
  - Light (up to 100 eggs/g).
  - Moderate (100–400 eggs/g).
  - Severe (>400 eggs/g).
- Intensity of urinary schistosomiasis:
  - Light to moderate (up to 50 eggs/10 mL) or severe (>50 eggs/10 mL).
- Serologic testing for antischistosomal antibody indicated for diagnosis for travelers or immigrants from endemic areas (antiadult worm antibody):
  - Serum at least 6–8 weeks after last exposure to potentially contaminated water; allow for full development of the parasite and antibody to the adult stage.
  - ELISA, radioimmunoassay, indirect hemagglutina-tion, Western blot, and complement fixation.
  - Extracts of adult worms, cercarial antigens, or egg extracts such as the *S. mansoni* soluble egg antigen (SmSEA).

- Most commercially produced antibody test assays are not species-specific; therefore these assays are gener-ally used as screening tests for schistosome infection (high sensitivity and low specificity).
- Antibody titer does not correlate with parasite burden.

Treatment

Praziquantel (PZQ) is the gold standard: effective with low toxicity (cure rates 90% with single treatment).
- Not recommended unless diagnostic microscopy and/or serology: not initiated before at least 6 weeks post-expo-sure (**full adult maturation as minimally efficacious in larval stages).**
- PZQ exposes parasite antigen to host immune responses (previously hidden); leads to cytokine and chemokine cascades.
- Adult disintegrating, dead worms can release eggs as they are being destroyed; PZQ kills worms but not eggs or larval stages; expulsion by peristalsis.
- Confirm cure with egg excretion surveillance 2–6 months.
- Repeat therapy if persistent egg excretion.
- MDA; aim to prevent morbidity in later life through regular treatment of school-age children.

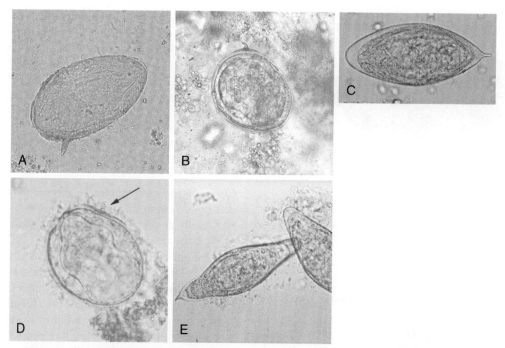

• **Fig. 35.22** Eggs of human schistosomes. Egg of *Schistosoma mansoni* (A) has a prominent lateral spine. Egg of *S. japonicum* (B) is more rounded and has a less prominent spine. Egg of *S. haematobium* (C) is larger with a terminal spine. Egg of *S. mekongi* (D) has an inconspicuous spine (*arrow*). Egg of *S. intercalatum* (E), like *S. haematobium*, has a terminal spine but has a central bulge. (From http://www.dpd.cdc.gov/dpdx/HTML/Schistosomiasis.htm. Part A courtesy of the Missouri State Public Health Laboratory.)

- Distinct aims of treatment:
  - Resolving acute/reversing early chronic pathology associated with developing life cycle.
  - Preventing complications of chronic long-term infection sequelae.

Globally we rely on a single drug for schistosoma treatment:

- Minimal resistance at present but may yet represent a problem in era of mass global treatment programs.
- *In vitro* resistance demonstrated and *in vivo* resistance noted in the field.
  - Most often in endemic areas of high worm burden, intense transmission with rapid re-infection.

Oral PZQ is available for human use in the United States and UK (unlicensed).

Control and Prevention

- Education.
- Sanitation.
- Careful molluscicide in endemic freshwater areas.
- Anthelminthic chemotherapy: single agent to treat all species of parasite that infect man: PZQ.
  - Mass treatment programs (MDA).
  - Regular treatment of all at-risk groups.
  - Areas of low transmission: aiming for interruption.
  - Global control programs: repeated treatment administration substantially diminishes schistosome-associated disease and accelerates the acquisition of a (partially) protective immunity.

Foodborne Trematodes (Fluke Infections)

Fasciola hepatica: worldwide distribution.

- Mollusc intermediate hosts.
- Sheep and cattle are the most important and common hosts for *F. hepatica*. Other hosts can include horses, camels, goats, deer, and rabbits (herbivorous mammals).
- Humans are incidental hosts. Infection commonly acquired through ingestion of contaminated aquatic plants (e.g., watercress).

Clinical Manifestations

- Acute: 6–12 weeks after metacercariae ingestion.
  - Symptoms correlate with early phase migration through the liver: fever, right upper quadrant pain, hepatomegaly, and jaundice.
  - Anorexia, nausea, vomiting, myalgia, cough, and urticaria.
  - Peripheral blood eosinophilia.
  - Symptoms may continue for many weeks.
- Chronic infection; develops 6 months postexposure and can persist for many years.
  - Biliary colic, cholangitis, cholelithiasis, obstructive jaundice, and secondary pancreatitis.
  - Prolonged and/or heavy infection can also result in sclerosing cholangitis and biliary cirrhosis.
- Extrahepatic manifestations may result from worm migration to ectopic sites through soft-tissues and/or hematogenously.

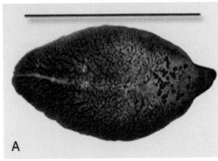

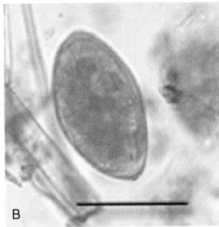

• **Fig. 35.23** Fasciola hepatica. (A) Adult (size 30 × 15 mm). The bar represents 30 mm. (B) Egg (size 130–150 × 60–90 μm). The bar represents 100 μm. (Courtesy of DPDx, Division of Parasitic Diseases, National Center for Infectious Diseases, Centers for Disease Control and Prevention.)

- Extrahepatic sites can include abdominal wall (most common), pulmonary, cardiac, brain, genitourinary tract, eyes, and skin.
- Pharyngeal fascioliasis ("halzoun" syndrome), majority from the Middle East and associated with the consumption of raw liver.

Management

- Microscopy identification of eggs in stool, duodenal aspirates, or bile specimens (Fig. 35.23).
  - Eggs not detectable in acute early phase of infection.
- Serology does becomes positive during early phase migration.
  - CDC recommends enzyme immunoassays (EIA) with excretory-secretory (ES) antigens combined with confirmation of positive results by immunoblot.
- Radiographic demonstration of flukes is useful in clinical context, including CT, ultrasonography, cholangiography, ERCP, and MRI.

Treatment

- **Triclabendazole** is an imidazole derivative; effective against all stages of fascioliasis with a cure rate of >90%. Oral treatment for 1 or 2 days.
- No established alternatives.
- Routine follow-up approximately 3 months posttreatment: resolution of eosinophilia, eggs clearance, and reduction in serology titer.

- Triclabendazole is not commercially available (not FDA approved for this indication) for use in the United States; only obtained through the CDC under an investigational protocol.
- Unlicensed use in the UK.
- No commercially available vaccine.

Clonorchis sinensis (and *Opisthorchis* spp.): Chinese Liver Fluke

Clonorchis sinensis, *Opisthorchis felineus*, or *O. viverrini* parasites of fish-eating mammals.
- Notably dogs and cats are large reservoirs.
- Humans are incidental hosts.
- Infection by ingestion of encysted metacercariae within raw, salted, pickled, smoked, marinated, dried, undercooked, or poorly processed freshwater fish.
- Can be found in China, the Democratic People's Republic of Korea, the Republic of Korea, and Vietnam.
- Estimated more than 35 million people infected worldwide, with another 600 million at risk.
- *O. felineus* Southeast Asia and in Central and Eastern Europe, particularly in Siberia and other parts of the former Soviet Union.
- *O. viverrini* endemic in Thailand, Vietnam, Cambodia, and Laos.

Pathogenesis and Clinical Manifestations

- Metacercariae excyst in duodenum and worms migrate to reside in biliary ducts, gallbladder, and/or pancreatic ducts.
- Cell-mediated immunity does not develop; repeated infections will engender cumulative worm burden.
- Symptoms may increase with age and time from initial infection.
- *C. sinensis* and *O. viverrini* are generally considered together as similar pathological processes.
- Most infections are benign and asymptomatic; pathology again depends on intensity and duration of infection.
- **Acute**
  - Usually around 10-30 days postingestion; nonspecific vague symptoms such as fatigue, malaise, and dyspepsia.
  - Nonspecific symptoms, such as right upper quadrant pain, indigestion, diarrhea, flatulence, and fatigue.
  - Acute infective symptoms more common in *O. felineus* infection.
    - High-grade fever, anorexia, nausea, vomiting, abdominal pain, malaise, myalgia, arthralgia, malaise, urticaria, lymph nodes, and tender hepatomegaly. Acute infective symptoms are more common in *O. felineus*; fevers, nausea, vomiting and abdominal pain, tender lymphadenopathy, and hepatomegaly.
  - Symptoms persist around 2–3 weeks.
- High peripheral eosinophilia ± elevated liver enzymes/serum IgE, eggs often detectable in feces at 2–4 weeks.

- **Chronic:** secondary to protracted episodes of re-infection.
  - Chronic inflammation results in duct fibrosis and adjacent liver parenchymal destruction.
  - Physical bile duct obstruction by the adult flukes.
  - Nonfunctional gallbladder provides a nidus for dead flukes and stone formation.
  - Obstructive jaundice, pancreatitis, recurrent cholangitis, pyogenic liver abscesses, and cholangiohepatitis.
  - Chronic *C. sinensis* infection strongly associated with cholangiocarcinoma,

Management

- Identify eggs in stool, duodenal, or bile specimens.
- Chronic phase: some techniques, such as the Kato–Katz thick smear can quantify the intensity of infection.
- Adjunctive imaging: useful but will depend on clinical context.
- ELISA cannot reliably distinguish between current and past infection and also may cross-react with other parasites, molecular techniques not used clinically.
- **Treatment**
  - PZQ for 1 or 2 days (same dosing for children).
  - Alternatives albendazole for 7 days (or mebendazole).

Paragonimiasis (Lung Fluke)

- 50 species *Paragonimus* identified; 16 considered clinically important.
- Most important *P. westermani* (Oriental lung fluke).
- *P. westermani* can be found in China, Democratic People's Republic of Korea, Republic of Korea, Vietnam, Japan, the Philippines, and India. *P. africanus* occurs in West Africa; *P. mexicanus* occurs only in Central and South America.
- Note *P. kellicotti* has been rarely found in midwestern and southern US freshwater crayfish.
- Human infection by ingestion of raw or undercooked infected crab or crayfish.
- First and second intermediate hosts (snails and crabs or crayfish respectively).
- Estimated 20 million people infected worldwide and more than 290 million at risk.
- Infections may persist for 20 years in humans.

Pathogenesis

- Encyst in the muscles and viscera of freshwater crabs and crayfish.
- Uncooked, partially cooked, salted, pickled larval stages of the parasite are released when the crab or crawfish is digested.
- Intestinal transit via duodenum, intestinal wall, peritoneum and subsequent migration through the diaphragm on to the lungs.
- Adult worms live in encapsulated cystic cavities within lung parenchyma.
- Operculate (lid-like structure at terminal end) eggs pass into bronchioles and are coughed up, expelled either through sputum or swallowed (thus pass into feces) (Fig. 35.24).

- Eggs hatch to miracidia in water and penetrate the first intermediate host (melania snail) and undergo several rounds of asexual multiplication and develop into cercariae.
- Cercariae are shed into water and infect the second intermediate hosts (crabs and crayfish) and encyst in muscles/viscera.

Clinical Manifestations

- Asymptomatic majority infections
- Acute symptoms occur within 2 months:
  - Abdominal pain, nausea, diarrhea, cough, urticaria, fever, chest pain.
  - Associated with first egg production and larval migration within the peritoneal cavity.
  - Peripheral blood eosinophilia.
- Acute and chronic **pulmonary:**
  - Inflammatory reactions to egg-shedding and encapsulated adults; essentially chronic pathologically and clinically similar to bronchitis/bronchiectasis:
    - Chronic cough, profuse sputa and recurrent hemoptysis.
    - Radiographic manifestations: calcification, diffuse infiltration, pleural effusions, and nodules.
- **Extrapulmonary:**
  - Most commonly CNS: parasite-induced eosinophilic meningoencephalitis or cerebral infections.
  - Calcified cysts in CNS essentially act as space-occupying lesions with associated symptoms and signs.
  - Almost any other organ – hypersensitivity reactions and chronic inflammation (dead-end life cycle as no egg exit) – leading to fibrosis.
    - Abdominal viscera, heart, skin.
  - *P. skrjabini* often produces skin nodules, subcutaneous abscesses, or a type of creeping eruption known as "trematode larva migrans."

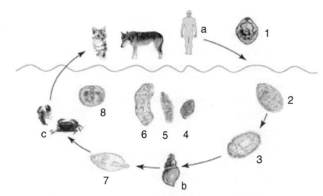

• **Fig. 35.24** The life cycle of *P. westermani*. In the definitive host (a), the adult worm (1) exists in the bronchioles of lungs. Eggs (2) are shed into the external environment via sputum and feces. Miracidia in water (3) penetrate the melania snail (b), the first intermediate host. Miracidia inside the snail go through several developmental stages [sporocysts (4), rediae (5, 6)] and develop cercariae (7), which are shed into water and seek the second intermediate hosts (crabs and crayfish) (c), in which the cercariae encyst as metacercariae (8) in the musculature or other organs. Ingestion of raw or undercooked infected crab or crayfish results in infection of the definitive host. (From Liu Q. Paragonimiasis: an important food-borne zoonosis in China. *Trends Parasitol.* 2008;24(7):318–323.)

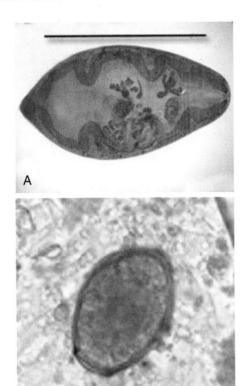

• **Fig. 35.25** *Paragonimus westermani*. (A) Adult (size 7–16 × 4–8 mm). The bar represents 10 mm. (B) Egg (size 80–120 × 50–60 μm), unstained wet mount. The bar represents 100 μm. (Courtesy DPDx, Division of Parasitic Diseases, National Center for Infectious Diseases, Centers for Disease Control and Prevention.)

Management

- Microscopic identification of eggs in sputa, feces, tissue biopsy (Fig. 35.25).
- Multiple samples may be necessary, especially in light/low worm burden infections.
- Serology useful in diagnosis particularly in presence of light infections; antibodies against selected *Paragonimus* proteins are detectable as early as 2–3 weeks after infection but may not decrease for up to 2 years following successful treatment.
  - ELISA is highly sensitive and specific (92% and >90% respectively) and can be performed on serum or CSF samples.
- **Treatment**
  - PZQ for 3 days: acceptable treatment for all species.
  - Triclabendazole as useful alternative, one or two doses.
  - Inflammatory reactions to dying worms requires concurrent corticosteroids in cerebral infections.

Fasciolopsiasis (Intestinal Trematode); *Fasciolopsis Buski*

- Largest intestinal fluke of humans; common in South and Southeast Asia.
- Infection through ingestion of contaminated aquatic plants; pigs are a major reservoir of infection.

- No direct person-to-person transmission; cercariae are released from the freshwater mollusc (*Segmentina* spp. intermediate host) and encyst as metacercariae on aquatic plants.
- Flukes are fully developed after 3 months, produce approximately 20,000 eggs/day, and adult lifespan is around 1 year.
- Adult flukes inhabit the duodenum and jejunum.
  - Most often asymptomatic.
  - Peripheral blood eosinophilia.
  - Abdominal pain, nausea, vomiting, and fever 1–2 months postexposure.
  - Local inflammation, edema, ulceration, and possible abscesses.
  - Intestinal obstruction and other complications.
- Allergic-type symptoms through hypersensitivity to worm antigens and metabolites more common in heavier infections.

Management

- Microscopic demonstration of egg or worms in the stool: eggs more difficult to identify than adult worms.
- **Treatment**
  - PZQ orally in three divided doses for 1 day (the dosage for children is the same).
  - Triclabendazole as alternative, one or two doses.
  - Again, treatment of cerebral disease usually requires a short course of corticosteroids together with PZQ to dampen inflammatory response associated with dying worms.

CESTODES

Taeniasis and Diphyllobothriasis (Tapeworms)

- Generally divide lifespan between two different hosts.
- Most common worldwide – *Taenia saginata* – beef tapeworm (Fig. 35.26) and *T. solium* – pork tapeworm (Fig. 35.27).
  - Cattle/pigs ingest contaminated vegetation containing eggs cysticerci/gravid proglottids.
  - Humans are the only definitive hosts.
- *Diphyllobothrium latum* and *D. nihonkaiense* (fish tapeworm).
  - Largest human tapeworm (up to 25 m length).
  - Transmission via consumption of a variety of freshwater fish containing infective plerocercoid cysts.
  - Most common worldwide is *D. latum*, frequently found in northern and eastern Europe, and Japan.
- Following ingestion, protoscolices are released from cysts and attach to the small intestinal wall.
  - Intestinal wall invasion by hatching embryos (oncospheres) with hematogenous migration to striated muscle.
  - Cysticerci thus develop within muscle tissue, where they can reside for many years.

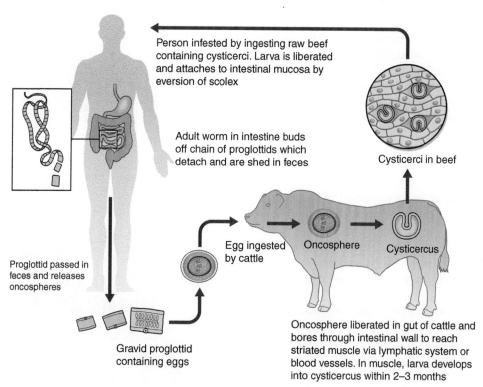

• **Fig. 35.26** Life cycle of *Taenia saginata*. (Courtesy Tropical Resources Unit, Wellcome Trust.)

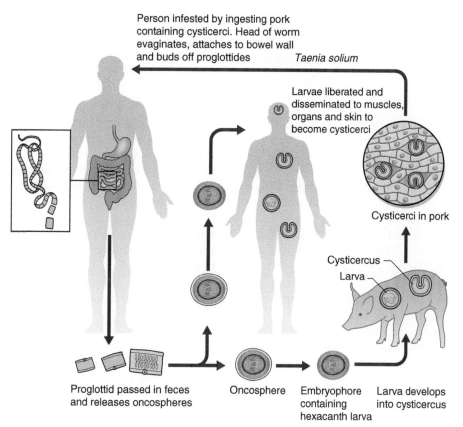

• **Fig. 35.27** Life cycle of *Taenia solium*. (Courtesy Tropical Resources Unit, Wellcome Trust.)

- Fully developed adult tapeworm develops within 8 weeks with often around 1–5 worms per human infection.
- The tapeworm adult is usually ≤5 m for *T. saginata* and 2–7 m for *T. solium.*
- Gravid proglottids ultimately detach from the adult worm thus to be passed in the stool and continue the cycle.
  - *T. saginata* adults around 1000 proglottids; each generating 100,000 eggs.
  - *T. solium* up to 2000 with 50,000 eggs.

Clinical Manifestations

Most infected individuals are asymptomatic or experience very few mild/moderate symptoms that may include (but not exhaustive):
- Nausea, anorexia, vomiting, epigastric/generalized abdominal pain, and nonspecific lethargy/malaise.
- Peripheral eosinophilia may be transient or unremarkable if present at all.
- Diphyllobothriasis can lead to fatigue, malaise, diarrhea, and hypersensitivity-type symptoms. Peripheral eosinophilia relatively uncommon in only 5-10% patients.
- Patients may pass adult proglottids/proglottid segments in the stool (live or dying/dead material) and be aware of foreign/active material; psychologically distressing.
- Mechanical obstruction of the intestine can occur if several worms become entangled.
- Proglottids can be aspirated or regurgitated, migration can cause cholecystitis or cholangitis.
- Specifically, diphyllobothriasis may lead to vitamin B_{12} deficiency with megaloblastic anemia; *D. latum* has a unique affinity for vitamin B_{12} and can compete with host for absorption.

Management

- Identify eggs (Fig. 35.28) and/or proglottids (Fig. 35.29) via simple microscopy of fecal material.
- Concentration techniques may be indicated (as low worm burden infections).
- *Taenia* spp. eggs are morphologically indistinguishable on microscopy; in contrast, proglottids and scolices are distinct and identifiable.
- In contrast, proglottids and scolices of *T. solium* and *T. saginata* are morphologically distinguishable and speciation may be useful for contamination tracing.
- **Treatment**
- Praziquantel single dose for both *Taenia* spp. and *Diphyllobothrium* spp. (children and adults).
- Niclosamide is acceptable alternative but not available in the United States (single dose); albendazole may also be effective.
  - Requires test of cure.

Cysticercosis: *T. solium*

Tissue infection with larval stages of *T. solium.*
- Estimated 50 million people worldwide infected, with 50,000 deaths per year (neurocysticercosis).
- Humans incidental dead-end hosts; essentially person-to-person transmission.

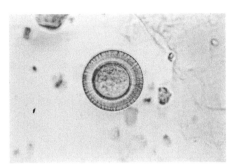

• **Fig. 35.28** *Taenia* ovum. Size usually 30–40 μm. (From the collection of Herman Zaiman, "A Presentation of Pictorial Parasites.")

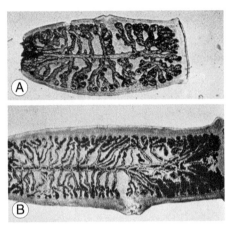

• **Fig. 35.29** (A) Taenia solium proglottid and (B) Taenia saginata proglottid (India ink-stained). (From Wittner M, White Jr AC, Tanowitz HB. Taenia and Other Tapeworm Infections. In Guerrant RL, Walker DH, Weller PF, eds. Tropical Infectious Diseases: Principles, Pathogens and Practice. 3rd ed. Elsevier; 2011.)

- Transmission by ingestion of *T. solium* embryonated eggs or gravid proglottids eggs shed in the stool of a human tapeworm carrier; asymptomatic household carrier (most common, or autoinfection).
- This is in contrast to humans ingesting cysticerci in porcine muscle, leading to adult tapeworms in human intestine.
- Following ingestion, embryos hatch in the small intestine (oncospheres), invade the mucosal wall, and disseminate hematogenously to brain, striated muscle, liver, and/or other tissues.
- Tissue cysticerci develop over around 3–8 weeks.
- Median incubation period prior to onset of symptoms is 3.5 years.

Clinical Manifestations Neurocysticercosis

- Intraparenchymal brain cysts: seizures and headache (important cause of adult-onset seizures in endemic areas), majority asymptomatic.
- Extraparenchymal cysts, including intraventricular or subarachnoid (racemose: older term, lobulated cysts without scolices); elevated intracranial pressure ± altered mental status.
- Hydrocephalus more common in adults than children (more likely to have parenchymal disease).

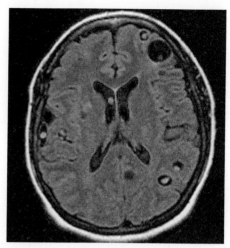

Fig. 35.30 MRI scan of the brain of a patient with multiple cysticerci. The scolex of the larval parasite can be seen within several cysticerci. There is also an intraventricular parasite in the frontal horn. (Courtesy Dr. T. Nash.)

- Other nonspecific clinical signs include mass effect, altered vision, focal neurologic signs, altered mental status, and meningitis.
- Typically no fever present.
- Extra-neural manifestations may involve a wide variety of tissues.
  - Muscle, subcutaneous tissue, spinal, or ocular involvement.
  - Cardiac cysts may be asymptomatic, cause dysrhythmias, and/or conduction abnormalities.

Diagnosis Neurocysticercosis

Range of clinical presentations, and natural history and prognosis vary with the number of cysticerci and degree of inflammation.
- Clinical presentation and radiographic imaging (usually MRI + non-contrast CT) (Fig. 35.30).
- Peripheral eosinophilia typically absent.
- Serology adjunct not necessary, negative does not exclude but ELISA recommended as confirmatory test.
- Screen for latent TB and *S. stercoralis* (prior to corticosteroid treatment).
- Funduscopy as standard.

Management

- Albendazole 10–14 days or albendazole together with PZQ.
- Dexamethasone used as adjunct in parenchymal neurocysticercosis to reduce inflammation associated with dying parasites (start 24 hours prior to anthelmintic).
- Neurosurgery may be indicated but evaluated on an individual basis ± follow-up radiological surveillance.

Prevention

- Prevent **human tapeworm** infection
  - Strict health and safety standards of pork production, processing and inspection.
  - Eliminate cysts visible in raw meat/discard meat.
  - Freeze or cook as above.
  - Improved sanitation.
- Prevent porcine cysticercosis
  - Eliminate access of pigs to human fecal material.
  - Interrupt transmission
    - Community and individual education.
    - Personal hygiene, sanitation.
    - Targeted carrier treatment and/or MDA.

Echinococcosis

- Four species of *Echinococcus* cause infection in humans:
  - Most common *E. granulosus* (hydatid disease/dog tapeworm) and *E. multilocularis*; **cystic echinococcosis** (CE) and **alveolar echinococcosis** (AE), respectively.
  - *E. vogeli* and *E. oligarthus* cause **polycystic echinococcosis** but much less frequent human infections.
  - Transmission by ingestion of viable infective eggs in contaminated food, water, or soil, or direct contact with animal hosts.
  - Humans are incidental intermediate hosts.
- *E. granulosus* (dog tapeworm): definitive host (usually dogs or related species) and an intermediate host (sheep, goats, camels, horses, cattle, and pigs).
- *E. multilocularis*: fox definitive host, other carnivores and small mammals (mostly rodents).
- Life cycle (Fig. 35.31): adult *E. granulosus* resides in the small bowel of definitive hosts, and gravid proglottids release eggs passed with feces into the environment.
- After ingestion by intermediate hosts (sheep, goats, cattle, horses, etc.), the egg hatches in the small bowel and releases an oncosphere.
- Oncospheres penetrate the intestinal mucosa and migrate through the circulatory system into various organs, especially the liver and lungs.
- The oncosphere develops into a cyst which gradually enlarges, producing protoscolices and daughter cysts that fill the cyst interior.
- Humans are infected by ingesting eggs, with resulting release of oncospheres in the intestine and the development of cysts in various organs.

Clinical Manifestations

E. granulosus
- Initial asymptomatic primary phase.
- Symptoms/signs depends on size and clinical site of cysts; almost any site of the body, either from primary inoculation or via secondary spread.
- Oncospheres penetrate mucosa and enter circulation, encyst in host viscera.
  - Most commonly affected is liver (approximately 50%–70% patients, right lobe most common, cysts up to 10 cm diameter before symptomatic) followed by pulmonary (25%; patients sometimes complain of expectoration of "salty" or saline-like sputum).

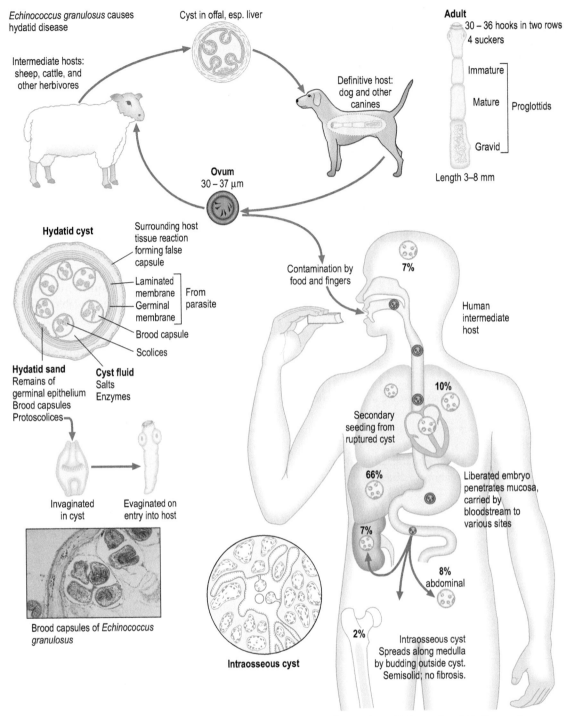

• **Fig. 35.31** Life cycle of *Echinococcus granulosus*. The adult *E. granulosus* (3–6 mm length) in the small bowel of definitive hosts (e.g., dogs). Gravid proglottids release eggs which are passed in the feces. Post-ingestion by a suitable intermediate host (e.g., sheep, goat, swine, cattle, horse, etc.), the egg hatches in the small bowel and releases an oncosphere that penetrates the intestinal wall and migrates through the circulatory system into various organs, especially the liver and lungs. In these organs, the oncosphere develops into a cyst that enlarges gradually, producing protoscolices and daughter cysts that fill the cyst interior. The definitive host becomes infected by ingesting the cyst-containing organs of the infected inter-mediate host. Postingestion, the protoscolices evaginate, attach to the intestinal mucosa and develop into adult stages in 32–80 days. (Data from the Centers for Disease Control and Prevention. DPDx – Laboratory Identification of Parasitic Diseases of Public Health Concern: Parasites – Echinococcosis. Last updated December 2012. https://www.cdc.gov/parasites/echinococcosis/). Moro PL. *Echinococcus* species: agents of echinococcosis. In: Long SS, Prober CG, Fischer M, eds. *Principles and Practice of Pediatric Infectious Diseases.* 5th ed. Elsevier; 2018.)

- Cysts can rupture into the biliary tree and produce biliary colic; obstructive jaundice, cholangitis, or pancreatitis often with associated right upper quadrant (RUQ) pain, vomiting, hypersensitivity reactions.
- Other solid organs include brain, muscle, renal, bone, cardiac, and pancreas.
- Single-organ involvement occurs in majority of patients, typically with a single cyst.
- Unfortunately cystic echinococcosis can relapse years after treatment.

  E. multilocularis
- More commonly symptomatic but rarely extrahepatic. Liver lesions have more mass-like appearance than cystic.

Management

- **Diagnosis** usually a combination of radiological imaging and serology; ultrasound scan (USS), CT, and/or MRI (Fig. 35.32).
  - Patients with liver cysts are more likely to be seropositive than those with lung cysts.
  - Serology sensitivity and specificity are greater for *E. multilocularis* than *E. granulosus*.
- **Treatment**: clear treatment guidelines dependent on size/location of cysts and presence of symptoms: see WHO treatment guidance. Options include:
  - Watch and wait.
  - Albendazole alone.
  - Albendazole ± percutaneous treatment (± modified catheterization) ± surgery (albendazole to reduce risk of recurrence or as primary treatment in inoperable cases).

- Note albendazole needs to be given at least 4 days prior to any attempted procedure to avoid fatal allergic reaction from cyst rupture and intraperitoneal spillage.
- Surgical resection usually follows installation of suitable cysticidal agent.
- Percutaneous treatment of the hydatid cysts with **PAIR** (**P**uncture, **A**spiration, **I**njection, **R**e-aspiration) technique.
- Modified catheterization techniques used to remove endocyst and daughter cysts from cavity.
  - Large-bore catheters and cutting devices together with an aspiration apparatus.
- Most procedures have potential for anaphylaxis and secondary spread of infection.

KEY FEATURES: SUMMARY (SEE TABLE 35.1)

- Autoinfection is unique to *Strongyloides*.
  - Other helminths that exhibit this include *Paracapillaria* and *Hymenolepis* (not covered in this chapter).
- Transient lung migration as part of life cycle: *Ascaris*, hookworm (*Ancylostoma*, *Necator*), *Strongyloides*, *Paragonimus*.
- Tissue nematodes: adult worms do not multiply in the human host – dead-end host.
- Helminth infections that usually do not require antiparasitic treatment: *Angiostrongylus* (antiparasitic drug is contraindicated), *Anisakis*, and *Toxocara*.
- Treatment: see Table 35.2.

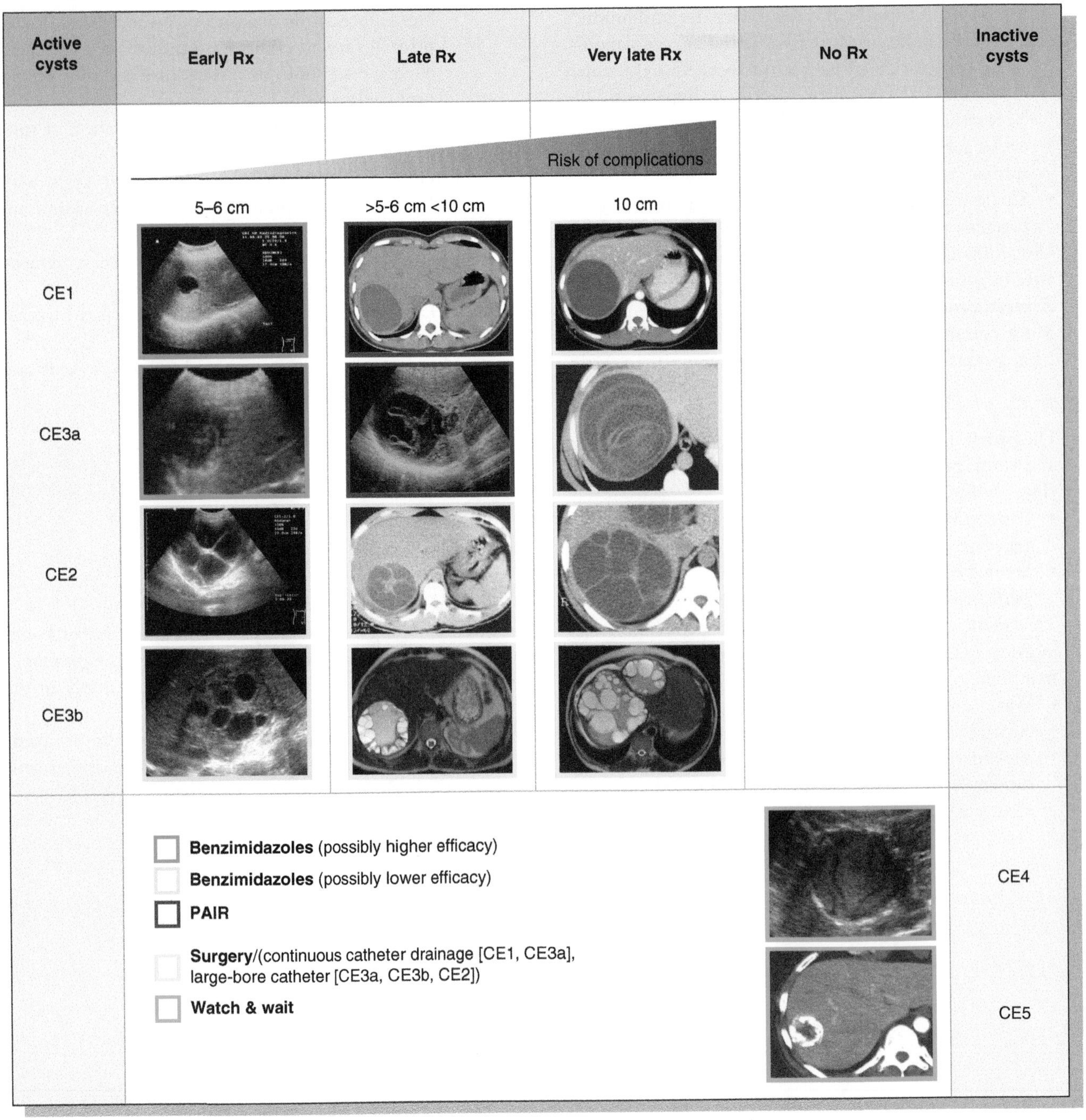

Active cysts	Early Rx	Late Rx	Very late Rx	No Rx	Inactive cysts

Risk of complications

5–6 cm | >5-6 cm <10 cm | 10 cm

CE1

CE3a

CE2

CE3b

☐ **Benzimidazoles** (possibly higher efficacy)
☐ **Benzimidazoles** (possibly lower efficacy)
☐ **PAIR**
☐ **Surgery**/(continuous catheter drainage [CE1, CE3a], large-bore catheter [CE3a, CE3b, CE2])
☐ **Watch & wait**

CE4

CE5

• **Fig. 35.32** Assignment of treatment modalities to individual CE (cystic echinococcosis) cyst stages and risk of complications in relation to cyst stage and size. Involution – CE cysts are driven from active cyst stages to inactive, dead cysts (natural involution). In the "watch and wait" approach (CE4 and CE5), natural involution is observed, and the patient is followed-up at regular intervals to detect complications and to ensure relapse-free. Benzimidazoles (albendazole usually) and percutaneous sterilizing techniques [mostly puncture – aspiration – injection – respiration (PAIR); in some centers continuous catheter drainage and large-bore catheters] – natural involution is accelerated. Surgery – parasitic material is completely removed from the patient either by removal of the parasite-derived cyst and part of the host-derived connective tissue capsule (pericyst): partial cystectomy; by removal of the parasite-derived cyst and the entire host-derived connective tissue capsule (pericyst): total cystectomy or by additional removal of part of the organ the CE cyst is embedded in: resection. Rx = treatment. (Images copyright © W. Hosch, Department of Radiology, Heidelberg University Hospital. Reproduced from Stojkovic M. Echinococcosis. In Farrar J, et al., eds. *Manson's Tropical Diseases*. 23rd ed. Elsevier; 2014.)

TABLE 35.1 Major Features of Globally Important Human Parasitic Helminths

Parasite (Common Name)	Zoonotic Host(s) or Vector	Transmission	Definitive Location Within Human Host	Key Pathological Manifestations[a,b]
Nematodes (Roundworms)				
Intestinal Roundworms				
Ascaris lumbricoides	-	Infective egg ingestion	Small bowel – free luminal	Transient pneumonitis, nutritional deficiencies, hepatobiliary obstruction, and secondary infection
Necator americanus (Hookworm)	-	Percutaneous penetration filariform larvae	Small bowel – attached	Iron deficiency anemia and protein malnutrition (blood loss)
Ancylostoma duodenale (Hookworm)	-	Percutaneous penetration filariform larvae	Small bowel – attached	Iron deficiency anemia and protein malnutrition (blood loss)
Trichuris trichiura (Whipworm)	-	Infective egg ingestion	Small bowel – superficial mucosa	Chronic abdominal pain, iron deficiency anemia, rectal prolapse, trichuris dysentery syndrome
Strongyloides stercoralis[c]	-	Filariform larvae percutaneous penetration/ autoinfection	Small bowel – embedded	Recurrent rashes, larval currens, hyperinfection, and disseminated strongyloidiasis syndromes
Enterobius vermicularis (Pinworm)[c]	-	Infective egg ingestion	Cecum, appendix, colon – free luminal	Local itch (usually perianal), uncommonly ectopic disease
Tissue Roundworms				
Trichinella spiralis	Pigs, horses, and other mammals	Ingestion of contaminated meat (encysted larvae)	Striated muscle	Prolonged GI irritation/ inflammation, periorbital/facial edema, fevers, malaise, rash, and conjunctivitis
Dracunculus medinensis (Guinea worm)	Freshwater crustaceans (copepods)	Ingestion copepods (infective larvae)	Subcutaneous tissue	Local inflammatory reactions with painful skin blistering and swelling
Wuchereria bancrofti (Lymphatic filariasis)	Anopheles, Culex, and Aedes spp.	Blood-feeding insect	Lymphatic system	Chronic lymphoedema (limbs), hydrocele, and orchitis, funiculitis
Brugia malayi (Lymphatic filariasis)	Anopheles, Culex, and Aedes spp.	Blood-feeding insect	Lymphatic system	Chronic lymphoedema (limbs), hydrocele, and orchitis, funiculitis
Loa loa (African eye worm)	Chrysops spp. (female tabanid redflies)	Blood-feeding insect	Subcutaneous tissue	Subcutaneous and conjunctival swelling
Onchocerca volvulus (River blindness)	Simulium spp. (blackflies)	Blood-feeding insect	Subcutaneous tissue/ muscle	Painless subcutaneous/ intramuscular nodules, dermatitis, atrophy, depigmentation, keratitis causing blindness (punctate followed by sclerosing)

Continued

TABLE 35.1	**Major Features of Globally Important Human Parasitic Helminths—cont'd**			

Parasite (Common Name)	Zoonotic Host(s) or Vector	Transmission	Definitive Location Within Human Host	Key Pathological Manifestations[a,b]
Trematodes (flukes)				
Schistosoma mansoni	*Biomphalaria* spp.	Percutaneous penetration cercariae	Mesenteric venules	Hepatosplenomegaly peri-sinusoidal egg granulomas, Symmers' pipe-stem periportal fibrosis, portal hypertension, rarely embolic CNS egg granulomas
Schistosoma japonicum	*Bulinus* spp.	Percutaneous penetration cercariae	Mesenteric venules	Hepatosplenomegaly peri-sinusoidal egg granulomas, Symmers' pipe-stem periportal fibrosis, portal hypertension, rarely embolic CNS egg granulomas
Schistosoma haematobium	*Oncomelania* spp.	Percutaneous penetration cercariae	Lower urinary tract venules	Fibrotic contracted bladder – calcified eggs and granuloma, complicating carcinoma bladder (SCC), damage to female genital tract
Fasciola hepatica (Liver fluke)	*Lymnaea* spp.	Ingestion contaminated watercress, other aquatic plants	Bile ducts	Urticaria, high fever, tender hepatomegaly, icterus, anemia, inflammation, and intermittent obstruction of bile ducts
Clonorchis sinensis (Chinese liver fluke)	*Bithynia* spp./ freshwater fish	Ingestion metacercariae-contaminated fish	Bile ducts, pancreatic ducts	Hepatomegaly, pigment stones, cholangitis, cholecystitis, liver abscesses, increased risk cholangiocarcinoma (hyperplastic biliary epithelium)
Opisthorchis spp.	*Bithynia* spp./ freshwater fish	Ingestion metacercariae-contaminated fish	Bile ducts, pancreatic ducts	Hepatomegaly, pigment stones, cholangitis, cholecystitis, liver abscesses, increased risk cholangiocarcinoma (hyperplastic biliary epithelium)
Paragonimus westermani (Oriental lung fluke)	*Semisulcospira, Oncomelania, Thiara* spp./ freshwater crabs, crayfish	Ingestion metacercariae-contaminated crabs, crayfish	Lung parenchyma	Pathological picture similar to chronic bronchitis and/or bronchiectasis
Fasciolopsis buski (Intestinal fluke)	*Segmentina* spp./ aquatic plants	Ingestion metacercariae-contaminated aquatic plants	Small bowel	Duodenal mucosal inflammation, ulceration, and abscesses
Cestodes (Tapeworms)				
Intestinal Tapeworms				
Taenia saginata (Beef tapeworm)	Cattle	Ingestion cysticerci in bovine muscle	Intraluminal bowel	Psychological distress and anxiety
Taenia solium (Pork tapeworm)	Pigs	Ingestion cysticerci in porcine muscle (larval cysts)	Intraluminal bowel	Cysticercosis (autoinfection with parasite eggs), psychological distress and anxiety

TABLE 35.1 **Major Features of Globally Important Human Parasitic Helminths—cont'd**

Parasite (Common Name)	Zoonotic Host(s) or Vector	Transmission	Definitive Location Within Human Host	Key Pathological Manifestations[a,b]
Diphyllobothrium latum (Fish tapeworm)	Cats, small mammals, wolves, bears	Ingestion of contaminated freshwater fish (plerocercoid cysts)	Intraluminal bowel	Megaloblastic anemia secondary to vitamin B12 deficiency (± concurrent folate deficiency)
Larval Tapeworms				
Larval *Taenia solium* (Cysticercosis)*	Pigs, humans	Ingestion of *T. solium* eggs (embryonated eggs or gravid proglottids) (human feces)	Tissue infection; commonly CNS	Neurocysticercosis; seizures, intracranial hypertension, intraparenchymal cerebral cysts, cerebritis, meningitis, hydrocephalus
Echinococcus granulosus (Cystic hydatid)	Dogs, sheep, goats, camels, horses, cattle, and pigs	Ingestion of infective eggs in contaminated food, water, or soil, or direct contact with animal hosts	Liver, lungs	Intrahepatic or lung cysts (also brain, heart, and bones); asexual budding forming "daughter cysts" – luminal obstruction and/or secondary bacterial infection (cyst leak/rupture)
Echinococcus multilocularis (Alveolar hydatid)	Foxes, other carnivores, and small mammals (mostly rodents)	Ingestion of infective eggs in contaminated food, water, or soil, or direct contact with animal hosts	Liver	Liver cysts asexual lateral budding; tumor-like tissue invasion and "metastasis" to ectopic sites; biliary obstruction, portal hypertension, and Budd–Chiari syndrome

[a]Generally accepted that the majority of parasitic helminth infections are rarely symptomatic.
[b]Many chronic severe helminth infections – either as single or co-infection, will lead to childhood growth retardation, impaired cognitive function, poor school performance, and ultimately contribute to decreased economic productivity and potential.
[c]Person-to-person transmission possible.

TABLE 35.2 **Summary of Antiparasitic Treatment**

Parasite	First-Line Treatment
Nematodes	Albendazole with the exception of: • *Strongyloides*: ivermectin • *Wuchereria*, *Brugia*: DEC • *Loa loa*: DEC (avoid in co-infection with *Onchocercus* and in high *L. loa* microfilaremia) • *Onchocercus*: ivermectin (avoid DEC)
Trematodes	PZQ with the exception of: • *Fasciola*: triclabendazole
Cestodes	Albendazole and/or PZQ

DEC, diethylcarbamazine citrate; PZQ, praziquantel.

Further Reading and Useful Resources

1. Bennett JE, Dolin R, Blaser MJ, eds. *Mandell, Douglas, and Bennett's Principles and Practice of Infectious Diseases*. Updated 8th ed. Elsevier; 2015.
2. WHO Neglected Tropical Diseases. Latest information regarding epidemiology, global treatment programs, eradication updates and current news: http://www.who.int/neglected_diseases/en/.
3. UpToDate (Wolters Kluwer). www.uptodate.com: Extensive repository of evidence-based resources.
4. Sanford Guide of Antimicrobial Chemotherapy: for US anti-helminth chemotherapy (use most up-to-date edition). https://www.sanfordguide.com/.
5. British National Formulary: for UK regimens, doses, and availability (use most up-to-date edition): https://bnf.nice.org.uk/drug/.

36

Natural History of HIV

STEFAN GEORGE

Epidemiology

History

- The first reported cases of human immunodeficiency virus (HIV) were in the early 1980s. Since then, roughly 76.1 million people have been diagnosed with HIV and around 35 million have died.
- The global incidence of HIV infections for adults aged 15–49 reached an estimated peak in 1997 of 0.11% and has declined since.
- The introduction of antiretroviral therapy (ART) in 1996 has resulted in a dramatic decrease in HIV-related morbidity and mortality. For example, Fig. 36.1 shows the effect of mortality in people with HIV of all ages following the introduction of ART in the United States.
- While the global incidence of HIV is now in decline, the introduction of ART has resulted in an overall increased prevalence of HIV, likely due to increased survival of people with HIV as more people access treatment. Fig. 36.2 illustrates this trend showing the increase in number of people aged 50 and over living with HIV by world region.

Global HIV Statistics

- In 2016 there were an estimated 36.7 million people living with HIV (PLWH). 17.8 million of these were women (around half) and 2.1 million were children (<15 years).
- Roughly 19.5 million PLWH (around 53%) were accessing ART.
- Fig. 36.3 shows the global prevalence of HIV by region in 2016.
- **Sub-Saharan Africa**
  - In 2016 there were 19.4 million PLWH in Eastern and Southern Africa and 6.1 million in Western and Central Africa, meaning roughly 5% of the adult population of this region is affected.
  - This accounts for nearly 70% of the global prevalence of HIV infection.
  - Women account for nearly 60% of these infections.
  - In Eastern and Southern Africa roughly 60% of PLWH were accessing ART in 2016, and in Western and Central Africa only around 35% were accessing ART.
- **Asia and the Pacific**
  - There were an estimated 5.1 million PLWH in Asia and the Pacific in 2016.
  - India has the highest number of PLWH in the region (around 2.1 million).
  - Prevalence is highest in Southeast Asia where commercial sex work, MSM, and injection drug use are the primary modes of transmission.
- **Latin America**
  - There were an estimated 1.8 million PLWH in Latin America in 2016, with nearly half of new infections occurring in Brazil, which has the highest prevalence in the area.
  - ART coverage has increased substantially in the region.
- **Eastern Europe and Central Asia**
  - There were an estimated 1.6 million PLWH in this region in 2016.
  - The epidemic here is being driven primarily by injection drug use, with heterosexual transmission also playing an important role.
- **Western and Central Europe and North America**
  - There were an estimated 2.1 million PLWH in this region in 2016.
  - High ART coverage in these regions has played a key role in the reduction of AIDS-related deaths, and numbers of PLWH in all countries have stayed steady or increased as people are living longer with the infection.
  - Men account for the majority of HIV infection here, with roughly 2.5 men with HIV for every woman.
  - In these high-income countries there is a significant ethnic disparity in HIV prevalence, with ethnic minority groups having a higher prevalence compared to the general population. In Western Europe approximately 35% of AIDS cases reported in 2006 were among migrants.

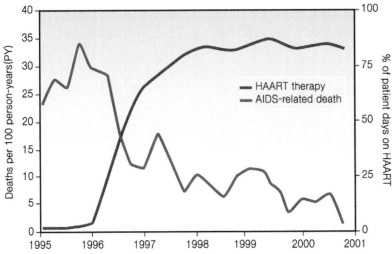

• **Fig. 36.1** Combination therapy and its impact on the AIDS-related deaths. (HAART = highly active antiretroviral therapy.) (From Ryu W-S. *Molecular Virology of Human Pathogenic Viruses.* Elsevier; 2016.)

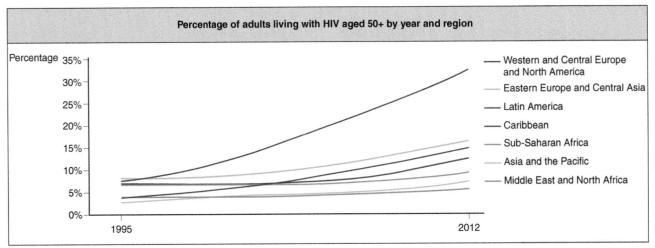

• **Fig. 36.2** Percentage of adults living with HIV aged 50+ by year and region. (From HIV and aging. A special supplement to the UNAIDS report on the global AIDS epidemic 2013. Figure 2. http://www.unaids.org/sites/default/files/media_asset/20131101_JC2563_hiv-and-aging_en_0.pdf.)

United States
- There were an estimated 1.1 million PLWH in the United States at the end of 2015.
- Men who have sex with men (MSM) are by far the most affected subpopulation (Fig. 36.4).
- As with other high-income countries, there is marked ethnic disparity in HIV prevalence in the United States, (Fig. 36.4), with African Americans and Hispanic Latinos being disproportionately affected.

Pathogenesis

Virology
- Human immunodeficiency virus is part of the *Lentivirus* genus belonging to the family *Retroviridae.*
- Two distinct species exist: HIV-1 and HIV-2. HIV-1 is responsible for the majority of infections globally. HIV-2

has a lower virulence and infectivity and is largely confined to West Africa.

Replication Cycle
- HIV targets the cellular immune system. Its specific targets include CD4+ T cells, macrophages, and dendritic cells.
- Fig. 36.5 depicts the stages involved in the HIV replication cycle.
- Glycoprotein (GP)-120 is the viral envelope protein which binds to the CD4 receptor on the target cell membrane allowing the viral capsid to enter the cell via endocytosis.
- Viral RNA is released into the host cell along with the *reverse transcriptase* enzyme which copies the RNA into viral DNA. This is transported to the cell nucleus and integrated into the host cell's genome using the *integrase* enzyme.

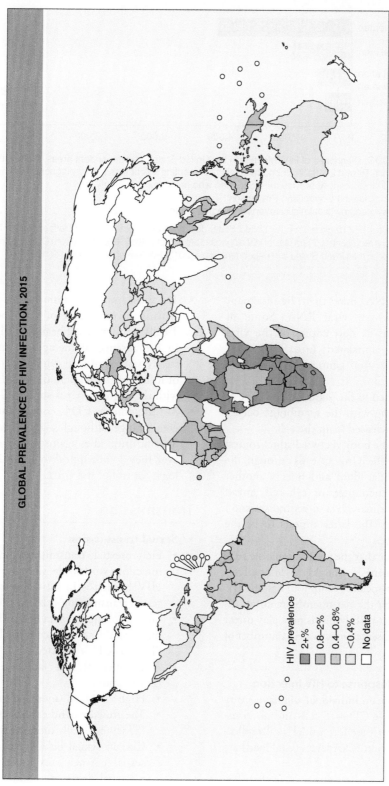

GLOBAL PREVALENCE OF HIV INFECTION, 2015

HIV prevalence
- 2+%
- 0.8–2%
- 0.4–0.8%
- <0.4%
- No data

• **Fig. 36.3** Global prevalence of HIV infection, 2015. Note: Data are estimates. Prevalence includes adults ages 15–49.) (From the Joint United Nations Programs on HIV/AIDS.)

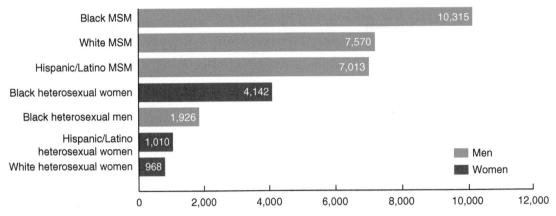

Source: CDC. Diagnoses of HIV infection in the United States and dependent areas, 2015. HIV Surveillance Report 2016;27. Subpopulations representing 2% or less of HIV diagnoses are not reflected in this chart. Abbreviation: *MSM*, men who have sex with men.
Centers for Disease Control and Prevention
https://www.cdc.gov/hiv/statistics/overview/ataglance.html

• **Fig. 36.4** New HIV diagnoses in the United States for the most-affected subpopulations, 2016. Note: Subpopulations representing 2% or less of HIV diagnoses are not reflected in this chart. (From CDC. Diagnoses of HIV infection in the United States and dependent areas, 2015. HIV Surveillance Report 2016; 27.)

• The integrated viral DNA may then lie dormant or be transcribed into new viral RNA. Some of this viral RNA functions as new copies of the viral genome and some is translated into HIV proteins, which package the viral genome creating new virions.

• New virions are transported to the plasma membrane of the host cell, and budding with the membrane occurs allowing the virus to be released from the cell.

• HIV can spread through the body via two distinct routes: cell-free spread whereby the virus spreads through the bloodstream or extracellular fluid and infects another host cell upon chance encounter, or cell–cell spread whereby the virus is disseminated via direct transmission from one cell to another. The latter appears to be the more efficient mechanism.

• There is emerging evidence that the gut microbiome may play a role in HIV pathogenesis. Roughly 60% of CD4+ T cells are found in gut-associated lymphoid tissue. HIV infection is known to alter the gut microbiota composition, and it is thought that this dysbiosis may play direct roles in mediating some disease processes via a number of potential mechanisms.

The Course and Immune Response to HIV Infection

• Following initial infection, an individual will have a very high number of susceptible CD4+ T cells and no virus-specific immune response; therefore initial viral replication is rapid and plasma viral RNA levels (viral load) are high (Fig. 36.6).

• The risk of transmission is highest during these first few weeks when the viral load peaks. This has significant clinical implications as the individual will often not know they are infected.

• The most important immunologic response to the HIV virus is the emergence of virus-specific CD8+ cytotoxic T-cells, and viral load begins to fall following this.

• In the absence of therapy, an individual will reach a steady state viral load (viral set point) within 6 months of infection (see Fig. 36.6), and this viral load correlates with the degree of virus-specific CD8+ T cells.

• At this point the CD4+ count returns to levels within reference range (although slightly lower than pre-infection).

• Specific antibodies against the virus are generated; however, they do not appear to be significant in the immunologic control of the virus.

Transmission

• **Sexual transmission**
  • Heterosexual transmission accounts for >80% of infections worldwide, since the majority of the world's HIV burden is in sub-Saharan Africa where heterosexual transmission is by far the most common route.
  • Outside of sub-Saharan Africa HIV is more prevalent in males reflecting the fact that MSM are 19 times more likely to be HIV-infected.
  • A number of risk factors increase likelihood of transmission:
    • High viral load (most important).
    • The presence of other sexually transmitted infections (STIs) (especially those causing genital ulcerations).
    • Certain sexual behaviors, such as the number of sexual partners, sex under the influence of recreational drugs, no condom use, and the type of sexual exposure – with receptive anal intercourse carrying the highest risk (Table 36.1).
  • Male circumcision ***reduces*** the risk of transmission.

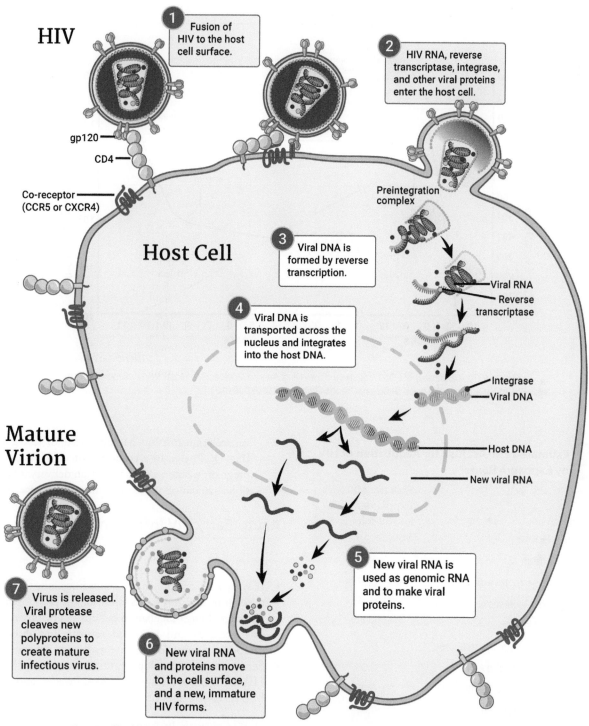

• **Fig. 36.5** The HIV replication cycle. (From National Institute of Allergy and Infectious Diseases. HIV replication cycle. https://www.niaid.nih.gov/diseases-conditions/hiv-replication-cycle.)

- **Parenteral transmission**
  - Outside of sub-Saharan Africa injection drug use accounts for roughly 30% of HIV infections.
- **Perinatal transmission**
  - Mother–child transmission is responsible for over 2 million infants with HIV annually, the majority in sub-Saharan Africa.
  - Transmission can occur in utero, at birth, or via breast feeding.

- Antiretroviral use can nearly eliminate this risk; however, very few women with HIV worldwide (25% or less) have access to appropriate treatment.
- Despite the substantial barriers, the introduction of ART during pregnancy, at delivery, and during breastfeeding has resulted in a significant decrease in perinatal transmission in resource-limited settings.
- In resource-rich settings this decrease has been far more dramatic. For example in the United States

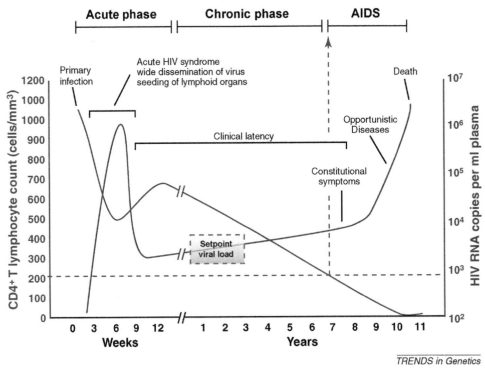

• **Fig. 36.6** Typical course of HIV-1 infection. (From Ping An and Winkler CA. Host genes associated with HIV/AIDS: advances in gene discovery. Trends Genet. 2010;26:119–131.)

TABLE 36.1	Estimated Per-Act Risk for Acquisition of HIV by Exposure Route[a]
Exposure Route	**Risk per 100 Exposures to an HIV-Infected Source**
Blood transfusion	90.
Needle-sharing injection-drug use	0.67
Percutaneous needlestick	0.3
Receptive anal intercourse	0.5
Receptive penile–vaginal intercourse	0.1
Insertive anal intercourse	0.065
Insertive penile–vaginal intercourse	0.05
Receptive oral intercourse	0.01
Insertive oral intercourse	0.005
Mother-to-child transmission (without breastfeeding)	30.
Breastfeeding for 18 months	15.

[a]Estimates of risk for transmission from sexual exposure assume no condom use.
Source: Smith DK, Grohskopf LA, Black RJ, et al. Antiretroviral post-exposure prophylaxis after sexual, injection-drug use, or other nonoccupational exposure to HIV in the United States: recommendations from the U.S. Department of Health and Human Services. *MMWR Recomm Rep.* 2005;54(RR-2):1–20; and Kourtis AP, Lee FK, Abrams EJ, Jamieson DJ, Bulterys M. Mother-to-child transmission of HIV-1: timing and implications for prevention. *Lancet Infect Dis.* 2007;6(11):726–732.

vertical transmission has decreased to less than 2% (Fig. 36.7) due to a combination of HIV testing in pregnant women, cesarean section delivery where possible, avoidance of breastfeeding, and access to ART.

Acute/Early HIV Infection

Time Course

- If symptoms are present in acute infection, they usually develop around 2–4 weeks following the point of infection (although longer incubation periods can be observed).
- The presence and increased severity and duration of symptoms appear to correlate with poor prognosis.
- Seroconversion (development of detectable antibodies to HIV antigens) occurs within 10–24 weeks, and the viral load drops to its set point.

Clinical Presentation

- Approximately 30% of individuals with acute HIV infection are asymptomatic.
- Symptoms mimic infectious mononucleosis caused by cytomegalovirus, Epstein–Barr virus, or *Toxoplasma*.
- When symptoms are present they are varied and non-specific. Potential manifestations include:
  - Constitutional: fever, malaise, myalgia, night sweats, weight loss.
  - Lymphadenopathy, particularly axillary, cervical, and occipital. Persistent generalized lymphadenopathy (PGL) is defined by lymphadenopathy in at least two areas for at least 3 months.

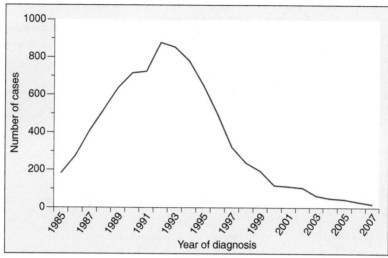

• **Fig. 36.7** Estimated number of perinatally acquired AIDS cases by year of diagnosis, United States, 1985–2007. (Courtesy DHAP, CDC, Pediatric HIV Surveillance.)

• Oropharyngeal: sore throat, painful mucocutaneous ulcers.
• Skin: generalized rash is common.
• Gastrointestinal symptoms: nausea, diarrhea, anorexia, weight loss.
• Neurologic: headache is common. More serious neurologic manifestations such aseptic meningitis, acute inflammatory demyelinating polyneuropathy, or mononeuritis multiplex can rarely occur.
• Recognition of symptoms is important as may provide an opportunity for early diagnosis of HIV. Early recognition can lead to earlier treatment and decreased disease progression and risk of viral transmission.

Long Term Nonprogressor HIV Infection

• A minority of people with HIV maintain a high CD4+ count and relatively low viral load despite remaining therapy-naive.
• Long-term nonprogressors (LTNP) are defined as HIV-infected individuals whose CD4+ count remains >500 cells/μL with a viral load <5000 copies/mL for at least 8 years despite not commencing ART.
• This group is thought to comprise somewhere between 1%–5% of people with HIV.
• Some LTNPs maintain a CD4+ count >500/μL for more than 10–15 years.
• LTNPs remain at increased risk of noninfectious complications of HIV infection (such as cardiovascular disease) in comparison to people without HIV.
• A small subgroup of LTNPs termed **elite controllers** maintain an undetectable viral load (i.e., plasma HIV-RNA remains <50 copies/mL) without commencing ART.
• A combination of host, genetic, and viral factors are thought to contribute to rate of HIV progression and whether someone will exhibit long-term nonprogression.

Diagnostics

When to Test

• HIV testing should be offered and recommended to any patient presenting to healthcare where HIV (including acute infection) enters the differential diagnosis (see section on acute HIV infection), or in any patient with risk factors for HIV infection (see section on transmission).
• Universal HIV testing is recommended in sexual health clinics, antenatal services, termination of pregnancy services, drug dependency programs, and any healthcare service for those diagnosed with tuberculosis, hepatitis B or C virus, or lymphoma.

Diagnostic Testing

• Fig. 36.8 shows the time course of the serologic events associated with acute HIV infection. The various stages of this process have been classified as the Fiebig stages I–VI, and these help explain the methods available for HIV diagnosis.
• The current recommended first line assay is a **fourth-generation test** which is an ELISA testing for both HIV-1/HIV-2 antibodies as well as the p24 antigen (a capsid protein of the virus).
• Because the p24 antigen is detectable before HIV antibodies (Fig. 36.8), fourth-generation tests can detect HIV infection earlier than tests that only detect HIV antibodies (third-generation tests).
• Fourth-generation tests will detect the majority of HIV-infected individuals within 4 weeks of initial exposure. An individual with a negative initial test should undergo repeat testing at around 12 weeks to exclude HIV infection.
• An individual who tests positive should undergo confirmatory testing with an HIV-1/HIV-2 antibody differentiation assay. If this is negative or indeterminate, an HIV-RNA test should be performed (Fig. 36.9).

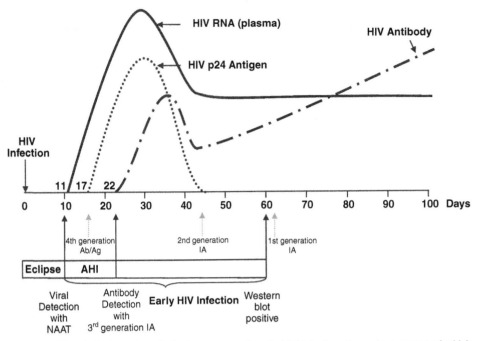

• **Fig. 36.8** The virologic and serologic time course of acute HIV infection, the various stages of which have been termed the Fiebig stages. The appearance of viral RNA at around day 3–8 represents stage I. This is followed by p24 antigen which becomes positive around day 7–14 (stage II). Anti-HIV IgM appears between 10–-17 days (stage III). An indeterminate Western blot develops by 15–23 days (Stage IV), develops a confirmatory pattern with p24 core and env antibody but no antibody to the p31/32 integrase by 47–130 days (Stage V) and then is followed by anti-p31/32 thereafter (Stage VI). (From Patel P, et al. for the CDC AHI Study Group. Rapid HIV screening: missed opportunities for HIV diagnosis and prevention. *J Clin Virol.* 2012;54:42–44.)

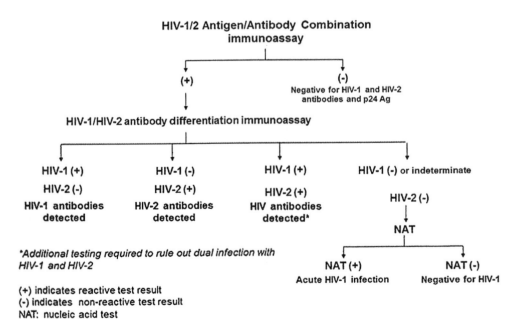

Additional testing required to rule out dual infection with HIV-1 and HIV-2

(+) indicates reactive test result
(-) indicates non-reactive test result
NAT: nucleic acid test

• **Fig. 36.9** Recommended HIV testing algorithm in the United States. If the fourth-generation test is positive, an HIV-1/HIV-2 antibody differentiation assay should be performed. If this is negative or indeterminate, an HIV-RNA (viral load) test should be performed. (From Smith C, McFarland E. Update on pediatric human immunodeficiency virus infection. *Adv Pediatr.* 2016;63(1):147–171.)

- HIV-RNA assays (viral load) are generally not recommended as screening tests.
- **Point of care testing (POCT)** is also available, which can give a result within minutes from a fingerprick or mouth swab sample. These have reduced sensitivity and specificity compared to fourth-generation tests, however, and should only be used in a clinical situation where a rapid result is vital, and all POCT tests should be followed up with a standard fourth-generation test.

Prevention

A number of strategies exist to help prevent the spread of HIV, and these focus around the various risk factors and mechanisms of HIV transmission.

- **Sexual transmission**
  - Comprehensive sexual education and encouraging a reduced number of sexual partners.
  - Promoting consistent use of barrier contraception.
  - Male circumcision is an effective method of reducing female–male HIV transmission.
  - Treatment and prevention of sexually transmitted infections (STIs).
- **Parenteral transmission**
  - Access to needle-exchange programs for intravenous drug users as well as comprehensive addiction treatment programs can help reduce the risk of parenteral HIV transmission.
  - Blood product and donor screening reduces the risk of transfusion-related transmission.
- **Vertical transmission**
  - Maternal testing and effective control of maternal infection.
  - Prenatal ART and treatment of the mother and infant during labor, delivery, and the neonatal period is recommended for mothers with HIV.
  - Breastfeeding should largely be avoided in mothers with HIV unless the local conditions make this unfeasible, unsustainable, or unsafe.
- **Prevention interventions for infected individuals**
  - Effective and early ART is the most effective mechanism of prevention of HIV transmission from individuals known to be infected.
  - Patients known to have HIV should be screened for high-risk behaviors and STIs and should be offered risk reduction counseling as well as partner counseling and referral services.
- **Pre/Postexposure prophylaxis (PEP/PrEP)**
  - PEP and PrEP are both effective tools in HIV prevention and are discussed in detail in Chapter 38.

37

Noninfectious Complications of HIV

LATESHA E. ELOPRE, JAMES HENRY WILLIG, GREER BURKHOLDER, BERNADETTE JOHNSON, AADIA RANA, EDGAR TURNER OVERTON

Neurologic Complications

- **HIV-associated neurocognitive disorders (HAND syndrome)** include changes in memory, concentration, attention, and motor skills that cannot be attributed to an alternative cause. Early after infection, human immunodeficiency virus (HIV) RNA is present in the cerebrospinal fluid (CSF) and may still be present even after viral suppression. This persistent immune response may be responsible for a spectrum of neurocognitive disorders. There are three levels of impairment in neuropsychologic testing, performance and function, including: (1) asymptomatic neurocognitive impairment, (2) mild neurocognitive disorder, and (3) HIV-associated dementia (HAD).
  - Epidemiology: in the postantiretroviral therapy (ART) era, HAD is not as prevalent; however, less severe levels of neurocognitive disease are more common. Risk factors include age >50 years and having metabolic syndrome.
  - Clinical features: classically, HAD symptoms will wax and wane over time, including cognitive deficits, behavioral and mood changes as well as motor symptoms. In mild neurocognitive disorders, patients may report primarily memory problems and generalized slowing in processing information. Overall, cognitive deficits may be described as mental slowing with impairment in higher executive functions leading to decreased ability to perform instrumental activities of daily living (IADLs). Mood disorders vary from apathy to frank psychosis and hallucinations. Motor signs typically result in slowness of movement, but can present on physical exam as hyperreflexia, frontal release signs, and dysdiadochokinesia.
  - Diagnosis is made through exclusion, with neurocognitive impairment found on exam. Work-up should include evaluation for progressive multifocal leukoencephalopathy, malignancy, nutritional deficiencies (vitamin B12 deficiency), endocrine disorders (thyroid or adrenal dysfunction), substance abuse, psychiatric disorders or other dementia syndromes. On imaging, cerebral atrophy may be seen in patient with HAD. Symmetric, periventricular hyperintense lesions on T2-weighted sequences are classically described on magnetic resonance imaging (MRI). In patients not receiving ART, nonspecific CSF findings may include an elevated protein and CSF HIV RNA.
- **Central nervous system (CNS) viral escape syndrome** occurs when there is HIV replication in the CNS leading to neurocognitive symptoms in patents who are virally suppressed on ART. Most patients have viral drug resistance in the CSF.
  - Treatment typically involves initiation of ART. Clinicians should avoid prescribing regimens with efavirenz. For patients with CNS escape syndrome, the CSF HIV RNA must be evaluated for resistance, and a tailored ART regimen is then chosen based on CSF profile.
- **Distal symmetric peripheral neuropathies** (DSPN) is a symmetric, bilateral pattern of diminished sensation and reflexes typically starting in the toes spreading proximally in the lower extremities.
  - Epidemiology: this is commonly seen in persons with advanced disease (CD4 <200 cells/µL and HIV RNA level >10,000 copies/mL), age >50 years, metabolic syndrome, and substance abuse. Historically, it was also associated with older nucleoside reverse transcriptase inhibitors (e.g., didanosine and stavudine). Other drugs associated with DSPN, include dapsone, isoniazid, ethambutol, nevirapine, thalidomide, and vincristine. There is no consensus of the role of coinfection with hepatitis C.
  - Clinical features include numbness and tingling in the lower extremities. On physical exam, decreased sensation in a stocking distribution and reduced deep tendon reflexes in the lower extremities may be present. Upper extremity findings are usually secondary to drug toxicity.
  - Diagnosis is made based on history and physical exam findings. If significant weakness is reported, further work-up is warranted with nerve conduction studies

or electromyography (EMG) to evaluate for other etiologies.

- Treatment includes initiation of ART and symptomatic management.
- **Vascular myelopathy** is a vacuolization of the lateral and posterior columns of the thoracic spine leading to a spastic paraparesis, loss of sensation, and urinary incontinence. The pattern is very similar in presentation to myelopathy from vitamin B12 deficiency.
- **Cerebrovascular disease** is commonly accepted to be more common in persons infected with HIV, both from chronic inflammation secondary to infection and certain ART regimens; however, there is very little supporting data for either. HIV-associated vasculopathies due to HIV infection, HIV-associated cardiac dysfunction leading to cardioembolism, and coagulopathy may all lead to an ischemic event. HIV-associated thrombocytopenia (discussed below) and/or vasculopathy may also lead to a hemorrhagic event. There is now evidence to suggest that long term ART use may also lead to increased risk of stroke due to endothelial toxicity and vascular dysfunction.

Dermatologic Manifestations

- **Acute HIV exanthem and enanthem** is typically a nonpruritic rash involving the upper trunk, proximal limbs, and potentially the palms and soles. It can be seen in up to half of patients with acute infection. It typically resolves in 1–2 weeks (Fig. 37.1).
- **Seborrheic dermatitis** may be severe on initial exam of people living with HIV (PLWH) with advanced disease and is very common. It is described as an eruption on the scalp and central areas of the face (Fig. 37.2).
  - Epidemiology: seborrheic dermatitis can be seen in up to half of patients presenting with advanced HIV infection.
  - Clinical manifestations: dermatitis with faint pink patches and waxy scales typically involve the facial brows and the nasolabial folds. It can also be more widespread and severe, involving the upper chest, axilla, and groin (intertriginous areas). Pruritus is generally absent or mild independent of severity of disease.
  - Pathogenesis is not typically from *Malassezia* infection.
  - Treatment does not differ from the general population and includes mild topical steroids, tar shampoos, and topical fungal creams (e.g., clotrimazole or ketoconazole) to treat inflammation and not actual fungal infection.
- **Eosinophilic folliculitis** is typically described in patients with advanced disease and is a pruritic skin eruption of follicular papules or pustules, predominantly located on the scalp, face, neck, and upper chest (Fig. 37.3).
  - Epidemiology: eosinophilic folliculitis has no gender predilection and is less prevalent since the ART era.

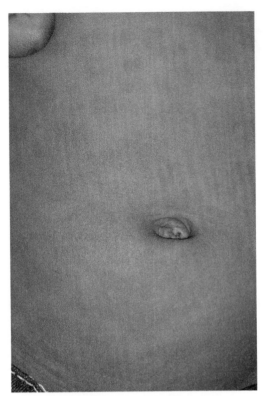

- **Fig. 37.1** Acute HIV exanthem: erythematous, edematous macules are present. (From Ramdial PK, Grayson W. Human immunodeficiency virus (HIV) and acquired immunodeficiency syndrome (AIDS)-associated cutaneous diseases. In: Calonje JE, Brenn T, eds. *McKee's Pathology of the Skin.* 4th ed. Elsevier; 2012.)

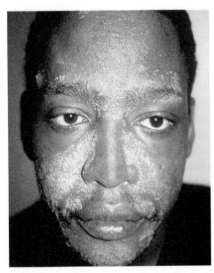

- **Fig. 37.2** Seborrheic dermatitis. (Courtesy William D. James, MD.)

- Pathogenesis: it is believed to be due to infection (with bacteria, *Pityrosporum* yeast, or *Demodex* mites) or an autoimmune reaction to sebocytes.
- Clinical manifestations include recurrent, pruritic, erythematous follicular papules and rare pustules (3–5 mm diameter) on locations of the body with more sebaceous glands. Lab work-up may reveal peripheral eosinophilia and high IgE levels.

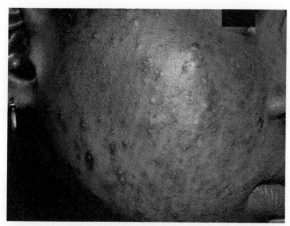

• **Fig. 37.3** HIV eosinophilic folliculitis. Numerous erythematous papules on the face. Excoriation, depigmentation, hyperpigmentation, and scarring are visible. (From Motswaledi M, Hendrick Visser W. The spectrum of HIV-associated infective and inflammatory dermatoses in pigmented skin. *Dermatol Clin.* 2014; https://doi.org/10.1016/j.det.2013.12.006.)

- Diagnosis is made by skin punch biopsy.
- Treatment includes initiation of ART (resulting in resolution for most) and symptomatic management with topical corticosteroids and oral antihistamines.
- **Psoriasis** is more common in PLWH with a similar silvery, plaque-like appearance with more wide distribution on extensor surfaces as well as potentially involvement of the palms, soles, axilla, and groin with associated arthritis. Treatment does not differ from the general population and may include potent topical steroids, ultraviolet light with or without tar, immunosuppressives (e.g., methotrexate), and retinoids.
- **Xerosis** or dry skin may be very severe in patients with advanced disease on presentation. In advanced disease, thickening of the skin can lead to an acquired ichthyosis. Distribution can be widespread but is primarily described on the anterior lower extremities. Risk factors include excessive bathing, and treatment includes emollients and topical corticosteroids.
- **Drug reactions** to trimethoprim–sulfamethoxazole (TMP–SMZ) are more common in persons infected with HIV. Typically drug reactions may be seen 1–2 weeks after initiation for *Pneumocystis jirovecii* pneumonia (PJP) prophylaxis or treatment as a maculopapular/morbilliform, urticarial rash beginning in the groin and pressure areas with subsequent generalized spread. However, more severe manifestations may include exfoliative erythroderma, fixed-drug eruption, erythema multiforme, and toxic epidermal necrolysis.
- **Kaposi sarcoma** (see malignancy section below).

Endocrinopathy

- **Adrenal gland** dysfunction may lead to electrolyte disturbances, hyper- or hypotension and changes in sex hormones. However, most patients are asymptomatic.

Patients with advanced disease presenting with hypotension and critical illness may need to be evaluated. Work-up should include a standard ACTH stimulation test, with high ACTH levels suggesting primary adrenal insufficiency from a potential infection infiltrating the adrenal glands. Steroids should be administered the same as in the general population.
  - Cushing's syndrome may result in patients given ritonavir and nasal or inhaled fluticasone.
  - Infections and cancers that may cause adrenal dysfunction discussed elsewhere may include, but are not limited to, cytomegalovirus (CMV), *Cryptococcus neoformans*, *Mycobacterium avium* complex (MAC), *M. tuberculosis*, toxoplasmosis, PJP, *Histoplasma capsulatum*, Kaposi sarcoma, and lymphoma.
- **Thyroid dysfunction** is common in persons infected with HIV, but there is insufficient evidence to recommend routine screening and most are asymptomatic. Persons with advanced disease are more likely to be diagnosed with hypothyroidism, with subclinical hypothyroidism being the most common abnormality. Subclinical hypothyroidism was particularly more common among patients taking stavudine (an older NRTI [nucleoside reverse transcriptase inhibitor]). Grave's disease has also been described as a consequence of immune reconstitution 1–2 years after initiation of ART. Management for hypo- and hyperthyroidism do not differ from the general population.
- **Gonadal dysfunction** is also very common among persons infected with HIV.
  - Male gonadal dysfunction can be primary (disease of the testes) or secondary (malfunction of the hypothalamus or pituitary gland). Lipodystrophy syndrome (described below) may also be a cause. Prevalence has decreased since the ART era.
  - Low serum testosterone level on lab work-up is typically associated with advanced disease, being on protease inhibitors (PIs) and co-infection with hepatitis C.
  - Clinical features may be fatigue, decreased libido, erectile dysfunction, muscle wasting, weight loss, and loss of body hair.
  - Diagnosis is made with testing testosterone levels between 08.00 and 10.00 hours, followed by a free testosterone assay for those with low levels. LH and FSH can then be checked to determine if the etiology is primary (increased levels) or secondary (normal or low levels).
  - Primary hypogonadism work-up should then include a prolactin level, iron studies, and evaluation of other hormones that reflect anterior pituitary dysfunction.
  - Secondary hypogonadism work-up should then include work-up for opportunistic infections with a scrotal ultrasound.
    - Initiation of ART may result in improvement in hypogonadism. If no improvement is seen, then

treatment with testosterone replacement therapy is indicated in symptomatic patients.

- **Pancreatic dysfunction** can present in patients infected with HIV manifesting as acute pancreatitis, diabetes mellitus, and/or insulin resistance.
  - **Acute pancreatitis** may be due to infection with HIV alone. However, historically it was due to patients on older ART therapy (particularly didanosine) and older regimens for PJP (e.g., pentamidine).
  - Diabetes mellitus and insulin resistance has been associated with several ART regimens, including PIs and older regimens like stavudine and indinavir. However, the chronic inflammation from HIV infection alone may also play a significant risk for development of insulin resistance.
- **Bone mineral dysfunction** due to suboptimal intake of calcium and vitamin D, cigarette smoking, and low testosterone levels may all contribute to ultimate development of osteopenia and osteoporosis in PLWH. Contributing factors, include:
  - Vitamin D deficiency with varying reports on its overall prevalence being higher when compared to the general population.
  - HIV infection which is independently associated with lower bone mineral densities due to proinflammatory cytokines increasing osteoclastic activity.
  - ART-exposure, particularly with tenofovir disoproxil fumarate (TDF) containing ART. This association is not as strong with tenofovir alafenamide (TAF).
- **Hypercalcemia and increased bone metabolism** may result from HIV infection alone or opportunistic infections causing granuloma formations or malignancy. In patients on TDF, higher levels of PTH and conversely lower levels of 25-hydroxy-vitamin D levels may also contribute. TDF use has also been associated with Fanconi syndrome (discussed below), leading to hypophosphatemia, which can lead to osteomalacia. Lastly, efavirenz has been associated with vitamin D deficiency.
  - Screening with a dual X-ray absorptiometry scan (DXA) is recommended in all HIV-infected postmenopausal women and men >50 years of age.
  - Treatment for osteoporosis and osteopenia includes initial evaluation of other causes by checking testosterone levels, PTH, TSH, 25-OH-vitamin D, and 24-hour urine calcium. Otherwise, treatment does not vary, with calcium and vitamin D supplementation if needed as well as bisphosphonate therapy for patients with osteoporosis. It is also suggested to discontinue TDF in patients diagnosed with low bone mineral density.
- **Osteonecrosis** is also more common in patients infected with HIV and classically presents with avascular necrosis of the hip; however, all joints may be infected. Etiology is secondary to insufficient circulation to the bone leading to unilateral joint pain. This is typically diagnosed with MRI of the joint and surgical repair is recommended.

Risk factors include white race, CD4 count <200 cells/µL, prior osteonecrosis, prior fracture, and having an AIDS-defining illness.

- **AIDS wasting syndrome** is still common among PLWH with advanced disease, and weight loss remains a predictor of mortality. It is defined as weight loss over 3 months of more than 10% body weight with a disproportionate loss of lean body mass and sparing of body fat. Hypertriglyceridemia is usually seen on lab work-up. Initiation of ART is essential for management.
- **HIV lipodystrophy syndrome** was more common prior to the ART era and is a constellation of symptoms, including severe wasting and decreased levels of cholesterol with multiple phenotypes described.
  - **Lipoatrophy** is primarily associated with the use of older ART, particularly the NRTIs stavudine and zidovudine. Concurrent use of other classes with NRTIs (i.e., efavirenz, rilpivirine, and PIs) may also increase risk for lipoatrophy.
    - Clinical features involve loss of subcutaneous fat in the face (buccal and/or temporal fat pads), arms, legs, abdomen, and/or buttocks. However, lean tissue mass is typically spared (Fig. 37.4).
    - Diagnosis is made through physical examination.
    - Treatment includes changing ART. In patients with diabetes mellitus, addition of thiazolidinediones has been shown to be beneficial in some studies.
  - **Fat accumulation** can occur to some degree with any ART regimen. It was initially thought to be more common with use of PIs, but this has since been disproven.
    - Clinical features include an excess of visceral adipose fat with normal subcutaneous fat resulting in increased abdominal girth. Fat accumulation may also occur around the dorsocervical area (i.e., "Buffalo hump"), trunk, and upper chest. This can also be seen in visceral organs like the liver.
    - Diagnosis is based on physical exam findings (abdominal circumference in men >102 cm and women >88 cm).
    - Treatment consists of diet, exercise, and treatment of type 2 diabetes mellitus. Metformin is the initial agent recommended unless the patient also has lipoatrophy, which can worsen with metformin.
  - **Metabolic abnormalities** with glucose and lipid metabolism can be associated with lipoatrophy and fat accumulation.
    - Pathogenesis: decreased levels of adiponectin are seen in PLWH who have peripheral lipoatrophy or fat accumulation. This is associated with insulin-resistant type 2 diabetes mellitus.
    - Dyslipidemia is also associated with fat accumulation in PLWH, particularly with increased triglycerides and decreased high-density lipoprotein (HDL) cholesterol.

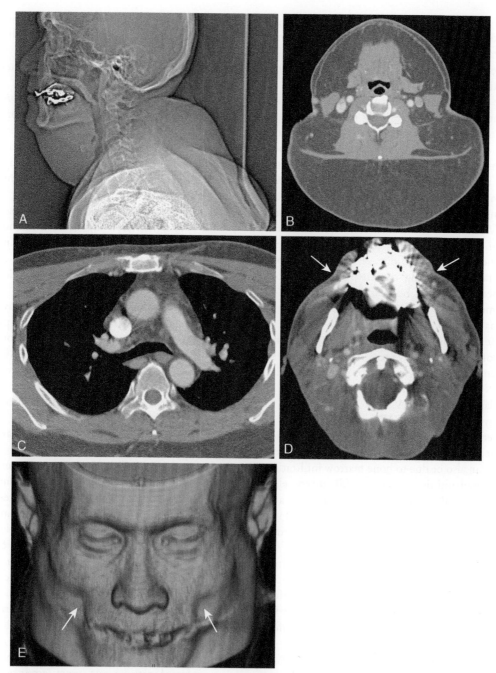

• **Fig. 37.4** (A) Lateral scout film shows the characteristic cervicodorsal hump and anterior cervical tissue prominence seen in HIV lipodystrophy. Axial CT image through the mid neck (B) shows the prominent fat with apparent mass effect on adjacent musculature; however, the amount of fat is markedly disproportionate to what is seen on the chest wall (C). This same patient had characteristic facial features of HIV lipoatrophy, with focal malar skin dimpling (*arrow*) seen on axial postcontrast-enhanced CT (D) and surface-rendered image of the face (E). (From Delman BN, Weissman JL, Som PM. Skin and soft-tissue lesions. In: Som PM, Curtin HD. *Head and Neck Imaging.* Elsevier; 2011.)

Hematologic Manifestations

- **Anemia** is the most common hematologic abnormality seen in patients with advanced HIV infection and is associated with increased mortality. Noninfectious causes include GI bleed, nutritional deficiencies, malignancy, and diminished erythropoiesis due to HIV infection.

Also many opportunistic infections can lead to anemia in patients with advanced disease.

- **Microcytic anemia** can be caused by iron deficiency anemia, intestinal malabsorption, and poor oral intake.
- **Normocytic anemia** can be due to chronic infection leading to hypoplastic anemia commonly from infections such as parvovirus B19 and MAC.

- Hemolytic anemias may also be normocytic (e.g., antibody-mediated, thrombotic thrombocytopenic purpura (TTP), hypersplenism, and drug toxicities in patients with glucose 6-phosphage deficiency).
- **Macrocytic anemia** is most commonly a side effect of drugs due to bone marrow suppression, in particular, zidovudine (which was historically used as a marker of adherence) and reported cases with stavudine and lamivudine. Other causes seen in patients with poor nutritional status such as thyroid dysfunction, vitamin B12, and folate deficiencies should be evaluated.
  - Diagnosis includes iron studies, with the understanding that ferritin can be slightly elevated due to HIV infection and may mask depleted stores of iron. Iron studies are commonly consistent with anemia of chronic disease (low serum iron, low total iron binding capacity, and normal or increased ferritin). If bone marrow aspiration is performed, common findings include a normocellular marrow.
  - Treatment depends on the underlying etiology and initiation of ART in naïve patients.
- **Neutropenia** is defined as an absolute neutrophil count (ANC) <1500/μL, and it can be common in persons diagnosed with HIV.
  - Etiology can be due to ART and drugs used in treatment of opportunistic infections such as zidovudine, TMP–SMX, ganciclovir, and hydroxyurea. It can also be due to bone marrow infiltration from opportunistic infections (discussed elsewhere), viral infections (e.g., parvovirus B12 and Epstein–Barr virus [EBV]), and malignancies. HIV infection may also play a role in effecting normal hematopoiesis.
  - Treatment should include initiation of ART (not including zidovudine), discontinuation of implicated medications, and treatment of possible infection or malignancy. G-CSF should be used only for patients with high risk of possible bacterial infections due to severe neutropenia.
- **Thrombocytopenia** is a very common finding in PLWH and is seen more frequently in patients as their disease progresses. Varying degrees can be found, and there are several etiologies.
  - **HIV-associated thrombocytopenia** is similar in presentation to immune thrombocytopenia purpura (ITP).
  - Noninfectious etiologies include (1) decreased platelet production and (2) reduced platelet survival. Opportunistic infections, malignancies, medications (e.g., heparin), and other comorbidities (i.e., liver cirrhosis) may also cause thrombocytopenia.
  - Decreased platelet production is seen due to the infection of megakaryocytes with HIV, leading to suppression of platelet production in the bone marrow.
  - Platelet survival is reduced due to the presence of antiplatelet antibodies because of the cross-reactivity of IgG with platelet glycoprotein complex (GP)IIb/IIIa and HIV envelope glycoproteins GP 120/120.
  - Clinical manifestations include low platelet counts on laboratory evaluation, but unlike ITP, splenomegaly may also be present on physical exam.
  - Diagnosis of exclusion after evaluation for other causes.
  - Treatment includes initiation of ART and treatment of the underlying disease if present. If thrombocytopenia does not improve after ART initiation and patient is symptomatic with an indication for treatment, then other therapies may be considered, including steroids, intravenous immune globulin, and anti-D immune globulin. In refractory cases, other regimens have reported success, including dapsone, interferon alfa, vincristine, and splenectomy.
- **HIV-associated TTP** was more common in the pre-ART era and in the post-ART era is exceedingly rare and only seen in advanced disease. Co-infection with hepatitis C is also associated.
  - Etiology is not clear, with some case studies showing only a fraction of PLWH presenting with TTP or hemolytic uremic syndrome (HUS) also having decreased levels of ADAMTS12. Another explanation is potentially the effect of HIV also infecting endothelial cells leading to release of von Willebrand factor and subsequent clearance of ADAMTS13.
  - Clinical manifestations are the same as the general population with typically thrombocytopenia, a microangiopathic hemolytic anemia (with presence of schistocytes), end-organ damage (typically renal dysfunction), and an elevated lactate dehydrogenase without another explanation.
  - Diagnosis is clinical and should include work-up for other etiologies like infection with Shiga toxin-producing organisms (*Escherichia coli* or *Shigella* species).
  - Treatment is currently plasma exchange for TTP and initiation of ART.
- **Coagulation abnormalities** are well described in HIV-infected patients, leading to higher likelihood to develop clots.
  - Venous thrombosis is more commonly seen in HIV-infected patients >45 years, advanced disease (lower CD4 counts and higher viral loads), acutely hospitalized, or have other malignancies. Etiologies may be due to:
    - Antiphospholipid antibodies.
    - Deficiency of proteins C and S.

Kidney Complications

- **HIV-associated nephropathy** (HIVAN) is a collapsing form of segmental glomerulosclerosis and can be seen after seroconversion and throughout disease progression, but is more common in patients with advanced disease.
  - Etiology can be due to HIV infection of the kidney's epithelial cells directly or other host factors leading to increased susceptibility.
  - Epidemiology: HIVAN is more common in African Americans. Overall incidence has declined with ART.

- Clinical manifestations include nephrotic range proteinuria (but lesser degrees can be present) and rapid decline in kidney function with most patients progressing to end-stage renal disease requiring dialysis. Other associated findings may include lower extremity edema and hypertension.
- Diagnosis is made by kidney biopsy.
- Treatment includes initiation of ART and possibly initiation of an angiotensin-converting enzyme (ACE) inhibitor or angiotensin II receptor blocker (ARB). Patients should also be referred to a nephrologist for management of their chronic kidney disease.
- **Immune complex-mediated glomerulonephritis** has been reported in patients with HIV and may be diagnosed instead of HIVAN with kidney biopsy, including membranous nephropathy, membranoproliferative and mesangial proliferative glomerulonephritis, "lupus-like" proliferative glomerulonephritis, IgA nephropathy, and HIVICK (HIV immune complex disease of the kidney). Although nonspecific, the pathologic finding of collapsing glomerulopathy (i.e., global collapse of capillary tufts) is commonly seen among PLWH. Other infectious causes of collapsing glomerulopathy include parvovirus B19 and CMV.
- **Fanconi syndrome** is a proximal renal tubular acidosis caused by generalized dysfunction of the proximal renal tubule leading to hypokalemia and hypophosphatemia from renal and phosphate and potassium wasting, renal glucosuria (even in the presence of normal serum glucose), aminoaciduria, and tubular proteinuria. In PLWH, cases have been reported secondary to TDF. Secondary rhabdomyolysis as a result of hypokalemia can occur.
- **Acute kidney injury** is common in patients infected with HIV with decreased incidence since introduction of ART. Older age and other comorbidities such as diabetes mellitus, chronic kidney disease, and liver disease are all risk factors. In patients with advanced disease, it can be associated with septicemia leading to acute tubular necrosis. A number of ART agents are also renally cleared and can lead to acute kidney injury (AKI), including protease inhibitors (e.g., indinavir and atazanavir) and TDF. These complications can be avoided with use of new regimens containing tenofovir alafenamide (TAF), a prodrug of TDF.
- **Chronic kidney disease** is more common in persons infected with HIV than the general population. Risk factors include hepatitis C co-infection, low CD4 count, and other comorbidities like diabetes mellitus and hypertension. Causes, outside of common comorbidities, can include HIVAN, glomerulonephritis from HCV co-infection, and immune complex-mediated glomerulonephritis.

Cardiovascular Complications

- **Cardiovascular disease** is becoming a very common problem in the post-ART era of HIV among aging patients, including increased risk for stroke, myocardial infarction, and sudden cardiac death. Contributing factors include ART, traditional cardiovascular risk factors (dyslipidemia, hypertension, diabetes, and cigarette smoking), and HIV infection in and of itself.
  - ART has been shown in many studies to have an association with myocardial infarction (MI); however, several studies also suggest viral suppression to be associated with decreased MI risk as well. In particular, interruption of ART has been associated with cardiovascular disease.
  - PIs, in particular lopinavir–ritonavir and indinavir, have been shown to have an association with cardiovascular events.
  - Abacavir has been associated with increased risk of MI.
  - ART associated with better lipid profiles include integrase inhibitors, rilpivirine, and first-line NRTIs like tenofovir and emtricitabine have not been shown to adversely affect lipid profiles.
- **Hypertension** is also more common in persons infected with HIV. This may be due to prolonged use of ART >5 years, but no specific ART regimens have been identified. Other common comorbidities also increase risk for cardiovascular disease, including cigarette smoking, substance abuse, diabetes mellitus, and hyperlipidemia.
- **Focal myocarditis** has been described on autopsies of PLWH. More contemporary data have shown signs on MRI of prior myocarditis. However, patients are typically asymptomatic.
- **AIDS cardiomyopathy** is not a very common manifestation of HIV, even prior to the ART era. But when present, the clinical presentation and treatment is similar to the general population.
- **Pericarditis** was very common prior to the ART era and patients with advanced disease. Clinical signs and symptoms are consistent with a pericardial effusion and most patients are asymptomatic. Etiology is usually infectious and may be due to bacterial infection, neoplasm, and fungal infections. A pericardiocentesis or biopsy is usually recommended for work-up, and management varies based on the etiology.

Pulmonary Complications

- **Chronic obstructive pulmonary disease (COPD)** is more common in PLWH with a smoking history. It typically presents at a younger age and is more prevalent among African Americans. Possible etiologies include chronic inflammation from HIV infection and increased likelihood due to ART.
  - Clinical features are the same for persons not infected with HIV.
  - Diagnosis is based on spirometry results showing a reduction in FEV_1, FVC, and FEV_1/FVC ratio.
  - Treatment does not differ from the general population.
- **HIV-associated pulmonary hypertension** is more common in persons infected with HIV and overall risk increases with age. It typically progresses to heart failure within 1–2 years of diagnosis despite therapy.

- Pathogenesis: Primary pulmonary hypertension is thought to result in part from vascular changes resulting in remodeling of the media and adventitia of the arterial pulmonary tree, the extracellular matrix and plexiform lesions induced by infection with HIV-1. However, secondary pulmonary hypertension may be due to other comorbidities like COPD, interstitial pulmonary disease, microembolism from drug use, essential hypertension, chronic thromboembolism, and valvular heart disease.
- Clinical features include dyspnea on exertion, fatigue, angina, presyncope or syncope, and peripheral edema.
- Diagnosis is made by cardiac catheterization to measure pulmonary artery pressure, cardiac output, and left ventricular filling pressure. Other findings may include cardiomegaly with enlarged central pulmonary arteries on chest imaging, right axis deviation of echocardiogram, and hypoxia on arterial blood gas.
- Treatment typically involves epoprostenol, inhaled prostacyclin, inhaled iloprost, bosentan, and sildenafil in addition to initiation of ART. Higher CD4 cell counts are associated with longer survival.
- **Nonspecific interstitial pneumonitis** (NIP) is primarily seen in PLWH with advanced disease (CD4 count <200 cells/μL). Histopathologic findings consistent with pneumonitis can also be found in patients who are asymptomatic.
- Epidemiology: the etiology for NIP is unknown and, given that it can be found in asymptomatic persons, prevalence is not really known.
- Clinical features when present include cough, fever, and shortness of breath. Imaging with chest X-rays and computed tomography (CT) scans may be normal or show diffuse interstitial infiltrates.
- Diagnosis is through exclusion of other pathogens. Biopsy is required and typically shows lymphoid aggregates.
- Treatment always includes initiation of ART with likely resolution of symptoms.
- **Lymphocytic interstitial pneumonitis** (LIP) is associated with HIV infection and autoimmune disease.
  - Clinical manifestations often include diffuse lymphadenopathy, peripheral CD8+ T lymphocytosis, and clubbing in children. Imaging findings vary in chest radiographs from normal to diffuse alveolar, nodular, or interstitial infiltration.
  - Diagnosis is based on exclusion of a pathogen on biopsy. Typically lymphocytic infiltration is seen and plasma cells. Septal infiltration differentiates LIP from NIP.
  - Treatment includes initiation of ART, which usually leads to resolution of symptoms.
- **Cryptogenic organizing pneumonia** (COP) typically is characterized by acute or subacute development of flu-like symptoms. On imaging, bilateral opacities are primarily seen, but nodular or linear opacities have also been described. CD8+ T lymphocytes, foamy macrophages,

and a slight increase in neutrophils, eosinophils, and mast cells can be seen on alveolar lavage representing an alveolitis. In this condition, steroids are required in addition of initiation of ART.

Gastrointestinal Manifestations

- **HIV-associated diarrhea** without identified infectious etiology in the post-ART era has been more commonly recognized. This is often due to
  - **ART-associated diarrhea** is historically associated with older classes of PIs. However, even with fixed-dose combination, single-dose ART, incidence in clinical trials of diarrhea varies from 8%–22%. However, most patients have improvement in side effects after 8–12 weeks.
  - Theorized etiologies include damage to the intestinal epithelial barrier and secretory diarrhea from alteration of intestinal chloride ion secretions.
  - **HIV enteropathy** from HIV infection of enterocytes, leading to loss of gastrointestinal mucosa and increased permeability. Also, faster intestinal transit times may result from HIV directly damaging the autonomic nerves of the intestine.
  - Diagnosis should begin with evaluation of infectious etiologies of diarrhea if patients are severely immunosuppressed.
  - Treatment of noninfectious diarrhea often involves dietary modifications and symptomatic management. In patients with no improvement, changing ART regimens may be required.
- **Aphthous ulcers** in PLWH in the oral, non-keratinized mucosa are commonly reported with unknown etiology. They are typically well-circumscribed ulcers with erythematous margins and appear to be exacerbated with stress. Ulcers are typically painful and do not resolve for several weeks. Only if ulcers persists or are atypical is further work-up required with biopsy to rule out infections such as histoplasmosis or malignancy. Treatment is usually successful with topical steroids mixed with an oral analgesic. For extensive ulceration throughout the gastrointestinal tract, oral systemic steroids may be necessary.
- **Salivary gland disease and xerostomia** can present with or without salivary gland enlargement and usually involves the parotid gland as well. Enlargement may be due to cysts, but often a lymphocytic infiltrative process is seen on histopathology (unlike the CD4 cell predominance seen in Sjögren's syndrome). The etiology is unknown. Therapy typically involves stimulation of the salivary glands.
  - **Diffuse interstitial lymphocytosis syndrome (DILS):** characterized by CD8+ T-cell infiltration of multiple organs can manifest with bilateral parotid gland enlargement described above. However, it also may affect multiple other organ systems. Primarily described with lung infiltration as a lymphocytic

interstitial pneumonia, other organ systems that may be affected include nervous system, liver, kidneys, and digestive tract.
- Treatment includes initiation of ART, and if this is not sufficient, steroids may be started.
- **Biliary tract disorders** that are noninfectious and associated with HIV infection include acalculous cholecystitis and AIDS cholangiopathy.
  - Acalculous cholecystitis is common in patients with advanced disease; however, it is more commonly associated with infection with CMV or *Cryptosporidium*.
  - AIDS cholangiopathy results in dilated intra- and extrahepatic biliary ducts and presents with right upper quadrant pain, icteric sclera, and elevated alkaline phosphatase. Infectious etiologies are not common in half of patients, but may include *Cryptosporidium*, microsporidiosis, and CMV when found.

Malignancies

- **Kaposi sarcoma** (KS) is a violaceous, low-grade vascular tumor associated with **HHV-8** infection and in the general population is rare and often limited to the lower extremities. In persons infected with HIV, this skin cancer can be very aggressive and invasive and include gastrointestinal as well as respiratory tract organ involvement in advanced stages. However, since the advent of ART, prognosis has been very good with high survival rates in patients with low disease burden.
  - Epidemiology: in the general population, KS most commonly is found in elderly men from the Mediterranean or Central/Eastern European ancestry. However, for persons infected with HIV, KS is considered an "AIDS-defining illness" and is typically seen in PLWH with advanced disease.
  - Clinical features: classically cutaneous disease is primarily reported; however, extracutaneous involvement may also be present in advanced disease.

- Cutaneous disease appears as red or violet macules, papules, or nodules in various sizes up to several centimeters in diameter.
- Extracutaneous involvement can be respiratory, mucosal, or GI and often takes months to years. However, case reports of other visceral involvement have been reported.
  - Oral involvement most commonly involves the palate or gingiva and is present in about a third of PLWH with KS.
  - When respiratory involvement is present, imaging with chest X-ray and chest CTs may show peribronchovascular nodules, consolidation, or diffuse infiltrates or may be normal. (Fig. 37.5) Symptoms may include hemoptysis, shortness of breath, fever, cough, or chest pain.
  - GI involvement can occur in the absence of cutaneous disease. Symptoms for GI involvement may include obstruction, abdominal pain, weight loss, and diarrhea. On endoscopy, hemorrhagic lesions can be found all along the GI tract.
- Diagnosis is made by biopsy. Radiographic evaluation is often not warranted, unless there are suggestive symptoms or associated lab abnormalities. Initial evaluation for visceral involvement may include checking the stool for occult blood and chest X-ray.
- Treatment always includes initiation of antiretroviral therapy. With initiation of ART, immune reconstitution inflammatory syndrome (IRIS) may occur within 2–8 weeks with worsening of symptoms. If there is evidence of rapid disease progression with visceral or respiratory involvement, chemotherapy with liposomal doxorubicin or liposomal daunorubicin may be indicated.
- **Multicentric Castleman's disease** is a lymphoproliferative disorder characterized by angiofollicular lymph node hyperplasia associated with HIV and **human herpesvirus 8 (HHV-8)** infection as well as other malignancies including concomitant KS. Multicentric Castleman's

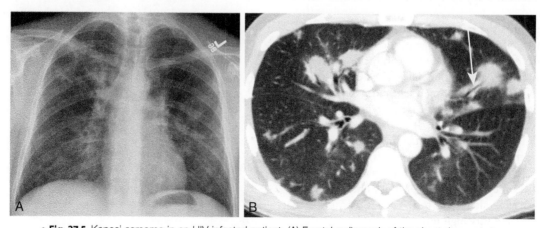

• **Fig. 37.5** Kaposi sarcoma in an HIV-infected patient. (A) Frontal radiograph of the chest demonstrates bilateral predominantly perihilar patchy opacities with poorly defined margins. (B) Axial computed tomography image from the same patient reveals multiple bilateral nodules in a peribronchovascular distribution, some of which demonstrate air bronchograms (*arrow*). (From Natcheva H. Pulmonary disease in the immunocompromised patient. In: Shepard J-AO. *Thoracic Imaging: The Requisites.* Elsevier; 2019.)

disease manifests with systemic symptoms including fever, fatigue, generalized lymphadenopathy, hepatosplenomegaly, and pancytopenia.

- Epidemiology: incidence has increased in HIV-infected patients since the advent of ART. It is more common among older (median age between 50 and 65), non-white men with nadir CD4 counts >200 cells/μL.
- Diagnosis is based on lung biopsy.
- Treatment to treat systemic disease usually requires corticosteroids. Chemotherapy, immune therapy, and radiation may also be necessary based on responsiveness and extent of disease. However, the gold standard for treatment includes rituximab.

- **Non-Hodgkin lymphoma** (NHL) is considered an AIDS-defining illness and overall rates have declined since the introduction of ART. Concomitant infection usually occurs with HHV-8 and/or EBV. In contrast to diffuse large B cell lymphoma in immunocompetent hosts, BCL-2 activation is generally not seen. Other genes affected include *p53* mutation, *bcl6* deregulation, and *c-MYC* overexpression. Prognosis is poor for primary pulmonary lymphoma.

  - Epidemiology: risk factors among PLWH for NHL include CD4 counts <100 cells/μL, high HIV viral loads, family history, and not being on ART. Also, persons co-infected with HIV and either hepatitis B or C are more likely to be diagnosed with NHL. A more favorable diagnosis is associated with PLWH who have a CCR5-32 deletion.
  - Clinical features for patients with pulmonary involvement may include shortness of breath, cough, chest pain, and B symptoms (fever, weight loss, and night sweats).
    - Lab findings include leukopenia, anemia, thrombocytopenia, and elevated serum lactate dehydrogenase (LDH) in persons who do not have primary pulmonary involvement.
  - Diagnosis requires biopsy, which is often achieved with bronchoscopy or percutaneous thoracic needle biopsy.
  - Treatment is the same for primary or secondary pulmonary NHL. Chemotherapeutic regimens often include cyclophosphamide, doxorubicin, vincristine (Oncovin), and prednisone (CHOP) or CHOP–rituximab (CHOP-R) with concurrent initiation of ART.

- **Primary effusion lymphoma** is a rare type of NHL that occurs exclusively in PLWH. It is also associated with HHV-8. This type of lymphoma grows in body cavities (pleural, pericardial, and peritoneal) as lymphomatous effusions that are not associated with a mass. Diagnosis is made based on cytology of the pleural fluid. In contrast to NHL, it lacks alterations to the genes *bcl2*, *bcl6*, *ras*, and *p53*. It has a very high mortality rate.

- **AIDS-related lymphomas** typically occur in patients with advanced disease and commonly include:
  - **Diffuse large B cell lymphoma**: tumors consisting of large, atypical lymphoid patterns that express pan-B cell antigens.

- **Burkitt's lymphoma**: have a "starry-sky" pattern with prominent cytoplasmic vacuoles in monomorphic, medium-sized cells with multiple nuclei.
- **Plasmablastic lymphoma**: rare lymphoma that typically presents in the oral cavity and is driven by HHV-8 infection. They are very aggressive and have a poor prognosis.
- **Hodgkin lymphoma** is very common and is classically defined by Reed–Sternberg cells (Fig. 37.6) among small lymphocytes, eosinophils, neutrophils, histiocytes, and plasma cells.

- **Primary central nervous system lymphoma** is also considered an AIDS-defining illness. Primary CNS lymphoma may present with confusion, memory loss, focal neurologic deficits, and seizures as well as B symptoms. On brain imaging with CT or MRI, solitary or multiple mass lesions may be seen, which differs from toxoplasma encephalitis where multiple lesions are usually found. Lesions also may be ring enhancing or have enhancement that is irregular or patchy. Other differences with toxoplasma encephalitis also include larger size (typically >4 cm) and location (typically not found in the posterior fossa).

  - Epidemiology: overall incidence for CNS lymphoma has declined with the ART era. CNS lymphoma is also more commonly found in HIV-infected patients with advanced disease (CD4 count <200 cells/μL). Prognosis varies with survival rates up to 44 months pending receipt of effective therapy.
  - Diagnosis varies depending on whether there is a lesion with mass effect present. If there is a lesion with mass effect, then lumbar puncture is contraindicated. Stereotactic brain biopsy is the gold standard for diagnosis. However, a trial of empiric therapy for toxoplasmosis may be considered if serologies indicate previous infection and the patient was not taking

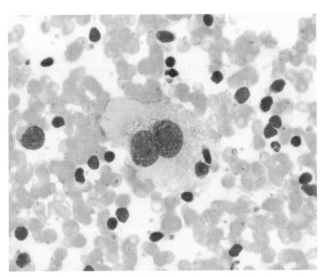

• **Fig. 37.6** Lymph nodes in Hodgkin lymphoma. Note the large mirror-image binucleated lymphoid cell of Reed–Sternberg type with a mixed population of lymphoid cells in the background (MGG). (From Skoog L, Tani E. Lymph nodes. In: Gray W, Kocjan G. *Diagnostic Cytopathology.* 3rd ed. Elsevier; 2010.)

Pneumocystis prophylaxis with TMP–SMX. If there is no focal mass lesion, then cerebral spinal fluid should be collected and sent for cytology, but this is helpful in only 15% of cases.

- Treatment usually consists of high dose methotrexate. Opinion on other chemotherapeutic regimens varies, and there is no evidence-based consensus on additional therapy.

- **Cervical cancer** is an AIDS-defining illness.
  - Epidemiology: cervical intraepithelial neoplasia (CIN) is more common in women living with HIV, as well as the risk for progression to cancer. Women with more advanced disease have the highest prevalence and are more likely to have high-risk HPV types.
  - Etiology: due to immunosuppression from infection with HIV, HPV infection is more commonly not cleared.
  - Screening: there is no consensus of Pap smear recommendations for women who have had hysterectomies.
  - Women <30 years: screening with cervical cytology is recommended at initiation of care (i.e., baseline) and at 12-month intervals for 3 years. If results remain normal during that time, then follow-up intervals become every 3 years.
    - Atypical squamous cells of undetermined significance (ASCUS) with positive HPV testing, colposcopy should be done with repeat cytology in 6–12 months.
    - Low-grade squamous epithelial lesions (LSIL) and higher, colposcopy should be performed.
  - Women ≥30 years: Cervical cytology with or without co-testing of HPV should be done at baseline and then at 12 months for three consecutive years if normal. Then, as above, follow-up intervals become every 3 years.
    - ASCUS with positive HPV, then management is the same as above.
    - LSIL and higher, then management is the same as above.
    - If co-testing was performed with cervical cytology:
      - Co-test negative: cervical cancer screening every 3 years.
      - Cytology-negative, HPV-positive: repeat co-testing in 1 year (unless genotypes 16 or 16/18 and then colposcopy). If abnormal at 1 year, then colposcopy should be performed.
  - Management: for women with colposcopic, biopsies showing CIN II/III or persistent CIN I, ablation and excision are acceptable treatments. If recurrence after ablation, then excision with cryosurgery, cone biopsy or loop electrosurgical excision procedure (LEEP) are acceptable.
  - Initiation of ART has been associated with regression of CIN.
  - If invasive cancer is found, surgical excision, chemotherapy, and radiation are all mainstays of therapy.
- **Anal cancer** is very common in HIV-infected patients reporting anal sex, particularly men who have sex with

men (MSM). The role of whether HIV directly impacts development of cancer or whether it is HPV alone is not clear. However, persons with greater immunosuppression from more advanced disease are more likely to have progression of anal intraepithelial lesions (AIN) to anal cancer.

- Clinical manifestations typically include itching, rectal bleeding or discharge, and tenesmus; however, most patients are asymptomatic.
- Screening: There is no consensus on screening guidelines, but the Infectious Diseases Society of America recommends screening for anal cytology among the following risk groups: MSM, women with history of anal intercourse or abnormal cervical Pap smears, and those with genital warts.
- Management: Referral for high-resolution anoscopy should be considered for any individuals with abnormal results.
- Treatment varies depending on size and severity:
  - Small lesions (<1 cm² base): topical therapy with trichloroacetic acid and imiquimod are reasonable. Intraanal imiquimod can also be used to treat SIL.
  - Larger lesions: infrared coagulation and anoscopy-directed lesion ablation can be used.
  - Invasive cancer includes chemotherapy, radiation, and excision.
- **Lung cancer** is more common in persons infected with HIV when compared to the general population. The most common type of lung cancer seen is adenocarcinoma, and other types also include small cell carcinoma, non-small cell carcinoma, and bronchoalveolar carcinoma.
  - Epidemiology: when compared to the general population, PLWH diagnosed with lung cancer usually present at a younger age. Males are more commonly affected compared to females. Cigarette smoking is still a significant risk factor and patients typically have a CD4 count <500 cells/μL. Mortality rates are also higher for PLWH.
  - Clinical features may include chronic cough, weight loss, shortness of breath, and/or chest pain.
  - Diagnosis is typically made with chest imaging consistent with the type of lung cancer and therefore can have varying patterns from a nodular or diffuse infiltrate, hilar or mediastinal lymphadenopathy, or pleural effusion. Biopsy is required for histologic diagnosis.
  - Treatment does not differ for PLWH and is determined by the type of lung cancer and staging at diagnosis.

Summary of Common HIV-Associated Conditions

Table 37.1 lists common noninfectious conditions associated with immunodeficiency in PLWH.

TABLE 37.1 **Degree of Immunodeficiency and Common Associated HIV Conditions**

Degree of Immunodeficiency	Noninfectious HIV-Associated Condition
Advanced (CD4 <200 cells/μL)	**Cancers** • Lung cancer • Kaposi sarcoma • Non-Hodgkin lymphoma • Primary CNS lymphoma • Cervical cancer **Pulmonary** • Nonspecific interstitial pneumonitis • Lymphocytic interstitial pneumonitis • COPD • Pulmonary HTN • Antiretroviral-induced respiratory disease **Neurologic** HIV-associated dementia Distal symmetric peripheral neuropathy Vascular myelopathy **Endocrinopathies** • Adrenalitis • Hypothyroidism • Male gonadal dysfunction • Avascular necrosis • AIDS wasting syndrome **Dermatology** • Seborrheic dermatitis • Eosinophilic folliculitis • Psoriasis **Hematology** • Cytopenia • HIV-associated thrombocytopenia (but can be seen at any CD4) • HIV-associated TTP **Renal** • HIVAN (but can be seen at any CD4) • CKD (but can be seen at any CD4) **Gastrointestinal** • AIDS cholangiopathy
Moderate (CD4 200–500)	**Cancers** • Lung cancer • Castleman's disease **Neurologic** • HAND
Normal (CD4 >500)	**Cancers** • Castleman's disease **Neurologic** • HAND – CSF viral escape **Endocrine** • Metabolic syndrome

CKD, chronic kidney disease; COPD, chronic obstructive pulmonary disease; HAND, HIV-associated neurocognitive disorders; HIVAN, HIV-associated nephropathy; HTN, hypertension; TTP, thrombocytopenic purpura.

Further Reading

1. Khoury MN, Tan CS, Peaslee M, Koralnik IJ. CSF viral escape in a patient with HIV-associated neurocognitive disorder. *J Neurovirol.* 2013;19(4):402–405.
2. Benjamin LA, Bryer A, Emsley HCA, Khoo S, Solomon T, Connor MD. HIV infection and stroke: current perspectives and future directions. *Lancet Neurol.* 2012;11(10):878–890.
3. Kibirige D, Ssekitoleko R. Endocrine and metabolic abnormalities among HIV-infected patients: a current review. *Int J STD AIDS.* 2013;24(8):603–611.
4. Warriner AH, Burkholder GA, Overton ET. HIV-related metabolic comorbidities in the current ART era. *Infect Dis Clin North Am.* 2014;28(3):457–476.
5. Yoong D, Naccarato M, Gough K. Extensive bruising and elevated rivaroxaban plasma concentration in a patient receiving cobicistat-boosted elvitegravir [published online March 1, 2017]. *Ann Pharmacother.* 2017;51(10):931–932.
6. Brecher ME, Hay SN, Park YA. Is it HIV TTP or HIV-associated thrombotic microangiopathy? *J Clin Apheresis.* 2008;23(6):186–190.
7. Clay PG, Crutchley RD. Noninfectious diarrhea in HIV Seropositive individuals: a review of prevalence rates, etiology, and management in the era of combination antiretroviral therapy. *Infect Dis Ther.* 2014;3(2):103–122.
8. Ghrenassia E, Martis N, Boyer J, Burel-Vandenbos F, Mekinian A, Coppo P. The diffuse infiltrative lymphocytosis syndrome (DILS). A comprehensive review. *J Autoimmun.* 2015;59:19–25.
9. Benifield T. *Clinical Respiratory Medicine.* 4th ed. Elsevier; 2012.
10. Letendre SL, Ellis RJ, Everall I, Ances B, Bharti A, McCutchan JA. Neurologic complications of HIV disease and their treatment. *Topics HIV Med.* 2009;17(2):46–56.

38
Antiretroviral Therapy

JANE A. O'HALLORAN

Antiretroviral Agents

- Approximately 30 agents are currently available for treatment of human immunodeficiency virus-1 (HIV-1) infection, although many are no longer used.
- With the exception of cobicistat (used as a pharmacokinetic enhancer), the remaining agents belong to one of six classes of antiretroviral therapy (Table 38.1).
- Each antiretroviral drug class targets a specific stage in the HIV life cycle (Fig. 38.1).

Nucleoside/Nucleotide Reverse Transcriptase Inhibitors (NRTIs)

Recommended Agents

Tenofovir

Only available nucleotide analog, two prodrugs currently available:

- Tenofovir disoproxil fumarate (TDF)
  - Associated with renal insufficiency, Fanconi's syndrome, proximal renal tubulopathy.
  - Reduced bone mineral density, osteomalacia.
- Tenofovir alafenamide (TAF)
  - Achieves higher intracellular active drug concentrations than TDF at lower oral doses, resulting in lower plasma concentrations and less drug exposure to kidney, bones, and other organs.
  - Can be substituted for TDF in the treatment of HIV and hepatitis B (HBV). Insufficient information for its use in pregnancy at present.
  - Not recommended for CrCl <30 mL/min.
  - **Discontinuation of TDF or TAF in people living with HIV (PLWH) with HIV/HBV co-infection can result in severe acute exacerbation of hepatitis.**

Lamivudine (3TC)/Emtricitabine (FTC)

- Considered clinically interchangeable. Should not be administered together.
- Limited toxicity. FTC can cause hyperpigmentation of the skin.

- **Discontinuation of 3TC/FTC in PLWH with HIV/HBV co-infection can result in severe acute exacerbation of hepatitis.**

Alternative Agents

Abacavir (ABC)

- For use in PLWH with CD4+ T-cell counts >200 cells/μL and HIV RNA <100,000 copies/mL unless paired with dolutegravir.
- **Hypersensitivity** reaction, including rash, fever, respiratory, gastrointestinal, or constitutional symptoms.
- Greater risk in PLWH positive for **HLA B*5701.**
- Associated with increased myocardial infarction risk in some cohort studies.

Zidovudine (AZT)

- Not recommended in treatment-naïve setting, rarely used except in pregnancy.
- Bone marrow suppression including neutropenia and macrocytic anemia, not thrombocytopenia.
- Dyslipidemia, insulin resistance, diabetes mellitus.
- Myopathy.

Nonnucleoside Reverse Transcriptase Inhibitors (NNRTIs)

Recommended Agents

No longer considered recommended (first line) agents in HIV treatment-naïve PLWH. Can be considered for use as alternative agents if INSTI or PIs not appropriate.

Alternative Agents

Efavirenz (EFV)

- Neuropsychiatric symptoms reported in up to 50%, including vivid dreams, dizziness, somnolence, insomnia, hallucinations, depression, and suicidality.
- Teratogenic in pregnant monkeys. Pregnancy registries do not indicate increased risk of teratogenicity in humans. Women who become pregnant while taking EFV and who are virally suppressed should continue their EFV-based regimen.

TABLE 38.1 Characteristics of Antiretroviral Drug Classes

	Mechanism of Action	Metabolism	Class Toxicity
Chemokine receptor antagonists	Attaches to CCR5 coreceptors on the cell surface, preventing strains of HIV that use CCR5 coreceptors from attaching to or entering the cell (Fig. 38.1 *1*)	Predominantly metabolized by CYP3A4	Maraviroc is the only drug in class. Minimal toxicity
Fusion inhibitors	Binds to gp41, preventing the fusion of the virion with the cell (Fig. 38.1 *2*)	Catabolized to its constituent amino acids	Enfuvirtide (T20) only drug in class. Injection site reactions
Nucleoside reverse transcriptase inhibitors (NRTIs)	Structural analogs of normal nucleosides or nucleotides that terminate HIV DNA synthesis by targeting reverse transcriptase (Fig. 38.1 *3*)	Variation within class. ABC: alcohol dehydrogenase and glucuronyl transferase TDF/FTC/3TC: renal excretion TAF: metabolized by the P-glycoprotein substrate, cathepsin A Not substrates of, or induced or inhibited by, the CYP 450 pathway	Lactic acidosis, hepatitis steatosis, lipoatrophy
Nonnucleoside reverse transcriptase inhibitors (NNRTIs)	Binds noncompetitively to reverse transcriptase and blocks polymerization of the viral DNA (Fig. 38.1 *4*)	Metabolized by CYP3A4; may also be inhibitors or inducers of CYP450 pathways	Rash, may cause Stevens–Johnson syndrome or toxic epidermal necrolysis
Integrase strand transfer inhibitors (INSTI)	Binds to HIV integrase and blocks the insertion of HIV pro viral DNA into host cells thus inhibiting HIV-catalyzed strand transfer (Fig. 38.1 *5*)	UGT1A1-mediated glucuronidation ETG (and to a lesser extent DTG) also metabolized through CYP3A4	Overall well tolerated. Rarely depression and suicidal ideation
Protease inhibitors (PI)	Binds to HIV protease preventing the packaging of virions (Fig. 38.1 *6*)	Metabolized by CYP3A4; also inhibitors of the pathway	Dyslipidemia, hyperglycemia, insulin resistance, lipodystrophy

TAF, tenofovir alafenamide; TDF, tenofovir disoproxil fumarate; 3TC, lamivudine; FTC, emtricitabine.

Rilpivirine (RPV)
- For use in PLWH with CD4 T-cell counts >200 cells/μL and HIV RNA <100,000 copies/mL.
- Should be taken with a meal of approx. 400 kcal (protein shake inadequate).
- Requires acid for absorption; concomitant use of proton pump inhibitors (PPIs) not recommended; H_2 antagonists should be taken 12 hours before or 4 hours after.
- Neuropsychiatric side effects (lesser extent than EFV); QTc prolongation.

Doravirine (DOR)
- Available on its own for use with other antiretrovirals or in a fixed dose combination with TDF and 3TC.
- Fewer drug–drug interactions than with other NNRTIs and can be taken with or without food.
- Fewer CNS side effects than with EFV and has a favorable lipid profile.

Integrase Strand Transfer Inhibitors (INSTIs)

Recommended Agents
Raltegravir (RAL)
- Originally only available as twice-daily dosing. Once-daily formulation now available (OD dosing not recommended in pregnancy or for use with rifampin).
- Elevated creatine kinase, muscle weakness, rhabdomyolysis.

Dolutegravir (DTG)
- A higher barrier to resistance than RAL or ETG.
- Requires twice-daily dosing if preexisting INSTI resistance.
- Polyvalent cations (including calcium, iron, and zinc, and antacids that contain these cations) reduce its efficacy and caution required regarding timing of administration.

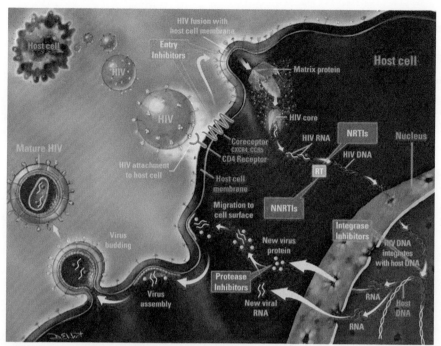

• **Fig. 38.1** Life cycle of HIV: Binding of HIV gp120 surface protein to CCR5, or less commonly, to CXCR4 coreceptors on the surface of CD4+ T cells is the first step in the HIV life cycle and allows the virus to enter host cells. Upon binding to the chemokine coreceptor, HIV gp120/gp41 undergoes a conformational change, resulting in a hairpin-like structure that promotes fusion between the cell membrane and the virion. Once inside the cytoplasm, the viral RNA undergoes reverse transcription using a virally encoded reverse transcriptase to become double-stranded DNA that is transported to the nucleus. On entering the nucleus, the double-stranded DNA integrates into the host chromosomal DNA, mediated by HIV integrase. Newly produced viral RNA is packaged in a virion along with structural proteins and enzymes. The virion then buds into the extracellular environment. The final infectious virion requires cleavage of structural proteins by HIV protease. (Courtesy of David H. Spach, MD, University of Washington.)

• Should be avoided in women who are contemplating pregnancy and if used need to ensure adequate birth control prior to starting women of child-bearing potential as recent concerns for increased rates of neural tube defects in babies conceived on DTG.

Bictegravir (BIC)
• Once-daily preparation that does not require boosting.
• Like DTG, has a high barrier to resistance with activity to most INSTI-resistant variants.
• Eliminated by hepatic metabolism with similar contributions of CYP3A4 and UGT1A1.

Alternative Agents
Elvitegravir (ETG)
• Only available in fixed dose combination.
• Requires **pharmacokinetic enhancing** or **"boosting,"** currently coformulated with cobicistat. Caution regarding drug–drug interactions.

Protease Inhibitors (PIs)

PI boosting with ritonavir or cobicistat is recommended.

Recommended Agents
Darunavir (DRV)
• Contains a sulfa moiety but is not contraindicated in sulfa allergic PLWH. Skin rash in 10% of PLWH. Erythema multiforme, Stevens–Johnson syndrome, or toxic epidermal necrolysis have occurred.

Alternative Agents
Atazanavir (ATV)
• Nephrolithiasis; cholelithiasis; PR prolongation.
• Indirect hyperbilirubinemia, clinically insignificant but may be cosmetically unacceptable to PLWH.
• Requires acid for absorption; concomitant use of PPIs not recommended.
• May be unboosted but boosting is preferred; must be boosted when administered with tenofovir.

Entry Inhibitors (Not Routinely Used)

Chemokine Receptor Antagonists
Maraviroc (MVC)
• Only drug currently available in this class and is not recommended in PLWH with dual/mixed- or CXCR4-tropic HIV-1 infection.

TABLE 38.2	Associated Side Effects for Infrequently Used Antiretroviral Agents	
Antiretroviral Agent	**Abbreviation**	**Associated Side Effects**
Nucleoside Reverse Transcriptase Inhibitors (NRTIs)		
Didanosine	DDI	Pancreatitis; peripheral neuropathy
Stavudine	d4T	Lipodystrophy; peripheral neuropathy; lactic acidosis; pancreatitis
Zidovudine	AZT	Anemia; myopathy; lipodystrophy
Nonnucleoside Reverse Transcriptase Inhibitors (NNRTIs)		
Delavirdine	DLV	Three times daily dosing
Etravirine	ETR	Rash; treatment-experienced only
Nevirapine[a]	NPV	Hepatotoxicity (women CD4 >250/μL, men CD4 >400/μL)
Protease Inhibitors (PIs)		
Fosamprenavir	FPV	Stevens–Johnson syndrome
Indinavir	IDV	Renal calculi
Lopinavir/r	LPV/r	Diarrhea
Nelfinavir[a]	NFV	Hepatotoxicity in moderate to severe liver disease; only unboosted PI
Saquinavir[a]	SQV	Arrhythmia
Tipranavir[a]	TPV	Intracranial hemorrhage; hepatotoxicity
Entry Inhibitors		
Enfuvirtide (fusion inhibitors	T20	Injection site reactions
Maraviroc (CCR5 antagonist)	MVC	Hepatotoxicity preceded by severe rash or system allergic reaction

[a]Inferior virologic activity.

- Well tolerated in general.

Fusion Inhibitors

Enfuvirtide (T20)
- Only fusion inhibitor currently available. Use limited by need for twice-daily injection.

Infrequently Used Antiretroviral Agents

Table 38.2 outlines side effects associated with antiretroviral agents that are not commonly used.

What, When, and Why of Antiretroviral Therapy

Guidelines for the management of HIV infection and, in particular, antiretroviral therapy are constantly changing. Up-to-date guidelines can be found at https://aidsinfo.nih.gov/guidelines or https://www.iasusa.org/guidelines.

When to Start ART?

- Recommended for **all individuals with HIV** (regardless of CD4+ T-cell count) to reduce morbidity and mortality as well as to prevent HIV transmission.
- Important to assess readiness of PLWH to start ART and educate them on the importance of adherence once treatment initiated so as to minimize the development of ART resistance.

What ART to Start? (Table 38.3)

There are a number of factors that need to be considered when choosing an ART regimen, including:
- Efficacy.
- Baseline resistance.
- Tolerability.
- Long-term toxicity.
- Drug–drug interaction.
- Convenience (pill burden, dosing frequency).
- HBV co-infection.

TABLE 38.3	Initial Regimens for Antiretroviral-Naïve Persons

Recommended Initial Regimens for Most PLWH

INSTI plus 2 NRTIs

- BIC/TAF/FTC
- DTG/ABC/3TC (HLA-B*5701 negative only)
- DTG plus TDF/FTC or TAF/FTC
- RAL plus TDF/FTC or TAF/FTC

Recommended Initial Regimens in Certain Clinical Situations

Boosted PI plus 2 NRTIs (boosted DRV preferred over boosted ATV)
- DRV/c or DRV/r plus TDF/FTC or TAF/FTC
- ATV/c or ATV/r plus TDF/FTC or TAF/FTC
- DRV/c or DRV/r plus ABC/3TC (HLA-B*5701 negative only)

NNRTI Plus 2 NRTIs
- DOR/TDF/3TC or DOR plus TAF/FTC
- EFV/TDF/FTC or EFV plus TAF/FTC
- RPV/TDF/FTC or RPV/TAF/FTC (if HIV RNA <100,000 copies/mL and CD4 >200 cells/μL)

INSTI Plus 2 NRTIs
- RAL plus ABC/3TC (HLA-B*5701 negative only)
- ETG/COBI/TDF/FTC or ETG/COBI/TAF/FTC

Regimens to Consider When ABC, TAF, or TDF Cannot Be Used
- DTG plus 3TC
- DRV/r plus RAL BID (if HIV RNA <100,000 copies/mL and CD4 >200 cells/μL)
- DRV/r plus 3TC

Source: Adapted from US DHHS guidelines. Last Updated October 25, 2018.

Why Do Regimens Fail?

Causes of failure of antiretroviral therapy regimens are summarized in Table 38.4.

When to Change

- Virological failure (inability to achieve or maintain HIV RNA <200 copies/mL).
  - Resistance testing should be performed while PLWH is taking the failing regimen or within 4 weeks of discontinuing.
  - New regimen should contain at least two active drugs but ideally three.
  - The addition of one new drug to a failing regimen is not recommended.
- **No benefit** to ART intensification or switching ART regimens in virally suppressed PLWH with poor CD4 recovery.

Antiretroviral Resistance

- In the United States 5%–15% of PLWH have transmitted resistance at baseline, with NNRTI mutations the most commonly identified.

TABLE 38.4	Causes of Virological Failure

ART Regimen-Related Factors
- Inadequate viral potency
- Impaired pharmacokinetics, e.g., poor absorption
- Drug–drug interactions
- Specific dietary requirement
- Low genetic barrier to resistance

HIV-Related Factors
- Higher HIV RNA pretreatment
- Preexisting drug resistance (transmitted or acquired)
- Inactivity of agent against the virus based on tropism
- Co-infection with HIV-2 infection
- Previous treatment failure

Patient-Related Factors
- Tolerability due to adverse drug effects
- Pill burden
- Dosing frequency
- Access to care and ART
- Psychosocial factors
- Substance abuse and mental health disorders

- Based on current resistance patterns, guidelines recommend performing resistance testing for PI and RT mutations routinely prior to initiation of ART in all PLWH. Assessment for INSTI mutations only recommended if there is a specific concern for transmission of INSTI resistant virus.
- Only replicating HIV virus can become resistant. If viral replication occurs while a PLWH is taking ART, a sufficient number of critical drug-resistance mutations is required to overcome the anti-HIV activity of the drug regimen, often referred to as the "genetic barrier" to resistance.
- Mutation nomenclature consists of a number and two letters:

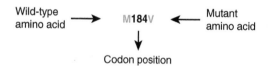

- In the absence of drug pressure, previously selected mutations may be missed or "archived" and only become apparent when treatment with ART is initiated.
- Deep sequencing can identify resistance mutations which are rare or in the setting of low viral loads.

Resistance Assays

- Genotypic resistance test
  - Looks for viral genetic mutations associated with specific HIV drugs.
  - Useful after 1st and 2nd virologic failure.
  - Requires interpretation. HIV drug resistance databases available to assist with interpretation https://hivdb.stanford.edu/.
  - Less expensive and more readily available than phenotypic resistance testing.

TABLE 38.5	Mutations Worth a Mention	
Mutation	**Selected by**	**Comments**
NRTI		
TAMS (thymidine analogue mutations) Type 1: M41L, L210W, T215F/Y Type 2: D67N, K70R, K219Q/E)	Zidovudine Stavudine	↓ susceptibility to all NRTIs Type 1 TAMS have greater impact on tenofovir, didanosine, and abacavir than type 2 TAMS
M184V/I	Lamivudine Emtricitabine	High-level resistance to lamivudine and emtricitabine ↓ susceptibility to abacavir ↑ susceptibility to tenofovir and zidovudine
K65R	Tenofovir Abacavir Didanosine Rarely lamivudine	High-level resistance to tenofovir ↓ susceptibility to abacavir, didanosine, and stavudine ↑ susceptibility to zidovudine
T69 insertion	Didanosine Stavudine	High-level resistance to tenofovir, abacavir, didanosine, and the thymidine analogs ↓ susceptibility to lamivudine and emtricitabine
Q151M	Didanosine Zidovudine	High-level resistance to abacavir, didanosine, and the thymidine analogs ↓ susceptibility to lamivudine, emtricitabine Low-level resistance to tenofovir
L74V	Abacavir Didanosine	High-level resistance to didanosine ↓ susceptibility to abacavir ↑ susceptibility to tenofovir and zidovudine
NNRTI		
K103N	Efavirenz Nevirapine	High level resistance to efavirenz and nevirapine Rilpivirine and etravirine remain susceptible
Y181C	Nevirapine	High level resistance to nevirapine ↓ susceptibility to efavirenz, rilpivirine, and etravirine (all NNRTI affected)
E138K	Rilpivirine	↓ susceptibility to rilpivirine and in combination with K101E can cause failure of rilpivirine-containing regimens
INSTI		
Q148R	Raltegravir Elvitegravir	High-level resistance to raltegravir and elvitegravir If present, administer dolutegravir twice-daily
N155H		High-level resistance to raltegravir and elvitegravir ↓ dolutegravir and bictegravir susceptibility in combination with Q148R
PI		
(resistance usually caused by accumulation of mutations rather than point mutations)		
I50L	Atazanavir	High-level resistance to atazanavir ↑ susceptibility to other Pi's

- Phenotypic
  - Measures viral replication in the presence of ART.
  - May be more instructive in heavily treatment-experienced PLWH with multiple resistance mutations on genotypic testing.
  - More expensive than genotypic resistance testing.

Table 38.5 provides further information regarding specific mutations.

Drug–Drug Interactions

Common ART drug interactions are outlined in Table 38.6 and pharmacokinetic mechanisms are illustrated in Fig. 38.2.

- **Pharmacokinetic enhancers (boosters)**
  - **"Boosting"** is the use of a drug to inhibit the enzymes that metabolize ART.

TABLE 38.6 Common ART Drug–Drug Interactions

Statins
Do Not Coadminister PIs with Simvastatin or Lovastatin

Atorvastatin	Start with lowest possible dose
Pitavastatin	No dose adjustment, monitor for side effect
Pravastatin	Does not rely on CYP3A4 for metabolism. Avoid with DRV/r
Rosuvastatin	Start with lowest possible statin dose

Antidepressants/Anxiolytics
Should be Monitored for Response and Titrated Appropriately

Benzodiazepines	PIs increase concentration of benzodiazepines, use with caution.
Bupropion	PIs and EFV decrease concentration, COBI may increase concentrations, monitor for response
Sertraline	PIs and EFV decrease concentration, COBI may increase concentrations, monitor for response

Acid Reducers
ATV and RPV Need Acid Environment for Absorption

PPIs	Coadministration not recommended with ATV or RPV
H_2 receptor antagonists	Administer ATV or RPV >10 h after the H_2 receptor antagonist

Anticonvulsants

Phenytoin	PIs reduced levels. Consider alternative anticonvulsant
Carbamazepine	Coadministration with PIs increases carbamazepine level and decreases PI levels
Phenobarbital	PI levels reduced substantially
Lamotrigine	Levels decreased with concurrent use of PIs. Titrate lamotrigine dose to effect

Antifungals (Azoles)
Azoles Have Significant Interactions with PIs and NNRTIs

Itraconazole	Coadministration of itraconazole and PIs or COBI may result in increased itraconazole or PI levels. Itraconazole level should be monitored for dose adjustments
Posaconazole	Posaconazole increases ATV level, monitor for adverse events
Voriconazole	Voriconazole level is reduced with concomitant use of RTV. Voriconazole is contraindicated to coadminister with standard dose EFV
Isavuconazole	Limited data available. Potential interaction with PIs and NNRTIs

Inhaled, Intranasal, and Intraarticular Steroids
Risk of Iatrogenic Cushing's Syndrome

Fluticasone budesonide Mometasone	Contraindicated with ritonavir boosted PIs and cobicistat
Triamcinolone	Contraindicated with ritonavir boosted PIs and cobicistat

Antimycobacterials
Rifamycins are p-gp Inducers. TAF Contraindicated as p-gp Substrate

Rifampin/rifapentine	Contraindicated with PIs, ETG/COBI containing regimens and MVC. DTG and RAL require twice-daily dosing. NNRTIs except EFV contraindicated. Monitor HIV RNA closely in patients receiving EFV
Rifabutin	Decrease dose of rifabutin if coadministered with PIs. Increase rifabutin dose if coadministered with NNRTIs. Avoid ETG/COBI, no change to RAL or DTG dosing

Hormonal Contraceptives

Ethinyl estradiol Norethindrone Levonorgesterol	Boosted PIs should be avoided although ATV/r may be used if the oral contraceptive contains at least 35 µg of ethinyl estradiol

Continued

TABLE 38.6	**Common ART Drug–Drug Interactions—cont'd**
Miscellaneous	
Methadone	PIs decrease the concentrations of methadone, titrate as necessary
Herbal preparations	St. John's wort decreases the level of PIs and should not be coadministered
Polyvalent cations	Administer compound containing polyvalent cations 2 hours before or 6 hours after INSTIs
Phosphodiesterase type 5 inhibitors	Concurrent use of PIs increases levels; start with lower dose and monitor for side effects

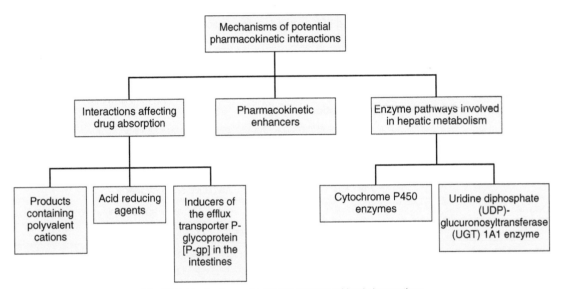

• **Fig. 38.2** Mechanisms of potential pharmacokinetic interactions.

- Two boosters currently available: **ritonavir**, a PI used at low dose (insufficient for viral suppression), and **cobicistat,** which has no antiretroviral activity.
- Both drugs are potent inhibitors of the CYP3A4 enzyme; however, they have different effects on other CYP and UGT-metabolizing enzymes as well as drug transporters. Therefore all ritonavir-related interactions cannot be extrapolated to cobicistat.

Special Considerations

Preexposure Prophylaxis (PrEP)

- ART taken **prior to potential HIV exposure** to prevent acquisition.
- Recommended as part of a package of measures to prevent HIV acquisition in sexually active adults and intravenous drug users at substantial risk of infection.
- Documentation of negative HIV status and assessment for acute infection required prior to initiating.
- Baseline assessment of renal function and hepatitis B status also recommended.
- TDF/FTC taken daily or just prior to and after a sexual encounter.

- Regular HIV and STI testing recommended while on PrEP. Monitor renal function 6-monthly while on TDF/FTC.
- Other oral antiretroviral agents including TAF, long-acting injectable antiretrovirals, microbicides, and antiretroviral topical formulations for use in PrEP under review.

Postexposure Prophylaxis (PEP)

Nonoccupational Exposure

- Offered for high-risk exposures (sexual or needle sharing) from a known HIV-positive source, presenting within 72 hours.
- High-risk exposure from a source with an unknown HIV status has to be individualized.
- Three-drug antiretroviral regimen is provided for 28 days.
  - Preferred: TDF/FTC *plus* RAL or DTG.
  - Alternative: TDF/FTC *plus* DRV/r.

Occupational Exposure

- Assess the exposure, type of fluid (transmission risk with blood or bloodstained fluid or genital secretions), volume of fluid, and timing of the exposure.

- If source is HIV-negative, PEP not required unless concern for acute infection.
- Baseline for HIV, hepatitis B (HBV) and C (HCV) testing for exposed healthcare personnel.
- ART should be initiated as soon as possible.
- Three-drug antiretroviral regimen is provided for 28 days.
- Preferred: TDF/FTC *plus* RAL or DTG.
- Testing of the exposed person should be performed at baseline, 6 weeks, 12 weeks, and 4 months provided a fourth-generation HIV Ag/Ab combination immunoassay is used. If not, testing should be extended to 6 months.

Acute HIV Infection

- ART recommended in acute HIV infection as shown to reduce symptoms and decrease transmission risk.
- As yet limited data available on the long-term clinical, virologic, or immunologic benefits of ART initiation in acute HIV.
- Treatment selected as per standard guideline. If baseline genotype is not available, a PI or DTG-based regime should be initiated.

ART in Pregnancy

- Recommended for prevention of mother to child transmission (MTCT) for all pregnant women.
- Women who present for prenatal care on a well-tolerated, fully suppressive ART regimen **(including those on efavirenz-based regimens)** should continue on their existing regimen.
- Resistance testing should be performed in women with untreated HIV or those with HIV RNA >500 copies/mL.
- In women who present with untreated HIV, initiating an ART regimen comprising two NRTIs and either a PI or INSTI is recommended. Preferred drugs include:
  - **NRTIs:** ABC, TDF, 3TC or FTC. Insufficient data on TAF.
  - **PIs:** ritonavir boosted ATV or DRV recommended; LPV/r alternative. Avoid cobicistat as no data in pregnancy.
  - **INSTIs:** RAL taken twice-daily. DTG was listed in guidelines as an alternative in pregnancy; however, recent data suggest increased rates of neural tube defects in women who conceived while on DTG, prompting regulatory authorities in May 2018 to advise avoiding DTG in women with HIV who are contemplating pregnancy and ensuring adequate

birth control prior to starting women of child-bearing potential on DTG pending further data.
- **Intravenous AZT** should be administered if HIV RNA is >1,000 copies/mL (or unknown HIV RNA) near delivery but is not required for women with HIV receiving ART regimens who have HIV RNA ≤1,000 copies/mL during late pregnancy.
- Scheduled cesarean delivery **at 38 weeks' gestation** is recommended for women who have HIV RNA >1,000 copies/mL near delivery.

HIV–TB Co-infection

- HIV co-infection does not change the recommended treatment regimen for management of TB; however, drug–drug interactions may need to be considered.
- Timing of ART initiation in PLWH with TB depends on the CD4+ T-cell count.
  - Within 2 weeks of TB treatment in CD4+ T-cell counts <50 cells/μL.
  - Can postpone to between 8–12 weeks in CD4+ T-cell count >50 cells/μL.
- Both ART and TB treatment should be continued in the setting of IRIS (immune reconstitution inflammatory syndrome).

HIV–HBV Co-infection

- When treatment is considered for HIV, a regimen that treats both viruses adequately should be constructed. Optimal HBV treatment should include two active agents, while three active agents are required for HIV treatment.
- ART with activity against HBV includes lamivudine, emtricitabine, and tenofovir (both TDF and TAF).
- HBV drugs, including entecavir have some activity against HIV. Use of entecavir monotherapy in co-infection may give rise to 3TC/FTC resistance and should be avoided.

HIV–HCV Co-infection (Table 38.7)

- HIV/HCV co-infected PLWH should be treated and re-treated the same as HCV monoinfected PLWH.
- Assessment of potential interaction between HCV therapy and ART is essential.

HIV-2 Infection

- No studies performed on the optimal timing of ART in HIV-2; however, consensus suggests that treatment should be initiated prior to clinical progression.
- Intrinsically resistant to NNRTIs and T20.

TABLE 38.7 Suitability of Commonly Used ART with Preferred HCV Treatment

	Ledipasvir/ Sofosbuvir	Sofosbuvir/ Velpatasvir	Elbasvir/ Grazoprevir	Glecaprevir/ Pibrentasvir	Sofosbuvir/ Velpatasvir/ Voxilaprevir
ABC	✓	✓	✓	✓	✓
3TC	✓	✓	✓	✓	✓
FTC	✓	✓	✓	✓	✓
TDF	✓ Monitor for TDF toxicity	✓ Monitor for TDF toxicity	✓	✓	✓ Monitor for TDF toxicity
TAF	✓	✓	✓	✓	✓
ATV/r or ATV/c	✓*	✓*	✗	✗	✗
DRV/r or DRV/c			✗	✗	✓*
EFV	✓*	✗	✗	✗	✗
RPV		✓	✓	✓	✓
RAL	✓	✓	✓	✓	✓
DTG	✓*	✓	✓	✓	✓
ETG/c	✗ Not with TDF OK with TAF	✓*	✗	✓*	✓*

*If coadministered with TDF, monitor for TDF toxicity.

39
Opportunistic Infections in HIV

JAMES CUTRELL, ANAND ATHAVALE

Definitions

Acquired immunodeficiency syndrome (AIDS): advanced stage of infection with human immunodeficiency virus (HIV) defined as an absolute CD4 count <200 cells/µL (CD4% <14%) or the diagnosis of an AIDS-defining illness in the context of HIV infection (Box 39.1).

HIV-related opportunistic infections (OIs): infections that are more frequent or severe from immunosuppression in persons living with HIV (PLWH).

Immune reconstitution inflammatory syndrome (IRIS): clinical findings associated with immune reconstitution in persons living with HIV who experience either paradoxical worsening of a known OI *or* unmasking of a previously undiagnosed OI after starting antiretroviral therapy (ART).

Primary prophylaxis: prophylaxis given prior to an OI to prevent its occurrence.

Secondary prophylaxis: prophylaxis or chronic maintenance treatment given after acute treatment to prevent OI recurrence.

Epidemiology

- The hallmark of untreated HIV infection is progressive immunosuppression with declining CD4 counts, which increases the risk of OIs.
- Prior to widespread use of combination ART, OIs were the primary cause of HIV-related morbidity and mortality.
- Use of chemoprophylaxis, vaccination, and better OI diagnosis and management improved survival in the early 1990s.
- Subsequent widespread use of combination ART, starting in 1996, profoundly decreased the incidence and mortality from OIs.
- Despite availability of ART, OIs continue to cause significant morbidity and mortality in the United States in three main groups:
  - People unaware of HIV infection (25% of all PLWH in United States), who often initially present with OIs.

- PLWH with poor adherence to ART or antimicrobial prophylaxis.
- PLWH with virologic or immunologic failure on ART.
- OIs occur as primary infection or reactivation of latent infection.
- **The critical determinant of the risk of developing a particular OI is the person's immune status** (based primarily on CD4 count).
  - Tuberculosis (TB), bacterial pneumonia, herpes zoster, oral candidiasis, Kaposi sarcoma (KS), and lymphoma occur even at CD4 >200 cells/µL.
  - *Pneumocystis* pneumonia (PCP), progressive multifocal leukoencephalopathy (PML), and esophageal candidiasis generally occur at CD4 <200 cells/µL.
  - Cerebral toxoplasmosis, cryptococcosis, and miliary TB generally occur at CD4 <100 cells/µL.
  - Disseminated *Mycobacterium avium* complex (MAC) and cytomegalovirus (CMV) chorioretinitis generally occur at CD4 <50 cells/µL.

Diagnostic Approach

- Given the breadth of OIs seen in AIDS it is imperative to pursue aggressively a microbiologic or histopathologic diagnosis to guide targeted therapy while limiting toxicity.
- Importantly, **PLWH may present with multiple concurrent OIs.** Additionally, PLWH develop community- or hospital-acquired nonopportunistic infections or noninfectious mimics that must be considered.
- Thorough history (focused on **ART and chemoprophylaxis adherence, current CD4 and HIV viral load and trends, prior OIs**, geographic location, and exposure history [e.g., sexual, travel-related, environmental]) and physical examination (focused on funduscopic, dermatologic, mucosal, anogenital, lymph node, and neurologic exam) provides initial clues for diagnostic work-up.
- A syndromic approach can ensure the diagnostic differential and work-up capture the most likely etiologies. A sample diagnostic algorithm based on clinical syndromes is provided in Fig. 39.1.

• BOX 39.1 Select AIDS-Defining Illnesses in Adults or Adolescents

- Candidiasis of bronchi, esophagus, trachea, or lungs
- Cervical cancer, invasive
- Coccidioidomycosis, disseminated or extrapulmonary
- Cryptococcosis, extrapulmonary
- Cryptosporidiosis, chronic intestinal (>1 month)
- Cystoisosporiasis, chronic intestinal (>1 month)
- Cytomegalovirus, retinitis, pneumonitis, or gastrointestinal disease
- Herpes simplex virus, chronic ulcers (>1 month), pneumonitis, esophagitis
- Histoplasmosis, disseminated or extrapulmonary
- Kaposi sarcoma
- Lymphoma, of Burkitt, immunoblastic, or primary central nervous system type
- *Mycobacterium tuberculosis* of any site, pulmonary, disseminated or extrapulmonary
- *Mycobacterium avium* complex or *Mycobacterium kansasii*, disseminated or extrapulmonary
- *Mycobacterium*, other or unidentified species, disseminated or extrapulmonary
- *Pneumocystis jirovecii* pneumonia
- Pneumonia, recurrent
- Progressive multifocal leukoencephalopathy
- *Salmonella* septicemia, recurrent
- Toxoplasmosis of the brain
- HIV wasting syndrome
- HIV-related encephalopathy

- Histopathology and culture from tissue or bone marrow biopsy have diagnostic value in cases of suspected disseminated OIs or hematologic involvement.

Treatment

- Specific treatment recommendations for common OIs are discussed below.
- While an etiologic diagnosis is pursued, empiric treatment may be indicated based on the patient's clinical status (e.g., sepsis, meningitis) or a high pretest probability of specific diagnosis (e.g., patient with dysphagia, thrush, and CD4 <50 cells/μL).
- Overlapping drug toxicities, tolerability, and drug–drug interactions with ART and other medications are of special concern in OI management. Comprehensive drug–drug interaction and adverse reaction tables in guidelines are useful, and consultation with HIV experts may be required.
- Important pharmacokinetic/pharmacodynamic considerations include weight-based dosing, renal and hepatic dose adjustments, drug absorption, and metabolism.
- Critical to avoiding OI relapses is the initiation and maintenance of effective ART for immunologic recovery.
- **Timing of ART initiation with acute OIs**: generally, patients with acute OIs not previously on ART should have ART started within 2 weeks, which demonstrated a survival benefit in AIDS Clinical Trial Group A5164 study (excluding TB).

- Some OIs without effective treatment (e.g., cryptosporidiosis, microsporidiosis, PML) require ART initiation as soon as possible to promote immune recovery.
- OIs in the central nervous system (CNS) (e.g., TB or cryptococcal meningitis) warrant delay in ART initiation due to risks of severe IRIS leading to increased intracranial pressure (ICP).
- **Nonmeningeal TB infections**: ART initiation is recommended within 2 weeks of starting TB therapy for CD4 <50 cells/μL or within 8 weeks of starting TB therapy for CD4 >50 cells/μL.
- Clinical judgment regarding drug toxicity, pharmacokinetics, and patient readiness to take ART consistently must be weighed.
- For patients with acute OIs already on ART, it should be continued unless drug absorption, toxicities, or interactions are prohibitive.

Prevention

- The paramount strategy for preventing HIV-related OIs is early diagnosis and initiation of ART prior to significant immunosuppression.
- The landmark START trial definitively established that early ART initiation regardless of CD4 count, compared to delayed ART initiation for CD4 <350 cells/μL, significantly reduced the risk of death, serious AIDS-related or non-AIDS-related events by 57%, driven primarily by prevention of AIDS-related OIs and malignancies.
- Antimicrobial prophylaxis either as **primary prophylaxis** (to prevent an OI from occurring) or as **secondary prophylaxis** (to prevent an OI recurrence) is a highly effective adjunctive prevention strategy, in accordance with OI guidelines (Table 39.1).
- Appropriate immunizations should follow HIV-specific published vaccine schedules. **Importantly, the live attenuated vaccines (measles, mumps, and rubella [MMR]; varicella; and herpes zoster) are contraindicated with CD4 <200 cells/μL.**
- Preventive counseling regarding sexual exposures, injection drug use, environmental exposures, pets, food- and water-related exposures or travel are also important and discussed in guidelines.

OVERVIEW OF KEY OPPORTUNISTIC INFECTIONS

Fungal Infections

Pneumocystis Pneumonia (PCP) (see Chapter 27)

Overview and Clinical Presentation

- PCP is caused by ubiquitous fungi, *Pneumocystis jirovecii*, either from new infection or latent reactivation.

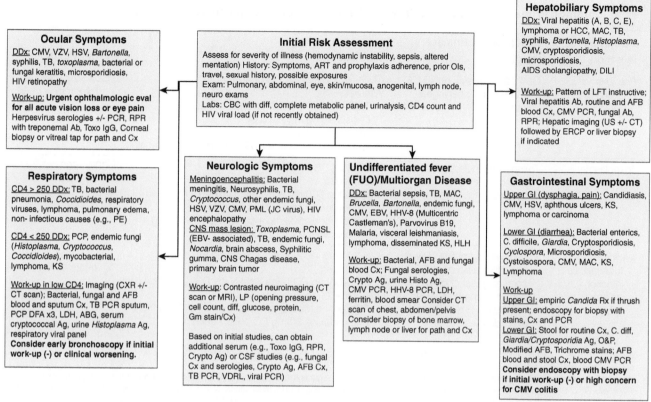

Initial Risk Assessment
Assess for severity of illness (hemodynamic instability, sepsis, altered mentation) History: Symptoms, ART and prophylaxis adherence, prior OIs, travel, sexual history, possible exposures
Exam: Pulmonary, abdominal, eye, skin/mucosa, anogenital, lymph node, neuro exams
Labs: CBC with diff, complete metabolic panel, urinalysis, CD4 count and HIV viral load (if not recently obtained)

Ocular Symptoms
DDx: CMV, VZV, HSV, *Bartonella*, syphilis, TB, *toxoplasma*, bacterial or fungal keratitis, microsporidiosis, HIV retinopathy

Work-up: **Urgent ophthalmologic eval for all acute vision loss or eye pain** Herpesvirus serologies +/- PCR, RPR with treponemal Ab, Toxo IgG, Corneal biopsy or vitreal tap for path and Cx

Hepatobiliary Symptoms
DDx: Viral hepatitis (A, B, C, E), lymphoma or HCC, MAC, TB, syphilis, *Bartonella*, *Histoplasma*, CMV, cryptosporidiosis, microsporidiosis, AIDS cholangiopathy, DILI

Work-up: Pattern of LFT instructive; Viral hepatitis Ab, routine and AFB blood Cx, CMV PCR, fungal Ab, RPR; Hepatic imaging (US +/- CT) followed by ERCP or liver biopsy if indicated

Respiratory Symptoms
CD4 > 250 DDx: TB, bacterial pneumonia, *Coccidioides*, respiratory viruses, lymphoma, pulmonary edema, non- infectious causes (e.g., PE)

CD4 < 250 DDx: PCP, endemic fungi (*Histoplasma, Cryptococcus, Coccidioides*), mycobacterial, lymphoma, KS

Work-up in low CD4: Imaging (CXR +/- CT scan); Bacterial, fungal and AFB blood and sputum Cx, TB PCR sputum, PCP DFA x3, LDH, ABG, serum cryptococcal Ag, urine *Histoplasma* Ag, respiratory viral panel
Consider early bronchoscopy if initial work-up (-) or clinical worsening.

Neurologic Symptoms
Meningoencephalitis: Bacterial meningitis, Neurosyphilis, TB, *Cryptococcus*, other endemic fungi, HSV, VZV, CMV, PML (JC virus), HIV encephalopathy
CNS mass lesion: *Toxoplasma*, PCNSL (EBV- associated), TB, endemic fungi, *Nocardia*, brain abscess, Syphilitic gumma, CNS Chagas disease, primary brain tumor

Work-up: Contrasted neuroimaging (CT scan or MRI), LP (opening pressure, cell count, diff, glucose, protein, Gm stain/Cx)

Based on initial studies, can obtain additional serum (e.g., Toxo IgG, RPR, Crypto Ag) or CSF studies (e.g., fungal Cx and serologies, Crypto Ag, AFB Cx, TB PCR, VDRL, viral PCR)

Undifferentiated fever (FUO)/Multiorgan Disease
DDx: Bacterial sepsis, TB, MAC, *Brucella, Bartonella*, endemic fungi, CMV, EBV, HHV-8 (Multicentric Castleman's), Parvovirus B19, Malaria, visceral leishmaniasis, lymphoma, disseminated KS, HLH

Work-up: Bacterial, AFB and fungal blood Cx; Fungal serologies, Crypto Ag, urine Histo Ag, CMV PCR, HHV-8 PCR, LDH, ferritin, blood smear Consider CT scan of chest, abdomen/pelvis Consider biopsy of bone marrow, lymph node or liver for path and Cx

Gastrointestinal Symptoms
Upper GI (dysphagia, pain): Candidiasis, CMV, HSV, aphthous ulcers, KS, lymphoma or carcinoma

Lower GI (diarrhea): Bacterial enterics, C. difficile, *Giardia*, Cryptosporidiosis, *Cyclospora*, Microsporidiosis, Cystoisospora, CMV, MAC, KS, Lymphoma

Work-up
Upper GI: empiric *Candida* Rx if thrush present; endoscopy for biopsy with stains, Cx and PCR
Lower GI: Stool for routine Cx, C. diff, *Giardia/Cryptosporidia* Ag, O&P, Modified AFB, Trichrome stains; AFB blood and stool Cx, blood CMV PCR
Consider endoscopy with biopsy if initial work-up (-) or high concern for CMV colitis

• **Fig. 39.1** Syndromic approach to suspected opportunistic infection in HIV. AFB, acid-fast bacilli; ABG, arterial blood gas; ART, antiretroviral therapy; CBC, complete blood count; CMV, cytomegalovirus; DFA, direct fluorescent antibody; DILI, drug-induced liver injury; EBV, Epstein–Barr virus; ERCP, endoscopic retrograde cholangiopancreatography; FUO, fever of unknown origin; HCC, hepatocellular carcinoma; HHV-8, human herpes virus 8; HLH, hemophagocytic lymphohistiocytosis; HSV, herpes simplex virus; KS, Kaposi sarcoma; LDH, lactate dehydrogenase; LP, lumbar puncture; MAC, *Mycobacterium avium* complex; O&P, ova and parasite; PCNSL, primary CNS lymphoma; PCP, *Pneumocystis* pneumonia; PCR, polymerase chain reaction; PE, pulmonary embolism; PML, progressive multifocal leukoencephalopathy; RPR, rapid plasma reagin; TB, tuberculosis; US, ultrasound; VDRL, venereal disease research laboratory test; VZV, varicella-zoster virus.

• Prior to ART and chemoprophylaxis, PCP occurred in almost 80% of persons living with AIDS.
• Significant decline in incidence but still one of most common OIs seen.
• **Risk factors:** CD4 <200 cells/µL, history of oral thrush, or prior PCP.
• **Presentation:** subacute dyspnea, fever, nonproductive cough, and pleuritic chest pain.
• Exam shows **exertional oxygen desaturation** and diffuse dry rales.

Diagnosis

• Chest X-ray findings range from normal to the classic bilateral, butterfly-pattern ground-glass interstitial infiltrates (Fig. 39.2). Atypical presentations include nodules, blebs, cysts, or asymmetric disease, but pleural effusion or cavitation is unusual.
• **Spontaneous pneumothoraces in a PLWH should raise high suspicion for PCP.**
• High-resolution computed tomography (CT) scan shows ground glass attenuation even with normal chest X-ray.
• Elevation of lactate dehydrogenase (LDH) more than 500 mg/dL is common but nonspecific.

• Arterial blood gas (ABG) documenting degree of hypoxemia and alveolar–arterial (A–a) oxygen gradient is important to triage patients and determine if adjunctive steroids are needed.
• Definitive diagnosis requires microscopic visualization of the organism on respiratory specimens using silver, Giemsa, or direct fluorescent antibody (DFA) staining (Fig. 39.3). **Induced sputum only has 60% sensitivity while bronchoscopy with bronchoalveolar lavage or transbronchial biopsy provides sensitivity >90%–95%.**
• 1,3-β-D-glucan is elevated in PCP but nonspecific so a positive test is less useful but a **negative test has a high negative predictive value.**

Treatment and Prophylaxis

• First-line treatment is trimethoprim–sulfamethoxazole (TMP–SMX) for 21 days. Treatment recommendations based on severity are listed in Table 39.2.
• **Adjunctive corticosteroids are recommended for patients with a room air PaO_2<70 mmHg or A–a gradient ≥35 mmHg.**

TABLE 39.1	Common Primary Prophylaxis to Prevent First Episode of an Opportunistic Infection		
Opportunistic Infection	**Indication for Primary Prophylaxis**	**Medications**	**Discontinue Prophylaxis**
Pneumocystis pneumonia (PCP)	CD4 <200 cells/μL *or* CD4% <14% *or* oropharyngeal candidiasis	TMP–SMX DS or SS PO daily Alternatives[a]: TMP–-SMX DS PO three times weekly Dapsone 100 mg PO daily Atovaquone 1500 mg PO daily Aerosolized pentamidine 300 mg via nebulizer monthly	CD4 >200 cells/μL for 3 mth
Toxoplasmosis	*Toxoplasma* IgG-positive patients with CD4 <100 cells/μL	TMP–SMX DS PO daily Alternatives: Dapsone 200 mg + pyrimethamine 75 mg + leucovorin 25 mg) PO once weekly Atovaquone 1500 mg + pyrimethamine 25 mg + leucovorin 10 mg) PO daily	CD4 >200 cells/μL for 3 mth
Mycobacterium tuberculosis infection (i.e., treatment of LTBI)	Patient without active TB who has either a positive LTBI screening test *or* close contact with person with infectious TB regardless of screening test result	INH 300 mg + pyridoxine 25–50 mg PO daily Alternatives: INH 900 mg PO twice weekly (by DOT) + pyridoxine 25–50 mg PO daily Rifapentine (dosed by weight) + INH 900 mg PO + pyridoxine 50 mg PO once weekly[b]	Completion of LTBI treatment

[a]Patients who are *Toxoplasma* seropositive should receive PCP prophylaxis with activity against both pathogens, while those on treatment for toxoplasmosis do not need additional PCP prophylaxis.
[b]Rifapentine-based regimens can only be used in efavirenz or raltegravir-based regimens in combination with abacavir/lamivudine or tenofovir/emtricitabine.
TMP–SMX DS or SS, trimethoprim–sulfamethoxazole double-strength or single-strength; LTBI, latent tuberculosis infection; INH, isoniazid; DOT, directly observed therapy; MAC, *Mycobacterium avium* complex.

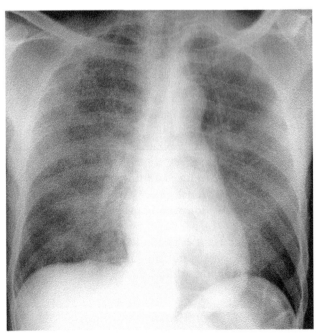

• **Fig. 39.2** Diffuse bilateral perihilar infiltrate due to *Pneumocystis* pneumonia seen on chest X-ray. (Courtesy Dr. Joel E. Fishman, University of Miami.)

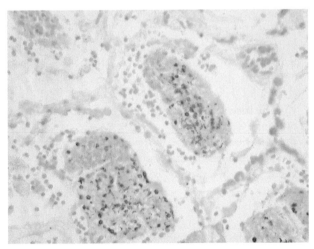

• **Fig. 39.3** *Pneumocystis jirovecii* seen on Giemsa stain (GMS) from lung tissue biopsy. (From Harris K, Maroun R, Chalhoub M, Elsayegh D. Unusual presentation of pneumocystis pneumonia in an immunocompetent patient diagnosed by open lung biopsy. *Heart Lung Circ.* 2012;21(4):221–224. © 2011 Australian and New Zealand Society of Cardiac and Thoracic Surgeons and the Cardiac Society of Australia and New Zealand.)

TABLE 39.2   Treatment Regimens for *Pneumocystis* Pneumonia (PCP)

Disease Severity	Preferred Therapy	Alternative Therapies
Mild-to-moderate PCP (Able to take orals, PaO_2 >70 mmHg on room air)	TMP–SMX DS two tabs PO q8h	Primaquine 30 mg (base) PO daily + Clindamycin 450 mg PO q6h Atovaquone 750 mg PO BID
Moderate-to-severe PCP (Acutely ill, not able to take orals, or PaO_2 <70 mmHg or A–a gradient >35 mmHg on room air)	TMP–SMX (5 mg/kg of TMP component per dose) IV q6–8h, with switch to PO once clinical improvement	Pentamidine 4 mg/kg IV daily infused over 60 min Primaquine 30 mg (base) PO daily + Clindamycin 600 mg IV q6h

Additional comments:
1. All treatments are for 21 days' duration and then secondary prophylaxis started after completion until the CD4 >200 cells/µL for more than 3 months.
2. Indications for corticosteroids include PaO_2 <70 mmHg or A–a gradient > 35 mmHg on room air. Prednisone taper: 40 mg BID for 5 days, 40 mg daily for 5 days, then 20 mg daily for 11 days.
3. IV pentamidine is associated with serious reactions including pancreatitis, nephrotoxicity, hypoglycemia, hypotension, and cardiac arrhythmias.
TMP–SMX, trimethoprim-sulfamethoxazole; A–a gradient, alveolar–arterial oxygen gradient; PaO_2, arterial partial pressure of oxygen.

- Median time to PCP clinical improvement is 4–8 days, beyond which treatment failure and treatment modification should be considered.
- Glucose-6-phosphate dehydrogenase (G-6-PD) deficiency should be excluded prior to use of alternative regimens with dapsone or primaquine due to hemolytic anemia risk.
- Mortality up to 60% occurs in patients requiring ICU admission and mechanical ventilation.
- ART initiation should be within 2 weeks of PCP diagnosis in those not already on therapy.
- Primary prophylaxis criteria are listed in Table 39.1. Secondary prophylaxis with similar regimens should be given indefinitely or until CD4 >200 cells/µL for 3 months.
- Routine MAC prophylaxis for people with CD4 <50 cells/mm3 is not longer recommended in patients initiating suppressive ART.

Cryptococcosis (see Chapter 27)

Overview and Clinical Presentation

- Cryptococcosis is most common systemic fungal infection in PLWH worldwide.
- *Cryptococcus neoformans* is most common species although *Cryptococcus gattii* is seen in Pacific Northwest and Australia.
- Before ART, 5%–8% of PLWH developed disseminated cryptococcosis, but incidence has substantially declined.
- Most cases occur with CD4 <100 cells/µL; other risks include exposure to bird droppings although it is ubiquitous in environment.
- **Presentation**: Subacute meningoencephalitis with fever, headache, lethargy, and progressive altered mentation. Meningismus only seen in minority.
- Disseminated disease can involve any organ with predilection for the lungs, skin (umbilicated lesions mimicking molluscum; Fig. 39.4), bone, and prostate. **CNS involvement must be ruled out in all nonmeningeal presentations in PLWH.**

Fig. 39.4 Nodular, umbilicated skin lesion secondary to *Cryptococcus neoformans*. (From Negroni R. Disseminated cryptococcosis with a nodular ulcerated skin lesion in an AIDS patient. *Clin Dermatol.* 2012;30(6):599–609.)

Diagnosis

- Lumbar puncture (LP) with cerebrospinal fluid (CSF) analysis typically demonstrates elevated protein, low-to-normal glucose, and lymphocytic pleocytosis. **A low or normal CSF cell count is a poor prognostic marker.**
- Opening pressure (OP) should be measured and is elevated ≥25 mmHg in 60%–80% of cases. Elevated OP requires serial, large-volume (25–30 mL) CSF drainage to reduce complications from elevated ICP. Other measures such as steroids, mannitol, or acetazolamide are **not effective.**
- Diagnostic gold standard is positive CSF culture for *C. neoformans.*
- However, **cryptococcal antigen (CrAg) testing by latex agglutination or lateral flow assay** is highly sensitive and specific in both serum and CSF in PLWH, providing a rapid screening and diagnostic tool.

Treatment and Prophylaxis

- Treatment of meningitis and other extrapulmonary sites occurs in three phases: induction (2 weeks), consolidation (8 weeks), and maintenance therapy (minimum 12 months).
  - **Induction phase:** While historically amphotericin B deoxycholate (0.7–1.0 mg/kg per day IV daily) was used, growing evidence shows lipid formulations of amphotericin B are equally effective with less nephrotoxicity. A typical regimen is **liposomal amphotericin B** (3–4 mg/kg per day IV) plus **flucytosine** (5-FC) 100 mg/kg per day PO divided over 4 doses for **at least 2 weeks and until clinical improvement with negative CSF culture on repeat LP.**
  - Addition of 5-FC more rapidly sterilizes the CSF and reduces relapse but drug monitoring is required to avoid bone marrow toxicity (goal peaks of <100 µg/mL 2 hours after dose).
  - For patients intolerant of amphotericin B, alternative induction with combination of fluconazole 400–800 mg daily plus 5-FC may be used for 4–6 weeks.
  - **Consolidation phase:** Fluconazole 400 mg PO daily for 8 weeks is preferred.
  - **Maintenance phase:** Fluconazole 200 mg PO daily for at least 1 year and continued indefinitely or until CD4 >100 cells/µL and undetectable HIV viral load on ART for >3 months.
- Other extrapulmonary or severe pulmonary cryptococcosis should be treated like meningitis; mild-to-moderate isolated pulmonary disease is treated with fluconazole 400 mg PO daily for at least 12 months.
- Timing of ART initiation is controversial in cryptococcal meningitis, but guidelines recommend **between 2 and 10 weeks after antifungal therapy starts** with close monitoring for IRIS.
- While primary prophylaxis is not currently recommended in the United States due to low disease prevalence, some experts recommend screening asymptomatic, newly diagnosed HIV patients with CD4 <100 cells/µL with serum CrAg.
- A positive screening test prompts fungal blood cultures and CSF evaluation, which if positive warrants meningitis treatment. If negative CSF evaluation, patients with asymptomatic antigenemia receive fluconazole 400 mg PO daily until CD4 >100 cells/µL for 3 months.

Candidiasis (see Chapter 27)

Overview and Clinical Presentation

- Oropharyngeal candidiasis is most common OI in PLWH and key indicator of immunosuppression (usually CD4 <200 cells/µL).
- *Candida albicans* is the most common species worldwide, but non-*albicans Candida* species are increasing, especially in patients with prior antifungal exposure.

- **Presentation:** oropharyngeal candidiasis (thrush) presents as white, creamy plaque-like lesions on mucosa or palate that easily scrape off. Esophagitis presents with retrosternal burning or odynophagia.
- Females living with HIV can have severe, recurrent vulvovaginal candidiasis.

Diagnosis

- Oropharyngeal candidiasis is diagnosed by characteristic clinical appearance and ability to scrape off mucosa, distinguishing from oral hairy leukoplakia.
- Esophagitis can be presumed by response to empiric treatment or confirmed by endoscopic visualization of lesions. Histopathology with fungal culture may be used in atypical cases or where antifungal resistance is suspected.

Treatment and Prophylaxis

- Oral fluconazole 200 mg loading dose followed by 100 mg PO daily for 7–14 days is first-line treatment for oropharyngeal candidiasis. Topical antifungals are alternatives although less effective in severe disease or advanced AIDS.
- Oral fluconazole 400 mg loading dose followed by 200 mg PO daily for 14–21 days is preferred in esophagitis. Those cases refractory to fluconazole can be treated with a different azole (voriconazole or posaconazole) or an IV echinocandin.
- Treatment failures require evaluation for other esophagitis pathogens such as CMV or herpes simplex.
- Primary prophylaxis is not recommended.

Coccidioidomycosis (see Chapter 27)

Overview and Clinical Presentation

- Infection due to soil-dwelling dimorphic fungi, *Coccidioides immitis* and *Coccidioides posadasii.*
- Most cases occur in endemic areas in southwestern United States, Mexico, and other parts of Latin America.
- **Risk factors:** CD4 <250 cells/µL, pregnancy, large inoculum exposure.
- **Presentations:** focal pneumonia in PLWH with high CD4 counts; diffuse pulmonary disease or disseminated disease (with predilection for skin, bone, or CNS involvement) occurs more commonly in AIDS.
- Asymptomatic patients may have elevated coccidioidal serologies.

Diagnosis

- Diagnosis confirmed by culture or demonstration of **characteristic spherule form on histopathology.**
- More commonly, presumptive diagnosis is made by serologic testing with compatible clinical syndrome.

- Complement fixation IgG serologies are frequently positive in the CSF with meningitis. Coccidioidal serum or urine antigen can be useful in disseminated disease.

Treatment and Prophylaxis

- Oral azole therapy preferred for focal pneumonia or mild disease, but amphotericin B formulations preferred in severe or disseminated disease with step-down to azole maintenance after clinical improvement.
- Coccidioidal meningitis requires expert management and may require CSF shunting for hydrocephalus or intrathecal antifungals in addition to systemic treatment.
- Secondary prophylaxis for mild infection can be stopped after at least 1 year of therapy and CD4 >250 cells/μL on suppressive ART.
- Unlike other mycoses, **secondary prophylaxis for severe or meningeal coccidioidomycosis is lifelong, regardless of CD4, due to high relapse rates.**
- While primary prophylaxis is not recommended, fluconazole 400 mg PO daily is recommended for patients living in endemic areas, with newly positive serology and CD4 <250 cells/μL until immune reconstitution occurs.

Histoplasmosis

Overview and Clinical Presentation

- Caused by the dimorphic fungi *Histoplasma capsulatum*, endemic in south–central United States and in Ohio and Mississippi river valleys.
- In endemic regions, incidence approached 5% prior to ART.
- Disease occurs from dissemination during primary infection or latent reactivation, usually in PLWH with CD4 <100 cells/μL.
- **Presentation: progressive disseminated histoplasmosis** (PDH) presents with fevers, systemic symptoms, hepatosplenomegaly, and pulmonary symptoms (50% of cases).
- Less frequently, causes cutaneous, gastrointestinal (GI), or CNS involvement (subacute meningitis or brain mass) or septic shock with acute respiratory distress syndrome and/or adrenal insufficiency.
- At higher CD4 counts, PLWH may have isolated or chronic pulmonary disease.

Diagnosis

- Marked elevation of LDH (>600 mg/dL) or serum ferritin seen in PDH but are nonspecific.
- Definitive diagnosis occurs by isolation of *H. capsulatum* in culture from blood, bone marrow, tissue, or respiratory cultures. Histopathology from tissue demonstrates **characteristic 2–4 μm, budding intracellular yeast forms.**
- Serologic testing useful in PLWH with isolated pulmonary disease and intact immune system.

- *Histoplasma* antigen detection from blood or urine is highly sensitive for PDH in persons with AIDS but may cross-react with other dimorphic fungi.

Treatment and Prophylaxis

- Preferred treatment for severe PDH is induction with liposomal amphotericin B 3 mg/kg per day IV for 2 weeks followed by oral itraconazole 200 mg PO twice daily for at least 12 months. Less severe disseminated or isolated pulmonary histoplasmosis can be treated with oral itraconazole alone.
- **Itraconazole levels must be monitored on treatment** with goal serum concentrations of itraconazole + hydroxyitraconazole >1 μg/mL.
- Secondary prophylaxis with itraconazole should be continued until all of the following are met:
  - Minimum 1 year of antifungal therapy.
  - Negative fungal blood cultures and *Histoplasma* serum antigen <2 units.
  - CD4 >150 cells/μL on suppressive ART for 6 months.
- ART should begin as soon as possible since *Histoplasma* IRIS is rarely seen.
- Primary prophylaxis with itraconazole 200 mg PO daily can be considered in PLWH with CD4 <150 cells/μL at high occupational risk or living in a hyperendemic area for histoplasmosis

Talaromycosis (formerly Penicilliosis)

- Caused by dimorphic fungi *Talaromyces marneffei* (formerly *Penicillium marneffei*).
- Rare in United States but **common AIDS-defining OI in Southeast Asia** (Thailand, Vietnam, China).
- **Presentation:** disseminated, multiorgan disease similar to histoplasmosis with characteristic skin lesions and hepatic involvement with marked elevation in serum alkaline phosphatase.
- Treatment involves liposomal amphotericin B for 2 weeks followed by oral itraconazole therapy until immune reconstitution.
- Primary prophylaxis with itraconazole offered to PLWH with CD4 <100 cells/μL with residence or extended visit to hyperendemic regions.

Bacterial Infections

Mycobacterium Tuberculosis (MTB)
Overview and Clinical Presentation

- For comprehensive review of tuberculosis, please refer to Chapter 32, Tuberculosis.
- **TB is the leading cause of HIV-related morbidity and mortality worldwide.**
- Infection occurs after inhaling aerosol droplets with *M. tuberculosis*, but the immune system usually controls, establishing condition of latent TB infection (LTBI).

- Active TB disease develops either during primary infection or from reactivation of LTBI.
- Annual risk of reactivation in untreated HIV is 3%–16% annually, which approximates the **lifetime risk** in persons with LTBI but without HIV.
- In United States, the dominant risk factor for TB infection is birth or residence outside the US.
- Risk of conversion to active TB is highest in PLWH with lower CD4 counts and in the first year following new HIV or LTBI diagnosis.
- **Presentation:** varies based on patient immune status. PLWH with CD4 >350 cells/μL present with classic upper lobe cavitary lung disease with fevers and constitutional symptoms.
- PLWH with CD4 <200 cells/μL present with lower lobe disease, no cavitation, and, more commonly, extrapulmonary TB involving any organ system. Most common extrapulmonary sites are lymphadenitis, genitourinary tract, bone marrow, and CNS.

Diagnosis

- Initial evaluation should include chest X-ray, even in absence of pulmonary symptoms if TB is suspected. However, normal X-ray does not exclude active TB.
- Sputum acid-fast bacillus (AFB) smears and culture should be submitted in all symptomatic patients or those with extrapulmonary TB even though up to 50% of PLWH have smear-negative TB.
- MTB nucleic acid amplification testing (NAAT) on at least one sputum is recommended due to its improved sensitivity over AFB smear and the ability to rapidly identify TB, particularly in smear-positive disease.
- AFB stains and culture should be performed on blood, other tissue, or body fluids from other sites that may be clinically involved.
- Culture remains an important tool for drug-susceptibility testing to guide treatment and reduce transmission of drug-resistant TB.

Treatment and Prophylaxis

- After appropriate specimen collection, empiric TB treatment may be warranted in patients with suggestive clinical and radiographic presentations.
- For details of TB treatment, refer to Chapter 32. Generally, empiric TB treatment in PLWH is the same as HIV-negative, with initial 4-drug combination therapy of isoniazid, a rifamycin, ethambutol, and pyrazinamide followed by two-drug therapy with INH and rifamycin if drug-susceptible TB.
- Important drug interactions exist between several ART drug classes and antimycobacterial drugs, particularly the rifamycins, so reference to treatment guidelines or a treatment expert is often necessary.
- **The preferred cotreatment regimen for HIV-related TB includes ART with efavirenz and two nucleoside(tide) analogs**; this ART regimen can be used with rifampin-containing TB regimens with excellent outcomes and low rates of serious toxicity.

- Alternative ART regimens include raltegravir or dolutegravir-based ART regimens, although the doses may need to be increased if used with rifampin-containing TB regimens.
- When protease inhibitor or nonnucleoside reverse transcriptase inhibitor-based ART is needed, **rifabutin may be used instead in TB regimens** due to rifampin's potent cytochrome CYP3A induction, which lowers the concentrations of both ART classes.
- The following drugs are contraindicated with the use of rifampin: rilpivirine, etravirine, and elvitegravir-cobicistat; **tenofovir alafenamide should not used with any rifamycins.**
- **Directly observed therapy regimens given 5–7 days per week** are recommended in HIV co-infection as opposed to intermittent dosing.
- Duration of treatment for drug-susceptible TB varies by disease location: pulmonary (6 months, extended to 9 months if culture-positive after 2 months), extrapulmonary bone or joint (6–9 months), CNS (9–12 months), and other extrapulmonary (6 months).
- **TB–IRIS**, either paradoxical or unmasking type, is commonly seen and can be treated with NSAIDS or corticosteroids in moderate-to-severe cases while excluding other causes of deterioration like TB drug resistance or nonadherence.
- Timing of ART initiation is discussed above.
- **LTBI:** all PLWH require screening for LTBI at diagnosis and annually and should complete treatment if positive (defined as **positive interferon-gamma release assay** [preferred in HIV] or **tuberculin skin test with induration of >5 mm**) (Table 39.1).

Mycobacterium avium Complex (MAC)

Overview and Clinical Presentation

- Disseminated MAC, most commonly from *M. avium*, causes multiorgan disease in PLWH with CD4 <50 cells/μL.
- Prior to ART or chemoprophylaxis, incidence of disseminated MAC was 20%–40%.
- **Presentation:** in persons living with AIDS off ART, MAC presents with fevers, night sweats, weight loss, chronic diarrhea accompanied by hepatosplenomegaly and diffuse lymphadenopathy.
- PLWH with higher CD4 counts or immune reconstitution present with localized disease including lymphadenitis, pneumonia, osteomyelitis, soft-tissue abscesses, or CNS disease. Paradoxical or unmasking IRIS is also well described.

Diagnosis

- Common lab abnormalities include cytopenias and elevated alkaline phosphatase.
- Definitive diagnosis requires compatible clinical syndrome plus positive cultures from blood, bone marrow, or normally sterile tissue, which can take weeks to grow. Specific DNA probes can distinguish MAC from other mycobacteria once sufficient growth occurs.

Treatment and Prophylaxis

- First-line treatment is combination of **clarithromycin** 500 mg PO twice daily plus **ethambutol** 15 mg/kg PO daily for at least 12 months. **Azithromycin** 500–600 mg PO daily may be substituted if drug interactions or intolerance preclude clarithromycin use. For further details, refer to Chapter 33.
- A third agent (rifabutin 300 mg PO daily) can be considered in severe cases but increases potential drug toxicity and interactions.
- ART initiation should be as soon as possible after the first 2 weeks of mycobacterial treatment.
- Moderate-to-severe IRIS from disseminated MAC is treated with NSAIDS or corticosteroids.
- Regimens and discontinuation criteria are listed in Table 39.1.
- Secondary prophylaxis can be stopped after at least 12 months of MAC treatment and CD4 >100 cells/μL for >6 months.

Syphilis

- For comprehensive review of syphilis, please refer to Chapter 21.
- While HIV may modify the natural history or clinical presentation of syphilis, the diagnosis and management principles are similar to those applied in the general population.
- In PLWH primary syphilis may present with atypical chancres or progress more rapidly to secondary syphilis.
- Neurosyphilis can occur at any syphilis stage but is more likely to manifest clinically in PLWH. All PLWH with neurologic signs or symptoms regardless of stage warrant CSF evaluation.
- CSF venereal disease research laboratory (VDRL) test is highly specific but not sensitive so a negative test cannot exclude neurosyphilis, especially if CSF cell count and protein are abnormal.
- Prior guidance to perform LP on all PLWH with CD4 <350 cells/μL and RPR titer ≥1:32 is not currently recommended since it is not associated with improved clinical outcomes in asymptomatic patients.

Bartonellosis

Overview and Clinical Presentation

- *Bartonella* spp. causes cat-scratch disease, trench fever, endocarditis, and bacillary angiomatosis (BA) and bacillary peliosis hepatis in immunocompromised hosts.
- *B. henselae* is specifically linked to cat exposure, while *B. quintana* is linked to homelessness and body lice.
- BA is caused by either species and typically seen in AIDS (CD4 <50 cells/μL).
- Presentation: BA causes vascular proliferative cutaneous lesions (Fig. 39.5) that are clinically indistinguishable

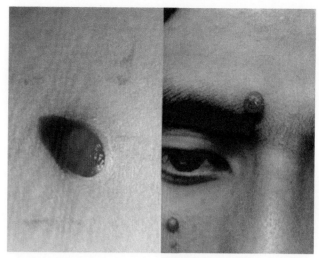

- **Fig. 39.5** Erythematous nodular skin lesions secondary to bartonellosis. (From Maguiña C, Guerra H, Ventosilla P, et al. Bartonellosis. *Clin Dermatol.* 2009;27(3):271–280.)

from KS. BA lesions may spread to distant organs including bone, lymph nodes, bone marrow, GI tract, and CNS.
- Peliosis hepatis causes angiomatous masses in the liver and spleen.
- *Bartonella* also is a major cause of fever of unknown origin and culture-negative endocarditis in AIDS.

Diagnosis

- Diagnosis usually requires Warthin–Starry stain of affected tissue on biopsy or culture in enriched media from biopsy specimens or blood collected using ethylenediaminetetraacetic acid (EDTA).

Treatment and Prophylaxis

- First-line treatments include either **erythromycin** or **doxycycline** for at least 3 months. Azithromycin or clarithromycin are alternatives. For further details on treatment, refer to Chapter 31.
- Severe or CNS bartonellosis should be treated with IV doxycycline, with or without a rifamycin, initially.
- Secondary prophylaxis should continue until minimum 3 months of treatment completed and CD4 >200 cells/μL for at least 6 months.

Bacterial Enteric Infections

- Gram-negative enteric infections occur at 10-fold higher rates in PLWH, with greatest risk in AIDS.
- Most common pathogens include nontyphoidal *Salmonella*, *Shigella*, *Campylobacter*, diarrheagenic *E. coli*, and *Clostridioides difficile*.
- **Recurrent *Salmonella* bacteremia** is an AIDS-defining illness.
- **Presentation:** self-limited gastroenteritis, more prolonged dysentery, or bacteremia with extraintestinal involvement all occur.

- **Diagnosis:** routine stool cultures, *C. difficile* testing, and blood cultures should be sent in all PLWH with diarrhea and fever (Fig. 39.1).
- **Treatment:** empiric fluoroquinolone treatment can be given in PLWH with clinically severe or febrile diarrhea but consider recent travel and enteric antibiotic resistance rates in the region. Third-generation IV cephalosporins are alternatives.
- Pathogen-directed therapy is similar to the general population although longer duration may be required in persons living with AIDS with bacteremia or metastatic complications.
- Based on limited supporting evidence, secondary prophylaxis may be considered in PLWH with recurrent *Salmonella* bacteremia.

Rhodococcus equi

- Although bacterial pneumonia occurs more frequently in PLWH regardless of CD4, certain unusual pathogens have a predilection for disease in AIDS.
- *Rhodococcus equi*, a gram-positive branching filamentous rod, causes cavitary lung lesions (Fig. 39.6) or abscesses in AIDS. It also can disseminate hematogenously to extrapulmonary sites.
- While an association with **exposure to horses or other livestock** has been reported, only about one-third of patients report such exposure.
- Treatment involves combination antibiotics with a macrolide or fluoroquinolone and at least one other active agent for at least 2 months.
- ART to improve the immune status is a critical adjunct to therapy.

Protozoal Infections

Toxoplasmosis

Overview and Clinical Presentation

- Toxoplasmic encephalitis (TE) caused by reactivation of the protozoan *Toxoplasma gondii* occurs in PLWH with CD4 count <100 cells/μL and is the **most common cause of CNS mass lesions in persons living with AIDS.**
- Prior to ART era, annual incidence was 33% among persons living with AIDS who were seropositive for *T. gondii* and not taking chemoprophylaxis.
- All PLWH should be screened for *toxoplasma* seropositivity at diagnosis and counseled to avoid exposure if seronegative.
- **Presentation:** fever, headaches, seizures, and focal deficits due to CNS mass lesions. Rarely, can disseminate to other organs including heart, lungs, or eye.

Diagnosis

- Contrasted neuroimaging with CT or magnetic resonance imaging (MRI) classically shows multiple ring-enhancing lesions in the cortical or basal ganglia grey matter (Fig. 39.7).

- Primary differential diagnosis for ring-enhancing brain lesions is primary CNS lymphoma, although other possibilities exist (see Fig. 39.1).
- PLWH with TE almost uniformly are seropositive for anti-*toxoplasma* IgG antibodies so a negative IgG makes this diagnosis unlikely though not impossible.
- Positron emission tomography (PET) or single-photon emission computed tomography (SPECT) scans may help distinguish between TE and primary CNS lymphoma.

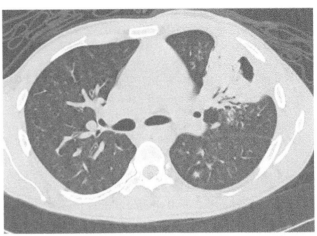

- **Fig. 39.6** Pulmonary consolidation and cavity in lingula due to *Rhodococcus equi*. (From Sax PE, Ard KL. Pulmonary manifestations of human immunodeficiency virus infection. In: Bennett JE, Dolin R, Blaser MJ, eds. *Mandell, Douglas, and Bennett's Principles and Practice of Infectious Diseases*. Updated 8th ed. Elsevier; 2015.)

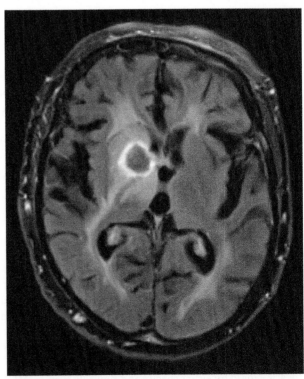

- **Fig. 39.7** Magnetic resonance imaging of *Toxoplasma gondii* ring-enhancing lesion of the right anterior putamen with vasogenic edema and mass effect. (From Greenway M, Sacco KA, Burton MC. Deep cerebral toxoplasmosis. *Am J Med*. 2017;130(7):802–804.)

- If safe, LP can be performed for CSF polymerase chain reaction (PCR) for *T. gondii*, which has very high specificity (>95%) but poor sensitivity (50%) especially after therapy has started.
- Definitive diagnosis requires stereotactic brain biopsy with demonstration of the *T. gondii* tachyzoites or cysts in tissue or positive PCR (Fig. 39.8).
- Often, empiric treatment for TE will be started in a *Toxoplasma*-seropositive person living with AIDS with compatible clinical syndrome and neuroimaging, with brain biopsy reserved for patients who fail to have an objective clinical and radiographic response within 14 days.

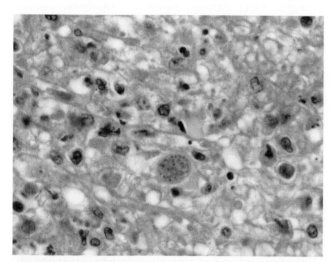

- **Fig. 39.8** *Toxoplasma gondii* cyst seen on brain biopsy (H&E, ×1000). (From Protozoal infections. In: Procop G, Pritt B, eds. *Pathology of Infectious Diseases*. Elsevier; 2015.)

Treatment and Prophylaxis

- First-line and alternative treatment regimens for TE are listed in Table 39.3.
- Adjunctive corticosteroids are added for significant cerebral edema or mass effect, and anticonvulsants are used in patients with seizure history.
- Guidelines suggest ART initiation within 2–3 weeks of TE diagnosis based on expert opinion alone.
- All *Toxoplasma*-seropositive PLWH with CD4 count <100 cells/µL should receive primary prophylaxis, with regimens and discontinuation criteria listed in Table 39.1.
- Chronic maintenance therapy should be given until completion of TE therapy and clinical resolution occurs as well as CD4 >200 cells/µL for 6 months.
- **Prevention**: seronegative patients should be counselled on avoiding transmission from ingestion of raw meat or shellfish or ingesting oocysts shed in cat feces.

Cryptosporidiosis

Overview and Clinical Presentation

- Chronic diarrheal illness caused by protozoan parasite *Cryptosporidium* (4–6 µm diameter; Fig. 39.9), of which the most common human pathogen is *C. parvum*.
- Causes self-limited disease in immunocompetent hosts but life-threatening, chronic diarrhea in PLWH with CD4 <100 cells/µL due to electrolyte abnormalities and wasting.
- **Presentation**: cholera-like diarrhea, nausea, vomiting, abdominal pain, and weight loss. Fulminant and extraintestinal disease, including sclerosing cholangitis and pancreatitis, may occur with prolonged disease in PLWH with CD4 counts <50 cells/µL.

TABLE 39.3	Treatment Regimens for Toxoplasmosis	
Disease Stage	**Preferred Therapy**	**Alternative Therapies**
Acute infection (At least 6 weeks treatment but longer if incomplete response)	Pyrimethamine 200 mg load followed by: If <60 kg, pyrimethamine 50 mg daily + sulfadiazine 1000 mg q6h + leucovorin 10–25 mg daily If >60 kg, pyrimethamine 75 mg daily + sulfadiazine 1500 mg q6h + leucovorin 10–25 mg daily Clindamycin 600 mg IV or PO q6h can be used in place of sulfadiazine if patient intolerant	Pyrimethamine (weight-based dosing) + leucovorin 10–25 mg daily + atovaquone 1500 mg BID TMP–SMX (TMP 5 mg/kg and SMX 25 mg/kg) IV or PO BID
Chronic maintenance therapy (Until complete clinical resolution and CD4 >200 cells/µL for 6 mth)	Pyrimethamine 25–50 mg daily + sulfadiazine 2000–4000 mg daily (in 2–4 divided doses) + leucovorin 10–25 mg daily	Clindamycin 600 mg q8h + pyrimethamine 25–50 mg daily + leucovorin 10–25 mg daily TMP–SMX DS 1 tab daily or BID a tovaquone 750–1500 mg BID

Additional comments:
1. TMP–SMX can be used in place of pyrimethamine–sulfadiazine if pyrimethamine is unavailable or delayed in obtaining drug.
2. Corticosteroids are used for significant mass effect or cerebral edema, and anticonvulsants are used for history of seizures.
3. Sulfa desensitization should be performed in cases of sulfa allergy.
TMP–SMX, trimethoprim–sulfamethoxazole.

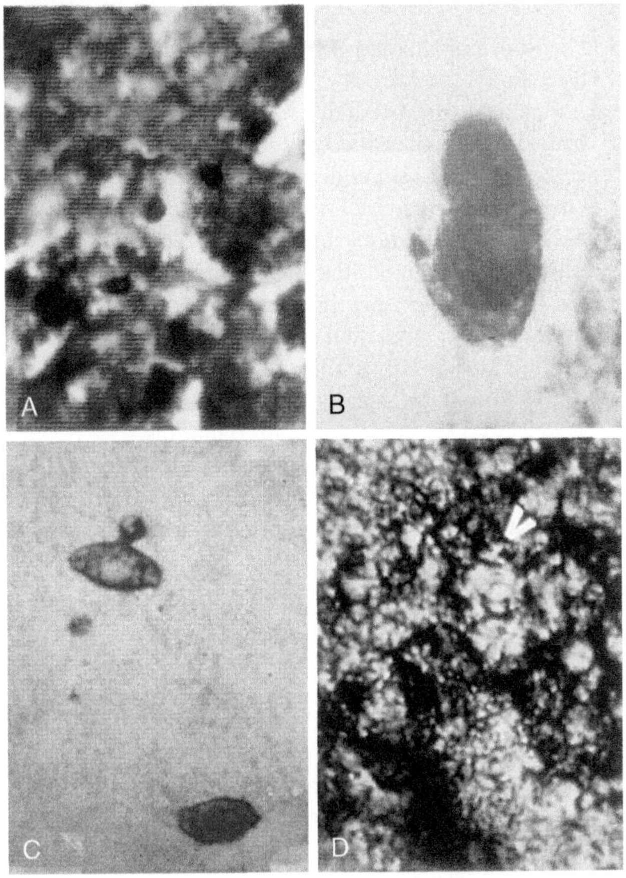

• **Fig. 39.9** Acid-fast protozoan and other causes of diarrhea in AIDS. (A) Acid-fast *Cryptosporidium* in fecal specimen. (B) Acid-fast *Cystoisospora belli* in stool of patient with diarrhea. (C) *Cystoisospora belli* and *Cryptosporidium* in PLWH with diarrhea. (D) Acid-fast *Mycobacterium avium–intracellulare* in stool of PLWH with diarrhea. (Panel A from Guerrant RL, Bobak DA. Bacterial and protozoal gastroenteritis. *N Engl J Med.* 1991;325:327. © 1991 Massachusetts Medical Society. All rights reserved. Panels B and C courtesy of Drs Rosemary Soave and Medelein Boncy; panel D courtesy Dr Cynthia Sears.)

Diagnosis

- Lab chemistries frequently show electrolyte abnormalities from chronic diarrhea and cholestatic liver function abnormalities.
- Ultrasonography can demonstrate gallbladder thickening or biliary dilation.
- Immunofluorescence staining, antigen detection, or PCR in the stool are diagnostic.

Treatment and Prophylaxis

- Since no proven therapy for cryptosporidiosis exists, immediate ART initiation to achieve immune restoration is imperative.
- Supportive care with rehydration and electrolyte repletion are a mainstay of therapy. A trial of nitazoxanide may provide some benefit but only in conjunction with ART initiation.
- Given no effective chemoprophylaxis, early ART initiation before severe immunosuppression develops and behavioral measures to reduce exposure are recommended.

Microsporidiosis

- Caused by protists related to fungi, these zoonotic, waterborne pathogens are the smallest in size (1–5 μm diameter) of the diarrheal pathogens.
- Two major genera in PLWH (CD4 <100 cells/μL):
  - *Enterocytozoon bieneusi*: causes 90% of intestinal disease and cholangiopathy due to microsporidiosis.
  - *Encephalitozoon* spp.: *E. cuniculi* and *E. hellem* cause disseminated disease to lungs and CNS, with the latter also causing keratoconjunctivitis. *E. intestinalis* typically causes chronic diarrhea.
- **Diagnosis**: Microscopic examination of tissue biopsy, corneal scraping, or stool with modified trichrome stain useful. Gold standard involves transmission electron microscopy of biopsy tissue.
- **Treatment**: Albendazole 400 mg PO twice daily for 2–4 weeks is recommended except for disease caused by *E. bieneusi*. Treatments for this species are fumagillin or its synthetic analog TNP-470, which are not available in the United States.
- **All patients with microsporidiosis should be treated with ART as soon as possible to promote immune reconstitution.**

Cystoisosporiasis

- Waterborne or foodborne illness due to *Cystoisospora belli* (formerly *Isospora*) that causes chronic diarrhea and wasting similar to cryptosporidiosis in PLWH (CD4 <50 cells/μL).
- Worldwide but more common in tropical and subtropical regions.
- **Diagnosis:** visualization of thin-walled, ellipsoidal oocysts (22–23 × 10–19 μm oval shape; Fig. 39.9) on stool modified AFB stains.
- **Treatment:** TMP–SMX DS 1 tablet PO twice daily for 10 days followed by secondary prophylaxis until CD4 >200 cells/μL for 6 months.
- Use of TMP–SMX for PCP prophylaxis also provides protection against this pathogen.

Cyclosporiasis

- Waterborne or foodborne diarrheal illness which can be protracted in persons living with AIDS. Caused by the acid-fast coccidian *Cyclospora cayetanensis*.
- Worldwide distribution but commonly reported from Latin America, India, and Southeast Asia.
- **Diagnosis:** visualization of oocyst forms (8–10 μm diameter) on stool modified AFB stains.
- **Treatment**: TMP–SMX DS 1 tablet PO twice daily for 14 days, followed by secondary prophylaxis with TMP–SMX DS three times weekly.

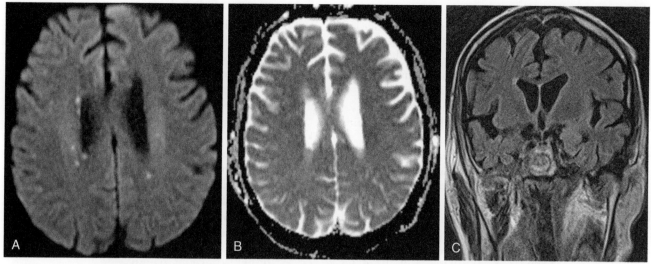

• **Fig. 39.10** Magnetic resonance imaging (MRI) of the brain of patient with CMV periventricular encephalitis. Axial diffusion weighted (DWI) (A) and apparent diffusion coefficient (ADC) (B) sequences with multiple subependymal and periventricular restricted diffusion lesions. (C) Coronal fluid-attenuated inversion recovery (FLAIR) sequences with thin curvilinear high-signal intensity lesions along the walls of both lateral ventricles. (From Renard T, Daumas-Duport B, Auffray-Calvier E, et al. Cytomegalovirus encephalitis: Undescribed diffusion-weighted imaging characteristics. Original aspects of cases extracted from a retrospective study, and from literature review. *J Neuroradiol.* 2016;43(6):371–377.)

Other Protozoal Infections

- Although not endemic in most of the United States, several important worldwide protozoal or parasitic infections cause significant disease burden in endemic countries where HIV is also prevalent. These infections include:
  - Malaria.
  - Leishmaniasis.
  - Chagas disease (American trypanosomiasis).
- HIV clinicians should be aware that PLWH who are returning travelers or immigrants from endemic countries may present with acute infection or latent reactivation from these pathogens.
- Guidelines discuss both clinical presentations and treatments of these infections in PLWH.

Viral Infections

Cytomegalovirus (CMV)
Overview and Clinical Presentation

- CMV is a double-stranded DNA herpesvirus that causes disseminated or localized end-organ disease in PLWH (typically CD4 <50 cells/μL).
- CMV disease usually occurs by reactivation, and risk of death or end-organ disease is associated with high CMV viremia measured by PCR.
- **Presentation**: CMV viremia can be asymptomatic, present with febrile CMV syndrome, or may affect one or more end-organs discussed further below (eye, CNS, GI disease, hepatitis).

Diagnosis

- **CMV chorioretinitis**: most common CMV manifestation in HIV, it presents with decreased visual acuity, "floaters," or vision loss in AIDS. Plasma CMV PCR may be negative, but funduscopic exam shows characteristic fluffy, yellow-white retinal lesions with perivascular exudate and hemorrhages ("scrambled eggs and ketchup" appearance).
- **CMV neurologic disease**: presents with periventricular encephalitis (Fig. 39.10), mononeuritis multiplex, or polyradiculopathy. Typically diagnosed by neurologic exam, MRI brain and spinal cord, and positive CMV PCR or stains from either CSF or peripheral nerve biopsy.
- **CMV gastrointestinal disease**: colitis represents 5%–10% of cases of CMV end-organ disease, presents with fever, diarrhea, abdominal pain, and even perforation. Diagnosis by colonoscopy with characteristic "owl eye" CMV inclusions on biopsy since plasma PCR may be negative. Esophagitis requires upper endoscopy with biopsy for diagnosis.
- **CMV pneumonitis**: unlike transplant recipients, **true CMV pneumonitis is distinctly uncommon in HIV.** Often requires lung biopsy to diagnose by histopathology since CMV PCR in respiratory specimens is frequently positive but not truly pathogenic.

Treatment and Prophylaxis

- Treatment of CMV chorioretinitis is individualized based on location and severity of lesions, immune status, and adherence to therapy in consultation with an experienced ophthalmologist.

- For sight-threatening lesions, intravitreal injections of ganciclovir or foscarnet (up to 4 doses) plus valganciclovir 900 mg PO twice daily for 14–21 days, followed by valganciclovir 900 mg PO daily maintenance therapy. IV anti-CMV antivirals are alternatives to valganciclovir.
  - For peripheral lesions, oral valganciclovir for 3–6 months without intravitreal injections is given.
  - Immune reconstitution uveitis (IRU) may require temporary periocular or systemic steroids.
- For proven gastrointestinal disease or rigorously diagnosed pneumonitis, IV ganciclovir is given for at least 21 days but can transition to PO valganciclovir once improving and tolerating orals.
- Proven neurologic disease is treated with combination IV ganciclovir plus IV foscarnet initially while optimizing ART.
- Chronic maintenance valganciclovir is continued in all patients with CMV chorioretinitis until all of the following:
  - CMV treatment for minimum 3–6 months.
  - All retinal lesions inactive and cleared by ophthalmologist.
  - CD4 >100 cells/µL for 3–6 months on ART.
- All PLWH with CD4 <50 cells/µL require biannual screening ophthalmologic examination for CMV retinitis.

Herpes Simplex Virus (HSV)

Overview and Clinical Presentation

- For comprehensive review of genital HSV disease, refer to Chapter 21: Sexually Transmitted Infections.
- HSV type 1 and HSV type 2 are double-stranded DNA herpesviruses that are frequently shed from mucosal surfaces.
- Approximately 70% of PLWH are seropositive for HSV-2 and 95% seropositive for either HSV-1 or -2.
- HSV-2 increases the risk of HIV acquisition and increases HIV RNA in blood and genital secretions of co-infected patients.
- **Presentation**: orolabial herpes (predominantly HSV-1) and genital herpes (predominantly HSV-2) are most common presentations. HSV also causes proctitis in men who have sex with men (MSM).
- Nonmucosal presentations including HSV keratitis, encephalitis, esophagitis, hepatitis, or disseminated disease are rare but can occur in AIDS.
- HSV retinitis manifests as **acute retinal necrosis (ARN) with rapidly progressive vision loss.**

Diagnosis

- Diagnosis of mucosal lesions involves **HSV type-specific DNA PCR and viral culture from affected lesions.** HSV DNA PCR from other body fluids including blood and CSF can diagnose nonmucosal disease.
- Type-specific serologies are most useful in asymptomatic patients for counselling regarding risk of transmission to sexual partners.

Treatment and Prophylaxis

- Orolabial and genital HSV are treated with oral aciclovir, valaciclovir, or famciclovir for 5–10 days for episodic therapy. Chronic suppressive therapy can be considered for frequent recurrences or to reduce transmission.
- Severe mucocutaneous HSV lesions and all forms of disseminated HSV should be treated initially with IV aciclovir.
- Failure of HSV mucosal lesions to resolve within 7–10 days raises concerns of aciclovir-resistant HSV, which should be confirmed with susceptibility testing. IV foscarnet is the drug of choice for drug-resistant HSV.
- Primary prophylaxis against HSV is not recommended, but barrier protection should be encouraged to reduce sexual transmission to seronegative partners.

Varicella-Zoster Virus (VZV)

Overview and Clinical Presentation

- VZV causes primary infection known as varicella as well as latent reactivation known as herpes zoster.
- Herpes zoster occurs at 15-fold higher rate in PLWH compared to age-matched controls.
- VZV reactivation can occur at any CD4 count, but most complications and disseminated disease occur at CD4 <200 cells/µL.
- **Presentations**: primary varicella infection (chickenpox) has a characteristic viral exanthem but can disseminate with significant morbidity in PLWH. Herpes zoster may present with a typical dermatomal shingles outbreak, but multidermatomal or dissemination can occur.
- A primary organ involved by VZV reactivation is the CNS. VZV-related neurologic complications include CNS vasculitis, ventriculitis, myelitis, aseptic meningitis, optic neuritis, cranial nerve palsies, and focal brain stem lesions.
- Three ocular complications of VZV in HIV warrant attention:
  - **Herpes zoster ophthalmicus**: reactivation along V1 of the trigeminal nerve, which can lead to keratitis and retinitis.
  - **Acute retinal necrosis (ARN)**: necrotizing retinopathy characterized by anterior uveitis, retinal vasculitis, and optic disc papillitis. This can occur at any CD4 count and is caused by VZV, HSV, or CMV.
- **Progressive outer retinal necrosis (PORN)**: necrotizing retinopathy caused only by VZV and seen in PLWH with CD4 <100/µL. Retina shows rapidly coalescing multifocal necrotic lesions, but minimal vitritis or vasculitis unlike ARN. Both PORN and ARN result in high rates of vision loss.

Diagnosis

- Typical varicella or zoster can be diagnosed clinically. Atypical lesions should be swabbed or biopsied from fresh lesions for viral PCR or culture.

- Histopathologic diagnosis or PCR from other body fluids and tissue can aid in diagnosis of visceral VZV dissemination.

Treatment and Prophylaxis

- Uncomplicated varicella infection is treated with oral valaciclovir, famciclovir, or aciclovir for 5–7 days; localized dermatomal zoster is treated similarly for 7–10 days.
- Extensive cutaneous or disseminated disease in either primary infection or reactivation should be treated with IV aciclovir.
- ARN requires aggressive systemic treatment with IV aciclovir 10 mg/kg every 8 hours for 10–14 days followed by 6 weeks of oral valaciclovir, in conjunction with ophthalmology.
- Optimal treatment of PORN remains undefined, but combinations of IV and intravitreal ganciclovir and foscarnet, guided by an experienced ophthalmologist, with optimization of ART has been used, although visual prognosis remains poor.
- **Postexposure prophylaxis with varicella-zoster immunoglobulin** (VariZIG) can be given to susceptible PLWH as soon as possible after close contact with a person with active varicella or zoster.
- Live attenuated varicella vaccine is safe to give PLWH with CD4 >200 cells/μL.

Human Herpesvirus 8 (HHV-8)

- HHV-8 is the causative agent KS as well as **primary effusion lymphoma** (PEL) and **multicentric Castleman's disease** (MCD). KS is discussed below under AIDS-associated malignancies.
- HHV-8 seroprevalence in the general population is 1%–5% but ranges from 20% to 70% in MSM population.
- KS and PEL usually occur in PLWH with CD4 <200 cells/μL, while MCD can occur at any CD4 count.
- **Presentations**: PEL is an uncommon AIDS-related lymphoma presenting as effusions of pleural, pericardial, or abdominal spaces rather than discrete masses.
- MCD is a lymphoproliferative disorder that presents with fevers, constitutional symptoms, generalized lymphadenopathy, and hepatosplenomegaly and can progress to multiorgan failure from interleukin-6 mediated cytokine storm. KS commonly coexists with MCD.
- **Diagnosis:** PEL is diagnosed by fluid cytology showing high-grade malignant lymphocytes that are immunohistochemical-stain positive for HHV-8. MCD is diagnosed on tissue biopsy by histology and immunologic cell markers.
- **Treatment:** for PEL, overall prognosis is poor and treatment experience is limited, so patients should be referred for clinical trials. All PLWH should receive ART, typically given with combination chemotherapy regimens for lymphoma.

- For MCD, patients should be referred for clinical trials if available; otherwise, combination therapies with the **monoclonal anti-CD20 antibody rituximab plus IV ganciclovir plus chemotherapy with etoposide** in addition to ART has shown early promise.

Progressive Multifocal Leukoencephalopathy (PML)

Overview and Clinical Presentation

- Opportunistic CNS infection caused by JC polyoma virus leading to demyelination of the deep white matter.
- Prior to ART era, PML developed in 3%–7% of persons living with AIDS and was universally fatal.
- Incidence has declined substantially with ART but remains a morbid disease.
- Reactivation occurs mainly in PLWH with CD4 <200 cells/μL but can occur at higher CD4 counts or in PLWH on other immunosuppressive agents (e.g., natalizumab or rituximab).
- **Presentation:** insidious and progressive onset of focal neurologic deficits (paresis, vision or speech defects) due to demyelinating lesions over weeks to months; seizures occur in 20% of cases.

Diagnosis

- Compatible clinical findings and neuroimaging on MRI showing discrete white matter lesions which are not contrast-enhancing and hypointense on T1-weighted and hyperintense on T2-weighted sequences and fluid-attenuated inversion recovery (FLAIR) sequences (Fig. 39.11).
- Magnetic resonance (MR) spectroscopy and diffusion-weighted imaging help distinguish PML from other lesions.
- CSF PCR testing for JC virus has approximately 80% sensitivity and 95% specificity in PLWH not on ART but is less sensitive in PLWH on ART. In atypical cases, brain biopsy is required to confirm the diagnosis.

Treatment and Prophylaxis

- No specific proven therapy exists for JC virus or PML.
- Immediate initiation of ART is strongly recommended and reduction or cessation of other immunosuppression may be useful.
- Other targeted therapies have been tested (e.g., cidofovir, cytarabine, 5HT2a serotonin receptor blockers), but none demonstrates consistent clinical benefit.

Parvovirus B19

- Parvovirus B19 is DNA erythrovirus that causes the childhood illness erythema infectiosum (fifth disease) and spread by respiratory, hematogenous, or vertical transmission.

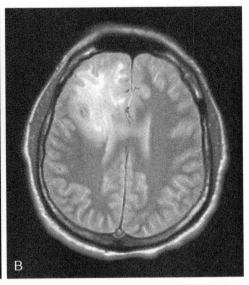

• **Fig. 39.11** Magnetic resonance imaging of progressive multifocal leukoencephalopathy (PML) lesion showing low signal intensity without contrast enhancement on T1-weighted images (A) compared to high signal intensity on T2-weighted images (B). (From Boren EJ, Cheema GS, Naguwa SM, et al. The emergence of progressive multifocal leukoencephalopathy (PML) in rheumatic diseases. *J Autoimmun.* 2008;30(1–2):90–98.)

• Although causing only self-limited febrile illness with rash or arthralgias in immunocompetent hosts, chronic infection in persons living with AIDS can lead to a **pure red cell aplasia with severe anemia and paradoxically low reticulocyte count.**
• **Diagnosis:** since serologies are less useful in immunosuppressed patients, parvovirus DNA PCR is the diagnostic test of choice.
• **Treatment:** PLWH with parvovirus B19-related pure red cell aplasia should be treated with **intravenous immunoglobulin (IVIG)** 1–2 grams/kg per day for 2–5 days with lower dose maintenance IVIG every 4 weeks for relapses.

Hepatitis B Virus (HBV)

• For comprehensive review of HBV, refer to Chapter 22: Viral Hepatitis.
• HBV is a DNA virus, which is the leading cause of liver disease worldwide, and chronically infects approximately 10% of PLWH.
• Like HIV, HBV can be transmitted through sexual contact, bloodborne exposure, or perinatal vertical transmission. Risk of progression to chronic HBV varies by age of acquisition (highest in perinatal transmission).
• HIV/HBV co-infection leads to higher HBV DNA levels and accelerated progression of liver disease compared to monoinfection.
• **Diagnosis:** All PLWH should be screened for chronic HBV. Initial serologic testing includes hepatitis B surface antigen (HBsAg), core antibody (anti-HBc total), and surface antibody (anti-HBsAb).

• Chronic HBV is defined as persistent HBsAg positivity for more than 6 months. Patients with chronic HBV should be further tested for hepatitis B e-antigen (HBeAg), antibody to e-antigen (anti-HBe), and HBV DNA levels.
• Isolated hepatitis B core antibody (anti-HBc) positivity, which is more common in PLWH could indicate a false-positive test, past infection with loss of anti-HBsAb, or occult chronic HBV with undetectable HBsAg titers. Routine HBV DNA testing is not recommended but HBV vaccination is.
• **Treatment: all persons with HIV/HBV co-infection, regardless of CD4 count or HBV viral load, should be treated with ART active against both viruses.** Preferred ART regimens contain two active drugs against HBV, with either tenofovir disoproxil fumarate (TDF) or tenofovir alafenamide (TAF)-based ART regimens.
• If a tenofovir-containing regimen cannot be used, entecavir should be added to a fully suppressive ART regimen.
• Importantly, monotherapy with emtricitabine (FTC) or lamivudine (3TC) for HBV is not recommended due to the high rate of drug resistance development.
• Monitoring on therapy should include aminotransferases (ALT) and HBV DNA every 3–6 months to evaluate response. Sustained loss of HBsAg is considered a complete response but rarely occurs (<1% per year).
• **HBV flares:** acute rises in serum aminotransferases or clinical signs of acute hepatitis may develop and can be due to **several scenarios that must be carefully distinguished** including:
  • HBV-IRIS or reactivation with immune reconstitution, usually 6–12 weeks after starting ART.

- Discontinuation or nonadherence to HBV-active ART medications.
- Emergence of HBV drug resistance.
- Drug-induced liver injury from ART or other drugs, including alcohol.
- Other infectious causes of acute hepatitis (e.g., acute hepatitis A, C, D, or E; CMV, HSV).
- **Prevention**: all PLWH without chronic HBV or without documented immunity (anti-HBsAb <10 IU/ml) should be vaccinated although those with lower CD4 counts may have poor response, requiring revaccination with a higher dose series.
- **Long-term follow-up**: PLWH with chronic HBV infection, both with cirrhosis and in other high-risk groups, require surveillance for hepatocellular carcinoma (HCC) with liver ultrasound every 6–12 months. Since HIV confers an increased HCC risk, some experts recommend HCC screening in all HBV co-infected PLWH over 40.

Hepatitis C Virus (HCV)

- For comprehensive review of HCV, refer to Chapter 22.
- HCV is a single-stranded RNA virus, with a worldwide prevalence of about 3% and approximately 3.5 million chronically infected persons in the United States.
- Both HIV and HCV can be transmitted via percutaneous exposure to blood or blood products, sexual intercourse, or mother-to-child transmission.
- Due to these shared transmission routes, approximately 20%–30% of PLWH in the United States are co-infected with HCV.
- All PLWH should undergo routine HCV screening at diagnosis and then annually if indicated by ongoing exposure risk.
- **HIV is an important risk factor for HCV progression**, with higher rates of fibrosis, decompensated liver disease, and liver-related morbidity and mortality in co-infected patients. CD4 count <200 cells/μL is associated with higher rates of liver disease progression and HCC.
- **Presentation**: most patients are asymptomatic until cirrhosis develops, at which time the complications of chronic liver disease may present. Extrahepatic manifestations of HCV include mixed cryoglobulinemic vasculitis, membranous glomerulonephritis, and porphyria cutanea tarda.
- **Diagnosis**: initial screening is performed by sensitive immunoassay to detect antibodies to HCV (anti-HCV) in the blood. Quantitative plasma HCV RNA level is then checked in all seropositive individuals or if clinical suspicion for HCV infection is high.
- Seven HCV genotypes exist, and a patient's HCV genotype has important implications for treatment.
- **Treatment**: the overall goals, treatment regimens, and monitoring in HIV/HCV co-infection are similar to those for HCV monoinfection. Given the development of direct acting antivirals (DAAs) and rapid evolution of treatment guidelines, clinicians should refer to the most recent HCV treatment guidelines for the latest recommendations (http://www.hcvguidelines.org).
- Importantly, treatment of HCV may require adjustment to a patient's ART due to drug–drug interactions.
- **Prevention**: since no effective HCV vaccine or postexposure prophylaxis exists, prevention involves behavioral risk reduction targeting injection drug use or high-risk sexual practices.
- **Long-term follow-up**: after successful cure of HCV (sustained virologic response, or SVR), patients should be counseled about avoiding other hepatic insults (alcohol, hepatotoxic drugs, HBV) and continue to be monitored for HCV re-infection if engaged in ongoing high-risk behaviors.
- Patients with underlying cirrhosis also require screening for HCC with liver ultrasound every 6–12 months and monitoring for complications of chronic liver disease.

Human Papillomavirus (HPV)

- HPV is a common sexually transmitted viral infection that causes cervical cancer, the fourth most common cancer in women worldwide. It is also the causative agent of oral and genital warts as well as anal, vulvar, and some oropharyngeal squamous cell cancers.
- PLWH are at higher risk to acquire HPV infection, and there is a direct relationship between CD4 count and cervical cancer risk. **Invasive cervical cancer is an AIDS-defining illness in women living with HIV.**
- There are over 100 different HPV serotypes, but HPV serotypes 16 and 18 account for the majority of cervical cancer while serotypes 6 and 11 cause 90% of benign genital warts.
- Cervical cancer screening via Pap smear and HPV co-testing is recommended in all women, but the frequency and intensity of screening intervals is slightly different in PLWH compared to the general population.
- Three FDA-approved HPV vaccines (bivalent, quadrivalent, and 9-valent) have been shown to prevent HPV 16 and HPV 18 infections and precancerous lesions. The quadrivalent and 9-valent vaccines also prevent genital warts due to HPV 6 and HPV 11 infections.
- Current immunization schedules recommend that all PLWH, both adults and adolescents, males and females, receive a 3-dose series of a HPV vaccine up to age 26.

HIV-Associated Malignancies

Kaposi Sarcoma (KS)

- Caused by HHV-8, also known as Kaposi sarcoma-associated herpesvirus.
- Most common HIV-associated malignancy, seen mainly in MSM population.
- **Presentation**: Multifocal purplish nodules (Fig. 39.12) on skin or mucous membranes (especially intraoral). Localized cutaneous disease seen at higher CD4 counts, while dissemination with lymphatic, pulmonary or GI involvement seen in persons living with AIDS.

Cutaneous Kaposi sarcoma lesions

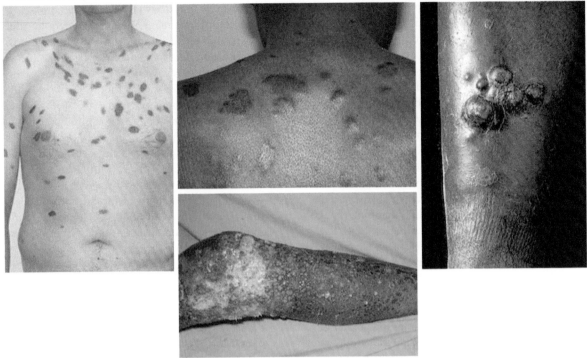

• **Fig. 39.12** Cutaneous Kaposi sarcoma skin lesions. (From Williams J, Bower M. AIDS-related malignant disease. *Medicine*. 2013;41(8):430–434.)

- **Diagnosis**: Biopsy shows characteristic whorls of spindle-shaped cells and abnormal vascular proliferation with positive immunohistochemical staining for HHV-8.
- **Treatment**: Varies by site and extent of disease. Local therapy includes radiotherapy, cryotherapy, or intralesional chemotherapy for limited disease while systemic chemotherapy is preferred for visceral or advanced KS.
- **All PLWH with KS should be started on ART as soon as possible since immune recovery alone may lead to lesion regression.**

Non-Hodgkin Lymphoma (NHL)

- Heterogeneous group of malignancies usually of B-cell origin and that can occur at widely variable CD4 counts. **Often associated with oncogenic viruses such as Epstein–Barr virus (EBV) or HHV-8.**
- Intermediate to high-grade NHL is an AIDS-defining illness, occurring at 200-fold higher rate than the general population.
- **Presentation**: systemic "B" symptoms (fevers, weight loss, night sweats), lymphadenopathy common but also frequently seen with extranodal disease to bone marrow, GI, liver, or CNS.
- **Treatment**: standard systemic chemotherapy regimens used, but ART is critical to support immune recovery if possible.

Primary CNS Lymphoma (PCNSL)

- Primary B-cell lymphoma of the CNS most commonly seen in PLWH (CD4 <50 cells/μL) and almost universally associated with EBV.
- **Presentation**: systemic "B" symptoms accompanied by focal or nonfocal neurologic signs of confusion, lethargy, hemiparesis, or seizures.
- **Diagnosis**: single or multiple ring-enhancing mass lesions seen on brain MRI suggestive in person living with AIDS. Since major differential diagnosis is cerebral toxoplasmosis, anti-*Toxoplasma* serologies and an empiric trial of *Toxoplasma* therapy often performed.
- **CSF EBV DNA PCR and SPECT imaging may be helpful in distinguishing PCNSL from other etiologies,** but brain biopsy may still be required in equivocal cases.
- Optimal therapy still to be defined, but whole-brain radiation and steroids along with early ART initiation are mainstays of current therapies.

Immune Reconstitution Inflammatory Syndrome (IRIS)

- Syndrome of worsening clinical findings from OIs with immune reconstitution and enhanced inflammation in PLWH after initiation of ART. Occurs in two forms:
  - Paradoxical IRIS: worsening or relapse of known OI despite effective microbiologic treatment success (most common in mycobacterial or cryptococcal infections).

- Unmasking IRIS: symptoms from previously occult OI "unmasked" by immune recovery with ART.
- The likelihood and severity of IRIS is correlated with the nadir CD4 count prior to ART initiation and the degree of viral suppression and CD4 recovery after ART initiation.
- No universal diagnostic criteria exist for IRIS; however, typically cases of IRIS should meet most or all of the following:
  - Positive virologic and immune recovery response to ART, usually starting from CD4 count <100 cells/μL.
  - Clinical worsening of OI signs or symptoms consistent with inflammatory response and not explained by drug resistance, adverse drug effects, superimposed infection, or inadequate drug levels due to nonadherence or poor absorption.
  - Temporal association between ART initiation and onset of clinical worsening.
- The most common pathogens associated with IRIS include TB, MAC, PCP, *Cryptococcus*, CMV, JC virus (PML), HBV, and HHV-8.
  - Mycobacterial IRIS (TB or MAC) typically involves recrudescence of fevers, weight loss, and worsening inflammatory response in either pulmonary or extrapulmonary sites, classically with lymphadenitis.
  - PCP IRIS is less common with routine use of corticosteroids for moderate to severe disease but manifests as recurrent fevers, cough, hypoxia, and pulmonary infiltrates similar to initial infection.
  - Cryptococcal IRIS presents with signs of recurrent meningoencephalitis and elevated ICP, but lumbar puncture studies show significantly higher opening pressures and CSF WBC counts while the CSF cultures usually remain sterile.

- CMV IRIS of the eye, also termed immune recovery uveitis, manifests with worsening eye symptoms and intense inflammatory response on funduscopic exam.
- PML IRIS differs from classic PML with lesions that progress more rapidly and show mass effect, edema, and contrast enhancement.
- **Management of IRIS**: ART should generally be continued in cases of IRIS unless severe or life-threatening sequelae require cessation (e.g., increased ICP). Non-steroidal antiinflammatory drugs (NSAIDs) or corticosteroids can reduce symptoms in moderate to severe IRIS cases.

Further Reading

1. Centers for Disease Control and Prevention. Appendix A: AIDS-defining conditions. *MMWR Morbid Mortal Wkly Rep.* 2008;57(RR-10):9.
2. Panel on Opportunistic Infections in HIV-Infected Adults and Adolescents. Guidelines for the prevention and treatment of opportunistic infections in HIV-infected adults and adolescents: recommendations from the Centers for Disease Control and Prevention, the National Institutes of Health, and the HIV Medicine Association of the Infectious Diseases Society of America. http://aidsinfo.nih.gov/contentfiles/lvguidelines/adult_oi.pdf.
3. Panel on Antiretroviral Guidelines for Adults and Adolescents. Guidelines for the use of antiretroviral agents in adults and adolescents living with HIV. Department of Health and Human Services. http://www.aidsinfo.nih.gov/ContentFiles/AdultandAdolescentGL.pdf.
4. Zolopa A, Andersen J, Powderly W, et al. Early antiretroviral therapy reduces AIDS progression/death in individuals with acute opportunistic infections: a multicenter randomized strategy trial. *PloS ONE.* 2009;4(5):e5575.
5. INSIGHT START Study. Lundgren JD, Babiker AG, Gordin F, Emery S, Grund B, et al. Initiation of antiretroviral therapy in early asymptomatic HIV infection. *NN Engl J Med.* 2015;373(9):795–807.

40

Infections in Patients with Cancer and Immunosuppressive Therapy

ANDREA J. ZIMMER, ALISON G. FREIFELD

Febrile Neutropenia (FN)

- Typically occurs following cytotoxic chemotherapy.
- Nonspecifically targets cell proliferation and therefore results in collateral damage.
  - Myelosuppression due to marrow toxicity.
  - Damage to mucosal surfaces of the mouth, gut, and respiratory tract (barrier breeches).

Definition
- **Temperature** of ≥38.3 × 1 or ≥38.0 sustained for 1 hour.
- ANC (absolute neutrophil count) of ≤500 neutrophils/µL at time of fever or <1000 neutrophils/L with anticipated drop to ≤500 neutrophils/L within next 48 hours.

Risk for Developing FN
- First cycle of chemotherapy.
- FN during previous cycles of chemotherapy.
- Type of malignancy
  - Hematologic malignancies (HM) are highest risk; acute myelogenous leukemia (AML), acute lymphoblastic leukemia (ALL), myelodysplastic syndrome (MDS), lymphoma, multiple myeloma.
  - Solid tumors that are >20% risk for FN
    - Bladder, kidney.
    - Breast, ovarian, testicular.
    - Melanoma.
    - Sarcoma.
    - Small cell lung cancer.
  - High disease burden increases rate of FN.
  - Bone marrow involvement.
  - Chemotherapy regimen
    - High dose regimens.
    - Curative intent.
- Comorbidities
  - Age >65.
  - Liver or kidney dysfunction.
  - Recent surgery.
  - Prior chemo or radiation therapy.

Complications Due to FN
- **MASCC score:** stratifies FN patients' risk for morbidity and mortality. (MASCC = Multinational Association of Supportive Care in Cancer.)
- Score of ≥21 is considered low risk, <21 is high risk (Table 40.1).
- Serious complications include:
  - Hypotension requiring vasopressor support.
  - Need for mechanical ventilation.
  - Sepsis.
  - Death.

Infection Risk
- Correlates to depth (ANC <100 neutrophils/µL) and duration of neutropenia.
- **Low risk** in patients with anticipated neutropenia of <7 days.
  - Solid tumor patients.
- **Intermediate risk** in patients with anticipated neutropenia of 7–10 days.
  - Lymphoma.
  - Multiple myeloma.
  - CLL.
  - Autologous hematopoietic stem cell transplant (HSCT).
- **High risk** in patients with anticipated neutropenia of >10 days.
  - Acute leukemia.
  - Allogeneic HSCT.

Causes of FN
- Infectious etiology identified only in about 50% of FN.
  - 10%–20% with bacteremia.
  - 20%–30% are clinically documented infections (i.e., pneumonia, colitis, skin/soft tissue infection).

Work-up
- Complete H&P (history and physical), including history of previous infections and social history.

TABLE 40.1	Score Derived from the Logistic Equation of the MASCC Predictive Model	
Characteristic		**Points**
Burden of illness		
No or mild symptoms		5
Moderate symptoms		3
No hypotension		5
No chronic obstructive pulmonary disease		4
Solid tumor or no previous fungal infection in hematological cancer		4
Outpatient status		3
No dehydration		3
Aged <60 years		2
Threshold: score ≥21 (maximum 26) predicts <5% of severe complications		

From Klasterksy J, Awada A, Paesmans M, Aoun M. Febrile neutropenia: a critical review of the initial management. *Crit Rev Oncol Hematol.* 2011;78(3):185–194.

- Blood cultures × at least 2 sets, ideally one from each catheter lumen and one peripheral.
- Complete blood count (CBC) w/differential, complete metabolic panel (CMP).
- Urinalysis and urine cultures (if symptoms or other clinical concern).
- Chest X-ray ±sputum culture or respiratory viral panel for respiratory symptoms.
- *Clostridioides difficile* assay, enteric pathogen panel for diarrhea.
- Abdominal imaging with CT or ultrasound for abdominal or rectal pain.
- CT or MRI head with lumbar puncture (LP) for CNS symptoms.
- CT sinus or MRI orbit with ENT or ophthalmologic evaluation for sinus or periorbital pain.
- Aspiration or biopsy of concerning skin lesions for pathologic examination, Gram stain, and culture.

Antimicrobial Prophylaxis
- **Bacterial:** used in many centers for intermediate and high-risk patients.
  - Often with levofloxacin or other fluoroquinolone, targeting enteric gram-negatives (GNR).
  - Decreases rates of FN and infection (in some studies), **but no benefit on mortality.**
  - Associated with increased antimicrobial resistance, particularly fluoroquinolone resistance in *E. coli.*
  - Some institutions moving away from using prophylaxis for this reason.
- **Fungal**: often used in intermediate and high-risk patients.
  - Prophylaxis against *Candida* with fluconazole or micafungin often used in intermediate risk and ALL (due to significant interaction between other azoles

and vincristine, an agent commonly used in ALL regimens).
  - Prophylaxis against *Candida* and molds with voriconazole, posaconazole, and micafungin typically used in high-risk patients.
  - Prolonged duration of neutropenia (>10–14 days).
  - High dose steroid use.
  - AML or MDS.
- **Viral**: Used during active therapy in intermediate to high risk patients or in patients with history of herpes simplex virus (HSV) reactivation.
  - Directed against HSV and varicella-zoster virus (VZV) (aciclovir, famciclovir, valaciclovir).

Empiric Treatment
- Empiric broad-spectrum antibiotics including antipseudomonal coverage, based on institutional susceptibility patterns and prior infections of the individual.
  - Low-risk patients (high MASCC score, solid tumor) can be considered for oral antibiotics. **Not recommended in patients receiving fluoroquinolone prophylaxis.**
    - Ciprofloxacin + amoxicillin/clavulanate.
    - Moxifloxacin.
    - Levofloxacin.
  - High-risk patients (low MASCC score) typically treated with IV beta-lactam monotherapy.
    - Cefepime.
    - Piperacillin/tazobactam.
    - Meropenem.
    - Imipenem/cilastatin.
    - Ceftazidime; **has less efficacy against gram-positive organisms**.

Indications to Expand Initial Empiric Therapy
- Consideration for adding dual gram-negative coverage with an aminoglycoside, polymyxin B, or fluoroquinolone (if not recently used for prophylaxis) in patients with hemodynamic instability or concern for resistant organism.
  - Tailor therapy to patient's previous infections and susceptibilities as well as institutional antibiogram.
- Consider choosing an agent with anaerobic coverage in patients with abdominal pain or diarrhea.
- No benefit to add **empiric vancomycin** except for the following indications:
  - Soft tissue or catheter site infection.
  - Blood cultures positive for gram-positive bacteria, awaiting identification and susceptibility testing.
  - Known colonization with MRSA or cephalosporin-resistant streptococci.
  - Hemodynamic instability or shock pending culture results.
  - In combination with aztreonam with true beta-lactam allergy.

Modifications to Initial Therapy

- Guided by clinical and microbiologic data.
  - Therapy should be modified to appropriately cover identified pathogens based on susceptibility data.
  - Escalation in coverage for patients with decompensation.
  - Persistent fever in an otherwise stable patient is not an indication to modify antibiotics.
  - **If vancomycin or other gram-positive coverage was empirically started, it may be stopped after 48 hours if no gram-positive infection identified.**
  - **If fevers persist despite 4–7 days of broad-spectrum antibiotic coverage, work-up should be expanded with imaging and consider use of empirical antifungal coverage.**
  - If no infection identified, antibiotics can be stopped upon recovery of ANC to ≥500.

Bloodstream Infections

- **Gram-positive cocci (GPC)** now account for at least 50%, likely due to prophylaxis use and indwelling catheters.
  - **Coagulase-negative *Staphylococci*.**
  - ***Staphylococcus aureus*** (including MRSA).
  - ***Enterococcus* spp.** (including VRE)
    - VRE requires treatment with daptomycin or linezolid.
    - VRE colonization is a risk for systemic infection; consider empiric treatment while awaiting culture data in patients with known colonization or prior infection.
  - ***Viridans* group *Streptococcus***
    - Associated with oral **mucositis**, can cause severe sepsis and/or pneumonia with acute respiratory distress syndrome in neutropenic patients; looks clinically like gram-negative rod (GNR) sepsis.
    - May **break through fluoroquinolone prophylaxis.**
    - **Penicillin and cephalosporin resistance** has been noted (indication for empiric vancomycin in patients with hemodynamic instability or known colonization).
  - ***Streptococcus pneumoniae*.**
- **Gram-negative rods (GNR)** are associated with higher morbidity and mortality than GPCs; most common source is gut translocation. Historically GNR were more common but incidence is influenced by prophylaxis use.
  - ***Escherichia coli*.**
  - ***Klebsiella* spp.**
  - ***Enterobacter* spp.**
  - ***Pseudomonas aeruginosa***
    - Only accounts for about 5% of infections, but associated with much higher morbidity and mortality, particularly with delayed treatment.
  - ***Citrobacter* spp.**
  - ***Stenotrophomonas*.**

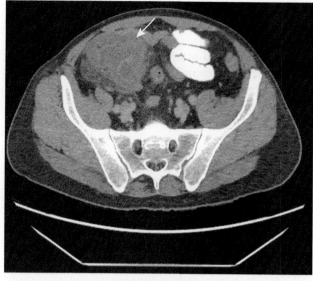

- **Fig. 40.1** Typhlitis.

- Multidrug-resistant GNR including extended spectrum beta-lactamases (ESBLs) or carbapenemases are becoming increasingly common and attention to institutional antibiograms is important.
- **Anaerobes**: infrequently isolated, but most common source is gut translocation.
- ***Candida*** also rather infrequent, likely due to azole prophylaxis.
- Catheter should be removed in central line-associated bloodstream infections (CLABSI) when due to *S. aureus*, *Pseudomonas*, *Stenotrophomonas*, and *Candida* spp. (see also Chapter 14 for indications of catheter removal for CLABSI).

Neutropenic Colitis

- Also known as typhlitis, classically involves ileocecal region (Fig. 40.1).
- Occurs following cytotoxic chemotherapy, likely as a result of damage to mucosal lining in the setting of prolonged neutropenia allowing enteric organisms to invade and translocate bowel wall.
- **Symptoms**
  - Abdominal pain, cramping: typically right lower quadrant.
  - Fever.
  - Diarrhea.
  - Hematochezia.
- **Work-up**
  - Computed tomography (CT) abdomen/pelvis with oral and IV contrast.
  - Blood cultures.
  - Testing for *C. difficile*.
- **Complications**
  - Sepsis, especially with translocation of enteric organisms into the bloodstream.
  - Bowel necrosis and perforation.
  - High mortality, some reports as high as >50%.

- **Management**
  - Broad-spectrum antibiotics that include coverage against *Pseudomonas aeruginosa*, enteric gram-negative organisms, and anaerobes.
  - Preferred regimens include:
    - Piperacillin-tazobactam.
    - Cefepime + metronidazole (also empirically treats *C. diff*).
    - Meropenem or imipenem-cilastatin.
  - Consider addition of antifungal agent if persistently febrile ×72 hours or hemodynamic instability.
  - Antimicrobial therapy should be continued through recovery of neutrophils and clinical recovery.
  - IV fluids.
  - Bowel rest for severe cases.
  - Close observation and frequent examinations.
  - Surgery
    - Try to avoid or delay due to significant neutropenia and thrombocytopenia.
    - May be necessary in perforation or clinical deterioration.

Pneumonia

- **Work-up**
  - Blood and sputum cultures (neutropenic patients may be unable to produce sputum even in the setting of pneumonia).
  - Chest X-ray (**infiltrates may be subtle during neutropenia and worsen with recovery of ANC**) or CT chest (more sensitive).
  - Urine *Legionella* and pneumococcal antigen tests.
  - Nasal wash with molecular respiratory pathogens panel.
  - Consider bronchoscopy with bronchoalveolar lavage (BAL), especially with diffuse infiltrates, unresponsive to initial empiric therapy or if patient unable to produce a sputum sample.
  - Serum ±BAL galactomannan and/or 1,3 beta-D-glucan in patients at high risk for mold infections (in patients with prolonged neutropenia including hematologic malignancy or HSCT).
- **Management**
  - Based on initial presentation and work-up, but recommend treating empirically for bacterial pneumonia unless viral or other etiology identified.
    - Empiric therapy consists of antipseudomonal beta-lactam + either respiratory fluoroquinolone or azithromycin. This should be guided by patient's previous cultures and institutional antibiogram (see Chapter 13).
    - Therapy should be tailored based on work-up and culture data but if patient worsens or failing to improve, further diagnostics should be pursued and treatment escalated to cover for resistant organisms and/or possible fungal pathogens.

Etiologies
- **Bacterial**
  - Typical presentation is acute onset with fever, productive cough, and focal infiltrates (although the latter two may be blunted in neutropenia).
  - Most likely etiology particularly in patients with neutropenia of <7 days
    - Enterobacteriaceae (*E. coli*, *Klebsiella*, etc.).
    - Pseudomonas.
    - *Staphylococcus aureus.*
    - *Streptococcus viridans.*
  - Usually occurs with mucositis following **cytotoxic chemotherapy.**
  - Can cause ARDS or severe sepsis.
  - **Atypical bacteria** particularly in community-acquired (*Mycoplasma*, *Legionella*, *Chlamydia*); may cause atypical presentation with dry cough and diffuse infiltrates.
- **Viral**
  - Typically presents with acute onset dyspnea, dry cough, ± fever (almost always present in influenza), and diffuse bilateral infiltrates.
  - Pay attention to respiratory viruses circulating in the community.
  - **Winter months**
    - **Influenza A, B**
      - Should be treated with a neuraminidase inhibitor, typically oseltamivir, consider extending duration to 10 days in patients who are significantly immunocompromised.
      - IV peramivir is an alternative treatment option.
    - **Respiratory syncytial virus (RSV)**
      - Treatment with oral or inhaled ribavirin may be considered in patients with acute leukemia or HSCT recipients.
      - Note: inhaled formulation is expensive and technically difficult to administer, so many centers no longer use it.
    - **Human metapneumovirus** (hMPV).
    - **Coronavirus** (more commonly cause upper respiratory illness).
  - **Summer months**
    - **Rhinovirus** (more commonly cause upper respiratory illness).
    - **Parainfluenza.**
  - **Year-round**
    - **Adenovirus** (Adv); more severe presentation in patients with impaired cellular immunity, include HSCT recipients.
      - In severe infections treatment with cidofovir is often used (awaiting availability of brincidofovir).
    - CMV pneumonitis is uncommon outside of the allogeneic HSCT population but can occur occasionally in patients receiving alemtuzumab or other lymphocyte-depleting agents.
      - Typically has high serum viral load.
      - Diagnosis is confirmed if pathology demonstrates cytopathic effect with viral inclusions on immunohistochemistry.

- **Fungal** (see Chapters 27 and 29)
  - **Mold infections** should be considered in patients with prolonged (>10–14 days), profound neutropenia (ANC <500) who are not improving with initial antibiotic regimen (see below).
  - *Pneumocystis jirovecii* typically occurs in patients with impaired cellular immunity.
    - Presentation is usually subacute with dry cough, dyspnea, and hypoxia; often more severe illness than what typically occurs in people with human immunodeficiency virus (HIV) with *Pneumocystis jirovecii* pneumonia (PJP).
    - Classic radiographic findings are bilateral diffuse ground glass opacities.
    - Cannot be cultured; diagnosis typically made via cytology on BAL.
    - Will have very high 1,3 beta-D-glucan levels.
    - Treatment is with high-dose trimethoprim–sulfamethoxazole (TMP–SMX) (5 mg/kg TMP q8) and, based on data extrapolated from HIV population, corticosteroids are typically given to patients with significant hypoxia (PaO_2 <70 mmHg on room air).
  - *Cryptococcus* typically occurs in patients with impaired cellular immunity.
    - Presentation is variable from asymptomatic to cough and fevers.
    - May present with lung nodules or consolidations.
    - Diagnosis may be made with respiratory cultures, pathology, or serum cryptococcal antigen.
    - Patient should also be evaluated for disseminated or CNS infection.
    - Mild pulmonary infection alone can be treated with fluconazole; severe, systemic, or CNS infection should be initially treated with liposomal amphotericin B and flucytosine.

Noninfectious Etiologies

- **Diffuse alveolar hemorrhage (DAH)**: occurs in hematologic malignancy patients.
  - Risks include recent chemotherapy (causing mucosal damage) and prolonged thrombocytopenia.
  - Treated with high-dose steroid, platelet transfusions, and reversal of any coagulopathy.
- **Drug-induced pneumonitis**
  - Various chemotherapy agents are known to cause lung injury, in particular
    - Bleomycin.
    - Gemcitabine.
    - Epidermal growth factor receptor (EGFR) tyrosine kinase inhibitors (TKI).
    - Bcr-Abl tyrosine kinase inhibitor: imatinib, dasatinib.
      - Can cause pleural effusions.
    - PD-L1 inhibitors: pembrolizumab, nivolumab.
  - Antimicrobials.
    - Daptomycin-induced eosinophilic pneumonitis.
- **Radiation pneumonitis**

- Causes a spectrum of presentations depending on timing of onset from the radiation (hours to months postradiation).
  - Often treated with steroids.
- **Pulmonary edema.**
- **Malignancy**
  - Myeloid sarcoma in AML presents as a mass-like lesion.
  - Lymphatic spread of tumor often causes diffuse multifocal infiltrate.
  - Metastatic solid tumor typically causes nodules.

Invasive Mold Infections (see Chapter 29)

- Highest risk oncology populations are those with active AML or MDS due to neutropenia and/or neutrophil dysfunction. Other at-risk populations include patients with hematologic malignancies with prolonged neutropenia (>10–14 days) and/or receiving prolonged steroids (i.e., ALL), allo-HSCT recipients, especially delayed engraftment or in patients with graft versus host disease (GVHD).
- **Aspergillosis**
  - Aspergillus is the **most common cause of invasive mold infections** in the oncology population.
  - Typically the lungs are the primary site of infection but is also known to cause sinusitis.
  - Radiographic imaging is usually the first step in work-up.
  - Classic CT chest findings include:
    - Mass-like consolidation.
    - Pulmonary nodule.
    - **Halo sign** (solid infiltrate surrounded by ground glass opacities) (Fig. 40.2).

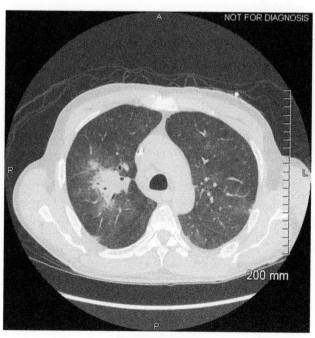

• **Fig. 40.2** Halo sign.

- Cavitary lesion.
- Air crescent sign (often once neutrophils recover).
- Biopsy of involved tissue is the diagnostic study of choice but often not an option due to thrombocytopenia.
  - Pathology demonstrates **septated acute angle branching hyphae**, but other *Aspergillus*-like molds can also have this appearance.
  - Cultures or PCR is required to determine species of mold.
- Other diagnostic testing only has sensitivities of 50%–70%.
  - Fungal respiratory cultures (BAL > sputum).
  - Galactomannan from serum or BAL fluid; can be positive in other molds, except for mucormycosis.
  - 1,3 beta-D-glucan (Fungitell); can be positive in other fungal infections, including PJP and *Candida*, but is negative in mucormycoses.
  - Molecular testing directly on tissue is also a new modality, but formal recommendations for its use have not been established.
- **Treatment**
  - Mold active triazoles are first line (voriconazole, posaconazole, isavuconazole).
  - Liposomal amphotericin B or echinocandins are options for salvage therapy.
  - Surgery can be considered for localized disease that is readily accessible for debridement in patients who are surgical candidates.
  - Reversal of underlying immunodeficiency.
- **Mucormycosis (zygomycosis)**
  - Includes organisms in the *Rhizopus*, *Mucor*, *Rhizomucor*, *Absidia*, and *Cunninghamella* genera.
  - Most common presentation is rhino-orbital-cerebral infection, but can also affect lungs and other organs/tissue.
  - In addition to active disease and prolonged, profound neutropenia, uncontrolled diabetes, iron overload or deferoxamine therapy are also risk factors for mucormycosis.
  - Radiographic imaging is usually the first step in work-up.
  - **Pulmonary infection**
    - CT chest findings are nonspecific and may include
      - Mass-like consolidation.
      - Pulmonary nodule.
      - Cavitary lesion.
      - **Reverse halo sign** (ground glass opacities surrounded by dense consolidation) (Fig. 40.3).
  - **Rhino-orbital-cerebral infection**
    - CT sinus findings may demonstrate sinusitis or bone erosion, in severe cases with extension into brain or orbits.
    - Requires urgent and aggressive surgical debridement down to healthy tissue.
    - Direct evaluation by ENT with nasal endoscopy may be helpful in patients in which diagnosis is uncertain.

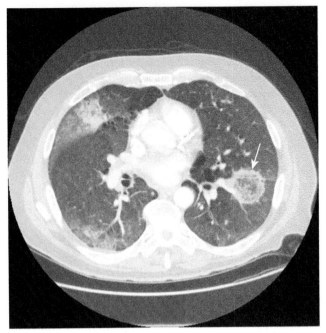

• **Fig. 40.3** Reverse halo.

- Biopsy of involved tissue is the diagnostic study of choice.
  - Pathology demonstrates pauciseptated (few septates) right-angle branching ribbon-like hyphae, which is specific for mucormycosis.
- Galactomannan and 1,3 beta-D-glucan (Fungitell) will be negative in mucormycosis, but culture is positive in ~50% of cases.

Treatment
- In addition to aggressive **surgical debridement, liposomal amphotericin B** is first line for treatment.
- Posaconazole or isavuconazole are often used for stepdown or salvage therapy (voriconazole and itraconazole have no activity against mucormycosis).
- Reversal of underlying condition is also essential.
  - Due to suboptimal sensitivity and specificity in testing, mold infections are difficult to diagnose. Definitions are set forth to aid in diagnosis.
- **Proven**
  - Requires recovery of mold by culture of a sterile site (i.e., blood, CSF, pleural fluid) *or* demonstration of invasive hyphae with associated tissue damage on histopathology or cytopathology.
- **Probable**
  - Requires host factor, clinical criteria, and mycologic criteria.
- **Host factor**
  - Recent or ongoing neutropenia with ANC <500 for at least 10 days.
  - Recipient of allogeneic HSCT.
  - Prolonged high-dose corticosteroid treatment (at least 0.3 mg/kg per day) for >3 weeks.
  - Treatment with agents that impair T-cell function.

- **Clinical criteria**
  - Radiographic signs including pulmonary nodule ± halo or reverse halo sign, cavitation, or air crescent sign in the lungs, sinusitis, or CNS lesion.
  - Bronchoscopy demonstrating tracheobronchitis.
- **Mycologic criteria**
  - Recovery of pathogenic mold by culture from nonsterile sources (including sputum, BAL fluid sinuses).
  - Positive antigen test with galactomannan or 1,3 beta-D-glucan (both will be negative in Mucormycoses).
- **Possible**
  - Requires host factor and clinical criteria in the absence of mycologic criteria.

Unique Infection Risks in Patients With Hematologic Malignancies

- **Chronic lymphocytic leukemia (CLL)**
  - Inherent humoral and cellular immunodeficiencies due to disease itself due to lymphocytes dysfunction.
- **Hypogammaglobulinemia**
  - May require IVIG replacement in IgG levels of <400 and frequent infections.
  - Decreased complement levels.
  - Neutrophil and monocyte deficiency and dysfunction.
  - Infection risk influenced both by CLL and its treatment
    - Typical bacterial infections especially involving the upper and lower respiratory tract.
    - Respiratory viral infections.
    - Cryptococcus.
    - Pneumocystis.
- **Acute myelogenous leukemia (AML)** and **myelodysplastic syndrome (MDS)**
  - Have prolonged neutropenia and neutrophil dysfunction.
  - Increased risk for bacterial and fungal (mold) infections.
  - Patients with refractory or relapsed disease are at highest risk.
  - Intensive chemotherapy required to put disease in remission.
    - Results in prolonged and profound neutropenia.
    - Damage to mucosal surfaces.

Infections Associated With Other Chemotherapy Agents

- **Fludarabine** (purine analog)
  - Fluorinated adenine analogue that is lymphotoxic, particularly affecting CD4 cells.
  - Used for treatment of various hematologic malignancies, including CLL and conditioning prior to HSCT, typically in combination with other chemotherapy.

- Causes profound, prolonged lymphopenia.
- Infection risk increases when combined with other immunosuppressants or chemotherapy agents.
  - *Pneumocystis*: prophylaxis with TMP–SMX is often used.
  - Herpesviruses (HSV, VZV, CMV): prophylaxis with aciclovir.
  - Listeria.
- **Bortezomib** (proteasome inhibitor)
  - Used to treatment multiple myeloma, lymphomas, and amyloidosis.
  - Infection risk
    - Herpesviruses (HSV and VZV): antiviral prophylaxis with aciclovir typically used.
    - *Listeria.*
    - *Toxoplasma.*

Infections Associated With Immunosuppressants

Lymphocyte Depleting Agents
- **Alemtuzumab** (Campath, Lemtrada)
  - Monoclonal antibody, targets CD52, depletes T and B cells.
  - Used in treatment of multiple sclerosis and B- and T-cell leukemias, as well as induction immunosuppression in SOT, as part of a conditioning regimen in allogeneic HSCT, treatment of graft rejection, or GVHD.
  - Increased infection risk
    - Herpesvirus, especially CMV: at risk patients typically receive prophylaxis or preemptive monitoring.
    - Epstein–Barr virus (EBV)/post-transplant lymphoproliferative disorder (PTLD).
    - BK virus.
    - **Progressive multifocal leukoencephalopathy (PML).**
    - *Pneumocystis*: should receive prophylaxis for 6–12 months after last dose.
    - *Cryptococcus.*
    - Endemic fungi (*Histoplasma, Blastomyces, Coccidioides*).
- **Rituximab** (Rituxan)
  - Monoclonal antibody, targets CD20.
  - Used for treatment of B-cell malignancies, PTLD, humoral rejection, chronic GVHD, rheumatoid arthritis (RA), and other autoimmune diseases.
  - Can cause severe mucocutaneous reactions such as Stevens–Johnson syndrome or toxic epidermal necrolysis (TEN).
  - Impairs immune response to vaccinations.
  - Infection risk
    - **Hepatitis B reactivation**: all patients should be screened prior to initiation of treatment and monitored during treatment.
    - **Progressive multifocal leukoencephalopathy (PML).**

- *Pneumocystis* when given in combination with other therapies or with certain diseases.
  - Prophylaxis recommended in patients with CLL, granulomatosis with polyangiitis (GPA), and microscopic polyangiitis (MPA).
- **Antithymocyte globulin** (ATG, thymoglobulin, Atgam)
  - T-cell depleting agent with multiple targets, particularly CD3.
  - Most frequently used as induction immunosuppression in SOT, as part of a conditioning regimen in allogeneic HSCT, or treatment of graft rejection or GVHD.
  - Impair B-cell, T-cell, and NK-cell function.
  - Causes prolonged lymphopenia (typically 3–12 months).
  - Can cause febrile reactions and serum sickness.
  - Increased infection risk
    - **Herpesvirus**, especially CMV: at-risk patients typically receive prophylaxis or preemptive monitoring.
    - EBV/PTLD.
    - BK virus.
    - *Pneumocystis*: should receive prophylaxis for 6–12 months.
    - Cryptococcus.
    - Endemic fungi (*Histoplasma*, *Blastomyces*, *Coccidioides*).

Steroids

- Multiple antiinflammatory effects.
- Suppression of leukocyte migration and function of neutrophils, lymphocytes, and monocytes.
- Effects increased when given in combination with other immunosuppressing agents.
- Higher dose and duration increase risk of infection.
  - Bacterial
    - TB reactivation.
    - Other typical organisms.
  - Herpesvirus reactivation (HSV, VZV).
  - Fungal.
    - Candida.
    - Pneumocystis: prophylaxis recommended in patients on prednisone equivalent of >20 mg for >2 weeks.
    - Endemic fungi.
    - Mold infections (less common except in setting of GVHD).

Cytokine Blocking

- **Tumor necrosis factor (TNF) inhibitors**: golimumab, infliximab, adalimumab (longer lasting effect >> certolizumab, etanercept)
- Used for autoimmune diseases, including RA, inflammatory bowel disease (IBD), and psoriatic arthritis.
- Increased risk for lymphoma and other malignancies.
- Break down granulomas.
- Risk for infections, particularly due to intracellular organisms, risk increases when used in combination with other immunosuppressants.

- **Mycobacterial**
  - Nontuberculosis mycobacteria (NTM).
  - **Tuberculous (TB)**
    - TB screening, rule out active TB.
    - Initiate treatment of latent TB prior to starting therapy.
- **Fungal**
  - *Aspergillus*.
  - Endemics (*Histoplasma*, *Blastomyces*, *Coccidioides*).
  - *Pneumocystis*.
  - *Cryptococcus*.
  - *Candida*.
- **Viral**
  - Hepatitis B
    Screen all patients prior to starting an agent and monitor during treatment.
  - Herpesviruses (particularly **VZV, HSV**).
- **Bacterial**
  - *Listeria*.
  - *Legionella* (black box warning).
  - *Nocardia*.
  - *Salmonella*.
  - *Staphylococcus aureus* joint infections in RA.
- **Parasites**
  - *Leishmania*.
  - Malaria.
  - *Babesia*.
  - *Strongyloides*.

Interleukin Receptor Antagonists

- **IL-1 inhibitors:** anakinra, canakinumab, rilonacept
  - Prevents B-cell and T-cell activation, febrile response, and cytokine activation.
  - Use to treat RA and other inflammatory diseases.
  - May cause neutropenia, increased risk of malignancies, including lymphoma.
  - Infection risk
    - TB reactivation
      - Test for and treat latent TB prior to starting therapy.
- **IL-2 inhibitors:** basiliximab (Simulect), daclizumab
  - Anti-CD25 monoclonal antibody, blocks IL-2 receptor.
  - Prevents proliferation, differentiation, and activation of B, T, and NK cells.
  - Used for induction immunosuppression in SOT and treatment of acute GVHD.
  - Effects typically last up to 3 months.
  - Infection risk less than other induction immunosuppression.
    - Reactivation of **herpesviruses**.
- **IL-6 inhibitor:** tocilizumab
  - Prevents fever, acute phase response, and cytokine production.
  - Used for treatment of cytokine release syndrome due to chimeric antigen receptor T-cell therapy (CAR T cells), RA, and giant cell arteritis.

- Infection risk
  - Reactivation of TB
    - Should test for TB and initiate treatment of latent TB prior to starting medication.
  - Fungal
    Candida.
    Aspergillus.
    Pneumocystis.
    Endemic mycoses.
  - Viral
    - Reactivation of **herpesviruses**.

T-Cell Costimulation Blockade: Abatacept, Belatacept

- Inhibits T cell activation by blocking CD28 interaction between antigen-presenting cells (APCs) and T cells.
- Increased risk of malignancies, including lymphoma and lung and skin cancer.
- Infection risk increases in patients receiving concomitant immunosuppression, particularly TNF antagonists.
  - Belatacept used as prophylaxis against rejection in SOT (typically used in combination with other immunosuppressants, which may account for increased rate of infections).
    - PTLD.
    - PML.
    - Herpesvirus reactivation.
      - **CMV** prophylaxis recommended for >3 months.
    - ***Pneumocystis:*** prophylaxis recommended.
    - TB reactivation.
    - Hepatitis B reactivation.
  - Abatacept for RA or psoriatic arthritis
    - TB reactivation.
    - Hepatitis B reactivation.

Adhesion Blocking: Natalizumab, Vedolizumab

- Humanized monoclonal antibody against integrin, inhibits T-cell migration.

- Used for multiple sclerosis (MS) and inflammatory bowel disease (IBD).
- Associated with hypersensitivity reactions, including anaphylaxis.
- Infection risk.

Complement Inhibitor: Eculizumab

- Humanized monoclonal antibody that binds C5 and inhibits terminal complex C5b-9.
- Used for atypical hemolytic uremic syndrome and paroxysmal nocturnal hemoglobinuria.
- Infection risk, particularly due to encapsulated bacteria.
  - **Severe meningococcal infection**.
  - Should receive meningococcal vaccine at least 2 weeks prior to treatment.
  - *Streptococcus pneumoniae.*
  - *Haemophilus influenza.*

Further Reading

1. Freifeld AG, Bow EJ, Sepkowitz KA, et al. Clinical practice guideline for the use of antimicrobial agents in neutropenic patients with cancer: 2010 update by the Infectious Diseases Society of America. *Clin Infect Dis.* 2011;52(4):e56–e93.
2. Baden LR, Swaminathan S, Angarone M, et al. Prevention and treatment of cancer-related infections, Version 2.2016, NCCN clinical practice guidelines in oncology. *J Natl Compr Canc Netw.* 2016;14(7):882–913.
3. Averbuch D, Orasch C, Cordonnier C, et al. European guidelines for empirical antibacterial therapy for febrile neutropenic patients in the era of growing resistance: summary of the 2011 4th European Conference on Infections in Leukemia. *Haematologica.* 2013;98(12):1826–1835.
4. Winthrop K, Mariette K, Silva JT, et al. ESCMID Study Group for Infections in Compromised Hosts (ESGICH) Consensus Document on the safety of targeted and biological therapies: an infectious diseases perspective. *Clin Microbiol Infect.* 2018;24(suppl 2):S21–S40.
5. Klasterksy J, Awada A, Paesmans M, Aoun M. Febrile neutropenia: a critical review of the initial management. *Crit Rev Oncol Hematol.* 2011;78(3):185–194.

41

Infections in Solid Organ Transplant Recipients

CARLOS A.Q. SANTOS, IGE A. GEORGE

Introduction

Infections are among the leading causes of morbidity and mortality in solid organ transplant recipients. Early and specific diagnosis of infection accompanied by timely and appropriate treatment is essential to achieving good clinical outcomes.

The management of infectious diseases in the solid organ transplant population consists of:
- Risk assessment for infectious disease.
- Donor and recipient screening.
- Prophylactic antiinfective administration and vaccinations.
- Timely diagnosis and management of infectious complications.

Risk Assessment for Infectious Disease

- Risk assessment should include identifying:
  - Any current and past immunosuppressive therapies.
  - Mucocutaneous barrier integrity, such as the presence of any catheters or drains.
  - Neutropenia or lymphopenia.
  - Underlying immune deficiencies.
  - Metabolic conditions, such as uremia, malnutrition, diabetes mellitus, or cirrhosis.
  - Viral co-infections, such as cytomegalovirus (CMV), hepatitis B (HBV), or hepatitis C (HCV).
- Greater infectious risk is associated with:
  - Induction therapy with lymphocyte-depleting agents.
  - High-dose corticosteroid therapy or plasmapheresis.
  - High rejection risk, early graft rejection, or graft dysfunction.
  - Technical complications, such as anastomotic leak, bleeding, wound infection, or poor wound healing.
- Lower infectious risk is associated with:
  - Immunologic tolerance.
  - Good HLA match.

- Technically successful surgery and good allograft function.
- Appropriate antiinfective prophylaxis and vaccination.

Donor and Recipient Screening

Frequently Utilized Serologic Tests for Screening of the Donor and Recipient

- Commonly obtained tests
  - Human immunodeficiency virus (HIV) antibody.
  - Herpes simplex virus (HSV) IgG antibody.
  - Cytomegalovirus (CMV) IgG antibody.
  - Hepatitis C virus (HCV) antibody.
  - Hepatitis B virus surface antigen (HBsAg).
  - Hepatitis B virus core antibody (HBcAb IgM and IgG or total core antibody).
  - Hepatitis B virus surface antibody (HBsAb).
  - Rapid plasma reagin (RPR).
  - *Toxoplasma* IgG antibody.
  - Epstein–Barr virus (EBV) antibody (EBV VCA IgG, IgM).
  - Varicella-zoster virus (VZV) antibody.
- Other screening measures.
  - Interferon-gamma release assay (IGRA) for latent tuberculosis in recipients.
  - *Strongyloides* serology (for recipients from endemic areas).
  - *Coccidioides* serology (for recipients from endemic areas).
  - Serologies for tetanus, diphtheria, measles, mumps, and pneumococcal titers as an aid to pretransplant immunization (at some centers).
- **Note** that any prospective donors with encephalitis or meningitis of unclear etiology should not be considered for organ donation given the possibility of undiagnosed viral, bacterial, mycobacterial, or fungal infection.

TABLE 41.1	Recommendations for Pretransplant Screening Results			
Pathogen	**Donor Antibody**	**Recipient Antibody**	**Recommendations for Transplant**	**Comment**
HIV	Positive	Negative	Reject donor	
	Negative	Positive	Proceed if HIV is well controlled	
	Positive	Positive	Reject	Being studied
CMV	+ or −	Positive	Proceed	CMV prevention guidelines in Table 41.2
	Positive	Negative	Accept, higher risk	
EBV	+ or −	Positive	Proceed	
	Positive	Negative	Accept, higher risk	
Toxoplasma	+ or −	Positive	Proceed	TMP–SMX for prevention
	Positive	Negative	Accept, higher risk	
HCV	Positive	Positive	Accept?	Reserve for sick patients
	Positive	Negative	Reject	Being studied
Syphilis (RPR)	Positive	+ or −	Accept	Treat with penicillin
HBV	HBsAb+	+ or −	Accept	
	HBsAg+	+ or −	Reject	
	HBcAb+	HBsAb−	Accept	Lamivudine for prophylaxis
	HBcAb+	HBsAb+	Accept	Monitor
TB		IGRA +	Proceed	Isoniazid treatment
Strongyloides		Positive	Proceed	Ivermectin treatment
Coccidioides		Positive	Proceed	Fluconazole treatment
CNS viral pathogen (e.g., LCMV, rabies, WNV)	Clinical suspicion		Reject	

CNS, central nervous system; LCMV, lymphocytic choriomeningitis virus; TMP–SMX, trimethoprim–sulfamethoxazole; WNV, West Nile virus.

Recommendations for Results of Screening Serologies

Recommendations for results of pretransplant screening serologies are outlined in Table 41.1.

Human Immunodeficiency Virus (HIV)

- If the donor antibody screen is positive, and the recipient is HIV-negative, the organ cannot be accepted for transplantation.
- If the donor antibody screen is negative, and the recipient is HIV-positive, the organ can be accepted for transplantation; typical requirements for transplant listing in people with HIV are CD4 count greater than 200 cells/µL, an undetectable viral load, and absence of incurable opportunistic infections such as progressive multifocal leukoencephalopathy (PML) or advanced *Cryptosporidium*; past opportunistic infections such as *Pneumocystis* or *Cryptococcus* are allowable as long as it is cured or well controlled.
- If the donor antibody screen is positive, and the recipient is HIV-positive, the organ cannot be accepted for transplantation; however, the HOPE in Action study is being performed to assess the efficacy and safety of this approach to increase the donor pool.

Cytomegalovirus (CMV)

- CMV disease is associated with increased risk of allograft loss and death and should be prevented.
- Greatest risk factor for CMV infection and disease is organ transplant from seropositive donors to seronegative recipients (D+/R−), followed by seropositive recipients (R+) (Table 41.2).

TABLE 41.2	CMV Prevention Strategies
Risk Category	**Recommendation**
D+/R−	*Prophylaxis* is strongly preferred • Valganciclovir orally daily for at least 6 months; lung transplant recipients can be given prophylaxis for as long as 12 months *Preemptive treatment* is an alternative • Weekly nucleic acid testing for 3 months, then PO valganciclovir, ganciclovir intravenously upon detection of active CMV infection (thresholds vary) for at least 21 days, and until repeat CMV nucleic acid testing is negative
R+	*Prophylaxis* is preferred • Valganciclovir for 3 months *Preemptive treatment* (as above) is an alternative
D−/R−	*No specific CMV prevention strategies* are recommended • Aciclovir orally for 3 months to prevent herpes simplex virus infection

- If the recipient is CMV-seropositive, preventive therapy with either prophylactic valganciclovir or preemptive treatment upon the detection of asymptomatic CMV viremia is indicated.
- If the donor is CMV-seropositive and the recipient is CMV-seronegative, the patient is at high risk of CMV disease, and prophylactic valganciclovir for at least 6 months is preferred.
- If both the donor and recipient are CMV-seronegative, the patient is at minimal risk for CMV disease posttransplant and no specific preventive anti-CMV treatment is indicated.

Epstein–Barr Virus
- Associated with posttransplant lymphoproliferative disease (PTLD).
- If the donor is EBV-seropositive and the recipient is EBV-seronegative, then the patient is at higher risk for PTLD; this more commonly occurs in pediatric transplant recipients; there is no specific preventive anti-EBV treatment, although aciclovir and ganciclovir have activity *in vitro*.

Toxoplasma gondii
- Rare opportunistic infection in solid organ transplant recipients; more frequently found in heart transplant patients.
- If the donor is *Toxoplasma*-seropositive and the recipient is *Toxoplasma*-seronegative, the patient is at higher risk of developing disease.
- Trimethoprim–sulfamethoxazole (TMP–SMX) has activity against *Toxoplasma* and can be used as prophylactic therapy.
- Atovaquone can be used as second-line prophylactic therapy for patients who cannot tolerate TMP–SMX.

Hepatitis C Virus (HCV)
- If the recipient is chronically infected with HCV, the patient can receive an organ from a HCV-seropositive donor; outcomes may be poorer, however, and such transplants should be reserved for the sickest patients.
- If the donor is HCV-seropositive and the recipient is HCV-seronegative, the organ must be rejected.

Syphilis
- A positive RPR in the donor is not a contraindication for transplantation; benzathine penicillin G should be administered to the recipient posttransplant

Hepatitis B Virus (HBV)
- If the donor is vaccine-immune to HBV, the organ can be accepted.
- If the donor is chronically infected with HBV, the organ must be rejected.
- If the donor is seropositive for hepatitis B core antibody and the recipient is not immune to HBV, prophylactic lamivudine will need to be administered posttransplant.
- If the donor is seropositive for hepatitis B core antibody and the recipient has vaccine immunity, the patient will need to be monitored for HBV replication every 3 months and may need prophylactic lamivudine posttransplant.
- If the donor is seropositive for hepatitis B core antibody and the recipient has natural immunity, the patient will not need prophylactic lamivudine but will need to be monitored for HBV replication every 3 months.

Mycobacterium Tuberculosis
- If the recipient has latent tuberculosis, treatment with isoniazid for 9 months is required; latent tuberculosis treatment can be provided posttransplant if it cannot be tolerated pretransplant.
- If the donor has latent tuberculosis and will participate in living organ donation, treatment with isoniazid for at least 6 months is ideal prior to transplantation.
- Indeterminate IGRAs (interferon gamma release assay) commonly occur; in these cases, risk stratification for tuberculosis will need to be individualized.

Strongyloides stercoralis
- Can cause hyperinfection syndrome posttransplant.
- Endemic to tropical areas, and is also present in the Southeastern United States.
- If seropositive for *Strongyloides*, recommended to administer two doses of ivermectin 1 week apart before transplant.

Coccidioides immitis
- Can cause catastrophic infection posttransplant.
- Screening should be performed for patients from the desert portions of the Southwestern United States and Mexico.
- If *Coccidioides*-seropositive, fluconazole prophylaxis would need to be administered.

TABLE 41.3	**Routine Adult Vaccines**			
Vaccine	**Inactivated or Live Attenuated**	**Recommended Pretransplant**	**Recommended Posttransplant**	**Monitor Vaccine Titers**
Influenza	I	Yes	Yes	No
	LA	No	No	No
Hepatitis B	I	Yes	Yes	Yes
Hepatitis A	I	Yes	Yes	Yes
Tetanus	I	Yes	Yes	No
Pertussis (Tdap)	I	Yes	Yes	No
Pneumovax	I	Yes	Yes	Yes
PCV13	I	Yes	Yes	Yes
Menactra	I	Yes	Yes	No
Rabies	I	Yes	Yes	No
HPV	I	Yes	Yes	No
Varivax	LA	Yes	No	No
Zostavax	LA	Yes	No	No
Shingrix	I	Yes	Yes	No
Smallpox	LA	No	No	No

TABLE 41.4	**Travel Vaccines**			
Vaccine	**Inactivated or Live Attenuated**	**Recommended Pretransplant**	**Recommended Posttransplant**	**Monitor Vaccine Titers**
Vibrio cholerae	I	Yes	Yes	No
	LA	Yes	No	No
Yellow fever	LA	Yes	No	No
Japanese encephalitis	I	Yes	Yes	No
Salmonella typhi Typhim Vi, IM	I	Yes	Yes	No
Salmonella typhi Vivotif, oral	LA	Yes	No	No

Unusual Donor Infections and Typical Presentations

- Lymphochoriomeningitis virus (LCMV): encephalitis, multiorgan failure.
- Rabies: encephalitis, unreported bat bite.
- *Trypanosoma cruzi:* fever of unknown origin, myocarditis.
- *Acanthamoeba:* encephalitis.
- *Balamuthia:* encephalitis.
- West Nile virus (WNV): meningoencephalitis, flaccid paralysis.
- *Cryptococcus:* graft failure, meningoencephalitis, skin and soft tissue infection.

Vaccinations

Immune response after transplantation and during end-stage organ disease is generally poor; immunization should be provided pretransplant if possible (Tables 41.3 and 41.4); live attenuated vaccines are generally contraindicated after transplantation.

Timely Diagnosis and Management of Infectious Complications

Timeline of Infections after Transplantation

Less than 4 Weeks Posttransplant
- Pneumonia
  - Diagnosis often confounded by noninfectious causes of pulmonary infiltrates, such as pulmonary edema or drug-induced pneumonitis.
  - Empiric antimicrobial therapy should include coverage for anaerobic bacteria since aspiration is a common cause.

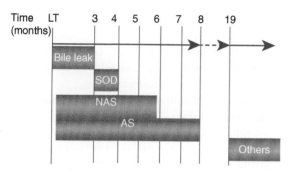

• **Fig. 41.1** Timeline of complications following liver transplantation. LT, liver transplantation; SOD, sphincter of Oddi dysfunction; NAS, non-anastomotic stricture; AS, anastomotic stricture; others, biliary stones, sludge, casts. (Modified from Ayoub WS, Esquivel CO, Martin P. Biliary complications following liver transplantation. *Dig Dis Sci.* 2010;55(6):1540–1546.)

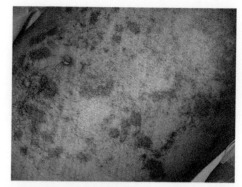

• **Fig. 41.2** Purpuric and petechial rash on a patient's thigh with disseminated strongyloides hyperinfection syndrome. (From Basile A, Simzar S, Bentow J, et al. Disseminated *Strongyloides stercoralis*: hyperinfection during medical immunosuppression. *J Am Acad Dermatol.* 2010;63(5):896–902. Copyright © 2009 American Academy of Dermatology, Inc.)

- Bronchoalveolar lavage may be helpful in determining the causative organism.
- Line infection
  - Indications for line removal include sustained bacteremia >72 hours, hemodynamic compromise, evidence of metastatic disease (e.g., septic pulmonary emboli, epidural abscess), endocarditis, tunnel infection, infection with *Staphylococcus aureus*, *Pseudomonas aeruginosa*, multidrug-resistant bacteria, mycobacteria, fungus.
- Urinary tract infection
  - Especially important in kidney transplant recipients.
  - Enterobacteriaceae are still the most common causative pathogens; however, the widespread use of prophylactic TMP–SMX has led to the emergence of *Enterococcus* species as causative agents.
- Surgical site infection
  - Bilious drainage from the surgical site of a liver transplant recipient portends an anastomotic leak. Hepatic artery thrombosis (1%–2%) (bile ducts are solely supplied by the hepatic artery) could lead to non-anastomotic biliary strictures and liver abscess.
  - Perinephric collections (lymphoceles) occasionally get infected after kidney transplantation and infected urinomas due to leak from ureterocystostomy is another complication.
  - Heart and lung transplant surgical complications include mediastinitis and pleural space infections. Complications following liver transplant are depicted in Fig. 41.1.
- *Clostridioides difficile* colitis
  - Common given antibiotic use posttransplant.
  - Unexplained leukocytosis and fever without diarrhea may represent paralytic ileus and concomitant *C. difficile* colitis.
- Donor-derived infections.
  - Suspect in early-onset infections occurring within 1–2 months of transplant with atypical presentations.
  - Prospective donors with encephalitis or meningitis of unclear etiology should not be considered for organ donation given the possibility of undiagnosed viral, bacterial, mycobacterial, or fungal infection; exceptions are documented and appropriately treated

bacterial meningitis (24–48 hours of effective therapy before procurement); recipients of donors with bacterial meningitis are usually treated with 2 weeks of antimicrobials after transplantation.
- Salient information include residence in or travel to endemic regions (e.g., coccidioidomycosis, tuberculosis), donor exposures (rodents – LCMV, mosquitos – WNV), organ transplanted (heart – Chagas disease), and validity of screening tests (e.g., *Trypanosoma cruzi* screening test lacks sensitivity).
- Recipient-derived infections
  - Stems from colonization.
  - Especially important in lung transplant recipients, with *Aspergillus* and *Pseudomonas* colonization of the native airway.
  - Preemptive therapy with antiinfectives may be warranted.

Between 1 and 6 Months Posttransplant
- *Mycobacterium* tuberculosis (see Chapter 32)
  - Isoniazid, rifampin, and pyrazinamide are hepatotoxic and can be problematic in liver transplant recipients.
  - Pyrazinamide is the most hepatotoxic.
  - Rifampin is associated with early-onset cholestatic hepatitis and increases the metabolism of calcineurin inhibitors.
  - Isoniazid causes delayed-onset hepatitis.
- *Strongyloides stercoralis* (see Chapter 35)
  - Transplant recipients can present with *Strongyloides* hyperinfection syndrome (Fig. 41.2).
  - Ivermectin is the treatment of choice.
  - Especially common in residents of tropical areas; however, also present in the Southeastern United States.
- BK polyomavirus
  - Causes BK virus nephropathy and leads to renal allograft failure and loss.
  - Monthly nucleic acid testing for BK virus in the blood should be performed posttransplant; if positive, then immunosuppressive therapy should be preemptively decreased.

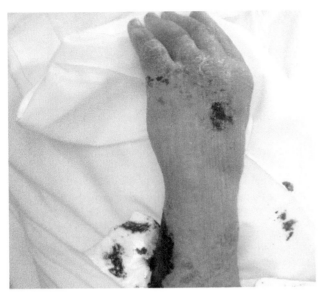

• **Fig. 41.3** Disseminated cryptococcosis presenting as cellulitis with eschar in a renal transplant recipient.

- BK viruria is nonspecific and does not immediately portend BK virus nephropathy.
- *C. difficile* colitis
  - Especially common in this period because of high usage of antibiotics.
  - Hepatitis C virus (see Chapter 22).
  - Almost always reactivates after liver transplant, but not a contraindication to transplantation since outcomes are no worse for liver transplants for other indications.
  - Direct-acting antivirals are now being used to successfully treat HCV before or after transplant.
- Respiratory viral infections
  - Can be severe posttransplant.
  - Includes influenza, parainfluenza, respiratory syncytial virus, adenovirus, rhinovirus, and human metapneumovirus.
- *Cryptococcus neoformans* (see Chapter 27)
  - Rare but deadly; often has atypical manifestations posttransplant. Nonmeningeal presentations are more common, including pneumonia and skin and soft tissue infections (Fig. 41.3).
  - Liposomal amphotericin B and 5-flucytosine are used for induction therapy, and fluconazole is used for consolidation and maintenance therapy.
  - Fluconazole inhibits the metabolism of calcineurin inhibitors, so levels need to be monitored closely (see Chapter 7).
  - Management of intracranial pressure is important but often missed.
- Without prophylaxis
  - *Pneumocystis jirovecii* (TMP–SMX).
  - HSV (aciclovir).
  - VZV (aciclovir).
  - CMV (valganciclovir).
  - EBV (no proven antiviral therapy; aciclovir and ganciclovir are active *in vitro*).
  - HBV (entecavir, tenofovir, or lamivudine).

Greater than 6 Months Posttransplant

- Urinary tract infections
  - Ciprofloxacin and TMP–SMX are drugs of choice.
  - Asymptomatic bacteriuria should not be treated.
- Community-acquired pneumonia
  - Watch out for antibiotic-immunosuppressive therapy drug interactions.
  - In general, beta-lactams, vancomycin, azithromycin, clindamycin, and ciprofloxacin are safe to use.
  - Avoid erythromycin and clarithromycin since they decrease the metabolism of tacrolimus, sirolimus, and cyclosporine.
- *Aspergillus, Mucor,* other molds (see Chapter 29)
  - Voriconazole is the drug of choice for aspergillosis; consider combination therapy with an echinocandin for severe disease; voriconazole impairs the metabolism of calcineurin inhibitors.
  - Liposomal amphotericin B is the drug of choice for mucormycosis; isavuconazole is the second line drug.
- Late viral infections
  - CMV disease can occur after prophylaxis is stopped; typically presents as CMV syndrome or tissue-invasive gastrointestinal disease.
  - HBV or HCV reactivation can cause recurrent cirrhosis.
  - Respiratory viral infections can occur late after transplant.
  - JC polyoma virus can present as progressive multifocal leukoencephalopathy.

Specific Infections or Clinical Syndromes

Bacterial Infections

- Early infections depend on the organ transplanted and complications related to surgery and hospitalization.
- Commonly identified sources include UTI in kidney transplant recipients, abdominal, and biliary infections in liver transplant recipients (especially with Roux-en-Y, bile leaks, and longer surgical times), pneumonia in heart and lung transplant recipients, and UTI and surgical site infections in pancreatic transplant recipients.
- The risk of invasive *Streptococcus pneumoniae* infection is 12 times higher than that observed in immunocompetent hosts; presentations include pneumonia, bacteremia, peritonitis, and meningitis.[6]
- *Listeria monocytogenes* is a gram-positive rod that can present as a bacteremic illness; patients with bacteremia should have a cerebrospinal fluid examination even if overt signs of meningitis are absent; suspect *Listeria* if "diphtheroids" are reported in spinal fluid along with involvement of the cerebellum and brainstem (rhombencephalitis); treatment is with ampicillin with or without gentamicin for 3–6 weeks.
- *Nocardia* is a gram-positive rod that is partially acid-fast; often presents with pulmonary and skin nodules; given its predilection for infecting brain parenchyma, imaging to evaluate for brain abscess is indicated; TMP–SMX is the treatment of choice.

Viral Infections

Cytomegalovirus

- Tends to invade the allograft; has been implicated in acute and chronic graft injury and increased risk of graft rejection.
- Most common type of CMV disease is a mononucleosis syndrome of fever, malaise, leukopenia, and thrombocytopenia, accompanied by detectable viremia.
- Tissue-invasive disease commonly manifests as hepatitis, pneumonitis, or colitis; rarely can manifest as encephalitis, retinitis, or adrenalitis; CMV colitis may not have accompanying viremia, and diagnosis is made by biopsy.
- Treatment with IV ganciclovir until symptoms resolve and viremia is undetectable (typically 2–4 weeks) is indicated.
- Treatment with oral valganciclovir is a reasonable alternative for mild to moderate CMV disease.
- If there is no clinical or virologic response after 2 weeks of therapy, ganciclovir resistance may be present; treatment alternatives include foscarnet or cidofovir; UL97 mutations confer resistance to ganciclovir, whereas UL54 mutations confer resistance to ganciclovir, cidofovir, and foscarnet.

Epstein–Barr Virus and Posttransplant Lymphoproliferative Disorder (PTLD)

- PTLD typically occurs within the first year of transplant.
- Risk factors for PTLD include primary EBV infection, young age, CMV infection or disease, and receipt of antilymphocyte antibodies.
- Small intestine and lung transplant patients are at highest risk, with an incidence of up to 32%, whereas kidney transplant recipients are at lowest risk, within an incidence of 1%–2%.
- Can present as a mononucleosis syndrome with fever and lymphadenopathy, or diffuse polymorphous B-cell infiltration of visceral organs preceded by a mononucleosis-like episode; can also involve the CNS and the transplanted organ.
- Treatment requires reducing immunosuppression for mild cases and the use of rituximab with or without chemotherapy for severe cases; antivirals are not effective.

BK Polyomavirus (BKV) and Nephropathy (BKVN)

- Primary BKV infection is usually asymptomatic and occurs in the first decade of life; latent infection is usually established in uroepithelial and renal cells.
- BKVN is usually asymptomatic and presents as an unexplained rise in serum creatinine in kidney transplant recipients; up to 10% of kidney transplant patients may be affected; typically occurs within the first year of transplant.
- One-third of kidney transplant patients with high-level BK viruria progress to viremia and nephropathy.
- Definitive diagnosis is made by kidney histopathology; viruria has poor specificity for nephropathy but has a high negative predictive value; BKV DNA is detected

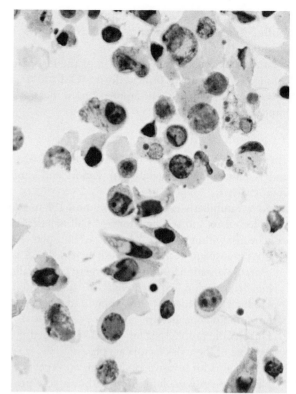

• **Fig. 41.4** Decoy cells in fresh urine – degenerating epithelial cells with high nuclear:cytoplasmic ratio showing peripheral clumped chromatin, intranuclear ground glass viral inclusions (Papanicolaou stain). (From Chantziantoniou N, Joudeh A, Hamed R, Al-Abbadi M. Significance, cytomorphology of decoy cells in polyomavirus-associated nephropathy. *J Am Soc Cytopathol.* 2016;5(2):71–85.)

in the urine and plasma in nearly all cases of BKVN (Fig. 41.4).
- Treatment requires reducing immunosuppression; antiviral therapy with leflunomide or cidofovir has been used in conjunction with decreasing immunosuppression with limited evidence.
- The presentation of BKV is very different in patients with bone marrow transplants (see Chapter 42).

Adenovirus

- Adenovirus commonly causes upper or lower respiratory tract infection but can also cause conjunctivitis, hepatitis, enteritis, and hemorrhagic cystitis in transplant recipients.
- In liver transplant recipients, adenovirus results in hepatitis. In lung transplant recipients, it can result in flu-like illness, necrotizing pneumonia, or chronic changes like bronchiolitis obliterans. Hemorrhagic cystitis and renal allograft nephropathy are described in renal transplant recipients.
- Diagnosis is made by PCR testing and with quantitative viral loads shown to predict clinical response and prognosis, while histopathological examination remains the gold standard for diagnosis.
- Detection of adenovirus at two or more sites is predictive of disseminated disease.

- Asymptomatic viremia is common (6.5%–22.5%), and routine screening for adenovirus DNAemia is not recommended.
- Treatment options include cidofovir, or the newer lipid conjugated derivative brincidofovir (CMX001) and IVIG. Decreasing immunosuppression, if possible, is important.

Invasive Fungal Infections (IFI)

- The type of IFI depends on the organ transplanted and is influenced by medical risk factors and surgical complexity.
- Invasive candidiasis is the most common IFI in transplant recipients and accounts for over half of cases; typically occurs within the first 3 months of transplant.
    - Liver transplant recipients are at increased risk with re-transplantation, prolonged surgery, renal failure, high transfusion requirement (>40 units of blood products), choledochojejunostomy, and *Candida* colonization preoperatively.
    - Fluconazole prophylaxis for 4 weeks is advised if two or more of these risk factors are present.
    - Risk factors for invasive aspergillosis are repeat transplant, *Aspergillus* colonization within a year pre- or posttransplant, and induction with alemtuzumab or thymoglobulin; risk factors specific to lung transplant recipients include allograft rejection and augmented immunosuppression, early airway ischemia and a vulnerable anastomotic site, and bronchiolitis obliterans; risk factors specific to heart transplant recipients are prior invasive aspergillosis and CMV disease.
    - Liver and lung transplant recipients are at higher risk for cryptococcosis; clinical presentation is often less typical (pneumonia, skin, and soft tissue infections) which can result in delayed diagnosis and worse prognosis compared to people with HIV.

Toxoplasmosis (see Chapter 34)

- *Toxoplasma gondii* infection occurs worldwide but is more common in patients from endemic regions including France and tropical areas of Latin America and sub-Saharan Africa.
- Latent infection in donor myocardium during cardiac transplantation is the most common method of donor-related transmission.
- Seronegative heart transplant patients receiving organs from seropositive donors have a 57%–75% risk of developing symptomatic infection without prophylaxis
- Clinical manifestations include fever, myocarditis, lymphadenopathy, chorioretinitis, and pneumonitis; usually presents within 3 months of transplant; pulmonary disease may be indistinguishable from *Pneumocystis jirovecii* pneumonia, but *Toxoplasma* tachyzoites are identified in bronchoalveolar lavage fluid instead.
- Treatment involves sulfadiazine and pyrimethamine.

Strongyloidiasis

- Endemic to the tropics and subtropics; has been reported from temperate areas including the southeastern United States.
- Infection may be donor-derived or from reactivation of latent disease; HTLV-1 co-infection is a risk factor.
- Mortality rate approaches 50% for hyperinfection syndrome and 70% for disseminated infection.
- Suspect in a patient from the southeastern United States or another endemic area who presents with sepsis syndrome, multiorgan (predominantly pulmonary and gastrointestinal) involvement and gram-negative intestinal bacteremia; absence of eosinophilia does not rule out disease in the recipient or donors.
- The treatment of choice is ivermectin.

Clinical Syndromes

Fever with Unclear Focus

- Early posttransplant (<1 month)
    - Surgical site infections, catheter-related infections; hospital-acquired infections (UTI, CDI), and consider donor-derived infections.
- Late posttransplant (>1 month): broad
    - Viral: CMV, human herpesvirus 6 (HHV-6), adenovirus, parvovirus, EBV.
    - Bacterial: along with routine: consider TB, NTM, *Nocardia, Ehrlichia.*
    - Fungal: cryptococcosis, endemic mycosis, PCP, *Aspergillus.*
    - Parasitic: toxoplasmosis, *Strongyloides.*

Meningitis/Encephalitis

- Bacterial: *Listeria, Pneumococcus, Haemophilus influenza,* syphilis, mycobacteria, and *Nocardia.*
- Viral: CMV, HSV, VZV, WNV, enterovirus.
- Fungal: *Cryptococcus, Coccidioides, Histoplasma, Candida.*
- Donor derived: WNV, LCMV, *Balamuthia,* rabies.
- Noninfectious: drug-induced (TMP–SMX), posterior reversible encephalopathy syndrome (PRES) due to calcineurin inhibitors (CNIs).

Focal Brain Abscess or Space-Occupying Lesions

- Bacterial: septic emboli, invasion from parameningeal foci (gram positive, negative and anaerobes), nocardia, TB, *Listeria,* and *Actinomyces.*
- Fungal: *Aspergillus, Mucor, Cryptococcus.*
- Others.
- *Toxoplasma,* neurocysticercosis, CNS PTLD
    - Subacute cognitive decline with white matter changes on MRI.
    - Progressive multifocal leukoencephalopathy (PML): subacute motor, sensory, visual, or cognitive decline. JC virus DNA PCR + in CSF.

Pneumonia

- Community-acquired: *Pneumococcus, Haemophilus, Legionella, Mycoplasma,* respiratory viruses.

- Nosocomial: gram-negative bacilli, *Staphylococcus aureus* (MRSA).
- Opportunistic pathogens:
  - Fungal: *Aspergillus*, PJP, *Cryptococcus*, endemic fungi.
  - Viral: CMV, adenovirus, HSV, VZV.
  - Bacterial: TB, other mycobacteria, *Nocardia*, *Toxoplasma*.
  - Noninfectious causes: PTLD, sirolimus hypersensitivity pneumonitis, rounded atelectasis.

Enteritis/Colitis

- Bacterial: *Salmonella, Shigella, Campylobacter, Listeria, C. difficile.*
- Viral: norovirus, adenovirus, CMV, EBV (PTLD).
- Parasitic: *Entamoeba, Giardia, Strongyloides.*
- Others: bacterial overgrowth after Roux-en-Y (liver transplant).

Hepatitis

- Viral: HBV, HCV, and CMV, HSV, VZV, adenovirus, and HHV-6.
- Others: part of a disseminated bacterial, mycobacterial, or fungal infection.
- Noninfectious: rejection, graft ischemia for liver transplants, drug-induced liver injury.

Skin and Soft Tissue

- Cellulitis: *Staphylococcus, Streptococcus*, occasional gram-negatives. Consider mycobacterial, cryptococcosis, and histoplasmosis in persistent lesions.
- Papulo-nodular lesions: Disseminated fungal (*Candida*, cryptococcal, histoplasma) infections, *Nocardia*, and atypical mycobacterial.
- Vesicular/crusted lesions: HSV, VZV, *Staphylococcus, Streptococcus.*
- Eschar/ecthyma/necrotic lesions: *Pseudomonas, Meningococcus, Aspergillus, Mucor*, endovascular septic infections, shock, and DIC.

Other Important Points

Infectious Disease Mimics in SOT (See Chapter 48)

- Posterior reversible encephalopathy syndrome (PRES) is a rare neurologic side effect of calcineurin inhibitors (CNIs), and patients manifesting with seizures and confusion could mimic encephalitis.
- Acute graft-versus-host disease (GVHD) is a rare but fatal complication after SOT and can present with skin rash, diarrhea, and pancytopenia usually within the first 8 weeks of transplant. Diagnosis is made based on clinical and histologic evidence, supported by chimerism studies showing donor HLA alleles in the recipient bone marrow or blood.

Drug Interactions

- Antimicrobials can have significant interactions with commonly used immunosuppressive agents; CINs such as tacrolimus and cyclosporine, and mTOR inhibitors such as sirolimus are metabolized via the cytochrome CYP3A4 system.
- All macrolide antibiotics with the exception of azithromycin and azole antifungal agents (itraconazole and posaconazole > voriconazole, fluconazole) are moderate to strong inhibitors of CYP3A4 and can induce profound increases in serum concentrations of immunosuppressants.
- Rifamycins are strong inducers of CYP3A4 and can dramatically decrease plasma levels of immunosuppressants.

Side Effects of Immunosuppressive Medications

- Tacrolimus: increased creatinine, hypertension, posterior reversible encephalopathy syndrome.
- Mycophenolate: leukopenia, mouth ulcers.
- Sirolimus: poor wound healing, pneumonitis.
- Eculizumab (used for prevention of antibody-mediated rejection in kidney transplant recipients and in atypical hemolytic uremic syndromes): predisposes to meningococcal sepsis and infections with other encapsulated bacteria; patients should receive prophylactic antibiotics and meningococcal vaccination at the start of therapy.

Further Reading

1. Fischer SA, Lu K, Practice ASTIDCo. Screening of donor and recipient in solid organ transplantation. *Am J Transplant.* 2013;13(suppl 4):9–21.
2. Santos CA, Brennan DC, Chapman WC, Fraser VJ, Olsen MA. Delayed-onset cytomegalovirus disease coded during hospital readmission in a multicenter, retrospective cohort of liver transplant recipients. *Liver Transplant.* 2015;21(5):581–590.
3. Ayoub WS, Esquivel CO, Martin P. Biliary complications following liver transplantation. *Dig Dis Sci.* 2010;55(6):1540–1546.
4. George IA, Santos CAQ, Olsen MA, Powderly WG. Epidemiology of cryptococcosis and cryptococcal meningitis in a large retrospective cohort of patients after solid organ transplantation. *Open Forum Infect Dis.* 2017;4(1):ofx004.
5. Origuen J, Lopez-Medrano F, Fernandez-Ruiz M, et al. Should asymptomatic bacteriuria be systematically treated in kidney transplant recipients? Results from a randomized controlled trial. *Am J Transplant.* 2016;16(10):2943–2953.
6. Kumar D, Humar A, Plevneshi A, et al. Invasive pneumococcal disease in solid organ transplant recipients – 10-year prospective population surveillance. *Am J Transplant.* 2007;7(5):1209–1214.
7. Humar A, Kumar D, Mazzulli T, et al. A surveillance study of adenovirus infection in adult solid organ transplant recipients. *Am J Transplant.* 2005;5(10):2555–2559.

42

Infections in Bone Marrow Transplant Recipients

JADE LE, ADRIENNE D. WORKMAN

Definitions

Hematopoietic cell transplantation (HCT): the collection of stem cells from bone marrow, peripheral blood, or umbilical cord to re-establish the immune system and provide a new source for hematopoiesis.

Allogeneic transplantation (Allo HCT): stem cells are acquired from a donor other than oneself, related or matched-unrelated.

Autologous transplantation (Auto HCT): stem cells are acquired from oneself.

Conditioning regimen: treatment used to prepare a patient for stem cell transplantation. Includes chemotherapy, radiation, or monoclonal antibody therapy.

Engraftment: incorporation of grafted tissue into the body of the host.

Graft versus host disease (GVHD): condition following allogeneic HCT caused when the cells from donated stem cells attack the normal tissue of the transplant recipient, including the immune system, skin, liver, lungs, and intestinal tract.

Neutropenic fever: temperature >38°C associated with an absolute neutrophilic count of <500 cells/mm³.

Neutropenia: condition in which there is a decrease in circulating neutrophils.

Severe neutropenia: absolute neutrophil count of <500 cells/mm³.

Epidemiology

HCT is a treatment option for patients with malignancies, disorders of bone marrow failure, severe immunodeficiencies, some solid tumors, and a limited number of autoimmune diseases. HCT involves the intravenous delivery of hematopoietic stem cells (from peripheral blood, bone marrow, or umbilical cord blood) to a recipient whose hematopoietic and immune system has been ablated or altered by a conditioning regimen, with the end result of engraftment of these transplanted cells.

Risk for infection in HCT is dependent on numerous factors.

Underlying Disease Process

- Risk for infection in patients with immune deficiencies (e.g., severe combined immunodeficiency [SCID]) >> leukemia/lymphoma/chronic granulomatous disease >> solid tumors.

Conditioning Regimen

- Immunosuppressive and cytotoxic chemotherapy ± radiation.
- Myeloablative vs. reduced intensity (aka nonmyeloablative or "mini" transplants) depending on how much of the hematopoietic/immune system is ablated.
  - Myeloablative regimens → most infections early after transplant, with a similar risk of infections late after transplantation due to GVHD.
- Biologic agent antithymocyte globulin (ATG) eliminates T cells and is extremely immunosuppressive, as are antilymphoid antibodies such as alemtuzumab and rituximab.
- Total body irradiation causes mucositis → bacterial translocation across the gut wall.

Donor Source/Type of Transplant

Autologous or allogeneic donor source, peripheral stem cell vs. umbilical cord blood transplant.

- **Umbilical cord blood transplants (UCB)**
  - Prolonged neutropenia (due to the low dose of stem cells) → increased risk of bacterial and fungal infections.
  - Lack of antigen-specific memory T cells → increased viral and other opportunistic infections.
  - Less GVHD.

- **Peripheral blood stem cell transplants (PBSC)**
  - Shorter neutropenia due to faster engraftment than UCB but more chronic GVHD (cGVHD).
- **Auto HCT**
  - Less risk of infections than Allo HCT.
  - Immune reconstitution occurs more rapidly than Allo HCT.
- **Allo HCT**
  - More HLA mismatch → more immunosuppression required → delayed immune reconstitution, prolonged engraftment, increased risk of GVHD, and higher risk of infections related to T-cell immunodeficiency such as *Pneumocystis jirovecii* pneumonia (PCP), cytomegalovirus (CMV), Epstein–Barr virus-associated posttransplant lymphoproliferative disorder (EBV-PTLD), fungal infections.
  - Engraftment and immune reconstitution delayed more than autologous or syngeneic HCT → increased risk of infections.
- **Syngeneic HCT** = transfer of stem cells from one identical twin to the other.
  - Less risk of infections than Allo HCT. Similar to Auto HCT.

Presence of GVHD

- The most important cause of mortality after HCT, due to complications from infections.
- Affects 40%–80% of Allo HCT recipients.
- Predisposes to infections by:
  - Disruption of the GI tract → mucositis → bacterial translocation.
  - Alterations in both humoral/cellular immunity → delayed immune reconstitution.
  - Functional hyposplenism and poor response to vaccinations → pneumococcal infections, fungal infections, and CMV reactivation.
  - Prophylaxis of GVHD via immunosuppressive agents (cyclosporine, methotrexate, corticosteroids, mycophenolate mofetil (MMF), or tacrolimus) for approx. 6 months to 1 year after HCT → increases risk of opportunistic infections.
  - Acute GVHD treated with high-dose corticosteroids or other immunosuppressive regimens → increased risk of fungal infections and viral reactivation.

Pretransplant Exposure History

- Screening tests below are center-dependent:
  - Cytomegalovirus (CMV) serologies.
  - Herpes simplex virus (HSV) serologies.
  - Varicella-zoster virus (VZV) serologies.
  - Epstein–Barr virus (EBV) serologies.
  - Hepatitis B serologies.
  - Hepatitis C antibody.
  - *Toxoplasma gondii* serologies.
  - Tuberculin skin test (TST, aka PPD) or interferon-gamma release assay (Quantiferon-Gold or TB-spot).
  - Human immunodeficiency virus (HIV)-1/2 antigen/antibody.
  - Human T-lymphotrophic virus (HTLV)-I/II serologies.

Time Period after Transplantation

Time period after transplantation = intensity of immunosuppression.

- **Prior to Engraftment**
  High-risk patient characteristics
  - Age >40.
  - Prior HCT.
  - Underlying condition: acute myelogenous leukemia (AML), aplastic anemia, or non-first remission malignancy.
  - Degree of immunosuppression.
    - Allo HCT >> Auto HCT.
    - Antithymocyte globulin (ATG).
    - Methotrexate: causes increased mucosal injury and prolonged time to neutrophil engraftment → increased risk for fungal and herpesvirus infections.
  - Exposure to CMV, HSV, EBV, VZV.
  - Mucositis → bacterial translocation → infections with enteric gram-negative bacteria as well as gram-positive bacteria.
  - Use of central venous catheters (CVCs) → increases risk of bacteremia with gram-positive bacteria.
  - Myeloablative conditioning.
  - Prolonged neutropenia → increases risk of bacterial, viral, and fungal (*Candida*, early aspergillosis) infections.

  Low-risk patient characteristics
  - Chronic phase of chronic myelogenous leukemia (CML).
  - Age <19.
  - Nonmyeloablative conditioning.
- **Engraftment**
  Type of transplantation and degree of HLA similarity.
  - High risk.
    - Allo unrelated matched HCT, Allo related mismatched HCT.
    - CMV reactivation.
  - Low risk: Allo-related matched HCT, Auto HCT.
  Other high-risk factors.
  - CD34 infused <2.0 ×10⁶/kg.
    - These are the most primitive stem cells. Usual dose of infusion of nucleated cells for stable long-term engraftment is approximately 2.0 ×10⁸/kg. Lower quantity leads to delay of engraftment.
  - T-cell depletion (ATG).
    - Causes higher risk for graft rejection, neutropenic infections, herpesvirus, and invasive fungal infections.
- **Postengraftment**
  High-risk factors.
  - CD4 <200/μL.
  - Glucocorticoids >1 mg/kg per day.
  - Exposure to CMV, HIV, human herpesvirus 6 (HHV-6), and human herpesvirus 7 (HHV-7).
  - CMV reactivation increases risk of invasive aspergillosis.

- Presence of Grade 2–4 GVHD.
- Graft failure.
- Skin breakdown.
- Organ dysfunction.
  - Severe mucositis, renal failure, liver insufficiency, pulmonary insufficiency.
- Pathogen exposure.
  - Reactivation of CMV, HSV, EBV, and VZV.
- Healthcare setting.
  - Risk of nosocomial infections such as methicillin-resistant *Staphylococcus aureus* (MRSA), vancomycin-resistant *enterococcus* (VRE), *Clostridioides difficile* colitis, and other multidrug-resistant organisms (MDRO).

Prophylaxis

Lack of appropriate prophylaxis for pathogens at highest risk during the different periods posttransplantation increases risk of infections. Please note that the actual antibiotic/antiviral selected for prophylaxis and the duration of prophylaxis vary with each institution.

- **Bacterial infections**
Prophylactic antibiotics (fluoroquinolones) when absolute neutrophil count (ANC) << 500/mm³ until neutrophil recovery.
  - Auto HCT: duration approx. 2 weeks – 30 days.
  - Allo HCT: duration approx. 30–90 days.
    - Longer duration of prophylaxis in Allo HCT recipients due to prolonged duration of neutropenia.
  - Reduces mortality.
  - Protects against gram-negative bacteria (Enterobacteriaceae and non-lactose-fermenting gram-negatives such as *Pseudomonas, Stenotrophomonas,* and *Acinetobacter*) as well as some gram-positive bacteria (*Streptococcus viridans*).
  - No role for prophylaxis for MRSA or coagulase-negative staphylococcus or VRE.
- **Viral infections**
HSV reactivation common; 80% of seropositive recipients.
  - Prophylaxis = aciclovir/valaciclovir.
    - Covers VZV.
    - For HSV or VZV seropositive patients.
    - Auto HCT: prophylaxis may be up to 1 year post-HCT.
    - Allo HCT: prophylaxis while on immunosuppression may be prolonged in the setting of GVHD.
CMV reactivation in 20%–40% of CMV seronegative HCT recipients who have seropositive donors; CMV reactivation in up to 80% of CMV seropositive HCT recipients.
  - Consider CMV prophylaxis for high-risk patients who are CMV seropositive, depending on transplant center protocol.
    - Universal prophylaxis posttransplantation: high-risk patients placed on prophylaxis with valganciclovir post HCT.
    Concerns over prolonging neutropenia with valganciclovir.

- Preemptive therapy: CMV PCR weekly or bi-weekly monitoring in high-risk patients and initiation of CMV treatment with IV ganciclovir/IV foscarnet, or treatment dose valganciclovir when positive. More late-onset CMV disease with this strategy.
- Recipient CMV IgG+ are at highest risk of infection:
  - D–/R+ > D+/R+ >> D+/R– > D–/R–.
  - Use CMV seronegative blood products for CMV R– patients.
- CMV prophylaxis: oral valganciclovir due to high bioavailability.
  - Some centers do not use valganciclovir due to risk of prolonging the duration of neutropenia.
- Letermovir 240 mg orally once daily was approved by the FDA 11/2017 for the prevention of CMV infection and disease in adult CMV seropositive recipients of Allo HCT.
- **Fungal infections**
Candidemia increases with mucositis, neutropenia.
  - Prophylaxis = fluconazole.
  - Usually for Auto HCT.
  - Duration: usually until ANC >500 (approx 15–30 days).
Late-onset *Aspergillus* or other fungal infections (mucormycosis, *Fusarium, Scedosporium,* etc.). Highest risk in Allo HCT.
  - Prophylaxis = voriconazole, posaconazole. Some centers use echinocandins if cannot tolerate azoles.
  - Duration: until at least day +75 or longer if still neutropenic, + cGVHD, or low CD4 count.
- ***Pneumocystis jirovecii***:
  - High risk secondary to steroids, immunosuppressants.
  - Prophylaxis = trimethoprim–sulfamethoxazole (TMP–SMX).
    - Note: may prolong neutropenia, so some centers use nebulized pentamidine monthly but breakthrough pneumocystis infections may occur.
  - Other alternatives: dapsone (if G6PD normal), or atovaquone.
  - Auto HCT: duration until day +180 or until CD4 >200/µL.
  - Allo HCT: duration until day +180 or until CD4 >200/µL, off immunosuppression, and no cGVHD.

Infections Encountered After HCT

Risk of infection is stratified according to time period pre- or postengraftment (see Fig. 42.1).

Preengraftment: Time of Transplantation (Day 0) through Day 30

- Associated with leukopenia with risk for neutropenia and lymphocytopenia. Overall risk, type of infection, and organisms similar to neutropenic patients due to chemotherapy.
- Neutropenic fever.
- Source identified <30% of time.

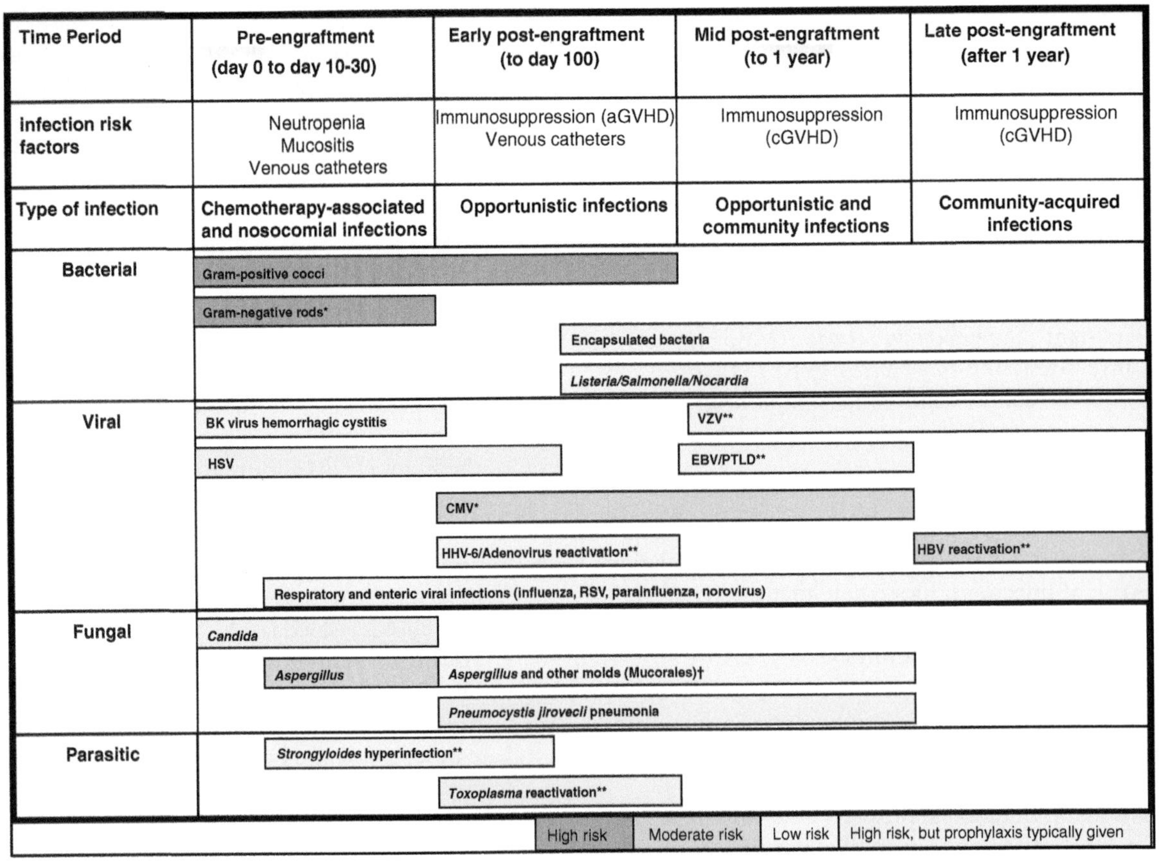

Time Period	Pre-engraftment (day 0 to day 10-30)	Early post-engraftment (to day 100)	Mid post-engraftment (to 1 year)	Late post-engraftment (after 1 year)
Infection risk factors	Neutropenia Mucositis Venous catheters	Immunosuppression (aGVHD) Venous catheters	Immunosuppression (cGVHD)	Immunosuppression (cGVHD)
Type of infection	Chemotherapy-associated and nosocomial infections	Opportunistic infections	Opportunistic and community infections	Community-acquired infections
Bacterial	Gram-positive cocci / Gram-negative rods*		Encapsulated bacteria / Listeria/Salmonella/Nocardia	
Viral	BK virus hemorrhagic cystitis / HSV / CMV* / HHV-6/Adenovirus reactivation** / Respiratory and enteric viral infections (influenza, RSV, parainfluenza, norovirus)		VZV** / EBV/PTLD**	HBV reactivation**
Fungal	Candida / Aspergillus / Pneumocystis jirovecii pneumonia	Aspergillus and other molds (Mucorales)†		
Parasitic	Strongyloides hyperinfection** / Toxoplasma reactivation**			

Legend: High risk | Moderate risk | Low risk | High risk, but prophylaxis typically given

• **Fig. 42.1** Infections following hematopoietic cell transplantation. (From O'Shea DT, Humar A. Life threatening infections in transplant recipients. *Crit Care Clin.* 2013;29(4):953–973.)

Bacteria
- Bacteremia most common complication.
  - Cause of infection in approximately 20% of neutropenic patients.
  - **Risk factor:** CVCs, mucositis.
  - Higher risk with severe neutropenia or prolonged neutropenia >7 days.
  - Gram-positive organisms > gram-negative organisms.
- **Gram-positive bacteria**
  - **Risk factors:** neutropenia, CVCs, mucositis.
  - *Staphylococcus aureus.*
  - *Staphylococcus epidermidis* or coagulase-negative *staphylococcus* most commonly isolated in bloodstream infections, especially patients with CVCs.
  - Oropharyngeal or GI pathogens: *Streptococcus pyogenes, Streptococcus viridans,* and *Enterococcus faecalis, Enterococcus faecium* isolated in patients with poor dental hygiene, mucositis, or HSV-induced oral ulcerations.
  - *Corynebacterium* isolated in patients with CVCs.
- **Gram-negative bacteria**
  - Enterobacteriaceae and the non-lactose fermenters are the next most frequently isolated bacterial pathogens in neutropenic HCT patients.
  - **Risk factors:** neutropenia, mucositis, GVHD, and presence of CVCs.
  - Cause significant morbidity and mortality, especially secondary to *Pseudomonas.*

- *Escherichia coli, Klebsiella* species.
- Emergence of drug-resistant pathogens: *Pseudomonas aeruginosa, Stenotrophomonas maltophilia,* and *Acinetobacter baumannii.*
- **Anaerobic bacteria**
  - Rare but consider in settings of oral mucositis, perirectal, or intraabdominal infections.

Fungi
- **Candida**
  - **Risk factors:** neutropenia, mucositis from chemotherapy or GVHD, presence of indwelling catheters, overgrowth due to the use of broad-spectrum antibiotics or corticosteroids.
  - **Prophylaxis:** fluconazole; however, rise of fluconazole-resistant candidal species such as *C. krusei, C. glabrata* is of concern.
  - **Diagnosis:** culture of the blood or other tissues. Biopsy with histopathology. Beta-D-glucan antigen assay detects beta-D-glucan (present in cell walls of fungi) but not specific for *Candida.*
- Aspergillus, late onset, is uncommon (5%).

Viruses
- **Herpes simplex virus.**
  - Reactivation occurs in 80% of seropositive patients (5% if on prophylaxis).

- **Clinical:** oropharyngeal ulcerations, esophageal ulcerations, or perianal ulcerations. Rarely, encephalitis, hepatitis, or Bell's palsy.
- **Diagnosis:** viral culture, HSV DFA, HSV PCR.
- **Prophylaxis:** aciclovir/valaciclovir.

Early Postengraftment: Days 31 to 100

- Often associated with GVHD.

Bacteria

- **Bacterial infections:** gram-positive (*Enterococcus*, coagulase-negative staphylococci) or enteric gram-negatives.
  - Risk factors: indwelling CVC, mucositis from GVHD.

Viruses

- **HSV** reactivation, similar to preengraftment period.
  Cytomegalovirus
- Reactivation 20%–40% of CMV seropositive HCT recipients, but CMV disease is decreasing due to preventive strategies.
- Reactivation depends on the serostatus of the recipient (R) and donor: D–/R+ > D+/R+ >> D+/R– > D–/R–.
  - **Risk factors:** acute or chronic, GVHD, lymphopenia, high dose corticosteroid use, T-cell depletion, mismatched or unrelated donor status, umbilical cord transplant in CMV seropositive recipient, use of alemtuzumab.
- CMV is an immunomodulatory virus → predisposes to other bacterial and fungal infections.
- CMV indirect effects: reactivation associated with increased transplant-related mortality and decreased overall survival, increased incidence of GVHD, increased mortality due to bacterial and fungal infections.
- **Clinical:** CMV infection (fever + CMV viremia) vs. CMV disease (pneumonia, enteritis, bone marrow suppression, and rarely retinitis).
  - **CMV pneumonitis:** patients may present with fever, dyspnea, nonproductive cough, hypoxia.
    - Chest X-ray/CT chest may show interstitial infiltrates (Fig. 42.2).
    - Most serious manifestation with mortality rate up to 50%.
    - More often seen in late disease due to widespread use of preemptive therapy strategy.
    - **Diagnosis:** bronchoalveolar lavage (BAL) or lung biopsy + CMV by immunohistochemical stain or viral culture (Fig. 42.2).
    - **Note:** CMV polymerase chain reaction (PCR) presence in BAL specimen in absence of clinical symptoms is not proof of CMV pneumonia, as pulmonary shedding of CMV is common in HCT; however, approx. 60% may develop CMV pneumonia. Negative CMV PCR in BAL, however, can rule out CMV pneumonia.

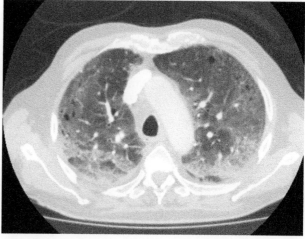

- **Fig. 42.2** Predominantly diffuse pattern ground glass opacities: CMV lung infection. (From Bommart S, Bourdin A, Makinson A, et al. Infectious chest complications in haematological malignancies. *Diagnost Intervent Imaging*. 2013;94(2):193–201.)

- **CMV enteritis:** most common presentation (up to 70%–80% of CMV disease) and may affect any portion of the gastrointestinal tract.
  - Endoscopy: may see ulcers extending into submucosal layers.
    Difficult to distinguish on visualization from GVHD or adenovirus.
    May lead to enteric perforation.
  - Diagnosis relies on CMV + immunohistochemical staining on biopsy samples.
  - Note CMV PCR in the serum may be negative in patients with CMV enteritis (not reliable in ruling out CMV enteritis).
- **CMV retinitis:** very uncommon, unlike in acquired immune deficiency (AIDS) patients.
  - Common complaint is blurry vision, floaters → call ophthalmology consult.
- CMV hepatitis is rare, but may be suspected in patients with fever, rising transaminases, and positive CMV PCR in the serum.
- **Diagnosis:** quantitative CMV PCR testing should be considered weekly post-HCT regardless of prophylaxis as screening for at least 100 days or longer in the presence of GVHD.
- **Prevention:** if CMV seronegative, use CMV-safe blood products (leukoreduced), can consider valganciclovir or letermovir prophylaxis.
- **Treatment:** IV ganciclovir/oral valganciclovir ± CMV immune globulin.
  - CMV resistance due to the *UL97* or *UL54* gene mutations may be treated with foscarnet or cidofovir.
  - Resistance arises in up to 15% of patients, especially high-risk.
  - Suspect CMV resistance if CMV viremia fails to improve after 2 weeks of appropriate anti-CMV therapy or if CMV end-organ disease occurs during prolonged anti-CMV therapy.

TABLE 42.1	*UL54* Mutation and Effect on Treatment of CMV Infection		
	Ganciclovir	**Cidofovir**	**Foscarnet**
UL54 mutation	Ganciclovir and cidofovir cross-resistance (rare foscarnet cross-resistance)	Cidofovir resistance and ganciclovir cross-resistance (rare foscarnet cross-resistance)	Foscarnet resistance (rare ganciclovir/cidofovir cross-resistance)

Adapted from Drew WL. Cytomegalovirus resistance testing: pitfalls and problems for the clinician. *Clin Infect Dis.* 2010;50(5):733–6.

- Send blood for CMV genotypic analysis for resistance and can switch to foscarnet and reduce immunosuppression if possible.
- *UL97* mutation confers ganciclovir/valganciclovir resistance.
  - If >5 fold ganciclovir EC50 (i.e., M460V, H530Q, A594V, L595S, C603W, and L595F) continue foscarnet monotherapy and consider adding leflunomide (adjunct and later as maintenance).
  - If <5 fold GCV EC50 (M460I, C592G, L595W) *and*
  - No CMV disease confirmed can resume ganciclovir and increase dose by 2× to 7.5–10 mg/kg twice daily (renally adjusted) and consider ½ dose of foscarnet (90 mg/kg IV q24h).
  - CMV disease present continue foscarnet and consider adding leflunomide (adjunct and later as maintenance).
- *UL54* mutation: depends on current treatment (Table 42.1).

Varicella-Zoster Virus
- **Clinical**: localized zoster (shingles), disseminated zoster, hemorrhagic pneumonia, hepatitis, abdominal pain, encephalitis, and retinal necrosis.
  - Strong association of disseminated VZV with GVHD.
- **Diagnosis**: viral culture, VZV DFA, VZV PCR.
- **Prophylaxis**: Oral aciclovir/valaciclovir.
- **Treatment**: IV aciclovir for severe disease.

Epstein–Barr Virus
- Most EBV reactivation is subclinical.
- **Risk factors**: EBV-negative serostatus recipient of HCT from EBV-seropositive donor is the most important risk factor; treatment for GVHD, mismatched transplant recipients, and UCB, treated with ATG, or who received T-cell depleted grafts.
  - EBV posttransplant lymphoproliferative disease (EBV-PTLD) is a spectrum of lymphoid proliferations (up to high-grade B-cell lymphoma) that arise in the setting of persistently high EBV viral loads (Table 42.2).
- **Clinical manifestations**
  - Acute primary EBV infection (mononucleosis).
  - Spectrum of disease varies and relies on pathologic identification.
  - Limited nodular lesions (>65%–80% present with extranodal disease: gastrointestinal (GI), liver, lungs

TABLE 42.2	Categories of Posttransplant Lymphoproliferative Disease (PTLD)

Early lesions[a]
    Plasmacytic hyperplasia
    Infectious mononucleosis-like lesion

Polymorphic PTLD

Monomorphic PTLD (classify according to lymphoma they resemble)
    B-cell neoplasms
        Diffuse large B-cell lymphoma
        Burkitt lymphoma
        Plasma cell myeloma
        Plasmacytoma-like lesion
    T-cell neoplasms
        Peripheral T-cell lymphoma, NOS
        Hepatosplenic T-cell lymphoma
        Other[b]

Classic Hodgkin lymphoma-like PTLD

[a]Some mass-like lesions in the posttransplant setting may have the morphologic appearance of florid follicular hyperplasia or other marked but non-IM-like lymphoid hyperplasias.
[b]Indolent small B-cell lymphomas, arising in transplant recipients are not included among the PTLD.
From Post-transplant lymphoproliferative disorders. In: Swerdlow SH, Campo E, Harris NL, et al., eds. *WHO Classification of Tumors of Haematopoietic and Lymphoid Tissues.* 4th ed. Geneva: WHO Press; 2008:343–4.

most involved, central nervous system (CNS), skin are other sites).
- GI manifestations: GI bleeding, weight loss, low albumin, bowel obstruction, bowel perforation. Usually aggressive. Treatment with resection confers better prognosis.
- Lung manifestations: pleural effusions, pulmonary nodules.
- CNS presentations: altered mental status, focal neurologic deficits in setting of CNS mass lesions. Very poor prognosis.
- Disseminated disease (especially in HCT recipients): early posttransplant (within few months) with fever, lymphoproliferation and multiorgan failure, and frequently CNS involvement → very poor prognosis.
- Late EBV-PTLD (after one year post-HCT): older patients, usually extranodal (CNS/head and neck/bowel) mass lesions, presentation similar to

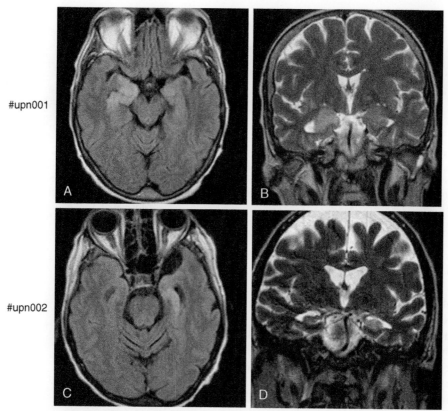

• **Fig. 42.3** Acute limbic encephalitis. Magnetic resonance imaging (MRI) findings in two patients (upn001 and upn002). (A and C) Axial section of T2-weighted fluid-attenuated inversion recovery MRI showing asymmetrical signal hyperintensity in the limbic system (insular and hippocampal region). (B and D) Coronal section of T2-weigthed MRI in the same patients. (From Greco R, Crucitti L, Noviello M, et al. Human herpesvirus 6 infection following haploidentical transplantation: immune recovery and outcome. *Biol Blood Marrow Transplant.* 2016:22(12);2250–2255.)

non-Hodgkin's lymphoma, fewer constitutional symptoms, fatal in >70% although course may progress slowly.
- Note some late PTLD may be EBV-negative.
- Rare: EBV-associated hemophagocytic syndrome, most often in primary EBV infection.
- **Diagnosis**: high index of suspicion + EBV PCR serum + pathology consistent with PTLD.
- **Prevention**
  - Monitor high-risk patients with EBV PCR although EBV viremia does not always predict PTLD, and lack of EBV viremia does not always rule out PTLD.
  - No role for routine antiviral prophylaxis with aciclovir/valaciclovir or ganciclovir/valganciclovir.
  - Reduce immunosuppression if feasible per institutional protocol.
  - No data to support prophylactic intravenous immunoglobulin (IVIG) or CMV-IG in HCT recipients.
  - Rituximab is commonly used as part of preemptive therapy.
- **Treatment**
  - Reduction of immunosuppression is the cornerstone of therapy.
  - Rituximab may offer survival benefit.

- Depending on the presentation, chemotherapy plus rituximab, or surgery, or radiation therapy.
- Role of antivirals (ganciclovir/aciclovir) is uncertain.
- Role of IVIG is uncertain.
- Some centers offer EBV-specific cytotoxic T-cell therapy.

HHV-6, HHV-7, HHV-8
- **HHV-6**
  - Reactivation occurs in up to 46% of HCT recipients, especially UCB transplant; most cases are asymptomatic without clinical significance.
  - Associated with meningoencephalitis, bone marrow suppression, interstitial pneumonitis, rash, GVHD, thrombocytopenia, and posttransplant acute limbic encephalitis (PALE) (Fig. 42.3).
  - **Diagnosis**: HHV-6 PCR of blood.
  - **Treatment**: ganciclovir or foscarnet with variable success.
- **HHV-7**: no current association with clinical syndromes.
- **HHV-8**: implicated in the development of Kaposi sarcoma in HCT, but rare.

BK Virus
- **Clinical**: hemorrhagic cystitis, but not BK-induced nephropathy as is seen in renal transplant recipients (see Chapter 41).

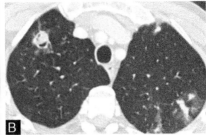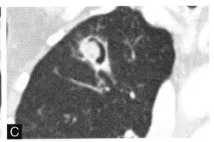

• **Fig. 42.4** (A) Axial CT image in a leukemic patient showing a right upper lobe nodule surrounded by mild ground glass attenuation. (B; and C) Axial and coronal CT images acquired 3 weeks later showing an "air crescent" sign surrounding a focal opacity. This feature is similar to aspergilloma but is relevant to a necrotic lung fragment in an angio-invasive form of aspergillosis. (From Chabi ML, Goracci A, Roche N, et al. *Pulmonary aspergillosis. Diagnost Intervent Imaging.* 2015;96(5):435–442.)

• **Diagnosis**: BK virus PCR of urine and blood.
• **Treatment**: reduction immunosuppression, cidofovir.

Parvovirus B19

• Rare incidence of infection post-HCT compared to renal transplant recipients.
• **Clinical**: anemia/thrombocytopenia/leukopenia, flu-like symptoms, rarely hepatitis, myocarditis, pneumonitis, collapsing glomerulopathy, CNS vasculitis, hemophagocytic lymphohistiocytosis.
  • Suspect in patients with refractory anemia, especially with low reticulocyte count, associated leucopenia/thrombocytopenia not responding to usual therapies.
  • Patients post-HCT may develop GVHD-like rash.
• **Diagnosis**: parvovirus B19 PCR, parvovirus serologies, bone marrow examination (giant pronormoblasts, red cell aplasia, PCR +), if rash present (skin biopsy with parvovirus PCR).
• **Treatment**: IVIG.

Fungi

Candida (see Chapter 27)

• Visceral or hepatosplenic candidiasis arises at the point of neutrophil recovery → multiple liver/spleen micro abscesses.
• **Treatment**: fluconazole, echinocandins, or liposomal amphotericin B for drug-resistant *Candida.*

Aspergillosis (see Chapter 29)

• Most common invasive fungal infection, since the advent of fluconazole prophylaxis, with incidence ranging from 4% to 15% in HCT recipients.
• Infection occurs via inhalation of spores into the respiratory tract → sinus and lung infections (pulmonary nodules, fungal balls, infiltrates), dissemination → skin nodules, brain abscesses.
  • Suspect in patients with febrile neutropenia not responding to antibiotics. Computed tomography (CT) chest scan may reveal pulmonary nodules with halo sign, air crescent sign, tree-in-bud nodules (Figs. 42.4 and 42.5).
• Infections occur at specific time points after transplantation: peak 1 at 2–3 weeks, peak 2 at 3–4 months, and peak 3 late, during treatment for chronic GVHD.

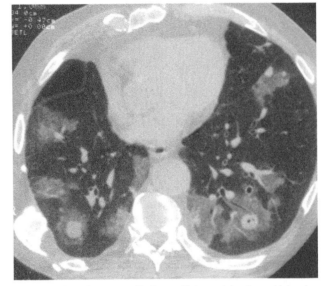

• **Fig. 42.5** Invasive aspergillosis, multiple nodular form. Halo sign. (From Bommart S, Bourdin A, Makinson A, et al. Infectious chest complications in haematological malignancies. *Diagnost Intervent Imaging.* 2013;94(2):193–201.)

• **Risk factors**: prolonged neutropenia is one of the most important risk factors, chronic GVHD, older age, construction in hospital vicinity, CMV, respiratory virus infection, and multiple myeloma.
• **Diagnosis**: fungal culture from respiratory samples or tissue samples, histopathology + for mold with septated narrow-branching hyphae, and *Aspergillus* galactomannan assay (antigen in *Aspergillus* cell wall) (Fig. 42.6).
• **Treatment**: voriconazole ± echinocandin for salvage, isavuconazole, posaconazole, or liposomal amphotericin. Note the azoles are the most effective treatment for invasive aspergillosis, in combination with recovery of neutrophils.

Late Postengraftment: >100 Days Until Normal Immunity (c. 18–36 Months After HCT)

• Risk persists in Auto HCT: 6–12 months.
• Risk persists in Allo HCT: 12–24 months.
• cGVHD delays immune recovery.

- Use of immunosuppressants to treat cGVHD → lymphocyte and macrophage dysfunction with abnormal antibody function.
- UCB and unrelated donor transplants impair immune recovery → late infections.

Bacteria

Encapsulated bacteria

- *Streptococcus pneumoniae, Haemophilus influenzae, Neisseria meningitides.*
- Otitis, sinusitis, bronchitis, pneumonia.
- **Risk factor**: cGVHD → functional asplenia, asplenia from underlying disease.
- Life-threatening sepsis.
- **Prevention**: pneumococcal vaccination and penicillin, macrolide, or fluoroquinolone antibiotics in patients with cGVHD.

Intracellular Bacteria

- *Legionella* infections rare: causes pneumonia or pulmonary nodules.
- *Listeria monocytogenes* infections rare: causes meningitis, bacteremia.

Filamentous bacteria

- *Nocardia* infections are rare but risk increases with GVHD.
  - **Clinical presentations**: pneumonia or pulmonary nodules, brain abscesses (Figs. 42.7–42.9). Note in any patients with pulmonary *Nocardia* infections, need to obtain brain imaging (CT or MRI) to rule out brain abscesses given predisposition to CNS disease.
  - **Prophylaxis**: TMP–SMX provides some coverage.
  - **Treatment** may require surgical debridement in addition to sulfonamide therapy ± cephalosporin, carbapenem, or aminoglycoside antibiotics for synergy.
- Mycobacteria (see Chapters 32 and 33 for further discussion).
  - Rare, but problematic in that identification of the species may take many weeks; difficult to treat and no uniform drug regimen.
  - Rapidly growing mycobacteria: *Mycobacterium abscessus, Mycobacterium chelonae,* and *Mycobacterium fortuitum* associated with CVC exit site infections, bacteremia (*Mycobacterium mucogenicum*), or pneumonia.
  - **Diagnosis**: acid-fast bacilli (AFB) culture, Mycobacterial DNA probes available for some species.
  - *Mycobacterium tuberculosis* is a significant pathogen in areas of high endemicity (countries with high prevalence).
  - Screening with tuberculin skin test or interferon gamma release assay (IGRA).
  - **Prophylaxis**: isoniazid (INH) + pyridoxine.
  - **Treatment** of mycobacterial infections prolonged (6–12 months) depending on the species and site/severity of infection. Some infections require surgical resection.

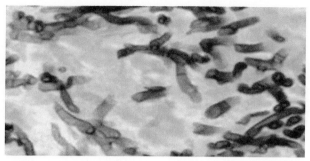

• **Fig. 42.6** Invasive aspergillosis. Lung tissue section. Fungi (branched, septated hyphae), morphologically compatible with *Aspergillus* are identified with Gomori methenamine stain (GMS), consistent with *Aspergillus* infection. (From Qualter E, Satwani P, Ricci A, et al. A comparison of bronchoalveolar lavage versus lung biopsy in pediatric recipients after stem cell transplantation. *Biol Blood Marrow Transplant.* 2014;20(8):1229–1237.)

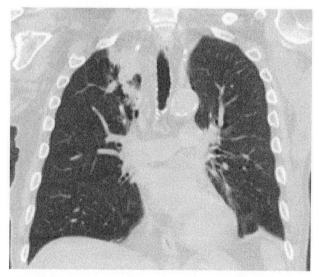

• **Fig. 42.7** Invasive nocardiosis. Coronal, contrast-enhanced chest CT, upper lobe mass. (From Lee LE, Blyth DM, Barsoumian AE, et al., Invasive nocardiosis in patients intolerant to trimethoprim/sulfamethoxazole after allogeneic stem cell transplantation. *Biol Blood Marrow Transplant.* 2016;22(3):S168–S169.)

Viruses

- Respiratory infections predominate.
- Influenza virus, parainfluenza virus, respiratory syncytial virus (RSV), rhinovirus, adenovirus, coronavirus, and the recently identified metapneumovirus and bocavirus are significant pathogens in HCT recipients within the first 3 months after transplant.
- Mostly in winter; however, parainfluenza infects year-round.
- **Clinical**: upper respiratory symptoms → pneumonia → respiratory failure and death.
- Progression from upper to lower respiratory tract infections promoted by lymphopenia.
- Predispose patients to secondary bacterial or fungal infections.
- **Diagnosis** varies from viral DFA to PCR testing, and treatment regimens vary depending on the virus.

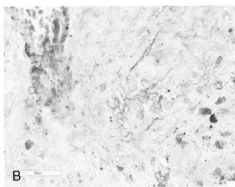

• **Fig. 42.8** Invasive nocardiosis. H&E sections of the lung (A) and thigh biopsy (B) demonstrated mixed inflammation and hemorrhage. The Gomori methenamine silver stain highlights filamentous bacteria morphologically consistent with the cultured *Nocardia* species (GMS ×400). (From Lee LE, Blyth DM, Barsoumian AE, et al., Invasive nocardiosis in patients intolerant to trimethoprim/sulfamethoxazole after allogeneic stem cell transplantation. *Biol Blood Marrow Transplant.* 2016;22(3):S168–S169.)

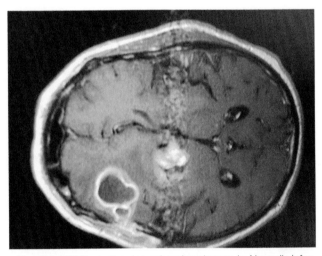

• **Fig. 42.9** MRI illustrating ring-enhancing abscess in *Nocardia* infection. (From Farran Y, Antony S. Nocardia abscessus-related intracranial aneurysm of the internal carotid artery with associated brain abscess: A case report and review of the literature. *J Infect Publ Health.* 2016;9(3):358–361.)

- **Treatment:** antivirals may be effective for some respiratory pathogens. Reduction of immunosuppression if feasible.
  - Influenza: oseltamivir, zanamivir (inhaled), or peramivir (IV).
  - RSV: ribavirin (IV, nebulized, or oral) have been utilized, in combination with palivizumab (monoclonal antibody), steroids, IVIG. Protocols vary according to center. There is no evidence that nebulized ribavirin is superior to oral; however, it is significantly more expensive and has toxicity to healthcare workers.
  - Parainfluenzavirus: DAS181 is a novel antiviral that has emerged for the treatment of parainfluenzavirus in transplant recipients.
  - Adenovirus: cidofovir.
  - Metapneumovirus: ribavirin may be considered, ± IVIG.
- **Prevention of infection:** strict observance of proper hand hygiene measures and cough etiquette. Vaccination of family members and close contacts for influenza.

Adenovirus
- **Risk factors:** GVHD, lymphopenia, recipients of unrelated donor, or UCB transplants.
- **Clinical:** hemorrhagic cystitis, pneumonitis, enteritis, hepatitis, and nephritis.
- **Diagnosis:** adenovirus DFA, adenovirus PCR, or viral culture of blood, urine, stool, sputum, or tissues.
- **Treatment:** no effective therapy is proven, although cidofovir may be used.

Other viral infections
- VZV and CMV reactivation may occur in patients with GVHD not on antiviral prophylaxis.

Fungi
Pneumocystis jirovecii (see Chapter 27)
- Formerly *Pneumocystis carinii.* Now identified as a fungus.
- Causes pneumonia.
- **Diagnosis:** *Pneumocystis* DFA testing of sputum or respiratory samples. *Pneumocystis* PCR not widely available. Beta-D-glucan assay detects *Pneumocystis.*
- **Prophylaxis:** TMP–SMX, dapsone, atovaquone, or inhaled pentamidine.
- **Treatment:** TMP–SMX (strongly preferred), clindamycin + primaquine, intravenous pentamidine.

Non-*Aspergillus* mold infections (see Chapter 29)
- *Fusarium, Scedosporium, Rhizopus, Mucor, Alternaria,* etc.
  - More prevalent in the setting of empiric voriconazole prophylaxis in HCT recipients.
  - Cause clinical syndromes similar to *Aspergillus.*
  - *Fusarium:* disseminated fusariosis with positive blood cultures and skin lesions and occasionally endophthalmitis (Fig. 42.10).
  - *Mucor* or *Rhizopus:* invasive fungal sinusitis, brain abscesses, and pneumonias, often requiring surgical removal plus the addition of antifungal agents such as liposomal amphotericin or posaconazole. Recovery of neutrophils is imperative for treatment success.

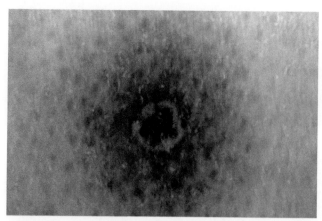

• **Fig. 42.10** Cutaneous lesions caused by *Fusarium solani*. (From Jossi M, Ambrosioni J, Macedo-Vinas M, Garbino J. Invasive fusariosis with prolonged fungemia in a patient with acute lymphoblastic leukemia: case report and review of the literature. *Int J Infect Dis.* 2010;10(4):e354-e356.)

- **Diagnosis**: culture, histopathology. Wide angle branching nonseptated hyphae are characteristic (Fig. 42.11).
- **Treatment**: liposomal amphotericin, azoles such as isavuconazole or posaconazole depending on susceptibilities. Echinocandins usually not effective.
  Dimorphic fungi (see Chapter 28)
- Coccidioidomycosis, histoplasmosis, and blastomycosis.
- Reactivation disease or new infections are rare in HCT recipients, even in hyperendemic areas.
- **Diagnosis**: fungal serology, or urine antigen testing, fungal cultures.
- **Treatment**: liposomal amphotericin ± flucytosine for severe infections, followed by itraconazole.
  Non-Candidal yeasts
- *Cryptococcus neoformans*: rarely causes infection (meningitis) in HCT recipients, likely due to the use of fluconazole as prophylaxis.
- *Malassezia furfur*: associated with catheter-related fungemia, necessitating removal of the catheter and use of antifungals.

Parasites

- Most parasitic infections after HCT in the United States are due to reactivation of disease.
- *Toxoplasma gondii* is the most common parasitic infection, although only in 2%–7% of HCT recipients.
  - **Risk factors**: GVHD suppression of cell-mediated immunity, ATG, UCB transplants, and unrelated donor mismatched transplants.
  - Highest risk period from 2 to 8 weeks after HCT.
  - **Clinical**: encephalitis, fever, pneumonitis, or myocarditis.
  - **Diagnosis**: identification of the parasites in tissue culture, toxoplasma PCR.
  - **Treatment**: TMP–SMX provides some toxoplasmosis prophylaxis.
- Other parasitic infections reported in HCT recipients include Chagas disease, malaria, strongyloidiasis, giardiasis, cryptosporidiosis, schistosomiasis,

Clonorchis infection, and *Acanthamoeba* and *Trichomonas* meningoencephalitis.

Infections: Summary

A summary of infections that may be encountered after HCT is presented in Table 42.3.

Clinical Presentation

- Fever is usually the most common clinical presentation of infection post-HCT; however, some patients may not mount a high fever due to immunosuppression. Neutropenic fever is a clinical emergency and warrants immediate evaluation.
- Work-up will depend on the associated symptoms and localization of the infection. In addition to fever, are there pulmonary, gastrointestinal, or neurologic symptoms? Was the patient on appropriate antimicrobial coverage?
- **Initial work-up should include:**
  - Blood cultures ×2 (both peripherally drawn, separate sticks).
  - Detailed physical examination with a focus on CVCs for signs of exit site infection, oral examination for severe mucositis, skin examination for skin lesions suggestive of invasive fungal infections, lung exam for rhonchi or signs of pneumonia, and abdominal examination for signs of enteritis.
  - Chest X-ray, with consideration of CT scan of the chest without contrast if a pulmonary source of infection is suspected, especially if the patient remains febrile despite broad-spectrum antibiotics.
  - Urinalysis and culture especially if patient has dysuria.
  - Consideration of beta-D-glucan assay if patient is not on antifungal prophylaxis in setting of prolonged neutropenia, or consideration of empiric antifungals.
  - Additional infectious work-up or radiographic tests to be ordered based on the risk factors for particular infections and clinical suspicion based on timing of infection pre- or postengraftment, prophylactic medications, and clinical suspicion for particular infections.
    - Algorithm for work-up of neutropenic figure (see Fig. 42.12).
    - Differential diagnosis of infectious and noninfectious causes of respiratory symptoms (see Table 42.4) and diarrhea (see Table 42.5) in HCT depend on the timing of infection pre- or postengraftment.

Approach to HCT Recipients With Pneumonia

- In patients with fever, cough, shortness of breath, hemoptysis, chest pain.
- 2/3 of pneumonia post-HCT is infectious.
- Most common infection posttransplant.

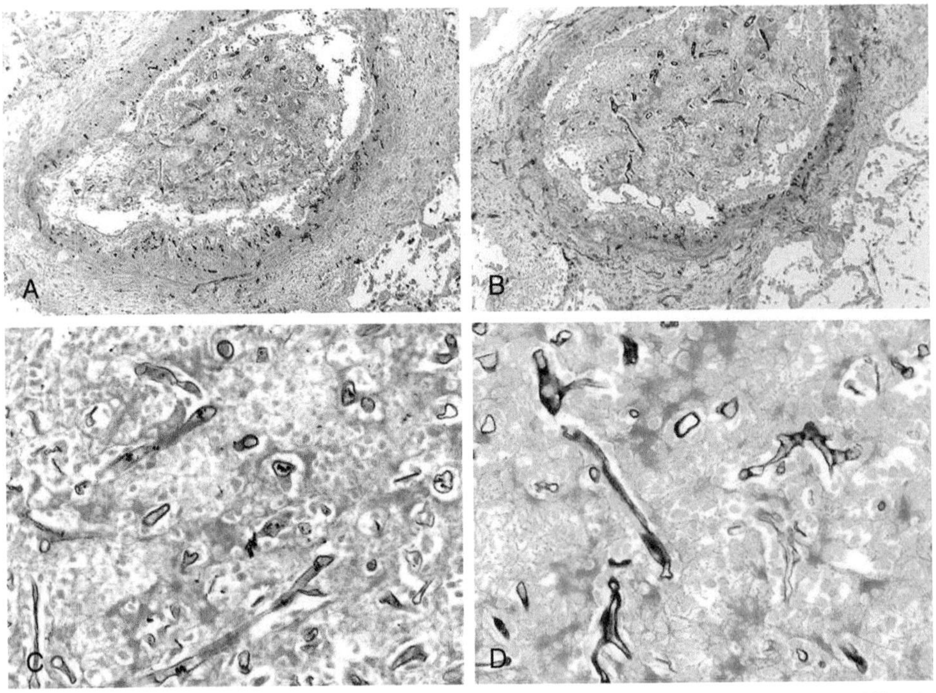

• **Fig. 42.11** (A and B) Angioinvasive Mucorales infection with an intraluminal infected clot. (A) H&E stain ×200; (B) Gomori methenamine silver stain ×200. (C and D) High-power morphology of hyphae on patient 1 demonstrating nonseptate, ribbon-like hyphae with right-angle branches. Also note the "bubble-like" appearance of hyphae seen in cross-section. (C) H&E stain ×600; (D) Gomori methenamine silver stain ×600). (From Lekakis J, Lawson A, Prante J, et al. Fatal *Rhizopus* pneumonia in allogeneic stem cell transplant patients despite posaconazole prophylaxis: two cases and review of the literature. *Biol Blood Marrow Transplant.* 2009;15(8):991–995.)

TABLE 42.3 Types of Infections Encountered After HCT

	Period		
	Preengraftment	**Early Postengraftment**	**Late Postengraftment**
Risk factors for decreased host defense	Neutropenia Mucositis Lymphopenia Neutropenia Hypogammaglobinemia	Lymphopenia Hypogammaglobinemia Decreased cell-mediated immunity	Decreased cell-mediated immunity
Type of Pathogen			
Bacteria	Gram-negative bacteria Gram-positive bacteria *Clostridioides difficile*	Gram-positive bacteria Gram-negative bacteria	Encapsulated bacteria *Nocardia*
Viruses	HSV, respiratory viruses	CMV, EBV, BK virus, respiratory viruses, HHV-6, HHV-7	CMV, VZV, EBV, respiratory viruses, HHV-6, HHV-7
Fungus	*Candida*	*Aspergillus, Pneumocystis jirovecii* Molds	*Aspergillus, Pneumocystis jirovecii* Molds

Modified from Wingard JR, Hsu J, Hiemenz JW. Hematopoietic stem cell transplantation: an overview of infection risks and epidemiology. *Infect Dis Clin North Am.* 2010;24:257.

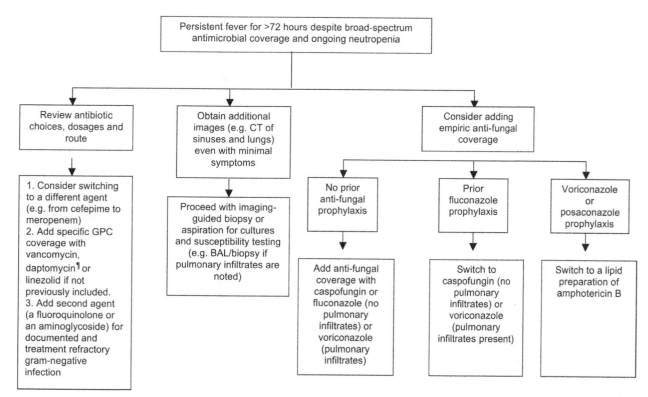

• **Fig. 42.12** Evaluation of febrile neutropenia. (From Rizvi SA, Sohail MR. Neutropenic fever. *Hosp Med Clin*. 2014;3(2):e218–e234.)

Diagnosis
- CT imaging is essential: higher sensitivity and specificity over CXR.
- Would obtain blood/sputum cultures, check *Aspergillus* galactomannan, obtain respiratory PCR nasal swab.
- Bronchoscopy with BAL or CT-guided biopsy should be pursued in transplant recipients with lower respiratory tract infections, when feasible.

Differential diagnosis (Table 42.4)
- **Community-acquired**
  - Respiratory viruses: influenza, RSV, parainfluenza, metapneumovirus, adenovirus, rhinovirus.
  - Bacterial pneumonias: *Streptococcus pneumoniae*, *Legionella*.
- **Nosocomial**
  - Prolonged intubation and ventilator-associated pneumonia (VAP): *Pseudomonas*, MRSA, *Klebsiella*, *Acinetobacter*, *Stenotrophomonas*.
  - Line-associated infection with secondary pneumonia: MRSA, coagulase-negative *Staphylococcus*, *Escherichia coli*, *Pseudomonas* and other gram negative pathogens, *Candida*.
- **Environmental exposure**
  - Soil: *Aspergillus*, *Nocardia*, *Mucormycosis*.
  - Water: *Pseudomonas*, *Legionella*.
- **Transmission**
  - Donor-derived transmission: TB, *Cryptococcus*, *Strongyloides*.
- **Reactivation**
  - Viruses: CMV, HSV, parvovirus, HHV-6, HTLV-1/2.
  - Parasites: toxoplasmosis, *Strongyloides*.
  - *Mycobacteria*.
  - Fungi: *Cryptococcus*, histoplasmosis, coccidiomycosis.
- **Noninfectious**
  - Pulmonary emboli.
  - Acute respiratory distress syndrome (ARDS).
  - Hemorrhagic alveolitis.
  - Engraftment syndrome: usually occurs within 5 days of engraftment. Fever ± rash, pneumonitis, hyperbilirubinemia, diarrhea. Consider CT. Treatment with short-course high-dose steroids.
  - Bronchiolitis obliterans with organizing pneumonia (GVHD).

Treatment
- **Rapid initiation of appropriate therapy is crucial.**
  - Empiric antibiotics depend on risk factors for MRSA, *Pseudomonas*, etc., and local antibiogram.
  - Consider antivirals based on imaging findings and risk factors: CMV? Influenza, etc.?
  - Reduction of immunosuppression (if feasible) may be crucial: EBV-PTLD, respiratory viral infections, *Strongyloides* hyperinfection syndrome.

Approach to HCT Recipients With Diarrhea
- Infectious causes occur in <15%.
- In the history determine if there is fever, abdominal pain and where, nature of the diarrhea (large volume, bloody, small volume but frequent), associated nausea/vomiting?

TABLE 42.4 **Differential Diagnosis of Infectious and Noninfectious Causes of Respiratory Symptoms**

Type of Infiltrate	Source	Preengraftment	Early Post-engraftment	Late Postengraftment
Localized	Noninfectious	Aspiration PE Micronodules from chemotherapy		
	Infectious	Bacterial pneumonia	Bacterial pneumonia	Bacterial pneumonia
		Aspergillus, mold	*Aspergillus*, mold, or *Nocardia*	*Aspergillus*, mold, or *Nocardia*
Diffuse	Noninfectious	ARDS CHF Fluid overload Hemorrhagic alveolitis	Idiopathic interstitial pneumonitis Hemorrhagic alveolitis	Bronchiolitis obliterans or bronchiolitis obliterans with organizing pneumonia
	Infectious	Respiratory virus	CMV Respiratory virus PCP Adenovirus	CMV Respiratory virus PCP Adenovirus

ARDS, acute respiratory distress syndrome; CHF, congestive heart failure; CMV, cytomegalovirus; PCP, *Pneumocystis jirovecii* pneumonia; PE, pulmonary embolism.
Modified from Wingard JR, Hsu J, Hiemenz JW. Hematopoietic stem cell transplantation: an overview of infection risks and epidemiology. *Infect Dis Clin North Am.* 2010; 24:257.

TABLE 42.5 **Infectious and Noninfectious Causes of Diarrhea**

Preengraftment	Early Postengraftment	Late Postengraftment
Mucosal injury from conditioning regimen Sinusoidal obstruction syndrome	GVHD	cGVHD EBV-PTLD
Neutropenic enterocolitis	*C. difficile* enterocolitis	*C. difficile* enterocolitis
C. difficile enterocolitis	CMV	CMV
Enteric viruses	Adenovirus, enteric viruses	Adenovirus, enteric viruses

Modified from Wingard JR, Hsu J, Hiemenz JW. Hematopoietic stem cell transplantation: an overview of infection risks and epidemiology. *Infect Dis Clin North Am.* 2010; 24:257.

Any travel or food exposures? Review the medication list carefully (mycophenolate mofetil). At risk for GVHD or GVHD symptoms present in other organ systems?
- Stool studies may be unrevealing or may take time (depending on whether or not PCR vs. culture assays are available).

Differential Diagnosis (Table 42.5)
Bacterial
- *C. difficile* is common post-HCT, especially in patients receiving broad-spectrum antibiotics.
- Neutropenic enterocolitis: *C. septicum.* Usually right-sided. Fever, nausea, vomiting, right-sided pain, shock. CT shows bowel-wall thickening. Treatment is bowel rest, broad-spectrum antibiotics, consider surgery if suspect perforation or clinical deterioration.
- Rare: intestinal mycobacteria, *Aeromonas*, enterohemorrhagic *E. coli*.

Viral
- CMV >>> HSV.
- Norovirus, astrovirus, rotavirus, coxsackievirus.
- Adenovirus: enteritis ± hepatitis, hemorrhagic cystitis, pneumonitis.
- EBV-PTLD: patients may develop watery or bloody diarrhea.

Fungal
- Intestinal overgrowth (*Candida*).

Parasites
- *Cryptosporidium* (mimics GVHD).
- *Strongyloides.*
- *Giardia, Isospora, Blastocystis hominis.*

TABLE 42.6	Etiologies of Focal Lesions vs. Meningoencephalitis in Central Nervous System Infections in HCT Recipients	

Focal Lesions	Meningitis/ Meningoencephalitis
Aspergillus	Cryptococcus
Zygomycetes	Herpesviruses (HHV-6 >> CMV > VZV
Dematiaceous fungi	Polyomavirus (JC, BK)
Nocardia	West Nile virus
Toxoplasma	Other viruses (adenovirus, measles, parvovirus)
EBV-PTLD	Listeria
PRES	Amoeba

From Bowden RA, Ljungman P, Snydman DR. *Transplant Infections*, 3rd ed. Lippincott, Williams and Wilkins/Wolters Kluwer; 2010. Courtesy DR Snydman.

Noninfectious

- Most common cause of diarrhea posttransplant.
- **Medications**
  - Magnesium salts.
  - Promotility drugs or effects of drugs (macrolides, tacrolimus, sirolimus).
  - Mycophenolate mofetil mucosal toxicity is a common cause of diarrhea.
- **GVHD**: a common cause of profuse watery diarrhea with protein loss, protracted nausea/vomiting, abdominal pain, ileus, gastrointestinal bleeding.
- **Mucosal injury from myeloablative conditioning**
  - >13.2 Gy total body irradiation.
  - Cytarabine.
  - High-dose melphalan.
  - Mucosal injury may last up to 20–30 days post-transplant.

Diagnosis

- Would obtain stool *C. difficile* testing (PCR may be too sensitive and detect colonization), stool ova and parasite screen, stool culture, stool norovirus testing (PCR preferred), CMV PCR serum, stool *Giardia* antigen test, and if available multiplex GI panels may be helpful.
- CT abdomen/pelvis to delineate the area of infection: small bowel, colon. Is there enteritis, abscess, fistulas, etc.?
- Consider GI consult for endoscopy if feasible.

Treatment

- Treatment: depends on the diagnosis:
  - *C. difficile*: oral vancomycin or fidaxomicin.
  - Adenovirus: cidofovir.
  - *Strongyloides*: ivermectin.

- Norovirus: nitazoxanide, oral IVIG have been utilized. Reduction of immunosuppression if feasible and supportive therapy. Note prolonged duration of symptoms in HCT recipients.

Approach to HCT Recipients With CNS Disease

- Patients may present with seizures, altered mental status, focal neurologic deficits, headaches, with or without fever.
- Brain imaging (CT head or MRI head) is crucial.
- Lumbar puncture (LP) (check opening pressure if possible): send for cell count with differential, protein, glucose, Gram stain and culture, and depending on risk factors and LP characteristics: cryptococcal antigen, CMV PCR, EBV PCR, HHV-6 PCR, VZV PCR, HSV PCR, toxoplasma PCR.
- Ultimately brain biopsy (if CNS lesions present) may be warranted.
- Incidence 2%–15% in HCT, but mortality is high (36%–67%).
  - Unrelated Allo 39% > related Allo 21% > Auto 11%.

Differential Diagnosis
Infectious

- Fungal pathogens (*Aspergillus*) are the most common causes of CNS infections in HCT (up to 70%).
- *Toxoplasma* ring-enhancing lesions.
- *Nocardia* ring-enhancing lesions.
- HHV-6-associated encephalitis (seizures) >> CMV > VZV.
- Polyomaviruses (JC, BK).
- EBV-encephalitis or PTLD (CNS mass lesions).
- *Listeria*.
- *Streptococcus*.
- Brain abscess: oral flora.
- Amoebic granulomatous encephalitis: *Acanthamoeba* or *Balamuthia mandrillaris*.

Noninfectious

- Metabolic encephalopathy.
- Medication adverse reaction or side effect.
- Total body irradiation (>1200 cGy) associated encephalopathy (w/i 100 days posttransplant).
- Posterior reversible encephalopathy syndrome (PRES) secondary to calcineurin inhibitors.
- Busulfan: seizures, Wernicke-like encephalopathy.
- GVHD.

Treatment

- Depends on the differential (and the diagnosis).

Approach to the HCT Recipient With Skin Lesions

- Dermatologic diseases are common post-HCT: infectious (75% of transplant recipients) to noninfectious manifestations.

- Routine dermatologic screening is essential and dermatologic consultation for a neutropenic patient with new onset skin lesions is warranted for evaluation with biopsy and cultures.
- Diagnosis relies on biopsies with cultures: consider sending bacterial, fungal, acid-fast bacillus, and *Nocardia* cultures depending on the clinical presentation (skin nodules vs. cellulitis).

Differential Diagnosis

Bacterial (during period of neutropenia)
- Surgical wound infections.
- Nosocomial catheter-associated: MRSA.
- Gram-positives: *Staphylococcus, Streptococcus.*
- Rarely necrotizing fasciitis (especially pediatric).
- Nontuberculous mycobacteria (usually skin nodules): rare (0.5% of HCT), usually early post-HCT. Can be associated with CVC infections, rapidly growing mycobacteria predominate.
- *Nocardia* (draining mycetoma, cutaneous/subcutaneous nodules, abscess or cellulitis with sporotrichoid pattern), very rare incidence 0.3% of HCT, median time 7 months post HCT.

Fungal
- 2%–15% of HCT recipients with strong association with neutropenia. Confer significant morbidity and mortality.
- *Cryptococcus*: primary infection, or secondary to dissemination → subcutaneous abscess, nodules, ulcers, cellulitis → necrotizing fasciitis (not responding to antibiotics).
- Disseminated candidiasis: maculopapular skin lesions.
- Aspergillosis: nodules, abscess, ulcers → necrotic and purpuric with central eschar.
- Mucormycosis: rare, but prolonged neutropenia is risk factor. Rapidly progressive necrotic eschar is a clue. Usually fatal without surgical debridement.
- Histoplasmosis: very rare. Tender nodules or plaque-like cellulitis. Usually secondary to dissemination.

Viral
- HSV: rare on prophylaxis. Oral herpetic lesions, genital HSV lesions: shallow painful ulcers.
- CMV: rare in HCT, usually within 2 months post-HCT. Localized ulcerations (perianal, genital), rarely exanthematous maculopapular rash.
- VZV: early, within 6 months. Reactivation with shingles more common, rarely dissemination (5%).
- HHV-6: rare. Fever + rash.

Parasites
- Rare in HCT; more common in foreign countries.
- *Leishmaniasis*: nodules → ulcers.
- *Strongyloides*: maculopapular/urticarial eruption on buttocks/lower extremities.

Noninfectious
- Skin neoplasms.
- GVHD of the skin.
- Steroid acne.
- Sirolimus and delayed wound healing.

Approach to the HCT Recipient With Transaminitis

- Would verify HSV, CMV, hepatitis B and C serostatus.
- Determine if patient has traveled overseas and is at risk of hepatitis A/B.
- Go over the medication list as medications are a common cause of transaminitis.
- Consider ultrasound of liver or CT abdomen/pelvis.
- May need liver biopsy for final diagnosis.

Differential Diagnosis

Viral
- CMV.
- HSV.
- VZV.
- HHV-6.
- EBV: hemophagocytic lymphohistiocytosis.
- Adenovirus.
- Hepatitis B: reactivation or new infection if not immune.
- Hepatitis C.

Fungal
- *Candida*: Consider hepatosplenic (visceral) candidiasis in patients with fever/transaminitis during periods of neutrophil recovery.

Noninfectious
- GVHD.
- Drug-induced liver toxicity: antibiotics, antifungals (azoles), cyclosporine, tacrolimus (elevated bilirubin), total parenteral nutrition (TPN).
- Veno-occlusive disease (aka sinusoidal obstruction syndrome): incidence 5%–50%.
- Iron overload: up to 30%–60% Allo HCT recipients.

Treatment
- Depends on the diagnosis. Try to reduce or remove hepatotoxins.

Further Reading

1. Bowden RA, Ljungman P, Snydman DR. *Transplant Infections.* 3rd ed. Lippincott, Williams and Wilkins/Wolters Kluwer; 2010.
2. Ljungman P. Respiratory virus infections in stem cell transplant patients: the European experience. *Biol Blood Marrow Transplant.* 2001;7:5S–7S.
3. Tomblyn M, Chiller T, Einsele H, et al. Guidelines for preventing infectious complications among hematopoietic cell transplant recipients: a global perspective. *Bone Marrow Transplant.* 2009;15:1143–1238.
4. De La Rosa GR, Champlin RE, Kontoyiannis DP. Risk factors for the development of invasive fungal infections in allogeneic blood and marrow transplant recipients. *Transplant Infect Dis.* 2002;4:3–9.
5. Bodey GP. Infections associated with malignancy. In: Gorbach SL, Bartlett JG, Blacklow NR, eds. *Infectious Diseases.* 3rd ed. Philadelphia: Lippincott Williams & Wilkins; 2004:1106–1111.

6. O'Shea DT, Humar A. Life-threatening infections in transplant recipients. *Crit Care Clin.* 2013;29(4):953–973.

7. Rizvi SA, Sohail MR. Neutropenic fever. *Hosp Med Clin.* 2014;3(2):e218–e234.

8. Wingard JR, Hsu J, Hiemenz JW. Hematopoietic stem cell transplantation: an overview of infection risks and epidemiology. *Infect Dis Clin North Am.* 2010;24:257.

9. Zinner SH. Treatment and prevention of infections in immuno-compromised hosts. In: Gorbach SL, Bartlett JG, Blacklow NR, eds. *Infectious Diseases.* 3rd ed. Philadelphia: Lippincott Williams & Wilkins; 2004:1141–1150.

10. Guidelines for preventing opportunistic infections among hematopoietic stem cell patients. *CDC MMWR.* 2000/49(RR10);1–128. https://www.cdc.gov/mmwr/preview/mmwrhtml/rr4910a1.htm.

11. Mannick J, Ellison RT. Infections associated with bone marrow transplantation. In: Gorbach SL, Bartlett JG, Blacklow NR, eds. *Infectious Diseases.* 3rd ed. Philadelphia: Lippincott Williams & Wilkins; 2004:1123–1128.

43

Primary Immunodeficiency Disorders

BLACHY J. DÁVILA SALDAÑA, CARLOS R. FERREIRA LOPEZ

Definition

- An innate disorder due to a genetic mutation, in which part of the immune system is missing or does not function normally.
- Over 350 such defects have been described, most in the last 15 years.
- Defective white blood cells result in repeated infections and poor immune surveillance. This is part of the reason why many are cancer predisposition syndromes (particularly lymphomas).
- Poor immune function results in loss of discrimination of self vs. nonself. This predisposes patients to autoimmunity, allergy, and autoinflammation.
- Presenting symptoms are typically secondary to the specific function missing within the immune system.
- "Classic" (complete lack of function) defects present very early in life. Atypical (hypomorphic, partially functioning) mutations may present later in childhood or even adulthood. They are much more common than previously thought, though overall still quite rare.

Presentation

- Epidemiology: extremely rare. Overall, around 30–50 per 100,000 patients are found to have some sort of primary immunodeficiency (PID). B-cell defects remain the most commonly identified (Table 43.1).
- Presents as increased predisposition to infections (Table 43.2).

T Cell Defects

Severe Combined Immunodeficiency (SCID)
- Most common *severe* PID (1/60,000 live births).
- Fully absent or mostly absent T-cells that do not work.
- Laboratory definition of classic SCID = Absolute T-cell count of <300/μL and an absence of T-cell responses to mitogens (<10% response as compared to control).

- Hypomorphic SCID = Reduced number of CD3+ T cells for age (or normal with reduced diversity) with <30% T-cell function as compared to control.
  - Omenn syndrome (erythroderma, desquamation, organomegaly with eosinophilia) is a clinical diagnosis that can be caused by hypomorphic mutations in several SCID genes, though it is most commonly associated with *RAG1/RAG2* defects.
- Uniformly fatal in early life unless definitive treatment given.
- Many genetic defects results in SCID.
- B and Natural Killer (NK) cells may or may not be present depending on the genetic defect. Hypomorphic defects may also result in aberrant T-cell production. Because of this, a normal absolute lymphocyte count (ALC) does *not* rule out SCID.
- Regardless of presence of B cells, these require T-cell activation in order to function, so *all SCID patients are functionally B-cell-deficient as well.*
- >90% of the US population covered for SCID newborn screening (TREC assay).
  - TREC = T-cell receptor excision circles. A marker of T-cell receptor development. Does not screen for immunodeficiencies where normal amount of T-cell receptors are created but is >99% sensitive for classic and hypomorphic forms of SCID.

Wiskott–Aldrich Syndrome (WAS)
- Epidemiology: 4/1,000,000 births.
- Due to mutations in the WAS protein (WASP).
- Expressed in all hematopoietic cells.
- Important for cell mobility, cell–cell interactions, and platelet function. Defective interaction causes poor T-cell function.
- Famous triad: thrombocytopenia (with decreased MPV), eczema (Fig. 43.1), recurrent infections.
- High predisposition to malignancy and autoimmunity.
- Hypomorphic mutations cause X-linked thrombocytopenia (XLT). Classic mutations result in WAS.
- Autoimmunity and/or malignancy are diagnostic of classic WAS and are associated with increased morbidity and mortality early in life.

TABLE 43.1	**Classic Presentation of Immune Defects**			
	T-Cell Defects	**B-Cell Defects**	**Phagocytic Defects**	**Complement Defects**
Main issue	Cellular Immunity	Antibodies	Dysfunctional phagocytosis	Opsonization, cell lysis
Age at presentation	Infancy (<6 mo. if classic)	6–12 months (after waning of maternal ab)	First 2 years of life	Childhood (opsonization) to adulthood (terminal complement)
Most common organisms	Intracellular, viruses, fungi, protozoa (*Herpesviridae*, *Pneumocystis*, *Candida*, *Cryptococcus*, *Histoplasma*)	Encapsulated bacteria (*Staphylococcus*, *Streptococcus pneumoniae*, *Haemophilus influenzae*)	Catalase positive bacteria + fungi (*Staphylococcus*, *Serratia*, *Aspergillus*, *Nocardia*)	Bacteria (*Neisseria*, *Streptococcus*)
Most common affected organs	Systemic, failure to thrive (FTT)	Respiratory (sinus, pneumonias), gastrointestinal (diarrhea)	Skin, gastrointestinal, genitourinary, dental	Central nervous system (meningitis)

- Mean age of death for WASP-negative patients: 6–8 years.
- Improved survival if partial expression, but with high morbidity (bleeding, infections).

CD40 Ligand Deficiency

- Most common etiology for the hyperimmunoglobulin (Ig) M syndrome.
- X-linked (most other versions of Hyper IgM syndrome are autosomal recessive); expressed mainly on *activated* CD4+ T cells.
- It is pivotal for B-cell survival, growth, and differentiation (CD40 is expressed on all B cells).
- Laboratory hallmark is high IgM (but may be normal) with low/absent IgG, IgA, IgE due to inability to class switch. There is a lack of specific IgG production.
- While CD4+ count is normal, they are nonfunctioning. Thus they present as CD4+-deficient patients.
- Because cells are not activated to proliferate, these patients *lack germinal centers* and have no lymphadenopathy. This is different from autosomal recessive manifestations of Hyper IgM, which may have excessive lymphadenopathy since the production defect is downstream.
- Most common presentation is *Pneumocystis jirovecii* (see Chapter 27) pneumonia. Other common infections include *Cryptosporidium* (see Chapter 34) and *Cryptococcus* (see Chapter 27).
- Gastrointestinal disease (diarrhea, liver dysfunction) is common and frequent reason for morbidity. Liver involvement is typically associated with a higher risk of mortality.
- High risk of malignancy, particularly lymphomas and liver cancers.

GATA2 Deficiency

- Age of onset from teenage years to late adulthood (median age of onset: 20 years).

- Hematologic findings include decreased B and NK cells and monocytopenia (>80%) with occasional CD4 lymphopenia and neutropenia (50%).
- Most common reported infections are viral (recalcitrant, severe HPV) and disseminated nontuberculous mycobacteria. Epstein–Barr virus (EBV) viremia and herpes simplex virus (HSV) outbreaks are also commonly reported.
- Associated with antibody-negative pulmonary alveolar proteinosis (PAP).
- High predisposition to hematologic malignancies (myelodysplastic syndrome/acute myelogenous leukemia).
- Sensorineural hearing loss and lymphedema also commonly seen.

Familial Hemophagocytic Lymphohistiocytosis (HLH)

- A reactive process caused by autoinflammation.
- Prolonged, excessive activation of antigen-presenting and cytotoxic cells due to an inability to clear the inciting pathogen lead to uncontrolled, systemic hyperinflammation
- The high degree of inflammation is due to hypercytokinemia (i.e., cytokine storm) caused by the antigen-presenting cells.
- Typically diagnosed when patients meet 5 of 8 criteria (all associated with inflammation)
  - Fever.
  - Splenomegaly.
  - Cytopenias (Hgb <9, Plt <100, ANC <1,000).
  - High triglycerides (>265).
  - Low fibrinogen (<150).
  - High ferritin (>500).
  - High soluble IL-2 receptor (>2400), a marker of T-cell activation.
  - Low or absent NK-cell activity.
  - Hemophagocytosis noted on pathology.

TABLE 43.2   Increased Predisposition to Specific Infections

Infection	Condition	Inheritance	Manifestations
Mycobacterial	Interleukin-12 deficiency Interleukin-23 deficiency Interferon-gamma receptor deficiency	AR AR AR/AD	Disseminated infections with mycobacteria, *M. tuberculosis*, and *Salmonella*
Invasive candidiasis	CARD9 deficiency	AR	Familial candidiasis
Chronic mucocutaneous candidiasis (CMC)	Interleukin-17 deficiency	AR	CMC affecting skin, scalp, mucosae, or nails; sometimes *Staphylococcal* skin infections
	Autoimmune polyendocrine candidiasis ectodermal dystrophy (APECED) syndrome	AR/AD	CMC, Addison disease, hypoparathyroidism, metaphyseal dysplasia
Cryptosporidium	Interleukin-21 receptor deficiency	AR	Chronic cholangitis and hepatic cirrhosis due to *Cryptosporidium* infection
EBV	ITK deficiency MAGT1 deficiency STK4 deficiency CD27 deficiency Coronin-1A deficiency	AR XL AR AR AR	Chronic EBV viremia, EBV-associated lymphoproliferative disorder, dysgammaglobulinemia
HPV	Epidermodysplasia verruciformis	AR	Disseminated flat, wart-like papules, malignant potential
	CXCR4 deficiency (warts, hypogammaglobulinemia, immunodeficiency, myelokathexis [WHIM] syndrome)	AD	Myelokathexis (retention of neutrophils in bone marrow), hypogammaglobulinemia, warts
	DOCK8 deficiency	AR	Hyperimmunoglobulin E, eosinophilia, severe viral skin infections, recurrent staphylococcal infections, lack of connective tissue or skeletal involvement
	GATA2 deficiency	AD	Monocytopenia and NK-cell deficiency, myelodysplasia, predisposition to HPV, fungal and mycobacterial infections, lymphedema, pulmonary alveolar proteinosis
HSV	Toll-like receptor 3 deficiency	AD	Herpes encephalitis, incomplete penetrance
	Caspase 8	AR	Mucocutaneous HSV
Neisseria	Terminal complement deficiency	Codominant	Recurrent invasive *Neisseria* infections
Granulibacter bethesdensis *Chromobacterium violaceum* *Francisella philomiragia* *Burkholderia cepacia* *Nocardia* (not in the setting of high dose steroids) *Aspergillus fumigatus* (non-neutropenic patient)	Chronic granulomatous disease (CGD)	X-linked, AR	Severe infections by these catalase-positive organisms are highly suspicious for CGD

AR, autosomal recessive; AD, autosomal dominant; CGD, chronic granulomatous disease; HPV, human papilloma virus; HSV, herpes simplex virus; NK, Natural Killer; XL, X-linked.

- Other common associations that are not part of criteria: Marked transaminitis with hepatosplenomegaly.
- All known genetic reasons for familial HLH are due to a problem in the cytotoxic function of T and NK cells
- Most common "triggers" include viral (EBV, *Herpesviridae*), bacterial, and fungal infections.
- Nonfamilial, or secondary HLH, can occur in states of high inflammation despite lack of genetic mutations. Most common associations include malignancies and uncontrolled autoimmune diseases. In the latter, the disease may also be called *macrophage activation syndrome (MAS)*.

B Cell Defects

IgA Deficiency
- The most commonly found primary immune deficiency, particularly among the Caucasian population.
- Incidence perhaps as high as 1 in every 500 Caucasians.
- In general, may be the mildest form of genetic immunodeficiency.
- Defined as undetectable level of Ig A in the blood and secretions but no other immunoglobulin deficiencies.
- Most affected people have no illness as a result.
- 25%–50% of affected patients that come to medical attention will have recurrent infections, particularly involving mucosal surfaces (ear infections, sinusitis, bronchitis, pneumonias).
- Gastrointestinal manifestations and chronic diarrhea may also occur.

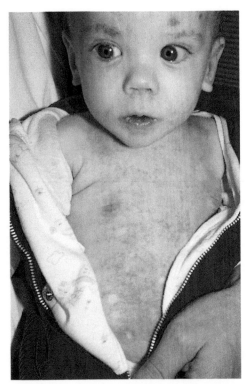

- **Fig. 43.1** Eczema in a child with Wiskott–Aldrich syndrome. (From Chong H, Green T, Larkin A. Allergy and Immunology. In Zitelli B, McIntire S, Nowalk AJ, eds. Zitelli and Davis' Atlas of Pediatric Physical Diagnosis. Elsevier; 2018.)

- Autoimmune diseases are more common in patients that seek medical help (20%–30% incidence).
- Allergies may be more common in this subgroup as well.
- No specific treatment; tailored antibiotics for recurrent infections may be required.

X-Linked Agammaglobulinemia
- The first described primary immunodeficiency.
- Due to deficiencies in Bruton's Tyrosine Kinase (*btk*), which lies on the X chromosome.
- Absent protein results in severely decreased B-cell numbers and absence of serum immunoglobulins.
- Bacterial respiratory and gastrointestinal infections most common manifestation: *H. influenza, S. aureus, S. pneumonia* most common.
- Chronic enteroviral infections a big problem, may cause meningoencephalitis.
- Monoarticular arthritis is frequently observed. It is most commonly aseptic and responds to high-dose gamma-globulin treatment.

Common Variable Immune Deficiency (CVID)
- Very common (1/25,000 individuals), mainly in adults.
- Characterized by low levels of serum immunoglobulins *with decreased specific antibody responses.*
- Must exclude defined causes of hypogammaglobulinemia (drug-induced, infections, malignancy, among others). These are more common than CVID.
- A small subset have minor T-cell defects as well.
- Presumed genetic, but cause unknown most of the time. Several new genetic defects have identified subsets of these patients.
- Present mainly with recurrent respiratory and gastrointestinal tract infections.
- A subset present with autoimmunity, including inflammatory bowel disease, granulomatous formation, and endocrinopathies. Autoimmunity typically heralds a worse outcome compared to those that are only antibody-deficient.
- Some patients with CVID, particularly those with autoimmune manifestations, are at a higher risk of developing cancer (mostly lymphomas).

Phagocytic Defects

Chronic Granulomatous Disease (CGD)
- Nicotinamide adenine dinucleotide phosphate (NADPH) oxidase defects.
- Inability to produce superoxide anions.
- Diagnosed by DHR (dihydrorhodamine) testing.
- Incidence: 4–5/1,000,000
- X-linked (*CYBB*) most common and most severe.
- Without diagnosis: fatal in first decade of life.
- With diagnosis and adequate prophylaxis:
  - X-linked: median life expectancy 20–25 years.
  - AR: 30–40 years.
- Inflamed tissue around the uncleared pathogen creates the granulomas.

- Most common is gastrointestinal disease (can mimic colitis, IBD) (Fig. 43.2).
- Fungal (mainly *Aspergillus*) lesions are ubiquitous and most common cause of death.
- Sepsis from uncommon catalase-positive organisms (*Granulibacter bethesdensis, Chromobacterium violaceum, Francisella philomiragia*) is virtually pathognomonic of CGD.
- Other phagocytic defects are presented in Table 43.3.

Complement Defects

- Inherited complement defects are extremely rare, biggest estimates are around 25 per 100,000 people.
- Patients with deficiency of a complement pathway protein are susceptible to recurrent sinopulmonary infections, bacteremia, and/or meningitis.

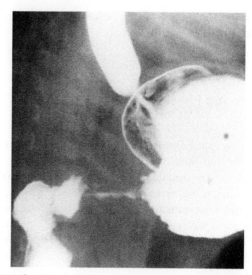

• **Fig. 43.2** Gastric antral stricture secondary to granuloma formation in a patient with chronic granulomatous disease. (From Chong H, Green T, Larkin A. Allergy and Immunology. In Zitelli B, McIntire S, Nowalk AJ, eds. Zitelli and Davis' Atlas of Pediatric Physical Diagnosis. Elsevier; 2018.)

- The pathogens most commonly implicated are encapsulated bacteria, such as *Streptococcus pneumoniae, Haemophilus influenzae* type b, and *Neisseria meningitidis*.
- Consider screening in patients with recurrent *Neisseria* infections at any age, as well as strong family history of *Neisseria* infections.
- These infections may be recurrent but clinically mild-to-moderate.
- May also be considered in recurrent pyogenic infections when other components of the immune system are normal.
- A substantial number of patients, particularly those deficient in early components of the classic pathway, are prone to develop systemic lupus erythematosus (SLE).
- Partial deficiencies in complement regulatory proteins (Factor H, Factor I, etc.) result in predisposition to atypical hemolytic uremic syndrome (aHUS).

Folate Metabolism Defects

Hereditary Folate Malabsorption
- Defects in the proton-coupled folate transporter.
- Decreased intestinal absorption of folate and folate intake through blood–brain barrier.
- Megaloblastic anemia is primary manifestation.
- Subsequent pancytopenia causes T-cell lymphocytopenia, leading to SCID-like infections (*Pneumocystis* most common).
- Also hypogammaglobulinemia.
- Other symptoms include diarrhea, oral mucositis, failure to thrive, developmental delay, and frequently seizures.
- Diagnosed via low serum and cerebrospinal folate concentrations.
- Treatment with parenteral folinic acid.
  - Avoid folic acid as it interferes with active folinic acid transport.

TABLE 43.3	Other Phagocytic Defects			
Condition	**Inheritance**	**Age Onset**	**Manifestations**
Severe congenital neutropenia	AD	Variable; typically childhood	Severe neutropenia, cyclic neutropenia, with neutropenic infections (bacterial, fungal). High susceptibility to MDS/leukemia
X-linked neutropenia (XLN)	AR	Childhood	Gain-of-function mutations in Wiskott gene (*WAS*). Myeloid maturation arrest
Shwachman–Diamond syndrome	AR	0–18 years	Neutropenia, pancytopenia, exocrine pancreatic insufficiency, skeletal anomalies
Leukocyte adhesion deficiency (LAD)	AR	Infancy	Delayed umbilical cord separation, omphalitis, gingivitis, periodontitis, bacterial/fungal mucous membrane infections without pus (Figs. 43.3 and 43.4)

AD, autosomal dominant; ARE, autosomal recessive; MDS, myelodysplastic syndrome.

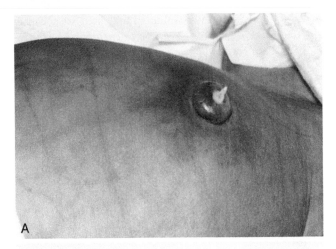

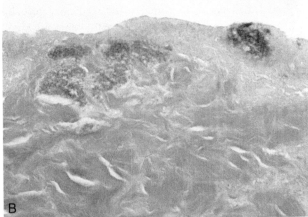

• **Fig. 43.3** (A) Omphalitis in a newborn with leukocyte adhesion deficiency (LAD) type 1. (B) H&E staining of scalp abscess showing lack of inflammatory infiltrate despite bacterial (basophilic) infiltrate. (From Chong H, Green T, Larkin A. Allergy and Immunology. In Zitelli B, McIntire S, Nowalk AJ, eds. Zitelli and Davis' Atlas of Pediatric Physical Diagnosis. Elsevier; 2018.)

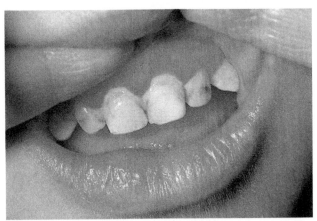

• **Fig. 43.4** Periodontitis and gingivitis in a patient with LAD type 1. (From Uzel G, Holland SM. Phagocyte deficiencies. In Rich R, Fleisher T, Shearer W, et al, eds. Clinical Immunology. Saunders, 2013.)

Methylenetetrahydrofolate Dehydrogenase (MTHFD1) Deficiency

- SCID.
- Megaloblastic anemia.
- Atypical hemolytic uremic syndrome in some.

- Serum folate levels are normal, but total homocysteine can be increased.

Hyper IgE (Job's) Syndrome

- Autosomal dominant condition caused by mutations in *STAT3*.
- Newborn eosinophilic pustulosis followed by eczematoid dermatitis.
- "Cold" skin abscesses lacking inflammatory reaction.
- Formation of pneumatoceles following lung infections (Fig. 43.5).
- High IgE levels and eosinophilia.
- Nonimmune features, including retained primary teeth, scoliosis, fractures under minimal trauma, joint laxity, increased nasal width (Figs. 43.5 and 43.6, Table 43.4).

Additional Note

- Immunodeficiency-like syndromes also exist and can present in adulthood (see Table 43.4).

Assessment

History and Physical Findings to Suggest Defects

- T-cell defects: failure to thrive, skin rash, diarrhea, opportunistic infections in early age.
- B-cell defects: respiratory/GI symptoms after maternal antibodies wane, enterovirus meningoencephalitis, recurrent sinusitis, recurrent pneumonias, bronchiectasis.
- Phagocytic defects: cellulitis without pus, granulomas, IBD, liver abscesses, prolonged attachment of cord.
- Complement defects: *Streptococcus*, *Neisseria*, rheumatoid disorders.
- If T-cell defect suspected:
  - Obtain lymphocyte subsets and absolute lymphocyte count (ALC).
  - If ALC low in young age, *strongly consider SCID* (this is an immunologic emergency!).
  - If ALC normal, evaluate T-cell function (mitogens, antigens).
    - If normal, consider defect in another part of immune system.
    - If abnormal, consider other T-cell defects (immunology consultation recommended).
- If B-cell defect suspected:
  - Obtain lymphocyte subsets and ALC.
  - If low ALC, may be combined immune deficiency, and consider further evaluation of T-cell defects as above.
  - If ALC normal, obtain B-cell number, quantitative immunoglobulins, and antibody responses to vaccines.
    - If B-cell number/function absent in early age, this is likely XLA.
    - If B-cell number/function abnormal, consider XLA, Hyper IgM syndromes, or CVID (immunology consult recommended).

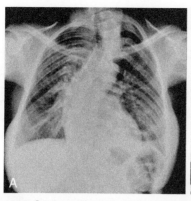
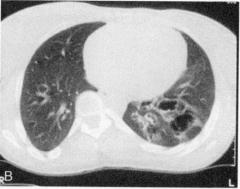

• **Fig. 43.5** Scoliosis (A) and multiple pneumatoceles (B) in a patient with Hyper IgE syndrome. (From Uzel G, Holland SM. Phagocyte deficiencies. In Rich R, Fleisher T, Shearer W, et al, eds. Clinical Immunology. Saunders, 2013.)

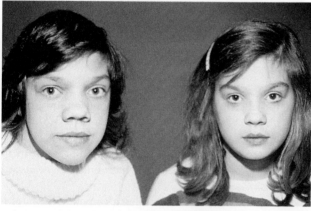

• **Fig. 43.6** Wide nasal bridge, wide nasal base, widely spaced eyes and prognathism in a girl with Hyper IgE syndrome (*left*), compared to her unaffected sister (*right*). (From Chong H, Green T, Larkin A. Allergy and Immunology. In Zitelli B, McIntire S, Nowalk AJ, eds. Zitelli and Davis' Atlas of Pediatric Physical Diagnosis. Elsevier; 2018.)

- If onset in adult age, consider CVID.
- If phagocytic defect suspected:
  - Obtain CBC and absolute neutrophil count (ANC).
  - If low ANC, consider cyclic neutropenia, autoimmune neutropenia, and/or referral to hematology for consideration of bone marrow biopsy.
  - If normal ANC, consider CGD (DHR burst testing), leukocyte adhesion defects (CD11/CD18 flow cytometry).
- Consider screening for complement defects in recurrent *Neisseria* infections, or in recurrent pyogenic infections if other components of the immune system are normal.
  - CH50 is the best screening test; classic deficiencies result in undetectable values.
  - If abnormal, specific complement testing is indicated.

Treatment

Conventional Therapy

- Prophylaxis

- *Pneumocystis* prophylaxis is standard for all PIDs with low CD4 count (SCID) or those with CD4 dysfunction despite normal numbers (i.e., CD40L deficiency).
- Antifungal prophylaxis against *Candida* is standard for severe T-cell defects (SCID).
- Broader antifungal prophylaxis is recommended for patients at high risk of *Aspergillus* (CGD). Consider as well in prolonged, nonbenign neutropenia.
- CGD patients also require antibacterial prophylaxis (typically with trimethoprim–sulfamethoxazole) as well as interferon-gamma (which has been proven to decrease frequency and severity of infections).
- Live vaccines are *absolutely contraindicated* in severe T-cell defects.
- Immunoglobulin supplementation is standard for all B-cell defects.
- Note B-cells are nonfunctional in severe T-cell defects due to lack of activation, therefore all severe T-cell defects also require immunoglobulin supplementation.
- Antibiotic prophylaxis may be required in patients with B-cell defects, particularly in those with structural damage (bronchiectasis), or in those with repeated infections despite optimal Ig supplementation.
- With prophylaxis, survival is improved:
  - B-cell defects may have normal life expectancy if started on treatment before organ damage.
  - Neutrophil defects result in improved but still very decreased survival (average 30–40 years for CGD).
  - Severe T-cell defects still result in high mortality (>90%) in first years of life without definitive treatment despite prophylaxis.

Definitive Treatments

- **Allogeneic bone marrow transplantation (BMT)** is standard of care for all patients with severe T-cell defects (SCID, WAS, familial HLH).
  - Mortality is associated with age at onset and infections. If transplanted early in life without infections, survival is excellent.

TABLE 43.4	Immunodeficiency-Like Syndromes Presenting in Adulthood		
Condition	**Inheritance**	**Age Onset**	**Manifestations**
Good's syndrome	Unknown	40–70	Hypogammaglobulinemia with thymoma, severe opportunistic infections (CMV, PJP)
Atypical hemolytic uremic syndrome (aHUS)	AD, AR, autoimmune	10–60	Fever with hemolytic anemia, thrombocytopenia, renal failure
Pulmonary alveolar proteinosis (PAP)	Autoimmune	20–40	Antibodies to GM–CSF, cryptococcal meningitis, *Nocardia*, PAP
Adult-onset susceptibility to mycobacteria	Autoimmune	30–60	Antibodies to IFN-gamma, mycobacterial, fungal, *Salmonella*, VZV infections

AD, autosomal dominant; AR, autosomal recessive; CMV, cytomegalovirus; GM-CSF, granulocyte-macrophage colony-stimulating factor; IFN, interferon, PCP, Pneumocystis jirovecii pneumonia; VZV, varicella-zoster virus.

- SCID newborn screening (currently in 45 US states + the District of Columbia) has greatly decreased time to diagnosis and earlier interventions.
- B-cell defects are *not* recommended for bone marrow transplantation since IVIG supplementation ameliorates most issues.
- Due to markedly decreased survival, consider referral to BMT for phagocytic defects, particularly those with fully absent function.
- The biggest hurdle to transplant is finding an appropriate donor. This is highly dependent on ethnicity (Caucasians > Asian Americans > African Americans > Mixed Ancestry) as HLA genes cluster among ethnicities and the vast majority of registered donors are Caucasian.
- Infectious prophylaxis and improved supportive care measures have resulted in drastic improvement in survival for those who undergo bone marrow transplantation.
- Graft versus host disease and infections due to immunosuppression can cause significant morbidity in transplanted patients. Those with mismatched donors are at higher risk of these complications.
- **Gene therapy** is becoming a promising new option.
  - Trials exist for several diseases, including several subtypes of SCID, WAS, and CGD, and will likely continue to expand over the next years.
- Initial gene therapy trials were hampered by a risk of insertional leukemogenesis (leukemias related to the modified genes).
- Better selection of viral vectors and improvements in DNA insertional technology have greatly decreased this risk.
- Treatment involves chemotherapy in order for autologous transduced cells to engraft, though typically at lower doses than those required by BMT.

Further Reading

1. Ochs HD, Smith E, Puck JM. *Primary Immunodeficiency Diseases.* 2nd ed. Oxford: Oxford University Press; 2007.
2. Buckley RH, Immune Deficiency Foundation. *Diagnostic and Clinical Care Guidelines for Primary Immunodeficiency Diseases.* 2nd ed. Towson, MD: Immune Deficiency Foundation; 2009.
3. Shearer WT, Dunn E, Luigi D, et al. Establishing diagnostic criteria for SCID, leaky SCID, and Omenn syndrome: the primary immune deficiency treatment consortium experience. *J Allerg Clin Immunol.* 2014;133(4):1092–1098.
4. Bousfiha AA, Jeddane L, Ailal F, et al. A phenotypic approach for IUIS PID classification and diagnosis: guidelines for clinicians at the bedside. *J Clin Immunol.* 2013;33:1078–1087.
5. Jordan MB, Allen CE, Weitzman S, et al. How I treat Hemophagocytic lymphohistiocytosis. *Blood.* 2011;118:4041–4052.

44

Infection Control and Prevention

JUSTIN F. HAYES, RACHAEL A. LEE

Definitions

- **Standardized Infection Ratio (SIR)**: statistic used to track healthcare-associated infections (HAIs) over time at a local, state, or national level.
  - Compares the actual number of HAIs at each hospital to the predicted number of infections.
  - Predicted infection is calculated based on 2015 national HAI aggregate data and adjusted for each facility using variables found to be significant predictors of HAI incidence.
    - Calculated for central line-associated bloodstream infection (CLABSI), catheter-associated urinary tract infections (CAUTI), surgical site infections (SSI), *C. difficile* infections (CDI), methicillin-resistant *Staphylococcus aureus* (MRSA), and ventilator-associated events (VAE).
    - SIR >1.0 indicates more HAIs were observed than predicted.
    - SIR <1.0 indicates that fewer HAIs were observed than predicted.
- **Surveillance**: used to determine the endemic rates of infection.
  - Allows for identification of an outbreak.
  - Targeted to areas of the hospital that have higher rates of infection and/or antibiotic resistance.
- **Outbreak**: identified when the rate of occurrence of an infection is significantly higher than the endemic rate of that particular infection.
- **Vertical interventions**: method of infection prevention aimed at reducing infection due to a single pathogen.
  - Example: Surveillance cultures used to isolate patients with resistant organisms, such as MRSA.
- **Horizontal interventions**: method of infection prevention aimed at reducing infection due to all pathogens transmitted by the same mechanism.
  - Example: Hand hygiene.

Outbreak Investigation

- An outbreak is the occurrence of more cases of disease than expected in a given area or among a specific group of people.

- Examples: See Table 44.1.
- A cluster is an aggregation of cases in a given area over a particular period of time.
- A case definition is a standard set of criteria for deciding whether an individual should be classified as having the health condition of interest.
  - Example: Person (e.g., age group, sex, occupation), place (e.g., geographic location, facility), time (e.g., illness onset), clinical features (e.g., pneumonia), laboratory features (e.g., cultures, serology).
- Epidemic curve: provides a visual display of an outbreak's magnitude and time trend.

Types

- **Point-source epidemic**: persons are exposed to the same source over a relative brief period (steep upslope). All cases occur within one incubation period.
- **Continuous common-source epidemic**: exposure is prolonged, occuring over multiple incubation periods (curve has a plateau instead of a peak).
- **Intermittent common-source epidemic**: exposure to the causative agent is sporadic over time (irregularly jagged curve).
- **Propagated epidemic**: spread from person-to-person with increasing numbers of cases one incubation period apart (series of progressively taller peaks)

Infection Prevention Programs

- **Primary role** is to reduce the risk of a hospital-acquired infection and promote a culture of safety.
- **Functions**
  - Surveillance.
  - Isolation.
  - Outbreak investigation.
  - Education.
  - Employee health.
  - Monitoring and management of antibiotic use and resistance trends.
  - Development of policies and interventions.
  - Environmental hygiene.
  - Assistance with quality improvement and patient safety.

TABLE 44.1	Examples of Organisms and Associated Outbreaks	
Organism	**Related Infection(s)**	**Source Responsible**
Exserohilum rostratum	Fungal meningitis	Compounded steroids
Serratia marcescens	Surgical wound infections	Propofol
Atypical mycobacteria	Surgical wound infections	Heater–cooler units
Salmonella spp.	Gastroenteritis, bacteremia	Eggs, chicken
Listeria spp.	Gastroenteritis, bacteremia, meningitis	Soft cheese, dairy products, deli meat

Standard Precautions

- Based on the assumption that any patient may be colonized or infected with organisms that are transmissible.
- Use personal protective equipment whenever there is an expectation of possible exposure to infectious material.
  - Example: Surgical mask prior to lumbar puncture.
- Hand hygiene, protective personal equipment, and safe needle practices apply to standard precautions and apply to all patients.

Hand Hygiene
- The **single most important method** to prevent transmission of nosocomial pathogens.
- Numerous methods have been implemented for improving compliance.
- Organisms spread by hands can be divided into two groups:
  - Resident flora: organisms of low virulence (i.e., coagulase-negative staphylococci).
  - Transient flora: organisms associated with HAIs (i.e., MRSA).
    - Acquired primarily by contact.
- Alcohol-based hand rubs are frequently used.
- Soap and water are recommended if hands are visibly soiled and in the setting of *Clostridioides difficile* infection.
- Hand hygiene recommended:
  - Before contact with patients.
  - Before any aseptic task.
  - After any contact with the patient's body fluid.
  - After patient contact.
  - After contact with patient surroundings.

Transmission-Based Precautions

- Organisms vary by size, by how long they survive on surfaces or in the air, and by how they can be transmitted.
  - Example: influenza lasts 1–2 days on surfaces, norovirus up to 7 days, and *C. difficile* up to 7 months.
- Transmission-based precautions apply to selected patients based on a suspected or confirmed clinical syndrome, a specific diagnosis, or colonization or infection due to epidemiologically important organisms.
- Implemented along with standard precautions.
- Three major types of transmission-based precautions:
  - Airborne.
  - Droplet.
  - Contact.

TABLE 44.2	Airborne Isolation Duration: Recommendations by Disease	
MERS	Airborne and contact for duration of illness	
Measles	4 days after onset of rash*	
Monkeypox	Until confirmed and smallpox excluded, contact until lesions are crusted	
SARS	Airborne + droplet + contact × 10 days after resolution of fever	
Smallpox	Airborne + contact, duration of illness[a]	
Tuberculosis (pulmonary and laryngeal)	Until 3 consecutive negative smears	
Varicella-zoster (disseminated)	Airborne + contact, until lesions dry and crusted[a]	

[a]Susceptible healthcare workers should not enter room if immune caregivers are available.
MERS, Middle East respiratory syndrome; SARS, severe acute respiratory syndrome.

Airborne Precautions
- Designed to prevent the transmission of diseases by airborne droplet nuclei (≤5 mm size) or dust particles carrying an infectious agent.
- These droplet nuclei and particles can travel long distances and remain suspended in the air.
- If inhaled by a susceptible host, can lead to infection.
- Patients placed on airborne precautions should be placed in a private room with monitored negative air pressure in relation to surrounding areas.
- All individuals entering the room should wear N95 masks (UK = FFP3).
- Limit movement of patient outside room to medically necessary purposes; if necessary, patient should wear surgical mask and observe cough etiquette.
- Clinical syndromes that require empiric airborne precautions include vesicular rashes with unknown etiology, rash concerning for measles, or symptoms consistent with tuberculosis.
- Airborne isolation recommended as shown in Table 44.2.

Droplet Precautions
- Used to prevent transmission of large-particle droplets.
  - Generated by coughing, sneezing, and talking.
  - Do not remain suspended in the air for long periods of time or travel long distances (up to 6 feet/2 meters).

TABLE 44.3	Droplet Isolation Duration: Recommendations by Disease
Adenovirus (pneumonia)	Droplet + contact for duration of illness
Diphtheria (pharyngeal)	Droplet until off antimicrobial treatment and culture-negative
Group A Streptococcus	24 hours after initiation of effective therapy, contact if skin lesions present
Haemophilus influenzae type b (epiglottitis, pneumonia, and meningitis)	For 24 hours after effective therapy
Influenza	Duration of treatment
Mumps	9 days after onset of swelling
Mycoplasma pneumonia	Duration of illness
Neisseria meningitidis (sepsis, meningitis, pneumonia)	Until 24 hours after initiation of effective therapy
Parvovirus B19	Duration of hospitalization in immunocompromised patient
Pertussis	5 days after initiation of effective therapy
Poliomyelitis	Duration of illness
Rhinovirus	Duration of illness
Rubella	7 days after onset of rash
Viral hemorrhagic fevers	Droplet + contact, duration of illness
Yersinia pestis (pneumonic)	48 hours

TABLE 44.4	Contact Isolation Duration: Recommendations by Disease
Clostridioides difficile	Duration of illness
Congenital rubella	Until 1 year of age
Diphtheria (cutaneous)	Until off antimicrobial therapy and culture-negative
Hepatitis A	>14 years of age, 1 week after onset of symptoms
Herpes simplex, mucocutaneous	Until lesions are crusted
Human metapneumovirus	Duration of illness
Lice	Until 24 hours of effective therapy
MDRO	
Norovirus	48 hours after resolution of symptoms
Parainfluenza	Duration of illness
Poliomyelitis	Duration of illness
Respiratory syncytial virus	Duration of illness
Rotavirus	Duration of illness
Scabies	24 hours
Staphylococcal scalded skin syndrome	Duration of illness
Vaccinia	Until lesions crusted, scabs separated
Varicella zoster (localized disease only)	Until lesions crusted

MDRO, multidrug-resistant organisms.

- A susceptible host may become infected if the droplets land on the mucosa of the nose, mouth, or eyes.
- Patients require isolation in private rooms but not in a negative-pressure room.
- Individuals entering the room should wear a surgical mask.
- Limit movement of patient outside room to medically necessary purposes; if necessary, patient should wear surgical mask and observe cough etiquette.
- Clinical syndromes that necessitate empiric droplet precautions include meningitis and viral respiratory infections.
- Recommended for patients suspected or confirmed to have infections as shown in Table 44.3.

Contact Precautions

- Implemented to prevent spread of epidemiologically significant organisms from an infected or colonized patient to another individual through direct and/or indirect contact.
- Preferable to place patients in a private room.
- Healthcare workers (HCW) should don both gowns and gloves when entering the room.
- Gowns and gloves should be removed before exiting the room, and hand hygiene should be performed.
- Clinical syndromes that require empiric contact isolation include acute diarrhea with likely infectious cause, viral respiratory infections in young children, or a draining wound that cannot be covered.
- Contact precautions are indicated for the conditions listed in Table 44.4.

Catheter-Associated Urinary Tract Infections (CAUTI)

- One of the most common HAIs and a leading cause of secondary bacteremia in acute care facilities (see Chapter 19).
- Account for more than 12% of infections reported by acute care hospitals.
- **Duration of catheterization** is the major risk factor for CAUTI.
- Catheter trauma and catheter obstruction can be precipitating events for CAUTI.
- Other risk factors for CAUTI:
  - Female sex.
  - Severe underlying illness.
  - Age greater than 50 years.
  - Catheter insertion outside operating room.
  - Diabetes mellitus.
  - Renal impairment.

Prevention Opportunities

- The **most important intervention** to prevent CAUTI is to **avoid use** of an indwelling urinary catheter.
- Other opportunities for prevention include:
  - Removal of catheters when no longer indicated.
  - Proper education.
  - Insertion of catheters under aseptic conditions.
  - Using the smallest possible catheter.
  - Adherence to hand hygiene.
  - Use of a bundled system of care.
- Antimicrobial prophylaxis

- Antimicrobial prophylaxis selects for resistant pathogens with limited evidence of a decrease in bacteriuria.

Central Line-Associated Bloodstream Infections (CLABSI)

- CLABSIs have been associated with **increased length of hospital stay** along with increased costs.
- A CLABSI is defined as a laboratory-confirmed bloodstream infection (BSI) where a central line was in place for **greater than 2 calendar days** before the blood culture is drawn, provided that the same BSI is not related to an infection at another site.
- Major risk factors
  - Insertion with less than maximum sterile barriers.
  - Placement in an old site via **guidewire exchange.**
  - Heavy cutaneous colonization at the catheter hub.
  - **Duration** of catheter greater than 7 days.

Prevention

- Use and implementation of **prevention bundles** have been shown to be effective.
- Education of healthcare personnel involved in insertion of central venous catheters (CVCs) as well maintenance and care of patients with CVCs in place has reduced the incidence of CLABSI.
- Checklists have also been used and allow institutions to ensure adherence to infection prevention practices.
- **Avoidance of femoral vein** catheterization is advised.
- Full sterile barrier precautions are recommended during the insertion of CVCs.
- Exchange of catheter over a guidewire is associated with increased risk for infection.
- **Chlorhexidine-based antiseptics** allow for **prolonged antimicrobial activity** on the skin surface after a single application.
- Use of antiseptic and antimicrobial-impregnated catheters.
  - Recommended in three scenarios:
    - Hospital units or patient populations have CLABSI rates above institutional goals despite compliance with basic CLABSI principles.
    - Patients have limited venous access and a history of recurrent CLABSI.
    - Patients are at risk of severe sequelae from CLABSI.

Surgical Site Infections

- Surgical site infections (SSIs) are considered one of the most common and costly HAIs.
- A large proportion are considered preventable.
- Classification of SSIs is based on depth of infection.
  - Superficial incisional infection
    - Involves only the skin and subcutaneous tissues.
    - Can often be managed in the outpatient setting.
  - Deep incisional infections
    - Involve the fascia and/or muscular layers.

- Can be further broken down into primary (involves primary incision) or secondary (involves secondary incision).
- Organ/space infections
  - Involve any part of the body opened or manipulated during a procedure, excluding skin incision, fascia, or muscle layers.
- Risk factors are identified in Table 44.5.

Prevention

- Guidelines have been well established for the prevention of SSIs.
- Guidelines for prevention focus on **proper hair removal**, **glycemic control postoperatively**, and **maintenance of normothermia.**
- Perform skin preparation in the operating room using an alcohol-based agent, unless contraindicated.
- Administer a fraction of inspired oxygen during surgery and after extubation in the immediate postoperative period for patients with normal pulmonary function receiving general anesthesia and undergoing endotracheal intubation.
- Education is the key to prevention within the hospital.

Antimicrobial Prophylaxis

- Prophylactic antibiotics should be administered within **1 hour prior to incision** (2 hours for vancomycin and fluoroquinolones).
- Antibiotics should be given prior to the skin incision for cesarean sections.
- Additional antimicrobial prophylaxis should not be used after the surgical incision is closed in the operating room for clean and clean-contaminated procedures, even if drains are left in place.
- **Prolonged use of antibiotics leads to increased resistance, higher rates of *C. difficile*, and higher rates of acute kidney injury.**

TABLE 44.5	**Intrinsic and Extrinsic Risk Factors Associated With Surgical Site Infections**	
Intrinsic Patient-Related Factors	**Extrinsic Procedure-Related Risk Factors**
Age	Surgical scrub
History of radiation at a surgical site	Skin preparation
Previous history of skin infection	Antimicrobial prophylaxis
Glycemic control	Avoidance of blood transfusion
Obesity	Minimizing operative time and operative room traffic
Smoking cessation	Sterilization of surgical equipment according to published guidelines
Avoidance of immunosuppressive medications perioperatively	
Hypoalbuminemia	

Clostridioides difficile infection

- *Clostridioides* (formerly *Clostridium*) *difficile* is a well-known hospital pathogen.
- *C. difficile* infection (CDI) is a leading cause of infectious diarrhea among hospitalized patients.
- CDI is defined as a case of clinically significant diarrhea or toxic megacolon without other known etiology in which: a stool sample yields a positive result of *C. difficile* toxin; *or* pseudomembranous colitis is seen on endoscopic examination; *or* pseudomembranous colitis is seen on histopathologic examination.
  - Community-Onset (CO): collected in an outpatient location or an inpatient location ≤3 days after admission to the facility.
  - Healthcare Facility-Onset (HO): collected >3 days after admission to the facility (i.e., on or after day 4).
- CDI surveillance is based on positive results for a laboratory test for *C. difficile* toxin A and/or B, *or* a toxin-producing *C. difficile* organism detected in the stool specimen by culture or other laboratory means.
- Testing should only be done when patients present with diarrheal illness.
- Two-step diagnostic testing recommended (Table 44.6):
  - Glutamate dehydrogenase (GDH) + toxin.
  - GDH + toxin, arbitrated by NAAT.
  - NAAT + toxin.
- The spore-forming nature of *C. difficile* presents challenges for hand hygiene and environmental disinfection practices since **spores are resistant to the effects of alcohol.**
  - **Chlorine-based agents** should be used (at least 1,000 ppm available chlorine).
- Full barrier precautions and hand hygiene are successful interventions to prevent transmission.
- As mentioned earlier, **contact precautions** are recommended up to **48 hours after resolution of diarrhea.**
- **Effective antimicrobial stewardship** is essential along with infection prevention for successful prevention of CDI in hospitals. Restriction of high-risk antibiotics, such as fluoroquinolones, has been successful in stewardship efforts.

Ventilator-Associated Pneumonia

- Ventilator-associated pneumonia (VAP) incidence is difficult to determine as surveillance definitions have changed over the years.
  - VAP used to be defined by clinical, radiographic, and microbiologic criteria, but these signs were neither sensitive nor specific compared to histology.
  - The US Centers for Disease Control and Prevention (CDC) created a three-tiered approach called ventilator-associated events (see Box 44.1).

Creutzfeldt-Jakob Disease (CJD)

- Iatrogenic transmission of CJD has been reported globally.
  - Cases were linked to use of contaminated human growth hormone, dura mater, or corneal grafts; or neurosurgical equipment.

BOX 44.1 Ventilator-Associated Events in a Nutshell

- Ventilator-associated conditions (VAC): deterioration in oxygenation after stable or improving period.
- Infection-related ventilator-associated conditions (IVAC): VAC plus temperature or altered white cell count plus new antibiotic.
- Ventilator-associated pneumonia (VAP): IVAC plus positive sputum/BAL microscopy or culture.
- Mortality of VAP varies based on patient factors.
- Primary route of infection is by microaspiration of endogenous or exogenously acquired organisms via endotracheal tube leakage around the cuff.
- Impaired host defenses also play a role.
- Risk factors and efforts at prevention for VAP have been identified (Box 44.2).

TABLE 44.6 Clostridioides difficile Diagnostic Testing Methods

Test	Sensitivity	Specificity
Toxigenic culture	High	Low
Nucleic acid amplification tests (NAAT)	High	Low/moderate
Glutamate dehydrogenase (GDH)	High	Low
Cell culture cytotoxicity neutralization assay	High	High
Toxin A and B enzyme immunoassays	Low	Moderate

BOX 44.2 Ventilator-Associated Pneumonia

Risk Factors

First few days of mechanical ventilation
Overall duration of mechanical ventilation

Prevention

Avoidance of intubation by use of noninvasive positive-pressure ventilation
Avoidance of prolonged sedation
Daily spontaneous breathing trials
Minimization of pooling of secretions above the endotracheal tube cuff
Elevation of the head of the bed to 30–45 degrees

- There is no evidence of person-to-person spread by close contact.
  - Isolation of the patient is not required; standard precautions suffice.
  - Body secretions and fluids are low risk.
- Classification of tissue:
  - High infectivity tissues (brain, spinal cord, cranial nerves, and eyes).
  - Medium infectivity tissues (spinal ganglia and olfactory epithelium).
  - Low infectivity tissues (cerebrospinal fluid, kidneys, liver, lungs, lymph nodes, spleen, olfactory epithelium, and placenta).
- WHO recommends destruction of heat-resistant surgical instruments that come into contact with high-infectivity tissues of patients with suspected or confirmed CJD.
- If this is not practical or cost-effective, stringent sterilization methods are listed within WHO guidance. **Effective decontamination** is paramount in reducing the risk of surgical transmission of CJD.
  - Disposable instruments should be disposed of by **incineration.**
  - Surfaces and heat-sensitive re-usable instruments should be decontaminated with NaOH with a normality of 2N or undiluted sodium hypochlorite for 1 hour and rinsed with water.
  - In the UK: instruments used on medium or high infectivity tissue in a patient with definite or probable CJD may be **quarantined for re-use exclusively on the same patient.** They may not be used for any other patient.

Surveillance for HAIs

- Surveillance of HAIs is key to their control; measurement is needed to assess impact of interventions.
- Essential elements
  - Standardized definitions.
  - Identification of at-risk patient populations.
  - Statistical analysis.
  - Feedback of results to caregiver.
- **In the United States**, the CDC use the National Healthcare Safety Network (NHSN), which is a widely used HAI tracking system.
  - Reports include national and state progress in preventing CLABSI, CAUTI, select surgical site infections, hospital-onset *C. difficile* infections, and hospital-onset MRSA bacteremia and MDROs.
- **In the UK**, Public Health England run national surveillance programs on HAIs.
  - **Mandatory** surveillance of:
    - MSSA and MRSA bacteremia.

- *E. coli, Klebsiella*, and *Pseudomonas aeruginosa* bacteremias.
- *C. difficile* infection.
- Surgical site infection for orthopedic surgical categories.
  - **Voluntary** surveillance of:
    - Surgical site infection for 13 other surgical categories, including but not limited to cardiac surgery, gastric surgery, spinal surgery.
- Both the UK and US run intermittent HAI point-prevalence surveys. These data are used to identify trends in the prevalence of HAI and to inform national policy.

Employee Health

- Infection prevention programs work closely with employee health services at hospitals.
- Deal with issues related to exposures to bloodborne pathogens and other communicable diseases.
- Employee health is charged with ensuring that healthcare employees are fit for duty and free of communicable diseases.
- Employee health should work to ensure compliance with baseline and periodic testing for latent tuberculosis as well as delivering a system that encourages compliance with annual influenza vaccination (Table 44.7).

Antimicrobial Stewardship

- Antimicrobial stewardship committees (ASC) have been established to prevent the emergence of antimicrobial resistance, improve patient outcomes, and reduce costs.
- CDC has developed seven core elements for hospital antimicrobial stewardship programs to adhere to:
  - Leadership commitment
  - Accountability
  - Drug expertise
  - Action
  - Tracking
  - Reporting
  - Education
- Allows for implementation of programs that focus on both pre- or postprescription methods.
- These programs can be both active (i.e., formulary restriction, preauthorization) or passive (i.e., education, feedback of antimicrobial utilization data).
- Infection prevention programs can work along with the ASC to utilize data regarding increasing trends of antimicrobial resistance to inform new policies and interventions.
- Further work can also be done to elucidate whether resistant isolates are **nosocomial** or **community-acquired.**

TABLE 44.7 Preexposure, Work Restrictions, and Postexposure Guidelines for Select Pathogens for Employees

Disease	Preexposure	Work Restrictions	Postexposure
Hepatitis B	Determine infection status, vaccination recommended for all HCW	Positive HbsAg: No restriction if not performing exposure-prone invasive procedures HCW should not perform exposure-prone invasive procedures until they have sought counsel from expert review panel	Source HBsAg+ Unvaccinated HCW: HBIG ×1, initiate HB vaccine Known responder: no treatment Known nonresponder: HBIG ×1 and initiate revaccination Source HbSAg– Unvaccinated: HB series Responder: no treatment Nonresponder: no treatment
Influenza	All HCW should receive annual influenza vaccination	Exclude from duty if sick until afebrile >24 hours	
Measles	History of disease no longer considered adequate presumptive evidence of measles or mumps Laboratory confirmation of disease is acceptable presumptive evidence of immunity	Active: exclude from duty 4 days after rash appears Postexposure: exclude 5 days after first exposure through 21 days after last exposure; and/or 4 days after rash appears	See Ch. 45
Mumps	2 doses should be recommended for all HCW who lack evidence of immunity	Active: exclude from duty 5 days after onset of parotitis Postexposure: from 12th day after exposure through 25th day; those with evidence of immunity do not need to be excluded	Vaccine is not recommended for PEP
Rubella	1 dose should be recommended for all HCW who lack evidence of immunity	Active: exclude from duty 7 days after rash appears Postexposure: for those without immunity: 7 days after first exposure through 23 days after last exposure and/or 7 days after rash appears	Neither postexposure vaccination nor immune globulin is effective for PEP
Pertussis	All HCW, regardless of age, should receive single dose of Tdap as soon as feasible if they have not previously	Active: exclude from duty from beginning of catarrhal stage through 3rd week after onset of paroxysms or until 5 days after effective antimicrobial therapy Postexposure: exclude from duty symptomatic personnel for 5 days after start of antimicrobial therapy	Data for PEP in Tdap-vaccinated HCW are inconclusive. PEP is recommended for HCW who have unprotected exposure and are likely to expose a patient at risk for severe pertussis (e.g., Neonatal ICU). Other HCW should either receive PEP or be monitored for 21 days and treated if symptoms develop
Varicella	Evidence of immunity: – documentation of 2 doses of vaccine – laboratory evidence of immunity – diagnosis of history of varicella by HCW	Active: exclude from duty until all lesions dry and crust Postexposure: for those without immunity: exclude from duty unless receipt of second dose within 3–5 days after exposure, otherwise 8th day through 21st day	HCW who have received 2 doses of varicella should be monitored daily HCW with 1 dose of varicella: receive 2nd dose within 3-5 days of exposure Unvaccinated HCW: vaccinate within 5 days of exposure, but are still furloughed. Varicella IG is recommended for pregnant or immunocompromised (see Ch. 20 and 45)
Herpes zoster		Localized immunocompetent: cover lesions, restrict from care of high-risk patient until lesions crust Disseminated: exclude from duty until crusting	See above

Continued

TABLE 44.7	Preexposure, Work Restrictions, and Postexposure Guidelines for Select Pathogens for Employees—cont'd		
Disease	**Preexposure**	**Work Restrictions**	**Postexposure**
Meningococcal	Anatomic or functional asplenia *or* HIV *or* persistent complement component deficiencies should receive 2 dose series		Antimicrobial prophylaxis advised for all persons who had intensive, unprotected contact (no mask, endotracheal intubation/management), regardless of vaccination status
Tuberculosis	All HCW should undergo baseline TB screening, with an individual TB risk assessment, symptom evaluation and either TST or IGRA The UK also then offer BCG if tests negative and if not contraindicated	None	Symptom evaluation for all exposures. For HCW with negative TB test, perform either IGRA/TST. If negative, repeat test 8-10 weeks after last exposure
Hepatitis C		Circulating HCV viral burden of greater than 1000 copies should be restricted from general surgery	Serologic testing at baseline, repeated at 6 weeks, 3 months, 6 months
HIV		US: Circulating HIV viral load >500 copies should be restricted UK: must have plasma viral load <200 copies/mL and be on cART; or be an elite controller, to be able to perform EPPs	PEP with ART within 72 hours of exposure, continued for 4 weeks. HIV testing should be done at baseline, 6 weeks after exposure, and 4 months after exposure

ART, antiretroviral therapy; cART, combination antiretroviral therapy; EPP, exposure-prone procedure; HBIG, hepatitis immunoglobulin; HCW, healthcare worker; IGRA, interferon gamma release assay; PEP, post-exposure prophylaxis; PPD, purified protein derivative.

Further Reading and Resources

1. Lesson 6: Investigating an Outbreak, Section 2: STEPS of an Outbreak Investigation. http://www.cdc.gov/ophss/csels/dsepd/ss1978/lesson6/section2.html.
2. CDC. Guideline for Isolation Precautions: Preventing Transmission of Infectious Agents in Healthcare Settings; 2007. http://www.cdc.gov/infectioncontrol/pdf/guidelines/isolation-guidelines.pdf.
3. epic3: National Evidence-Based Guidelines for Preventing Healthcare-Associated Infections in NHS Hospitals in England. https://improvement.nhs.uk/resources/epic3-guidelines-preventing-healthcare-associated-infections/.
4. Immunization of Health-Care Personnel: Recommendations of the Advisory Committee on Immunization Practices (ACIP). https://www.cdc.gov/mmwr/preview/mmwrhtml/rr6007a1.htm.
5. CDC. Urinary tract infection (catheter-associated urinary tract infection [CAUTI] and non-catheter-associated urinary tract infection [UTI]) and other urinary system infection [USI]) events. https://www.cdc.gov/nhsn/pdfs/pscmanual/7psccauticurrent.pdf.
6. *Clostridium Difficile* Infection: How to Deal With the Problem. https://www.gov.uk/government/uploads/system/uploads/attachment_data/file/340851/Clostridium_difficile_infection_how_to_deal_with_the_problem.pdf.
7. Clinical Practice Guidelines for *Clostridium Difficile* Infection in Adults and Children: 2017 Update by IDSA and SHEA. https://doi.org/10.1093/cid/cix1085.
8. SHEA guideline for MANAGEMENT of healthcare workers who are infected with hepatitis B virus, hepatitis C virus, and/or human immunodeficiency virus. http://www.shea-online.org/images/guidelines/BBPathogen_GL.pdf.

45

Adult Immunization

HEMA SHARMA

Definitions

Immunization: a process that renders an individual immune to an infectious disease.

Active immunization: induction of immunity following antigen exposure whereby antibodies are created by the host.

Passive immunization: induction of immunity by transfer of antibodies to the nonimmune host.

Vaccine: a biological preparation that stimulates immunity to a disease, typically containing a substance resembling a causative microorganism, often made from inactivated or attenuated forms of the microbe, its toxins, or one of its surface proteins.

Live, attenuated vaccines: contain a living microorganism that has been altered to reduce its virulence.

Inactivated vaccines: contain killed microorganisms.

Subunit vaccines: contain only the microbial antigens that stimulate the immune system.

Toxoid vaccines: contain inactivated microbial toxins.

Conjugate vaccines: contain a poor antigen attached to a strong antigen to enhance immunogenicity.

DNA vaccines: contain genetically engineered DNA that produces foreign antigens in host cells that stimulate immunity.

Recombinant vector vaccines: DNA encoding an antigen that stimulates immunity is inserted into a bacterial or mammalian cell that produces the antigen, which is then purified and formed into a vaccine.

VACCINES USED IN ADULTS

- **Universal contraindication**: do not administer any vaccine to individuals that report **anaphylaxis** to a previous dose of that vaccine or any of the vaccine components.
- **Dosing**: please refer to individual vaccine instructions for precise dosing schedules as vaccine types and dosing may vary according to vaccine manufacturer.

Bacille Calmette–Guérin (BCG) Immunization against Tuberculosis

- **Type**: live attenuated.

- Derived from *Mycobacterium bovis.*
- **Dosing**: 1 dose administered intradermally into the deltoid.
  - This may be repeated after 2–3 months if the tuberculin skin test remains negative.
  - The expected reaction is local induration followed 2 weeks later by development of a papule into a localized lesion. This may ulcerate. Should heal over weeks to months to leave a small, flat scar. Regional lymphadenopathy may develop (but <1 cm).
- **Indications**
  - US: as per CDC recommendations, BCG is not generally recommended for use in the United States. May be considered in certain high risk scenarios.
  - UK: Majority relate to children <16 years.
  - Adults (UK only): only in those who have **occupational risk** of exposure to TB:
    - Healthcare workers, laboratory workers, veterinary practices, prison staff, staff in elderly care homes, workers in hostels for homeless people, refugees, and asylum seekers.
  - All individuals must have a negative tuberculin skin test and be aged less than 35 years old.
- **Contraindications**: previous history of tuberculosis, previous BCG immunization, tuberculin skin test result >6 mm, pregnancy, immunocompromise, human immunodeficiency virus (HIV), and cancer invading the bladder wall.
- **Efficacy**
  - 60%–80% efficacy against severe TB in children, especially effective against meningitis.
  - Poorly protective against pulmonary disease in adolescents and adults.
- **Adverse reactions**: persistent local abscess, suppurative regional lymphadenopathy, disseminated BCG disease (rare).
- **BCG as treatment for bladder cancer**: BCG is used as intravesical immunotherapy for early-stage bladder cancer. BCG inserted into the bladder has a direct effect on tumor cells and also activates the host's immune response leading to tumor cell destruction through nonspecific and specific cell-mediated mechanisms.

Haemophilus influenzae Type b (Hib) Immunization

- **Type: conjugate polysaccharide** vaccine delivered as combined vaccine (DTaP/IPV/Hib) or Hib/MenC conjugate.
- **Dosing:** 1 dose for asplenia, 3 doses in hematopoietic stem cell transplantation patients at monthly intervals following transplantation, 1 more dose may be required for boosting.
- **Indications**
  - **Clinical risk groups:** anatomical or functional asplenia, sickle cell anemia, and elective splenectomy or complement deficiency.
- **Contraindications:** see universal contraindication.

Hepatitis A Virus (HAV) Immunization

- See also Chapter 22.
- **Type**
  - Vaccine: **inactivated** vaccine may be given as a single or combination vaccine with recombinant hepatitis B.
  - Immunoglobulin: human normal immunoglobulin (HNIG), made from the **pooled plasma of non-UK donors.**
- **Dosing**
  - Vaccine: 2–3 doses depending on vaccine used and indication.
  - HNIG: intramuscular dose of 500 mg can be administered to individuals aged >10 years old.
- **Indications**
  - Clinical risk groups: chronic liver disease, recreational and injecting drug use, hemophiliacs, hepatitis A contacts in outbreak settings, men who have sex with men, travelers to countries with a high or intermediate prevalence or endemic hepatitis A.
  - Occupational risk groups: hepatitis A laboratory workers, staff at residential institutions, sewage workers.
- **Contraindications: egg allergy** (for certain vaccine types, check manufacturer's information).
- **Special groups:** close contacts of international adoptees from a country with high or intermediate level of hepatitis A should receive vaccination within the first 60 days of arrival of the adoptee.
- **Postexposure prophylaxis** of HAV
  - Household or sexual contacts (adults)
    - Within 14 days of exposure:
      - Offer HAV vaccine to all.
      - Also give HNIG if >60 years, HIV with CD4 <200/µL or other immunosuppression.
    - Within 28 days of exposure:
      - Offer HNIG and HAV vaccine if chronic liver disease or chronic hepatitis B/C infection to attenuate disease.
    - Within 8 weeks of exposure:
      - Offer HAV vaccine if >1 close contact within the household to prevent tertiary infection.

Hepatitis B Virus (HBV) Immunization

- See also Chapter 22
- **Type**
  - Vaccine: HBV component is **recombinant.** May be single, in combination with inactivated hepatitis A, or in a hexavalent combination vaccine (DTaP/IPV/Hib/HepB). Now included in routine childhood immunization programs in both UK and United States.
  - Immunoglobulin: hepatitis B immunoglobulin (HBIG), made from the **pooled plasma of non-UK donors.**
- **Dosing**
  - Vaccine: 3 doses at **0, 1, 6 months** (2 months for end-stage renal failure). Booster doses for healthcare workers should be administered 5 years after primary vaccination.
  - HBIG: one dose of 500 IU, intramuscularly. Used for **rapid protection** until vaccine-induced immunity develops in individuals exposed to hepatitis B in high or unknown risk situations. It is administered at the same time as vaccine, ideally within 24 hours of the exposure but can be given up until 1 week following the exposure.
- **Indications**
  - **Clinical risk groups**
    - **Sexual** exposure: partners of people with hepatitis B, people with multiple sexual partners, people seeking assessment or treatment for sexually transmitted infections, men who have sex with men, people with HIV.
    - **Percutaneous/mucosal exposure** to blood: recreational and injecting drug users, household contacts of people with hepatitis B, residents and staff in prisons, healthcare, social care institutions, in accommodation for those with learning difficulties, individuals with diabetes, individuals receiving regular blood/blood products and their carers, and laboratory staff.
    - Adults with **chronic liver disease:** people with hepatitis C, cirrhosis, fatty liver disease, alcoholic liver disease, autoimmune hepatitis, and an alanine aminotransferase (ALT) or aspartate aminotransferase (AST) level greater than twice the upper limit of normal.
    - Adults with **end-stage renal failure:** hemodialysis, peritoneal dialysis.
    - Travelers to regions with high or intermediate levels of endemic HBV.
    - Families **adopting** children from countries with high or intermediate prevalence of hepatitis B, foster carers.
- **Special groups**
  - **Vaccine nonresponders** (anti-HBs <10 mIU/mL) after primary HBV vaccine series should repeat the vaccination course in the first instance. If these individuals fail to respond they should be given HBIG if they are exposed together with hepatitis B vaccine.

TABLE 45.1   Guidelines for Postexposure Prophylaxis[a] of Persons With Nonoccupational Exposure to Blood or Body Fluids that Contain Blood, by Exposure Type and Vaccination Status

Exposure	Treatment	
	Unvaccinated Person	**Previously Vaccinated Person**
Source with Hepatitis B		
Percutaneous (e.g., bite or needlestick) or mucosal exposure to HBsAg-positive blood or body fluids	Administer hepatitis B vaccine series and HBIG	Administer hepatitis B vaccine booster dose
Sex or needle-sharing contact of a person with hepatitis B	Administer hepatitis B vaccine series and HBIG	Administer hepatitis B vaccine booster dose
Victim of sexual assault/abuse by a perpetrator with hepatitis B	Administer hepatitis B vaccine series and HBIG	Administer hepatitis B vaccine booster dose
Source with Unknown Hepatitis B Status		
Victim of sexual assault/abuse by a perpetrator with unknown hepatitis B status	Administer hepatitis B vaccine series	No treatment
Percutaneous (e.g., bite or needlestick) or mucosal exposure to potentially infectious blood or body fluids from a source with unknown hepatitis B status	Administer hepatitis B vaccine series	No treatment
Sex or needle-sharing contact of person with unknown hepatitis B status	Administer hepatitis B vaccine series	No treatment

[a]When indicated, immunoprophylaxis should be initiated as soon as possible, preferably within 24 hours. Studies are limited on the maximum interval after exposure during which postexposure prophylaxis is effective, but the interval is unlikely to exceed 7 days for percutaneous exposures or 14 days for sexual exposures. From Centers for Disease Control and Prevention. Postexposure prophylaxis to prevent hepatitis B virus infection. *MMWR Recomm Rep.* 2006;55 (No. RR-16).

- Patients with **end-stage renal failure** experience a reduced efficacy of the vaccine and a rapid decline in postvaccination anti-HBs titer associated with uremia. Thus they should have their antibody levels checked regularly and be given a booster if their anti-hepatitis B surface antigen (anti-HBs) antibody levels fall below **10 mIU/mL.**
- **Postexposure prophylaxis** (Table 45.1)
  - **Efficacy**
    - Multiple HBIG doses alone and 1st dose initiated within 1 week of exposure: 70%–75%.
    - HBV vaccine series alone: 70%–75%.
    - HBIG and HBV vaccine series in combination: 85%–95%.

Herpes Zoster Immunization

- **Type**
  - Vaccine: **live attenuated** varicella vaccine (VAR) for protection against chickenpox and herpes zoster vaccine (HZV) for protection against shingles.
  - Immunoglobulin: varicella-zoster immunoglobulin (VZIG), made from the **pooled plasma of non-UK donors.**
- **Dosing**
  - Vaccine
    - 2 dose VAR regime, ideally 4–8 weeks apart.
    - 1 dose of HZV vaccine is required for vaccination against shingles.

- VZIG: 1 dose is given intramuscularly within 10 days of exposure.
- **Indications**
  - Varicella vaccine
    - Clinical risk groups: healthy susceptible household contacts of immunocompromised patients.
    - Occupational risk groups: susceptible healthcare workers, virology laboratory workers, workers in infectious diseases units.
    - Those with a definite history of chickenpox or herpes zoster may be considered immune.
    - Those with uncertain status should be serologically tested, and vaccine offered to those without varicella-zoster virus (VZV) antibody.
  - Shingles (zoster) vaccination
    - All adults >60 years old (United States) or >70 years old (UK).
- **Contraindications**: lymphoma, leukemia, individuals receiving systemic immunosuppression, HIV with a CD4 cell count less than 200 cells/μL, pregnancy.
- **Special groups**
- Women should avoid pregnancy for 1 month following the last dose of vaccine.
- People with HIV: nonimmune individuals with a CD4 cell count >200 cells/μL should be given 2 doses of varicella vaccine 3 months apart.
- Patients anticipating immunosuppressive therapy should be vaccinated with zoster vaccination at least 2 weeks before the start of treatment.

- **Postexposure prophylaxis**
  - VZIG prophylaxis recommended within 10 days of exposure for individuals with all three of the following:
  - **Significant exposure to chickenpox or herpes zoster** as determined by type of varicella zoster contact with index case: chickenpox, disseminated zoster, exposed lesions in immunocompetent individuals, immunosuppressed patients with localized zoster anywhere (greater viral shedding).
  - **Timing of exposure** in relation to rash onset in index case:
    - Chickenpox or disseminated zoster: 48 hours prior onset of rash until lesions crust over.
    - Localized zoster: day of rash onset until lesions crust over.
  - **Closeness and duration of contact**: same room for 15 minutes or more, face-to-face contact, patients on open wards.
  - **Clinical condition** with increased risk of varicella: immunosuppressed, neonates, pregnancy.
  - VZV nonimmune (VZV IgG negative).
  See Chapter 20 for management of varicella exposure in pregnancy.

Human Papilloma Virus (HPV) Immunization

See also Chapters 21 and 50.

These vaccines offer potential protection from strains causing 90% of cases of anogenital warts (HPV genotypes 6 and 11), 90% of cervical cancers (genotypes 16, 18, 31, 33, 45, 52, 58), 90% of anal cancers (genotypes 16 and 18), and significant proportions of oropharyngeal, vulvar, vaginal, and penile cancers.

- **Type**: subunit vaccine
  - Currently bivalent (HPV genotypes 16 and 18), quadrivalent (genotypes 6, 11, 16, 18), and 9-valent (genotypes 6, 11, 16, 18, 31, 33, 45, 52, 58) options available.
- **Dosing**: 3 doses at 0, 1–2 and 4–6 months.
  - Currently offered at 11–13 years.
  - May begin as early as 9 years.
- **Indications**
  - Nonimmune females aged up to 26 years and non-immune males aged up to 21 years old.
  - **Clinical risk groups**: defects of cell-mediated or humoral immunity, B-lymphocyte antibody deficiencies, complete or partial T-lymphocyte defects, people with HIV, malignant neoplasm, transplantation, autoimmune disease and immunosuppressive therapy, men who have sex with men up to the age of 45 years old.
- **Contraindications**: pregnancy.
- **Special groups**: pregnant women. If pregnancy occurs after vaccination initiation, delay any remaining doses until after pregnancy, no other intervention required.

Influenza Immunization

See also Chapter 13.
- **Type**: inactivated, recombinant, and live attenuated vaccines are available.
  - The live attenuated vaccine has been **cold-adapted**, so that the virus can only replicate at the lower temperatures of the nasal passage and cannot replicate efficiently elsewhere in the body.
- **Dosing**: one dose annually.
  - Based on annual global epidemiology, the WHO make recommendations as to which strains should be included in the vaccine for the northern and southern hemispheres.
  - Most are **trivalent** (2A, 1B), but quadrivalent (2A, 2B) vaccines are now available.
- **Indications**
- All individuals >6 months of age in clinical risk groups.
- Those age 2–17 years or ≥65 years without contraindications.
- **Clinical risk groups**: chronic lung/heart/liver/neurologic/or kidney disease, patients with diabetes mellitus, immunosuppression, anatomical or functional asplenia, pregnant women, and morbid obesity (body mass index >40 kg/m^2).
- **Occupational risk groups**: health and social care workers, residents of long-stay residential homes, and carers of elderly or disabled persons.
- **Contraindications**
  - The live attenuated vaccine should not be administered to individuals with severe immunodeficiency, leukemia, lymphoma, cellular immunodeficiency, people with HIV who are antiretroviral treatment-naïve, those receiving high-dose corticosteroids or salicylate therapy (other than topical treatment), and individuals with severe asthma or active wheezing.
- **Efficacy**
  - Vaccine efficacy varies between 40%–60% depending on how well matched the vaccine is to circulating influenza strains. Vaccine efficacy is assessed at the end of each influenza season.
- **Special groups**
  - Pregnancy and breastfeeding: the inactivated vaccine is safe and effective in any trimester of pregnancy.
  - Patients with **egg allergy** may be given an ovalbumin-free vaccine, or an inactivated vaccine with an ovalbumin content of <0.12 µg/mL providing they have never required admission to the intensive therapy unit due to their allergy.

Tetanus, Diphtheria, Acellular Pertussis, and Inactivated Polio Immunization

- **Type**
  - Immunoglobulin: passive immunization with tetanus immunoglobulin (IgG).

TABLE 45.2 Tetanus and Diphtheria-Containing Vaccines

Vaccine	Where Used	Diphtheria Toxoid	Tetanus Toxoid	Acellular Pertussis	Inactivated Polio
Td	US	+	+	–	–
Tdap	US	+	+	+	–
Td/IPV	UK	Low dose	+	–	+
DTaP/IPV	UK	High dose	+	+	+
DTaP/IPV	UK	Low dose	+	+	+

+ a component of this vaccine; – not included in this vaccine.

- Vaccine (Table 45.2).
- **Contraindications**: anaphylaxis to neomycin, streptomycin, or polymyxin B.
- **Dosing**
  - Adults with unknown or incomplete primary vaccination history: 3 doses of vaccine (DTaP/IPV) with 1st and 2nd doses 4 weeks apart and 3rd dose 6–12 months following the 2nd dose.
  - Other indications: single dose.

Tetanus

- **Indications**
  - Incomplete primary vaccination schedule.
  - UK: once 5 doses received, no further routine immunization required.
  - United States: booster every 10 years recommended.
  - **Intravenous drug users (IDUs)**: at greater risk of tetanus; every opportunity should be taken to ensure fully protected; give booster if any doubt about status.
  - **Travelers**: give booster if none in last 10 years and traveling to areas without readily accessible medical facilities.
  - Wound management
    - Tetanus-prone wounds include wounds or burns: with sepsis; that require surgical intervention delayed by more than 6 hours; that show significant devitalized tissue with contact with soil or manure; that contain foreign bodies; or with compound fractures.
    - Tetanus vaccine given at the time of injury may not boost immunity early enough to be of benefit. The opportunity may be taken to start/complete the immunization schedule to ensure future immunity.
  - Tetanus IgG for prevention of tetanus
    - Usually 250 IU of tetanus IgG by intramuscular injection.
    - 500 IU if risk of heavy contamination or >24 hours since injury sustained.
    - Clean wounds do not require human tetanus immunoglobulin.

Diphtheria

- **Indications**
  - Incomplete primary vaccination schedule.

- Travelers to epidemic or endemic areas, depending on nature of travel and activity, e.g., living and working with local people.
- Occupational risk groups: microbiology laboratory workers, workers in infectious diseases units. Check antibody levels at 3 months postdose and give 10-yearly boosters.

Pertussis

- **Indications**
  - Incomplete primary vaccination schedule.
  - **Pregnant women** should be given 1 dose of a pertussis-containing vaccine regardless of prior vaccine history. This should ideally be at **16–32 weeks of gestation** for maximal fetal benefit but may also be any time until 2 months postnatally to reduce risk of exposure to the infant.

Polio

- **Indications**
  - Incomplete primary vaccination schedule.
  - Occupational risk groups: microbiology laboratory workers. Staff regularly handling fecal samples that are likely to be exposed to polio viruses should be offered 10-yearly boosters.
  - Travelers to epidemic or endemic areas, depending on nature of travel and activity, e.g., living and working with local people. Give booster if final dose received >10 years previously.

Measles, Mumps, and Rubella (MMR) Immunization

See also Chapters 20 and 23.
- **Type**: live, attenuated vaccine (MMR) or measles immunoglobulin (intravenous immunoglobulin [IVIG] or human normal immunoglobulin [HNIG]).
- **Dosing**
  - MMR: 2 doses at least 4 weeks apart.
    - Can be given simultaneously with VZV vaccines or at least 28 days apart, otherwise there may be an attenuated response to the second vaccine given.

- **MMR should not be given on the same day as yellow fever vaccine**; a 4-week minimum interval should be observed.
  - If possible, MMR should be delayed until 3 months after receiving blood products as they may contain a significant amount of measles antibody.
  - **Tuberculin skin testing should be delayed until 4 weeks** after MMR as it may reduce the hypersensitivity response.
- Measles immunoglobulin
  - Should be given within 6 days of exposure.
  - Made from the pooled plasma of non-United Kingdom donors (due to theoretical risk of new variant Creutzfeldt–Jakob disease).
  - Can be given intravenously (IVIG) or intramuscularly (HNIG).
- **Indications**
  - Clinical risk groups: travelers to endemic regions, seronegative women of childbearing age, and contacts of measles cases in outbreak settings.
  - Occupational risk groups: healthcare workers (for personal benefit and to assist in protecting patients), students on entry into college or university; entry into prison or into military service.
  - Adults with no evidence of immunity to measles, mumps, or rubella:
    - Born **1980–1990**: May have received vaccination to measles and rubella but not to mumps, thus **MMR is indicated.**
    - Born **1970–1979**: May have received vaccination to measles but not mumps or rubella. These individuals may have immunity due to prior exposure to mumps or rubella. These individuals can be assessed and offered MMR if at risk.
    - Born **before 1970 (UK) or 1957 (US)**: These individuals are likely to have had all infections naturally and may be offered vaccine on request or if at risk.
- **Contraindications**: severe immunodeficiency, lymphoma, leukemia, systemic immunosuppression, cellular immunodeficiency, pregnancy, neomycin allergy, gelatin allergy, or blood product administration in the last 3 months.
- **Special groups**
  - **People with HIV**: Individuals with a CD4 cell count **>200 cells/µL for at least 6 months** duration and nonimmune to measles, mumps, or rubella should receive the MMR vaccination.
- **Postexposure prophylaxis**
  - Nonimmune contacts of measles cases should be vaccinated with **MMR within 3 days of exposure** or HNIG within 6 days if the MMR vaccine is contraindicated.
  - **The vaccine is not useful in rubella or mumps outbreaks** as antibody responses do not develop quickly enough to afford protection.
  - HNIG is unlikely to confer additional benefit in those who have detectable measles antibodies. Its use is restricted to those known or likely to be measles antibody-negative.
  - Immunoglobulin (IM or IV) should be considered in pregnancy and immunosuppression; all exposed infants <6 months of age should be given intramuscular IG as passive maternal immunity may either have waned, or may interfere with a response to MMR.

Meningococcal Immunization

- **Type**
  - Conjugate vaccines, either bivalent meningitis serotype C *with Haemophilus influenzae* B capsular polysaccharide (HiB/MenC), or quadrivalent meningitis serotypes A, C, W, Y (MenACWY); recombinant multicomponent meningitis B vaccine (MenB-4C or MenB-FHbp).
  - MenB-4C and MenB-FHbp are not interchangeable: the same vaccine should be used for all doses to complete a series.
- **Dosing**
  - UK
    - 1 dose of HiB/MenC followed 1 month later by 1 dose of MenACWY; and
    - 2 doses of MenB vaccine at least 1 month apart.
    - Boosters not currently recommended as need and timing not yet determined.
  - United States
    - 1 or 2 doses of MenACWY at least 2 months apart, with additional boosters every 5 years; and
    - 2 doses of MenB-4C at least 1 month apart or 3 doses of MenB-FHbp at 0, 1–2 months and 6 months.
- **Indications**
  - Not routinely required as an adult, even if primary course not complete.
    - Adults up to 25 years may be offered a single dose of MenACWY in the UK.
    - Adults up to 23 years may be offered MenB immunization in the United States.
  - Clinical risk groups: anatomical or functional **asplenia**, **complement** disorders, **eculizumab therapy** (monoclonal antibody that inhibits the terminal complement pathway), sickle cell anemia, HIV.
  - Travelers to a country with hyperendemic or epidemic meningococcal disease (MenACWY).
  - Evidence of MenACWY vaccination required for visa to travel to Saudi Arabia for pilgrims and workers.
  - Occupational risk groups: laboratory workers, military recruits, 1st year university students (MenACWY), if not vaccinated as a teenager.
- **Special groups**
  - Patients undergoing an elective splenectomy or treatment with eculizumab should be vaccinated with MenACWY and MenB at least 2 weeks before the procedure or start of treatment.
  - HIV
    - In the UK, BHIVA recommends that adults with HIV follow general indications for immunization. However, recommended dosing is affected, with 2 doses of MenACWY at 2-month interval recommended to increase immunogenicity and for booster doses every 5 years if ongoing risk.

- In the United States, **all adults with HIV should be offered vaccination with MenACWY**; there is no current recommendation for MenB vaccination in this population.
- **Postexposure prophylaxis**
  - MenACWY and Hib/MenC may be offered to all close contacts of any age, if any previous meningococcal vaccine was more than 1 year before.
  - MenB vaccines are not currently recommended in the UK for close contacts of an index case.
  - **Administration of vaccine should not delay antibiotic chemoprophylaxis, which is the single most important intervention.**
  - The risk of vaccination in pregnancy is unknown and may be considered if there is risk of meningococcal infection.

Pneumococcal Immunization

- **Types**
  - Pneumococcal conjugate vaccine (PCV13) and pneumococcal polysaccharide vaccine (PPSV23).
  - Both contain capsular polysaccharide; those in PCV13 are conjugated to protein to increase immunogenicity in young children.
  - **PCV13 and PPSV23 should not be administered together.**
    - PCV13 should be given first. PPSV23 should be given >2 months later.
    - If PPSV23 has been administered first, PCV13 should be given at least 1 year later (theoretical risk of serotype-specific hyporesponsiveness).
- **Dosing**: UK and US schedules differ significantly.
  - United States
    - PCV13: a single dose is recommended:
      - <65 years if underlying condition predisposes to pneumococcal disease.
      - At ≥65 years otherwise.
    - PPSV23:
      - A single dose to adults >65 years old; ≥2 months after PCV13.
      - At-risk adults aged 19–64 years should receive a single dose of PPSV23.
      - Boosters are recommended in some at-risk groups (up to 3 doses of PPSV23 may be administered).
      - The interval between doses of PPSV23 should be ≥5 years.
  - UK
    - At-risk adults aged 19–64 years should receive a single dose of PPSV23.
      - For most, no additional dose is needed.
      - Patients with splenic dysfunction or chronic kidney disease should receive boosters of PPSV23 at 5-yearly intervals.
    - Severely immunocompromised individuals should also receive a single dose of PCV13, ideally prior to their PPSV23.

TABLE 45.3	Indications for Pneumococcal Immunization
Clinical Risk Group	**Underlying Medical Condition**
Immunocompetent – chronic condition	Alcoholism Chronic heart/liver/lung diseases Cigarette smoking Diabetes mellitus
Immunocompetent – structural abnormality	Cochlear implants CSF leaks (including leakage after trauma or neurosurgery, and all CSF shunts)
Asplenia	Congenital or acquired asplenia: Splenectomy Sickle cell disease/other hemoglobinopathies 30% of patients with celiac disease have defective splenic function (correlates with duration of exposure to gluten)
Immunocompromised	Congenital or acquired immunodeficiency: B-/T-lymphocyte or complement Phagocytic disorders (excluding chronic granulomatous disease) HIV Malignancy Leukemia, lymphoma, Hodgkin disease, generalized malignancy, and multiple myeloma Renal disorders Chronic renal failure (CKD 4/5), nephrotic syndrome, renal dialysis Iatrogenic immunosuppression Solid organ transplant recipients, patients receiving long-term systemic corticosteroid and radiation therapy
Occupational risk groups	Welders or workers subject to metal fume exposure

CKD, chronic kidney disease; CSF, cerebrospinal fluid.

- Bone marrow transplant, acute or chronic leukemia, multiple myeloma, genetic immune disorders.
- All adults ≥65 years should be offered a single dose of PPSV23 if not already received one.
- **Indications** (see Table 45.3)
- **Efficacy**
  - PCV13: approximately 75% protection against invasive pneumococcal disease and 45% against pneumonia caused by vaccine serotypes.
  - PPSV23: 50%–80% protection against invasive disease caused by vaccine serotypes.

TABLE 45.4 Adult Immunization Recommendations by Clinical Risk Group

Vaccine	Pregnancy	Immuno-compromise (excluding HIV)	HIV CD4+ Count (cells/µL)		Asplenia, Splenic Dysfunction, Complement Deficiency	Chronic or End-Stage Kidney Disease	Chronic Liver Disease	Diabetes Mellitus	HCW	MSM
			<200	>200						
BCG	X	X	X	X	X	✔	✔	✔	✔	✔
Hib	✔	✔	✔	✔	✔	✔	✔	✔	✔	✔
HepA	✔	✔	✔	✔	✔	✔	✔	✔	✔	✔
HepB	✔	✔	✔	✔	✔	✔	✔	✔	✔	✔
HZV	X	X	X	✔	✔	✔	✔	✔	✔	✔
HPV	X	✔	✔	✔	✔	✔	✔	✔	✔	✔
Influenza	✔	✔	✔	✔	✔	✔	✔	✔	✔	✔
MMR	X	X	X	✔	✔	✔	✔	✔	✔	✔
MenACWY	✔	✔	✔	✔	✔	✔	✔	✔	✔	✔
MenB	*	✔	✔	✔	✔	✔	✔	✔	✔	✔
PCV13/ PPSV23	✔	✔	✔	✔	✔	✔	✔	✔	✔	✔
DTaP/IPV	✔	✔	✔	✔	✔	✔	✔	✔	✔	✔
VAR	X	X	X	✔	✔	✔	✔	✔	✔	✔

X, contraindication; ✔, safe to administer if indicated according to age or clinical risk category; * see text on meningococcal immunization. HCW, healthcare workers; MSM, men who have sex with men.

- **Special groups**
  - Elective splenectomy: administer vaccine **ideally 4-6 weeks before**, but up to 2 weeks before procedure; **otherwise delay until at least 2 weeks after** procedure if vaccination not possible in advance.
  - Chemotherapy or radiotherapy: administer vaccine 2 weeks before therapy or delay until **3 months after** treatment.
  - Leukemia patients: PCV13 may be given **6 months after** the completion of chemotherapy.
  - Bone marrow transplantation patients: PCV13 may be given **9–12 months** following transplantation.
  - Anatomical or functional asplenia and chronic kidney diseases: administer PPSV23 **every 5 years.**

Immunization Recommendations Summary

A summary of adult immunization recommendations for clinical risk groups is offered in Table 45.4

Further Reading

1. Public Health England. The Green Book. https://www.gov.uk/government/collections/immunisation-against-infectious-disease-the-green-book#the-green-book.
2. Centers for Disease Control and Prevention. *Recommended Adult Immunization Schedule for Ages 19 Years or Older*, United States. 2019. https://www.cdc.gov/vaccines/schedules/hcp/adult.html.

46

General Principles of Travel Medicine

GERMAN HENOSTROZA, MARTIN RODRIGUEZ

Pretravel Consultation

Considerations when evaluating travelers should include the following.

Risk Assessment

- **Medical history**: includes current medical conditions, medications, immune status, up-to-date immunization records, allergies, pregnancy/breastfeeding, birth control methods, and plans for pregnancy in the near future.
- **Specific itinerary**: countries to visit, regions (rural vs. urban), departure date (ideally 4–6 weeks before departure), length of stay, visiting friends and relatives, single visit vs. multiple visits, altitude.
- Travel **activities**: adventure travel, hiking, night-time exposure to insects, medical or aid missions, mass gatherings, dietary habits, potential for new sexual partners, accessing health care while away, e.g., dialysis.
- **Lodging**: staying with friends and relatives, rural lodge or hotel, air conditioning or not.
- Traveler's risk **tolerance**: adventurer traveler vs. risk-averse traveler.

Office Interventions

Vaccinations

See Table 46.1.

- Update **routine age-appropriate** vaccines including all childhood and adolescent vaccines:
  - Tetanus, diphtheria, pertussis, polio, MMR (or history of measles, mumps, and rubella disease), pneumococcal, hepatitis B (HBV), influenza.
  - United States only: varicella-zoster virus (VZV) (or history of disease).
  - UK only: meningococcal B and C.
- Update routine vaccines based on **comorbidities** such as immunosuppression, chronic disease, etc.: *Haemophilus influenzae* type b (HiB), pneumococcal polysaccharide (PPV), meningococcal B and ACWY, hepatitis A (HAV), HBV.

- **Routine traveler's vaccinations**: HAV, typhoid.
- **Itinerary-specific travel-related vaccines**
  - Initial administration or boosters depending on the vaccine.
  - Complete series before departure if time allows.
  - Yellow fever, Japanese encephalitis, HBV, rabies, polio, meningococcal ACWY, cholera, dengue, tick-borne encephalitis (the last two not available in the United States). See Fig. 46.1 for the global distribution of flaviviruses.
  - Consider accelerated vaccination schedule for people departing soon (HBV, Japanese encephalitis).
- Watch for **contraindications** (i.e., live vaccines in some immunocompromised patients).

Specific Vaccine Issues

Yellow Fever

- Yellow fever (YF) vaccine is a **live attenuated vaccine** grown in chick eggs.
- Single dose confers protective immunity in 95%–100% recipients.
- Suboptimal response if given simultaneously with MMR – give 28 days apart.
- Should be given minimum of 10 days before travel to endemic area.
- Contraindicated in travelers with primary or acquired immunodeficiency; with a thymus disorder; egg anaphylaxis.
  Complications
- Vaccine-associated encephalitis
  - Infants under 9 months.
  - Risk inversely proportional to age.
  - **Infants <6 months should never be vaccinated.**
- Yellow fever vaccine-associated neurologic disease (YEL-AND)
  - Onset 4–23 days after vaccine with fever and headache.
  - May progress to confusion, focal neurologic deficit, Guillain–Barré, or coma.
  - Increased incidence in first-time vaccine recipients >60 years age.

TABLE 46.1	Vaccines Considered During Pretravel Evaluation		
Vaccine	**Schedule**	**Duration of Protection**	**Recommended for/When Travel to**
Available in the United States			
Cholera (live attenuated)	Single dose	3–6 mth	Ongoing outbreaks of cholera
Hepatitis A	2 doses: 0 and 6 mth	>20 yr	Worldwide
Hepatitis B	3 doses: Day 0, 1 mth and 6 mth	>30 yr	Worldwide depending on activities and length of stay
Influenza			
Recombinant	Annual	1 yr	Worldwide, seasonal
Quadrivalent (live attenuated)	Annual	1 yr	Worldwide, seasonal
Japanese encephalitis	2 doses: Days 0 and 28	1–2 yr after 1st dose; >6 yr if boosted at 1–2 yr	Asian countries and parts of Western Pacific
MMR (live attenuated)	2 doses: Days 0 and 28	Lifelong after 2 doses	Worldwide
Meningococcal disease	1 dose	3–5 yr	Africa's meningococcal belt
Poliomyelitis	1 dose (if received in primary childhood series)	Lifelong, after primary series plus boost at 18 years old	Aid, refugee healthcare workers going to high-risk countries. Afghanistan, Pakistan, Guinea, Laos, Madagascar, Nigeria, Saudi Arabia for Hajj/Umrah pilgrimage
Rabies	3 doses: Days 0, 7, and 21–28		Long-stay travelers going to high-risk countries (Africa, Asia, Central and South America). Short-stay travelers where no rabies immunoglobulin (RIG) available, substantial outdoor exposure (occupational or adventure)
Tdap (tetanus, diphtheria, and pertussis)	1 dose (if received in primary childhood series)	10 yr; 5 yr for high-risk travelers (adventure travel, risk of wounds, or lack of appropriate medical care)	Worldwide
Typhoid			
Bacterial cell wall polysaccharide	1 dose	2–3 yr	Worldwide
Live attenuated bacteria	4 capsule series: one every other day	5 yr	Worldwide
Yellow fever (live attenuated)	1 dose	Lifelong as of July 11, 2016. Some countries could still require every 10 yr, or in setting of ongoing outbreak	South America, Africa
Not available in the United States			
Dengue	1 dose		
Tickborne encephalitis	3 doses: day 0, 1–3 mth and 5–12 mth	3 yr	Areas in Europe and Asia, from eastern France to northern Japan and from northern Russia to Albania

- Complete recovery is expected.
- Yellow fever vaccine-associated viscerotropic disease (YEL-AVD)
  - Onset 2–7 days after vaccine.
  - Fever and multiorgan failure.
  - Death in >60% reported cases.

- Increased incidence in >60 years age and even higher >70 years.
- Only after first dose of vaccine.

Malaria Prophylaxis

- Required if risk exists according to itinerary.

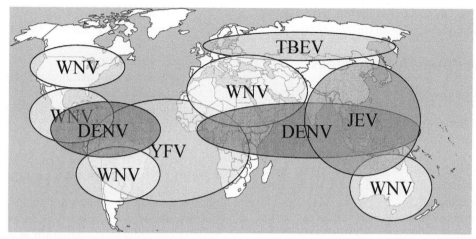

• **Fig. 46.1** Worldwide distribution of flaviviruses. (From Ishikawa T, Yamanaka A, Konishi E. A review of successful flavivirus vaccines and the problems with those flaviviruses for which vaccines are not yet available. *Vaccine.* 2014; 32 (12):1326–1337.)

- Individualize to itinerary, patients' medical conditions, and side effect tolerance.
  - For **all malaria species in all malarial areas**: atovaquone/proguanil.
    - Alternative drugs (all species): mefloquine, doxycycline.
    - Chloroquine in sensitive malaria areas.
- Consider terminal prophylaxis (2 weeks when finishing the trip) with primaquine for prolonged exposures in *Plasmodium vivax* or *Plasmodium ovale* areas, to eradicate hypnozoites.
- Watch for drug interactions.

Travelers' Diarrhea

- **Education** about potential risks and ways to try to limit risk (water, meals)
  - Peel fruit; avoid salad and raw vegetables.
  - Boiled, bottled, treated, or carbonated drinks; check seals.
  - Avoid ice cubes.
  - Meals in private home less risk than restaurant; street vendors especially risky.
- Oral rehydration.
- Loperamide.
- Bismuth subsalicylate (as prophylaxis)
  - Reduces attack rates of travelers' diarrhea.
  - Avoid if allergic to salicylates.
  - Interferes with absorption of doxycycline.
- **Antibiotic self-treatment** (single dose may be sufficient)
  - Azithromycin.
  - Ciprofloxacin or levofloxacin.
  - Rifaximin.
  - Consider prophylaxis with antibiotics only if high risk (i.e., immunocompromised and high risk for disease – rifaximin advised).

Patient's Pretravel Education – Targeted to Itinerary Areas

- **Vectorborne diseases**: education targeting traveler's protection against dengue, chikungunya, Zika, African sleeping sickness, Japanese encephalitis, filariasis, leishmaniasis, rickettsial diseases such as African tick bite fever. Practicing insect bite avoidance is key.
- **Other travel diseases**
  - Tuberculosis and respiratory infections: if high likelihood of exposure to active tuberculosis (TB) patients, advise **PPD/IGRA before travel** (medical mission trips, orphanages, healthcare workers) and **repeat 3 months posttravel.**
  - Sexually transmitted infections: HIV, syphilis, chlamydia, gonorrhea, HBV, HSV.
  - Exposure to fresh water, mud: leptospirosis (worldwide), melioidosis (Southeast Asia in particular), schistosomiasis (Africa, Southeast Asia, some areas in the Americas).
  - Blood clots: DVT/PE associated with lack of mobility, prophylaxis if high risk (graduated compression stockings), advise leg exercises when flying, to walk around aircraft or stand up every 3–4 hours. Avoid sleeping pills while flying if taking birth control pills or history of previous DVT.
  - High altitude sickness: when ascending rapidly over **2500 m** (8200 feet) above sea level, low dose acetazolamide best option but educate traveler about the need to start 24 hours before ascent and the potential side effects (paresthesia, increased urination, taste changes).
  - Rabies and animal-associated diseases.
  - Snake bites, spider bites, scorpions, sea creatures.
- Medical care while traveling
  - Medical kit: bandages, antiseptic ointment, skin glue, thermometer, antifever medications, antifungal creams, cough/cold drugs, condoms, sunscreen and insect repellent (DEET >30% or picaridin for exposed skin, consider permethrin for clothes).
- Carry all medicines in prescription bottles.
- Carry list of medical conditions, allergies, and current medications with respective dosages.
- Obtain reliable medical travel insurance and evacuation insurance.

- Keep information about local consulate (according to traveler's nationality) in case of an emergency.

Travelers With Special Health Needs

Travelers With Diabetes

- **Diabetes management**
  - Monitor blood glucose more frequently while travelling.
  - Insulin should be protected from **temperature variations**: use insulated bag/flask; do not put in aircraft hold as may freeze.
  - Advise travelers to avoid obtaining insulin overseas as great variation.
  - Monitoring equipment may be affected by environmental factors such as humidity, heat, and altitude.
- **Vaccines**: routine immunizations, including pneumococcal and influenza for those with a chronic medical condition.
- **Malaria**: check drug interaction and renal function with choice of malaria prophylaxis.

Traveling in Pregnancy

See also Chapter 20.

Commercial air travel is considered safe up to 36/40 weeks in uncomplicated pregnancy, and 32/40 weeks in multiple pregnancy.

- **Zika**
  - Risk of congenital Zika syndrome.
  - Pregnant women should postpone nonessential travel to Zika-endemic areas until no longer pregnant.
- **Malaria**
  - Up to 50% DEET considered safe.
  - **Increased risk of developing severe malaria and death** from malaria compared to nonpregnant women.
  - Diagnosis may be more difficult due to parasite sequestration in placenta.
  - Chloroquine and proguanil are safe in all trimesters (take folic acid 5 mg).
  - Doxycycline is usually contraindicated in pregnancy.
  - Mefloquine may be used in 2nd and 3rd trimesters; possibly use with caution in 1st trimester if risk–benefit assessed.
  - Atovaquone/proguanil safety in pregnancy not established. Use not advised, but in practice may be considered in 2nd and 3rd trimesters.
- **Vaccines**
  - Inactivated vaccines can be given if indicated.
  - **Live vaccines are usually avoided**; if high risk of disease, a careful risk–benefit analysis should be performed.
- Pregnancy increases the risk of **venous thromboembolism.**
  - For travel >4 hours:
    - Wear properly fitted compression stockings.

- Mobilize regularly.
- Consider low molecular weight heparin prophylaxis if additional risk factors.
- Food and water health.
  - Risk of serious complications if contract hepatitis E, listeriosis, toxoplasmosis.
  - **Ciprofloxacin and loperamide are not recommended in pregnancy.**

Traveling While Immunosuppressed

Travelers who are immunosuppressed are at **greater risk of severe illness** from infections acquired while travelling; they may also suffer an **exacerbation or worsening of their underlying condition**.

- Advise comprehensive travel insurance is obtained with full disclosure of medical history.
- Conditions include:
  - Bone marrow transplant (BMT) recipients (until 12 months after treatment completed, or longer if GVHD).
  - Chemotherapy and radiotherapy.
  - HIV depending on CD4 count and disease activity.
  - Solid organ transplant recipients on immunosuppressive therapy.
  - Primary immunodeficiency syndromes.
  - Asplenia.
  - Chronic medical conditions, and those on immunosuppressive medications.
- Take care to take a full drug history, including ones that are only received every few weeks/months.
- **Vaccines**
  - Inactivated vaccines may be given but **may not be as effective.**
  - **Live vaccines usually contraindicated**, especially if heavily immunosuppressed as risk of replication of viral strain causing severe or fatal infection:
  - e.g., TB (BCG), oral typhoid, MMR, nasal influenza, VZV, yellow fever, shingles, and rotavirus.
  - Travelers who are heavily immunosuppressed should be advised to avoid travelling to yellow fever risk areas as the vaccine is contraindicated; a medical letter of exemption may be issued if required.
  - Public health guidance, e.g., from Centers for Disease Control and Prevention (CDC) or Public Health England (PHE) guidance should be checked.
  - BMT recipients should be considered for a re-immunization program of all standard vaccines, as likely to lose any natural or immunization-derived protective antibodies.
- **Malaria and other infections**
  - At greater risk of **severe infection** with malaria, Chagas, visceral leishmaniasis.
  - Check drug interactions carefully.
  - Respiratory fungal infections should be considered, and risk activities such as caving or exposure to bat or bird droppings avoided.

Posttravel Evaluation

Evaluation of patients with a probable travel-related illness should include the following.

- **Severity** of illness: always assess for life-threatening infection, malaria, meningitis, severe respiratory syndrome, hemorrhagic fever; any of these requires immediate action and may require involvement of public health authorities.
- Travel **itinerary** and duration of travel: it is of extreme importance to formulate a differential diagnosis; knowing the places/regions visited will allow the clinician to exclude infections and, in consequence, unnecessary testing. Fever in a returning traveler from a malaria-endemic country needs to be evaluated immediately.
- Timing of onset of illness: most travel-related infections have a short **period of incubation**; ill travelers will usually seek medical attention within 1 month of return. Some infections could manifest months or years after travel completion.
- Past medical history and medications.
- History of pretravel encounter
  - Travel-specific **immunizations**: all vaccination received prior to travel. Most common vaccine-preventable diseases in returned travelers are enteric fever (typhoid and paratyphoid), viral hepatitis, and influenza.
  - **Malaria prophylaxis adherence**: drug prescribed and treatment completion.
- Traveler **exposures**
  - Accommodation: air conditioning facilities vs. camping in rural areas, bed nets availability.
  - Insect precautions used: bug spray with DEET >30% or other effective repellents, bed nets used.
  - Drinking water sources: bottled water (filtered, boiled) vs. tap water; ice in drinks.
  - Food ingestion: raw vegetables/salad or uncooked food eaten during travel (raw meat, seafood/shellfish), unpasteurized products.
  - Insect/arthropod bites.
  - Animal bites and scratches.
  - Body fluid exposures (tattoos, sexual activity).
  - Activities, e.g., safari, caving, freshwater exposure (swimming, rafting).
  - Work in hospitals or refugee camps.

In order to establish an appropriate diagnosis, it is important to have a syndromic approach in the returning traveler that could narrow possible etiologies. The most common clinical presentations after traveling to developing countries include fever, diarrheal disease, and dermatologic conditions.

Fever Within 10 Days of Return

- Fever with **nonspecific** symptoms: dengue, Zika, chikungunya, rickettsial diseases (scrub typhus, spotted fevers, African tick bite fever), leptospirosis, viral hemorrhagic fevers.
- Fever with **central nervous system (CNS)** involvement: meningococcal meningitis, arbovirus encephalitis (Japanese encephalitis, tickborne encephalitis), eosinophilic meningitis (i.e., angiostrongyliasis).
- Fever with **respiratory** symptoms: influenza, bacterial or viral pneumonia, histoplasmosis, coccidioidomycosis, legionella, tularemia, pneumonic plague, Middle East respiratory syndrome coronavirus (MERS-CoV), severe acute respiratory syndrome (SARS), avian flu.
- Fever and **skin rash**: dengue, chikungunya, Zika, measles, varicella, spotted fevers, Lyme disease.

Fever Between 10 and 21 Days

- Bacterial: enteric fever (typhoid and paratyphoid), leptospirosis, brucellosis, Q fever.
- Fungal: histoplasmosis, coccidioidomycosis.
- Viral: cytomegalovirus (CMV), Epstein–Barr virus (EBV), human immunodeficiency virus (HIV), viral hemorrhagic fever (VHF).
- Parasitic: malaria, African trypanosomiasis (*rhodesiense*), acute Chagas disease.

Fever After 21 Days

- Bacterial: brucellosis, tuberculosis.
- Fungal: histoplasmosis, blastomycosis.
- Viral: HIV, viral hepatitis A–E, rabies.
- Parasitic: malaria, amebic liver abscess, African trypanosomiasis *(gambiense)*, visceral leishmaniasis, acute schistosomiasis.

Returning Travelers Presenting With Diarrhea

- Most cases of travelers' diarrhea are bacterial and self-limited (<14 days).
  - Majority = enterotoxigenic *Escherichia coli* (ETEC).
  - *Shigella, Campylobacter, Salmonella, Aeromonas, Plesiomonas*, and noncholera *Vibrio* species also responsible.
- >90% occur within first 2 weeks of travel.
- 1% require hospitalization.
- Prolonged diarrheal illness could represent immunosuppression, sequential infection with other pathogen or protozoan parasites.
  - Consider *Giardia, Cryptosporidium, Cyclospora*, and *Entamoeba histolytica*.
- Bloody diarrhea: consider *Shigella, Salmonella*, amoebiasis.

Returning Travelers Presenting With Dermatologic Conditions

Common rashes and skin lesions are listed in Table 46.2.

- Assessment of a travel-associated skin condition should also involve:
  - Location: exposed vs. unexposed skin areas.
  - Exposure history: freshwater, ocean, insects, animals, or human contact.

TABLE 46.2	**Skin Lesions in Returned Travelers**	
Linear	Cutaneous larva migrans (*Ancylostoma* spp.)	Pruritic serpiginous lesions that advance slowly
	Larva currens	Urticarial linear lesions moving faster due to cutaneous migration of *Strongyloides stercoralis* filariform larvae
	Phytophotodermatitis	Noninfectious lesion due to interaction of natural psoralens (in lime juice spilled on skin) that interacts with UV radiation
Macular	Generalized	Consider drug reactions
	Localized	Consider tinea corporis or tinea versicolor
	Leprosy	Hypopigmented macular lesions with hypoesthesia or peripheral nerve enlargement
Maculopapular	With fever	Arbovirus: dengue, chikungunya, measles, rubella, parvovirus, EBV, CMV, HIV, syphilis VHF Rickettsial infection
Nodular	Bacterial skin infection (staphylococcal/streptococcal)	May follow bug bites; pyoderma, impetigo, abscess formation, erysipelas, cellulitis, lymphangitis, or ulceration
	Gnathostomiasis	Migratory panniculitis common in Southeast Asia, less in Africa and Latin America
	Myiasis	Painful "boil"-like lesions in Africa (*Cordylobia anthropophaga)*; or Latin America (*Dermatobia hominis*)
	Tungiasis (*Tunga penetrans*)	Nodular pale subcutaneous lesion with central dark spot
Papular	Bug bites = most common	Grouped papules due to bed bug and flea bites
	Endemic mycoses	Histoplasmosis, penicilliosis
	Onchocerciasis (sub-Saharan Africa)	Generalized pruritic papular dermatitis
	Scabies	Regional or generalized pruritic papular rash
Ulcerative	Anthrax	Necrotic ulcer surrounded by edema
	Buruli ulcer (*Mycobacterium ulcerans*)	Destructive ulcer with undermining edges
	Chancre	*Trypanosoma brucei rhodesiense*: occurs 48 hours after tsetse fly bite; itchy, painful red/purple nodule, 2–5 cm diameter which ulcerates, with surrounding edema and associated lymphadenopathy
	Cutaneous leishmaniasis	Chronic, usually painless ulcer unless superinfected, with heaped-up margins on exposed skin surfaces, in travelers from high-risk areas, including Latin America, Mediterranean, Middle East, Asia, and parts of Africa
	Rickettsial infection such as African tick-bite fever or scrub typhus	Eschar: dark, scabbed lesion at site of insect bite
	Ulceroglandular tularemia	Papule develops at site of inoculation with fever onset; becomes vesicular and pustular, then ulcerates. Tender, associated with painful lymphadenitis

CMV, cytomegalovirus; EBV, Epstein–Barr virus; HIV, human immunodeficiency virus; UV, ultraviolet; VHF, viral hemorrhagic fever.

TABLE 46.3	Eosinophilia in the Returned Traveler
Syndrome: Eosinophilia with...	**Infection**
Fever/ respiratory symptoms	Acute schistosomiasis Coccidioidomycosis or paracoccidioidomycosis Löeffler's syndrome due to *Ascaris*, hookworms, or *Strongyloides* Paragonimiasis Tropical pulmonary eosinophilia due to *Wuchereria bancrofti* or *Brugia malayi* Visceral larva migrans due to *Toxocara* spp.
Gastrointestinal symptoms	Ascariasis Hookworms (*Ancylostoma duodenale* and *Necator americanus*) Schistosomiasis (*Schistosoma mansoni* and *S. japonicum*) Strongyloidiasis Tapeworms (*Taenia solium* and *T. saginata*) Trichinellosis
RUQ pain	Fascioliasis Liver flukes (*Clonorchis sinensis* and *Opisthorchis* spp.) Liver hydatid disease
Neurologic symptoms	Coccidioidomycosis (chronic meningitis in the immunosuppressed) Eosinophilic meningitis due to *Angiostrongylus* or *Gnathostoma* Neurocysticercosis due to *T. solium*
Skin changes	Gnathostomiasis (intermittent pruritic edematous subcutaneous swellings) Loiasis (Calabar swellings) Lymphatic filariasis (lymphadenitis and edema) Onchocerciasis (diffuse, pruritic dermatitis) Strongyloidiasis (larva currens)

- Symptoms associated: fever, pain, pruritus.
- Location and duration of travel.
- Time of onset: during or after travel.

Eosinophilia in the Returning Traveler

Eosinophilia, defined as peripheral blood eosinophil count of >0.45 ×10^9/L, is occasionally seen in returned travelers. A differential diagnosis is provided in Table 46.3.

47
Bioterrorism

JOANNA PETERS

Background

The malicious use of biological agents to control, harm, and potentially destroy whole populations is a modern threat, even more so in the age of global terrorism.

After the Twin Towers attacks of 11th September 2001, CDC recommended enhanced surveillance for **unusual disease presentations** or **high numbers** of cases which could be consistent with release of biological agents. Shortly after this, 22 cases of anthrax, both inhalational and cutaneous, were described in New York and Florida leading to five deaths. Environmental sampling and investigation pointed toward the intentional contamination of letters sent to major news organizations and two US Senators. This was propounded by one "homegrown" individual. Since then the "new age of bioterrorism" has begun, assisted by increasingly advanced biotechnology. Research into biological weapons is not new, however, and was conducted extensively during the world wars of the 20th century. Intentional release of plague in China was used as a bioweapon. More recently, use of chemical weapons on populations in Syria has heightened the threat of widespread use of biological weapons.

Syndromic Awareness

The first clinical case(s) in a bioterrorism event may be unheralded and present to any local medical provider. As such, there is a need for all physicians to hold an awareness of how biological agents may present, and to consider them in their differential (Table 47.1).

Categorization of Biological Agents

The Centers for Disease Control and Prevention (CDC) assigns various biological agents into categories (see Table 47.2), depending on:
- Ability to disseminate.
- Transmissibility.
- Potential harm.
- Public health and social impact in the event of release.

TABLE 47.1	Syndromes and Biological Agents to Consider in Differential Diagnosis	
Syndrome	Specific Biological Agents to Consider	Differential Diagnosis
Fever and shock ± bleeding	VHFs Anthrax VTEC-producing *E. coli* Tularemia Glanders Melioidosis	Meningococcal Staphylococcal/ streptococcal sepsis/ toxic shock syndrome Gram-negative sepsis
Fever and rash	Smallpox	Measles Mumps Rubella Parvovirus B19 Scarlet fever VZV HSV Molluscum contagiosum Monkeypox Hand, foot, and mouth
Fever and skin signs	Cutaneous anthrax Tularemia Bubonic plague Melioidosis Glanders	Cellulitis Impetigo Orf Cowpox LGV/chancroid Tick/spider bites
Fever and chest signs	Inhalational/ pulmonary anthrax Plague Tularemia Melioidosis Ricin poisoning Glanders	Lobar pneumonia COPD exacerbation Atypical pneumonia Empyema Tuberculosis SARS
Neurologic signs	Botulism	Stroke Guillain–Barré syndrome Polio Transverse myelitis Myasthenia gravis Organophosphate poisoning

TABLE 47.2	Categorization of Biological Agents					
Category	Dissemination	Transmission	Morbidity	Mortality	Other	Examples
A	High	High	High	High	Special measures required	Anthrax Botulism Plague Smallpox Tularemia Viral hemorrhagic fevers (VHFs)
B	Moderate	Low	Moderate	Low		Brucellosis *Clostridium perfringens* toxin Food safety threats (*Salmonella*, *Shigella* spp, *E.coli* O157) Glanders Melioidosis Psittacosis Q fever Ricin toxin Staphylococcal enterotoxin B Typhus fever Viral encephalitis alphaviruses Water safety threats
C	Potentially high	Potentially high	Potentially high	Potentially high	Potential threat based on availability and capacity to engineer	Emerging infectious diseases such as Nipah and Hantavirus

Management of incidents involving these organisms is more complex for higher-category agents and requires expedient and comprehensive discussion with CDC.

Category A Organisms

Category A organisms are the six pathogens that are deemed to pose the highest threat to the public through their potential use as biological weapons.

Anthrax

See also Chapter 31, Infections Associated with Animal Exposure.

Epidemiology

- Anthrax is a zoonosis.
  - *Bacillus anthracis* spores reside naturally in the environment.
  - Infection occurs in grazing sheep, cattle, and goats by **ingestion** of soil-derived spores.
- Human infection occurs most commonly after contact with infected animals or animal products.

- The majority of human infections are **cutaneous** in nature, after spores inoculate small breaks in the skin.
- Transmission can also occur via **inhalation of spores** or ingestion of contaminated meat.
- Secondary cutaneous cases can arise after contact with primary lesions, but transmission to other people from cases with inhalational disease has not been reported.
- Incubation period (IP) usually 24 hours to 7 days, but injectional disease occurs within 48 hours.

Anthrax as a Bioweapon

- Spores can be disseminated over large areas and can lie **dormant** for **many years.**
  - High resistance to temperature, pressure, pH, ionizing radiations.
- Naturally available in soil so potential to be developed by many sources.
  - Easy to produce and store.
- Can be **aerosolized** but also sent directly via various communication methods.
  - Inhalational and cutaneous disease are therefore the most likely result of use of anthrax as a bioweapon.
- Disease phenotype severe with **high case fatality.**
  - Early diagnosis of inhalational anthrax difficult due to similarity to influenza.

Clinical Features

Anthrax has four main presentations depending on route of transmission

Inhalational

- Shortly after inhalation of spores, an **influenza-like illness** occurs with fever, myalgia, headache, vomiting/nausea, then cough and **onset of severe shortness of breath 48 hours** afterward.
  - Respiratory failure develops frequently.
- Characteristic radiographic appearances are of a **widened mediastinum** (due to lymph node dissemination and hemorrhagic mediastinitis) and **pleural effusions.**
  - Lung parenchyma appearance may be normal.
- Germinating spores then disseminate via the bloodstream correlating with severe systemic instability.
- Meningitis and parenchymal brain infection must be considered (≤50% patients).

Cutaneous

- Local skin lesions occur where contact has occurred.
  - Usually on the head, neck, hands, and forearms.
- An itchy raised lesion develops into a papule then vesicle, with **prominent edema** surrounding the lesion, which then develops a **black eschar** centrally over a few days (Fig. 47.1).
  - The **swelling** is often **disproportionate** to the size of the skin lesion itself and is **painless.**
  - Local lymphadenopathy is common.

Gastrointestinal and injectional forms are also described but less likely to result from use of anthrax as a bioweapon. (See Chapter 31.)

Immediate Management

- Patients most likely to present to the emergency department.
- **Awareness** and assessment for the potential forms of the disease and transmission **risk factors** (i.e., postal workers, military or political personnel) is key to early recognition and investigation.

- **CDC case definition:** If one specific symptom related to anthrax is present, or two more nonspecific factors with risk factors, then immediate notification to CDC should take place.
- The risk of transmission from cases to healthcare personnel is negligible as it is the spores and not the vegetative form of the bacteria that is infectious.
- **IPC (infection, prevention, and control) precautions** such as gloves, gown, and mask should be employed when collecting patient samples for diagnostic purposes.
- **Patient isolation not required.**

Diagnosis

- Anthrax is caused by the gram-positive nonmotile, spore-forming rod, *Bacillus anthracis.*
- It is a **Biosafety level 3 organism** that needs to be handled in appropriate approved laboratories.
- Blood cultures, nasal swabs, respiratory samples, cerebrospinal fluid, and skin swabs can be cultured on standard media.
- Clotted and EDTA blood for serology and polymerase chain reaction (**PCR**) should be collected.
- Demonstration of a **four-fold rise in titers** of IgG between acute and convalescent samples is diagnostic.
- Skin biopsies of cutaneous lesions should be sought as histology and PCR can be useful to confirm diagnosis in absence of positive cultures.
- Gram stain and colony appearance is characteristic (see Figs. 47.2 and 47.3).
- Other routine investigations to aid diagnosis: full blood count (high WCC), renal and liver function, arterial blood gases (hypoxia), chest radiograph/CT scan (lymphadenopathy, pleural effusions).

Treatment

- Suspected systemic anthrax or meningitis: use combination of quinolone + beta lactam + protein synthesis inhibitor.

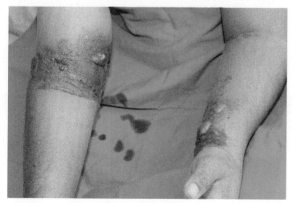

- **Fig. 47.1** Cutaneous anthrax with hemorrhagic blistering and surrounding edema. (From Doganay M, Metan G, Alp E. A review of cutaneous anthrax and its outcome. *J Infect Publ Health.* 2010;3(3):98–105.)

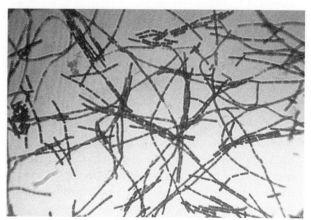

- **Fig. 47.2** Gram stain of *Bacillus anthracis* showing large gram-positive rods arranged in chains. (Courtesy Centers for Disease Control and Prevention Public Health Image Library.)

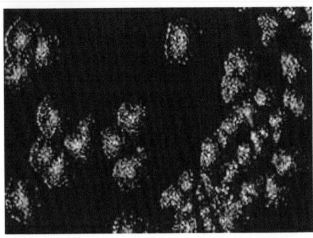

• **Fig. 47.3** *Bacillus anthracis* colonies on blood agar are grey/white with a "medusa head" appearance. (From Hall GS, Woods GL. Medical bacteriology. In: McPherson RA, Pincus MR, eds. *Henry's Clinical Diagnosis and Management by Laboratory Methods*. 23rd ed. Elsevier; 2017.)

- E.g., ciprofloxacin 400 mg TDS IV + meropenem 2 g TDS IV + linezolid 600 mg BD IV.
- **Due to variable β-lactam resistance and need for good CNS penetration.**
  - The beta-lactam can be stopped if meningitis is excluded.
- Antitoxin therapy is also recommended for inhalational or systemic anthrax.
  - Antitoxins counteract extracellular toxins; prevent binding and translocation.
  - Recombinant or anthrax immune globulin available.
  - Limited data available, but suggest improved survival with combination antimicrobial/antitoxin therapy.
  - Potential benefit outweighs potential risk.
  - If supplies limited due to mass casualties, prioritize those who do not respond to antimicrobials or who present with more severe illness.
- Cutaneous disease without systemic upset: ciprofloxacin or doxycycline can be used.
- Duration of treatment: up to 3 weeks for systemic disease and 60 days for cutaneous diseases associated with bioterrorism.
- If strains are cultured and found to be penicillin-sensitive, then high-dose penicillin or oral amoxicillin may be used in place of the quinolone treatment.

Public Health Management and Postexposure Prophylaxis

- Notify public health officials as soon as diagnosis suspected as it is likely to indicate deliberate release of the organism and more cases would be expected.
- Empiric prophylactic regimens: **oral ciprofloxacin or doxycycline for up to 3 months.**
  - Long duration due to spores which may be retained in lungs after initial exposure.
- Anthrax postexposure vaccine can be used for those who respond acutely to a deliberate release.

Botulinum Toxin

Epidemiology

- Botulism is caused by *Clostridium botulinum*, a grampositive spore-forming anaerobe.
  - Spores reside in soil and marine environments.
  - Can contaminate food production processes and infect wounds.
  - Disease is due to botulinum toxin, a potent neurotoxin.
  - Toxin could be aerosolized or directly introduced into food and water supplies.
    - Inhalational botulism is not a natural form.
    - Toxin is destroyed by common water treatment processes, such as chlorination or boiling.
- IP depends on exposure route
  - Inhalation: 1–3 days.
  - Foodborne toxin: 6 hours to 8 days.
  - Ingestion of spores: unknown.
- There is **no person-to-person spread**.

Botulinum Toxin as a Bioweapon

- Botox can be aerosolized with potential to disseminate widely and cause numerous cases.
- Could also be released to contaminate **food or water supplies.**
  - Either as spores or as toxin.
- Severe disease phenotype with high mortality if not recognized quickly.
- Available within the environment.
- Cases would **require prolonged care** placing significant strain on services in the event of deliberate release.

Clinical Features

- **Acute symmetric flaccid paralysis with bulbar palsies** prominent.
  - All forms share a common illness pathway regardless of infective route.
  - Disease is notable for the **absence of fever and lack of sensory deficit.**
- Symptoms include difficulty with swallowing and speaking and double vision.
- Signs start centrally with ptosis and facial weakness, dysarthria, diplopia, and dysphonia.
- Gastrointestinal symptoms may complicate foodborne disease.

CLINICAL PEARL

- Progression from symmetrical, severe, and bilateral cranial nerve signs to a descending flaccid paralysis, respiratory failure, and autonomic instability, is characteristic.

- Death occurs due to respiratory muscle paralysis.
- Onset and progression to later signs can be rapid especially when high levels of toxin are inhaled.

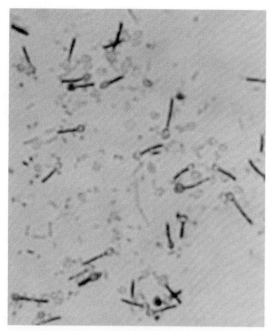

Fig. 47.4 Gram stain showing large gram-positive bacilli with terminal spores. (From Thwaites CL. Botulism and tetanus. *Medicine*. 2014;42(1):11–13.)

Immediate Management

- Expedient discussion with infectious diseases and neurology to establish diagnosis is important.
- Public heath must be notified immediately.
- Isolation is not required.
  - If aerosol exposure is suspected, the patient's clothing must be removed and the patient shower and be decontaminated immediately to prevent additional exposure to the patient or others.
- Assessment for potential risk factors and occupational exposures is important.
- Serum samples and other samples depending on nature of disease, wound swabs, respiratory secretions should be collected.
- Central nervous system imaging and CSF samples should be obtained to look for other etiologies.

Diagnosis

- Initially based on clinical history and examination followed by lab confirmation.
- Antitoxin antibodies can be detected from acute serum (prior to antitoxin).
- *Clostridium botulinum* may be cultured from stool, wound, or food.
  - *C. botulinum* has characteristic Gram and colonial appearance on blood agar (Fig. 47.4).
- Direct toxin detection in serum, stool, or food may be performed at reference laboratories.

Treatment

- **Antitoxin** must be administered **as soon as diagnosis is suspected**, after taking a serum sample. This will always

be before confirmation of disease but is key in preventing disease progression and death.
- Supportive care is vital.
- Patients should be cared for in a critical care environment from the beginning of their illness and monitored for reduction in vital capacity and hypercarbia.
- Ventilation may be needed for a prolonged period while awaiting neurologic recovery.
- Secondary infection is common and should be treated as per hospital guidelines.

Public Health Management and Postexposure Prophylaxis

- Laboratory staff working with the organism on a regular basis are given toxoid vaccine.
- No prophylaxis is required for contacts.

Pneumonic Plague

See also Chapter 31, Infections Associated with Animal Exposure.

Epidemiology

Plague is a zoonosis caused by the bacteria *Yersinia pestis*. Fleas spread the disease to humans from the natural rodent reservoir. There are still thousands of naturally occurring cases worldwide each year, particularly in Madagascar, parts of Asia, and also the Western United States.
- Infected flea bites lead to **bubonic** plague; inhalation of the organism causes **pneumonic** plague.
- Progression of either form can lead to septicemic plague.
- Person-to-person spread of pneumonic plague can occur.
- Other forms of the disease are not considered infectious.
- **Occupational risk factors**: laboratory workers, animal trappers or hunters in endemic areas.
- IP period depends on form of disease
  - 2–8 days for bubonic plague.
  - 2–4 days for pneumonic plague.

Plague as a Bioweapon

- Severe disease phenotype: fatal unless treated early.
- **Person-to-person spread** giving secondary cases.
- Available to engineer as a bioweapon as many natural cases per year.

Clinical Features

Bubonic Plague
- Fever and lymph node swelling in the groin, cervical, or axillary region depending on the site of the flea bite. See Chapter 31.

Pneumonic Plague
- Presents abruptly with nonspecific symptom of fevers, sweats, malaise, headache, then progressive shortness of breath, **bloody sputum**, and **chest pain** are characteristic.
- Disease rapidly progresses to acute respiratory distress syndrome (ARDS) and respiratory failure and can be rapidly fatal without institution of antibiotic treatment.

- Septicemic plague is a feature of progression from the bubonic and pneumonic phase of the illness. Hallmarks of this stage of the disease include disseminated intravascular coagulation, shock, and widespread purpura.

Immediate Management/Isolation Precautions

- Isolate patient in side room and enforce **barrier and airborne precautions**.
- Inform CDC and liaise with infectious diseases team.
- **Isolate for 72 hours** from start of antibiotic treatment.
- Take blood cultures, sputum, lymph node aspirates, bronchial washing, and serum samples.

Diagnosis

- Samples should be handled in a Biosafety level 2 facility.
- Gram stain of samples may reveal **fat gram-negative bacilli with bipolar staining** arranged singly or in short chains.
- Blood agar or broth cultures should culture the organism (Fig. 47.5).
- The organism is not fastidious but grows slowly.
- The classical bipolar, **"safety-pin"** appearance may be more evident in older cultures.
- Colonies on blood agar at 48 hours are small, grey/white/yellow in color and have an irregular surface.
- Formal identification would usually be done at a CDC facility.
  - PCR or immunofluorescent antibodies can also be used to identify culture-negative samples or postmortem specimens.
  - Demonstration of a serologic response to *Yersinia* with acute and convalescent samples is also possible.
  - Radiographic appearances of lungs include multilobar consolidation and bilateral pleural effusions.

Treatment

- Initial treatment: IV gentamicin and IV ciprofloxacin, minimum 2 weeks.

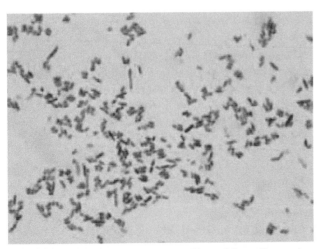

- **Fig. 47.5** *Yersinia pestis* Gram stain and bacterial growth on selective media. (From Drancourt M. Plague. In: Magill AJ, Hill DR, Solomon T, Ryan E, eds. *Hunter's Tropical Medicine and Emerging Infectious Diseases.* 9th ed. Elsevier; 2013.)

- Oral ciprofloxacin is used for mild disease or as a step down with clinical improvement.

Public Health Management and Postexposure Prophylaxis

- For healthcare staff, laboratory workers, and close contacts of cases of pneumonic plague, ciprofloxacin or doxycycline is given for 7 days postexposure.
- No postexposure vaccine available.

Smallpox

Epidemiology

Eradication of smallpox was declared by WHO in 1980 after a global vaccination campaign. The last outbreak of the disease in the United States had been in 1949. Two laboratories in the United States and Russia securely hold the virus.

- Smallpox is caused by the variola virus, part of the *Orthopox* genera and family *Poxviridae*.
- Transmitted by **airborne droplets** and **direct contact** with vesicles and respiratory secretions.
- Person-to-person transmission occurs frequently with **attack rates of 25%.**
  - Smallpox is a human disease that does not affect other animals.
- Mortality is increased at extremes of age; up to 1/3 of cases in epidemic conditions die from the disease.
- **Infectious period** is from onset of fever in the prodromal illness to the last scab separation from the skin.
- IP is 10–16 days.

Smallpox as a Bioweapon

- Highly infectious with large numbers of secondary cases likely.
- Person-to-person spread.
- Unvaccinated populations with no immunity.
- No known effective treatment.
- Severe disease with 25% mortality.

Clinical Features

- A short prodromal illness (3 days) with abrupt fever, severe body aches, headache, malaise, and vomiting is followed by development of mouth sores, and then rash affecting the face, then body and extremities (3 days).
- The rash evolves from widespread erythema to a maculopapular rash, which becomes vesicular then pustular.

> **CLINICAL PEARL**
>
> - Characteristic **deep tense pustules** particularly affect the **extremities and face**, then scab and heal (10 days) (Fig. 47.6).
> - Overall scabs take about 6 days to fall off.
> - Chickenpox, in contrast, has relative sparing of extremities; vesicles crop together and are superficial with quick scabbing and healing (Fig. 47.7).

- Long term effects include significant **scarring** on the face and **blindness.**

Immediate Management/Isolation Precautions

- If suspected, patient should be isolated in a single room as soon as possible and given a surgical mask.
- **Barrier and respiratory precautions** should be employed and transport and areas used by the patient should be isolated.
- As the virus can be transmitted by fomites, bedding and sheets associated with the patient environment will be infected and must be handled with caution and incinerated.
- CDC notification as soon as possible to guide further management.

Diagnosis

- Clinical recognition is key but vesicular fluid and viral throat swabs should be taken for nucleic amplification detection.
- Samples must be processed in a **Biosafety level 4 laboratory.**

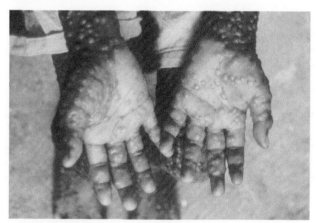

• **Fig. 47.6** Smallpox lesions on the hands. Face and extremities are particularly affected with deep hard blisters. (Courtesy Centers for Disease Control and Prevention Public Health Image Library. ID#: 5163. Photograph taken in 1972 by Dr. Paul B. Dean.)

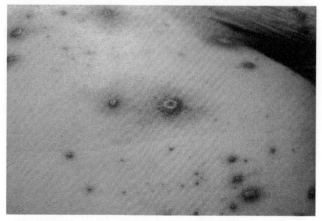

• **Fig. 47.7** Chickenpox vesicles becoming pustules on the trunk. Vesicles are more superficial and characteristically "crop" with lesions at different stages of development.

- Major and minor criteria for diagnosis have been developed by the CDC to aid for differentiating smallpox from other etiologies, and also define the risk of a febrile, vesicular rash illness being smallpox.
- Major criteria include:
  - **Severe** prodromal illness with high fever 1–4 days prerash.
  - Deep, **hard, well circumscribed** vesicles/blisters.
  - All vesicles at **same stage** of development.

Treatment

- There is no known effective antiviral treatment.
- A few antivirals have *in vitro* activity against smallpox, are known to be safe to use *in vivo*, and could be used in the event of cases.
- Cidofovir; tecovirimat (stocks are held by the CDC).
- Management consists of **supportive care**, particularly to replace fluid losses and prevent secondary bacterial infection.

Public Health Management and Postexposure Prophylaxis

- Smallpox vaccine is made from live vaccinia virus, a different pox virus that causes a mild illness.
- Vaccine should be given as soon as possible after exposure to prevent or reduce severity of infection.
  - More effective the earlier it is given (**≤3 days ideally**).
  - Should still be offered within 4–7 days of exposure.
- **"Ring vaccination"** would be employed in a deliberate-release event where contacts of confirmed cases and contacts of contacts are vaccinated.
  - This method was used in the eradication of smallpox campaign to good effect.
- Smallpox vaccine
  - >95% develop neutralizing antibodies after primary vaccination.
  - Vesiculation and pustule formation must occur for a "take" (positive vaccine reaction) to have occurred.
  - Mild to severe adverse effects are well recognized
    - 1/3 mild symptoms requiring time off work/school.
    - Death, progressive vaccinia, generalized vaccinia, postvaccinial encephalitis, and eczema vaccinatum.

Tularemia

See also Chapter 31, Infections Associated with Animal Exposure.

- Caused by *Francisella tularensis.*
- Stockpiled by the US military in the late 1960s.
- IP likely 3–5 days (range 1–14).

Tularemia as a Bioweapon

- Pros: **extreme infectivity** (as few as 10 organisms required for infective dose); could be aerosolized; high mortality rates if untreated; initial symptoms nonspecific so frequently misdiagnosed at first presentation.
- Cons: no human-to-human transmission.

Treatment

- Aminoglycosides (streptomycin or gentamicin); alternatives include doxycycline or ciprofloxacin; 10–14 days required to prevent relapse.

Public Health Management and Postexposure Prophylaxis

- 14 days of doxycycline or ciprofloxacin if early after exposure; otherwise advise fever-watch.
- No postexposure vaccination available.
- No isolation required for patient.
- Significant risk of laboratory-acquired infection; manipulation of cultures which may generate aerosols should be done in BSL-3 conditions.
- Bodies can be handled with normal precautions, but avoid autopsy procedures that may generate aerosols.

Viral Hemorrhagic Fevers

See Chapter 3, Virology.
- Diverse group of RNA viruses.
- Ebola, Marburg, Lassa fever, New World arenaviruses (e.g., Junin), and Crimean–Congo hemorrhagic fever viruses transmit person-to-person naturally.

VHFs as a Bioweapon

- Pros: high infectivity; high morbidity and mortality; lack of effective treatment or vaccination; could be aerosolized for mass dissemination.
- Cons: no airborne transmission onward from infected individuals; routine infection control may be sufficient to halt spread; difficult to acquire, plus unstable in environment, and production of aerosols for weaponry would probably be too challenging to be likely.

Category B Organisms

Coxiella burnetii (Q fever)

See also Chapter 31, Infections Associated with Animal Exposure.
- Transmission primarily by **inhalation** of infected dust/droplets/aerosols.
- IP 18–21 days.
- **Patient isolation not required.**

Coxiella as a Bioweapon

- Pros: **contaminated aerosols may disseminate several kilometers.**
- Cons: person-to-person transmission rare; fatality rate <1%; effective available treatment (doxycycline).

Glanders

Epidemiology

- Caused by *Burkholderia mallei.*
- Zoonosis; primarily a disease of horses, donkeys, or mules.

- Does not persist in the environment.
- Low infective dose; all people considered susceptible.
- Transmission by contact with broken skin or mucous membranes; or by inhalation.
- IP variable – may be as short as 1–2 days with inhalation.

Clinical Features

- Varies from asymptomatic infection to life-threatening disease.
- Ulcerative necrosis of the tracheobronchial tree with regional (neck and mediastinal) lymphadenopathy.
- Respiratory infection with pneumonia, lung abscesses, effusions, or miliary infection.
- Bacteremia with multiple disseminated abscesses including pustular skin lesions.

Immediate Management/Isolation Precautions

- Not considered to be very contagious person-to-person.
- Standard precautions with bodily fluids should be sufficient.

Diagnosis

- By culture of *B. mallei* from blood, exudates, or pus.
- Culture on standard media.
- May be misidentified as a *Pseudomonas* species.

Treatment

- Extrapolated from experience with *Burkholderia pseudomallei.*
- Initial intensive therapy: ceftazidime, meropenem, or imipenem.
- Eradication therapy: trimethoprim–sulfamethoxazole or amoxicillin–clavulanic acid.
  - Required for several months to prevent relapse.

Postexposure Prophylaxis

- No vaccine available.
- Efficacy not established.
- Recommended drugs are trimethoprim–sulfamethoxazole or co-amoxiclav.

Psittacosis

- Caused by *Chlamydophila psittaci* (formerly *Chlamydia psittaci*).
- Usual exposure is through inhalation of dried avian secretions or feces.
- IP 1–4 weeks.

Chlamydophila psittaci as a Bioweapon

- Pros: untreated mortality 15%–20%; availability; usual route of transmission is aerosol.
- Cons: available, effective treatment (doxycycline); mortality <1% with appropriate treatment; no person-to-person onward transmission.

Treatment

- Treatment of choice is doxycycline.
- Can relapse; continue for >10–14 days after fever settles.
- No postexposure treatment required.

Epidemic (Louse-Borne) Typhus

- Caused by *Rickettsia prowazekii*. Caused >30 million cases of typhus during and immediately after World War I, with 3 million deaths attributed.
- Usually louseborne.
- Laboratory-acquired infections due to aerosolization.
- IP 7–14 days.

Epidemic Typhus as a Bioweapon

- Pros: environmental stability, aerosol transmission possible, low infectious dose, high associated morbidity and mortality (untreated case fatality rate 40%).
- Cons: difficult to produce; no onward transmission between human hosts without louse vector; widely available effective treatment.

Clinical Features

- Sudden onset of fever, headache, malaise, severe myalgia, and tachypnea.
  - Rash appears 5–6 days later.
  - Often associated with confusion or drowsiness.
- May get late relapse (Brill–Zinsser disease) decades later.
  - Usually much less severe, but may initiate a reemerging outbreak.

Treatment

- 1st line: doxycycline.
- Alternative: chloramphenicol.
- Usually respond well within 48 hours; consider alternative diagnosis if not.

Further Reading and Resources

1. Health Protection Agency. *CBRN Incidents: Clinical Management and Health Protection.* Biological Agents: Syndromes and Differential Diagnosis. V3.0; 2008. https://tinyurl.com/y6ttlewe.
2. Update: Investigation of anthrax associated with intentional exposure and interim public health guidelines, October 2001. *MMWR Weekly.* 2001;50(41):889–893.
3. Madad J. Bioterrorism: an emerging global health threat. *J Bioterrorism Biodefense.* 2014;5:1.
4. Biosafety in Microbiological and Biomedical Laboratories (BMBL). 5th ed. HHS Publication No. (CDC) 21-1112 Revised December 2009.
5. C.D.C. Emergency. Preparedness and Response. https://emergency.cdc.gov/bioterrorism/index.asp.
6. Public Health England. Guidance: unusual illness: investigation and management of outbreaks and incidents. https://tinyurl.com/y6426yjb.
7. World Health Organization. Public health response to biological and chemical weapons – WHO Guidance. Annex 3: Biological agents. http://www.who.int/csr/delibepidemics/annex3.pdf.

48

Syndromes that Mimic Infectious Diseases

CHRIS KOSMIDIS, GEROME ESCOTA

Introduction

- Certain noninfectious conditions can present with symptoms or signs suggestive of infection, such as fever, chills, sweats, or lymphadenopathy. Laboratory findings may include elevated white cell count and raised inflammatory markers.
- May lead to unnecessary antibiotic use and prolonged hospital stays before a diagnosis is made.
- Conditions mimicking infections are due to a variety of causes, including vasculitic, autoinflammatory, neoplastic, drug-induced, or of unknown etiology.
- It can also be useful to consider them by the predominant features of the presenting clinical syndrome.

Fever as Principal Feature

Systemic Lupus Erythematosus (SLE) and Other Autoimmune Diseases

- Together with vasculitic disorders, SLE and other autoimmune diseases are called **"the great mimics"** as they can manifest with symptoms that masquerade as almost any disease entity; they often elude diagnosis for a good period of time; **neoplastic diseases (particularly lymphoma)**, **tuberculosis**, **syphilis**, and **brucellosis** also share this moniker.
- It is not uncommon for infectious disease providers to be consulted on patients with fever of unknown origin (FUO) who end up having a rheumatologic diagnosis.
- A full discussion of these entities is beyond the scope of this book, but Table 48.1 offers details of tests that can aid in diagnosing autoimmune diseases.

Vasculitis

Giant Cell Arteritis (Large Vessel Vasculitis)

- The most common rheumatologic cause of FUO.

- Consider in a patient older than 50 years with **FUO**, **headaches**, visual disturbances, anemia, high erythrocyte sedimentation rate (ESR), jaw claudication.
- Leads to extensive work-up for infection, including endocarditis.
- Useful investigations include **temporal artery biopsy** and positron emission tomography–computed tomography (PET–CT).
- Biopsy positive in ~40%; increased positivity with abnormal clinical examination such as tenderness, absent temporal pulse, or an enlarged temporal artery.

Kawasaki Syndrome (Medium Vessel Vasculitis)

- Worldwide
  - African-American and Asian ethnicities disproportionately affected.
  - Most <5 years old.
- Diagnosis: fever of at least 5 days plus any 4 of the 5 clinical criteria below (classic Kawasaki):
  - Bilateral conjunctival injection.
  - Erythema of lips and oral mucosa with strawberry tongue (Fig. 48.1A).
  - Rash (polymorphous).
  - Cervical lymphadenopathy.
  - Edema and erythema of hands and feet, followed by desquamation (Fig. 48.1B).
- Patients with fever but meeting <4 criteria are classified as **incomplete Kawasaki.**
- <100 cases of Kawasaki **in adults** reported in literature; adults tend to present more commonly with cervical adenopathy, elevated liver enzymes, arthralgia; they tend to have a lower prevalence of coronary aneurysm.
- Can be confused with childhood infectious exanthems such as measles, adenovirus, Epstein–Barr virus (EBV), scarlet fever; **also mimics toxic shock syndrome, streptococcal scarlet fever.**

TABLE 48.1	Autoantibodies Associated With Autoimmune Diseases	
Autoantibody	**Autoimmune Disease**	**Features**
ANA	SLE >>> systemic sclerosis, Sjögren, mixed connective tissue disease	Very sensitive but not specific
Anti-double-stranded DNA	SLE	Very specific test
Anti-Smith	SLE	Most specific test (>99%)
Anti-U1-RNP	Mixed connective tissue disease	
Anti-Ro/SSA; anti-La/SSB	Sjögren	
Rheumatoid factor	Rheumatoid arthritis	Can be false +ve in hepatitis C
Anticyclic citrullinated peptide	Rheumatoid arthritis	Can be +ve in patients with negative rheumatoid factor
Anti-Scl-70 and anti-centromere	Systemic sclerosis	
Antihistone	Drug-induced lupus	
Anti-Jo-1	Myositis, antisynthetase syndrome	
c-ANCA (antiproteinase-3)	Granulomatosis with polyangiitis (see below)	
p-ANCA (antimyeloperoxidase)	Eosinophilic granulomatosis with polyangiitis (see below)	

ANA, antinuclear antibodies; ANCA, antineutrophil cytoplasmic antibodies.

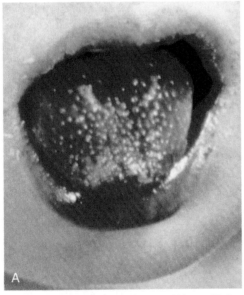
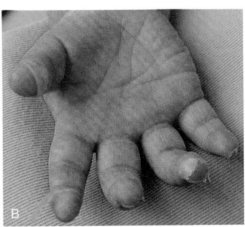

• **Fig. 48.1** Clinical manifestations of Kawasaki disease. (A) Strawberry tongue and (B) desquamation of fingers. (From Kato H. Kawasaki disease. In: Crawford MH, Marco JP, Paulus WJ, eds. *Cardiology.* 3rd ed. Elsevier; 2010.)

- Treatment = **high dose intravenous immunoglobulin (IVIG)** plus **aspirin.**
- **Coronary artery aneurysms** in 25% untreated; drops to 5% with prompt treatment.
- Macrophage activation syndrome is another rare complication.

Other Vasculitides

Takayasu arteritis (large vessel vasculitis)

- Patient presents with fever, arthralgia/myalgia, **extremity claudication, weak pulses**, and discrepant blood pressure measurements.

Polyarteritis nodosa (medium vessel vasculitis)

- Patient presents with fever, peripheral neuropathy, arthralgia/myalgia, abdominal pain, cutaneous disease (**nodules, ulcers, palpable purpura**).
- Also characterized by **multiorgan ischemia** (GI ischemia manifesting as abdominal pain, intestinal bleeding/perforation, ischemic skin; renal ischemia with renal insufficiency; stroke-like manifestations); **mimics infective endocarditis with septic embolization.**
- A classic finding is the demonstration of **multiple aneurysms** and irregular arterial constrictions on mesenteric/renal arteriography; can mimic **mycotic aneurysm.**

Granulomatosis with polyangiitis (GPA)

- Formerly Wegener's granulomatosis; small vessel, ANCA-positive vasculitis.
- Patients present with fever and other constitutional symptoms, **upper respiratory tract disease** (sinusitis, nasal discharge, nasal ulcers, saddle nose deformity), **lower respiratory tract disease** (tracheal stenosis, **chronic pneumonia**), and renal manifestations (glomerulonephritis).
- On biopsy, **granulomas (sometimes necrotizing)** are visualized, thus mimics other infectious granulomatous diseases (e.g.; mycobacterial and fungal infections).

Eosinophilic granulomatosis with polyangiitis (EGPA)

- Formerly Churg–Strauss; small vessel, ANCA-positive vasculitis.
- Patients present with fever, peripheral blood **eosinophilia**, and symptoms that arise from eosinophilic organ infiltration (**chronic pneumonia**, eosinophilic gastroenteritis, glomerulonephritis, heart failure).
- Prior to the development of fever (marks the vasculitic phase of the disease), the patient has had a long history of **refractory asthma.**
- On biopsy, **granulomas** are also seen.

Behçet syndrome

- Recurrent and painful oral/genital ulcers (**mimics HSV infection).**
- Patients can present with fever and other constitutional symptoms.
- Patients have characteristic **pathergy** (papular or pustular reaction that occurs 48 hours after a skin injury, including a needlestick).
- Also mimics infectious causes of chronic and acute meningitis and encephalitis (neuro-Behçet).

IgA vasculitis (formerly Henoch–Schonlein purpura)

- Majority of cases are <20 years old.
- **Rash (palpable purpura) located in the lower extremities (any pressure or gravity-dependent area)**, arthritis/arthralgia, recurrent abdominal pain (can be severe; intussusception may occur), glomerulonephritis.

- **Testicular pain is common (mimics infectious epididymitis).**

Relapsing polychondritis

- Although not technically classified as vasculitis, can accompany and manifest similarly as vasculitic disorders.
- Recurrent ear involvement (pain, tenderness, redness, sparing the ear lobes) **mimics ear infection.**
- Like GPA, can present with recurrent upper respiratory tract disease.
- Can present as FUO.

Neoplastic Disorders

Lymphoma

- May present the same way as tuberculous lymphadenitis, even with the classic triad of fever, sweats, and weight loss.
- Fine-needle aspiration of a lymph node may not be enough to rule out lymphoma; tissue diagnosis may be required via **excisional biopsy.**
- **Pel–Ebstein fever** (cyclic, regular high fever episodes that last for weeks) is classically described in patients with Hodgkin lymphoma although it can occur in other infections and causes of FUO.

Renal Cell Carcinoma

- Can present with intermittent fever (20%), sweats, weight loss.
- Investigations: CT abdomen and tissue for histology; may require nephrectomy to make diagnosis.

Leukemias

- Myelodysplastic disorders, multiple myeloma, and myeloid leukemia may present with fever.
- Aleukemic leukemias have a normal or low peripheral white cell count.
- Diagnosis by bone marrow biopsy.

Atrial Myxoma

- Uncommon, but one-third have fever. Diagnosis by echocardiogram.

Autoinflammatory Diseases

These diseases are caused by **aberrant activation of the innate** immune system. They differ from autoimmune conditions as they are antigen-independent and involve inflammatory mechanisms rather than adaptive immune responses. The majority present with **recurrent fevers and systemic inflammation**, but particular clinical features may dominate, such as rashes or lymphadenopathy. These phenotypes may be used to classify the more heterogeneous disorders.

Hereditary Periodic Fever Syndromes

- Very rare apart from familial Mediterranean fever (FMF) and Periodic Fever with Aphthous Stomatitis, Pharyngitis, and Adenitis (PFAPA syndrome).
- Present with recurrent fevers, **usually in childhood** but about 10% start after the age of 30.
- Often a therapeutic trial with colchicine, steroids, or IL-2 blockage is effective. Genetic testing can contribute.
- If untreated, can lead to secondary amyloidosis.
- **Useful discriminators** include:
  - Duration and periodicity of symptoms.
  - Ethnicity and family history.
  - Associated clinical features.
  - See Table 48.2.

FMF

- The most common periodic fever syndrome; **fever with serositis**, synovitis, and/or rash.
- Autosomal recessive.
- Highest prevalence in people of Turkish, Armenian, Jewish, and Arab descent. Also, Southern Italy, Greece, North Africa. 1/1000 in Turks, 1/250 in Sephardic Jews.
- Starts in childhood, most cases by 20 years of age.
- Clinical features
  - Fever lasts 1–3 days.
  - Abdominal pain with signs of **peritonitis** on exam, which may lead to unnecessary surgery, and **pleuritic** type pain.
  - Rash = typical erysipelas-like erythema on legs.
  - Monoarticular large joint arthritis.
- **Attacks may be precipitated** by stress or menstrual cycle.
- Characteristically **responds to prophylactic colchicine**, which is used in high prevalence areas as diagnostic criterion. Colchicine prevents the emergence of amyloidosis.

TNF-Receptor-Associated Periodic Syndrome (TRAPS)

- Also known as familial Hibernian fever.
- Autosomal dominant with incomplete penetrance.
- Any ethnicity may be affected.
- Presents around 4 years of age, but 10% after the age of 30.
- Fever lasts for 5 days to 2 weeks; may be nearly continuous.
- **Eye involvement common** (periorbital edema, conjunctivitis), also **migratory rash**, muscle and abdominal pains, large joint arthritis.
- **Responds to high-dose steroids**, with maintenance IL-1 inhibitors.

Mevalonate Kinase Deficiency (Hyper IgD Syndrome, HIDS)

- Autosomal recessive.
- Usually presents in 1st year of life. Can be **triggered by vaccinations.**
- Fever lasts 3 to 7 days. Abdominal pain, vomiting, diarrhea, maculopapular rash. 90% have palpable lymphadenopathy, commonly cervical.
- **Elevated IgD** and usually also IgA levels.

Cryopyrin-Associated Periodic Syndrome (CAPS)

- Autosomal dominant.
- Mildest form is also called familial cold autoinflammatory syndrome, presenting with brief episodes of fever, red eyes, and urticarial rash after cold exposure.
- More severe form of neonatal onset can cause meningitis, hearing loss.
- IL-1 inhibition effective.

Periodic Fever with Aphthous Stomatitis, Pharyngitis, and Adenitis (PFAPA Syndrome)

- Relatively common. Age of onset 2–3 years.
- Manifest similarly to the autoinflammatory syndromes, although no genetic defect has been identified yet.
- Symptoms last for 3–6 days and recurs every 3–4 weeks with **regularity.**
- Rapid response to steroids.
- Usually **symptoms abate over time, and patients develop normally.**
- Need to exclude cyclic neutropenia.

TABLE 48.2 Comparison of Hereditary Periodic Fever Syndromes

	Inheritance	Trigger	Length of Attack	Skin	Specifics
FMF	Recessive	Stress; menstrual cycle	1–3 days	Erysipelas-like	Serositis
TRAPS	Dominant	–	>7 days	Migratory rash	Orbital edema
HIDS	Recessive	Vaccinations	4–6 days	Erythematous macular rash	Cervical lymphadenopathy
CAPS	Dominant	Cold	Continuous	Urticaria	Conjunctivitis
PFAPA	Polygenic	No – occur with clockwork regularity	3–6 days	Aphthous ulcers	Abate over time

CAPS, cryopyrin-associated periodic syndrome; FMF, familial Mediterranean fever; HIDS, hyper IgD syndrome; PFAPA, periodic fever, aphthous stomatitis, pharyngitis, adenitis; TRAPS, TNF (tumor necrosis factor) receptor-associated periodic syndrome.

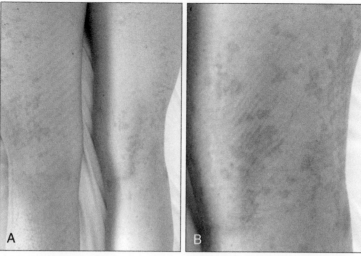

• **Fig. 48.2** Adult onset Still's disease. Example of the typical salmon-pink maculopapular rash affecting the extremities (A) and in more detail (B). (From Alonso ER, Olive A. Adult-onset Still disease. In: Hochberg M, Silman A, Smolen J, et al. *Rheumatology*. 6th ed. Elsevier; 2014.)

Fever and Rash

Adult Onset Still's Disease

- Worldwide; young adults (3/4 patients <35 years at onset).
- Rare, waxing and waning disease.
- Spiking daily fevers >39 °C
  - Classically described as **quotidian** (daily recurring spikes) or **double quotidian** (two spikes per day).
- Sore throat.
- **Evanescent salmon-pink rash** (usually occurs with fever spike) (Fig. 48.2).
- Arthritis, arthralgia, myalgia.
- Cervical lymphadenopathy.
- Hepatomegaly, elevated liver enzymes.
- **Very high ferritin** (>5× upper limit normal). (See Box 48.1.)
- Diagnosis of pattern recognition and exclusion; no specific diagnostic test.
- Differential may include parvovirus B19, viral hepatitis, HIV, bacteremia or endocarditis.
- 1/3 develop chronic arthritis.
- Initial treatment: non-steroidal anti-inflammatory drugs (NSAIDs) or steroids. Methotrexate may be added.
- Severe disease may be life-threatening. Refractory disease may require biologics (IL-1 or IL-6 inhibitors).

Schnitzler's Syndrome

- Presents later in life, usually in the **6th decade.**
- Acquired syndrome, caused by the presence of an IgM paraprotein, although mechanism unclear.
- Daily fevers, chronic **urticarial rash, skeletal hyperostosis on imaging, lymphadenopathy.**
- Most respond well to IL-1 inhibition.
- 15% of cases progress to hematological malignancy.

> **• BOX 48.1 Very High Ferritin Level, Differential Diagnoses**
>
> Think of the following in patients with fever of unknown origin (FUO) and very high ferritin (especially ≥2000 µg/L):
> 1. Adult Still's disease (less sick).
> 2. Hemophagocytic syndrome (sicker patients).

Sweet's Syndrome (Acute Febrile Neutrophilic Dermatosis)

- Abrupt onset of painful skin nodules (Fig. 48.3).
- Idiopathic, paraneoplastic, or drug-induced (typically caused by G-CSF).
- Differential includes bacterial, fungal, or mycobacterial skin infection.
- May be associated with fever, ocular involvement, and leukocytosis.
- Pathergy may occur (lesions develop at sites of cutaneous injury).
- Biopsy and dramatic response to steroids confirm the diagnosis.
- **Can manifest after receipt of granulocyte colony-stimulating factor.**

Drug Reaction With Eosinophilia and Systemic Symptoms (DRESS)

- Rare, drug-induced, potentially life-threatening drug reaction.
  - Fever (38–40 °C).
- Skin rash (rapidly progresses to diffuse and confluent erythema; **>50% body surface** area involved; **facial edema** in 50% cases) (Fig. 48.4).
- **Eosinophilia** (can be absent in some cases); and atypical lymphocytes.

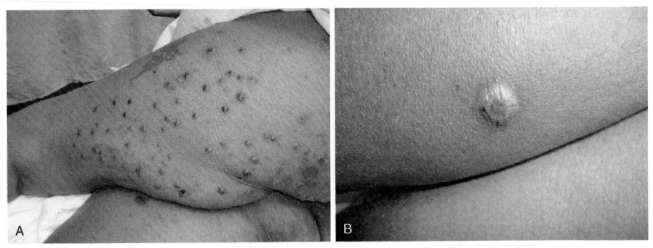

• **Fig. 48.3** Characteristic skin lesions of Sweet's syndrome. (A and B) Multiple tender erythematous papules with a distinct mammillated appearance were seen distributed over bilateral upper and lower extremities. (From Ilias Basha H, Towfiq B, Krznarich TS. Sweet's syndrome as a dermatological manifestation of underlying coronary artery disease. *J Cardiol Cases*. 2012;6(1):e8-e12.)

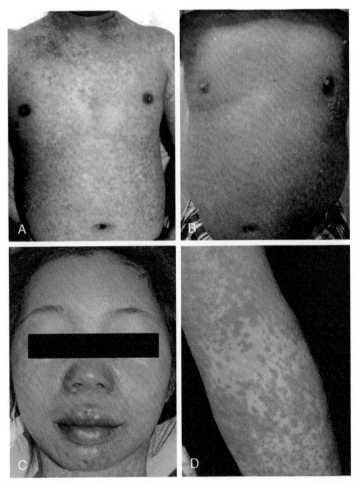

• **Fig. 48.4** Clinical presentations of DRESS/DIHS. (A) The skin rash of DRESS usually begins as a nonspecific morbilliform eruption, which is indistinguishable from other less severe drug reactions, but it can then progress to (B) a generalized infiltrated form or even to exfoliative dermatitis (erythroderma). Typical skin lesions for DRESS are (C) facial edema and (D) confluent and infiltrated plaques. (From Chen YC, Cho YTs, Chang CY et al. Drug reaction with eosinophilia and systemic symptoms: a drug-induced hypersensitivity syndrome with variable clinical features. *Dermatologica Sinica*. 2013;31(4):196–204.)

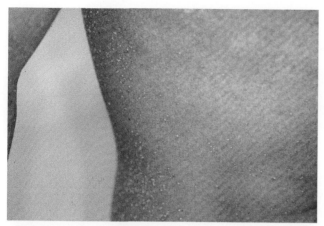

• **Fig. 48.5** Acute generalized exanthematous pustulosis. Note the pinhead-sized nonfollicular pustulosis surrounded by erythematous skin. (From Brinster NK, Liu V, Diwan A, Hafeez MD, McKee P. *Dermatology: High-Yield Pathology.* Elsevier; 2011.)

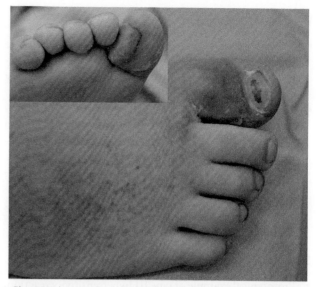

• **Fig. 48.6** Loxoscelism. Patient's right foot showing petechial skin rash and a dermonecrotic lesion in the right big toe with swelling, redness, and an erythematous halo around the necrotic area with the typical gravitational spread of the venom. (From Levin C, Rozemman D, Sakran W, et al. Severe thrombocytopenia and dermonecrosis after *Loxosceles* spider bite in a 3-year-old child. *J Pediatr.* 2013;163(4): 1228–28.e1.)

- • **Lymphadenopathy** (diffuse, tender).
  - • Liver and renal involvement.
- • Begins 2–6 weeks after introduction of drug.
  - • **Antiepileptics** (also known as anticonvulsant hypersensitivity syndrome) and sulfonamides most frequent causes.
  - • May relapse even if causative drug stopped.
- • Associated with reactivation of herpes family viruses (especially EBV, human herpesvirus [HHV] 6 and [**sometimes used as a marker of severe DRESS**] HHV-7).
- • Treatment: **discontinuation of offending drug**; systemic steroids for DRESS with organ involvement.
- • Usually recover within 6–9 weeks, but may last several months with series of relapses.

Acute Generalized Exanthematous Pustulosis (AGEP)

- • Acute and sudden eruption of **pinhead-sized nonfollicular sterile pustules** accompanied by fever; surrounding skin is commonly edematous and erythematous (Fig. 48.5).
- • Drugs (e.g., aminopenicillins, macrolides, quinolones, tetracyclines, **diltiazem**) are the most common inciting agent; rarely, can result from spider bite, or infection (e.g., *Mycoplasma*, parvovirus B19).
- • Diagnosis: clinical and histopathologic.
- • Treatment: **discontinuation of offending drug** (clinical resolution occurs in 2 weeks); **systemic steroids are not indicated.**

Acute Pustular Psoriasis of von Zumbusch

- • A rare subclassification of pustular psoriasis.
- • **Very similar presentation as AGEP** with acute and sudden eruption of pustules on a background of erythematous skin associated with fever and other constitutional symptoms.
- • **"Lake of pus"** can sometimes happen when tiny pustules coalesce.

- • **30%–70% of patients have a history of another form of psoriasis** (usually plaque psoriasis).
- • **Withdrawal of systemic or topical steroids** can precipitate disease.
- • Other precipitation factors: pregnancy (disease is also known as **impetigo herpetiformis**), immunomodulating agents, antimicrobials (e.g., amoxicillin, terbinafine).

Loxoscelism

- • Systemic symptoms (fever, nausea, vomiting, myalgia, malaise) that accompany the bite of recluse spiders.
- • Secondary to the recluse spider venom sphingomyelinase D which activates complement and incites neutrophil chemotaxis.
  - • **Severe manifestations**: acute hemolytic anemia, disseminated intravascular coagulopathy, rhabdomyolysis.
  - • Often, patients will present with **symptoms of loxoscelism** and a necrotic or nonnecrotic **skin lesion** on exam (degree of systemic symptoms does not correlate with the extent of the bite); note that patients do not always remember a spider bite or seeing spiders in the vicinity (in this situation, maintain a high index of suspicion). (See Fig. 48.6.)
- • Treatment is supportive.
  - • **Dapsone has no role** in treating bite necrosis and should be avoided.
  - • Early surgical debridement is also not recommended.
  - • **Antivenom** (not available in the United States) is used for severe loxoscelism.

Weber–Christian Disease

- A broad term that encompasses the acute, subacute appearance of deep-seated nodules and plaques associated with **systemic symptoms including fever**; biopsy often shows **lobular panniculitis.**
- The term is no longer used; cases of Weber–Christian disease reported in the literature have been reclassified into specific disease entities (i.e., pancreatic panniculitis, lymphoma panniculitis, alpha-1-antitrypsin panniculitis, etc.).
- Can mimic a wide variety of infectious diseases, including cellulitis, systemic fungal and mycobacterial infections, leprosy (lepra reactions).

Serum Sickness Syndrome

- Prototypical example of type III hypersensitivity reaction.
- **Triad of fever**, **rash**, and **polyarthralgia/polyarthritis** that occur days after introduction of the offending agent (antimicrobial toxins such as equine antirabies, vaccines, monoclonal antibodies, antibiotics, specifically **cefaclor**, sulfa, and penicillin).
- **Other causes: insect bites**, **bee stings**, **infectious agents associated with circulating immune complexes** (e.g., **acute hepatitis B infection**, **infective endocarditis**).
- Symmetric arthritis involving the **metacarpophalangeal joints**, wrists, knees, and shoulders.
- Treatment: discontinuation of offending agent; systemic steroids in severe cases.

Fever, Muscular Rigidity, Mental Status Change

Serotonin Syndrome

- Occurs by (1) interaction between serotonergic agents and monoamine oxidase inhibitors; (2) overdose of serotonergic agents; (3) concomitant use of multiple serotonergic agents.
- Onset <24 hours.
- Clinical features (closely resemble neuroleptic malignancy syndrome, see Box 48.2):
  - Mental status changes (e.g., confusion, anxiety, restlessness, euphoria).
  - Autonomic manifestations (e.g., **fever, tachycardia, tachypnea**, hypertension, **diaphoresis**, **GI symptoms**).
  - Neuromuscular hyperactivity (e.g., tremor, hyperreflexia, muscle rigidity, clonus).
  - Leukocytosis and DIC may occur.
- Supportive management, usually self-limited with removal of offending agent; **cyproheptadine** in severe and refractory cases.

Neuroleptic Malignant Syndrome

- **Life-threatening** neuroleptic-induced catatonia.

> • BOX 48.2 | **Clinical Features of Serotonin Syndrome and Neuroleptic Malignant Syndrome**
>
> **Common to Both**
> - Fever (or hyperthermia), mental status change, muscular rigidity with elevated creatinine kinase, leucocytosis, metabolic acidosis, elevated AST, and ALT.
>
> **Unique Features**
> - Serotonin syndrome: tremors, hyperreflexia, myoclonus are very common.
> - Neuroleptic malignant syndrome: tremors, hyperreflexia, myoclonus are *rare*; hyporeflexia and bradykinesia are common.

- Usually within 2 weeks of starting the offending drug, but idiosyncratic.
- Drugs implicated: neuroleptics (e.g., haloperidol, chlorpromazine, risperidone, olanzapine) and antiemetics (e.g., metoclopramide, promethazine).
- May also be seen after withdrawal/change of treatment in Parkinson's.
- Clinical features (onset over 1–3 days), closely resemble serotonin syndrome, see Box 48.2:
  - Mental status change (mutism, stupor).
  - Autonomic dysfunction (**fever**, tachycardia, hypertension, tachypnea**).
  - **Rigidity.**
  - Raised **creatinine kinase (CK);** >4× upper limit of normal.
  - Leukocytosis common.
- Treatment: supportive; bromocriptine and dantrolene also used.

Malignant Hyperthermia

- Also manifests as hyperthermia, rigidity with elevation of creatinine kinase, metabolic acidosis.
- Occurs in predisposed individuals after receipt of volatile anesthetics (e.g., halothane) or succinylcholine.
- Treatment: supportive, **dantrolene.**

Anticholinergic Poisoning

- Acetylcholine blocked at both central and peripheral muscarinic receptors.
- Clinical features
  - Fever ("hot as a hare"), flushing ("red as a beet"), anhidrosis ("dry as a bone"), nonreactive mydriasis ("blind as a bat"), altered mental status ("mad as a hatter"), urinary retention ("full as a flask"), tachycardia.
  - **Muscular rigidity is not present, but anticholinergic overdose may be mistaken for serotonin syndrome, neuroleptic malignant syndrome, or malignant hyperthermia.**

- Numerous agents in overdose may cause the syndrome, including:
  - Plants (e.g., deadly nightshade); atropine and related agents; antispasmodics; antiparkinsonian drugs; topical mydriatics; antihistamines (e.g., chlorphenamine); antipsychotics (e.g., clozapine).

Fever and Cytopenia

Hemophagocytic Lymphohistiocytosis (HLH)

- A **life-threatening disorder** of excessive immune activation and inflammation with tissue destruction.
- May be single or recurrent episodes.
- Can be precipitated by infection, usually viral (particularly **EBV**), but other infections have precipitated HLH as well (e.g., *Histoplasma*, *Ehrlichia*, tuberculosis, parvovirus B19, and many others).
- Can usually mimic FUO, severe sepsis with multiorgan failure, acute hepatitis, acute encephalitis/meningitis.
- Criteria for diagnosis (**5 of 8 criteria should be met**):
  - Fever.
  - Splenomegaly.
  - Blood cytopenia (Hgb <9 g/dL, platelet <100,000/µL, absolute neutrophil count <1000/µL).
  - Hypertriglyceridemia (fasting triglyceride >265 mg/dL) and/or hypofibrinogenemia (fibrinogen <150 mg/dL).
  - Demonstration of hemophagocytosis on liver, lymph node, spleen, or bone marrow biopsy (**this histopathologic finding is not enough by itself to diagnose HLH**).
  - Low or absent natural killer cell activity.
  - High soluble CD25.
  - Ferritin >500 ng/mL (**usually even higher**; see Box 48.1).
- Treatment: involves the use of etoposide, dexamethasone, with or without intrathecal methotrexate; stem cell transplant in refractory cases.

Thrombotic Thrombocytopenic Purpura

- Occurs as a result of a decrease in the function of ADAMTS13, a protease that inactivates von Willebrand factor; **thrombotic microangiopathy** results (i.e., platelet-rich plugs present in small vessels).
- Classically manifests as the pentad of fever, microangiopathic hemolytic anemia (**schistocytes** on blood smear [Fig. 48.7], see Box 48.3), thrombocytopenia, renal abnormalities, and neurologic findings (seizure, stroke, coma, mental status change).
- But pentad rarely seen now with earlier diagnosis and treatment; most common presentations now are microangiopathic anemia, thrombocytopenia, neurologic and renal manifestations; 50% will have normal creatinine; fever is less common, and frank renal failure is rare.

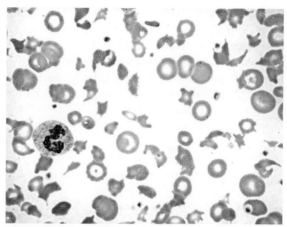

• Fig. 48.7 Schistocytes in microangiopathic hemolytic anemia (peripheral smear). (From Hudnall SD. *Haematology: A Pathophysiologic Approach.* Elsevier; 2012.)

• BOX 48.3 Causes of Microangiopathic Hemolytic Anemia With Presence of Schistocytes

Schistocytes are a hallmark of microangiopathic hemolytic anemia (i.e., Coombs-negative intravascular hemolysis, low haptoglobin, indirect hyperbilirubinemia, high LDH).
Causes:
- Thrombotic thrombocytopenic purpura
- Disseminated intravascular coagulation
- Hemolytic uremic syndrome
- Defective mechanical heart valve
- Catastrophic antiphospholipid antibody syndrome (see below).

- People with HIV and autoimmune diseases are predisposed to developing TTP.
- Treatment: **plasma exchange** and steroids.

Pneumonia Mimics

Organizing Pneumonia

- Presents with cough, mild dyspnea, fever, and weight loss of a few weeks' duration.
- Moderate leukocytosis and raised C-reactive protein.
- Symptoms are indistinguishable from those of an infectious pneumonia. The usual clue is lack of response to antibiotics.
- Most cases are cryptogenic, although connective tissue disease or medications may play a role.
- Lung biopsy establishes the diagnosis: characterized by buds of intraalveolar granulation tissue.
- Reversible with corticosteroids.

Acute Interstitial Pneumonia (Hamman–Rich Syndrome)

- Rare but represents the **most acute, fulminant, and progressive** kind of idiopathic interstitial pneumonia.

- Prodromal illness of about 1–2 weeks occurs before a rapid deterioration of respiratory function; heralded by cough, fever, and progressive dyspnea.
- Differential diagnoses would include rapidly progressive infectious pneumonia, hypersensitivity pneumonitis, drug-induced alveolar damage, radiation-induced pneumonitis, eosinophilic pneumonia.
- Diagnosis: acute respiratory distress syndrome-picture, lung biopsy showing diffuse alveolar damage in the absence of inciting agents mentioned above.
- Treatment: supportive, high-dose steroids.

Hypersensitivity Pneumonitis

- Mimics acute, subacute, and chronic forms of infectious pneumonia.
- Mimics true fungal and mycobacterial pneumonia in that **lung biopsy often demonstrates granulomas** (however, **almost always noncaseating** in contrast to true infectious granulomas that are usually caseating).
- Triggers: moldy hay (fungal elements; **"farmer's lung"**), water/ventilation-associated (**"hot-tub lung"** caused by *Mycobacterium avium* complex), bird excreta (**"bird fancier's lung"**), cotton mill dust (byssinosis or **"brown lung"**).
- Diagnosis: known and consistent exposure (**abrupt onset of signs and symptoms with exposure [no prodromal symptoms]** unlike the gradual development of symptoms within days for true infectious pneumonia). Bronchoalveolar lavage (BAL) can demonstrate lymphocyte-predominance with **low CD4 to CD8 ratio**, biopsy with noncaseating granuloma, inhalation challenge.
- Treatment: discontinuation of exposure to offending agents, supportive, steroids.
  - *Mycobacterium avium* complex-associated hypersensitivity pneumonitis may need antimycobacterial agents if symptoms persist after avoidance of exposure and steroid therapy.

Daptomycin-Induced Eosinophilic Pneumonia

- A syndrome of fever and dyspnea that occurs with the use of daptomycin.
- The median duration of onset is 2–3 weeks; onset of symptoms is not dose-dependent.
- **Peripheral eosinophilia is common (80%) although not required for diagnosis**; BAL usually demonstrates **>25% eosinophils.**
- Treatment: discontinuation of daptomycin; adjunctive steroids in more severe cases; improvement occurs 1–7 days after.
- Should be entertained in any patient who develops respiratory symptoms **while receiving** daptomycin (note that **breakthrough bacterial pneumonia** can occur as well

given that daptomycin only covers gram-positive organisms and that the drug is significantly inactivated by pulmonary surfactant).

Lymphadenopathy

Sarcoidosis

- Multisystem granulomatous disorder; unknown etiology.
- Characterized by noncaseating granulomata.
- Common features = hilar lymphadenopathy, lung infiltrates (Fig. 48.8), eye, skin, and joint lesions.
- In the absence of extrapulmonary findings, sarcoidosis presenting with hilar or mediastinal lymphadenopathy is difficult to distinguish clinically from mycobacterial infection, lymphoma, and fungal infection.
- Diagnostic uncertainty may lead to empirical treatment for tuberculosis before steroids are considered.

Kikuchi's Disease

- Etiology unknown, but thought to be due to T-cell and histiocyte response to an infective organism.
- Presents as **fever (usually low grade, 35%) and cervical lymphadenopathy (100%)** typically in a young female (classically described mostly in women of Asian descent; but Caucasians and other races can be significantly affected as well).
- Differential may include toxoplasmosis, mononucleosis, or tuberculosis.
- Can sometimes **overlap with SLE** (some patients develop SLE over time).
- Diagnosis is by excision biopsy with characteristic **histology** (will show **necrosis and significant histiocytic infiltration**).
- Treatment: steroids.

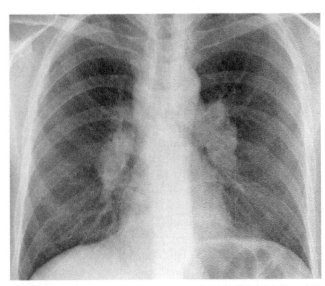

• **Fig. 48.8** Sarcoidosis. (From Hansell DM, Lynch DA, McAdams HP, Banker AA. Mediastinal and aortic disease. In: *Imaging of Diseases of the Chest.* Elsevier; 2010.)

Gastrointestinal Syndromes

Inflammatory Bowel Disease (IBD)

- IBD of the ileum and cecum may mimic tuberculosis.
- Distal disease can mimic sexually transmitted infection such as *N. gonorrhoeae*, LGV, or HSV.
- Acute presentations of IBD may mimic *Salmonella*, *Shigella*, *Campylobacter*, *Yersinia*, amebiasis, or CMV infection.

Cellulitis Mimics

Wells Disease (Eosinophilic Cellulitis)

- Characterized by the development of erythematous plaques and swelling that mimics infectious cellulitis (Fig. 48.9); can be painful or pruritic; blisters, bullae, papules, nodules can also be seen.
- Fever, malaise, arthralgia are common.
- Does not respond to antibiotics.
- A helpful clue is the presence of **peripheral eosinophilia although present only in 2/3 of cases.**
- Biopsy demonstrates eosinophilic infiltration.
- Treatment: steroids (oral > topical).
- Note: **Shulman's disease** is another eosinophilic skin disorder that solely involves the fascia (eosinophilic fasciitis); **not accompanied by fever or any systemic symptoms**; manifests acutely or subacutely with **symmetric swelling** of the extremities.

Pyoderma Gangrenosum

- Characterized by the development of a pustule that rapidly progresses to form an ulcer with undermined border and purulent base (Fig. 48.10); **lesions are painful** and patients may or may not have fever.
  - Characterized by **pathergy** (i.e., lesions typically appear in sites of trauma such as peripheral IV sites, puncture/surgical wounds) (see Box 48.4).
  - Strong association with inflammatory bowel disease, hematologic malignancies, inflammatory arthritis, other autoimmune diseases.
  - Diagnosis: skin biopsy demonstrates **neutrophilic dermatoses** (i.e., intense neutrophilic infiltration of **all layers of the skin** in the absence of infection); **multiple bacterial/fungal/mycobacterial cultures are negative.**
- Can occur with other manifestations in certain genetic conditions:
  - **PAPA syndrome**: pyogenic arthritis, pyoderma gangrenosum, acne.
  - **PAPASH syndrome**: pyogenic arthritis, pyoderma gangrenosum, acne, suppurative hidradenitis.
- **Treatment**: surgical debridement should be reserved for necrotic lesions only (lesions tend to get worse with surgery because of pathergy); systemic steroids.

Erythromelalgia

- Characterized by the intermittent development of redness, warmth, and pain, usually of the distal lower extremities (Fig. 48.11).

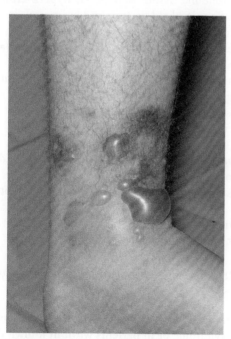

• **Fig. 48.9** Wells disease. Note the blisters and erythema that can be mistaken for cellulitis. (From Alwan W, Benton E, Coulson I. Wells syndrome. In: Lebwohl MG, Heymann WR, Berth-Jones J, Coulson IH, eds. *Treatment of Skin Disease: Comprehensive Therapeutic Strategies*. 5th ed. Elsevier; 2018.)

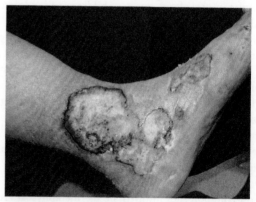

• **Fig. 48.10** Pyoderma gangrenosum. Note the undermined border and purulent base. (From Callen JP, Jackson JM. Pyoderma gangrenosum: an update. *Rheum Dis Clin North Am.* 2007;3(4):787–802.)

• BOX 48.4 Causes of Pathergy

- Sweet's syndrome
- Pyoderma gangrenosum
- Behçet syndrome (skin lesions)
  Note: they all demonstrate neutrophilic dermatosis on skin biopsy.

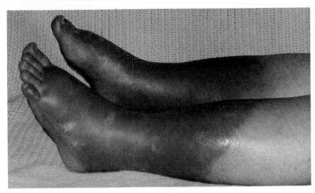

• **Fig. 48.11** Erythromelalgia. (From Mørk C, Kvernebo K. Erythromelalgia. In: Lebwohl MG, Heymann WR, Berth-Jones J, Coulson IH, eds. *Treatment of Skin Disease: Comprehensive Therapeutic Strategies.* 5th ed. Elsevier; 2018.)

- **Increase in ambient temperature and exercise** are known precipitating factors; **patients report cooling the area with cold shower causes symptom relief.**
- Although **intermittent**, can be continuous for several days to months.
- **Classically associated with myeloproliferative diseases.**
- Treatment: no cure; supportive and symptom relief only; treatment of underlying disease.

Osteomyelitis Mimics

Chronic Recurrent Multifocal Osteomyelitis (CRMO)

- An inflammatory condition with incompletely understood pathogenesis.
- Occurs most often among children and adolescents, although seen in adults as well.
- As the name implies, it is characterized by **relapsing and remitting bone pain** associated with **fever** over a course of **several months to years; patients are usually asymptomatic between episodes.**
- Often, but not always, **more than two noncontiguous sites/bones** are involved.
- Associated with elevated inflammatory markers; **magnetic resonance imaging (MRI) demonstrates features suggestive of osteomyelitis**; cultures are negative.
- Does not respond to antibiotics.
- Most common sites involved are the **metaphyseal areas of long bones** (e.g., distal tibia, femur, clavicle, mandible, spine).
- Diagnosis: exclusion of infection; MRI, radionuclide bone scan; pathology shows nonspecific inflammation.
- Treatment: supportive; pain control with NSAIDs; occasionally steroids.

Synovitis, Acne, Pustulosis, Hyperostosis, Osteitis (SAPHO) Syndrome

- An autoinflammatory condition; exact mechanism is unknown but thought to involve genetic factors and immune dysregulation.

- **Unlike CRMO, affects mostly adults in the 3rd to 5th decade of life.**
- Like CRMO, one of the major manifestation is **recurrent bone pain with elevated inflammatory markers ± fever**; imaging will show synovitis, osteitis, and hyperostosis (late manifestation; bony overgrowth and sclerosis).
- Cutaneous lesions are commonly acneiform and various degree of pustulosis; skin biopsy often demonstrates evidence of **neutrophilic dermatosis.**
- **"Bull's head" sign** (Fig. 48.12): classic bilateral and symmetric sternoclavicular increased uptake seen on radionuclide bone scan.
- Treatment: supportive; NSAIDs, methotrexate, immunomodulating agents.

Other ID Mimics

Anti-NMDA Receptor Encephalitis

- Mimics acute/subacute viral encephalitis.
- **Relatively common disease**; in the California Encephalitis Project, the largest cohort study of the epidemiology of encephalitis, **anti-NMDA receptor encephalitis rivals viral etiologies as a cause of encephalitis.**
- Occurs more commonly among **young females**, of whom **50% have associated unilateral or bilateral ovarian teratoma**; older women can be affected, but only 10% have demonstrable neoplasm; other kinds of neoplasms have been reported as well.
- Autoimmune encephalitis characterized by:
  - Autonomic dysfunction (fever, **hyperthermia**, fluctuations in blood pressure and heart rate).
  - Prominent psychiatric manifestations (e.g., **bizarre behavior**, **disorganized speech**, **agitation/anxiety**, **hallucinations**).
  - Unusual motor dyskinesia (e.g., dystonia, **catatonia**, rigidity, opisthotonus), echolalia, mutism, memory loss.
  - Seizure.
- CSF with lymphocyte-predominant pleocytosis.
- **Brain MRI and EEG are nonspecific and often normal.**
- Diagnosis: demonstration of anti-NMDA receptor antibody in the serum or CSF.
- Treatment: resection of tumor if found; steroids and other immunosuppressive agents.

Catastrophic Antiphospholipid Antibody Syndrome

- Occurs in patients with known antiphospholipid antibody syndrome **or in patients without known disease.**
- Characterized by the rapid development of thrombotic infarctions of at least three organ systems associated with systemic signs and symptoms (leukocytosis, fever, elevated inflammatory markers).

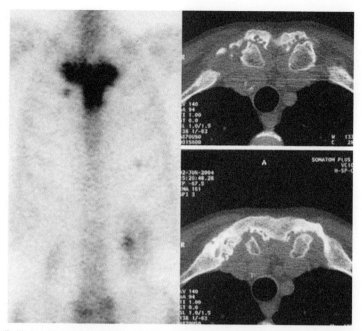

• **Fig. 48.12** "Bull's head" pattern. Radionuclide bone scintigraphy demonstrating the characteristic "bull's head" pattern of tracer uptake in the left sternoclavicular region; axial computed tomography images showing erosive change of both sternoclavicular regions with hyperostosis in the right sternocostal region. (From Depasquale R, Kumar N, Lalam RK, et al. SAPHO: what radiologists should know. *Clin Radiol.* 2012;67:195–206.)

- Similar to thrombotic thrombocytopenic purpura and disseminated intravascular coagulation, also characterized by microangiopathic hemolytic anemia (i.e., demonstrable schistocytes on peripheral blood smear) (see Box 48.3).
- Also mimics severe sepsis, multiorgan dysfunction syndrome, acute infective endocarditis, vasculitis.
- Diagnosis: ruling out disseminated intravascular coagulation, thrombotic thrombocytopenic purpura; demonstration of multiple infarcts on biopsy or imaging; **positive antiphospholipid antibody work-up** (e.g., **lupus anticoagulant, anticardiolipin antibody, anti-beta-2 glycoprotein 1 antibody**).

IgG4-Related Diseases

- A new entity that now encompasses a growing list of disease entities and manifestations that were previously thought to be separate entities.
- Characterized by a proliferative, tumor-like infiltration of multiple organ systems by a **lymphoplasmacytic-predominant, IgG4-rich, cell population** leading to organ dysfunction.
- Common syndromes that can mimic infections:
  - Thoracic or abdominal aortitis (Fig. 48.13).
  - Pulmonary IgG4-related disease, including interstitial pneumonitis.
  - Chronic pachymeningitis.
  - Diffuse lymphadenopathy.

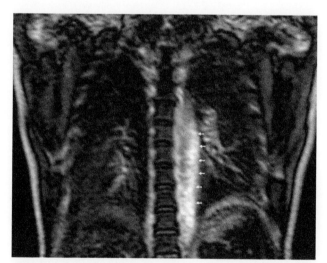

• **Fig. 48.13** Sclerosing periaortitis, presented as a hyperintense circumferential periaortic mass around the thoracic aorta, as it was assessed by late gadolinium-enhanced T1 imaging in a patient with IgG4-related cardiovascular involvement. (From Mavrogeni S, Markousis-Mavrogenis G, Kolovou G. IgG4-related cardiovascular disease: the emerging role of cardiovascular imaging. *Eur J Radiol.* 2017;86:169–175.)

  - Salivary gland enlargement.
  - Others: skin manifestation, prostatitis, constrictive pericarditis, midline-destructive lesions.
- Enters in the differential diagnosis for chronic mycobacterial (especially tuberculosis) and fungal infections.
- Diagnosis: **serum IgG4 usually elevated**; biopsy showing **IgG4-rich plasma cells.**

49
High Yield Biostatistics

MARGARET A. OLSEN

Introduction

Knowledge of basic statistical methods and interpretation is essential in infectious diseases just as it is in all of medicine. This chapter will focus on an overview of study designs commonly used in studies of infectious diseases, discussion of statistical tests used for bivariate analyses of categorical and continuous data, strategies for development of multivariable models, and performance characteristics of diagnostic tests. The chapter is designed as a brief introduction to the concepts and methods, with the understanding that more in-depth studies of statistical methods is necessary for those who plan to interpret published studies or analyze data on their own. Some of the topics are not tested on boards, but they are important for understanding and interpreting the data for the rest of your career. The topics that lend themselves well to testing on the boards will be highlighted.

Definitions

Incidence: number of new cases of a disease in a time period/number in population at risk.

Prevalence: number of existing cases of a disease/total population.

Types of variables
    Dependent: outcome.
    Independent: risk factor, exposure.
    Nominal: categorical variable, cannot be ordered (e.g., gender).
    Ordinal: categorical variable, can be ordered. Distance may not be equal between categories (e.g., Glasgow Coma Scale).
    Continuous: quantitative data that can be measured, with no restriction on values within a selected range (e.g., height, weight, serum creatinine).

Independent samples: samples are not dependent on each other (i.e., cannot determine the members of one sample with information from the other). Matched pairs are dependent samples.

Parametric test: test based on the assumption of normal distribution of the data. The parameter tested is the mean, assuming it is the appropriate measure of central tendency. If this is not true, nonparametric tests, which do not assume that the data follows a specific distribution, should be used.

Errors and power
    Type 1: error that occurs when the null hypothesis is rejected when it is true. In most instances we allow a 5% chance of a type 1 error (i.e., $\alpha = 0.05$).
    Type 2: error that occurs when the null hypothesis is not rejected, but it is false. The type 2 error = ß.
    Power is the probability of rejecting the null hypothesis when it is false, equal to 1-ß. It can also be reworded as the probability of detecting a significant difference when it truly exists. In most studies power = 0.80 is considered sufficient. A nonsignificant finding in a study with lower power is not sufficient to conclude lack of an association.

Confounder: an additional factor B that distorts the relationship between an outcome and an exposure A. A confounding variable is associated with both the outcome and exposure A.

Common Study Designs in Infectious Diseases

Cross-Sectional

- Exposures and outcome assessed simultaneously.
- Cannot determine causation since temporality cannot be established.

Example
- National Health and Nutrition Examination Survey. Used to identify risk factors for methicillin-resistant *Staphylococcus aureus* (MRSA) colonization in screened participants.

Ecological

- Exposures and outcomes compared in aggregate data.
- Weakest study design.
- No inferences can be made about individuals from aggregate data.

- Cannot determine causation.
- Inability to control for potential confounders.

Examples
- Comparison of regional sexually transmitted disease incidence and condom sales.
- Comparison of state cigarette excise taxes and prevalence of periodontitis.
- Comparison of prevalence of antibiotic-resistant infections by country-level consumption of antibiotics.

Case–Control

- Always retrospective.
- Cases with disease identified and controls without disease selected for comparison.
  - Optimal case:control ratio 1:4 to achieve maximum power and efficiency.
  - Information from cases and controls must be collected in the same way to avoid information bias.
  - Controls must be selected from the same population as the cases (i.e., controls have to have opportunity to be a case).
- Odds ratio is used to measure association of exposure with disease.
- Advantage: efficient design for diseases with low incidence.
- Disadvantages
  - May have recall bias, since information collected about potential risk factors after determination of disease status.
  - Inability to calculate incidence, due to lack of information on the entire population.

Examples
- Cases with surgical site infection (SSI) compared to sample of uninfected persons after spine surgery to identify risk factors for SSI.
- Cases with gastroenteritis after eating in hospital A cafeteria compared to sample of uninfected persons who ate in hospital A cafeteria in the same time frame.

Cohort

- Prospective cohort is the strongest observational study design.
  - Classic design involves selection of all individuals with particular exposure compared to those without the exposure.
  - Can also include all patients in a defined population, e.g.,
    - Framingham Study.
    - Olmstead County residents.
    - Follow individuals for a predefined time for development of outcome.
  - Advantages of prospective cohort:
    - Clear establishment of temporal relationship between exposure and outcome.

- Ability to calculate incidence of disease.
- Relative risk used to measure association of exposure with disease.
  - In some cohort studies odds ratio calculated. Important to remember that the odds ratio only approximates the relative risk when the outcome is rare (usually defined as <10%).
- Can also be done retrospectively.

Examples
- Prospective: Multicenter AIDS Cohort Study of >7000 men begun in 1984 to study the epidemiology of HIV/AIDS in the male homosexual/bisexual community (aidscohortstudy.org).
- Retrospective: all patients who underwent lung transplant at Center A from 1990 to 2005 to study incidence and risk factors for nontuberculous mycobacterial infections.

Randomized Controlled Trial

- The randomized controlled trial (RCT) is the strongest study design in terms of establishing causation.
  - Eligible participants randomized to treatment (e.g., treatment A vs. B, treatment A vs. placebo).
    - Optimal design will include blinding of investigators and participants to treatment assignment.
  - Assuming adequate design and sample size, measured and unmeasured confounders equally distributed among the groups.
- Allows for calculation of the average effect of treatment in the population (i.e., what would happen if participants eligible for treatment were treated?).
- RCTs result in the strongest internal validity (accurate determination of differences between groups in the study).
  - External validity (generalizability of results to the broader population) may be poor, particularly if stringent inclusion criteria used to identify eligible participants.
- RCTs should follow CONSORT (Consolidated Standards of Reporting Trials) guidelines.

Types of Statistical Tests for Independent Samples

Choice of Statistical Tests for Categorical and Continuous Variables (see Table 49.1)

- For categorical variables basic tests include Chi-square, Fisher's exact, and logistic regression.
- Collect continuous data as continuous whenever possible to avoid loss of information.
  - Gives maximum flexibility in analysis.
- Check frequencies of all variables before starting analyses.
  - Missing data: figure out why it is missing and correct if possible.

TABLE 49.1	Choice of Statistical Tests for Categorical and Continuous Variables	

		Dependent Variable (Y)	
		Categorical	Continuous
Independent Variable (X)	Categorical	X², Fisher's exact, logistic regression	Student's t-test, one-way ANOVA
	Continuous	Logistic regression	Scatterplot, Pearson correlation, linear regression

- May need to use imputation if truly missing.
- Outliers: correct if possible.
- For nominal/ordinal data, if some categories have small numbers may have to collapse categories for analysis.
- Check 2 × 2 tables (or larger for variables with >2 categories). Determine if numbers in cells sufficient for comparison.
- Graphical representation of data
  - Categorical: bar charts, pie charts.
  - Continuous: box plots, histogram, scatterplot.

Types of Statistical Tests

Parametric Tests for Continuous Variables (see Table 49.2)

- For continuous variables the assumptions for the statistical model must hold (e.g., assumptions for Student's t-test are statistical independence between groups, data normally distributed in the population, and equal population variances).
- Comparable tests available for matched samples.
  - Easiest way is to visualize the data by plotting the histogram (eyeball test).
  - Kolmogorov–Smirnov test. KS test is very sample size-dependent, so visualization may be better in large samples.
- Parametric–nonparametric equivalents (Table 49.2).
- Most commonly have dichotomous-dependent variable (e.g., infection yes/no, treatment successful yes/no).

Logistic Regression

- Use when dichotomous dependent variable, equal follow-up time.
- Approximate rule: one independent variable for every 10 outcomes.

Example

- For dependent variable SSI within 90 days after surgery, if have 54 SSI can include up to 5 independent variables in model.

Cox Proportional Hazards

- Time to event model. Use if do not have equal follow-up time in the population.
- Same approximate rule for number of independent variables in model (1 per 10 outcomes).

TABLE 49.2	Parametric and Nonparametric Test Equivalents	
Type of Variable	Parametric Test	Nonparametric Test
Nominal	N/A	X², Fisher's exact
Ordinal	N/A	X², Spearman correlation, Kruskal–Wallis test
Continuous (2 groups)	Pearson correlation, Student's t-test	Spearman correlation, Mann–Whitney U test
Continuous (> = 3 groups)	One-way ANOVA	Kruskal–Wallis test

- Censor at loss to follow-up, participant withdrawal, or end of study. Assumption is outcome still possible at time of censoring (i.e., truly lost to follow-up, noninformative censoring).
  - When censoring is informative (e.g., death, another competing outcome), may need to treat censor time as competing risk with analysis of cause-specific hazards.
  - Example of competing risk: dependent variable death due to infection; death due to other causes is a competing risk.

How to Approach Creation of a Multivariable Model

- Perform bivariate analyses of all potential independent variables with the dependent variable.
- Include independent variables in model based on:
  - Clinical knowledge of risk factors for outcome.
  - Variables associated with outcome in bivariate analysis.
    - Remember that potential confounders do not have to be significantly associated with both the outcome and another exposure. For this reason the threshold for inclusion of potential risk factors to be included in initial multivariable models is often higher ($\alpha = 0.1$ or higher) to ensure adjustment for confounding variables.
- Do not include variables with small cell sizes (<5) in bivariate analysis.

- Check independent variables for collinearity. Highly collinear variables (e.g., recent cancer and treatment with chemotherapy) will create instability in the model.
  - Use clinical knowledge to select the most relevant among collinear variables for inclusion.
  - Example: What is likely the true reason for increased risk of infection: the underlying malignancy or the treatment with chemotherapy?
- Inclusion of continuous variables in multivariable model.
  - Inclusion of continuous independent variable assumes a linear response in the logit (i.e., for every unit increase in the independent variable there is an equal increase [or decrease] in the odds ratio).
  - If linearity in the logit is not the case, have to determine different modeling strategy for the continuous variable (e.g., splines, categorization).
- Use of stepwise regression
  - Forward: add variables one at a time based on significance. Does not take into account all potential confounding variables.
  - Backward: include a set of variables based on preset criteria, with removal one at a time based on significance.
  - The process is myopic, since looking only one step forward or backward at any point. If use, do so carefully, thinking through model building from clinical perspective first.
- Bottom line: multivariable model has to make sense or it's worthless!

Evaluation of Diagnostic Tests

Evaluation of diagnostic tests is commonly tested in boards questions.

Measures Used to Evaluate Diagnostic Tests

- Data used to calculate diagnostic test evaluation measures (see Table 49.3):
- Sensitivity = # positive by test / # with disease = $a/(a+c)$.
- Specificity = # negative by test / # without disease = $d/(b+d)$.
- Positive predictive value (PPV) = probability person has disease given that they test positive = $a/(a+b)$.
- The PPV is a function of the prevalence of disease and therefore depends on the specific population in which the test is performed.
- A test may perform well in a high prevalence population but not in a low prevalence population.
  - In a low prevalence population, the number of false-positive test results may be higher than the true positive test results.
  - Basis of two-stage testing for some infectious diseases (e.g., RPR as screening test for syphilis with more specific test (e.g., FTA-ABS) used for confirmation.

TABLE 49.3	Data Used to Evaluate a Diagnostic Test	
Test Result	Diseased	Not Diseased
Positive	a	b
Negative	c	d

- Negative predictive value (NPV) = probability person does not have disease given that they test negative = $d/(c+d)$.

Predictive Values Calculated Based on Bayes' Theorem

- Calculate probability of event based on prior knowledge (i.e., conditional probability).
- If prevalence of disease known in a population can use together with the sensitivity and specificity of a test to calculate positive and negative predictive values.

$$PPV = \frac{sensitivity \times prevalence}{(sensitivity \times prevalence) + ((1-specificity) \times (1-prevalence))}$$

$$NPV = \frac{sensitivity \times (1-prevalence)}{((1-sensitivity) \times prevalence) + (specificity \times (1-prevalence))}$$

- To put in context, suppose you have developed a new diagnostic test for *Chlamydia*, with sensitivity = 90% and specificity = 95%. You plan to use this test in a population of pregnant women with a prevalence of *Chlamydia* of 2%. Given this information:
  - Using Bayes' theorem, the PPV for this new test in this population = 0.27 (i.e., 27% of the time a positive test is associated with true *Chlamydia* infection).
  - If, however, the test is used in an STD clinic with prevalence of *Chlamydia* infection of 20%, the PPV = 0.82 (i.e., 82% of the time a positive test is associated with true *Chlamydia* infection in the STD clinic).
  - This follows from Bayes' theorem, since in the setting of a higher pretest probability of *Chlamydia* infection, the test performs better with higher PPV than in the low prevalence setting.

Likelihood Ratios (LR) and Diagnostic Tests

- Positive LR = true-positive rate/false-positive rate = sensitivity/(1-specificity).
  - Positive LR is the likelihood that a person will test positive given that they have disease, compared to a person without disease. The positive LR should be >1 since we expect a person with a positive test will have greater likelihood of disease than a person with a negative test.
- Negative LR = false-negative rate/(true-negative rate) = (1-sensitivity)/specificity.

- Negative LR is the likelihood that a person will test negative given that they have disease, compared to a person without disease. The negative LR should be <1 since we expect a person with a negative test will have a lower likelihood of disease than a person with a positive test.

Receiver-Operator Curve (ROC) and Diagnostic Tests

- The ROC plots the sensitivity on the *y*-axis vs. 1-specificity (i.e., false-positive rate) on the *x*-axis for a diagnostic test (Fig. 49.1).
- Used to identify diagnostic threshold (i.e., cutpoint) for a positive test result, in order to optimize the sensitivity with the lowest false-positive rate.
- Overall interpretation: at a given point on the ROC plot, the value represents the probability that, for two randomly selected individuals, a specimen from the person

with disease will have a higher test value than a specimen from a person without disease.

Meta-Analysis

- Statistical analysis of multiple studies, including methods to combine the results from the studies.
- Calculates average effect across studies.
- Increases power to detect an effect due to combining studies.
- Resolves association if heterogeneity exists in study results.
    - If results inconsistent, determine risk of bias in individual studies.
- Include systematic review to identify studies for inclusion in analysis.
    - Goal of systematic review is to identify all relevant information to answer research question.
    - Enlist help from librarian to find all relevant published and nonpublished results (including other languages).
    - May be difficult to find studies with negative results due to publication bias (i.e., more likely to publish results of study if findings are positive).
- Use PRISMA (Preferred Reporting Items for Systematic Reviews and Meta-Analyses) guidelines.

Further Reading

1. Gordis L. *Epidemiology*. 5th ed. Philadelphia: Elsevier; 2014. **Excellent discussion of validity of diagnostic tests.**
2. Rothman KJ, Greenland S, Lash TL. *Modern Epidemiology*. 3rd ed. Philadelphia: Lippincott Williams & Wilkins; 2008.
3. Hosmer DW, Lemeshow S, Sturdivant RX. *Applied Logistic Regression*. 3rd ed. Hoboken, NJ: John Wiley & Sons; 2013.
4. Moher D, Hopewell S, Schulz KF, et al. CONSORT 2010 explanation and elaboration: updated guidelines for reporting parallel group randomised trials. *BMJ*. 2010;340:c869.
5. Liberati A, Altman DG, Tetzlaff J, et al. The PRISMA statement for reporting systematic reviews and meta-analyses of studies that evaluate health care interventions: explanation and elaboration. *PLoS Med*. 2009;6:e1000100.

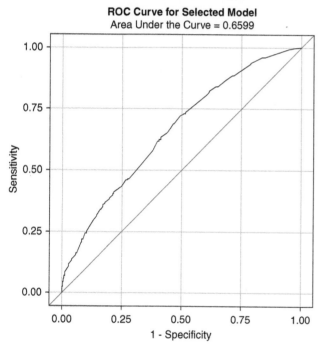

• **Fig. 49.1** ROC curve for selected model.

50
Commonly Encountered Skin Manifestations in Infectious Disease

RONNIE M. GRAVETT, JAMES HENRY WILLIG

BACTERIAL SKIN DISEASES

See also Chapter 25.

Impetigo

Infection of **superficial epidermis** with initial **vesicles** that subsequently crust over (Fig. 50.1).

- Pustular lesions that are often pruritic.
- Primarily caused by **group A streptococci**.
- Bullous impetigo is caused by *Staphylococcus aureus* toxin production (exfoliative toxins A/B).
- Treat with penicillinase-resistant penicillins, antistaphylococcal cephalosporins.
- Should also treat with anti-MRSA agent when high prevalence in community.
- Topical mupirocin or retapamulin ointments also may be effective.

Ecthyma

Infection extending from epidermis into **superficial dermis**. Leads to crusting ulcerations deeper than impetigo. Commonly on lower extremities.
- Usually caused by group A streptococci.
- Treat ecthyma as impetigo.
- **Ecthyma gangrenosum** is a consequence of **bacteremia and perivascular infection** by bacteria leading to local ischemia, classically *Pseudomonas aeruginosa* (Fig. 50.2), but other bacteria (i.e., MRSA) can cause this.
- **Angioinvasive molds** can cause similar lesions (i.e., *Mucor*, *Aspergillus*, dematiaceous molds, etc.) (see Chapter 29).

Folliculitis

Small pustular papules surrounding hair follicle.
- Most often caused by *S. aureus*.

- Think *Pseudomonas* and *Aeromonas* when exposed to water or jacuzzi ("hot tub folliculitis").
- Treat with topical antimicrobials (mupirocin).

Furuncle/Carbuncle

Purulent nodular infection that extends deeper into the subcutaneous tissue. Furuncles (Fig. 50.3) coalesce to form deeper more serious infections called carbuncles.
- May lead to systemic illness via bacteremia, seeding of distal foci (i.e., endocarditis, discitis, etc.).
- Main pathogen is almost always *S. aureus*.
- Treatment starts with **drainage of pus** (may need surgical assistance for carbuncles). If surrounding induration, cellulitis or signs of systemic illness, then treat with antistaphylococcal penicillin or cephalosporin for MSSA or agent for MRSA (i.e., trimethoprim–sulfamethoxazole [TMP–SMX], doxycycline).

Necrotizing Soft Tissue Infections

Necrotizing fasciitis and myositis involve infection extending down into deeper structures facilitated by proteolytic enzyme production by bacteria.
- Key physical exam findings include:
  - **Pain out of proportion** to expected physical exam findings with cellulitis due to ischemic nature of pain with compression of blood vessels by edema within fascia.
  - Rapidly advancing cellulitis borders.
  - Woody induration.
- Different eponyms related to location:
  - Fournier's gangrene: involves perineum and adjacent areas.
  - Ludwig's angina: involves head and neck.
- Causative organisms:
  - Type I: polymicrobial with mixed aerobes and anaerobes.
  - Type II: monomicrobial with group A streptococcus, *Aeromonas*, or *Vibrio vulnificus*.

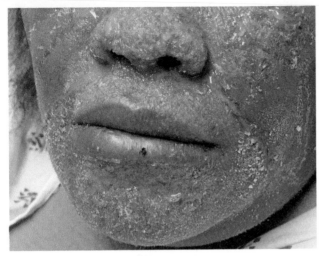

• **Fig. 50.1** Impetigo.

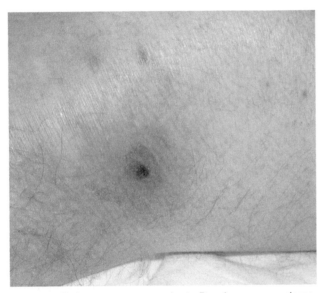

• **Fig. 50.2** Ecthyma gangrenosum due to *Pseudomonas aeruginosa*.

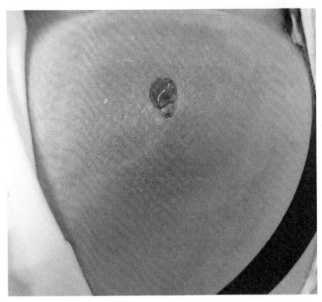

• **Fig. 50.3** Draining furuncle.

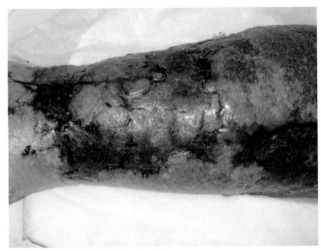

• **Fig. 50.4** Necrotizing cryptococcal cellulitis in solid organ transplant recipient.

- Diagnosis with high clinical suspicion but ultimately is a **surgical diagnosis.**
  - Cultures may be helpful to identify causative pathogens, but they should not delay surgical treatment.
- **Treatment is with surgery primarily**
  - Empiric antibiotics should be broad and aimed to cover gram-positive organisms, primarily streptococci and staphylococci (including MRSA), as well as gram-negative and anaerobic organisms.
  - **Clindamycin** may be helpful to **stop toxin production.**
- Necrotizing cellulitis (Fig. 50.4): gradual onset of pain, swelling, and skin changes of darkening color and drainage. Infection remains superficial to the fascia and muscle. In solid organ transplant recipients, cryptococcal cellulitis can be necrotizing.
- Meleney's synergistic gangrene: rare postoperative infection characterized by slowly expanding indolent ulceration confined to superficial fascia (*S. aureus* and microaerophilic streptococci typically involved).

Cutaneous Anthrax (Woolsorter's Disease) (see Chapter 31)

Manifests as a **nontender eschar with associated edema** (can be significant as *malignant edema*).

- Caused by *Bacillus anthracis.*
- Typically seen in farmers and cattle and sheep handlers as well as those who work with the hides of these animals.
- Regional lymphadenopathy can be tender.
- Diagnosed clinically, supported by direct Gram or Giemsa stain in samples from the skin.
- ELISA serologic assay useful only retrospectively.
- Treatment is with ciprofloxacin, doxycycline, or levofloxacin. In cases of anthrax associated with bioterrorism, concern for inhalation spores and developing systemic involvement leads to recommendation to more prolonged treatment as long as 60 days.
- Cutaneous lesions can progress to systemic illness.

Corynebacterium spp.

Corynebacterium spp. can cause a "trinity" of cutaneous patterns.

- **Trichomycosis axillaris**: presence of tan concretions on hair follicles in axilla.
- **Erythrasma**: with moisture and occlusion, *Corynebacterium minutissimum* proliferates in stratum corneum in intertriginous areas and feet.
  - Clinically indistinguishable from dermatophyte and fungal infections in these areas, but exhibit **coral red fluorescence** under Wood's lamp in affected areas.
  - False-negative if patient took shower before your exam and washed away coproporphyrin III produced by organism!
  - Obesity, immunosuppression, and diabetes can predispose.
    - Treat with topical or oral erythromycin.
- **Pitted keratolysis**: malodorous feet with small indented pits on hyperkeratotic soles.
- Associated with increased sweating (favors proliferation of bacteria that release proteinases that destroy stratum corneum).
- Etiologic considerations include *Corynebacterium* spp., *Kytococcus sedentarius*, and *Actinomyces* spp.
- Treat by keeping feet dry and using topical antibiotics (clindamycin, erythromycin, or mupirocin).

Erythema Marginatum (see Chapter 15)

- One of the five major manifestations of rheumatic fever.
- Painless, nonpruritic, transient ring-shaped lesions that spread on trunk and limbs.
- Serpiginous, reddened edges are sharp on the outside with a diffuse inner edge.
- Does not usually involve face.
- Rarely seen in adults.

Erythema Migrans (see Chapter 24)

- Caused by untreated infection with *Borrelia* spp.
- Occurs in 70%–80% of those infected.
- Expanding lesions develop at site of tick bite, within 3–30 days.

Rocky Mountain Spotted Fever (RMSF) (see Chapter 30)

Caused by *Rickettsia rickettsii*, transmitted by infected tick bite.

- Classic rash appears **day 3–5** of illness (Fig. 50.5).
  - ~90% patients overall develop rash.
  - Delay in onset or absence of rash may delay diagnosis.
  - Starts around **wrists and ankles** before generalizing; may include palms and soles (late).
  - Initially discrete, macular lesions; **becomes petechial.**

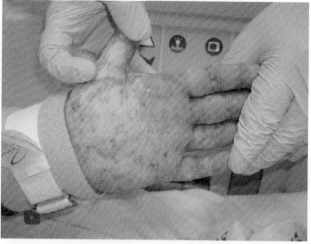

• **Fig. 50.5** Rocky Mountain spotted fever (RMSF), *Rickettsia rickettsii.*

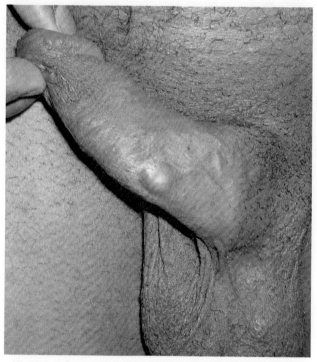

• **Fig. 50.6** Primary syphilis with multiple chancres in person with HIV.

- Skin necrosis or gangrene in 4% due to direct damage by Rickettsiae to microcirculation.
- Rash fades with residual hyperpigmentation.

Treponema pallidum (see Chapter 21)

Primary Syphilis
- Classic pattern is **single painless chancre** with an incubation period of 3 weeks at site of exposure.
  - Bacterial superinfection might make lesion painful.
  - Immunosuppressed hosts may develop multiple chancres (Fig. 50.6).
  - Chancre(s) usually accompanied by regional lymphadenopathy.

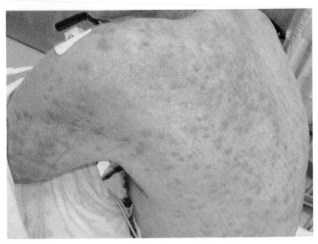

• **Fig. 50.7** Secondary syphilis rash.

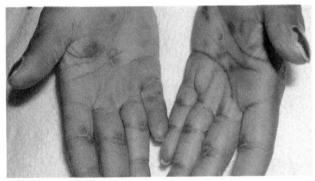

• **Fig. 50.8** Secondary syphilis rash involving palms and soles: coin-shaped lesions crossing life lines.

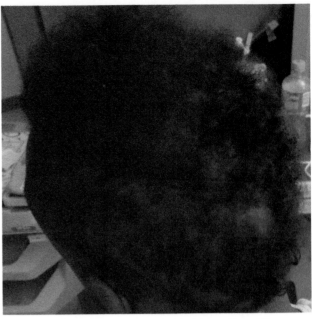

• **Fig. 50.9** Moth-eaten cranium hair loss with syphilis.

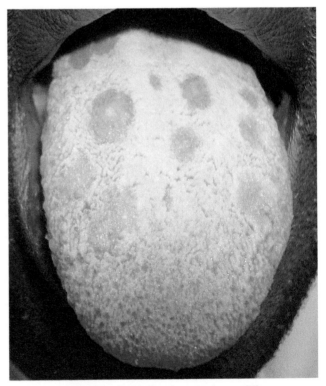

• **Fig. 50.10** Oral lesions in secondary syphilis.

- Without treatment, the lesion will **heal spontaneously in 3–6 weeks**, but it is not saying, "goodbye," it is saying, **"see you in a bit as secondary syphilis!"**

Secondary Syphilis
- 3–10 weeks after primary chancre, hematogenous and lymphatic spread lead to multiple cutaneous manifestations.
- Classic pattern is of a generalized **papulosquamous nonpruritic rash** (Fig. 50.7).
  - Includes the **palms and soles** (Fig. 50.8).
  - Hair loss, patchy alopecia described as a "**moth-eaten cranium**" (Fig. 50.9).
  - Mucosal lesions including oral lesions (mucous patches, if former confluent form serpiginous "**snail track**" **ulcers**, leukoplakia-like lesions, stomatitis [Fig. 50.10], etc.) and condyloma lata (ulcers, gray-colored plaques).
  - Keratoderma blenorrhagicum or thickened skin of palms/soles (Fig. 50.11) (also seen in reactive arthritis).
- Malignant syphilis or lues maligna (predominantly associated with human immunodeficiency virus [HIV]) is a rare presentation consisting of generalized papules, nodules, pustules, or ulcers with thick overlying crusts (Fig. 50.12).

- Nonspecific systemic symptoms may accompany any of these patterns (fever, weight loss, malaise, lymphadenopathy, myalgias, etc.).
- Secondary syphilis findings typically resolve spontaneously after 3–12 weeks; but it is not saying "goodbye," it's saying, "see you in a bit as either a relapse or tertiary syphilis with CNS, heart, bone, or other involvement!"

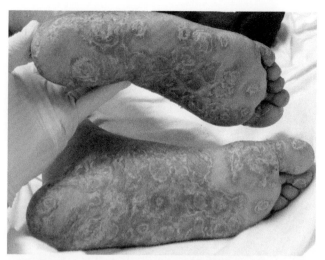

• **Fig. 50.11** Keratoderma blenorrhagicum in syphilis, also seen in reactive arthritis.

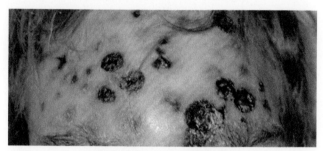

• **Fig. 50.12** Lues maligna lesions.

Mycobacterial Skin Diseases

See also Chapter 33.

Buruli Ulcer

Large, cutaneous ulcer caused by *Mycobacterium ulcerans*.
- It is the third most common mycobacterial infection (after tuberculosis and leprosy).
- More common in tropical regions, especially West Africa (named for Buruli region of Uganda), but it is also seen in Latin America as well as Australia and Asian Pacific region.
- **Transmission is not entirely clear** but associations with stagnant water have been suggested as well as possible vectorborne transmission via mosquitos in Australia.
- Pathogenesis is related to mycolactone toxin produced by *M. ulcerans* that leads to tissue necrosis and ulceration as well as downregulation of local host immune response.
- Presents initially as a **painless nodule** most often on the extremities and **slowly progresses** over weeks to months into the **hallmark ulcer with deeply undermined edges.**
  - Lesions are notably **painless.**
  - Usually no systemic illness unless wound becomes secondarily infected.

- **Osteomyelitis** can develop as superficial lesions extend deeper into bones.
  - WHO categories:
    - Category I: single nodules or papules or ulcers ≤5 cm.
    - Category II: single plaques or ulcers 5–15 cm.
    - Category III: single plaques or ulcers ≥15 cm, >1 lesion, or lesions involving joints or bone or other critical areas, i.e., face or genitals.
- Epidemiological exposures and exam aid diagnosis. AFB staining of scraping from undermined border, histopathology with polymerase chain reaction (PCR), and culture (swab purulent discharge from undermined ulcer edges) can help confirm diagnosis. Tuberculin skin test is often positive with progressive disease, but this should not be used in diagnostic criteria.
- Treatment varies by category.
  - Most regimens consist of a combination of rifampin and streptomycin and occasionally surgery.
  - Treatment length varies, with Category I treated for 4 weeks and occasional surgical excision whereas categories II and III are treated with antibiotics for 8 weeks with occasional surgical involvement.
  - Wound care is of paramount importance for ulcers to heal.

Leprosy (also called Hansen's Disease)

Infection of peripheral nerves by *Mycobacterium leprae* that leads to a spectrum of cutaneous manifestations. *M. lepromatosis* is a more recently described species, causes similar clinical manifestations, found in Northeastern and Northern Mexico.
- Incidence has dropped dramatically. Now it is seen almost exclusively in developing countries.
- Transmission is believed to be via respiratory route, although vast majority of people exposed do not develop disease. Immunologic defects and immunosuppression as well as older age seem to predispose to disease development. There is also a notable association with nine-banded armadillos.
- The spectrum of manifestations depends on host immune response and organism burden. Tuberculoid refers to high immune response with relatively few mycobacteria, whereas lepromatous leprosy is seen with lower immune response allowing for higher organism burden.
- Physical manifestations depend on degree of host response and may range from singular hypoesthetic or anesthetic plaque, to plaques over entire body with occasional punched out lesions. **Peripheral nerves (especially ulnar, great auricular, and common peroneal nerves may become thickened and palpable.** Weakness may be a late manifestation; wounds on extremities may be present due to neuropathy. Ridley–Jopling Classification denotes the following presentations:
  - Tuberculoid (TT): single or few, **anesthetic, usually hypopigmented macules within the same nerve distribution**; may have raised borders.

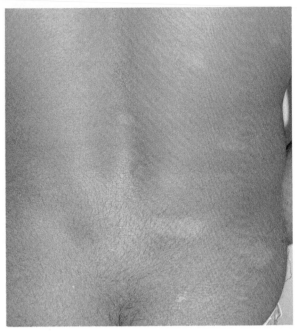

• **Fig. 50.13** Tuberculoid leprosy with hypopigmented and anesthetic patches.

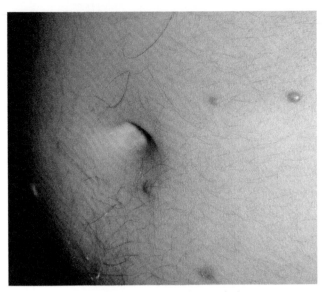

• **Fig. 50.14** Lepromatous leprosy lesion.

- Borderline Tuberculoid (BT): multiple macular lesions with central clearing areas that may appear as targets; more numerous than tuberculoid (Fig. 50.13).
- Mid-Borderline (BB): many macular or plaque lesions with "punched-out" areas.
- Borderline Lepromatous (BL): many erythematous, papular, or nodular lesions over entire body without as sharply demarcated borders.
- Lepromatous (LL): diffuse macules or papules (Fig. 50.14) but often infiltrated, thickened skin over body (Fig. 50.15) with **particular involvement of face and scalp**; hair loss is also associated. Can also involve nasal septum, eye brow ridges, or ear lobes. Visceral involvement with bacteremia or infiltration into the bone marrow can also be seen.
- Diagnosis by demonstration of acid-fast bacilli on biopsy of margin of lesion. Skin smears obtained from ear lobe, elbow, or knee cap (cooler regions of body) is alternative to biopsy.
- Treat TT and BT disease with dapsone and rifampin for 12 months.
- Treat BB, BL, and LL disease with dapsone, rifampin, and clofazimine for 24 months. Clofazimine can cause skin darkening, especially with sun exposure.
- Immune reactions can occur before or after treatment.
  - Type I reaction (also called reversal reaction): seen only in BT, BB, and BL and related to changes in cell-mediated immune response to pathogens and may lead to changing stage. Symptoms include worsening of existing lesions, worsening pain or neuritis, edema, and even ulceration of skin lesions. Treatment is with steroids.

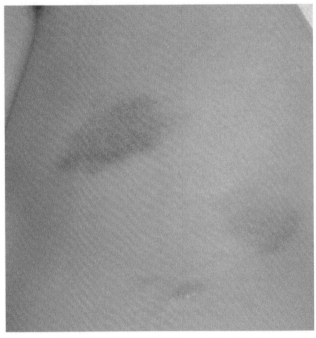

• **Fig. 50.15** Infiltrated skin in lepromatous leprosy.

- Type II reaction (erythema nodosum leprosum): seen only in BL and LL disease. Usually manifests as multiple painful nodules that can be deeper in the skin or even ulcerate. Treatment is also with steroids.

Mycobacterium marinum

Cutaneous infection causing nodular lesions that can spread via lymphatics.
- Most commonly seen on the extremities.
- Associated with water exposures including fresh and brackish/salt water as well as aquariums.
- Manifests as **nodular lesions that can ulcerate**; there may be single or multiple lesions spread via lymphangitic pattern (**sporotrichoid spread**).

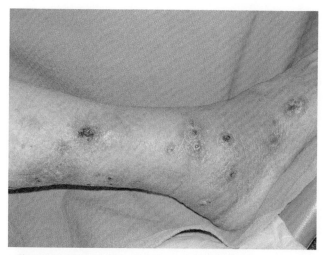

• **Fig. 50.16** *Mycobacterium chelonae* infection in immunocompromised host.

- Diagnosis is by biopsy with culture and histopathology of lesion. PCR may be helpful as well.
- Treatment is largely anecdotal with reports of success with clarithromycin, doxycycline, rifampin, or even TMP–SMX; treatment is often for several weeks (8 weeks) with extension of therapy even after resolution of lesion for some weeks.

Rapidly Growing Mycobacteria

Mycobacterium chelonae (Fig. 50.16), *M. abscessus*, and *M. fortuitum* can cause skin disease, although somewhat uncommonly, but they are becoming more relevant.
- Various exposures including nail salon foot spas, tattooing, and cosmetic surgery performed abroad. Immunosuppressed individuals can be affected.
- Manifests as nodular or furuncular diseases but can also develop chronic abscesses or draining sinus tracts.
- Diagnosis is by biopsy of lesion with culture and histopathology; PCR can be used as well.
- Treatment may vary but should be dependent on sensitivities of organism isolated. Empiric treatment may include TMP–SMX, doxycycline, or levofloxacin; clarithromycin can be considered for *M. chelonae* isolates but should be avoided in *M. fortuitum* or *M. abscessus* due to possibility of inducible resistance. Treatment should be given for several months, and may extend depending on clinical response.

FUNGAL SKIN DISEASES

See also Chapters 27–29.

Candida Intertrigo

Intertrigo is an inflammatory condition caused by rubbing of opposing skin surfaces in the presence of heat and moisture. This environment favors overgrowth of *Candida*.

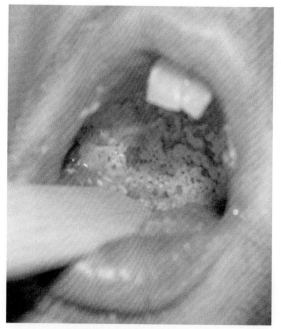

• **Fig. 50.17** Oral candidiasis in AIDS.

- Risk factors include obesity, excess moisture, tight clothing as well as immunocompromised conditions (diabetes, HIV, chemotherapy, etc.) and occupational exposures to moisture and sugar (bartenders, bakers, dishwashers, etc.).
- Clinically manifests as **erythematous and painful plaques** with peripheral, discrete erythematous macules (**satellitosis**) most frequently involving groin, axilla, inframammary region, pannus, and web spaces.
- Diagnosis is clinical, but the KOH Test (potassium hydroxide preparation, "KOH prep") can be helpful.
- Treatment is first with removing or correcting offending conditions combined with topical antifungal therapy. If patient has failed topical therapy or has extensive, severe disease, then can do oral, systemic therapy.

Oral Candidiasis (see Chapter 11)

Candida albicans is the most frequently causative species.
- Risk factors include xerostomia (medication related or after head/neck radiation), antibiotic therapy, inhaled corticosteroid use, diabetes, and immunosuppression (HIV/AIDS with low CD4, receiving immunosuppressive agents, leukemia, or other malignancies, etc.).
- May be classified as acute or chronic.
  - Most common presentation is acute pseudomembranous candidiasis (thrush), white plaques on oral mucosa (Fig. 50.17). Wiping these lesions off uncovers normal or erythematous mucosa.
  - Acute atrophic (erythematous) candidiasis is associated with a burning sensation.
  - Chronic plaque-like candidiasis occurs commonly in smokers or men >30 years.
  - May be a cause of angular cheilitis (perleche).

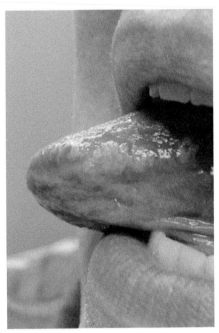

• **Fig. 50.18** Oral hairy leukoplakia in AIDS.

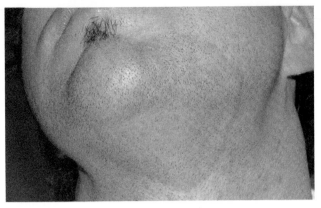

• **Fig. 50.19** Tinea barbae.

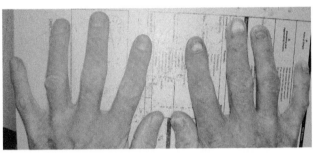

• **Fig. 50.20** Dermatophytes affecting nails (tinea unguium) and a single hand affected in two foot, one hand pattern.

- In people with HIV, oral candidiasis may need to be differentiated from oral hairy leukoplakia (OHL), benign Epstein–Barr virus (EBV)-associated white plaques typically on the lateral borders of the tongue that cannot be scraped off (Fig. 50.18).
- Treatment is with local (nystatin preparation) or systemic (fluconazole) therapy.

Erosio Interdigitalis Blastomycetica

- Interdigital candidiasis of the hands or feet, most likely in those at risk for chronic maceration of web spaces (i.e., launderers, dishwashers, etc.), obese and immunosuppressed patients (i.e., diabetes).
- Painful or pruritic, round or oval erythematous patches and plaques in web spaces of the hand, may have satellite pustules. Classic site is between middle and ring finger (third web space).

Dermatophyte Infections (see Chapter 29)

Dermatophytes – *Trichophyton*, *Microsporum*, and *Epidermophyton* – cause infection of hair, skin, and nails (keratinized tissue).
- Clinical syndrome may vary by location: tinea capitis (scalp), tinea barbae (beard, Fig. 50.19), tinea faciei (face without hair), tinea corporis (body, "ringworm"), etc.
- Acquired from contact with infected person, fomite, or other infected area.
- Scaling, erythematous, and circular plaque with central clearing spreads outward from center.
  - Tinea cruris (groin, aka "jock itch"):
    - Affects men much more than women.

- Can be made worse by moisture and obesity.
- Erythematous, itchy plaque with sharp borders in the groin.
- Tinea pedis (feet, aka "athlete's foot"):
  - Associated with young men, often contact with shower or locker room floors.
  - Itchy, scaling erosions, hyperkeratotic skin, or even vesicular lesions if very inflammatory.
  - Bilateral tinea pedis with accompanying tinea manuum or unguium has been described as the "two foot, one hand syndrome" (Fig. 50.20).
- Tinea unguium (nails) and onychomycosis:
  - Primarily dermatophyte infection, but onychomycosis can be caused by *Candida* spp. Risks include older age, immunocompromise, and diabetes among others.
  - Variable clinical presentations but discoloration to yellow or darker and thickening with subungual hyperkeratosis.
  - Distal lateral, proximal subungual and white superficial onychomycosis variants refer to site of infection. The latter two have been associated with significant immunocompromise such as AIDS.
- Majocchi's granuloma:
  - Deeper infection by dermatophytes into the dermis seen in immunocompromised hosts. Suspect if furuncular lesions suggestive of *S. aureus* infection that do not resolve with antibiotics.
- Diagnosis is largely clinical but may be reinforced by KOH prep demonstrating hyphae or even fungal culture to grow causative organisms.

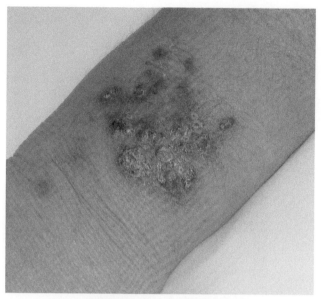

• **Fig. 50.21** Chromoblastomycosis.

• If clinically apparent dermatophyte infections in inter-triginous areas do not respond to antifungals, consider erythrasma (*Corynebacterium minutissimum*, see above).

Chromoblastomycosis

Chronic, progressive infection by pigmented molds, commonly *Fonsecaea* and *Cladophialophora* species.
• Most often in tropical and subtropical environments but can be seen worldwide especially in immunocompromised hosts.
• Typically occurs after **trauma involving plant debris or soil with inoculation** of pigmented mold. Progression is **indolent** and occurs over months to years.
• Protean manifestations, including nodular, verrucous, tumorous, cicatricial, and plaques (Fig. 50.21).
• Diagnosis by demonstration of fungal organisms with sclerotic bodies or "copper pennies" seen on KOH prep or skin biopsy.
• Treatment is with surgical excision for small individual lesions. Larger or multiple lesions require treatment with systemic itraconazole. Terbinafine can also be considered.

Dimorphic Mycoses (see Chapter 28)

Coccidioidomycosis

• Usually within weeks of primary infection.
• Only a minority (0.5%) of immunocompetent individuals develop disseminated infection beyond the lungs.
• Increased with cell-mediated immunodeficiency; tumor necrosis factor-alpha inhibitors; pregnancy.
• Skin is a common extrapulmonary site of infection. Variety of lesions including ulcers, maculopapular lesions, and subcutaneous abscesses. Can occur anywhere on the body.

Cutaneous Blastomycosis

• Skin lesions in >70% due to hematogenous spread.
• Painless ulcers or raised irregular, verrucous lesions, both arising from subcutaneous abscesses.
• Commonly face, arms, neck, and scalp.

Histoplasmosis

• Acute progressive disseminated infection: severely immunosuppressed adults; 10% have skin changes (maculopapular, petechiae or ecchymoses); may be crusted. Fungi may be seen intra- or extracellularly, or within an infiltrate of macrophages.
• Chronic progressive disseminated: previously healthy adults; 50% have an oropharyngeal ulcer that is deep, painless, indurated, and well-demarcated.

Mucocutaneous Paracoccidioidomycosis

• Painful ulcerated lesions which progress over weeks/months on gums, lips, tongue, or palate.
• Lesions may appear on facial skin **around mouth and nose**.

Talaromyces marneffei (previously known as *Penicillium marneffei*)

• Disseminated infection associated with cell-mediated immunodeficiency, especially people with HIV with CD4 <100 cells/μL.
• Skin lesions in 70%; papules on face, chest, extremities, which may umbilicate, resembling molluscum.

Sporotrichosis

• Most cases caused by *Sporothrix schenckii*.
• Disease usually limited to skin/subcutaneous tissues (= lymphocutaneous sporotrichosis).
• Worldwide in decaying matter with exposure due to minor injuries that inoculate contaminated soil into wound.
• Subacute/chronic course.
• Primary lesion at site of inoculation is papulonodular which usually ulcerates. Further lesions then appear proximally along lymphatic channels, nodular lymphangitis (Fig. 50.22).

VIRAL SKIN DISEASES

Varicella-Zoster Virus (VZV) (see Chapters 23 and 45)

Chickenpox (Primary Varicella Infection)

• Manifests primarily with fever and malaise followed by vesicular rash, which initially begins as a macule and then progresses through papule, vesicle, pustule, and eventual crusted pustule before healing.

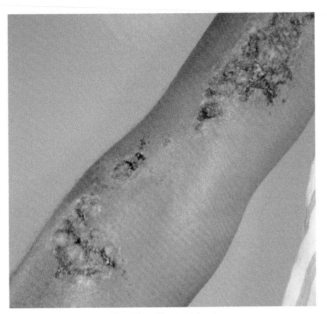

• **Fig. 50.22** Sporotrichosis.

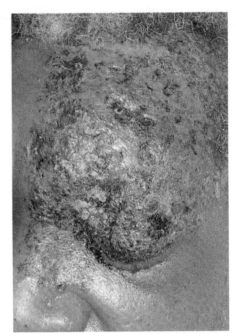

• **Fig. 50.23** Herpes zoster ophthalmicus.

- Lesions classically develop at different stages such that one patient may have a diffuse rash with lesions at different stages. (Key differentiator from smallpox where all lesions would be at concurrent stage of development.)
- Bacterial superinfection may complicate, including impetigo or deeper skin and soft tissue infections.

Herpes Zoster (Varicella Reactivation)

Cutaneous manifestations include very painful, vesicular rash limited to dermatomal distribution.
- Notable presentations
  - **Disseminated** disease defined by involvement of **≥2 noncontiguous dermatomes** or by presence of visceral or neurologic involvement.
  - **Herpes zoster ophthalmicus**: VZV reactivation with vesicular eruption along trigeminal ganglion distribution (V1).
    - Over 50% experience direct ocular involvement (keratitis to retinal involvement) and **may be sight-threatening** (Fig. 50.23).
    - Clues for possible retinal involvement include hyperemic conjunctivitis, Hutchinson's sign (vesicular lesion in nose signifying involvement nasociliary branch of the trigeminal nerve).
  - **Herpes zoster oticus (Ramsay–Hunt syndrome)**: combination of ipsilateral facial palsy, ear pain, and vesicles seen in external ear.

Herpes Simplex Virus (HSV)

Herpes Gladiatorum

Vesicular lesions seen on extremities and face most commonly, but can involve trunk also.

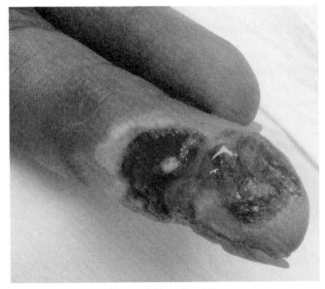

• **Fig. 50.24** Herpetic whitlow.

- Wrestlers, fighters, and contact sports participants seem to be at higher risk.

Herpes Whitlow

Lesion seen on fingers and seen more commonly in primary exposure, whether oral or genital (Fig. 50.24).
- Healthcare and dental workers are at higher risk.

Anogenital HSV

See Chapter 21.

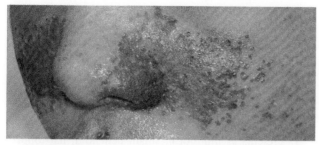

• **Fig. 50.25** Eczema herpeticum or Kaposi's varicelliform eruption.

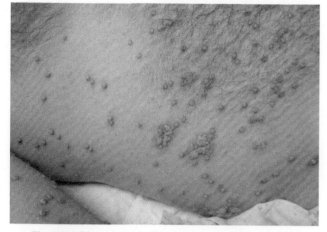

• **Fig. 50.26** Disseminated HSV in an immunosuppressed host.

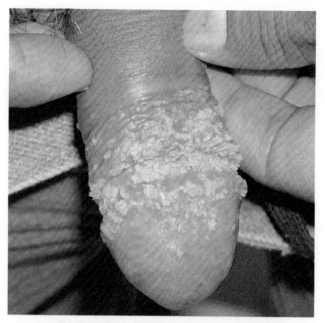

• **Fig. 50.27** Penile HPV lesions in person with HIV.

Eczema Herpeticum or Kaposi's Varicelliform Eruption

HSV (typically HSV-1) spreads to area of skin compromised by preexisting skin disease (i.e., atopic dermatitis, psoriasis, burns, contact dermatitis, etc.).
- New painful skin lesions (small ulcers, vesiculopustules which may be clustered, umbilicated, or even hemorrhagic with crusts on erythematous bases) develop, overlaid on preexisting dermatoses (which may make recognition more difficult) (Fig. 50.25).
- In immunosuppressed hosts, lesions can spread rapidly and lead to significant morbidity and even mortality, often related to viremia and bacterial superinfection with sepsis.

Disseminated HSV

Presents as widespread vesicles, pustules, or erosions.
- Cellular immunity is needed for containment HSV and without it, immunocompromised hosts are at risk for dissemination and involvement of diffuse cutaneous (Fig. 50.26) and visceral sites (i.e., fulminant hepatitis, pneumonia, esophagitis, acute retinal necrosis, etc.).

Recurrent Erythema Multiforme

- HSV-1 outbreaks have been associated with recurrent erythema multiforme. A classic image to remember this is that of a palm showing a target lesion held aloft by the patient's lips which in turn show a herpes labialis lesion.

Human Papilloma Virus (HPV)

Common Warts (Verruca vulgaris)

Flesh-colored, hyperkeratotic papules commonly caused by HPV-1, 2, and 4.
- Tiny black or red dots are best visualized if surface of lesions removed (represent thrombosed capillaries). Can also present as plantar warts and flat warts.
- Treatment is destruction with topical medications (5-fluorouracil, imiquimod, etc.) or directly (cryotherapy, CO_2 laser therapy, electrocautery, etc.).

Genital Warts (Condylomata acuminata) (Figs. 50.27 and 50.28)

- Over 40 subtypes can infect the genital tract. Benign anogenital warts are predominantly caused by HPV-6 and 11 (about 90% of lesions). HPV types (HPV-16 and 18 in particular) have been found to play an important role in causing cancer, notably cervical cancer (virtually all cases) but also vulvar/vaginal, penile, anal, and oropharyngeal cancers (tongue, tonsil, larynx).
- Treatment is destruction (medications or directly), similar to common warts.

Other Notable Patterns of HPV-Related Disease

- **Giant condyloma of Buschke-Lowenstein (GCBL):** rare, locally destructive anogenital tumor.
  - Over years will progress from a slow-growing warty plaque to a cauliflower-like mass without causing much discomfort.

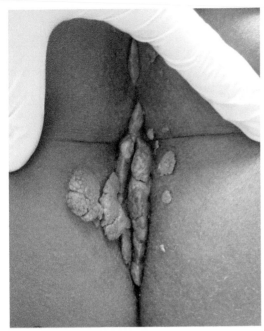

• **Fig. 50.28** Rectal condyloma acuminata lesions due to HPV infection in person with HIV.

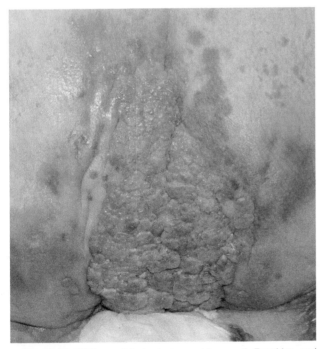

• **Fig. 50.29** HPV-associated giant condyloma of Buschke and Lowenstein.

- Later invasive stages lead to obstructions and strictures (urethral, anorectal, etc.), fistulas, and other complications (Fig. 50.29).
- For diagnosis, a deep biopsy is needed to differentiate a common condyloma from a GCBL which is considered a verrucous or well-differentiated variety of squamous cell carcinoma.

- Multidisciplinary oncologic management may include chemotherapy, radiotherapy, and surgical ablation for management.
- Recurrence is possible despite optimal therapy.
- **Bowenoid papulosis**: low-grade squamous cell carcinoma (SCC) in situ caused by HPV (typically subtypes 16, 18, 32, 33).
  - Affects genital or perianal areas.
  - Presents as multifocal, small, lichenoid, flat-topped, papules or plaques with sharp borders and color range from pale brown to black.
  - Considered transitional state between condyloma acuminata and SCC in situ (Erythroplasia of Queyrat is Bowen's disease or SCC in situ affecting glans or prepuce which presents as red, moist, smooth/velvety plaque).
- **Epidermodysplasia verruciformis**: rare, autosomal recessive condition where HPV-induced warts appear on skin surfaces with sun exposure at childhood and experience malignant transformation in about half of patients by adulthood.

Hand, Foot, and Mouth Disease (HFMD) (see Chapter 23)

HFMD is a syndrome characterized by combination of oral lesions and exanthema involving feet and hands ± other areas (Fig. 50.30).
- Caused by enterovirus infection, especially coxsackie A16 and enterovirus A71.
  - Worldwide, most commonly affects infants and preschool children.
  - Oral enanthem: multiple small haloed vesicles rupturing into ulcers (Figure 50.30 A,B).
    - Predominantly on tongue and buccal mucosa; may involve lips.
    - **Painful**: children complain of mouth pain or refuse to eat.
  - Exanthem: mix of macules, maculopapular, and vesicular lesions.
    - Nonpruritic, usually painless.
    - Hand (including palms), feet (including soles), buttocks, arms, and thighs (Figure 50.30 C).
    - Resolve in 3–4 days.

Associated with HIV/AIDS (see Chapters 37 and 39)

Kaposi Sarcoma (KS) (see Chapter 39)

Malignancy of endothelial vascular cells (vascular tumor) associated with human herpesvirus 8 (HHV-8) aka Kaposi sarcoma herpes virus (KSHV).
- Four forms that are morphologically and histologically indistinguishable:
  - AIDS-related (considered an AIDS-defining illness).
  - Endemic or African.

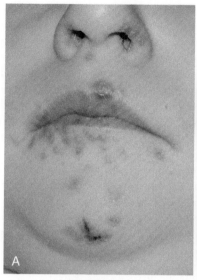
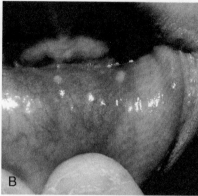
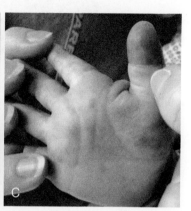

• **Fig. 50.30** Hand, foot, and mouth disease. A) Vesicular lesions on lip. B) Oral ulcers. C) Nodular, palm lesions. (From Mancini AJ, Shani-Adir A, Sidbury R. Other viral diseases. In: Bolognia JL, Schaffer JV, Cerroni L, eds. *Dermatology*. 4th ed. Elsevier; 2018.)

- Organ transplant-associated (thought to be associated with chronic immunosuppression).
- Classic (indolent disease affecting older Mediterranean men and Jewish origin).
- Corticosteroid usage and presence of opportunistic infections associated with AIDS have been associated with induction or worsening of existing KS.
- Cutaneous is most common presentation.
  - Whereas classic KS favors lower extremity involvement, AIDS-associated KS may affect multiple locations.
  - Varied colors (deep red, brown, purple, pink) and morphology (patches, plaques, nodules, fungating) on extremities, face, oral mucosa, and genitalia, etc. (Fig. 50.31).
  - Lesions are not painful, pruritic, or necrotic.
  - Lymphedema may occur in area of lesion distribution (obstructive lymphadenopathy and cytokines associated with KS pathogenesis contribute).
- Visceral presentation: has been seen in almost all visceral sites, most frequently reported in oral cavity, GI tract, and respiratory system.
  - Oral cavity KS.
  - Involvement in up to 1/3 of KS cases.
  - Dentists often identify first.
  - Palate then gingiva most commonly affected (Fig. 50.32).
  - If oral involvement, consider GI involvement.

Bacillary Angiomatosis (BA) (see Chapters 31 and 39)

Bartonella henselae (acquired from cat exposure, scratch) or *Bartonella quintana* (mostly in homeless persons with body lice) may affect patients with advanced immunosuppression due to HIV (AIDS).

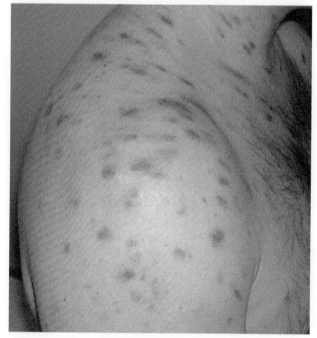

• **Fig. 50.31** Kaposi sarcoma

- **Angiomatous** (bacteria stimulate proliferation of endothelial cells) lesions affect skin or multiple internal organs.
  - Liver: peliosis hepatica, splenitis, bone: painful lytic lesions under skin lesions, respiratory tract, GI tract, lymph nodes, CNS; uncommon.
  - Can cause bacteremia (organisms difficult to isolate on blood culture) which may be associated with infective endocarditis and/or unexplained fever.
  - Has been associated with hemophagocytic lymphohistiocytosis (HLH), a rare and life-threatening syndrome due to hyperinflammatory immune response.

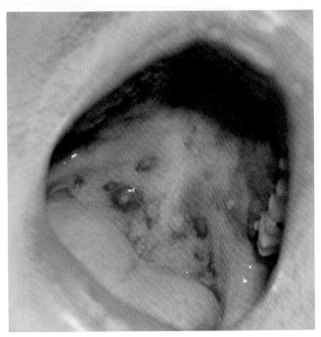

• **Fig. 50.32** One presentation of oral lesions in Kaposi sarcoma.

- May cause a variety of skin lesions, especially papular and plaque (hyperkeratotic or cellulitic) forms. May also present as subcutaneous nodules that can ulcerate, nodules, and large pedunculated lesions. Typically presents as single or multiple cutaneous lesions (rarely disseminated with over 1000 small lesions).
  - Papular lesions: differential diagnosis includes nodular KS, lobular capillary hemangioma (formerly pyogenic granuloma), verruga peruana (South America typically, infection with *Bartonella bacilliformis*).
  - Plaque and nodular forms: differential diagnosis includes mycobacterial and fungal (histoplasmosis, coccidioidomycosis, cryptococcosis, sporotrichosis, etc.) infections.
- Diagnosis can be challenging and often made with several tests.
  - Difficult to isolate on blood and tissue cultures. Chances to isolate organisms can be increased with changes to collection (get blood sample in pediatric or adult isolator tubes) and culture technique (changes to culture media to optimize chance of growth).
  - PCR testing for *Bartonella* from blood is increasingly important while serology (IFA and EIA) provide only supportive evidence of *Bartonella* infection.
  - Histopathology can show suggestive morphologic changes in tissue via standard hematoxylin and eosin staining (lobular vascular proliferations, etc., while the causative organisms may be visualized via the **Warthin–Starry stain** (show small, dark-staining bacteria) and electron microscopy.
- Treatment is typically with doxycycline or erythromycin (3 months in BA, 4 months if peliosis hepatica and/or osteomyelitis, endocarditis is 3 months doxycycline with gentamicin for first 14 days). Note that the optimal

treatment duration with concomitant HIV is unknown. Thus response to therapy is monitored via *Bartonella* IgG titers checked at baseline and every 6–8 weeks (goal is ≥4-fold titer decline). Therapy is extended for those without adequate clinical improvement. Suppressive therapy is used in those who relapse after completing 3 months of therapy (discontinue when CD4 >200 for 6 months).
- In those with HIV, start antiretroviral therapy (ART) at time of initiation of treatment for *Bartonella* infection, unless CNS or ophthalmologic disease where current recommendations are to delay ART 2–4 weeks (due to concern for additional morbidity with IRIS in these locations).

Eosinophilic Folliculitis (EF) aka Eosinophilic Pustular Folliculitis

Culture-negative folliculitis of currently unknown etiology.
- Variants include immunosuppression-associated EF (common in HIV, also seen in transplants and hematologic malignancies), eosinophilic pustular folliculitis in infancy (sterile pustules of unknown etiology, rare, self-limited), Ofuji disease (recurrent crops of follicular papular pustules atop erythematous plaques on normal skin, affects immunocompetent, more common in men, Japanese, peak incidence age 30, responds to indomethacin).
- Presents as **intensely pruritic crops of papules and pustules.**
  - Seems to favor areas with a high concentration of sebaceous glands (scalp, face, trunk, upper limbs, etc.).
  - Pruritus indicated by excoriations. Chronic pruritus and scratching can lead to prurigo nodularis (severely pruritic smooth dome-shaped nodules, hyperpigmented or violaceous, unknown etiology thought triggered by repetitive scratching) and hyperpigmentation.
- Treatment is mostly **symptomatic** targeting pruritus (topical steroids of varying potency, antihistamines, phototherapy with narrowband UVB, etc.). **Start ART.**

Some Quick Additional HIV and Skin Associations

- **Seborrheic dermatitis** is more extensive in HIV/AIDS, may regress with ART and may worsen as part of IRIS.
- Check for HIV in new diagnosis **psoriasis** as this may be the presenting sign of HIV infection. Also suspect new HIV in psoriatic patient whose symptoms worsen. Psoriasis and its complications (arthritis mutilans, etc.) are more pronounced in HIV.
- Proximal subungual onychomycosis and white superficial onychomycosis can be indicative of undiagnosed HIV infection. Test for HIV when you see these variants rather than the more common distal lateral onychomycosis.

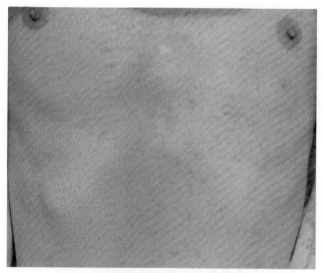

• **Fig. 50.33** Rash in acute HIV.

• Acute HIV infection can cause a generalized, nonspecific rash typically with pink to red, small macules or papules. Typically involves upper thorax, collar region, face, and less commonly extremities (Fig. 50.33).

PARASITIC SKIN DISEASES

Cutaneous Leishmaniasis

See also Chapter 34.
• Spectrum of cutaneous disease related to variability in parasite virulence and host immune response and may be characteristic for specific species.
• Transmitted by sandflies.
• Localized cutaneous leishmaniasis = LCL
  • Exposed areas of skin.
  • Papule → nodule → painless ulceration with indurated edge (Fig. 50.34).
• Leishmaniasis recidivans = LR
  • Uncommon; *Leishmania tropica* infection.
  • New papules form around healed scar margin.
  • Low parasite burden with strong granulomatous immune response on histology.
• Diffuse cutaneous leishmaniasis = DCL
  • Uncommon.
  • Initial localized lesion does not ulcerate.
  • Amastigotes disseminate, especially to face and extensor surfaces of limbs.
  • Soft nodules or plaques.
  • High parasite burden with sparse immune response on histology.

Cutaneous Helminthiasis

See also Chapter 35

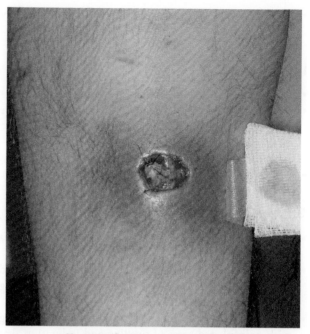

• **Fig. 50.34** Cutaneous leishmaniasis ulcer.

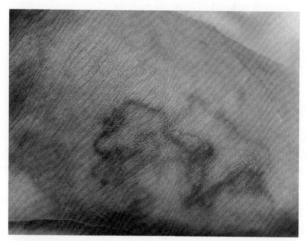

• **Fig. 50.35** Cutaneous larva migrans. (From Kincaid L, Klowak M, Klowak S, Boggild AK. Management of imported cutaneous larva migrans: a case series and mini-review. *Travel Med Infect Dis.* 2015;13(5):382–387.)

Cutaneous Larva Migrans

• **Serpiginous**, "creeping" pink or red rash usually on the extremities (Fig. 50.35) where there is contact with ground, particularly sand. Often **very itchy but rarely painful.**
• Caused by *Ancylostoma braziliense* larvae, dog hookworm, in the Americas and Caribbean. Humans are a dead-end host. Organism is found throughout tropical and subtropical regions.
• Clinical diagnosis. Biopsy rarely helpful as pathogen rarely at biopsy site.
• Can defer specific treatment as the larvae will not progress though life cycle in humans and will die. Often will regress in weeks to occasionally months.

- Can treat with mebendazole or ivermectin if intensely symptomatic.

Larva Currens

- Cutaneous manifestation of strongyloidiasis.
- Very rapid, migratory erythematous rash that can involve any part of the body but is often seen perianally due to larvae passed in the stool.
- Diagnosis is with stool studies to detect larvae or serology.
- Treat with ivermectin for strongyloidiasis.

Gnathostomiasis

- Migratory erythematous lesions, much slower than larva currens.
- Caused by *Gnathostoma* spp. larva from undercooked fish. Larvae migrate through various tissues, including both skin and visceral tissues.
- Presents most commonly with **intermittent swelling** with **painful, red** areas of swelling and induration that may **migrate** every few weeks.
- Treatment is with surgical excision of the worms or with systemic albendazole or ivermectin.

INFESTATIONS

Scabies

Cutaneous infection by *Sarcoptes scabiei* var. *hominis*, an eight-legged mite. Females burrow into the skin to lay eggs, and the host develops a delayed hypersensitivity reaction to the mite and eggs.
- Transmission is via **direct skin contact** with **infected host or with fomites**, particularly bedsheets, clothing, etc.
- Clinical presentation depends on immune status of host and mite burden. The chief complaint of scabies is **significant pruritus**, often worse at night.
- **Classic scabies**
  - Occurs in immunocompetent host. There are typically only a few mites. Small papules with occasional tracking erythema (along burrow track) and often associated with significant excoriations. Most commonly seen in the interdigital spaces, wrist flexor area, and waist, but can be seen anywhere
- **Crusted scabies**
  - Often associated with immunocompromise (i.e., AIDS, HTLV-1 infection, lymphoma, diabetes, steroid use, etc.). Thousands to millions of mites present. Pruritus and thick crusted plaques are common (Fig. 50.36). Can cause dystrophic nails, alopecia, erythroderma, etc. Diagnosis is often clinical but may be aided by identifying mite organisms or eggs from biopsy or scrapings. Also known as Norwegian scabies.

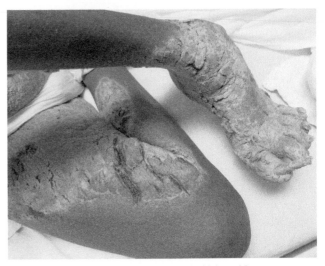

- **Fig. 50.36** Scabies crustosa thigh and foot

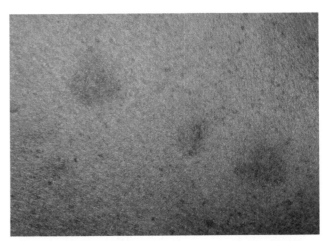

- **Fig. 50.37** Bedbug insect bites. (From Inflammatory papules. In: Marks JG, Miller JJ. *Lookingbill and Marks' Principles of Dermatology.* 6th ed. Elsevier; 2019.)

- Treatment of classic scabies is with topical permethrin or oral ivermectin once with a repeat treatment in 1–2 weeks afterward. Treatment of crusted scabies is with combination of topical permethrin and oral ivermectin for several days. Isolation and treatment of contacts important in crusted scabies.

Bedbug (*Cimex lectularius*) Bites (Fig. 50.37)

- Typically, 3–4 lesions ("breakfast, lunch, and dinner") grouped close together in somewhat **linear** pattern that happen after bedbug takes a blood meal. Individual variation in response leads to different lesions in those with same exposure, from no lesions to pruritic urticarial-like papules to large urticarial wheals.
- Treat symptomatically with topical steroids and oral antihistamines, will resolve in 1–2 weeks. Secondary bacterial infections would require antibiotics.

Cutaneous Myiasis

Self-limited fly larval infestation when ova are laid on skin or clothing by various species of fly of the order Diptera (i.e., *Cordylobia anthropophaga*, tumbu fly, sub-Saharan Africa; *Dermatobia hominis*, human botfly, found in the Americas, etc.).

- Furuncular (or papular) myiasis: develop after botfly or tumbu fly ova come in contact with human skin and **develop into larvae in the dermis.** Start as single or multiple small erythematous papules, enlarge to furuncles with distinct central punctum.
- Wound myiasis (*Cochliomyia hominovorax* and *Chrysomya bezziana* larvae) suspected with development of pain and bleeding in preexisting wounds. Fever, chills, leukocytosis with eosinophilia may be seen. Lesions in head concerning as larvae can burrow and cause sequelae such as blindness and systemic illness (i.e., sepsis).

- Diagnosis is suggested by history including geographic exposures and clinical exam. Suspicion confirmed with removal of the larva.
- Treat definitively with **mechanical removal of larvae** by a variety of means; larvae should be removed intact if at all possible.

SUMMARY OF CUTANEOUS MANIFESTATIONS OF INFECTION

This chapter has covered key infections involving the skin, common either in clinical practice or in exam questions, using a pathogen-dependent categorization. An alternative way of approaching this topic is via the particular cutaneous manifestation seen. Table 50.1 summarizes the common patterns of skin changes with a differential of the infections that may be associated.

TABLE 50.1 Cutaneous Patterns and Associated Infections

Cutaneous Patterns	Associated Infections
Umbilicated papules	• Cutaneous cryptococcosis (Fig. 50.38) • Histoplasmosis • Molluscum contagiosum (Fig. 50.39) • *Talaromyces marneffei*
Infection-related lesions on palms and soles	• Erythema multiforme (recurrent often triggered by HSV-1 outbreak) • Hand, foot, and mouth disease (coxsackieviruses especially A16, enterovirus 71, etc.) (Fig. 50.30) • Lesions associated with infective endocarditis (Fig. 50.40, Osler node, Janeway lesion) (Fig. 50.40) • *Neisseria gonorrhoeae* (disseminated gonococcal infection) • *Neisseria meningitidis* (Fig. 50.41, meningococcemia) • Rocky Mountain spotted fever (Fig. 50.5) • *Treponema pallidum* (secondary syphilis) (Fig. 50.8), keratoderma blenorrhagicum (reactive arthritis, syphilis) (Fig. 50.11)
Ascending lymphangitis aka "sporotrichoid spread"	• Cutaneous leishmaniasis (Fig. 50.34) • *Mycobacterium marinum* • Nocardiosis • *Sporothrix schenckii* (Fig. 50.22) • Systemic mycoses may present this way (coccidioidomycosis, blastomycosis, histoplasmosis)
Flexural lesions	• Candidal intertrigo • Dermatophyte infection • Erythrasma (*Corynebacterium minutissimum*)
Large cutaneous ulcers	• Cutaneous leishmaniasis (Fig. 50.34) • *Mycobacterium ulcerans* (Buruli ulcer) • Noma or cancrum oris (polymicrobial predominantly anaerobes like *Fusobacterium necrophorum*) • Sexually transmitted infections (STIs) (HSV particularly in immunosuppressed hosts, granuloma inguinale/donovanosis – *Klebsiella granulomatis*)

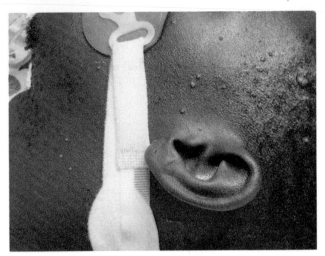

• **Fig. 50.38** Cutaneous lesions of cryptococcosis in intubated patient with AIDS.

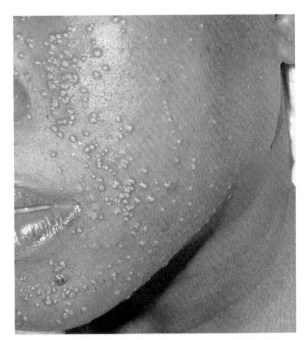

• **Fig. 50.39** Molluscum contagiosum in person with HIV: facial lesions associated with CD4 less than 100/μL.

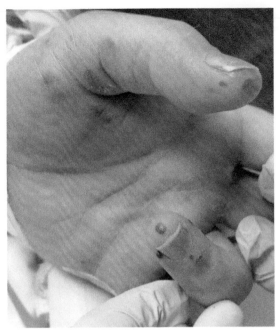

• **Fig. 50.40** Osler nodes in case of infective endocarditis due to MRSA.

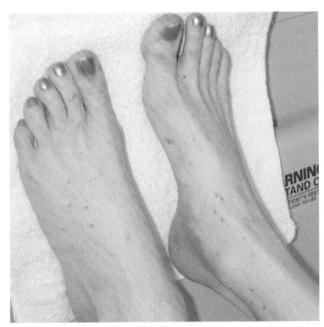

• **Fig. 50.41** *Neisseria meningitidis* infection with associated petechial rash.

Further Resources

1. DermNet NZ – All About the Skin. https://www.dermnetnz.org/.
2. Stevens DL, Bisno AL, Chambers HF, et al. Practice guidelines for the diagnosis and management of skin and soft tissue infections: 2014 Update by the Infectious Diseases Society of America. *Clin Infect Dis.* 2014;59(2):e10–52.
3. DPDx – Laboratory Identification of Parasites of Public Health Concern. Centers for Disease Control and Prevention. https://www.cdc.gov/dpdx/.
4. Mycoses Study Group Education and Research Consortium (MS-GERC) Doctor Fungus. http://msgercdoctorfungus.com/.

51

ID Memory Aids

CARLOS R. MEJIA-CHEW, GEROME ESCOTA, JANE A. O'HALLORAN

The items summarized here are not intended to be the sole indicators of disease. They only serve as clues and not proofs of specific infectious diseases. They are presented here to provide buzzwords for the board exam.

A–Z of Zoonoses

Animal-associated infections (quick DDX guide)	**P**lague
	Anthrax
"PATrick BBQs LeftoveRs"	**T**ularemia
	Brucellosis
	Bartonellosis
	Q fever
	Leptospirosis
	Rat bite fever
Armadillos	*Sporothrix schenckii* (sporotrichosis)
	Mycobacterium leprae (leprosy)
Bamboo rats	*Talaromyces marneffei* (formerly *Penicillium marneffei*)
Beavers	*Giardia lamblia*
Bat	*Histoplasma capsulatum*
	Rabies
Birds	*Chlamydophila psittaci* (psittacosis)
Cats	*Bartonella henselae* (cat scratch or bite)
	Coxiella burnetii (placental exposure)
	Pasteurella multocida (bite)
	Toxocara cati (cat feces)
	Toxoplasma gondii (cat feces)
Cattle	*Brucellosis abortus* (brucellosis)
	Coxiella burnetii (Q fever)
	Mycobacterium bovis
	Mycobacterium caprae
	Taenia saginata (beef tapeworm)
	Prions (variant CJD)
Chipmunk	La Crosse virus
Dogs	*Capnocytophaga canimorsus* (dog bite)
	Echinococcus granulosus (dog feces)
	Staphylococcus intermedius (dog bite)
	Toxocara canis (dog feces)
Elephants	*Mycobacterium tuberculosis*

Continued

Fish
(Direct contact/contaminated water or raw consumption)

Anisakis simplex (raw consumption)
Clonorchis sinensis (raw consumption)
Opisthorchis viverrini (raw consumption)
Diphyllobothrium latum (raw consumption)
Edwardsiella tarda
Erysipelothrix rhusiopathiae
Gnathostoma spinigerum (raw consumption)
Mycobacterium marinum (fish tank granuloma)
Streptococcus iniae

Fleas

Rickettsia typhi (murine/endemic typhus)
Yersinia pestis (plague)

Flying squirrels
Flies

Rickettsia prowazekii (Epidemic typhus)
Onchocerca volvulus (blackfly)
Leishmania spp. (sandfly)
Bartonella bacilliformis/Oroya fever (sandfly)
Trypanosoma brucei (tsetse fly)
Loa loa (deer fly)
Myiasis (fly larva)

Foxes
Goats

Echinococcus multilocularis
Brucellosis melitensis (brucellosis)
Coxiella burnetii (Q fever)

Hamsters
Horses
Iguanas and other reptiles
Jackals (wild carnivores and domestic dogs)
Kangaroo
Leeches
Lice (associated with homelessness,
    poor living condition)

Lymphocytic choriomeningitis virus
Rhodococcus equi
Salmonella spp.
Rabies
Coxiella burnetii (Q fever)
Aeromonas hydrophila
Bartonella quintana (trench fever)
Borrelia recurrentis (louse-borne relapsing fever)
Rickettsia prowazekii (epidemic fever)

Macaques (old world monkeys)
Mites

Herpes B virus
Rickettsia akari (rickettsialpox)
Orientia tsutsugamushi (scrub typhus)

Mosquitoes

Chikungunya virus
Dengue virus
Yellow fever virus
Zika virus
Plasmodium spp.
Encephalitis viruses (West Nile, St. Louis, Eastern equine, Western
    equine, La Crosse, Japanese encephalitis)
Wuchereria bancrofti (lymphatic filariasis)

Oysters

Vibrio parahaemolyticus
Vibrio vulnificus

Pigeons (droppings)

Cryptococcus neoformans
Histoplasma capsulatum

Pigs

Balantidium coli
Brucellosis suis (brucellosis)
Erysipelothrix rhusiopathiae
Hepatitis E
Nipah virus (encephalitis)
Taenia solium
Ingested cysts in undercooked meat (pork tapeworm)
Ingested eggs from feces (cysticercosis)

Poultry

Campylobacter spp.
Salmonella spp.

Prairie dogs	*Yersinia pestis*
	Monkeypox
Quack, quack (ducks)!	*Chlamydophila psittaci* (psittacosis) rare
Rabbits	*Francisella tularensis*
Raccoons	*Baylisascaris procyonis* (raccoon roundworm)
Rats	Hanta virus
	Lassa fever
	Leptospira interrogans (leptospirosis)
	Lymphocytic choriomeningitis virus
	Spirillum minus (rat bite fever)
	Streptobacillus moniliformis (rat bite fever)
	Yersinia pestis (plague)
Reduviid bug (kissing bug)	*Trypanosoma cruzi* (Chagas disease)
Seals	*Mycobacterium pinnipedii*
Sheep	*Brucellosis melitensis* (brucellosis)
	Coxiella burnetii (Q fever)
	Poxvirus (orf)
Squirrels	Bornavirus
Tick	
Dog tick (*Dermacentor variabilis*)	*Rickettsia rickettsii* (Rocky Mountain spotted fever)
	Francisella tularensis
Deer tick (*Ixodes scapularis*)	*Anaplasma phagocytophilum*
	Babesia microti
	Borrelia burgdorferi
	Borrelia miyamotoi
	Powassan virus
Lone Star tick (*Amblyomma americanum*)	*Ehrlichia chaffeensis*
	Francisella tularensis
	STARI
	Heartland virus
	Bourbon virus
Turtles	*Clostridium botulinum*
	Salmonella spp. (like other reptiles)
Urchins (a spiny marine creature)	*Vibrio alginolyticus*
Voles	*Mycobacterium microti*
Wild boars	*Trichinella spiralis* (trichinosis)
Yaks	*Echinococcus granulosus* (hydatid cyst)

Food Associations

Aquatic vegetation (e.g., watercress)	*Fasciola hepatica* (liver fluke)
Honey	*Clostridium botulinum* (infantile botulism)
Home-canned vegetables	*Clostridium botulinum*
Imported raspberries	*Cyclospora cayetanensis*
Oysters	*Plesiomonas shigelloides*
Potato or egg salad	*Staphylococcus aureus*
Peanut butter	*Salmonella* spp.
	Listeria monocytogenes
Raw crayfish/crabs	*Paragonimus westermani* or *Paragonimus kellicotti*
Slugs/snails	*Angiostrongylus cantonensis* (rat lungworm)
	Clonorchis sinensis
Rice (improperly cooked)	*Bacillus cereus*
Soft cheeses	*Listeria monocytogenes*

Continued

Uncooked meat	*Bacillus anthracis*
	Campylobacter spp. (chicken)
	Toxoplasma gondii
	Trichinella spiralis (pork and wild game)
	Shiga toxin producing *Escherichia coli*/Enterohemorrhagic *E. coli* (ground beef)
	Shigella spp.
	Salmonella spp.
Unpasteurized milk/dairy products	*Brucella* spp.
	Listeria monocytogenes
	Mycobacterium bovis
	Tickborne encephalitis
	Campylobacter
	Salmonella
	Yersinia
	Brainerd diarrhea (persistent diarrhea, unknown cause; occasional outbreaks, foodborne)
Water chestnuts/bamboo	*Fasciolopsis buski* (giant intestinal fluke)

Environmental Exposures

Abortion	*Clostridium sordellii*
Bird droppings/contaminated soil	*Histoplasma capsulatum*
Eucalyptus trees	*Cryptococcus gattii*
Heroin (black tar)	*Clostridium sordellii* (necrotizing soft tissue infection)
	Botulism
	Tetanus
Moist soil	*Blastomyces dermatitidis*
Mulch/plant debris	*Aspergillus* spp.
Rice paddies	*Talaromyces marneffei*
	Japanese encephalitis
	Schistosoma spp.
Rose gardening	*Sporothrix schenckii*
Semi-arid/dusty terrain	*Coccidioides immitis*
Spelunking/caving	*Histoplasma capsulatum*
Water-associated soft tissue infections	*Chromobacterium violaceum*
	Aeromonas species (brackish)
	Edwardsiella tarda (fish spines)
	Erysipelothrix rhusiopathiae (fishermen's hand)
	Vibrio vulnificus (brackish or salt water)
	Mycobacterium marinum (fish tank)
Warm water (aquatic sports)	*Naegleria fowleri*
Water parks	*Cryptosporidium parvum*

'I say..., you say...'

Abattoir (slaughterhouse) workers	*Brucella melitensis*
	Coxiella burnetii
Animal hides	*Bacillus anthracis* (anthrax)
Breast pumps	*Serratia marcescens*
Cabins/outhouses	Hantavirus
	Borrelia hermsii (tickborne relapsing fever)
Cardiac surgery	*Mycobacterium chimaera* (contaminated heater–coolers)

Central facial/nasal lesions

Bacteria
Leprosy (saddle nose deformity)
Endemic treponemal infection (e.g., pinta)
Congenital syphilis (saddle nose deformity)

Fungus
Paracoccidioidomycosis
Coccidioidomycosis
Mold infection
Blastomycosis

Parasite
Balamuthia
Mucocutaneous leishmaniasis

Malignancy
NK cell tumors

Autoimmune
Wegener's granulomatosis (saddle nose deformity)
Relapsing polychondritis (saddle nose deformity)

Others
Trigeminal trophic syndrome

Clothing dried on bushes	Tungiasis, myiasis
Contact lenses	*Acanthamoeba* spp.
Cosmetic surgery	*Mycobacterium abscessus*
Cruise ships	Norovirus
Delayed umbilical stump separation/cigarette paper scarring	Leukocyte adhesion deficiency type 1 (LAD-1)
Hot tubs	*Pseudomonas aeruginosa* (folliculitis) Nontuberculous mycobacteria (pneumonitis)
Intrauterine devices (IUDs)	*Actinomyces* spp. Group A streptococcus
Nail through sole of trainer	*Pseudomonas aeruginosa*
Near drowning	*Scedosporium prolificans*
Pedicures	Rapid growing nontuberculous mycobacterium (RG-NTM)
Pulpectomy (pediatric dental procedures)	*Mycobacterium abscessus*
Water coolers/fountains	*Legionella pneumophila*
Wound dehiscence	Chronic granulomatous disease
Reconstructive surgery	*Clostridium* spp.
Retained primary teeth	Hyper IgE syndrome (Job's syndrome)
Shepherds	*Echinococcus granulosus* (hydatid cyst) Orf
Triathlon, white water rafting	Leptospirosis

Disease Associations

Acute T-cell lymphoma	HTLV-1
Aplastic crisis in hemolytic anemia	Parvovirus B19
Bladder cancer (urothelial)	*Schistosoma haematobium*
Bullous myringitis	*Mycoplasma pneumoniae*
Brain and lung abscess	*Nocardia* spp.
Chronic granulomatous disease	*Aspergillus* spp. *Chromobacterium violaceum* *Francisella philomiragia* *Granulibacter bethesdensis* *Nocardia*

Continued

Cholangiocarcinoma	*Clonorchis sinensis/Opisthorchis viverrini*
Colon cancer	*Streptococcus gallolyticus* (formerly *S. bovis*)
	Clostridium septicum
Complement deficiency	*Neisseria meningitidis*
Cystic fibrosis	*Burkholderia cepacia*
Diabetic ketoacidosis	*Rhizopus/Mucor* spp. (mucormycosis)
Dysphagia as an ID clue	Tetanus
	Tick paralysis
	HTLV-1
	Enterovirus 71
	Botulism
	Guillain–Barré syndrome
	West Nile virus
	Polio
Ear lymphocytoma	Borreliosis (Lyme disease)
Ecthyma gangrenosum	*Pseudomonas aeruginosa*
Erythrasma	*Corynebacterium minutissimum*
Empyema necessitans	*Actinomyces* spp.
	Mycobacterium tuberculosis
Eosinophilic meningitis	*Angiostrongylus cantonensis*
	Baylisascaris procyonis
	Coccidioides spp.
	Gnathostoma spp.
	Strongyloides stercoralis
Eschar	Tickborne illnesses (tache noir):
	US: *Rickettsia akari* (rickettsialpox)
	Europe: *Rickettsia conorii* (boutonneuse fever)
	Asia: *Orientia tsutsugamushi* (scrub typhus)
	Africa: *Rickettsia africae* (African tick bite fever)
	North Asia: *Rickettsia sibirica* (North Asian typhus)
	Australia: *Rickettsia australis* (Queensland tick typhus)
	Anthrax
	Rat bite fever
	Tularemia
	Plague
	Ecthyma gangrenosum (secondary to a wide variety of infections including *Pseudomonas*, *Fusarium*, etc.)
	SPIDER BITE! Do not forget!
	Cowpox (part of evolution)
Fulminant liver failure on pregnancy	Hepatitis E
Gram negative meningitis (in patients without a history of neurosurgical procedure)	*Strongyloides stercoralis* Hypermucoviscous *Klebsiella pneumonia*
Hemorrhagic cystitis	Adenovirus
	BK virus
Human T-lymphotropic virus	*Strongyloides stercoralis*
Hyposplenism/splenectomy	*Babesia microti*
	Capnocytophaga canimorsus
	Haemophilus influenza
	Neisseria meningitis
	Streptococcus pneumoniae
	Salmonella spp.
Hypogammaglobinemia	*Mycoplasma* spp.
Ibrutinib	*Cryptococcus*

Iron overload syndromes	*Rhizopus/Mucor* spp. (mucormycosis)
	Vibrio vulnificus
	Mycobacterium haemophilum
	Yersinia pestis
	Aeromonas spp.
Lancinating pain	*Treponema pallidum* (syphilis, tabes dorsalis)
Lemierre's syndrome (septic thrombophlebitis)	*Fusobacterium* spp.
Löeffler's syndrome	Ascariasis
	Strongyloidiasis
	Hookworm
Madura foot	*Actinomyces* (bacterial) or fungal
Monomicrobial necrotizing fasciitis	Group A streptococcus
	Aeromonas spp.
	Vibrio vulnificus
	Cryptococcus neoformans (in immunocompromised)
Multiple myeloma	*Streptococcus pneumoniae*
Paralysis, ascending	Guillain-Barré syndrome
	Enterovirus D68
	Tick paralysis
	West Nile virus
Paralysis, descending	Botulism
Parkinson-like illness	Japanese encephalitis virus
Polio-like illness	West Nile virus
Postpartum toxic shock syndrome	*Clostridium sordellii*
Pulmonary alveolar proteinosis	*Nocardia* spp.
Rhombencephalitis (ataxia/nystagmus/cranial nerve palsies)	*Listeria monocytogenes*
	Enterovirus 71
Septic arthritis of shoulder	*Cutibacterium* (formerly *Propionibacterium*) *acnes*
Snowflake keratitis	*Onchocera volvulus*
Swimmer's itch (Great Lakes)	Avian schistosomiasis
Tropical spastic paraparesis	HTLV-1

Clinical Clues

Arthritis and rash syndrome	Acute rheumatic fever
	Subacute bacterial endocarditis
	Chronic meningococcemia
	Rat bite fever
	Relapsing fever (louse, tickborne)
	Henoch-Schönlein purpura
	Chronic parvovirus B19 (arthropathy similar to rheumatoid arthritis predominates)
	Lepra reaction from leprosy
Bilateral periorbital edema	*Trichinella spiralis* (Trichinellosis)
Polymyalgia rheumatic-like symptoms with normal or low ESR and CRP	*Trichinella spiralis* (Trichinellosis)
Bladder cancer, history of BCG vaccine	Disseminated BCG infection
Bloody ascites, pleural fluid	Kaposi sarcoma
	Bacillary angiomatosis
	Anthrax
Bull neck + gray pharyngeal pseudo membranes	*Corynebacterium diphtheriae* (Diphtheria)
Calf tenderness	Leptospirosis
Conjunctival suffusion	Leptospirosis
"Cotton balls" on funduscopy	*Candida* spp. endophthalmitis
Destructive ulcer with pizza-like borders	Leishmaniasis

Continued

Destructive ulcer with undermining edges

Ecthyma gangrenosum

Encephalitis + flaccid paralysis

Encephalitis + urinary symptoms

Evanescence rash

Genital elephantiasis (esthiomene = enlarged female genitalia; saxophone penis)

Hand tenosynovitis

Hutchinson's sign (vesicular lesions tip of nose)

Heart block

New onset hypercalcemia, in an endemic region

Koplik spots

Migratory panniculitis

Moth eaten head (patchy alopecia)

Muffled voice

Necrotic ulcer with surrounding edema

Olecranon bursitis, nonhealing after water exposure

Ovarian teratoma in a young encephalopathic female

Palms and/or soles involvement

Buruli ulcer (*Mycobacterium ulcerans*)

Pseudomonas aeruginosa

Angio-invasive molds (*Fusarium and Aspergillus* spp.)

West Nile virus

St. Louis encephalitis

Adult Still's disease

Lymphogranuloma venereum

Mycobacterium terrae complex

Disseminated gonorrheal infection

Herpes zoster ophthalmicus

Lyme disease (in the United States)

Chagas disease (in South America)

HTLV-1

Measles

Gnathostomiasis

Loa loa (calabar swellings)

Syphilis (secondary)

Epiglottitis

Anthrax

Cutaneous prototheceosis

Anti-NMDA encephalitis

Drugs

Stevens–Johnson syndrome/toxic epidermal necrolysis (SJS/TEN)

Infection

- Syphilis
- Rocky Mountain spotted fever (RMSF)
- Meningococcemia
- Coxsackie A16 (hand, foot, and mouth disease)
- Parvovirus B19 (papular pustular gloves and socks syndrome)
- Herpes simplex virus (HSV) and *Mycoplasma* (erythema multiforme)
- *Pseudomonas* (hot hand–foot syndrome)
- *Streptococcus* or *Staphylococcus* (toxic shock syndrome)
- Infective endocarditis

Noninfectious

- Bazex syndrome (GI squamous cell carcinoma)
- Tylosis
- Antisynthetase syndrome (dermatomyositis; mechanic's hand)
- Neutrophilic dermatoses of the dorsal hands
- Kawasaki disease
- Reiter's syndrome (keratoderma blenorrhagicum)

Painful genital ulcer

Painless genital ulcer

Paresthesia of mouth/lips

Parotitis + orchitis

Pneumonia, immunocompromised, especially posttransplant

"PANTT"

Preauricular lymphadenopathy + conjunctivitis

Proctitis

Haemophilus ducreyi (chancroid)

Herpes simplex virus (HSV)

Syphilis

Granuloma inguinale (*Klebsiella granulomatis*)

Paralytic shellfish poisoning

Mumps

Pneumocystis jirovecii

Aspergillus (think of other fungi as well: *Mucor*, dematiaceous molds, *Cryptococcus*, endemics like *Histoplasma*, *Blastomyces*, *Coccidioides*)

*N*ocardia

*T*oxoplasma

*T*uberculosis (and nontuberculous *Mycobacteria*)

Adenovirus

Lymphogranuloma venereum

Pustular rash, generalized

- THINK about DDX for vesicular rash as vesicles can exhibit pustulosis as well (i.e., herpes simplex virus, varicella zoster virus, eczema herpeticum, coxsackievirus, echovirus, small-pox, monkeypox, vaccinia)

Infection

Disseminated gonococcal infection

Chronic meningococcemia (usually presents as recurrent fever, pustular rash, arthralgia/arthritis, headache)

Moraxella bacteremia

Tuberculosis (rare, called tuberculosis cutis miliaris acuta general-isata acute pustular eruption in TB)

Noninfectious

AGEP

DRESS

Behçet

Generalized pustular psoriasis of von Zumbusch

Recurrent aseptic meningitis (Mollaret syndrome)	Herpes simplex virus type 2
Sacroiliitis	*Brucella* spp.
Salty sputum	Pulmonary *echinococcosis*
Serpiginous rash	Cutaneous larva migrans
	(*Ancylostoma braziliense*; *Necator americanus*)
	Larva currens (strongyloidiasis)
Shin pain, fever in a homeless patient	Trench fever (*Bartonella quintana*)
Sore throat + sand paper rash	Group A streptococcus (scarlet fever)
	Arcanobacterium haemolyticum
Sore throat + foul smelling breath	Vincent's angina (trench mouth)
Sore throat + oral + hand + foot vesicular lesion	Coxsackievirus (hand, foot, and mouth)
Sore throat + pharyngeal vesicular lesion	Coxsackievirus (herpangina)
Sporotrichoid-like lesions	*Sporothrix schenckii*
	Nocardia brasiliensis
	Mycobacterium marinum
	Leishmaniasis brasiliensis
	Francisella tularensis
Stellate maculopathy	Bartonella neuroretinitis
Strawberry cervix	Trichomoniasis
Strawberry tongue	Group A streptococcus
	Kawasaki disease
	Staphylococcus toxic shock syndrome
Testicular pain + back/joint pains in endemic areas	Brucellosis
Unilateral periorbital edema (Romaña sign)	Chagas disease
Vaginal pH >4.5	Bacterial vaginosis
	Trichomonas
Warty-like rash, diffuse	Epidermodysplasia verruciformis (HPV)
	Eczema herpeticum (HSV)
	Norwegian scabies
	Mycosis fungoides
	Langerhans cell histiocytosis
Warty-like rash, localized	Human papilloma virus (HPV) – of course!
	Tuberculosis verrucosa cutis
	Chromoblastomycosis
	Blastomycosis
	Histoplasma capsulatum var. *duboisii*
	Cancer
	Paracoccidioides

Continued

Hematology Hints

Amastigotes	Leishmaniasis
Maltese cross (RBC)	Babesiosis
Giant blue granules in neutrophils	Chediak–Higashi syndrome
Leukemoid reaction, lymphocytic	*Bordetella pertussis*
	Infectious mononucleosis
Morulae (neutrophils)	Anaplasmosis
Morulae (monocytes)	Ehrlichiosis
Trypomastigotes	Trypanosomiasis
Band-form trophozoites	*Plasmodium malariae*
Multiple ring-form trophozoites per cell	*Plasmodium falciparum*
Crescent-shaped gametocytes	*Plasmodium falciparum*
Low reticulocyte count and fever	Parvovirus B19
Schüffner's dots in RBCs	*Plasmodium vivax/ ovale*
Infections with positive blood smear	*Malaria*
(*My B*oy*F*riend is *ARAB*)	*Babesiosis*
	Filariasis
	• you will see microfilaria
	*A*merican trypanosomiasis (Chagas disease)
	• you will see trypomastigote
	*R*elapsing fever (tick- and louseborne)
	• you will see spiral bacteria
	*A*frican trypanosomiasis (sleeping sickness)
	• you will see trypomastigote
	*B*artonellosis (Oroya fever)
	• you will see intraerythrocytic bacteria
	Of course, don't forget *Ehrlichia* and *Anaplasma*

Micro Triggers

Safety pin on Gram stain	*Yersinia pestis*
	Vibrio parahaemolyticus
	Burkholderia pseudomallei
	Haemophilus ducreyi
	Klebsiella granulomatis
Weakly acid-fast	*Rhodococcus*
	Cyclospora cayetanensis
	Cystoisospora belli
	Cryptosporidium parvum
	Legionella micdadei
	Nocardia
	Gordonia spp.
	Tsukamurella spp.
	Dietzia spp.
School of fish on Gram stain	*Haemophilus ducreyi*
Salmon pink colonies	*Rhodococcus equi*
Odor and bacterial plates:	
Horse manure	*Clostridioides difficile*
Musty, earthy, dirt basement	*Nocardia, Burkholderia*
Grapes or corn tortilla	*Pseudomonas aeruginosa*
Butterscotch or caramel	*Streptococcus anginosus*
Bleach	*Eikenella corrodens*
Canoe-shaped conidia	*Fusarium* spp.
Copper pennies on KOH stain of skin	Chromoblastomycosis
Ciliated protozoa	*Balantidium coli*

Gram-negative bacteria
Glucose fermenter
Oxidase-negative, lactose-fermenting
"PEEKS"

Gram-negative bacteria
Glucose fermenter
Oxidase-negative, non-lactose-fermenting
"SHYPS"
Gram-negative bacteria
Glucose fermenter
Oxidase-positive

Gram-negative bacteria
Glucose nonfermenter
Oxidase-negative, non-lactose-fermenting
"SAB"
Gram-negative bacteria
Glucose nonfermenter
Oxidase-positive, non-lactose-fermenting
Streptococcus
Beta-hemolytic

Alpha-hemolytic
Gram-positive rods, branching
(also called branching filamentous organisms)

Gram-positive bacilli, aerobe
"CAREs for the LaB"

Gram-positive bacilli, anaerobe

Gram-negative coccobacilli

Providencia spp.
Enterobacter
Escherichia coli
Klebsiella
Serratia
Shigella
Yersinia
Proteus
Salmonella
Pasteurella
Vibrio
Aeromonas
Plesiomonas
Stenotrophomonas maltophilia
Acinetobacter baumannii
Burkholderia cepacia

Pseudomonas aeruginosa

Group A streptococcus (*S. pyogenes*)
Group B streptococcus (*S. agalactiae*)
Group C streptococcus (*S. dysgalactiae*)
Group D streptococcus (*S. bovis*)
Group F streptococcus (*S. milleri* group)
S. viridans
S. pneumoniae
Nocardia
Actinomyces
Streptomyces
Corynebacterium
Arcanobacterium
Rhodococcus
Erysipelothrix
Listeria
Bacillus
Clostridium
Cutibacterium
Lactobacillus
Moraxella
Yersinia
Bordetella
Francisella
Brucella
Pasteurella
HACEK organisms
   Haemophilus spp.
   Aggregatibacter spp.
   Cardiobacterium spp.
   Eikenella
   Kingella spp.
Legionella
Acinetobacter

Continued

Pathology Prompts

Acute-angle branched hyphae (45°)	*Aspergillus* spp.
Broad-based budding yeast (mother and daughter cells)	*Blastomyces dermatitidis*
Cigar-shaped yeast	*Sporothrix schenckii*
Clue cells	Bacterial vaginosis
Doughnut granuloma	*Coxiella burnetii*
	Epstein–Barr virus (EBV)
	Cytomegalovirus (CMV)
	Drug hypersensitivity
	Hodgkin lymphoma
Flower cells	HTLV-1
Foamy macrophages	*Tropheryma whipplei*
Lymphadenopathy, cervical; necrotizing histiocytes on pathology	Kikuchi–Fujimoto disease
Michaelis and Gutmann bodies	Malakoplakia
Negri bodies (brain tissue)	Rabies
Promastigotes	Leishmania
	Trypanosomes
Ship's wheel	Paracoccidioidomycosis
Spherules containing spores	Coccidioidomycosis
Stellate abscess	Lymphogranuloma venereum (LGV)
	Bartonella henselae (on Warthin–Starry stain)
Sulphur granules	*Actinomyces* spp.
Right-angle branched hyphae (90°)	*Zygomycetes* spp.
Intranuclear "owl's eye"	CMV

Radiological Reminders

Anterior–superior step-like erosion of the vertebra (Pedro–Pons sign)	*Brucella* spp.
Bear claw (kidney CT scan)	Xanthogranulomatous pyelonephritis
Cerebellar atrophy in HIV+ patients or other immunosuppressed patients with cerebellar signs and symptoms	JC virus granule cell neuronopathy
Feeding vessel sign (close to a nodule)	Invasive fungal infection (*Aspergillus*, *Mucor*)
	Septic embolization
Halo sign (solid infiltrated surrounded by ground-glass opacities)	Aspergillosis
Penumbra sign (high intensity rim lining of an abscess cavity on T1; aka Brodie's abscess)	Hematogenous spread subacute osteomyelitis (most commonly due to *Staphylococcus aureus*)
Pulvinar sign (bilateral hyperintensity)	Variant Creutzfeldt–Jakob Disease (vCJD)
Reverse halo sign (ground-glass opacities surrounded by solid consolidation)	Mucormycosis
Splendore–Hoeppli phenomenon	Botryomycosis
Rhombencephalitis	*Listeria*
Thumb print sign	Epiglottitis

Where in the World?

Brazil	Yellow fever
Jamaica, Japan	HTLV-1 associated diseases
Saudi Arabia (Hajj pilgrimage)	Meningococcal meningitis
Papua New Guinea	Kuru
India	Granuloma inguinale
Micronesia	*Bordetella holmesii*
Northern Australia	Melioidosis
Hawaii	Leptospirosis
Horn of Africa	*Mycobacterium canetti*
Southwest USA	Coccidioidomycosis
Tioman Island, Malaysia	Sarcocystis
Ohio and Mississippi river basin	Blastomycoses
Gulf of Mexico	*Vibrio vulnificus*
Thailand/China/Vietnam	*Talaromyces* (formerly *Penicillium*) *marneffei*
Thailand/Taiwan	Angiostrongyliasis
Haiti	Cholera
Yemen	Cholera
Madagascar	Plague
	Chromoblastomycosis
Latin America	Chagas disease
West Africa	HIV-2
	Lassa fever
Yosemite	Hantavirus

Miscellaneous Mishmash

Amphotericin resistance	*Candida lusitaniae*
	Candida auris (some isolates)
	Aspergillus terreus
	Fusarium (some species)
	Scedosporium (Lomentospora) prolificans
	Scedosporium apiospermum (some)
	Pseudallescheria boydii
	Sporothrix schenckii
Autoinfection	*Strongyloides*
	Paracapillaria
	Hymenolepis
Enterococci intrinsically resistant to vancomycin	*Enterococcus gallinarum*
	Enterococcus casseliflavus
Parasites that can penetrate intact skin	*Strongyloides stercoralis*
	Schistosoma spp.
	Hookworm
Gram-positives resistant to vancomycin	*Lactobacillus* spp.
	Leuconostoc spp.
	Erysipelothrix spp.
	Cutibacterium spp.
Fanconi's syndrome	Aminoglycoside
	Tenofovir disoproxil
	Cidofovir
Peppery tasting fish	Scombroid
Teeth feel loose	Ciguatera
Cells that look like "foot prints in the sand" seen in CSF	Mollaret's cells in HSV-2-associated recurrent meningitis (Mollaret's meningitis)

Continued

Bioterrorism	Smallpox
Person-to-person	Plague
Non-person-to-person	Viral hemorrhagic fever
	Anthrax
	Botulism
	Tularemia
Corynebacterium cutaneous diseases	Erythrasma
	Trichomycosis axillaris
	Pitted keratolysis
Free living amoebas	*Acanthamoeba* spp.
	Naegleria fowleri
	Balamuthia mandrillaris
	Sappinia pedata
Visceral larva migrans	*Toxocara cati* (cat roundworm)
	Toxocara canis (dog roundworm)
Neural larva migrans	*Baylisascaris procyonis* (raccoon roundworm)
Wolbachia spp.	Parasite of *Wuchereria bancrofti*
Chlorine-resistant organism	*Cryptosporidium* spp.
	Giardia lamblia
	Naegleria fowleri
Refractory nongonococcal urethritis	*Mycoplasma genitalium*
Stool exam showing parasite larva (not adult worm)	*Strongyloides stercoralis*

Key Antimicrobials-Associated Adverse Events

Antibacterials	
Fluoroquinolones	Tendinitis
Daptomycin	Myopathy/rhabdomyolysis
	Eosinophilic pneumonitis
Metronidazole	Peripheral neuropathy and encephalopathy
	Cerebellar toxicity (MRI: symmetric involvement of the dentate nuclei)
Vancomycin	Red man syndrome
	Linear IgA dermatitis (bullous lesion)
Aminoglycosides	Neuromuscular blockade (myasthenia gravis exacerbation)
Linezolid	Peripheral neuropathy
	Optic neuropathy (irreversible)
	Thrombocytopenia/anemia
	Lactic acidosis
Ceftriaxone	Hyperbilirubinemia
Cefepime	Akinetic seizures
Chloramphenicol	Idiosyncratic aplastic anemia
Tetracyclines	Photosensitivity
Minocycline	Vestibular toxicity
Sulfamethoxazole	Crystalluria
Trimethoprim	Hyperkalemia
Nitrofurantoin	Acute pneumonitis and pulmonary fibrosis
Colistin	Neurotoxicity
Dapsone	Methemoglobinemia (G6PD deficiency)
Antifungals	
Itraconazole	Heart failure (negative inotropic)
Voriconazole	Visual hallucinations
	Periostitis (bone pain/elevated alkaline phosphatase, fluoride toxicity)
	Skin cancer

Flucytosine	Bone marrow suppression
	Colitis (perforation)
Amphotericin	Chest/back pain during infusion

Antimycobacterials

Cycloserine	Neurotoxicity
Clofazimine	Skin/corneal discoloration
Pyrazinamide	Hyperuricemia (gout)
Ethambutol	Optic neuropathy

Antivirals

Aciclovir	Crystalline nephropathy
Oseltamivir	Neuropsychiatric symptoms
Foscarnet	Genital ulcerations
Peramivir	Exfoliative dermatitis

Antiretrovirals

Abacavir	Hypersensitivity syndrome (HLA B-157)
Atazanavir	Nephrolithiasis
Tenofovir disoproxil fumarate	Fanconi syndrome (proximal tubular acidosis)

Antiparasitics

Mefloquine	Neuropsychiatric symptoms
Quinine	Cinchonism (tinnitus, deafness, visual disturbances) and hypoglycemia
Primaquine	Methemoglobinemia and hemolytic anemia (G6PD deficiency)
Melarsoprol	Encephalopathy
Diethylcarbamazine (DEC)	Mazzotti reaction (pruritus, fever, arthralgia)
Pyrimethamine	Bone marrow suppression
Paromomycin	Cochlear and vestibular toxicity

Acronyms

MY SPACE – microorganisms with inducible AmpC	*Morganella* *Yersinia* *Serratia* *Pseudomonas/Proteus* (indole positive)/ *Providencia* *Aeromonas/Acinetobacter* *Citrobacter* *Enterobacter*
PROMOS – microorganisms to which colistin has no activity	*Providencia/Proteus* *Morganella* *Serratia*
ESKAPE – multidrug-resistant organisms	*Enterococcus faecium* *Staphylococcus aureus* *Klebsiella pneumoniae* *Acinetobacter baumannii* *Pseudomonas aeruginosa* *Enterobacter* spp.
CAKE produces gas – gas-producing microorganisms	*Clostridium* spp. Anaerobes *Klebsiella* spp. *Escherichia coli*
PEEKS - lactose-fermenting Enterobacteriaceae	*Providencia* spp. *Enterobacter* spp. *Escherichia coli* *Klebsiella* spp. *Serratia* spp.

Continued

ABCE – dematiaceous molds

Alternaria
Bipolaris
Curvularia
Exserohilum

FACE - antibiotics that exacerbate myasthenia gravis

Fluoroquinolones
Aminoglycosides
Colistin/Clindamycin
Erythromycin

VAcuuM – antibiotics associated with ototoxicity

Vancomycin
Aminoglycosides
Macrolides

DITCHERS – risk factors for TB disease

Diabetes
Intravenous drug use/Intestinal bypass
TNF-α inhibitors
Consistent CXR abnormalities
HIV (or other immunosuppression)
End-stage renal disease
Recent TB infection (exposure)
Silicosis

SwiRLL - medically important spirochetes

Syphilis
Relapsing fever (*Borrelia recurrentis*)
Leptospirosis
Lyme disease

TVM – pathogens requiring airborne isolation

Tuberculosis
Varicella/disseminated zoster
Measles

HI, My Mucous Requires Protection Please! – pathogens requiring droplet precautions

HiB (*Haemophilus influenza* B)
Influenza
Mycoplasma
Mumps/Meningococcus
Rubella
Pertussis
Parvovirus B19

Mr. Wiskott–Aldrich uses a TIE

Thrombocytopenia
Immunodeficiency
Eczema

CVID – common variable immunodeficiency

Cancer (lymphoma)
Vaccine (nonresponse)
Infections (sino-pulmonary and gastrointestinal)
Decreased immunoglobulins

Sample Questions

1. A 72-year-old man presented with a 6-month history of a chronic cough, occasional night sweats, and weight loss. He was known to have diabetes and hypertension. He had a smoking history of 60 packs per year (PPY), with occasional alcohol intake. He lived in Missouri, and was a truck driver with frequent visits to Phoenix, Arizona, and Michigan.

Investigations:

    CT chest: right upper lung lobe nodules and mediastinal lymphadenopathy

    PET scan: increased uptake in the lung nodule and lymphadenopathy

    Nodule biopsy histology: necrotizing granulomas on GMS stain

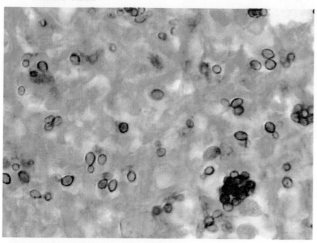

What is the most likely diagnosis?

A. Aspergillosis

B. Blastomycosis

C. Coccidioidomycosis

D. Cryptococcosis

E. Histoplasmosis

2. A 21-year-old man presented with new penile lesions. He had insertive vaginal and oral intercourse using a latex condom with a casual female partner 72 hours earlier. He denied any current medications, known past medical history, or allergies. He was a college student and worked part-time in a chemistry laboratory.

On examination, there were erythematous plaques over the shaft and glans penis.

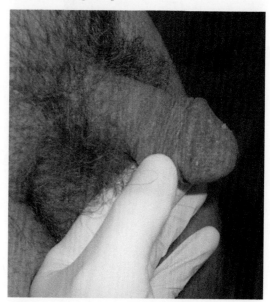

What is the most likely diagnosis?

A. Genital herpes

B. HIV

C. Latex allergy

D. Primary syphilis

E. Psoriasis

3. A 47-year-old man presented with a 1-week history of high fever and a painful left groin. He lived in a rural area in northern California. He reported sustaining tick bites during a recent hiking trip and multiple recent rodent and spider exposures since moving more rurally a few weeks ago. He had no significant travel history.

On physical exam, there was a lesion on his left leg, and he had very tender left inguinal lymphadenopathy.

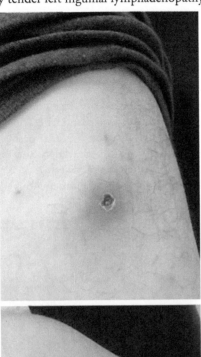

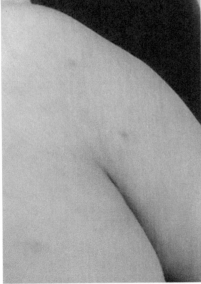

What is the most likely cause?

A. *Francisella tularensis*
B. Loxoscelism (recluse spider bite)
C. *Rickettsia conorii*
D. *Spirillum minus*
E. *Streptobacillus moniliformis*

4. A 72-year-old man was admitted with a 2-day history of fevers and worsening abdominal pain. He denied change in bowel habit. Past medical history included hypertension and type 2 diabetes mellitus controlled with oral hypoglycemic agents.

On examination, his temperature was 38.8°C, his blood pressure was 116/74 mmHg, and his heart rate was 94 beats per minute. He was tender in the right upper quadrant and he had normal bowel sounds.

Initial investigations:
C-reactive protein 330 mg/L (0–5)
Total white cell count 24.1 ×10^9/L (4.0–11.0)
Bilirubin 39 μmol/L (0–21)
Alkaline phosphatase 450 IU/L (40–129)
ALT 93 IU/L (5–35)
USS abdomen revealed gallstones
He was diagnosed with acute cholecystitis. Blood cultures were taken, and he was commenced on IV fluids, IV co-amoxiclav, and gentamicin.

Over the next 24 hours he failed to improve despite treatment, becoming hypotensive and tachycardic. On repeat examination his abdominal pain had become generalized and bowel sounds remained normal. An urgent abdominal X-ray was performed:

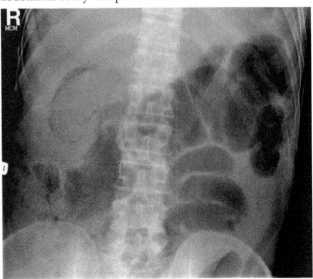

What is the most likely explanation for these findings?

A. Emphysematous cholecystitis
B. Gallbladder perforation
C. Gallstone ileus
D. Inadequate antibiotic therapy
E. Mirizzi syndrome

5. A 40-year-old man presented with neutropenic fevers and headache. He had finished induction therapy with cytarabine and daunorubicin 3 weeks ago after a new diagnosis of acute myeloid leukemia.

He had no other significant past medical history. He was a nonsmoker and only drank alcohol occasionally. He worked for a local chicken farm in Missouri.

On examination, his temperature was 39.8°C, his heart rate was 110 beats/minute, blood pressure 80/58 mmHg, and respiratory rate 18 breaths/minute with SPO$_2$ 95% on 2L. There was redness and tenderness over right subclavian Hohn catheter site. Lung exam showed decreased breath sounds on bilateral bases with scattered crackles. The Hohn catheter was removed, and he was started on vancomycin and cefepime.

Investigations:

Absolute neutrophil count 300 cells/μL

CXR: bibasilar scarring with no obvious consolidation

CT head: bilateral mild maxillary sinusitis

Blood cultures and catheter tip cultures: yeast

Serum galactomannan-negative

Serum cryptococcal antigen-positive with a titer of 1:64

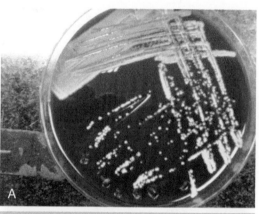

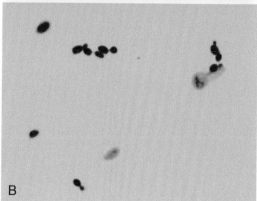

What is the most likely etiologic agent?

A. *Candida* sp.

B. *Cryptococcus neoformans*

C. *Histoplasma capsulatum*

D. *Rhizopus* sp.

E. *Trichosporon* sp.

6. A 54-year-old man was seen with a history of intermittent fevers over 6 weeks. He denied any other symptoms. He was being investigated for raised blood sugars and had a dental extraction 7 days earlier. He drank 35 units of alcohol per week. He returned from Malaysia 6 months ago following a 2-month stay with his family during the summer months.

On examination, his temperature was 38.9°C, and he had mild abdominal tenderness in his right upper quadrant. Investigations:

Total white cell count 17.2 ×10^9/L

CRP 230 mg/L

Alanine transaminase 152 U/L

Alkaline phosphatase 341 U/L

Urgent abdominal USS revealed a single large lesion in the right lobe of the liver consistent with an abscess. No biliary pathology was identified. He was commenced on fluids and IV co-amoxiclav

Blood cultures – no growth at 5 days

Liver aspirate MCS – mucoid colonies on blood and MacConkey agar. The organism did not react with oxidase or indole

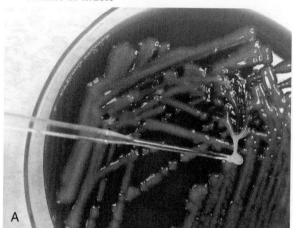

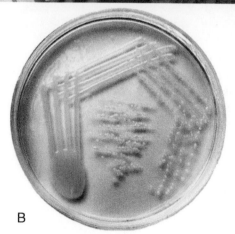

What is the most likely causative organism?

A. *Burkholderia pseudomallei*

B. *Entamoeba histolytica*

C. *Escherichia coli*

D. *Klebsiella pneumoniae*

E. *Streptococcus intermedius* (*S. milleri* group)

7. A 24-year-old man was brought in by ambulance with severe shortness of breath. He required immediate intubation for profound hypoxemia despite high flow oxygen. A collateral history was obtained from his brother. The patient came back from a trip to Colorado 2 weeks earlier where he helped his cousin renovate and clean an old farmhouse infested with rodents, cockroaches, and termites. The patient had tried drinking milk freshly squeezed from his cousin's cow a few times. His symptoms began a few days after coming back from the trip with flu-like symptoms that rapidly progressed to a dry cough and severe dyspnea.

His vital signs upon arrival were: temperature 39.1°C, blood pressure 60/40 mmHg, heart rate 120 beats/minute, and respiratory rate 30 breaths/minute.

Labs:

Total white cell count 15 ×10⁹/L (60% neutrophil with a significant amount of immature cells, 15% lymphocytes with a significant amount of atypical cells)

Hemoglobin 11.2 g/dL (hematocrit 64%)

Platelet count 62,000/μL

AST 24 U/L

ALT 25 U/L

Bilirubin 1 mg/dL

eGFR >60 mL/min/1.73 m²

Chest X-ray:

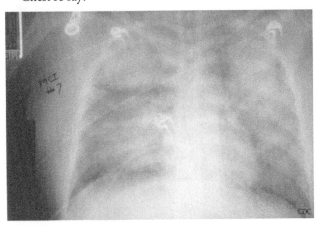

What is the most likely cause of his infection?

A. *Coccidioides immitis*

B. Hantavirus

C. Influenza

D. *Mycobacterium bovis*

E. PVL–*Staphylococcus aureus*

8.

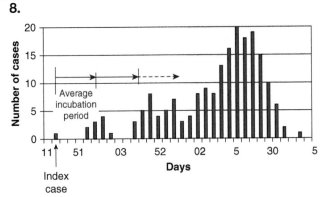

What type of outbreak is represented in the epidemic curve?

A. Common intermittent source

B. Common persistent source

C. Common point source

D. Intermittent outbreak

E. Propagated progressive source

9. A 19-year-old man was admitted with a three-day history of abdominal pain and fevers. He lived in New York City, but recently traveled to visit family in Malaysia. He did not seek pretravel counseling.

On physical examination, he appeared acutely ill. His blood pressure was 108/55 mmHg, his pulse rate was 114 beats/minute, and his temperature was 40°C. He had abdominal tenderness and was dyspneic at rest, with increasing oxygen requirements.

Investigations:

Hemoglobin level 8.3 mmol/L

Platelet count 56 ×10^9/L

Peripheral white cell 4.5 ×10^{9}cells/L

Blood smear revealed the following, with parasitemia to 3.8%.

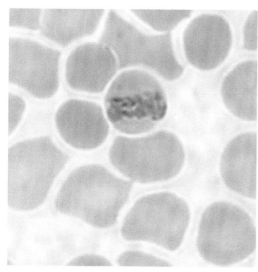

What pathogen is most likely to be responsible?

A. *P. falciparum*

B. *P. knowlesi*

C. *P. malariae*

D. *P. ovale*

E. *P. vivax*

10. A 25-year-old man presented with a 4-week history of a painful, hot, swollen left knee, low back pain with bilateral buttock pain, and left heel pain. There was no history of trauma. He had no fevers or other arthralgias. He had experienced some dysuria several weeks earlier without a noticeable discharge.

He was sexually active with other men, and engaged in oral and unprotected anal intercourse (insertive and receptive). He had not had any recent screening.

On examination, the patient was afebrile with conjunctival injection. There was a rash on his glans penis and his feet, and a large effusion of the left knee.

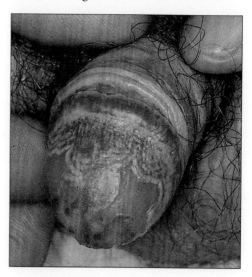

Investigations:

Total white cell count 7.3 ×10^9/L

ESR 60 mm/h

CRP 20 mg/dL

Joint aspiration:

Microscopy: no crystals seen

white cell count 1000

Gram stain negative

What is the most appropriate action?

A. Refer to orthopedics for arthroscopic washout

B. Repeat arthrocentesis with cultures and P16 RNA (16S ribosomal RNA)

C. Send urine for gonococcal/chlamydia NAAT

D. Start systemic antistaphylococcal antibiotics

E. Treat empirically for secondary syphilis

Sample Answers

1. E. Histoplasmosis

Presence of "B-symptoms" (fevers, night sweats, weight loss) and lung nodules suggests an active fungal infection. Considering epidemiology (from Missouri) raises concern for pulmonary histoplasmosis. GMS stain showing small narrow-base budding yeast confirms *Histoplasma* sp.

Aspergillosis occurs mostly in immunocompromised hosts, and the biopsy would show septate hyphae. Travel to southwestern United States suggests coccidioidomycosis, but there are no spherules on biopsy. Biopsy results are not consistent with *Coccidioides* (spherules) or *Blastomyces* (broad-based budding) or *Cryptococcus* (round yeast with a large capsule). Despite the name, *Histoplasma capsulatum* does not have a capsule.

(Image from Kauffman CA. Histoplasmosis. *Clin Chest Med*. 2009;30(2):217–225.)

2. E. Psoriasis

Genital psoriasis can cause significant distress and is often confused with sexually transmitted infections. It has been estimated that the first presentation of psoriasis is genital in as many as 2%–5% of cases, making it a diagnosis that Infectious Disease clinicians may encounter.

The lesions develop due to the Koebner phenomenon or "isomorphic response," which describes the development of skin lesions in sites of skin trauma (in this case friction associated with coitus) that may be seen in psoriasis.

There is no history of latex allergy in the setting of likely prior contact ("works in a laboratory," no history of food allergies), nor are the lesions or time course a good fit for primary syphilis, HIV, or HSV.

3. A. *Francisella tularensis*

Ulceroglandular tularemia is the most likely diagnosis, as it fits clinically and epidemiologically. Tularemia has been reported from all US states except Hawaii. All of the choices provided are differential diagnoses for eschar formation with regional lymphadenopathy except *Streptobacillus moniliformis*. However, geographically *Spirillum minus* is limited to Asia, and recluse spiders (leading to loxoscelism) are not found in northern California; *Rickettsia conorii* is found around the Mediterranean and causes Mediterranean spotted fever.

(Image from Cox JA, Visser LG. A family with African tick bite fever. *Travel Med Infect Dis*. 2015;13(3):274–275.)

4. A. Emphysematous cholecystitis

This scenario demonstrates an older man who fails to respond to treatment for acute cholecystitis. Urgent abdominal X-ray reveals air within the gallbladder which is diagnostic of emphysematous cholecystitis (EC). In addition, the patient has risk factors for this condition including his age (mean age of EC is 59 years) and diabetes. EC complicates 1% acute cholecystitis and is caused by gas-forming organisms (including clostridia). Definitive management is urgent cholecystectomy.

Dual agents (with different mechanisms of action) were chosen as empirical treatment. It is plausible that non-susceptible organisms are involved with this infection and broadening cover might be appropriate. However, in light of the radiologic findings, emphysematous cholecystitis is a more likely diagnosis, and surgery is the definitive treatment.

Mirizzi syndrome is a rare complication where a gallstone impacts the cystic duct or neck of the gallbladder, compressing the common bile duct or common hepatic duct, leading to obstruction and jaundice. There are no pathognomonic signs or symptoms, and this is usually diagnosed on USS.

Gallstone ileus is a rare cause of small bowel obstruction where a gallstone enters intestinal lumen (thought to be through a cholecystoenteric fistula) and obstructs the distal ileum. Diagnosis includes pneumobilia (air in the biliary tree), evidence of small bowel obstruction, and radioopaque gallstone on abdominal X-ray. In addition to the imaging, normal bowel sounds would go against obstruction.

Gallbladder perforation is a possibility but one would expect evidence of gas within the peritoneal cavity.

(Image from Dalrymple NC, Leyendecker JR, Oliphant M. *Problem Solving in Abdominal Imaging*. Mosby; 2009.)

5. E. *Trichosporon* sp.

Neutropenic fevers in immunocompromised patients have broad differential, including bacterial as well fungal etiologies.

Line-associated sepsis with blood culture positive for yeast could represent *Candida*, *Rhodotorula*, *Trichosporon*, or *Cryptococcus*.

Pseudohyphae with barrel-shaped arthroconidia and pleomorphic budding yeast favors *Candida* or *Trichosporon*. *Cryptococcus* are round yeast with no budding or pseudohyphae.

The positive cryptococcal antigen is likely to be a false-positive (*Cryptococcus* sp. would grow as a yeast) and raises the concern for infection with *Trichosporon*.

Management includes line removal and antifungal with amphotericin or voriconazole.

(Image from Lee W-S, Yu F-L, Ou T-Y. Breakthrough *Trichosporon asahii* fungemia during caspofungin therapy. *J Exp Clin Med.* 2014;6(3):108–109.)

6. E. *Klebsiella pneumoniae*

K. pneumoniae (K1 capsular serotype) is an emerging pathogen causing liver abscesses in the absence of hepatobiliary disease. It is found in SE Asia, in particular Malaysia. *K. pneumoniae* are oxidase-negative, lactose fermenting organism. The hypermucoviscous variant grows as very mucoid colonies and can be identified by a positive string test (stretching colonies forms a "string" of >5mm).

E. coli is a common causes of liver abscess, and the culture results would fit (although most *E. coli* are indole positive) but in the absence of hepatobiliary pathology and sterile blood cultures this would be unlikely.

E. histolytica commonly presents as an indolent infection and is endemic in rural areas of Malaysia. Against this diagnosis is no preceding colitis (one third) and *Entamoeba* do not grow on blood or MacConkey agar as they require supplemented media (usually egg yolk).

Melioidosis, caused by *B. pseudomallei*, is a condition causing large abscesses. *B. pseudomallei* is an environmental saprophyte found in aquatic environments and when cultured grows as mucoid colonies. Going against this as a diagnosis is that infections are most prevalent following the rainy season (rather than summer months when the patient traveled). Also, while it can be found in Malaysia is it more prevalent in Thailand and North Australia. Furthermore, *B. pseudomallei* are oxidase-positive.

Streptococcus intermedius is one of the *S. milleri* group, which are well recognized as causing deep-seated abscesses such as this. However, the colonial appearances on blood agar are not consistent with *S. intermedius*, and MacConkey agar does not support its growth.

(Image (*left*) reprinted with permission from Elsevier. The Lancet. From Prokesch BC, et al. Primary osteomyelitis caused by hypervirulent *Klebsiella pneumoniae. Lancet Infect Dis.* 2016;16(9):e190–e195. Image (*right*) from Rath S, Padhy RN. Prevalence of two multidrug-resistant *Klebsiella* species in an Indian teaching hospital and adjoining community. *J Infect Public Health.* 2014;7(6):496–507.)

7. B. Hantavirus

The clinical picture of a rapidly progressing respiratory failure associated with diffuse pulmonary edema, fever, leukocytosis with left shift and atypical lymphocytosis, thrombocytopenia, and elevated hematocrit, in the correct epidemiologic setting (Utah, Colorado, Arizona, New Mexico) and exposure history (rodents), is consistent with hantavirus pulmonary syndrome (Sin Nombre virus).

(Image from Shandro JR, Jauregui JM. Wilderness-acquired zoonoses. In Auerbach PS, Cushing TA, Harris NS, eds. *Auerbach's Wilderness Medicine.* 7th ed. Elsevier; 2017.)

8. E. Propagated progressive source

An epidemic curve is a visual display of the onset of illness during an outbreak. Point source epidemics involve a common source and occur over a brief period. Common persistent courses rise and fall, but the cases do not occur within a single incubation period. Propagated progressive sources occurs when there is an initial wave of infections followed by second or third waves. There are successively larger peaks. Intermittent outbreaks are separated by periods without evidence of infection.

9. B. *P. knowlesi*

The patient has manifestations of severe malaria, with high parasitemia and end-organ damage. *P. falciparum* is the most common cause of severe malaria. However, you are shown a band trophozoite on peripheral smear. This is consistent with *P. knowlesi*. Another clue is geographic. This patient is in an area where *P. knowlesi* is present. It is important, especially for your boards, to be able to differentiate between malaria species (see Fig. 30.13).

10. C. Send urine for gonococcal/chlamydia NAAT

Reactive arthritis can have multiple presentations beyond the common findings described in medical textbooks such as conjunctivitis, monoarticular arthritis, and urethritis. This particular patient is a sexually active young male engaging in high-risk sexual behavior, and in this case sexually transmitted infectious etiologies are more likely etiologic agents of reactive arthritis.

Clinical findings such as keratoderma blennorrhagicum can be found on the soles of the feet and less commonly on the palms of the hand. It is most commonly due to skin thickening. Circinate balanitis can also occur with a distinct serpiginous annular dermatitis of the glans penis.

Empiric therapy for secondary syphilis should not immediately be considered in this case given findings of conjunctivitis, urethritis, and a monoarticular arthritis. Testing for syphilis would not be incorrect in this situation, however.

Repeat arthrocentesis testing is not warranted in this case given negative Gram stain and negative culture result from the arthrocentesis fluid. Orthopedic evaluation is not warranted in this situation given the relatively benign appearance of arthrocentesis fluid studies.

(Image from Wu IB, Schwartz RA. Reiter's syndrome: the classic triad and more. *J Am Acad Dermatol.* 2008;59:113–121.)

Index

Note: Page numbers followed by "f" indicate figures, "t" indicate tables, and "b" indicate boxes.

Don't Forget Your Online Access to

ExpertConsult.com

Mobile. Searchable. Expandable.

ACCESS it on any Internet-ready device

SEARCH all Expert Consult titles you own

LINK to PubMed abstracts

ALREADY REGISTERED?

1. Log in at expertconsult.com
2. Scratch off your Activation Code below
3. Enter it into the "Add a Title" box
4. Click "Activate Now"
5. Click the title under "My Titles"

FIRST-TIME USER?

1. **REGISTER**
   - Click "Register Now" at expertconsult.com
   - Fill in your user information and click "Continue"
2. **ACTIVATE YOUR BOOK**
   - Scratch off your Activation Code below
   - Enter it into the "Enter Activation Code" box
   - Click "Activate Now"
   - Click the title under "My Titles"

For technical assistance:
email online.help@elsevier.com
call 800-401-9962 (inside the US)
call +1-314-995-3200 (outside the US)

Activation Code

ExpertConsult.com

Quiz 1

1. An 18-year-old man was reviewed with recurrent fevers. He was known to have relapsed acute lymphoblastic leukemia. He had been treated 6 months earlier for a Mediport infection with *Pseudomonas aeruginosa* and *Staphylococcus epidermidis* with cefepime and vancomycin. On this admission he was treated with gentamicin and meropenem for an ESBL-producing *Escherichia coli* bacteremia. Five days after meropenem was started, he spiked a fever to 38.5°C, and another blood culture was drawn. The blood culture signaled positive after 8 hours, and the Gram stain showed gram-negative rods.

What is the most likely pathogen?

A. *Burkholderia cepacia*
B. *E. coli* ESBL
C. *Morganella morganii*
D. *Pseudomonas aeruginosa*
E. *Stenotrophomonas maltophilia*

2. A 72-year-old man presented with a 6-month history of a chronic cough, occasional night sweats, and weight loss. He was known to have diabetes and hypertension. He had a smoking history of 60 packs per year (PPY), with occasional alcohol intake. He lived in Missouri, and was a truck driver with frequent visits to Phoenix, Arizona, and Michigan.

Investigations:

CT chest: right upper lung lobe nodules and mediastinal lymphadenopathy

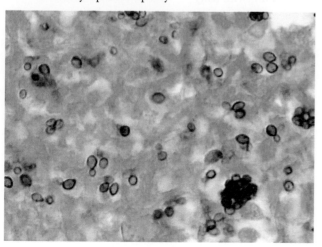

PET scan: increased uptake in the lung nodule and lymphadenopathy

Nodule biopsy histology: necrotizing granulomas on GMS stain

What is the most likely diagnosis?

A. Aspergillosis
B. Blastomycosis
C. Coccidioidomycosis
D. Cryptococcosis
E. Histoplasmosis

3. A 38-year-old man presented with a 3-day history of severe headache and a 1-day history of neck and shoulder pain, light and sound sensitivity, slight nausea, lower back pain, and a headache "all over." He denied any recent travel, tick bites, rashes, chest pain, or shortness of breath.

On examination, a faint erythematous rash was noted over his chest, he had a fever (38°C), and neck stiffness.

A lumbar puncture was performed and the following results were reported:

Total protein, CSF	53 (15–45 mg/dL)
Glucose, CSF	56 (40–70 mg/dL)
Xanthochromia	Absent
RBC, CSF	37/µL
Nucleated Cells, CSF	50 (0–5/µL)
PMN	14%
Lymphocytes	51%
Monocyte/ Macrophage	34%
Plasma cell	1%
Gram stain	PMNs seen, no organisms seen

What test is most likely to be diagnostic?

A. Bacterial culture of the CSF for Neisseria meningitidis
B. NAAT testing for Ebola virus
C. NAAT testing for West Nile virus infection from the blood
D. NAAT testing of the CSF for enterovirus
E. Streptococcus pneumoniae antigen test of the CSF

4. A 44-year-old woman presented with a 4-day history of fevers, malaise, and redness around the site of a long-term indwelling IV line in place for cancer chemotherapy. She had a history of metastatic cervical cancer. She had no known drug allergies.

On physical exam, some purulence was expressed from the IV line site.

Investigations:

Total white cell count 12.5 ×10⁹/L

Hemoglobin 8.5 g/dL

Platelets 55 ×10⁹/L

Creatinine 0.8 mg/dL

Gram-stain of exit site pus showed GPC in clusters
Blood cultures obtained through both the long-term indwelling IV line, as well from a peripheral vein, were positive for *Staphylococcus aureus*, with susceptibilities pending

What is the most appropriate initial empiric treatment of this patient's bacteremia?

A. Clindamycin

B. Dalbavancin

C. Linezolid

D. Oxacillin

E. Vancomycin

5. A 75-year-old woman was reviewed on the ward due to nausea and several diarrheal stools. She had recently sustained a cerebrovascular accident. She had no known drug allergies.

Investigations:

Total white cell count 22,000/mm³

Serum creatinine 2.5 mg/dL

Normal liver function tests

Blood and urine cultures were positive for
Pseudomonas aeruginosa, sensitivities pending

What is the most appropriate treatment?

A. Aztreonam IV

B. Ceftazidime IV

C. Ciprofloxacin PO

D. Imipenem–cilastatin IV

E. Tobramycin IV

6. A 35-year-old man presented with a seizure, having had well-controlled epilepsy for several years on levetiracetam. He had been diagnosed with an *Escherichia coli* urinary tract infection 1 week earlier for which he was started on trimethoprim–sulfamethoxazole (TMP–SMX). He had also started empiric treatment of *Mycobacterium abscessus* with imipenem–cilastatin, cefoxitin, and amikacin 2 weeks ago.

What medication is most likely to have precipitated his new seizure activity?

A. Amikacin

B. Cefoxitin

C. Imipenem–cilastatin

D. Levetiracetam

E. TMP–SMX

7. A 60-year-old woman presented to the clinic for a follow-up visit after receiving a diagnosis of pulmonary histoplasmosis. Two weeks prior, the patient had presented to the clinic with cough and fevers and received a diagnosis of pulmonary histoplasmosis. At this follow-up visit, the patient reported an improvement in the cough and resolution of fevers. The patient had no known drug allergies. The patient's comorbidities included hypertension and diabetes. Medications included the following:

Itraconazole 10 mg/mL oral solution – take 20 mL
by mouth twice daily (started 2 weeks ago)

Hydrochlorothiazide 25 mg by mouth once daily

Aspirin 81 mg by mouth once daily

Metformin 500 mg by mouth twice daily

Atorvastatin 10 mg by mouth once daily

Omeprazole 20 mg by mouth once daily

The patient denied any missed doses of medications
and reported taking the itraconazole solution on
an empty stomach.

Investigations:

Serum itraconazole 0.8 µg/mL

Serum hydroxyitraconazole 1.5 µg/mL

Creatinine 1 mg/dL

ALT 15 U/L

What is the most appropriate action?

A. Change to itraconazole capsules 200 mg by mouth twice daily

B. Change to posaconazole DR tabs 100 mg – take 3 tablets by mouth once daily

C. Continue itraconazole oral solution 200 mg by mouth twice daily

D. Educate the patient to take the itraconazole solution with food and repeat itraconazole serum concentration in 2 weeks

E. Increase itraconazole oral solution to 400 mg by mouth twice daily

8. A 43-year-old woman traveled to West Africa for a year-long research project. A few weeks into her trip she began to notice strange dreams followed by a paranoid feeling of people following her.

What prophylactic agent is most likely to be responsible?

A. Atovaquone/proguanil

B. Chloroquine

C. Coxycycline

D. Mefloquine

E. Primaquine

9. A 45-year-old man was reviewed with a 4-week history of daily fevers up to 38.2°C (100.9°F). The patient reported feeling otherwise fine except for some fatigue and denied any unintentional weight loss. An exhaustive history-taking and physical and a thorough baseline work-up was performed, all of which is unrevealing.

The baseline work-up included a complete blood count, basic metabolic panel, and hepatic panel, chest X-ray, blood cultures, urinalysis and urine culture, and HIV testing, which were not revealing.

What is the most appropriate action?

A. Bone marrow aspirate

B. Glucocorticoid therapy

C. Start empiric treatment for bacterial pneumonia

D. Wait and observe the patient

E. Whole body FDG/PET-CT

10. A 57-year-old man presented with a lump on the right side of his neck. He had been feeling well with no systemic symptoms. He had well-controlled diabetes (HbA1C of 6%) and no drug allergies.

On physical exam, the lump was nontender and easily moveable. It was not red or hot. He underwent a biopsy to evaluate for malignancy.

Investigations:

Direct microscopy: inflammatory cells and gram-positive branching rods seen

Culture: molar tooth-appearing colonies present on anaerobic plates

What is the most appropriate treatment?

A. Clindamycin

B. Doxycycline

C. Penicillin

D. Trimethoprim–sulfamethoxazole (TMP–SMX)

E. Surgical resection

11. A 74-year-old woman presented with headache and fever for 4 days. She had type 2 diabetes mellitus and hypertension, controlled with metformin and amlodipine. There was no recent travel. She lived at home with her partner. She had previously had a rash with penicillin. Her partner reported that she had been unsteady on her feet for the last 2 days.

On examination she was drowsy, with a reduced conscious level (GCS 14/15). Her temperature was 38.2°C, and her heart rate was 98 beats/minute. She had neck stiffness and was photophobic. She had nystagmus on left lateral gaze and a slight facial droop on the right. Peripheral nervous system examination was grossly intact, but difficult to assess formally as the patient was unable to follow commands.

In addition to ceftriaxone, what antibacterial agent should be given?

A. Amoxicillin/ampicillin

B. Chloramphenicol

C. Linezolid

D. Trimethoprim–sulfamethoxazole (TMP–SMX)

E. Vancomycin

12. A 21-year-old man was admitted to a detoxification center because of injection drug use with heroin. He complained of malaise but did not have fever or cough.

On examination his temperature was 37.1°C, blood pressure 162/82 mmHg, and pulse rate 100 beats/minute. On skin examination he had erythematous scarring on his hands and arms.

A tuberculin skin test was administered and read at 48 hours. The indurated area was 8 mm in diameter, and the erythema was 15 mm in diameter.

Bloodborne virus screening was negative.

What is the most appropriate management?

A. Chest radiography

B. Isoniazid

C. Isoniazid, rifampin, pyrazinamide, and ethambutol

D. Reassurance only

E. Repeat tuberculin skin testing in 2 weeks

13. A 33-year-old man presented with a week of fever and tachypnea. He was known to have HIV infection but had disengaged with care. He did not take antiretroviral therapies nor any prophylaxis for opportunistic infections. He had no recent CD4 count or HIV viral load result.

Investigations:

Blood gas analysis revealed a PaO_2 of 55 mmHg on room air (7.15 kPa)

CXR: bilateral alveolar infiltrates

BAL was positive for methenamine silver staining material

What is the most appropriate antimicrobial treatment?

A. Atovaquone

B. Clindamycin, primaquine, and leucovorin

C. Ganciclovir

D. Pentamidine

E. Trimethoprim–sulfamethoxazole (TMP–SMX)

14. A 58-year-old man presented with a 4-day history of low-grade fever, cough, and wheezing. He was known to have COPD. His chest X-ray showed no infiltrates. He was sent home with prescriptions for azithromycin and prednisone for treatment of presumed COPD exacerbation.

Two days later, his blood cultures returned positive.

What organism should prompt urgent re-evaluation?

A. *Bacillus* spp.

B. *Cutibacterium (Propionibacterium) acnes*

C. *Corynebacterium* spp.

D. *Staphylococcus aureus*

E. *Staphylococcus epidermidis*

15. A 24-year-old woman sought medical advice regarding long-term antibiotic prophylaxis. She was taking benzathine penicillin G every 3 weeks. She had been diagnosed and treated for rheumatic fever when she was 15 years old after developing subcutaneous nodules, polyarthritis, and carditis. Her last echocardiogram showed no residual valvular disease.

What is the most appropriate advice?
A. Change to oral antibiotic prophylaxis
B. Continue prophylaxis until age 25
C. Continue until at least age 40, and possibly lifelong
D. No indication for any further prophylaxis
E. Stop prophylaxis but give a rescue box of antibiotics for GAS pharyngitis

16. A 36-year-old man presented unwell with a 2-week history of fever and new-onset intense myalgia. He also initially had abdominal pain, diarrhea, and vomiting. He was usually well and did not take any regular medications. He was a nonsmoker and did not take any recreational drugs. He had arrived in the United States 3 weeks earlier from rural Mexico. For his farewell party his friends in Mexico prepared for him smoked boar meat.

On examination, his temperature was 38.5°C, his heart rate was 110 beats/minute, his respiratory rate was 26 breaths/minute, and his oxygen saturations were 93% on room air. He had periorbital edema and conjunctivitis, respiratory distress with bibasal crackles, and peripheral edema.

Investigations:
CPK 512 U/L
EKG: flat T waves in I, AVL, V5, and V6
Cardiac MR: gadolinium enhancement in the lateral and inferolateral epicardial areas

What is the most likely diagnosis?
A. Brucellosis
B. Enterovirus myocarditis
C. Influenza myocarditis
D. Lateral wall myocardial infarct
E. Trichinellosis

17. Several children admitted on the specialist pediatric gastroenterology ward developed loose stool. One 11-month child still in diapers had diarrhea and a fever >38°C; another 3-year child had diarrhea and vomiting; and one 5-year old child had vomiting only. All three had been on the unit for 3 weeks, with an underlying diagnosis of inflammatory bowel disease. Their symptoms began over a 48-hour period. Stool cultures for the 5-year-old were negative but were pending for the remaining two children. Blood results were unremarkable.

Two staff members also reported vomiting over the preceding 24 hours.

What is the most likely pathogen?
A. Adenovirus
B. *Bacillus cereus*
C. *Clostridioides difficile*
D. Norovirus
E. *Staphylococcus aureus*

18. A 68-year-old man presented with urosepsis. He had a history of poorly controlled type 2 diabetes. Urine cultures demonstrated a sensitive *Escherichia coli*. CT demonstrated gas within the left kidney and retroperitoneum. He was treated with oral ciprofloxacin but clinically deteriorated on day 3 of the admission with fever, tachycardia, and hypotension.

What is the most appropriate management?
A. Add an aminoglycoside
B. Check antimicrobial levels
C. Escalate to IV third-generation cephalosporin
D. Refer to endocrinology for optimization of glycemic control
E. Surgical referral for nephrectomy

19. A 27-year-old pregnant woman spent the day with her nephew at a family celebration. The following day he developed a widespread vesicular rash which was diagnosed as chickenpox (primary varicella-zoster virus infection). She contacted her obstetrician the same day concerned about the risks of chickenpox as she had never had this illness and had not been vaccinated. She was 34 weeks pregnant and had mild asthma.

What is the most appropriate action?
A. Administer varicella zoster immunoglobulin (VZIG)
B. Administer VZV vaccine
C. Reassurance only
D. Send serum for VZV IgG testing
E. Start postexposure prophylaxis with valaciclovir

20. A 19-year-old woman presented with vaginal discharge and odor for one week. She was sexually active with one regular male partner. She reported inconsistent condom use.

On pelvic examination, there were no external skin lesions. A thin, white to gray vaginal discharge was present. There was no cervical discharge or cervical motion tenderness.

A sample of vaginal fluid was collected. The pH of the fluid was 5.5, and a fishy odor was noted on addition of potassium hydroxide solution.

On wet prep of the specimen, epithelial cell borders were obscured by bacteria.

Urine NAAT for gonorrhea, chlamydia, and trichomoniasis were sent.

What is the most appropriate treatment?
A. Ceftriaxone 250 mg IM plus azithromycin 1g stat
B. Doxycycline 100 mg BD for 7 days
C. Fluconazole 150 mg oral stat
D. Metronidazole 500 mg BD for 7 days
E. Metronidazole 2 grams oral stat

21. A 29-year-old woman presented with lower abdominal pain and bleeding between menstrual periods. She also reported intermittent fevers to 101°F (38.3°C). She had appendicitis age 13 years and had no known drug allergies. She had had unprotected vaginal intercourse with two casual male partners in the past 3 months.

On examination, her temperature was 101.2°F (38.4°C), blood pressure 124/82 mmHg, pulse 80/minute, and respiratory rate of 14 breaths/minute, SaO_2 98% on room air.

A mucopurulent discharge was visible over the cervix, there was cervical motion and adnexal tenderness, and the cervix os bled easily upon application of pressure.

NAAT studies were sent for gonorrhea, chlamydia, and trichomoniasis.

What is the most appropriate empiric treatment?

A. Azithromycin 1 gram orally for one dose
B. Ceftriaxone 125 mg IM for one dose
C. Ceftriaxone 250 mg IM stat plus doxycycline 100 mg BID
D. Metronidazole 2 gram orally for one dose
E. Metronidazole 500 mg orally BID for 7 days

22. A 32-year-old woman was reviewed as part of contact tracing for an acute case of hepatitis A in a childcare center. She worked as a nursery nurse, had been born and brought up in the United States, and had no recent travel. She was asymptomatic. She was usually well and was not taking any regular medications.

What is the most appropriate action?

A. Give HAV-containing immunoglobulin
B. Give single-dose HAV vaccination
C. Reassurance only
D. Screen for underlying immunodeficiency or liver disorders
E. Test HAV IgG and IgG

23. A 43-year-old woman presented with a 9-month history of arthralgia and swelling of wrists and small joints of her hands bilaterally. Her symptoms had not resolved despite regular use of nonsteroidal antiinflammatories. She was otherwise fit and well and worked as a systems analyst for a large multinational company. She associated the start of her symptoms with a business trip to Brazil during which time she had a brief febrile illness with myalgia, a mild rash, and skin peeling from the palms of her hands.

What is the most likely infective cause?

A. Chikungunya virus
B. Erythrovirus (parvovirus B19)
C. HIV
D. Rubella virus
E. Zika virus

24. A 12-year-old boy was seen with an 8-week history of fever, fatigue, and painful, itchy lesions on both legs. He lived in a rural village in the Democratic Republic of Congo. His mother recalled that there was originally a single, raised lesion which appeared on the back of his leg, with several others appearing subsequently. The boy mentioned that several of his friends in his village had similar lesions.

On examination:

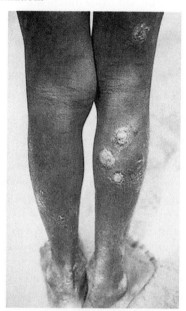

Clinical examination did not reveal any other cutaneous or mucosal lesions.
Investigations:
   CRP 56 mg/L (<5)
   VDRL (nontreponemal) positive
   TPHA (treponemal) positive
   He was treated with intramuscular benzathine penicillin G and lesions resolved within 2 weeks.

What is the most likely causative agent?

A. *Leishmania infantum*
B. *Treponema carateum*
C. *Treponema pallidum* subsp. *endemicum*
D. *Treponema pallidum* subsp. *pallidum*
E. *Treponema pallidum* subsp. *pertenue*

25. A 24-year-old woman presented with left arm pain and swelling for several hours. She was an active intravenous drug user.

On examination, there was minimal erythema in the left antecubital fossa and upper arm with significant pain on palpation.

Investigations:

    CT left arm: gas seen in fascial planes, suspicious
        for a necrotizing soft tissue infection

In addition to emergency surgical debridement, what would be the most appropriate antibiotic regimen?

  A. Cefazolin and metronidazole
  B. Ceftriaxone and metronidazole
  C. Ciprofloxacin and metronidazole
  D. Penicillin and clindamycin
  E. Piperacillin–tazobactam, vancomycin, clindamycin

26. A 26-year-old man presented with a 2-week history of dyspnea. His symptoms began as exertional dyspnea and dry cough but progressed to occurring at rest.

He had ulcerative colitis and gout and was on treatment with infliximab. He had previously developed a Stevens–Johnson syndrome in response to sulfasalazine. He had also required blood transfusions after taking a new gout medication, which he could not remember.

On examination, his respiratory rate was 32 breaths/minute, and his oxygen saturation 85% on room air. Fine crepitations were heard throughout all lung fields.

Investigations:

    Blood gas PaO_2 55 mmHg (7.3kPa)
    Chest X-ray

What is the most appropriate therapy?

  A. Atovaquone
  B. Clindamycin and primaquine
  C. Pentamidine
  D. Trimethoprim and dapsone
  E. Trimethoprim–sulfamethoxazole (TMP–SMX)

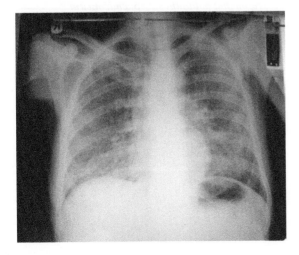

27. A 34-year-old man presented with chronic, painless swelling of his right foot. He was usually otherwise well and did not take any regular medications. Seven years earlier he developed a small wound after dropping a heavy box on his right foot. Several months later he developed swelling of the dorsum of the foot. Since then there had been intermittent drainage of pus from an area over the second metatarsal. He had received various courses of antibiotic treatment without improvement. He had no fevers and his weight was stable. He was visiting from India, where he worked as a farmer.

On exam, there was marked swelling and induration of the affected foot and a draining sinus tract.

X-ray showed no evidence of osseous involvement.

What is the most likely pathogen?

  A. *Madurella mycetomatis*
  B. *Pseudomonas aeruginosa*
  C. *Staphylococcus aureus*
  D. *Talaromyces marneffei*
  E. *Trichophyton rubrum*

28. A 33-year-old man presented with a 72-hour history of fever and malaise. He also had a mild headache and reported some loose stools and abdominal pain. He had returned 5 days earlier from a 6-week trip to Chad where he worked with locals to build a church. During the construction work, he was bitten by many mosquitoes. He also traveled throughout the region inspecting waterways. He had unprotected vaginal intercourse with 2 casual partners. He did not seek advice prior to his travels.

On examination, his temperature was 39.3°C, his heart rate was 88 beats/minute, and his blood pressure was 120/68 mmHg. He was flushed with reddened conjunctivae. He had tender hepatomegaly of 2 cm below the costal margin.

Investigations:

    Total WBC count 3.5 ×10^9/L
    Platelet count 150 ×10^9/L
    eGFR >60 mL/min/1.73 m^2
    Bilirubin 3 mg/dL
    AST 177 U/L
    ALT 89 U/L

What intervention would have prevented his condition?

  A. Atovaquone/proguanil prophylaxis
  B. Combined hepatitis A/typhoid immunization
  C. Doxycycline prophylaxis
  D. Hepatitis B immunization
  E. Yellow fever immunization

29. A 22-year-old man presented with fever, abdominal pain, nausea, vomiting, headache, and profound generalized weakness. He had no significant medical history. He denied alcohol drinking or drug use. He had returned from a 2-week trip to India. He reported a lot of flooding in the local village where he stayed. He also had a lot of mosquito bites and had eaten different local delicacies bought from the streets. Two of his roommates had become sick with fever and vomiting prior to his return. He had not taken any pretravel advice.

On examination, his temperature was 40.1°C, blood pressure 110/80 mmHg, heart rate 115 beats/minute, and respiratory rate 24 breaths/minute. He had icteric sclerae and muscle tenderness in his lower back and bilateral calves.
Investigations:
   Total white cell count 12 ×10⁹/L
   Platelet count 145,000/μL
   Hemoglobin 10 g/dL
   Aspartate aminotransferase 180 U/L
   Alanine aminotransferase 190 U/L
   Alkaline phosphatase 160 U/L
   Total bilirubin 15 mg/dL (predominantly conjugated)
   An ultrasound of the abdomen showed normal gall-bladder and liver.

What is the most likely route of acquisition of his illness?

  A. Floodwater exposure
  B. Food consumption
  C. Mosquito bite
  D. Sexual transmission
  E. Sick contact

30. A 44-year-old man presented with an 8-month history of right neck swelling. He also reported drenching night sweats and 10 lb weight loss but no fever or cough. He was originally from Mexico but had been living in Missouri for the past 10 years. He had been taking isoniazid for the past 5 months since a tuberculin skin test (TST) performed as part of a preemployment assessment demonstrated induration of 16 mm. He had a punch biopsy performed 3 months ago.

On physical exam there was an ulcerated right-anterior lymph node with a fistulous tract.

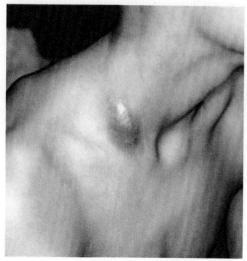

Investigations:
   Chest CT normal
   Total white cell count 5.7 ×10⁹/L
   Hemoglobin 145 g/L
   eGFR >60 mL/min/1.73 m²
   Histology of the punch biopsy from the skin lesion: granulomatous inflammation seen; Gomori and Ziehl–Neelsen stains negative
   A biopsy was arranged for bacterial, mycobacterial, and fungal cultures.

What is the most appropriate action?

  A. Change to RIF
  B. Change to RIF, EMB, PZA
  C. Continue INH to complete 9 months of therapy
  D. Do a confirmatory IGRA test
  E. Start voriconazole

31. A 56-year-old man presented with cough and dyspnea for 3 weeks. He had a history of gastro-esophageal reflux disease and a 40 pack-year smoking history.
Investigations:
   CXR: right upper lobe infiltrates
   Sputum MCS: mixed flora
   Sputum AFB smear negative; mycobacterial culture positive at 3 weeks with yellow colonies.

What is the most likely causative organism?

  A. *Mycobacterium abscessus*
  B. *Mycobacterium avium* complex
  C. *Mycobacterium chelonae*
  D. *Mycobacterium fortuitum*
  E. *Mycobacterium kansasii*

32. A 59-year-old man was seen with a recurrence of fevers and chills. He was on day 7 of a 2-week course of doxycycline (100 mg BID) for presumed Lyme disease. He was a deer hunter from Nantucket, who had first presented with a 5-day history of a circular rash on his back, associated with fevers and chills. The rash had cleared, and his systemic symptoms had settled on starting doxycycline.

What is the most appropriate treatment?

  A. Atovaquone and azithromycin PO for 7 days
  B. Ceftriaxone IV followed by doxycycline PO to complete 21 days
  C. Ceftriaxone IV for 21 days
  D. Clindamycin and chloroquine PO for 7 days
  E. Doxycycline PO for 21 days

33. A 19-year-old man presented with rectal prolapse. He had arrived in the UK 2 weeks earlier. He was normally resident in Vietnam. He reported recurrent intermittent episodes of mild abdominal pain for as long as he can remember. On examination he appeared small in stature, but otherwise the exam was unremarkable.

Feces microscopy for ova, cysts and parasites:

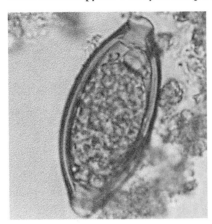

What is the most likely infective cause?

A. *Ascaris lumbricoides*
B. *Enterobius vermicularis*
C. *Giardia lamblia*
D. *Schistosoma mansoni*
E. *Trichuris trichiura*

34. A 27-year-old bisexual man presented with a request for postexposure HIV prophylaxis after sexual intercourse. He had not used barrier protection. He asked for advice about routes of transmission of HIV.

What poses the highest risk of HIV transmission?

A. Insertive anal intercourse
B. Insertive penile–vaginal intercourse
C. Receptive anal intercourse
D. Receptive oral intercourse
E. Receptive penile–vaginal intercourse

35. A 24-year-old man attended outpatient clinic for initiation of ART after a recent diagnosis of HIV infection. He was keen to get started on treatment.

Investigations:
    CD4 count 450 cells/μL
    HIV RNA 120,000 copies/mL
    No baseline resistance demonstrated on HIV genotyping
    HLA B*5701 negative

What is the most appropriate antiretroviral regimen?

A. Abacavir/lamivudine + boosted darunavir
B. Abacavir/lamivudine + rilpivirine
C. Abacavir/lamivudine + efavirenz
D. Tenofovir alafenamide/emtricitabine + boosted darunavir
E. Tenofovir alafenamide/emtricitabine/rilpivirine

36. A 25-year-old man presented with a 1-month history of fevers, cough, and hemoptysis. He was known to have untreated HIV.

Investigations:
    Sputum microscopy: numerous AFBs seen
        CD4 count 155 cells/μL
    He was started on 4-drug antimycobacterial therapy.

When is the most appropriate time to introduce ART?

A. 72 hours
B. 1 week
C. 4 weeks
D. 10 weeks
E. 16 weeks

37. A 45-year-old man presented with a 2-week history of substernal chest pain. He described it as burning and associated with swallowing solids and liquids. He had not had any vomiting, diarrhea, or blood in his stools. He was known to have HIV and intermittently took his antiretroviral therapy and prophylaxis treatments.

On oral examination there were white mucosal plaque lesions that easily scraped off but no ulcerations.

Investigations:
    CD4 count 65 cells/μL
    HIV-1 RNA viral load 22,150 copies/mL

What is the most appropriate treatment?

A. Aciclovir
B. Fluconazole
C. Ganciclovir
D. Nystatin
E. Pantoprazole

38. A 34-year-old man presented with one week of fevers, abdominal pain, and bloody stools. The patient reported 4–5 small volume bloody stools/day and bilateral lower abdominal pain. He was known to have HIV but only irregularly attended for follow-up and was not taking any ART.

On exam, his temperature was 38.3°C, his blood pressure was 105/65mmHg, and his pulse rate was 86 beats/min. There was bilateral lower quadrant tenderness without guarding.

Investigations:
    CD4 count 35 cells/μL
    HIV-1 RNA viral load 120,700 copies/mL

Routine stool culture, stool ova and parasite, and Clostridioides difficile testing all negative

What would be the most effective test to evaluate for cytomegalovirus (CMV) colitis?

A. CMV IgG serology
B. CMV plasma PCR
C. Colonoscopy with biopsies
D. CT scan of abdomen and pelvis
E. Viral stool culture

39. A 42-year-old man was brought in by ambulance with sudden onset fever and collapse. He was known to have acute myeloid leukemia and had received induction chemotherapy 10 days earlier. He was taking levofloxacin prophylaxis.

On examination his temperature was 38.5°C, his heart rate was 110 beats/minute, and his blood pressure was 84/42 mmHg. He was peripherally vasodilated. He had widespread inspiratory crackles on chest auscultation and mucositis on oral examination.
Investigations:

Neutrophil count 0.0 ×10^9/L
CXR: diffuse infiltrates bilaterally
Blood cultures: gram-positive cocci after 11 hours

What is the most likely causative organism?

A. *Enterococcus faecium*
B. *Staphylococcus aureus*
C. *Staphylococcus hominis*
D. Streptococcus pneumoniae
E. Viridans group streptococci

40. A 51-year-old woman was found to have a raised serum creatinine of 2.5 mg/dL. She had undergone a kidney transplantation 9 months earlier. She was asymptomatic. Her immunosuppressive medications included tacrolimus, mycophenolate, and prednisone. She had normal renal function on previous follow-up visits and had a baseline creatinine of 0.9 mg/dL. No changes were made to her medications recently. Her urinalysis was normal.

What is the most likely cause?

A. Acute pyelonephritis
B. Adenovirus nephritis
C. BK virus nephropathy
D. Cytomegalovirus nephritis
E. Nephrolithiasis causing urinary obstruction

41. A 3-year-old boy was recently diagnosed with osteomyelitis due to *Serratia marcescens*. He has a past medical history of pneumonia due to *Nocardia* and sepsis due to *Burkholderia cepacia*.

What is the most appropriate screening test?

A. Antibody responses to vaccines
B. CH50
C. Dihydrorhodamine (DHR) test
D. Lymphocyte subsets
E. Quantitative immunoglobulins

42. A 22-year-old woman was admitted to the ICU with suspected bacterial meningitis and was placed on empirical therapy with ceftriaxone and vancomycin. Cerebrospinal fluid culture grew *Neisseria meningitidis* on day 2. The patient had been on antibiotics for 48 hours.

What are the most appropriate infection prevention precautions?

A. Airborne precautions in a negative-pressure side room
B. Continue standard precautions
C. Airborne precautions
D. Contact precautions
E. Droplet precautions

43. A 42-year-old physician presented for new employee screening. She had recently volunteered as a provider at a homeless shelter. She was found to have 12 mm of induration around her PPD intradermal skin test at 48 hours after placement of the test. Her last PPD done one year ago was negative. Her chest radiograph was negative.

What is the most appropriate management?

A. Administer BCG vaccine
B. Perform an interferon gamma release assay
C. Repeat the PPD test in 8–12 weeks
D. Start RIPE therapy
E. Take a 6–9 month course of isoniazid

44. A 45-year-old healthcare worker received a needlestick injury. The recipient was known to be a hepatitis B vaccine non-responder despite two vaccination courses.

Recipient:	HBsAg negative
	Hepatitis B surface antibody 2 mIU/mL
	HBV cAb negative
Source:	HBsAg positive, HBeAg positive, HBeAb negative
	HBV DNA 62 million U/mL

What is the most appropriate treatment?

A. A single dose of hepatitis B vaccine
B. An accelerated course of hepatitis B vaccination
C. No prophylaxis required
D. Single dose of HBIG and an accelerated course of hepatitis B vaccine
E. Two doses of hepatitis B immunoglobulin (HBIG) 1 month apart

45. A 49-year-old man planned to travel to India for 10 days in Delhi. He was healthy, did not take any medications, and reported he received all his vaccines as a child. His last Tdap was 3 years prior, and he received annual influenza vaccination. He worked in sales.

In addition to typhoid and hepatitis A, what vaccination should be recommended to this patient?

A. Hepatitis B
B. Japanese encephalitis
C. MMR
D. No additional vaccinations needed
E. Rabies

46. A 45-year-old man presented with a 2-day history of rash and fever. He had returned 1 week before his symptoms began from a 4-week holiday in Nigeria visiting family. He worked as a postal worker.

On examination his temperature was 38.7°C, his heart rate was 110 beats/minute, and his blood pressure was 110/64 mmHg. He had a vesicular rash affecting predominantly his trunk, with many vesicles that were easy to burst. There are some macular lesions as well as the vesicles.

What is the most likely diagnosis?
- A. Bullous tinea corporis
- B. Chickenpox
- C. Hand, foot, and mouth
- D. Monkeypox
- E. Smallpox

47. An 18-year-old man presented with a 3-day history of fever, diffuse abdominal pain, and chest pain. His past medical history included exploratory laparotomy 2 years ago, and he was on no medications. These symptoms have occurred several times over a course of several years. He returned from Turkey 6 weeks previously where he visited relatives. He had a pet cat.

On examination, his temperature was 38.6°C. There were signs of peritonitis with rebound tenderness and guarding on abdominal examination. There were discrete erythematous plaques over his shins bilaterally.

What is the most likely diagnosis?
- A. Acute yersiniosis
- B. *Bartonella henselae* infection
- C. Familial Mediterranean fever
- D. Malaria
- E. Typhoid fever

48. Dr. Domagk is investigating the treatment of *Staphylococcus aureus* with a new compound. The compound is under heavy criticism because it does not appear to kill bacteria *in vitro,* but Dr. Domagk thinks it will work because it improves survival in *S. aureus*-infected mice. He is planning to do a study to prove that the new antibiotic should be used to treat *S. aureus* infections. In order to prove his theory, he needs a study design that provides the strongest evidence for causation.

What is the most appropriate study design?
- A. Ecological study
- B. Case control
- C. Prospective cohort
- D. Randomized controlled trial
- E. Meta-analysis

49. A 34-year-old man developed pustular, suppurative, nodular lesions over his arms that increased in size and quantity over 3 months. He had severe myasthenia gravis and had been taking prednisone 40 mg per day for 18 months. The lesions were unresponsive to a 14-day course of doxycycline and a subsequent 14-day course of oral trimethoprim–sulfamethoxazole.

On examination:

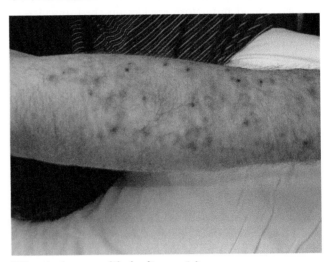

What is the most likely diagnosis?
- A. Ascending lymphangitis secondary to *Nocardia* spp. infection
- B. Community-acquired MRSA folliculitis
- C. HSV
- D. Nodular granulomatous perifolliculitis (Majocchi's granuloma)
- E. Pyoderma gangrenosum

Quiz 2

1. Based on the Gram stain, what is the most appropriate stain to perform?
A. Acid-fast
B. Giemsa
C. Modified acid-fast
D. Periodic acid–Schiff
E. Warthin–Starry

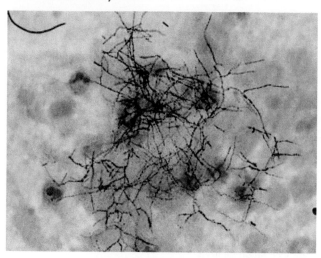

2. A 31-year-old man presented with fever, productive cough, lethargy, weakness, and malaise. He was known to have HIV but was not taking ART. He lived in Missouri. His respiratory status and mental status deteriorated, and he was transferred to the ICU.
Investigations:
HIV viral load 174,000 copies/mL
CD4 count 1 cell/μL
CXR: atelectasis and superimposed pneumonia
BAL: routine bacterial, fungal, and AFB cultures negative
BAL: PCR for adenovirus, CMV, and HSV negative
Pneumocystis DFA on BAL and induced sputum negative
Respiratory viral panel negative
Legionella urine antigen and *Legionella* antibody negative
Serum and CSF cryptococcal antigen negative
Histoplasma urine antigen negative

Antibodies for *Blastomyces*, *Coccidioides*, and West Nile virus negative

What is the most appropriate additional test to request?
A. Anaerobic culture on BAL
B. *Chlamydophila psittaci* PCR on BAL
C. *Legionella* culture on BAL
D. *M. pneumoniae* serology
E. West Nile virus antibody on CSF

3. A 26-year-old man presented with worsening headache, chills, fevers, and neck stiffness. He had no significant past medical history. He smoked 1 pack per day (PPD), and drank 2–3 beers every day. He reported unprotected sex with multiple male partners (around 5–6 partners in last 1 year). He lived in Phoenix, Arizona. He worked for a commercial painting company and had recently finished cleaning and painting an overpass.

On examination, his temperature was 39.4°C, pulse 110 beats/minute, blood pressure of 98/58 mmHg, and respiratory rate 18 breaths/minute. He was saturating 95% on room air. A lumbar puncture was performed after a neuroimaging.
Investigations:
CT head: no acute process or space-occupying lesions
LP opening pressure 40 cmH₂O
CSF white cell count 40/μL (30% polymorphonuclear cells and 70% mononuclear cells)
CSF glucose 30 mg/dL
CSF protein:70 mg/dL
Blood cultures negative at 24 hours

What diagnostic test should be performed to allow appropriate treatment?
A. *Coccidioides* antibodies
B. CSF cryptococcal antigen
C. CSF HSV PCR
D. CSF VDRL
E. Urine *Histoplasma* antigen

4. A 69-year-old man was admitted with MRSA pneumonia and bacteremia. He had a history of type 2 diabetes, controlled by diet alone.

On admission his serum creatinine was 2.4 mg/dL and BUN 40 mg/dL. The patient's most recent baseline serum creatinine and blood urea nitrogen were 1.3 mg/dL and 25 mg/dL, respectively.

What antistaphylococcal agent would be most vulnerable to drug accumulation and associated increased risk of adverse effects in this patient?

- A. Clindamycin
- B. Linezolid
- C. Minocycline
- D. Telavancin
- E. Tigecycline

5. A 55-year-old man was diagnosed with *Mycobacterium abscessus* infection. His combination therapy was to include amikacin IV.

What monitoring parameters would be most appropriate during this patient's course of therapy?

- A. Audiology exam
- B. Electrocardiogram
- C. Liver function tests
- D. Ocular examination
- E. Visual acuity testing

6. A 30-year-old patient was diagnosed with disseminated histoplasmosis. The patient was known to have HIV, well controlled on cobicistat/darunavir 150/800 mg and tenofovir alafenamide/emtricitabine 25/200 mg by mouth once daily. The patient did not take any other medications. Kidney and liver function were normal. The patient weighed 60 kg and had no known allergies.

What is the most appropriate medication regimen for empiric maintenance therapy for disseminated histoplasmosis?

- A. Itraconazole capsules 200 mg by mouth twice daily
- B. Itraconazole capsules 400 mg by mouth once daily
- C. Itraconazole oral solution 200 mg by mouth once daily
- D. Itraconazole oral solution 200 mg by mouth twice daily
- E. Liposomal amphotericin B 300 mg IV once daily

7. A 42-year-old man presented with a perianal lesion. He was known to have HIV infection (last CD4 count of 20 cells/μL, HIV-RNA viral load of 1.2 million).

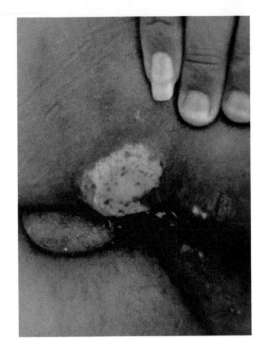

The lesion had been present for over 2.5 years and had previously responded to aciclovir or valaciclovir but had never completely healed. On this occasion, the painful ulcer had not responded to a 10-day course of oral valaciclovir 1 gram twice daily followed by a 14-day course of oral aciclovir 400 mg three times a day that was prescribed at the local STD clinic. The patient reported adherence to both regimens. DNA sequencing for resistance mutations cannot be obtained.

What is the most appropriate treatment?

- A. IV aciclovir
- B. IV foscarnet
- C. IV ribavirin
- D. PO famciclovir
- E. PO valganciclovir

8. A 57-year-old man was admitted with new onset confusion and a 2-day history of fevers. The fevers began during his return home from a month-long safari in South Africa. He was found to have severe *P. falciparum* malaria and treated with IV artesunate with significant improvement. Ten days later, he developed a sudden drop in hemoglobin and rise in bilirubin.

What is the most likely cause?

- A. Acute gastrointestinal bleeding
- B. Delayed postartesunate hemolysis
- C. Inadequate hematopoiesis
- D. Nutritional deficiency
- E. Persistent/relapsed malaria

9. A 64-year-old man was admitted to the hospital because of acute abdominal pain. He was found to be hypotensive, tachypneic, and confused. He was started on broad-spectrum antibiotics and brought to the ICU. A CT abdomen was done, which showed an inflamed sigmoid colon with an associated 5×5 cm rim enhancing fluid collection consistent with perforated sigmoid diverticulitis with abscess. Even after 48 hours and significant additional fluid therapy, the patient remained intermittently hypotensive.

What is the next appropriate step for this patient?

A. Broaden antibiotic therapy
B. Glucocorticoid therapy
C. Obtain blood cultures
D. Obtain chest X ray
E. Refer patient for guided drainage tube placement

10. A 26-year-old woman presented with fevers and a swollen right eyelid with a red eye, purulent drainage, tearing, and some blurriness. She was normally well and did not take any regular medications. She had no known drug allergies. She reported contact with a person that had recent smallpox vaccination as he had just joined the military.

On exam, she had periorbital edema and redness on the right eyelid with a cutaneous vesicle present. She had visual acuity of 20/40 on the right. There was no inflammation of the cornea. Right submandibular and preauricular lymphadenopathy were also present.
Conjunctival scrapings were sent for microbiology.

What is the best treatment option?

A. Azithromycin
B. Topical ciprofloxacin
C. Vaccinia immunoglobulin
D. Vaccinia immunoglobulin and topical trifluridine
E. Vancomycin and cefotaxime

11. A 52-year-old woman presented with a 3-day history of worsening headache. She had no past medical history of note but worked as an air hostess. Recent flights had been to New York, Los Angeles, and Paris. She was married with one teenage son and had not had any new sexual partners. She did not have any oral or genital ulceration on specific questioning. She had had similar illnesses on at least two other occasions.

On examination she was photophobic with mild neck stiffness. She was alert and cognitively intact.
Investigations:
Peripheral white cell count 7.1 ×10^9/L
CSF white cell count 342 ×10^6/L; 99% lymphocytes
CSF protein 1012 mg/L
CSF/plasma glucose 2.6/5.2 mmol/L
CSF microscopy: no organisms seen

What is the most likely causative organism?

A. *Borrelia burgdorferi*
B. Cytomegalovirus
C. Enterovirus
D. HSV-2
E. *Neisseria meningitidis*

12. A 42-year-old man was evaluated for a new pleural effusion. He had recently returned from a 2-year residence in Honduras. He described left-sided pleuritic chest pain and a nonproductive cough with a low-grade fever. His medical history was not remarkable.
Investigations:
CXR: moderate-sized left pleural effusion
A thoracentesis was performed

What pleural fluid investigation is most likely to establish the diagnosis?

A. Acid-fast bacilli stain
B. Adenosine deaminase measurement
C. Gram stain
D. LDH
E. pH

13. A 25-year-old woman presented with several days of fevers, rigors, and chest pain. She was an intravenous drug user, dependent on heroin. She had no other medical history. Physical exam revealed a regurgitant systolic heart murmur.
Investigations:
Blood cultures: Staphylococcus aureus, susceptible to methicillin
Transthoracic echocardiogram: poor visualization of valves due to body habitus.

What is the most appropriate treatment?

A. Cefazolin
B. Ceftazidime
C. Clindamycin
D. Trimethoprim–sulfamethoxazole
E. Vancomycin

14. A 32-year-old woman attended for a preoperative assessment 1 week before a scheduled tonsillectomy. She had a history of anxiety and mitral valve prolapse. She had a reported allergy to penicillin with transient rash and no other symptoms. She asked whether she needed antibiotic prophylaxis for endocarditis.

What is the most appropriate advice?

A. She does not require prophylaxis because she does not have a high-risk cardiac condition
B. She does not require prophylaxis because she is not undergoing a high-risk procedure
C. She requires a preoperative echocardiogram to inform the decision
D. She should receive prophylaxis with amoxicillin
E. She should receive prophylaxis with clindamycin

15. A 25-year-old woman presented with 2 days of bloody diarrhea. She worked as a school teacher and had led a school trip to a farm 4 days before her symptoms began. She had a history of mild asthma and used occasional salbutamol inhalers as needed. She had no known allergies. She had not received any recent steroids or antibiotics.

On admission she was dehydrated. Her temperature was 36.8°C, and she was diffusely tender on abdominal examination. She had a seizure shortly after admission and developed some motor weakness.
Investigations:
Creatinine clearance 42 mL/min
Peripheral white cell count 14.0 ×10⁹/L
Hemoglobin 8.2 g/dL
Platelet count 90,000/μL
CT scan abdomen findings consistent with pseudomembranous colitis
Supportive management with IV fluids was commenced

What is the most appropriate action?

A. CT cranial imaging
B. Endoscopy and biopsy
C. Request a surgical opinion
D. Send stool for enteric pathogens (culture/NAAT)
E. Start empirical ciprofloxacin and metronidazole

16. A 73-year-old woman presented with fever, bloody diarrhea, and right leg pain. Her symptoms had started 5 days earlier, and her diarrhea was starting to improve (frequency reduced to 2–3 stools/day). She was known to have peripheral vascular disease and hypertension. She kept reptiles as pets.
Stool cultures yielded a nontyphoidal *Salmonella* species.

What is a risk factor for invasive disease?

A. Age >5 years
B. Atherosclerotic disease
C. Bloody diarrhea
D. Hypertension
E. Stool frequency >3/day

17. A 56-year-old man presented with acute breathlessness, wheeze, and severe abdominal pain. He had a past medical history of allergic rhinitis which he controlled with antihistamines as required. One week earlier he had been diagnosed with temporal arteritis for which he started a course of high-dose oral prednisolone. He denied excessive alcohol use, smoking, or consuming any illicit drug use. He lived in Peru until age 18 years when he emigrated to the UK for work.

On examination the patient was unwell. Vitals revealed respiratory rate 28 breaths/minute, oxygen saturations 92% on 15 L/minute, blood pressure 104/62 mmHg, heart rate 124 beats/minute, and temperature 38.5°C. He had a diffuse wheeze throughout his chest and was unable to complete sentences. He had generalized abdominal pain with no guarding and normal bowel sounds.

Initial investigations:
Hemoglobin: 132 g/L (135–180)
Total WCC: 20.8 ×10⁹/L (4.0–11.0)
(neutrophils 15.2, lymphocytes 1.5, monocytes 1.1)
Platelets: 178 ×10⁹/L (150–450)
Urea: 9.2 mmol/L (2.8–8.1)
Creatinine: 112 μmol/L (62–106)
Amylase: 1250 U/L (60–180)
Cholesterol and triglycerides were normal
Urgent chest X-ray:

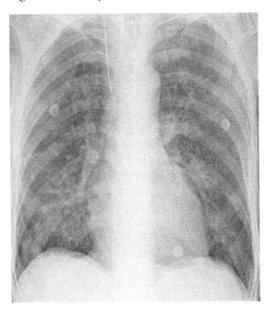

Urgent abdominal USS revealed sludge in a normal gallbladder but no gallstones or blockage of common bile or cystic duct.

What is the most likely diagnosis?

A. Acute cholangitis with SIRS response
B. Acute HIV infection
C. Adult-onset asthma
D. *Mycoplasma pneumoniae* infection
E. *Strongyloides stercoralis* hyperinfestation

18. A 37-year-old, 30-week pregnant (G1P0), woman presented for routine obstetric care. She denied any urinary frequency, dysuria, or suprapubic pain. She had no known drug allergies.

Urine culture was performed and demonstrated 10⁵ colony forming units per mL *Escherichia coli*. A second specimen confirmed the presence of *E. coli*.

What is the most appropriate treatment?

A. Amoxicillin
B. Cephalexin
C. Ciprofloxacin
D. No treatment required
E. Trimethoprim–sulfamethoxazole

19. A 23-year-old man presented with dysuria, urethral itching, and clear urethral discharge. He had been treated 1 week earlier with a stat dose of azithromycin 1 g for NGU. He had not had any sex since treatment.
Investigations:

Gram stain showed 5 PMNs per oil immersion field
NAAT for gonorrhea, chlamydia, and trichomoniasis were negative

What is the most likely cause?

A. *Chlamydia trachomatis*
B. Contact dermatitis
C. Herpes simplex virus type 2
D. *Mycoplasma genitalium*
E. *Neisseria gonorrhoeae*

20. A 35-year-old man attended for care. He was known to have HIV, HCV, and HBV infection related to previous intravenous drug use. He had previously been inconsistent in care but had completed a treatment program for his drug dependency 6 months and now attended regularly for follow up.
Investigations:

ALT 330 IU/L
CD4 430 cells/μL
HIV viral load: 90,000 copies/mL; no resistance on genotypic testing
HBV sAg positive, eAg positive, cAb positive; HBV eAb negative
HBV DNA: 22,000 IU/mL
HCV IgG positive, genotype 1; HCV viral load 600,000 IU/mL

What is the most appropriate treatment?

A. Abacavir, lamivudine, and efavirenz
B. Dolutegravir, darunavir, ritonavir, and ledipasvir
C. Entecavir and efavirenz
D. Entecavir, darunavir, ritonavir, and sofosbuvir
E. Tenofovir alafenamide, emtricitabine, and dolutegravir

21. A 28-year-old woman presented following contact with a child with a maculopapular rash. She was 24 weeks pregnant. The exposure occurred 24 hours previously.

In pregnancy, human normal immunoglobulin is used as postexposure prophylaxis for what infection?

A. Cytomegalovirus
B. Erythrovirus (parvovirus B19)
C. Herpes simplex virus
D. Measles virus
E. Rubella virus

22. A 60-year-old woman presented with progressive ataxia and dizziness. She gave a clear history of a flu-like illness and distinctive rash following a tick bite several years earlier in Slovenia.

A lumbar puncture was performed and showed a lymphocytic pleocytosis, raised protein, and oligoclonal bands. MRI imaging showed no lesions.

What is the most likely causative organism?

A. *Babesia microti*
B. *Borrelia afzelii*
C. *Borrelia garinii*
D. Tickborne encephalitis virus
E. *Treponema pallidum*

23. A 22-year-old man presented with a painful swelling on his thigh. He denied any associated fevers or chills. The patient had applied warm compresses to the site for the past two days with little improvement. He was normally well and did not take any regular medication.

On examination, there was a 3-cm lesion on his right inner thigh. The lesion was warm, tender, and fluctuant to palpation. The rest of his physical examination was unremarkable.

What is the most appropriate treatment?

A. Hold antibiotics pending results of a superficial swab MCS
B. Hospital admission for intravenous antibiotics
C. Incision and drainage at the bedside
D. List for urgent surgical debridement in an operating room
E. Oral antibiotics

24. A 71-year-old man presented with a 5-month history of drainage from his right total hip arthroplasty (THA) incision (completed 3 years prior). There were associated low-grade fevers, increasing fatigue, and lack of appetite. He was known to have hypertension, asthma, and depression. He was allergic to sulfa drugs, with previous anaphylaxis.

On examination, there was a sinus tract over the right hip with surrounding cellulitis.
Investigations:

X-ray of the right hip demonstrated periprosthetic lucency.
Blood cultures: MRSA sensitive to trimethoprim–sulfamethoxazole (TMP–SMX), linezolid, and vancomycin; resistant to clindamycin and doxycycline

What is the most appropriate surgical intervention?

A. Debridement, antibiotics, irrigation, and retention (DAIR)
B. Medical management with antibiotics
C. One-stage exchange
D. Permanent resection with arthrodesis
E. Two-stage exchange

25. A 78-year-old woman was reviewed in the intensive care with fever and hemodynamic instability. She was recently repatriated to a rehabilitation hospital in the United States from India, where she had been hospitalized for 3 months because of a cerebrovascular accident. She had a peripherally inserted central catheter for blood work, a percutaneous endoscopic gastrostomy tube for supplemental alimentation, and an indwelling urinary catheter. Five days earlier, she had developed fever, tachycardia, and hypotension. She was started on meropenem and fluconazole.

Investigations:

PICC and peripheral blood cultures: positive for *Candida haemulonii* after 72 hours; susceptibility as follows:

Agent	Minimum Inhibitory Concentration (MIC) or Mean Effective Concentration (MEC)	Interpretation
Fluconazole	128 µg/mL	Resistant
Amphotericin B	2 µg/mL	Resistant
Micafungin	0.5 µg/mL	Susceptible

What is the most likely correct identification of the organism?

A. *Candida auris*
B. *Candida glabrata*
C. *Candida haemulonii*
D. *Rhodotorula glutinis*
E. *Saccharomyces cerevisiae*

26. A 20-year-old man was reviewed with a 4-day history of fevers and hypotension despite empiric use of broad-spectrum antibiotics.

The man had presented to hospital 3 weeks earlier with profuse diarrhea and severe malnutrition. He had Crohn's disease with short gut syndrome secondary to multiple bowel resections. He was initiated at admission on total parenteral nutrition via central venous catheter.

His antimicrobials were changed to meropenem and micafungin.

Investigations:

Total white cell count 20 ×10⁹/L
Platelet count 50 ×10⁹/L
Blood cultures (central and peripheral) no growth after 3 days
CXR: bilateral airspace disease

What is the best next test to secure a diagnosis?

A. Blood culture inoculated onto Sabouraud dextrose agar
B. Blood culture on Sabouraud dextrose with olive oil
C. Panfungal PCR of whole blood
D. Serum 1,3-β-D-glucan
E. Serum cryptococcal antigen

27. A 19-year-old man presented with a 4-day history of sore throat, fever, headache, and myalgia. He had returned from a week-long trip to the Caribbean 6 days earlier. He was normally well and did not take any regular medications.

On physical examination, his temperature was 38°C (100.9°F), blood pressure 102/70 mmHg, heart rate 105 beats/minute, and respiratory rate 16 breaths/min. His pharynx was injected, but no exudate was seen. He had a maculopapular rash on his chest, back, and extremities, sparing the palms and soles.

Investigations:

Total white cell count 3.1 ×10⁹/L
Platelet count 81 ×10⁹/L

Hemoglobin 14.3 g/dL
Total bilirubin 1.3 mg/dL (22 µmol/L)
ALT 121 U/L
AST 163 U/L

What is the most likely diagnosis?

A. Dengue
B. Chikungunya
C. Leptospirosis
D. Malaria
E. Yellow fever

28. A 23-year old soldier presented with a 2-day history of sudden onset fever, marked prostration, cough with bloody sputum, and shortness of breath. He was previously well and did not take any regular medications.

On examination, his respiratory rate was 38 breaths/minute, his oxygen saturations were 84% on room air, and his blood pressure was 86/42 mmHg. There was no neck stiffness and no rash.

Investigations:

Total white cell count 21 ×10⁹/L
Platelet count 72,000/µL
CXR: widespread pulmonary infiltrates throughout the lung fields

Twenty other soldiers had also presented with similar complaints in the last week. Bioterrorism via an aerosol route was suspected with onward person-to-person transmission.

What organism is most likely to be responsible?

A. *Bacillus anthracis*
B. *Brucella melitensis*
C. *Coxiella burnetii*
D. *Francisella tularensis*
E. *Yersinia pestis*

29. A 25-year-old woman was referred for consideration of treatment for latent TB infection. She was asymptomatic. She had been born in Russia and recently moved to the United States. She had no past medical history and took no medications other than OTC vitamins. She worked in a retail store with alternating shifts. She did not smoke and drank alcohol occasionally, having stopped binge drinking one year ago.

On physical exam, she had a 12 mm TST induration on her forearm. Examination was otherwise unremarkable.

Investigations:

Interferon gamma release assay (*Tspot*) positive
CXR: normal appearances, clear lung fields
HIV Ag/Ab negative

What regimen would be most likely to ensure effective completion of therapy?

A. Isoniazid and rifapentine weekly for 3 months
B. Isoniazid daily for 9 months
C. Isoniazid daily for 6 months
D. Isoniazid twice a week for 9 months
E. Rifapentine daily for 4 months

30. A 26-year-old woman presented with fevers and night sweats for the last month with weight loss of 15 pounds during the same period. There was no cough or shortness of breath. She was known to have HIV but was nonadherent to her antiretroviral medications and did not engage regularly in care.
Investigations:
    CD4 count 15 cells/μL
    Blood cultures negative
    CXR: unremarkable
    CT chest, abdomen, and pelvis: diffuse lymphadenopathy above and below the diaphragm; mild splenomegaly
    Mycobacterial blood cultures negative
    Bone marrow biopsy: acid-fast bacilli seen on microscopy; mycobacterial cultures at 37 °C negative; subcultures at 30 °C positive

What is the most likely organism?

A. *Mycobacterium–avium* complex
B. *Mycobacterium fortuitum*
C. *Mycobacterium genavense*
D. *Mycobacterium gordonae*
E. *Mycobacterium haemophilum*

31. A 40-year-old man presented with a 2-week history of pain on defecation and hematochezia. He was known to have HIV but had declined previous antiretroviral treatment. A colonoscopy was performed.
Investigations:
    CD4 count 30 cells/μL
    Colonoscopy: ulcerated mucosa seen; biopsies taken
    Ulcer histology: amoebic trophozoites with a single nucleus and ingested red blood cells seen. No cysts seen

What organism is most likely to be responsible?

A. *Balantidium coli*
B. *Blastocystis hominis*
C. *Dientamoeba fragilis*
D. *Entamoeba histolytica*
E. *Giardia lamblia*

32. A 46-year-old man was reviewed with longstanding generalized abdominal pain. He had moved to the UK 4 years previously from Uganda where he had been born and brought up.
Clinical examination was unremarkable.
Investigations:
    Hemoglobin 9.5 g/dL
    MCV 69 fL
    Eosinophil count 0.5 ×10⁹/L
    Feces microscopy for ova, cysts, and parasites ×1: negative

What is the most appropriate initial treatment?

A. Albendazole
B. Diethylcarbamazine citrate (DEC)
C. Ferrous sulfate
D. Ivermectin
E. Pyrantel pamoate

33. A 26-year-old woman attended with flu-like symptoms. She had unprotected sexual intercourse with a casual partner 3 weeks before her symptoms began.
Investigations:
    Fourth-generation HIV test positive
    Confirmatory anti-HIV-1 and anti-HIV-2 antibodies negative
    HIV viral load 3 million copies/mL

In addition to HIV-1 and HIV-2 antibodies, what does a fourth-generation HIV test detect?

A. Co-receptor CXCR4
B. GP120
C. Integrase
D. p24 antigen
E. Reverse transcriptase

34. A 34-year-old woman attended for review after a positive pregnancy test. She was known to have HIV and was taking tenofovir disoproxil fumarate/emtricitabine/efavirenz. She reported ongoing compliance with her medication. She estimated that she was 7 weeks pregnant.
Investigations:
    CD4 count 550 cells/μL
    HIV viral load undetectable

What is the most appropriate management plan?

A. Advise her to consider termination due to the risk of teratogenicity
B. Continue current ART and routine monitoring
C. Stop ART and recommence during the 2nd trimester
D. Switch efavirenz to cobicistat-boosted darunavir
E. Switch to ritonavir-boosted darunavir, zidovudine, and emtricitabine

35. A 45-year-old woman presented with fevers and a neck lump. She had been started 6 weeks earlier on quadruple antituberculous treatment for TB lymphadenitis and combination ART. She had initially improved on treatment, but then her fevers returned, and she noticed worsening enlargement and pain at the site of the involved lymph node.
Investigations:
    Lymph node biopsy: granulomatous inflammation seen
    Lymph node culture: fully sensitive *Mycobacterium tuberculosis* isolated

	1st visit	2nd visit
CD4 count (cells/μL)	55	145
HIV viral load (copies/mL)	245,000	1,255

What is the most appropriate intervention?

A. Addition of a fifth anti-TB drug
B. Addition of a nonsteroidal antiinflammatory
C. Cessation of anti-TB therapy
D. Cessation of HIV antiretroviral therapy
E. Surgical excision of lymph node

36. A 54-year-old man presented with fevers, headaches, and altered mental status. He lived in Tucson, Arizona, and worked for a landscape management company. He was known to have HIV, atrial fibrillation, and hypertension but was not taking ART.

Investigations:

MRI brain: hydrocephalus and meningeal enhancement seen

CD4 count 95 cells/μL

HIV viral load undetectable

CSF microscopy: lymphocytic pleocytosis

CSF complement fixation IgG serology for *Coccidioides* positive 1:32

The patient was treated with IV fluconazole and intrathecal amphotericin B for 2 weeks with improvement in symptoms and MRI findings. The patient was then transitioned to oral fluconazole 400 mg daily upon discharge.

What duration of antifungal therapy should be recommended?

A. 6 months

B. 9 months

C. 12 months

D. 18 months

E. Indefinite

37. A 56-year-old woman presented with progressive headaches, confusion, and difficulty in walking. She was known to have relapsing–remitting multiple sclerosis and had been treated with monthly natalizumab for 3 years.

On examination she had bilateral lower extremity weakness. Sensation was intact. She had some word-finding difficulties. There was no photophobia or neck stiffness.

Investigations:

CT head: no mass effect seen. Asymmetric low attenuation foci in the periventricular and subcortical white matter.

What is the most appropriate treatment?

A. Aciclovir

B. Liposomal amphotericin and flucytosine

C. Pulsed methylprednisolone

D. Stop natalizumab and consider plasma exchange

E. Sulfadiazine and pyrimethamine

38. A 76-year-old man presented with a 2-day history of fever, fatigue, and occasional rigors. He had undergone deceased donor kidney transplantation for polycystic kidney disease 26 years ago and was on azathioprine and prednisone for maintenance immunosuppression. He had had recurrent episodes of fever, rigors, and sepsis for several months with blood cultures positive for *Escherichia coli*.

Investigations:

Blood cultures positive for *E. coli*

Urinalysis: +1 protein and trace blood; urine cultures no growth

An infected cyst was considered as a potential nidus of relapsing infection

What is the most sensitive diagnostic modality to detect cyst infection?

A. CT scan of the abdomen and pelvis

B. MRI of the abdomen and pelvis

C. Positron emission tomography scan

D. Tagged white blood cell scan

E. Ultrasound of the abdomen

39. A 45-year-old woman was reviewed with a 3-week history of fevers and a 1-week history of painful skin nodules. She was known to have a persistent neutropenia following an allogeneic stem cell transplant 4 weeks earlier for relapsed acute lymphoblastic leukemia. She had been taking levofloxacin, voriconazole, valaciclovir, and trimethoprim–sulfamethoxazole prophylaxis; the levofloxacin had been switched to intravenous cefepime 3 weeks earlier, but her symptoms had progressed.

On examination, her temperature was 103°F (39.4°C), her blood pressure was 110/68 mmHg, her heart rate was 116 beats/min, respiratory rate 18 breaths/min, and oxygen saturations 98% on room air. Cardiovascular and respiratory exams were unremarkable. There were multiple subcutaneous purplish popular and nodular lesions of various sizes scattered throughout her extremities, her neck, and her chest. Some of the lesions had central necrosis. She had pedal onychomycosis.

Investigations:

Total white cell count 0.2×10^9 /L (4–10)

Absolute neutrophil count 0.0×10^9 /L (2–8)

Hemoglobin 7.4 g/dL (13–17)

Platelets 43×10^9 /L (150–400)

eGFR>60 mL/min/1.73 m^2

Blood cultures at admission were negative, but repeat blood cultures at the point of review 3 weeks later were positive for a mold.

What is the most likely diagnosis?

A. *Aspergillus fumigatus*

B. *Candida tropicalis*

C. *Cryptococcus neoformans*

D. *Fusarium solani*

E. *Histoplasma capsulatum*

40. A 19-year-old woman developed meningococcemia. She had a history of systemic lupus erythematosus and had an episode of meningococcal meningitis at 12 years of age.

What is the most appropriate screening test?

A. Antibody responses to vaccines

B. CH50

C. Dihydrorhodamine (DHR) test

D. Lymphocyte subsets

E. Quantitative immunoglobulins

41. A 23-year-old woman sought medical advice after being bitten on the leg by a stray coyote. She had received all appropriate travel immunizations 5 months previously for an overseas trip, including a course of rabies vaccine. The wound had been cleaned thoroughly. The animal could not be captured.

What is the most appropriate action?

A. 2 doses of rabies vaccine

B. 4 doses of rabies vaccine and rabies immune globulin (HRIG)

C. 5 doses of rabies vaccine and rabies immune globulin (HRIG)

D. No further intervention is needed

E. Obtain a rabies serologic titer from the patient

42. A 27-year-old nurse presented for new employee screening. He was born and brought up in the UK. He was found to have 16 mm of induration around his PPD intradermal skin test at 48 hours after placement of the test. He had never received the BCG vaccine.

What is the most appropriate management?

A. Administer BCG vaccine

B. Perform an interferon gamma release assay

C. Repeat the PPD test in 8–12 weeks

D. Start RIPE therapy

E. Take a 6–9 month course of isoniazid

43. A 32-year-old woman sought travel advice for a 1-week trip to Zambia. Her departure date was in 1 month. She was 16-weeks pregnant. She intended to visit friends and relatives. She was given advice regarding mosquito bite avoidance.

What is the most appropriate malaria chemoprophylaxis?

A. Atovaquone–proguanil

B. Chloroquine

C. Doxycycline

D. Medical prophylaxis contraindicated due to pregnancy

E. Mefloquine

44. A 54-year-old woman presented with a productive cough as well as a painful swollen nose with copious discharge. She reported a biphasic illness, as the current symptoms had been preceded by recovery from a 1-week history of malaise, fever, headache, and myalgia. She had a history of osteoarthritis but did not take any regular medications. She worked as an equine vet.

On examination her temperature was 37.5°C, her respiratory rate was 18 breaths/minute, and her oxygen saturations were 97% on room air. Her nose and surrounding facial skin were moderately swollen, and she had palpable cervical lymphadenopathy.

Flexible nasal endoscopy was performed, followed by bronchoscopy, which revealed multiple necrotic ulcers in the mucosal lining of the tracheobronchial tree.
Investigations:

Biopsies were taken and sent for microscopy and culture
Results: gram-negative bacilli with rounded ends seen on direct microscopy
Chest X-ray was unremarkable

What is the most likely causative organism?

A. *Burkholderia mallei*

B. *Burkholderia pseudomallei*

C. *Coxiella burnetii*

D. *Francisella tularensis*

E. *Yersinia pestis*

45. A 5-year-old boy presented with recurrent fevers that lasted for 6 days. The episodes were very regular, appearing every 4 weeks. The fever was accompanied by sore throat and mouth ulcers. He was asymptomatic between episodes. There was no significant family history. His C-reactive protein and total white cell count were very elevated during each episode.

What is the most likely diagnosis?

A. Crohn's disease

B. Cyclic neutropenia

C. Familial Mediterranean fever

D. Periodic fever, aphthous stomatitis, pharyngitis, adenitis syndrome

E. Recurrent herpes simplex infection

46. A new diagnostic test has been developed for Lyme disease. Stored specimens from 1000 patients were tested with the new method, 80 of whom had previously been found to have Lyme disease by enzyme immunoassay/Western blot. The new test gave positive results in 60 of the previously identified individuals with Lyme disease, and gave positive results in 40 persons who were not previously identified with Lyme disease.

What are the sensitivity and positive predictive value of the new test compared to enzyme immunoassay/Western blot?

A. 55% and 60%

B. 60% and 55%

C. 60% and 75%

D. 75% and 55%

E. 75% and 60%

47. A 73-year-old man presented with a 3-month history of progressive, pruritic lesions primarily on his legs. He had a history of uncontrolled asthma and had taken oral prednisone multiple times in the preceding 4 months.

On examination:

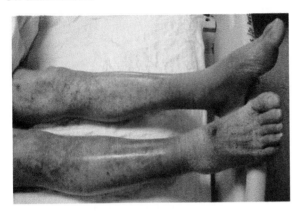

What is the most likely diagnosis?

A. Crusted scabies
B. Cutaneous T-cell lymphoma
C. Generalized pustular psoriasis
D. Kaposi's varicelliform eruption (eczema herpeticum)
E. Sweet's syndrome

48. A 21-year-old man presented with new penile lesions. He had insertive vaginal and oral intercourse using a latex condom with a casual female partner 72 hours earlier. He denied any current medications, known past medical history, or allergies. He was a college student and worked part-time in a chemistry laboratory.

On examination, there were erythematous plaques over the shaft and glans penis.

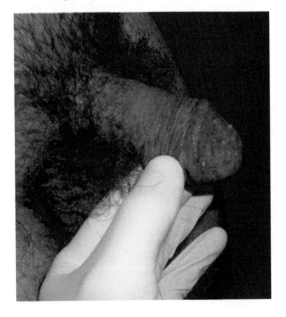

What is the most likely diagnosis?

A. Genital herpes
B. HIV
C. Latex allergy
D. Primary syphilis
E. Psoriasis

49. A 42-year-old man presented with a 3-month history of skin changes on his thighs. He reported that the lesions were occasionally pruritic. He had tried topical and oral antifungals without any response. He was known to have diabetes and was morbidly obese.

On examination there were multiple erythematous lesions over both thighs. The lesions were non-tender and cool to touch.

What is the most likely causative organism?

A. *Candida* spp.
B. Community-acquired MRSA
C. *Corynebacterium minutissimum*
D. *Malassezia furfur*
E. *Tinea rubrum*

Quiz 3

1. A 54-year-old woman was admitted with pneumonia following influenza A infection.

IV ceftriaxone was started empirically.

Investigations:

Sputum culture: *Staphylococcus aureus* isolated; resistant to clindamycin, sensitive to oxacillin, trimethoprim–sulfamethoxazole (TMP–SMX), and vancomycin

What is the most appropriate method for ceftriaxone susceptibility testing?

A. Broth microdilution
B. Gradient diffusion
C. Kirby–Bauer disk diffusion
D. Resistance can be inferred
E. Susceptibility can be inferred

2. A 52-year-old man presented with a 3-week history of a low-grade fever, myalgia, productive cough, and skin lesions on his left upper back that developed during the previous week.

He had a past medical history of poorly controlled diabetes (hemoglobin A1c 8.4) and hyperlipidemia. He was taking metformin, glipizide, aspirin, and atorvastatin.

He smoked 1 pack per day (PPD) and drank alcohol occasionally. He was a chiropterologist (bat expert) and frequently explored caves. He was from Wisconsin and had returned recently from a 1 month-long trip to Grand Canyon in Arizona, Death Valley in California, and Four Corners. On examination, his temperature was 38.4°C, heart rate was 90 beats/minute, blood pressure of 110/78 mmHg, and respiratory rate of 18 breaths/minute with SPO_2 95% on room air.

He had numerous erythematous plaques with minimal scaling and surrounding induration

Investigations:

CXR: normal appearances

Skin biopsy: changes consistent with a squamous cell carcinoma

Fungal cultures of skin biopsy: positive for mold after 14 days

What is the most likely organism?

A. *Blastomyces dermatitidis*
B. *Candida albicans*
C. *Coccidioides immitis*
D. *Cryptococcus neoformans*
E. *Histoplasma capsulatum*

3. A 22-year-old man presented with a 3-day history of subjective fever and sudden onset of behavioral changes and intermittent blurred vision. He also did not appear to fully recall the family members who brought him to the ED. He was never vaccinated against childhood diseases. He had no known exposures and did not endorse any insect bites, water, or animal exposures. The physical and neurologic exams were unremarkable.

Investigations:

CT brain: normal appearances

A lumbar puncture was performed: CSF was clear with normal glucose and elevated protein of 85 mg/dL (reference range 15–60 mg/dL)

CSF Gram stain: no organisms seen

CSF multiplex panel negative

CSF bacterial and viral cultures negative

Two days after admission the patient developed a myoclonic jerk and his cognitive function continued to decline.

An EEG showed period complexes occurring every 10 seconds. T2-weighted and fluid-attenuated inversion-recovery (FLAIR) sequences from magnetic resonance imaging (MRI) of the brain showed hyperintensity in the left frontal cortex.

MRI performed 15 days later showed bilateral progression of the lesion.

The patient continued to decline and died 60 days after admission.

What additional test result fits the diagnosis?

A. Bacterial culture positive for group A β-hemolytic streptococcus
B. IgM and IgG positive for West Nile virus in the serum and CSF
C. Increased measles IgG in the serum and CSF
D. Mumps IgG positive from serum
E. Respiratory viral panel positive for parainfluenza virus

4. A 60-year-old woman was diagnosed with methicillin-resistant *Staphylococcus aureus* pneumonia and bacteremia approximately 48 hours after recovering from a case of uncomplicated influenza. She had a history of hyperlipidemia and depression. She had no known drug allergies. Medications prior to admission were atorvastatin 20 mg daily and citalopram 20 mg daily.

Vancomycin 1250 mg IV q12 hours was initiated, with a serum trough concentration after the fourth dose of 16.1 μg/mL.

While receiving the fifth dose of vancomycin, the patient experienced face and neck flushing and redness.

What is the most appropriate action?

A. Change to daptomycin
B. Change to tigecycline
C. Change to linezolid
D. Decrease the vancomycin dose to 1250 mg q24 hours
E. Double the infusion time of subsequent vancomycin doses

5. A 55-year-old man presented with a foul-smelling right lower extremity soft tissue infection. He was obese and had a history of type 2 diabetes mellitus, anemia, hyperlipidemia, chronic obstructive pulmonary disease, and a recent deep vein thrombosis. He had no known drug allergies. Home medications were ferrous sulfate 325 mg PO TD, tizanidine 2 mg PO BD, theophylline 300 mg PO BD, warfarin 5 mg PO daily, and atorvastatin 40 mg PO daily.

On examination, he was afebrile with an infected ulcer on his right lower leg.

Investigations:

Total white cell count 9800 cells/mm^3
MRI: no evidence of underlying osteomyelitis
Wound swab culture: mixed organisms including *Pseudomonas* isolated
Plans were to treat the infection with ciprofloxacin PO and amoxicillin-clavulanic acid PO.

What medication would be most likely to interfere with the effectiveness of this planned antibiotic regimen?

A. Atorvastatin
B. Ferrous sulfate
C. Theophylline
D. Tizanidine
E. Warfarin

6. A 58-year-old man was diagnosed with *Mycobacterium avium* complex infection. His treatment regimen was to include azithromycin.

What monitoring parameters would need to be conducted on a routine basis?

A. Color discrimination test
B. Electrocardiogram
C. Ocular examination
D. Serum uric acid
E. Visual acuity testing

7. A 40-year-old woman presented to the hospital with a severe headache for the last week. The patient took no other medications and had no known drug allergies. The patient's weight and height were 80 kg and 66 inches, respectively.
Investigations:

Creatinine 0.8 mg/dL
ALT 20 units/L
CSF microscopy and culture negative
CSF cryptococcal antigen positive

What is the most appropriate treatment?

A. Caspofungin 70 mg IV × one dose, then 50 mg IV once daily
B. Fluconazole 800 mg IV once daily
C. Liposomal amphotericin B 8 mg IV once daily and flucytosine 500 mg by mouth four times daily
D. Liposomal amphotericin B 350 mg IV once daily and flucytosine 2000 mg by mouth four times daily
E. Voriconazole 480 mg IV twice daily for 2 doses, then 320 mg IV twice daily.

8. A 39-year-old woman was reviewed with a new diagnosis of HIV and hepatitis B co-infection. A pregnancy test was negative. Despite multiple educational meetings she declined HIV treatment but was interested in hepatitis B treatment.
Investigations:

AST 89 IU/L
ALT 98 units/L
CD4 count 434 cells/μL
HIV viral load 55,000 copies/mL
HBsAg positive
HBV viral load 540,000 IU/mL
Liver biopsy showed significant fibrosis but no cirrhosis

What is the most appropriate treatment to offer?

A. Lamivudine
B. Peginterferon alfa 2B
C. Peginterferon alfa 2B plus entecavir
D. Tenofovir
E. Tenofovir, emtricitabine, and dolutegravir

9. A 37-year-old man was reviewed for ongoing epigastric pain, nausea, vomiting, and diarrhea. He had been born and brought up in Thailand and had moved to the United States age 18.
Investigation:

Peripheral eosinophil count 1.4 ×10^9/L
Stool OCP ×3 negative
Strongyloides serology positive

What is the most appropriate treatment?

A. Albendazole
B. Ivermectin
C. Pentamidine
D. Praziquantel
E. Suramin

10. A 22-year-old man presented with acute vision loss on the left. His eye was not painful. There was no discharge from his eye. He had no past medical history. He reported unprotected sex with 3 male sexual partners in the last 6 months. He had never had an HIV test.

On examination there was a posterior uveitis of the left eye.
Investigations:
  Syphilis EIA positive
  RPR 1:128
  FTA-ABS positive
  HIV test pending

What is the next best test?

A. Conjunctival swab for *Gonorrhea* culture
B. Hearing test
C. HSV PCR of corneal scrapings
D. Lumbar puncture
E. Urine nucleic acid amplification testing for *Chlamydia*

11. An 82-year-old man presented with a 4-day history of fever and confusion. He had a history of atrial fibrillation, CABG 4 years ago, benign prostatic hypertrophy, and type 2 diabetes mellitus. He was a resident in a nursing home and had a long-term catheter in situ. He had been treated presumptively for a urinary tract infection but had deteriorated.

On examination his GCS was 13/15, his temperature was 38.1°C, and his heart rate was 112 beats/minute. His blood pressure was 128/68 mmHg. It was not possible to formally examine his neurologic systems, but his reflexes were universally brisk and his tone increased. There were no lateralizing signs. Pupils were equal and reactive to light.

He was admitted and treated with antibiotics for presumed urosepsis. Two days after his admission, he had a tonic clonic seizure on the ward. An urgent MRI showed temporal lobe enhancement, and a lumbar puncture showed a lymphocytic CSF with a raised red cell count. CSF PCR was positive for HSV-1.

Six months after discharge he was still suffering from significant cognitive impairment with behavioral abnormalities.

What factor in this case is associated with a poor outcome?

A. Delay in initiating aciclovir therapy
B. GCS score ≤13/15
C. Hemorrhagic CSF
D. MRI changes in the temporal lobes
E. Seizure activity

12. A 37-year-old woman presented with new onset speech disturbance, confusion, and left arm weakness. Her friend said that she had reported being unwell for 10 days with a mild headache and fever. She had been born and brought up in the Philippines. She was normally fit and well and was awaiting occupational health clearance to start work as a hospital nurse.

A lumbar puncture was performed after a CT head and clotting were checked.

Investigations:
  Peripheral white blood cell count 6.2 ×10⁹/L
  HIV Ag/Ab negative
  CSF white cell count 655 ×10⁶/L; 99% lymphocytes
  CSF protein 2910 mg/L
  CSF/plasma glucose 1.2/5.6 mmol/L
  CSF microscopy: no organisms seen
  A working diagnosis of TB meningitis (TBM) was made, and she was started on quadruple antituberculous therapy and dexamethasone.

What agent is the most critical at the start of TBM treatment?

A. Ethambutol
B. Isoniazid
C. Pyrazinamide
D. Rifampin
E. Streptomycin

13. A 70-year-old man presented with a 3-month history of weight loss, night sweats, and an increasing cough. He used to work as a miner and had been diagnosed in the past with pulmonary silicosis.

Investigations:
  Pulmonary function testing unchanged from the previous year
  CXR: multiple small nodules present through all lung zones but upper lobe predominant

What is the most appropriate intervention?

A. Bronchoscopy for AFB culture
B. High-resolution CT chest
C. Lung biopsy
D. Mantoux test
E. PET CT scan

14. A 50-year-old man presented with a worsening cough, shortness of breath, and fevers. He was known to have acute myeloid leukemia and had undergone a bone marrow transplant 3 months prior. He had occasionally required courses of corticosteroids to treat graft versus host disease.

Investigations:
  CXR: bilateral interstitial infiltrates, worse in the lower lobes
  Bronchoscopy: bacterial and mycobacterial cultures negative
  An open lung biopsy was performed
  Lung tissue histology: numerous cells seen which are several times larger than surrounding cells with a central inclusion

What would be the most appropriate treatment?

A. Cidofovir
B. CMV immune globulin
C. Foscarnet
D. Ganciclovir
E. Letermovir

15. A 65-year-old woman presented with a 5-day history of fevers. She had AML for which she was on induction chemotherapy. She had a tunneled intravenous catheter.

On examination, there were no signs of infection around her CVC site. There were two necrotic skin lesions on her right lower leg.

Investigations:

Neutrophil count 0.1 ×10^9/L

Blood and wound cultures grew gram-negative bacilli

What is the most likely causative organism?

A. *Bacteroides fragilis*
B. Escherichia *coli*
C. *Klebsiella pneumoniae*
D. *Pseudomonas aeruginosa*
E. *Stenotrophomonas maltophilia*

16. A 72-year-old man presented after a syncopal episode associated with firing of his implanted cardioverter-defibrillator (AICD). He had also had a 4-week history of fever and chills. He had undergone an AICD exchange 2 months earlier. He had a history of coronary artery disease and prior CABG, congestive heart failure, and had had an AICD for 15 years.

On examination his temperature was 38.4°C, heart rate was 105 beats/min, blood pressure was 110/80 mmHg, O$_2$ saturation 98% on room air. His AICD site had a well-healed incision with no erosion or discharge, but there was fluctuance over the AICD pocket.

He was started on vancomycin.

Investigations:

Total white cell count 15,000/mm^3

Blood cultures: gram-positive cocci in clusters seen

What is the most appropriate advice regarding echocardiogram?

A. Delayed transthoracic echocardiogram after AICD removal
B. No need for transthoracic echocardiogram as it will not change management because AICD needs to be removed anyway
C. Urgent transesophageal echocardiogram
D. Urgent transthoracic echocardiogram and if negative, OK to retain AICD generator and leads
E. Urgent transthoracic echocardiogram but AICD will require removal independent of results

17. A 36-year-old woman presented with a 1-day history of chest pain, 2 days of worsening dyspnea and fatigue, malaise, and upper respiratory symptoms for the preceding week. She had no significant medical history and did not take any regular medications.

On examination her heart rate was 115 beats/minute and her blood pressure was 124/72mmHg. Cardiac auscultation revealed an S3 gallop without any murmurs or rubs.

Investigations:

EKG: sinus tachycardia with nonspecific ST segment changes and T wave inversions

CPK 1000 U/L

CXR: bilateral pulmonary infiltrates and small pleural effusions

What is the most useful diagnostic test?

A. Cardiac MRI
B. Endomyocardial biopsy
C. Serial cardiac enzymes
D. Transthoracic echocardiogram
E. TSH

18. A 47-year-old man presented with a fever and constipation for 5 days. He had been nonspecifically unwell for 3 weeks. Two weeks before presentation, he had returned from a 6-month trip to India.

On examination he was systemically unwell with rigors and fever >38°C. He had palpable hepatosplenomegaly and generalized abdominal tenderness.

Investigations:

Total white cell count 3.0 ×10^9/L

Hemoglobin 10.2 g/dL

Platelet count 150,000/μL

Blood cultures negative at 24 hours

He was commenced on intravenous ceftriaxone therapy.

What further investigation would have the highest diagnostic yield?

A. Bone marrow culture
B. Computed tomography scan of the abdomen
C. Liver biopsy
D. Repeat blood cultures
E. Stool cultures

19. A 43-year-old man was admitted to hospital with a 7-day history of generalized abdominal pain and feeling intermittently sweaty. He stated he usually drank 42 units of alcohol each week although he had been abstinent from alcohol for the preceding 4 days as he had been confined to his house. He denied any other symptoms.

On examination, he was tremulous, and his GCS was 15/15. His temperature was 37.3°C. He had multiple spider nevi on his chest, bilateral Dupuytren's contracture, and he was icteric. His abdomen was distended, and shifting dullness was elicited, suggesting the presence of ascites.

Investigations:

Total white cell count 12.1 ×10^9/L (4.0–11.0)

Platelets 352 ×10^9/L (150–400)

INR 1.2 (<1.4)

Bilirubin 82 μmol/L (1–22)

ALT 95 U/L (5–35)

ALP 204 IU/L (40-129)

CRP 40 mg/L (0–5)

USS confirmed ascites and evidence of hepatic fibrosis

Ascitic fluid microscopy:

252 polymorphonuclear cells/mm^3 (≤250)

10,213 red blood cells/mm^3

low protein

normal glucose

Gram stain: gram-negative rods and gram-positive cocci in short chains

He was put on benzodiazepines, vitamin supplements for alcohol withdrawal, and IV piperacillin–tazobactam.

Ascitic fluid at 5 days: *Escherichia coli, Klebsiella pneumoniae,* and *Enterococcus faecium* isolated.

Blood cultures (taken prior to antibiotics) at 5 days: no growth.

What is the most likely diagnosis?

A. Monomicrobial nonneutrocytic bacterascites (MNBA)

B. Polymicrobial bacterascites (PMBA)

C. Secondary peritonitis

D. Spontaneous bacterial peritonitis (SBP)

E. Tertiary peritonitis

20. A 36-year-old woman presented with a 5-day history of smelly vaginal discharge. She was 16+2 weeks pregnant.

On examination she had a thin, grey vaginal discharge with strong odor.

Microscopy displayed clue cells and minimal lactobacilli.

The doctor recommended treatment as this condition is associated with adverse outcomes in pregnancy.

What complication is associated with this condition?

A. Chorioamnionitis

B. Intrauterine growth retardation (IUGR)

C. Miscarriage

D. Neonatal mortality

E. Oligoamnios

21. A 48-year-old woman presented for routine clinic review. She had insulin-dependent diabetes mellitus and was 4 years postrenal transplant. She denied urinary frequency, dysuria, or focal symptoms. Her graft function was excellent. Investigations:

Urine microscopy: 30 leucocytes per high-powered field

Urine culture: pure heavy growth of *Candida* species

What is the most appropriate management?

A. Fluconazole 1 week

B. Fosfomycin 3 g stat

C. Reassurance only

D. Repeat urine culture

E. Single dose fluconazole

22. A 50-year-old man presented with dysuria, urinary frequency, and fevers. He had a history of spinal injury and required intermittent self-catheterization. He had previously had recurrent urinary tract infections and ciprofloxacin-associated tendinopathy.

On examination he was unwell. His temperature was 38.5°C and his heart rate 120 beats/min. Rectal examination revealed a very tender prostate.

What is the most appropriate empiric treatment?

A. Co-amoxiclav

B. Ertapenem

C. Meropenem

D. Moxifloxacin

E. Single-dose ceftriaxone + azithromycin

23. A 19-year-old woman presented with fever, coryza, and a rash. She was in the first trimester of pregnancy. She had not traveled overseas in the last year. She was a college student in a rural area. She reports full vaccination.

On examination her temperature was 37.1°C. She had a widespread macular pink rash.

What is the most likely infective cause?

A. *Coxiella burnetii*

B. Measles virus

C. Parvovirus B19

D. Rubella virus

E. *Treponema pallidum*

24. A 22-year-old woman requested HPV vaccination. She reported sex with both men and women with five sex partners in the last year. She was tested annually for STIs and HIV. She tested positive for chlamydia 2 years ago and was treated with azithromycin 1 g. All STI tests were negative at her last screening 6 months ago.

What is the most appropriate action?

A. Do not vaccinate. Explain that she has likely already been exposed to HPV, and vaccination is not indicated

B. Do not vaccinate. She is too old to receive the vaccine

C. Test for presence of HPV using a vaginal swab. If HPV is present, do not vaccinate

D. Vaccinate with three-dose series

E. Vaccinate with two-dose series

25. A 27-year-old man presented with confusion. He had been discharged 3 days earlier after recovering from an episode of acute hepatitis and jaundice. He was an active intravenous drug user.

Investigations:

	Day 1	Day 7	Day 10
AST (IU/L)	1200	–	2200
ALT (IU/L)	1500	180	3000
INR	1.2	–	3.5
Total bilirubin (mg/dL)	0.9	–	5.4
Serology	HAV IgM negative HBV sAg positive HBV cAb IgM positive HCV Ab negative		HBV sAg positive HBV DNA positive HCV RNA negative HIV Ag/Ab negative

What is the most likely explanation?

A. Acute HCV superimposed on chronic HBV
B. Chronic HBV with HDV superinfection
C. Co-infection with HBV and HDV
D. Co-infection with HBV and HIV
E. Relapsing HAV

26. A 58-year-old man presented with a 48-hour history of rash. He had a background of polymyalgia rheumatica and was taking prednisolone 40 mg OD. The lesions first appeared over the left side of his face but had spread over the past 24 hours.

On examination his temperature was 38.5°C. There were vesicular lesions over his face, torso, and limbs.

What is the most appropriate investigation?

A. CMV viral load
B. Enterovirus PCR of lesion
C. Skin biopsy for histology
D. VZV PCR of lesion
E. VZV serology

27. A 22-year-old woman presented with a 3-day history of general malaise, high temperatures, and prostration. She returned from a holiday in Malaysia 2 weeks ago, where she spent one week on a multi-adventure trip including forest hiking, zip lining, lake kayaking, and snorkeling in the sea.

On examination, her temperature was 39°C, she was jaundiced, pale, and obtunded.
Investigations:
Total white cell count 3.2 ×10⁹/L
Neutrophils 2.2 ×10⁹/L
Hemoglobin 120 g/L
Platelets 227 ×10⁹/L
Na 128 mmol/L (135–145)
K 3.2 mmol/L (3.5–5)
Urea 9 mmol/L (2.5–6.7)
Creatinine 2.7 mg/dL (0.7–1.2)
ALT 350 IU/L
AST 247 IU/L
Bilirubin 30 μmol/L (3–17)
CXR: multiple lung infiltrates
Blood cultures on admission negative
HIV, hepatitis A + B + C, EBV, and CMV serology negative
She was transferred to the intensive care unit where she required hemofiltration.

What is the most likely diagnosis?

A. Acute hepatitis E
B. Crimean Congo hemorrhagic fever
C. Invasive group A streptococcal disease
D. Leptospirosis
E. Tularemia

28. A 30-year-old firefighter sustained third-degree burns to his forearms and hands. He was admitted to the burn unit and underwent wound debridement that evening. The next day, he developed significant erythema and induration involving his burn wounds.

What is the most likely causative organism?

A. *Acinetobacter baumannii*
B. *Candida albicans*
C. *Fusarium* spp.
D. *Pseudomonas aeruginosa*
E. *Staphylococcus aureus*

29. A 40-year-old man presented with fever, night sweats, dry cough, diarrhea, and 30 pound weight loss in 2 months. He lived in Indianapolis, IN.

On exam he was febrile to 38.3°C, had oral thrush, non-tender cervical and axillary adenopathy, a palpable spleen tip, and a diffuse papular rash.
Investigations:
Total white cell count 2 ×10⁹/L
Hemoglobin 80 g/L
Platelets 75 ×10⁹/L
AST 163 U/L
ALT 80 U/L
Alkaline phosphatase 400 U/L
CXR: bilateral reticulonodular infiltrates
HIV Ag/Ab positive
Absolute CD4 count 55 cells/μL
Blood cultures: blood smear shown below

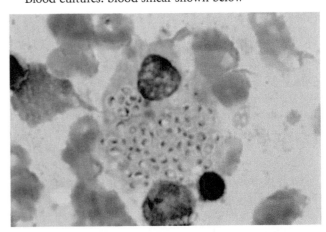

What is the most likely causative organism?

A. *Aspergillus fumigatus*
B. *Cryptococcus neoformans*
C. *Histoplasma capsulatum*
D. *Mycobacterium avium complex*
E. *Mycobacterium tuberculosis*

30. A 52-year-old woman with chronic myelogenous leukemia received an allogeneic hematopoietic stem cell transplant. Her course was complicated by multiple episodes of graft-versus-host disease. She received courses of methylprednisolone. She was on maintenance immunosuppression with cyclosporine. On day 132, she developed fever and patchy pulmonary infiltrates and rapidly progressed into respiratory failure. She was intubated and underwent bronchoscopy. Branched hyphae were noted on the wet mount from the bronchoalveolar lavage (BAL) fluid. The patient was commenced on liposomal amphotericin B (5 mg/kg daily).

Four days later the laboratory reported that the BAL culture grew *Scedosporium apiospermum*. The patient continued having fevers, and her respiratory status was not improving.

What is the most appropriate action?

A. Add caspofungin
B. Add terbinafine
C. Increase the dose of amphotericin B to 10 mg/kg daily
D. Switch to caspofungin
E. Switch to voriconazole

31. A 47-year-old man presented with a 1-week history of high fever and a painful left groin. He lived in a rural area in northern California. He reported sustaining tick bites during a recent hiking trip and multiple recent rodent and spider exposures since moving more rurally a few weeks ago. He had no significant travel history.

On physical exam, there was a lesion on his left leg, and he had very tender left inguinal lymphadenopathy.

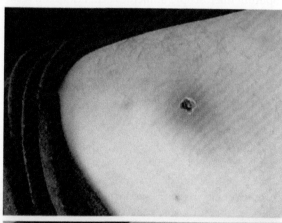

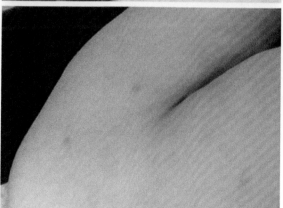

What is the most likely cause?

A. *Francisella tularensis*
B. Loxoscelism (recluse spider bite)
C. *Rickettsia conorii*
D. *Spirillum minus*
E. *Streptobacillus moniliformis*

32. A 63-year-old man presented with a 4-month history of lumbar back pain and night sweats. He was known to have a previous abdominal aortic aneurysm (AAA) repair and bladder cancer surgically removed and followed by intravesical BCG immunotherapy. He was born in the United States and was stationed in Vietnam for almost 2 years, but was TST negative while in the military.

Abdominal CT showed a 2-cm paraaortic mass contiguous to the AAA mesh concerning for vascular leak. An open surgical repair was undertaken, and biopsies sent for histology.

Investigations:

Histopathology of the tissue showed granulomatous inflammation

TST: positive at 11 mm

Interferon gamma release assay (QuantiFERON-TB Gold) negative

What agent should be avoided as part as the treatment regimen?

A. Ethambutol
B. Isoniazid
C. Pyrazinamide
D. Rifampin
E. Streptomycin

33. A 68-year-old man presented with subacute onset of multiple skin lesions all over his body. He had a history of lymphoma treated with high-dose steroids and periodic rituximab. The lesions were nodular with ulceration noted in some of them. There was no fever or respiratory symptoms. The patient had multiple pets at home including a cat, a dog, and a fish tank, but his wife took care of them.

Investigations:

Skin biopsy of the lesion: a granulomatous reaction was seen with positive AFB staining organisms

Mycobacterial cultures of the lesion biopsy: positive 5 days after inoculation

What is the most likely organism?

A. *Mycobacterium avium*
B. *Mycobacterium chelonae*
C. *Mycobacterium marinum*
D. *Mycobacterium simiae*
E. *Mycobacterium xenopi*

34. A patient was reviewed with a vague history of episodic abdominal symptoms including anorexia, nausea, and generalized pain.

Clinical examination was unremarkable.

Investigations:

Blood film: macrocytosis with anisocytosis, poikilocytosis, and hypersegmented neutrophils

What parasitic infection is most likely to be responsible?

A. *Diphyllobothrium latum*
B. *Necator americanus*
C. *Paragonimus westermani*
D. *Schistosoma japonicum*
E. *Taenia saginata*

35. A 35-year-old man attended for review after a new diagnosis of HIV. He had recently migrated from Nigeria and had been tested when he registered with a new primary care provider. He was asymptomatic.

Where is the highest prevalence of HIV globally?

A. Eastern and Southern Africa
B. Eastern Europe and Central Asia
C. Latin America
D. Western and Central Africa
E. Western and Central Europe and North America

36. A 38-year-old man presented with a 5-day history of myalgia of the lower extremities spreading proximally, increased fatigue, and polyuria. He was known to be HIV-positive, on treatment with tenofovir disoproxil fumarate/emtricitabine + raltegravir for the past year.

Investigations:

Sodium 135 mmol/L
Potassium 2.0 mmol/L
Glucose 90 mg/dl
Chloride 107 mmol/L
Bicarbonate 17 mEq/L
Phosphorus 1.4 mg/dl
Creatinine kinase 2015 U/L
Creatinine 2.1 mg/dL (previous baseline 1.2 mg/dL)
Urinalysis: protein 30 mg/d and glucose 500 mg/dL
Baseline genotype prior to initiating ART did not demonstrate resistance
HLA B*5701 negative
HBsAg positive

What is the most appropriate treatment regimen?

A. Abacavir/lamivudine/dolutegravir + entecavir
B. Abacavir/lamivudine + entecavir
C. Abacavir/lamivudine + raltegravir
D. No change in treatment
E. Tenofovir disoproxil fumarate/emtricitabine + darunavir/ritonavir

37. A 30-year-old woman attended care to discuss immunizations. She had recently been diagnosed with HIV and had started ART 2 weeks previously. She denied a history of chickenpox or measles as a child. She reported 10 lifetime sexual partners.

Investigations:

CD4 count 115 cells/mm^3
HIV-1 RNA viral load 145,000 copies/mL
Hepatitis B surface Ag negative
Hepatitis B surface Ab negative
Hepatitis B core Ab positive
Hepatitis B DNA <20 IU/mL
VZV IgG negative
Measles IgG negative

In addition to seasonal influenza vaccination, what immunizations should be offered?

A. Hepatitis B virus vaccine
B. Herpes zoster vaccine
C. Human papillomavirus vaccine
D. Measles, mumps, rubella vaccine
E. Varicella virus vaccine

38. A 24-year-old man presented with fever, productive cough, and weight loss. He was known to have HIV and was taking combination antiretroviral therapy with tenofovir-emtricitabine and darunavir boosted with ritonavir.

Investigations:

CXR: a single large cavitary lesion in the right upper lobe is seen, suspicious for pulmonary TB
Sputum microscopy: numerous acid fast bacilli seen. Direct PCR positive for *M. tuberculosis*
CD4 count 360 cells/μL
HIV viral load <20 copies/mL

What antimycobacterial drug is contraindicated?

A. Ethambutol
B. Isoniazid
C. Pyrazinamide
D. Rifabutin
E. Rifampin

39. A 35-year-old man was reviewed prior to treatment with eculizumab, a complement inhibitor. He was known to have paroxysmal nocturnal hemoglobinuria and had failed treatment with plasma exchanges.

What is the most important immunization to arrange before treatment?

A. *Haemophilus influenzae* type B
B. Influenza
C. Meningococcal ACWY and menB
D. Pneumococcal PSV23
E. Varicella

40. A 54-year-old man presented with sudden onset left flank pain, radiating to groin. He had a history of lung transplantation 9 months previously, and cerebral toxoplasmosis 3 weeks earlier. He was taking cyclosporine, prednisone, fluconazole, valganciclovir, sulfadiazine, and pyrimethamine.
Investigations:

Urine dipstick 3+ blood

CT kidney, ureter, and bladder: 7mm calcific density in the left proximal ureter with associated moderate hydronephrosis. Multiple 1–2 mm nonobstructing calculi also seen in the renal parenchyma

What is the most likely causative medication?

A. Cyclosporine
B. Fluconazole
C. Pyrimethamine
D. Sulfadiazine
E. Valganciclovir

41. A 24-year-old man presented with disseminated *Mycobacterium avium* complex (MAC) infection. He had a past medical history of recurrent nontyphoidal salmonellosis.
Investigations:

HIV Ag/Ab negative

HIV VL not detected

What is the most likely diagnosis?

A. A complement defect
B. A defect in the IL-12 or interferon-gamma pathway
C. A defect in the IL-17 pathway
D. A defect in the IL-21 pathway
E. A phagocyte defect

42. A 46-year-old man presented with a 5-day history of dyspnea and a nonproductive cough. Four weeks earlier he had returned from a holiday in West Africa where he had bought components for drums, which he then crafted himself. He had a history of hypertension, obesity, and type 2 diabetes.

On examination, he appeared ill. His blood pressure was 85/46mmHg, heart rate was 115 beats/minute, respiratory rate was 32 breaths/minute, and oxygen saturations were 86% on 4LPM oxygen. He required urgent intubation and transfer to the critical care unit.
Investigations:

CXR: small bilateral effusions seen with cardiomegaly

4 sets of blood cultures positive at 12 hours with gram-positive rods

What infection prevention intervention is most appropriate?

A. Contact precautions
B. Doxycycline prophylaxis for healthcare workers exposed to droplets
C. Immunization for all healthcare worker providing direct care
D. Respiratory isolation
E. Standard precautions only

43. A 55-year-old man presented with a 5-day history of fever, malaise, diarrhea, cough, and wheezing. He had returned 4 weeks earlier from a 3-week trip to Malawi. Prior to the trip he received HAV, typhoid, and Tdap vaccinations. He did not take malaria prophylaxis because he was concerned about possible side effects. During his trip he visited orphanages, participated in traditional baptism ceremonies in Lake Malawi, ate with locals, and visited a small hospital where he had contact with inpatients and outpatients.

On examination his temperature was 38.2°C, and he had a widespread urticarial rash.

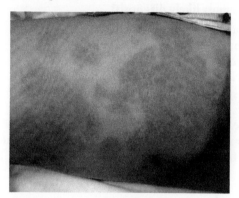

What is the most likely diagnosis?

A. Dengue fever
B. Malaria
C. Marburg fever
D. Measles
E. Schistosomiasis

44. A 25-year-old woman presented with a 2-day history of fever, headache, and malaise with a few-hour history of severe shortness of breath and chest pain. She was a laboratory worker.

On examination, the patient looked unwell. Her heart rate was 120 beats/minute, her blood pressure was 82/46 mmHg, and her respiratory rate was 38 breaths/minute, with oxygen saturations of 92% on 15 liters of oxygen.
Investigations:

Arterial blood gases showed type 1 respiratory failure

CXR: multilobar consolidation with bilateral small pleural effusions

Blood cultures: short gram-negative rods seen

What is the most appropriate treatment?

A. Benzylpenicillin + meropenem + linezolid
B. Ciprofloxacin
C. Doxycycline
D. Gentamicin and ciprofloxacin
E. Rifampicin + meropenem + linezolid

45. A 56-year-old woman presented with a 2-week history of fevers and painful skin nodules. She had a past medical history of immune neutropenia.

On examination, her temperature was 38.8°C, her blood pressure was 136/72 mmHg, her heart rate was 78 beats/minute, and her respiratory rate was 14 breaths/minute. There were several tender nodules over her forearms and dorsum of hands. The nodules were 1–2 cm in diameter and had a violaceous discoloration.

Investigations:

Total white cell count 46 ×10^9/L

What is the most likely diagnosis?

A. Disseminated cryptococcal infection
B. Ecthyma gangrenosum
C. *Fusarium* infection
D. Staphylococcal abscesses
E. Sweet syndrome

46. A 3-year-old boy presented with a 5-day history of fevers and rash and a 2-day history of swelling of the hands and feet. He had received all childhood vaccinations. He had no recent foreign travel and no sick contacts. He did not attend nursery and was a single child. On examination, his temperature was 38.4°C, he had bilateral nonpurulent conjunctivitis, cracked red lips, and a macular perineal rash.

What is the most likely diagnosis?

A. Kawasaki syndrome
B. Measles
C. Parvovirus B19 infection
D. Rubella
E. Stevens–Johnson syndrome

47. A survey is done to identify patients infected with hepatitis C virus in a community. Forty of the 1000 individuals surveyed in the community are found to be seropositive for HCV.

What is the most appropriate definition?

A. Incidence
B. Positive likelihood ratio
C. Positive predictive value
D. Prevalence
E. Sensitivity

Quiz 4

1. A 58-year-old man presented with 2 months of productive cough, shortness of breath, and a 15 lb weight loss. He was known to have COPD. He reported no sick contacts and no recent foreign travel. He lived in Omaha, Nebraska.

Investigations:

CXR: cavitary infiltrates

Interferon gamma release assay (IGRA) positive

Sputum AFB stain: 3+ AFB seen

Sputum Xpert MTB/RIF PCR assay: not detected

What organism is most likely to be the causative agent?

A. False-positive from lab contamination

B. *Mycobacterium abscessus*

C. *Mycobacterium kansasii*

D. *Mycobacterium marinum*

E. *Mycobacterium tuberculosis*

2. A 60-year-old woman presented with headache, fevers, and altered mental status. Her husband reported that she had been unwell 2 weeks earlier with fevers and dry cough which resolved spontaneously. She had returned 3 weeks ago from a 4-week trip to New Mexico. She normally lived in Chicago. She had no significant past medical history. She denied smoking and drank alcohol occasionally. She lived on a farm with 2 dogs and 10 chickens.

On examination, her temperature was 38.4°C, pulse 90 beats/min, blood pressure of 88/58 mmHg, and respiratory rate of 18 breaths/min with SPO_2 95% on room air (RA). Her CT head showed no acute process or space-occupying lesions.

Investigations:

Lumbar puncture showed:

Opening pressure 18 cmH_2O

CSF white cell count 60/μL (20% polymorphonuclear cells, 80% mononuclear cells)

CSF glucose 20 mg/dL

CSF protein 90 mg/dL

Blood cultures negative

HIV Ag/Ab negative

What test is most likely to be diagnostic?

A. CSF coccidioidal antibodies

B. CSF coccidioidal antigen

C. CSF cryptococcal antigen

D. Serum *Histoplasma* antibodies

E. Urine *Histoplasma* antigen

3. An 18-year-old man presented with fatigue, malaise, and sore throat, nausea, and anorexia. He could not recall any sick contacts.

On examination, there was an exudative pharyngitis and tender splenomegaly.

Investigations:

Group A streptococcus rapid antigen negative

CMV IgM positive

Heterophile antibody positive

EBV testing: VCA IgM positive

VCA IgG positive

EA IgG positive

EBNA IgG negative

What is the most likely etiologic agent?

A. CMV

B. EBV

C. HHV-7

D. HSV

E. *Streptococcus pyogenes*

4. A 74-year-old woman was diagnosed with healthcare-associated pneumonia. She was a nursing home resident with no drug allergies, type 2 diabetes, hypertension, and acute on chronic kidney disease.

Investigations:

Creatinine clearance 25 mL/min (baseline creatinine clearance 40 mL/min)

Sputum culture negative

Multiplex PCR respiratory virus panel negative

What antipseudomonal agent poses the greatest risk for neurotoxicity?

A. Aztreonam

B. Cefepime

C. Ceftazidime

D. Ceftolozane–tazobactam

E. Piperacillin–tazobactam

5. A 57-year-old man presented with increasing left lower extremity pain and swelling at the site of a minor trauma sustained 5 days prior. He had a history of bipolar affective disorder, alcohol abuse, and no drug allergies.

On examination, significant induration and erythema were noted, along with a temperature of 38.5°C and a white blood cell count of 18,000/mm³.

Broad-spectrum antimicrobial treatment was started with meropenem 1 gram IV q8hours. He was taken to the operating room, where necrotizing fascia and purulence were noted in the distal extremity. Cultures of multiple intraoperative specimens were positive for *Streptococcus pyogenes*. Antibiotic therapy was subsequently changed to penicillin G 4 million units IV q4 hours.

What agent would be most appropriate to add to penicillin to help control the pathogenicity of this infection?

A. Clindamycin

B. Doxycycline

C. Gentamicin

D. Metronidazole

E. Vancomycin

6. A 60-year-old man was diagnosed with pulmonary tuberculosis. Treatment with rifampin, isoniazid, pyrazinamide, and ethambutol was planned. He had atrial fibrillation and was taking warfarin 5 mg PO daily and multivitamins.

Investigations:

INR = 2.5

What drug–drug interaction should you be most concerned about?

A. Isoniazid and ethambutol

B. Isoniazid and warfarin

C. Pyrazinamide and rifampin

D. Rifampin and multivitamin

E. Rifampin and warfarin

7. A 50-year-old patient was diagnosed with pulmonary aspergillosis. The patient was a kidney transplant patient on the immunosuppressive regimen of tacrolimus, mycophenolate, and prednisone. Other medications included amlodipine. The patient was started on voriconazole 200 mg by mouth twice daily. One week later, the voriconazole trough serum concentration was 3.1 µg/mL, and the patient reported a "sunburn" despite being indoors most of the last week.

What is the most appropriate action?

A. Change to anidulafungin 100 mg by mouth once daily

B. Change to fluconazole 400 mg by mouth once daily

C. Change to posaconazole DR tablets 300 mg once daily

D. Continue voriconazole 200 mg by mouth twice daily

E. Decrease voriconazole to 200 mg once daily

8. A 20-year-old woman was reviewed 36 hours after sustaining a monkey bite to her arm from a wild macaque in Zambia. She had cleaned the wound immediately with soap and water and applied an OTC antimicrobial ointment. She took oral azithromycin to prevent bacterial superinfection and had returned to the United States for urgent medical care. Prior to her travel, she had received immunization for hepatitis A; combined tetanus, diphtheria, and pertussis; and typhoid. She was taking mefloquine for malaria prophylaxis.

On physical examination, she was anxious. Temperature was 37°C, pulse rate 84 beats/minute, and blood pressure 135/84 mmHg. The left upper arm had multiple scratches and deep bite marks, which were minimally inflamed.

In addition to rabies immunization, what is the most appropriate additional postexposure prophylaxis?

A. Cidofovir, single IV dose

B. Foscarnet, twice daily for one week

C. Reassurance only

D. Ribavirin PO q8h for 10 days

E. Valaciclovir 1 gram PO every 8 hours for 2 weeks

9. A 27-year-old woman presented with fever, pleuritic chest pain, and diarrhea. She had also noted recurrent but transient urticaria during this time. She had traveled with her family to Costa Rica 4 weeks earlier where she had eaten local food, which included raw shellfish. A diagnosis of paragonimiasis was confirmed by serology.

What is the most appropriate treatment?

A. Albendazole

B. Bithionol

C. Ivermectin

D. Nitazoxanide

E. Praziquantel

10. A 35-year-old developed fungemia with *Candida parapsilosis* during a prolonged hospital course in the ICU with nonischemic heart failure. Her central lines were removed, surveillance cultures were negative, and echocardiogram was unrevealing. She was treated initially with caspofungin followed by fluconazole once speciation and sensitivities returned. Two weeks later, she lost vision in her right eye. Dilated eye exam revealed fluffy vitreal lesions. She had an urgent vitrectomy with intravitreal antifungal injection.

What systemic agent would be preferred for treatment?

A. Amphotericin deoxycholate
B. Lipid formulation amphotericin
C. Micafungin
D. Terbinafine
E. Voriconazole

11. A 32-year-old woman was seen with a 4-month history of worsening gait disturbance, slurred speech, and mood swings. She had been low in mood and quick tempered and was sleeping poorly. This had not responded to a trial of antidepressant therapy. There had been no preceding illness or other associated symptoms. On physical exam, she demonstrated choreiform movements together with an ataxic gait. Detailed neuropsychologic assessment demonstrated impairment of memory, spatial judgment, verbal fluency, and language. She was not able to give the date or year. A diagnosis of new variant CJD was considered.

What test is most likely to be diagnostic?

A. CSF for 14-3-3 protein
B. EEG for pseudo-periodic sharp wave activity
C. Genotyping for codon 129 of the PrP gene
D. MRI for cortical ribboning
E. Tonsil biopsy for PrP^{SC} immunostaining

12. A 75-year-old woman presented with a 5-day history of worsening myalgia, restlessness, and sweating. Her jaw had been feeling tight for 2 days, and she felt unable to walk properly due to stiffness. She was a keen gardener. She had a history of hypertension, depression, and gastro-oesophageal reflux. She was taking bendroflumethiazide, sertraline, and ranitidine.

On examination she was sitting straight up in bed. Her blood pressure was 138/76 mmHg and her heart rate was 102 beats/minute. She was orientated to time, place, and person.
Her face was taut with a wide smile and tense masseters. She was sweating profusely. She had dilated but reactive pupils. Cardiovascular, respiratory, and abdominal examinations were unremarkable.
Her skin was intact except for a 6 cm healing laceration along her right shin.

Neurologic exam:
Diffusely increased tone and rigidity in all muscle groups. Occasional twitches visible.
Muscle power 5/5; reflexes brisk but equal; gag reflex elicited a bite.
Sensation intact.

What is the most likely diagnosis?

A. "Furious" rabies
B. Herpes meningoencephalitis
C. Neuroleptic malignant syndrome
D. Tetanus
E. Toxic shock syndrome

13. A 42-year-old man was admitted with a 2-day history of progressive dyspnea and a one-week history of fever, chills, and productive cough. The patient eventually required intubation and mechanical ventilation due to respiratory distress and hypoxemia.

A chest radiograph demonstrated consolidation in the left and right lower lobes and patchy airspace opacity in the right middle lobe. Blood cultures were taken and empirical antimicrobials started.

What is the most appropriate further investigation?

A. Bronchoscopy for AFBs
B. *Legionella* and *Streptococcus pneumoniae* urine antigen assays
C. NAAT for *Chlamydia* and *Mycoplasma pneumoniae* on throat swab
D. No further diagnostic testing required
E. Q fever serology

14. A 28-year-old woman presented with a third episode of recurrent cough along with a large amount of purulent sputum production. She was known to have common variable immunodeficiency and had multiple episodes of upper and lower respiratory infections. She was afebrile.

Investigations:
Chest X-ray: parallel linear opacities and a few ring-like shadows

What is the most likely diagnosis?

A. Bronchiectasis
B. *Mycoplasma* infection
C. Non-small-cell lung cancer
D. Pulmonary thromboembolism
E. Viral pneumonia

15. A 54-year-old man presented with a painful, red, purulent port site and fevers. He had pancreatic cancer and an implanted port for chemotherapy.

On exam, the port site was erythematous, with a central area of fluctuance, and some visible purulence. His temperature was 37.2°C, heart rate 98 beats/minute, and blood pressure 108/64 mmHg.

Investigations:

Neutrophil count 7.2 ×10⁹/L

Alkaline phosphatase 95 U/L

Empiric antibiotic therapy was started while plans were made for his port to be removed.

What antibiotic is an essential component of empirical treatment?

A. Cefepime

B. Ceftazidime

C. Doxycycline

D. Trimethoprim–sulfamethoxazole

E. Vancomycin

16. A 65-year-old man presented with fatigue, subjective fever and chills, and poor appetite. He had a history of hypertension, hyperlipidemia, diabetes, and CKD stage 4. He had no known drug allergies.

On examination he was found to have a new diastolic murmur. He was started empirically on vancomycin.

Investigations:

4/4 blood cultures positive for fully sensitive *Enterococcus faecalis*

Echocardiogram: a 5 mm vegetation of the aortic valve

Creatinine clearance 15 mL/min

What is the most appropriate treatment?

A. Ampicillin plus ceftriaxone

B. Ampicillin plus gentamicin

C. Daptomycin

D. Linezolid

E. Vancomycin

17. A 78-year-old man presented with dehiscence of his sternal wound with associated drainage of purulent material. He had undergone a 3-vessel CABG 3 weeks earlier after an episode of STEMI and abnormal cardiac catheterization that was not amenable to stenting.

On examination, his temperature was 100.2°F (37.8°C), his heart rate was 99 beats/minute, his blood pressure was 100/70 mmHg, and his respiratory rate was 20 breaths/minute.

Investigations:

CT chest: retrosternal fluid collection with associated stranding and cortical erosion in the sternal bone

Blood cultures: negative

What is the most appropriate management?

A. Aspiration of fluid via interventional radiology with culture and targeted antibiotics

B. Bedside debridement with surface culture and targeted antibiotics

C. Empiric broad-spectrum antibiotics for 6 weeks

D. Surgical intervention for wash out, operating room culture sampling, and targeted antibiotics

E. Wound care without need for antibiotics given negative blood cultures

18. An 18-year-old woman presented with new onset low-grade fever, sore throat, and painful joints. She had just recovered from a 2-week bout of diarrhea which she ascribed to eating some undercooked pork. She did not take regular medications and had no recent travel outside of the United States.

On exam, her throat was unremarkable. Her small and large joints were normal. Multiple tender nodules 3–4 cm in diameter were palpable over both shins.

Her serum TSH was noted to be elevated although she showed no signs of Graves' disease.

What is the most likely diagnosis?

A. *Campylobacter* spp.

B. Ciguatera poisoning

C. *Salmonella* spp.

D. *Streptococcus pyogenes*

E. *Yersinia enterocolitica*

19. A 52-year-old man presented with a 2-day history of fever, vomiting, and watery diarrhea. His symptoms developed 10 hours after a large meat feast. He had a history of hypertension and atrial fibrillation, controlled with bisoprolol.

On admission, his temperature was 38.4°C, his blood pressure was 92/46 mmHg, and his heart rate was 126 beats/min. He was markedly tender on abdominal exam.

Investigations:

Total white cell count 19.0 ×10⁹/L

Hemoglobin 12.2 g/dL

Platelet count 100,000/μL

Lactate 5 mmol/L

Computed tomography scan of the abdomen showed possible ischemic and edematous dilated segments of bowel.

What is the most likely diagnosis?

A. *Clostridioides difficile*

B. *Clostridium perfringens*

C. Perforated bowel

D. Volvulus

E. *Yersinia enterocolitica*

20. A 72-year-old man was admitted with a 2-day history of fevers and worsening abdominal pain. He denied change in bowel habit. Past medical history included hypertension and type 2 diabetes mellitus controlled with oral hypoglycemic agents.

On examination, his temperature was 38.8°C, his blood pressure was 116/74 mmHg, and his heart rate was 94 beats per minute. He was tender in the right upper quadrant, and he had normal bowel sounds.

Initial investigations:

C-reactive protein 330 mg/L (0–5)

Total white cell count 24.1 ×10⁹/L (4.0–11.0)

Bilirubin 39 µmol/L (0–21)

Alkaline phosphatase 450 IU/L (40–129)

ALT 93 IU/L (5–35)

USS abdomen revealed gallstones

He was diagnosed with acute cholecystitis. Blood cultures were taken, and he was commenced on IV fluids, IV co-amoxiclav, and gentamicin.

Over the next 24 hours he failed to improve despite treatment, becoming hypotensive and tachycardic. On repeat examination his abdominal pain had become generalized and bowel sounds remained normal. An urgent abdominal X-ray was performed:

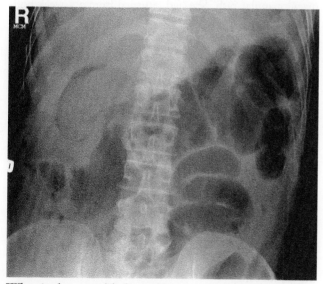

What is the most likely explanation for these findings?

A. Emphysematous cholecystitis
B. Gallbladder perforation
C. Gallstone ileus
D. Inadequate antibiotic therapy
E. Mirizzi syndrome

21. A 23-year-old woman was 40+2 weeks pregnant. She had a prolonged membrane rupture with multiple vaginal examinations.

On exam, her temperature was 39.2°C, and her heart rate was 118 beats/minute. Purulent amniotic fluid was noted.

What is the most likely causative organism?

A. *Bacteroides* spp.
B. *Escherichia coli*
C. *Gardnerella vaginalis*
D. *Mycoplasma hominis*
E. *Ureaplasma urealyticum*

22. A 35-year-old man presented unwell with fever, loin pain, and vomiting. He had no known allergies.

On examination, his temperature was 39.4°C, his blood pressure was 98/56 mmHg, and his heart rate was 115 beats/minute. He had right-sided renal angle tenderness.

Investigations:

Total white cell count 12 ×10⁹/L

Neutrophils 9 ×10⁹/L

eGFR >60 mL/min/1.73m²

What is the most appropriate empirical treatment?

A. Ceftriaxone + stat azithromycin
B. Ciprofloxacin + stat aminoglycoside
C. Fosfomycin
D. Nitrofurantoin
E. Vancomycin

23. A 31-year-old man attended for routine follow up. He was asymptomatic. He was known to have HIV and was taking a fixed-dose regimen of abacavir/dolutegravir/lamivudine He was last screened for STI 6 months previously. He was sexually active, and reported three casual male partners in the previous 3 months. He reported that he discloses his HIV status to partners. He engaged in anal receptive and oral insertive and receptive sex. He used condoms for anal sex most of the time.

On examination, his oropharynx was clear. His urogenital examination was without discharge, lymphadenopathy, or unusual skin findings. Rectal examination was performed, and no abnormalities were noted.

Investigations:

CD4 count 900 cells/mm³

HIV viral load undetectable

What screening tests should be performed?

A. No screening is recommended at today's visit. Screen annually
B. Urine and rectal screening by NAAT for *N. gonorrhoeae* and *C. trachomatis*, oropharyngeal screening by culture for *N. gonorrhoeae* plus syphilis serology
C. Urine, rectal, and oropharyngeal screening by NAAT for *N. gonorrhoeae* and *C. trachomatis*
D. Urine, rectal, and oropharyngeal screening by NAAT for *N. gonorrhoeae* and *C. trachomatis* plus syphilis serology
E. Urine screening by NAAT for *N. gonorrhoeae* and *C. trachomatis*

24. A 25-year-old woman presented with a malodorous, green-yellow vaginal discharge.
On cervical evaluation the cervix had an erythematous, punctate, and papilliform appearance.
Investigations:
  Microscopy of the vaginal fluid:

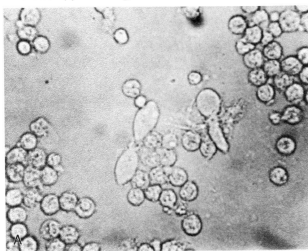

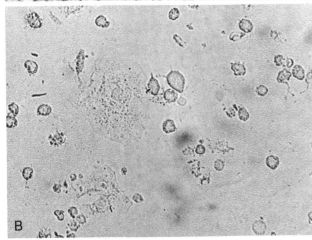

NAAT testing for gonorrhea and chlamydia negative
What is the most appropriate treatment?

    A. Azithromycin × 1 dose
    B. Ceftriaxone × 1 dose
    C. Doxycycline for 7 days
    D. Metronidazole × 1 dose
    E. Metronidazole for 14 days

25. A 47-year-old man was being treated for hepatitis C with ledipasvir/sofosbuvir.
Investigations:
  HAV IgG positive
  HBV cAb positive, HBV sAg negative, HBV sAb 0
  HBV DNA undetectable

HCV IgG positive, HCV genotype 1a
Liver biopsy showed grade 1 inflammation and stage 3 fibrosis with features of both chronic HCV and nonalcoholic steatohepatitis.

	Baseline	Week 4	Week 11
ALT (IU/L)	170	35	2250
AST (IU/L)	289	32	2970
HCV viral load (IU/mL)	1,200,000	Undetectable	Undetectable
INR			1.8
Total bilirubin (mg/dL)			7.2

What is the most likely reason for the worsening transaminases?
A. Acute alcoholic steatohepatitis
B. Drug reaction
C. Failure of ledipasvir/sofosbuvir
D. Immune reconstitution inflammatory syndrome
E. Reactivation of HBV

26. A 44-year-old woman presented with a 3-day history of low grade fever, malaise, itchy eyes, and a widespread itchy, maculopapular rash. She had returned from a 4-week holiday in the Caribbean 2 days before her symptoms began.
What vector is most likely to be responsible for her symptoms?

    A. *Aedes* mosquito
    B. *Anopheles* mosquito
    C. *Culex* mosquito
    D. *Triatoma* bug
    E. Tsetse fly

27. A 13-year-old girl was seen by a volunteering doctor as part of a vaccination campaign program in a rural area of Colombia. On clinical examination she was noted to have several hyperpigmented and hypopigmented papular lesions on her legs and arms. She was suspected to have pinta, a treponemal disease endemic in Latin America and the Caribbean.
What is the causative agent of pinta?

    A. *Treponema carateum*
    B. *Treponema denticola*
    C. *Treponema pallidum* subsp. *endemicum*
    D. *Treponema pallidum* subsp. *pallidum*
    E. *Treponema pallidum* subsp. *pertenue*

28. A 57-year-old man was brought into the Emergency Department in a state of collapse. He was known to have end-stage liver disease. He had been bitten on the calf by a neighbor's dog 5 days beforehand. He had not sought medical care immediately following the injury.

On examination, he was profoundly unwell. His temperature was 35.2°C, blood pressure 72/42 mmHg, heart rate 142 beats/min, GCS 14/15. There were multiple purpuric lesions over his torso and limbs. The bite injury was scabbed but clean, with no pus or erythema.

Investigations:

Creatinine clearance 30 mL/min

Lactate 4.6 mmol/L

What is the most likely causative organism?

A. *Capnocytophaga canimorsus*

B. *Eikenella corrodens*

C. *Fusobacterium necrophorum*

D. *Pasteurella multocida*

E. *Staphylococcus aureus*

29. A 28-year-old man presented with a 2-week history of fever, fatigue, myalgias, dry cough, and pleurisy. He was normally well and did not take any regular medications. He lived in Milwaukee, Wisconsin, but 4 weeks earlier had been on a 7-day biking trip through the Sonoran Desert in Tucson, Arizona.

Investigations:

Total white cell count 15 ×10⁹/L with 12% eosinophils

Blood cultures negative

HIV Ag/Ab negative

Chest X-ray: patchy infiltrate in the right lower lobe

What is the most likely causative organism?

A. *Blastomyces dermatitidis*

B. *Coccidioides immitis*

C. *Legionella pneumophila*

D. *Mycoplasma pneumoniae*

E. *Streptococcus pneumoniae*

30. A 37-year-old woman presented with a rash on her finger. It had been present for 2 months and had not improved. There was no history of fevers, and the rash was not painful or draining. She had a past medical history of type 2 diabetes. She lived in Chicago and had not travelled in recent years. She was a carpenter and recalled pulling a wooden splinter out of that finger about 1 month before the rash developed. She lived with her partner and 8-year-old son, who were both well. They had a pet dog and cat that were healthy and owned several exotic fish; the patient sometimes helped her son clean the tank.

On examination, there was an erythematous lesion that was not tender, warm, or fluctuant. There were no other skin lesions present.

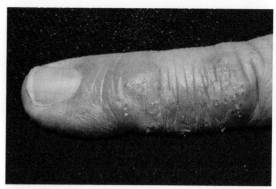

Investigations:

Plain radiograph of the hand showed no fracture or foreign body.

What is the most appropriate treatment?

A. Azithromycin

B. Clindamycin

C. Doxycycline

D. Clarithromycin plus ethambutol

E. Itraconazole

31. A 54-year-old woman presented with a 4-day history of fever, myalgia, and headache. She worked on a farm near Savannah, Georgia. Though she did not recall any recent rashes or illness, she removed at least two ticks from her skin in the past month. She had a history of hypertension and type 2 diabetes. She was taking losartan, metformin, and gliclazide.

On examination, the patient appeared ill. Her temperature was 39.3°C (102.7°F); other vital signs were normal.

Examination was otherwise unremarkable.

Investigations:

Total white cell count 2.3 ×10⁹/L

Platelet count 92 ×10⁹/L

ALT 84 U/L

Peripheral blood smear:

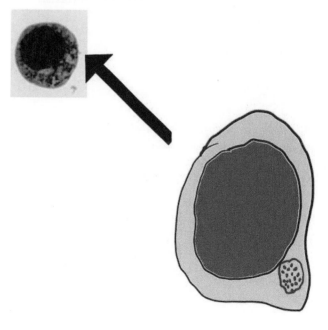

What organism is most likely to be responsible?

A. *Anaplasma phagocytophilum*
B. *Babesia microti*
C. *Borrelia hermsii*
D. *Ehrlichia chaffeensis*
E. *Rickettsia rickettsii*

32. A 27-year-old woman presented with a 2-week history of tingling in hands and feet. She had a history of well-controlled HIV and pleural tuberculosis. She was taking tenofovir alafenamide, emtricitabine, and dolutegravir, and was in the second month of continuation phase with RIF/INH. She was adherent with both her HIV and TB medications. She also took oral contraceptives.

Physical exam was unremarkable.

Investigations:

Hb 95 g/L, MCV 74.5fL
AST 21 IU/L
ALT 15 IU/L
Normal electrolytes, bilirubin, and albumin
Beta-human chorionic gonadotropin positive
CD4 count 520/mm^3
HIV viral load undetectable

What is the most likely cause of her symptoms?

A. Autoimmune disorder
B. Drug adverse effect
C. Drug–drug interaction
D. HIV
E. Pregnancy

33. A 29-year-old woman attended for pretravel advice. She was planning a 1-week trip to Haiti. She was 25 weeks pregnant, and it was her first pregnancy.

What is the most appropriate malaria prophylaxis?

A. Artemether–lumefantrine
B. Atovaquone–proguanil
C. Chloroquine
D. Doxycycline
E. None required

34. A 30-year-old man presented with a 1-week history of a painful right eye with blurry vision and photophobia. He wore contact lenses and had been using tap water to clean them.

On eye examination, a corneal ulcer was identified.

Investigations:

Microscopy of corneal scrapings: amebic cysts and trophozoites seen

What is the most likely agent?

A. *Acanthamoeba* sp.
B. *Balamuthia mandrillaris*
C. *Dientamoeba fragilis*
D. *Entamoeba histolytica*
E. *Giardia lamblia*

35. A 58-year-old man attended for review. He was known to have hypertension, chronic hepatitis B, and HIV. He had been started 3 months earlier on lisinopril 10 mg daily and rosuvastatin 20 mg daily as he had an elevated Framingham risk score due to elevated blood pressure and hypercholesterolemia. He was also taking hydrochlorothiazide, aspirin, multivitamins, and elvitegravir/cobicistat/emtricitabine/tenofovir alafenamide fumarate.

Investigations:

CD4 count 756 cells/µL
HIV viral load undetectable

	3 Months Earlier	Current Visit
Total cholesterol (mg/dL)	315	200
LDL (mg/dL)	197	80
HDL (mg/dL)	30	35
Triglycerides (mg/dL)	378	215
Total bilirubin (mg/dL)	0.9	1.1
Alkaline phosphatase (U/L)	45	46
ALT	34	116
AST	30	205

What is the most likely cause of the new onset hepatitis?

A. Drug–drug interaction with ACE-I
B. Drug–drug interaction with statin
C. Hepatitis B virus reactivation
D. Hepatitis D superinfection
E. Primary biliary cholangitis

36. A 45-year-old woman presented with a 3-month history of a productive cough, night sweats, and 20 lb weight loss. She was known to have HIV but was not on antiretroviral therapy. She was homeless, living on the streets and in hostels.

Investigations:

CXR: right upper lobe cavity
Sputum microscopy: AFB smear positive with *Mycobacterium tuberculosis* complex detected on DNA probe
CD4 count 45 cell/µL
HIV RNA 85,000 copies/mL
No HIV resistance mutations detected
HLA B*5701 negative
The patient was initiated on TB treatment with rifampin, isoniazid, pyrazinamide, and ethambutol pending sensitivities.

What antiretroviral regimen should be initiated?

A. Abacavir/lamivudine + ritonavir-boosted darunavir once daily
B. Tenofovir alafenamide/emtricitabine + efavirenz once daily
C. Tenofovir disoproxil fumarate/emtricitabine + raltegravir once daily
D. Tenofovir disoproxil fumarate/emtricitabine/cobicistat/elvitegravir once daily
E. Tenofovir disoproxil fumarate/emtricitabine/efavirenz once daily

37. A 45-year-old man presented with a 6-month history of decreased energy, weight loss, and diarrhea. He was known to have HIV but had not taken ART or attended clinic in over 10 years. He had previously discontinued ART due to nausea and vomiting. He had previously injected intravenous drugs but reported that he had been clean for 3 years. He was keen to restart antiretroviral therapy.

Investigations:

CD4 count 115 cells/μL

HIV viral load 200,000 copies/mL, dual tropic, M184V detected

HLA B*5701 negative

Creatinine 0.8 mg/dL

AST 65 units/L

ALT 96 units/L

Hepatitis A IgG positive

Hepatitis B sAg negative

Hepatitis C Ab negative

What would be the most appropriate antiretroviral regimen?

A. Abacavir/lamivudine/dolutegravir

B. Tenofovir alafenamide/emtricitabine/cobicistat/elvitegravir + darunavir

C. Tenofovir alafenamide/emtricitabine + rilpivirine + darunavir

D. Tenofovir disoproxil fumarate/emtricitabine + ritonavir-boosted darunavir

E. Tenofovir disoproxil fumarate + ritonavir-boosted darunavir + maraviroc

38. A 23-year-old man attended for a new patient appointment. He had recently been diagnosed with HIV and had a history of allergic asthma and sulfa allergy, which caused a blistering rash with oral lesions. The patient was leaving the country for a 3-month business trip in 2 weeks' time.

Investigations:

CD4 count 155 cells/mm³

HIV-1 RNA viral load 145,000 copies/mL

Toxoplasma IgG positive

Glucose-6-phosphate dehydrogenase 3.4 U/gram of Hgb (8.8–13.4)

In addition to starting combination antiretroviral therapy, what antimicrobial prophylaxis is most appropriate?

A. Aerosolized pentamidine once monthly

B. Atovaquone PO once daily

C. Azithromycin PO once weekly

D. Dapsone PO once daily

E. Trimethoprim–sulfamethoxazole PO once daily

39. A 45-year-old woman presented with 4 weeks of fevers, weight loss, and chronic diarrhea. The patient reported intermittent diffuse abdominal pain, 5 to 6 watery, nonbloody

bowel movements/day. She endorsed a 20 lb weight loss over this same duration. She was known to have HIV but was not taking HIV medications or antibiotic prophylaxis.

On examination there was diffuse abdominal tenderness but no peritoneal signs. Shotty axillary and inguinal lymphadenopathy was palpable.

Investigations:

CD4 count 30 cells/μL

HIV viral load 110,350 copies/mL

Mycobacterial blood cultures: positive with AFBs at 7 days; DNA probe negative for *Mycobacterium tuberculosis*

What is the most appropriate treatment?

A. Azithromycin, isoniazid, and pyrazinamide

B. Azithromycin, pyrazinamide, and rifabutin

C. Clarithromycin, ethambutol, and rifabutin

D. Clarithromycin, isoniazid, and rifabutin

E. Ethambutol, isoniazid, and rifabutin

40. A 32-year-old woman presented with fevers and abdominal pain. She had a recent diagnosis of acute myeloid leukemia and had received induction chemotherapy 12 days previously. She was taking aciclovir prophylaxis. She had no known allergies.

On examination, her temperature was 38.5°C, her heart rate was 104 beats/minute, and her blood pressure was 96/58 mmHg. She was tender in her right lower quadrant with localized guarding. Bowel sounds were normal.

Investigations:

Neutrophil count 0.1 ×10⁹/L

Blood cultures: pending

CT abdomen and pelvis: bowel thickening and inflammation in the ileocecal region

What is the most appropriate treatment?

A. Amoxicillin/clavulanate

B. Aztreonam and metronidazole

C. Cefepime and vancomycin

D. Ertapenem

E. Piperacillin–tazobactam

41. A 60-year-old man attended for pretravel advice. He had undergone heart transplantation 6 months previously. He was maintained on tacrolimus and prednisone for immunosuppression and had not had any episodes of allograft rejection. He intended to travel to Vellore, India, for 2 weeks and then on to Manila, the Philippines, for 2 weeks before returning home.

What treatment is contraindicated?

A. Hepatitis A vaccine

B. Influenza vaccine

C. Malaria prophylaxis

D. Oral typhoid vaccine

E. Polio vaccine (IPV)

42. A 21-year-old man had a history of frequent skin and upper respiratory bacterial infections.
Physical exam revealed silvery hair and findings consistent with Parkinsonism.
Investigations:
   Peripheral blood smear: giant granulocyte inclusions

What is the diagnosis?

A. A complement defect
B. Chediak–Higashi syndrome
C. Chronic granulomatous disease
D. Familial HLH
E. Griscelli syndrome

43. A 20-year-old college student was found unconscious by his college roommate. He was taken to the emergency room. Blood and cerebrospinal fluid cultures grew *Neisseria meningitidis*. His roommate received the quadrivalent meningococcal conjugate vaccine one year ago.

What is the most appropriate intervention for the roommate?

A. Booster vaccination with the conjugate vaccine
B. Chemoprophylaxis
C. No intervention needed
D. Treatment for meningococcal infection
E. Vaccination with the meningococcal serogroup b vaccine

44. A 23-year-old healthcare worker who was 12 weeks pregnant sought advice on the vaccinations she required before starting work.

What vaccination is contraindicated?

A. Combined tetanus, diphtheria, acellular pertussis, and inactivated polio vaccine (DTap/IPV)
B. Hepatitis A vaccine
C. Hepatitis B vaccine
D. Influenza vaccine
E. Varicella zoster vaccine

45. A 63-year-old woman was reviewed with a 4-week history of fever up to 39.2°C, headache, and generalized myalgias. She had been admitted 1 week earlier and treated empirically with piperacillin/tazobactam once blood cultures had been taken. She had a past medical history of diabetes and hypertension and was taking metformin and lisinopril. She had no recent travels. Her grandson had a viral illness 7 days before her admission. She had a pet dog.
Investigations:
   Blood cultures × 2 sets: no growth at 5 days
   C-reactive protein 212 mg/L
   CT chest, abdomen, and pelvis unremarkable
   Transthoracic echo showed no evidence of endocarditis

What is the most appropriate action?

A. Add clarithromycin
B. Change to meropenem and vancomycin
C. Order a transesophageal echo
D. Send a throat swab for influenza and start oseltamivir
E. Stop antibiotics and consider temporal artery biopsy

46. Dr. Smith has performed a small study looking at the association of St. John's wort with recurrent shingles. She has found a positive association and attempted to publish the paper. One of the reviewers is suggesting that this finding may have occurred due to chance alone.

What type of error is this?

A. Sensitivity
B. Type I
C. Type II
D. α (alpha)
E. β (beta)

47. A 42-year-old man was reviewed with new onset pustular lesions spreading through the legs, arms, and abdomen. He was on day 6 vancomycin and day 2 piperacillin/tazobactam for a right leg cellulitis which was slow to respond (*top image*). He had a history of chronic lymphedema due to obstructive sleep apnea with secondary pulmonary hypertension.
On examination the patient was well, his blood pressure was 138/72 mmHg, his heart rate was 92 beats/minute, and his temperature was 38.4°C. There were widespread skin lesions (*bottom image*).

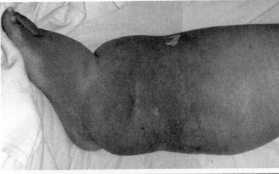

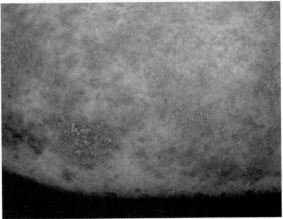

Investigations:

    Total white cell count 15 ×10⁹/L

    Absolute neutrophil count 13.2 ×10⁹/L

What is the most likely diagnosis?

  A. Acute generalized exanthematous pustulosis (AGEP)

  B. Generalized pustular psoriasis

  C. Necrotizing fasciitis

  D. Staphylococcal toxic shock syndrome

  E. Toxic epidermal necrolysis

48. A 27-year-old man presented with a new skin lesion which had developed over the preceding 3–4 weeks. It bled profusely with trauma but was not pruritic or painful. He had no other skin lesions or systemic symptoms. He had started antiretroviral therapy 2 months earlier for a new diagnosis of HIV and was taking tenofovir, emtricitabine, and dolutegravir boosted with ritonavir.

On examination:

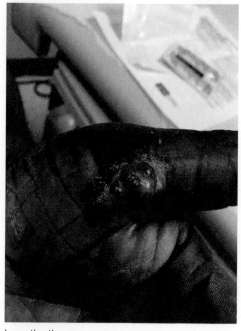

Investigations:

    HIV viral load undetectable

    CD4 count 493 cells/mm³

What is the most likely diagnosis?

  A. Acral lentiginous melanoma

  B. Glomus tumor

  C. Kaposi sarcoma

  D. Lobular capillary hemangioma (pyogenic granuloma)

  E. Longitudinal melanonychia

49. A 41-year-old man presented with fever and a new skin lesion. He was known to have had a prolonged neutropenia for at least 28 days following chemotherapy. He had a tunnelled line in situ which had been placed 10 days earlier.

On examination, his temperature was 38.7°C. He had an erythematous lesion with central necrosis on his left leg. It was nontender.

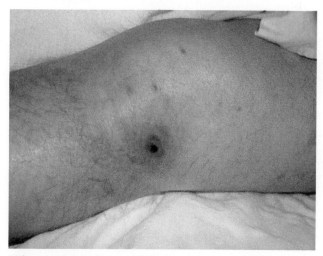

What organism is most likely to be responsible?

  A. *Candida albicans*

  B. *Corynebacterium minutissimum*

  C. *Escherichia coli*

  D. *Malassezia furfur*

  E. *Pseudomonas aeruginosa*

This page intentionally left blank

Quiz 5

1. A 33-year-old woman presented with a 1-day history of headache, myalgia, and fatigue. She had no recent travel, but she had competed in a triathlon 5 days prior.
Investigations:

    AST 80 U/L (reference range: 10–40 U/L)
    ALT 120 U/L (reference range: 7–56 U/L)
    Urine dipstick: 3+ hematuria

What is the most appropriate test?

A. *Leptospira* culture of blood
B. *Leptospira* culture of urine
C. *Leptospira* IgM
D. *Leptospira* IgM and IgG
E. Routine bacterial blood culture

2. A 40-year-old man presented with neutropenic fevers and headache. He had finished induction therapy with cytarabine and daunorubicin 3 weeks ago after a new diagnosis of acute myeloid leukemia.

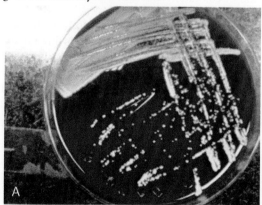

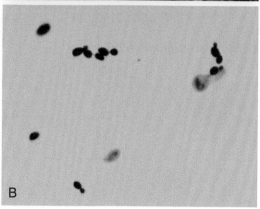

He had no other significant past medical history. He was a nonsmoker and only drank alcohol occasionally. He worked for a local chicken farm in Missouri.

On examination, his temperature was 39.8°C, his heart rate was 110 beats/minute, blood pressure 80/58 mmHg, and respiratory rate 18 breaths/minute with SPO_2 95% on 2L. There was redness and tenderness over right subclavian Hohn catheter site. Lung exam showed decreased breath sounds on bilateral bases with scattered crackles. The Hohn catheter was removed, and he was started on vancomycin and cefepime.
Investigations:

    Absolute neutrophil count 300 cells/μL
    CXR: bibasilar scarring with no obvious consolidation
    CT head: bilateral mild maxillary sinusitis
    Blood cultures and catheter tip cultures: yeast
    Serum galactomannan-negative
    Serum cryptococcal antigen-positive with a titer of 1:64

What is the most likely etiologic agent?

A. *Candida* sp.
B. *Cryptococcus neoformans*
C. *Histoplasma capsulatum*
D. *Rhizopus* sp.
E. *Trichosporon* sp.

3. A 35-year-old woman presented with a 3-week history of nausea, vomiting, and abdominal pain, and 10 days of jaundice. She was an active IV drug user.

On physical exam, she was jaundiced with right upper quadrant tenderness.
Investigations:

    ALT 2000 IU/mL
    AST 900 IU/mL
    HAV IgM negative, HAV PCR negative
    HCV IgG negative, HCV PCR negative
    HBVsAg positive, anti-HBs negative
    anti-HBc IgM positive, anti-HBc total positive
    HBe Ag positive, anti-HBe negative

What is the most likely diagnosis?

A. Acute hepatitis B
B. Acute hepatitis C
C. Chronic nonreplicating hepatitis B
D. Chronic replicating hepatitis B
E. Hepatitis A

4. A 26-year-old man presented with a fever of 39°C and disorientation. He had a history of myelomeningocele and a ventriculoperitoneal shunt. He had no drug allergies.

Investigations:

Head CT scan: consistent with ventriculitis

CSF microscopy: 250 nucleated cells with 85% neutrophils

CSF glucose 25 mg/dL

CSF protein 110 mg/dL

CSF culture positive for *Proteus mirabilis*, sensitivities consistent with extended-spectrum beta-lactamase (ESBL) production

What is the most appropriate treatment?

A. Cefotetan

B. Ceftriaxone

C. Gentamicin

D. Imipenem–cilastatin

E. Meropenem

5. A 48-year-old woman presented with a 3-day history of fever, chills, nausea, anorexia, myalgia, and fatigue. She had a history of colorectal cancer with biliary obstruction. She had no drug allergies.

Investigations:

Total white cell count 16,000/mm^3

Bicarbonate 19 mmol/L

Lactate 1.9 mmol/L

Bilirubin 5.5 mg/dL

Abdominal imaging revealed multiple collections in the liver, consistent with metastases versus abscesses.

One of the larger lesions was aspirated, revealing frank purulence. Cultures of this abscess were positive for *Citrobacter freundii* and *Enterococcus faecalis*, antibiotic sensitivities pending.

What empiric monotherapy agent would be most appropriate?

A. Ampicillin–sulbactam

B. Ertapenem

C. Imipenem–cilastatin

D. Meropenem

E. Piperacillin–tazobactam

6. A 64-year-old man presented with acutely altered mental status. The patient's family reported that the patient had been confused for 1–2 days and had been walking into walls. He had a history of hypertension, diabetes mellitus, hyperlipidemia, and poor dentition. He had no known drug allergies.

Physical exam revealed mild left hemiparesis and decreased left temporal visual field.

Investigations:

Total white cell count 13,300 cells/mm^3

Serum creatinine 1.05 mg/dL

Normal liver function tests

MRI brain: 4 ×3 cm rim-enhancing lesion in the right parieto-occipital region.

The patient was taken to the operating room, where frank pus was drained from the mass.

Gram-stain of the abscess fluid: abundant gram-positive cocci in pairs and chains on direct microscopy; culture revealed viridans group streptococci.

What beta-lactam would be most appropriate to include in this patient's antibiotic regimen?

A. Cefazolin

B. Cefepime

C. Cefotetan

D. Ceftazidime

E. Ceftriaxone

7. A 48-year-old woman was prescribed clofazimine as part of her treatment of *Mycobacterium tuberculosis* infection.

What adverse effect of clofazimine should this patient be made aware of prior to initiating therapy?

A. Hepatotoxicity

B. Nephrotoxicity

C. Neurotoxicity

D. Ocular changes

E. Skin discoloration

8. A 55-year-old patient was hospitalized in the surgical intensive care unit with septic shock following GI surgery. Comorbidities included atrial fibrillation, GERD, and hypertension. The patient had no known drug allergies. Medications included amiodarone, aspirin, cefepime, dabigatran, esomeprazole, heparin, vancomycin.

The patient's weight and height were 60 kg and 65 inches, respectively.

Investigations:

Fungal blood cultures grew *Candida*, speciation pending

Creatinine 2.1 mg/dL (baseline SCr 1.1 mg/dL)

ALT 15 units/L

EKG: QTc 480 ms

What is the most appropriate treatment?

A. Fluconazole

B. Micafungin

C. Posaconazole

D. Terbinafine

E. Voriconazole

9. A 36-year-old woman presented with a 2-day history of fever and tremor. She was an inpatient on the psychiatric ward for suicidal depression. She had recently been started on citalopram.

On physical exam, her temperature was 39°C (102.2°F). She had muscle rigidity but no other abnormalities.

What is the most appropriate management?

A. Give acetaminophen
B. Give haloperidol
C. Start empiric antibiotic therapy
D. Stop citalopram
E. Supportive management only

10. A 75-year-old man presented with fever, sepsis, and a painful left cheek. He had a history of diabetes treated with metformin. He had an ultrasound that revealed no abscess in the parotid. He was started on broad treatment with vancomycin and piperacillin/tazobactam along with volume resuscitation and was admitted to the ICU.

What is the most likely causative organism?

A. *Fusobacterium*
B. *Haemophilus influenzae*
C. *Pseudomonas aeruginosa*
D. *Staphylococcus aureus*
E. Viridans *Streptococcus*

11. A 72-year-old man presented with a 48-hour history of fever and confusion. He had a history of benign prostatic hypertrophy, chronic kidney disease, previous MI 3 years ago, and type 2 diabetes mellitus. His family reported that he had first complained of a headache, and they had noticed word finding difficulties.

On examination his GCS was 12/15, his temperature was 38.2°C, and his heart rate was 98 beats/minutes. His blood pressure was 116/64 mmHg. It was not possible to formally examine his neurologic systems, but his reflexes were universally brisk and his tone increased. There were no lateralizing signs.

An urgent CT with contrast was performed, followed by a lumbar puncture under sedation.

He was started empirically on ceftriaxone, amoxicillin, and aciclovir.

How does aciclovir usually cause nephrotoxicity?

A. Altered phospholipid metabolism
B. Direct tubular cytotoxicity
C. Increased cell membrane permeability by pore formation
D. Induction of arteriolar vasoconstriction
E. Tubular obstruction by crystal precipitation

12. A 65-year-old man presented with a 24-hour history of an excruciating headache, photophobia, and neck stiffness. The headache had been gradual in onset, progressing in severity. Seven days earlier he had returned from a 2-month holiday in Vietnam where he had been staying with family. He had a history of hypertension and osteoarthritis of his knees and took regular amlodipine.

Investigations:

Peripheral white blood cell count 7.3 ×10⁹/L
Peripheral eosinophil count 1.5 ×10⁹/L
CSF white cell count 346 ×10⁶/L; 30% eosinophils
CSF red cell count 22 ×10⁶/L
CSF protein 560 mg/L
CSF/plasma glucose 3.5/4.8 mmol/L
CSF microscopy: no organisms seen
CT head with contrast – mild leptomeningeal enhancement

What is the most likely source of the infecting organism?

A. Consumption of undercooked pork
B. Consumption of undercooked snails
C. Consumption of unwashed raw vegetables
D. Drinking contaminated water
E. Swimming in freshwater

13. A 56-year-old man presented with a 2-week history of fever, night sweats, and productive cough. He drank over 100 units of alcohol per week. He denied any intravenous drug use. He had a 10 pack-year smoking history. He had no recent travel. He had no other medical problems.

He had a negative HIV test.

Chest X-ray revealed a 2.4 cm cavitary lesion in the left lower lobe with an air–fluid level.

What is the most likely infective cause?

A. *Actinomyces* spp.
B. *Haemophilus influenzae*
C. *Mycobacterium tuberculosis*
D. *Mycoplasma pneumoniae*
E. *Streptococcus pneumoniae*

14. A 22-year-old man presented with complaints of rhinorrhea, cough, and nasal congestion for 4 days. He was not experiencing severe headaches or problems with his vision. On physical exam, his vital signs were stable, and he was afebrile. He had some sinus tenderness to palpation but no periorbital edema present.

What would be the most appropriate management for this patient?

A. Initiate nasal decongestants
B. Observation
C. Perform imaging of his sinuses
D. Prescribe antibiotic therapy
E. Refer for nasal endoscopy

15. A 42-year-old man with ESRD on hemodialysis and difficult intravenous access needed new intravenous access to be placed for daily administration of parenteral medications.

What type of intravenous catheter carries the highest risk of bloodstream infection?

A. Forearm peripheral IV

B. Nontunneled femoral CVC

C. Nontunneled subclavian CVC

D. Right upper arm PICC line

E. Tunneled internal jugular CVC

16. Catheter-retention in the setting of central line-associated bloodstream infection (CLABSI) is sometimes attempted depending on disease severity, alternative IV access options, and pathogenicity of the organism identified.

According to recommendations, long-term catheter retention may be attempted if blood cultures are positive for what organisms?

A. *Candida albicans*

B. *Micrococcus* spp.

C. *Mycobacterium mucogenicum*

D. *Staphylococcus aureus*

E. *Staphylococcus epidermidis*

17. A 62-year-old woman presented with subjective fevers without any localizing symptoms or signs. She had received a left ventricular assist device 6 months ago as destination strategy for chemotherapy-induced nonischemic cardiomyopathy on a background of breast cancer.

On examination, her temperature was 101.4°F (38.5°C), her heart rate was 100 beats/minute, and her blood pressure was 136/80 mmHg.

Investigations:

4/4 blood cultures positive for methicillin-susceptible *Staphylococcus aureus*, resistant only to penicillin on extended susceptibility testing (sensitive to oxacillin, ceftriaxone, cefazolin, vancomycin, TMP–SMX, doxycycline, and clindamycin)

CT chest/abdomen/pelvis: a large fluid collection surrounding the VAD pump with associated stranding and enhancement

Aspirate of collection fluid: MSSA isolated

She was deemed to be a poor candidate for open debridement and washout, and nor was she a candidate for pump exchange.

What is the most appropriate initial treatment?

A. Cefazolin

B. Dalbavancin

C. Daptomycin

D. Linezolid

E. Vancomycin

18. A 63-year-old woman developed flushing, blurring of vision, generalized itching, and perioral burning while eating at a restaurant. She had a salmon starter, followed by salad and swordfish, and had commented that her food was extremely spicy.

What is the most likely diagnosis?

A. *Bacillus cereus*

B. Ciguatera poisoning

C. Scombroid poisoning

D. Seafood allergy

E. *Staphylococcus aureus*

19. A 33-year-old man presented with a 5-day history of loose stool and fever. He was known to have bronchiectasis and required frequent admissions to hospital for chest infections. He had most recently been discharged 2 weeks earlier. He had severe abdominal pain and distension and was passing mucus per rectum.

Investigations:

Peripheral white cell count 22.0 ×10^9/L

Hemoglobin 14.2 g/dL

C-reactive protein 156 mg/L

Serum creatinine 195μmol/L

He was admitted and isolated in a single room.

What is the next step in his management?

A. Endoscopy and biopsy

B. IV ceftriaxone and metronidazole

C. Oral metronidazole

D. Oral vancomycin

E. Surgical review

20. A 54-year-old man was seen with a history of intermittent fevers over 6 weeks. He denied any other symptoms. He was being investigated for raised blood sugars and had a dental extraction 7 days earlier. He drank 35 units of alcohol per week. He returned from Malaysia 6 months ago following a 2-month stay with his family during the summer months.

On examination, his temperature was 38.9°C, and he had mild abdominal tenderness in his right upper quadrant.

Investigations:

Total white cell count 17.2 ×10^9/L

CRP 230 mg/L

Alanine transaminase 152 U/L

Alkaline phosphatase 341 U/L

Urgent abdominal USS revealed a single large lesion in the right lobe of the liver consistent with an abscess. No biliary pathology was identified. He was commenced on fluids and IV co-amoxiclav

Blood cultures – no growth at 5 days

Liver aspirate MCS – mucoid colonies on blood and MacConkey agar. The organism did not react with oxidase or indole

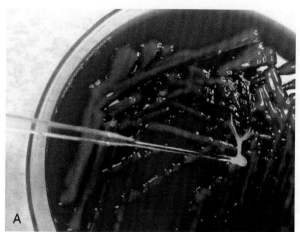

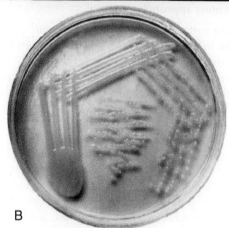

What is the most likely causative organism?

A. *Burkholderia pseudomallei*

B. *Entamoeba histolytica*

C. *Escherichia coli*

D. *Klebsiella pneumoniae*

E. *Streptococcus intermedius* (*S. milleri* group)

21. A 31-year-old woman (14/40; G1, P0) attending for routine antenatal check had a urine culture sent. She was generally well and had not experienced any dysuria or increased urinary frequency.

MSU: ≥10⁵ cfu/mL *Escherichia coli*, fully sensitive.

A repeat MSU was taken and the same organism was isolated again.

What is a recognized complication of this condition?

A. Cerebral palsy

B. Chorioamnionitis

C. Miscarriage

D. Neonatal mortality

E. Preterm delivery

22. A 34-year-old woman seroconverted for CMV infection during her second pregnancy after a febrile illness in her toddler. Antenatal ultrasound scans were normal. A healthy male infant was delivered at 39 weeks' gestation.

What is the most appropriate initial investigation of the baby to identify congenital CMV infection?

A. CSF CMV DNA PCR

B. Plasma CMV DNA PCR

C. Serum CMV IgG and avidity assay

D. Serum CMV IgM

E. Urine CMV DNA PCR

23. A 23-year-old man presented with 3 days of whitish-yellow urethral discharge. He reported that the discharge was staining his underwear. He also reported pain with urination. He had unprotected vaginal intercourse approximately 1 week ago.

On examination, there was white discharge at the meatus. There were no genital lesions and no inguinal lymphadenopathy.

Microscopy:

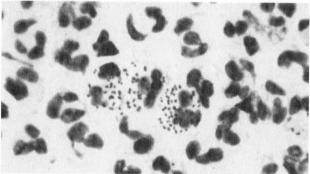

What is the most appropriate treatment?

A. Ceftriaxone 125 mg IM stat and azithromycin 1 gram stat

B. Ceftriaxone 250 mg IM stat and azithromycin 1 gram stat

C. Ciprofloxacin 500 mg stat

D. Doxycycline 100 mg BD for 7 days

E. Hold antibiotics pending NAAT results

24. A 35-year-old woman presented for STI screening prior to having condomless sex. She had a history of systemic lupus erythematosus. She had a regular male partner and used barrier contraception with condoms. She had two lifetime sexual partners. Physical examination, including the pelvic exam, was unremarkable.

Investigations:

HIV 4th-generation Ag/Ab negative

Rapid RPR reactive 1:4

Urine gonorrhea/chlamydia NAAT negative

What is the most appropriate action?

A. Perform a treponemal antibody test

B. Repeat the RPR

C. Send a blood sample for dark field microscopy

D. Treat for late latent syphilis with benzathine penicillin IM in 3 doses at 1 week intervals

E. Treat for primary syphilis with benzathine penicillin IM stat

25. A 25-year-old woman attended for antenatal care in her first trimester of pregnancy. She had a brother with HCV and was worried about her risk for developing liver disease.

Pregnant women are more susceptible to fulminant hepatitis from which virus?

A. Cytomegalovirus
B. Hepatitis A virus
C. Hepatitis B virus
D. Hepatitis C virus
E. Hepatitis E virus

26. A 4-year-old boy developed fever, coryzal symptoms, and a dry cough. 48 hours later he developed a widespread maculopapular rash. He lived in rural Uganda.

On examination his temperature was 39.5°C. He was noted to have bilateral conjunctivitis and white spots on his buccal mucosa.

What intervention has been shown to reduce mortality in such a child?

A. Calcium supplements
B. Iron supplements
C. Vitamin A supplements
D. Vitamin C supplements
E. Zinc supplements

27. A 32-year-old man presented with a 5-day history of fever, headache, rigors, and myalgia. He lived in a rural area and recalled that he cleared a rat infestation in his house basement 2 weeks previously.

On examination, he had hepatomegaly and conjunctival suffusion.
Investigations:
ALT 94 U/L
CRP 124 mg/L

What is the most likely etiologic agent?

A. *Francisella tularensis*
B. *Leptospira icterohaemorrhagiae*
C. *Salmonella enterica* serotype *Typhimurium*
D. *Spirillum minus*
E. *Streptobacillus moniliformis*

28. A 34-year-old woman was bitten by a Rhesus macaque on the forearm. The wound was thoroughly irrigated after the injury, and she was started on amoxicillin/clavulanate.

What other prophylactic agent should she be offered?

A. Aciclovir
B. Ciprofloxacin
C. Doxycycline
D. Foscarnet
E. Itraconazole

29. A 22-year-old woman with cystic fibrosis underwent bilateral lung transplant under alemtuzumab induction. The patient was known to be colonized with *Aspergillus fumigatus* preoperatively and received posttransplant antifungal prophylaxis with voriconazole. Her immediate postoperative course was complicated by acute kidney injury requiring hemodialysis. On postoperative day 18, the nurse noted a 4×6 cm left buttock decubitus wound with a black eschar. There was no surrounding erythema. Excisional debridement was performed. The underlying gluteus muscle was necrotic and liquefied. An organism grew on Sabouraud agar after 4 days of incubation. Microscopy demonstrated broad hyphae without septa. Rootlike hyphae were also noted.

What is the most appropriate action?

A. Continue voriconazole and add caspofungin
B. Decrease immunosuppression and perform serial wound debridements
C. Measure serum voriconazole concentration and adjust the antifungal dose accordingly
D. Switch to intravenous posaconazole
E. Switch to liposomal amphotericin B

30. A 28-year-old woman presented with a high fever and painful lesions on her lower leg. She was known to have acute myeloid leukemia, and she was day 17 of re-induction chemotherapy with fludarabine and doxorubicin. She had previously failed cytarabine and doxorubicin. She was born and brought up in the United States. A year ago, she had spent 2 months in the Dominican Republic on a mission trip. She worked in an office.

On examination, her temperature was 39.7°C. There were multiple tender nodules with central necrosis over her right shin.
Investigations:
Chest CT: a 2.3 cm right upper lobe pulmonary nodule surrounded by ground-glass opacity
Skin biopsy: septate, branching filamentous hyphae seen
Blood cultures: positive at 3 days; hyphae seen

What is the most likely pathogen?

A. *Aspergillus fumigatus*
B. *Fusarium solani*
C. *Histoplasma capsulatum*
D. *Lichtheimia corymbifera*
E. *Rhizomucor* spp.

31. A 27-year-old woman attended clinic for pretravel counseling. She was 18 weeks pregnant. She was planning a 2-week holiday to Kenya to visit her husband. It was her first pregnancy and had been uneventful to date. She was taking prenatal vitamins and was allergic to penicillin (rash only). She was given advice on mosquito bite avoidance and insect repellent.

What would be the most appropriate malaria chemoprophylaxis?

A. Atovaquone-proguanil

B. Clindamycin

C. Doxycycline

D. Hydroxychloroquine

E. Mefloquine

32. A 25-year-old woman presented with a new skin lesion. She was hiking in Provincetown, MA earlier during the week though she did not remember any tick bites. She was usually well and was only taking the oral contraceptive pill. She had no known drug allergies.

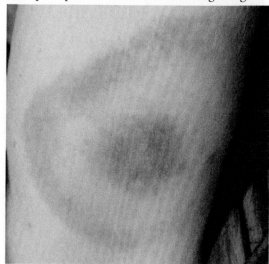

What is the most appropriate action?

A. Acute and convalescent serologies for *Borrelia burgdorferi*

B. *Borrelia burgdorferi* PCR testing

C. ELISA and Western blot for *Borrelia burgdorferi*

D. Start 14 days doxycycline

E. Take a skin biopsy

33. A 24-year-old man was brought in by ambulance with severe shortness of breath. He required immediate intubation for profound hypoxemia despite high flow oxygen. A collateral history was obtained from his brother. The patient came back from a trip to Colorado 2 weeks earlier where he helped his cousin renovate and clean an old farmhouse infested with rodents, cockroaches, and termites. The patient had tried drinking milk freshly squeezed from his cousin's cow a few times. His symptoms began a few days after coming back from the trip with flu-like symptoms that rapidly progressed to a dry cough and severe dyspnea.

His vital signs upon arrival were: temperature 39.1°C, blood pressure 60/40 mmHg, heart rate 120 beats/minute, and respiratory rate 30 breaths/minute.
Labs:

Total white cell count 15 ×10⁹/L (60% neutrophil with a significant amount of immature cells,

15% lymphocytes with a significant amount of atypical cells)

Hemoglobin 11.2 g/dL (hematocrit 64%)

Platelet count 62,000/μL

AST 24 U/L

ALT 25 U/L

Bilirubin 1 mg/dL

eGFR >60 mL/min/1.73 m²

Chest X-ray:

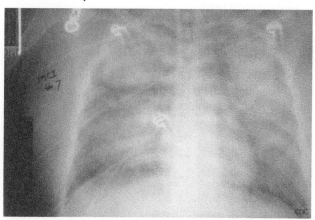

What is the most likely cause of his infection?

A. *Coccidioides immitis*

B. Hantavirus

C. Influenza

D. *Mycobacterium bovis*

E. PVL–*Staphylococcus aureus*

34. A 10-month-old boy was reviewed with a 2-month history of bloody diarrhea, intermittent vomiting, colicky abdominal pain, and recurrent fevers. He had been born in a refugee camp in Bangladesh and had arrived in the United States 1 week ago. He was breast fed until month 4 and since then had been fed with unpasteurized cow and goat milk when available. He had not received any vaccinations.
Investigations:

Stool culture and O&P ×3 negative

Gastric fluid microscopy: abundant acid-fast bacilli seen on ZN smear

What is the next best step in managing this patient?

A. Do a chest X-ray to rule out pulmonary involvement

B. Do a TST or IGRA to rule out TB disease

C. Give BCG vaccine to protect him from miliary TB

D. Give INH prophylaxis to all household contacts

E. Start treatment with RIF, INH, and PZA

35. A 74-year-old man presented with fever and malaise. His past medical history included severe aortic stenosis and ascending aortic aneurysm, for which he received concomitant aortic valve replacement and aortic root repair 2 years previously. The patient had well-controlled diabetes but no other comorbidities.

Physical exam revealed a new murmur.

Investigations:

Hemoglobin 8.2 g/dL

HIV Ag/Ab negative

Routine blood cultures ×3 pairs negative

Mycobacterial blood culture positive after 2 weeks of incubation

What organism is most likely to be responsible?

A. *Mycobacterium abscessus*

B. *Mycobacterium avium*

C. *Mycobacterium chimaera*

D. *Mycobacterium fortuitum*

E. *Mycobacterium kansasii*

36. An 80-year-old woman presented with a nonhealing ulcerative lesion on her left earlobe. She was from central Texas and spent many hours a day working on her ranch. The lesion had not responded to empiric cephalexin.

A biopsy of the lesion was performed.

Histology: histiocytes in the dermis are filled with small round structures that have both a nucleus and kinetoplast.

What is the most likely organism?

A. *Acanthamoeba* sp.

B. *Candida albicans*

C. *Histoplasma capsulatum*

D. *Leishmania mexicana*

E. *Trypanosoma cruzi*

37. A 28-year-old woman presented for a new patient appointment. She had been diagnosed with HIV 3 years earlier and was established on ART.

Investigations:

CD4 count 550 cells/μL

HIV viral load undetectable

Annual Pap smears for past 3 years: normal cytology

What is the most appropriate recommendation?

A. Continue annual Pap smear

B. Co-testing of HPV with next Pap smear

C. Offer HPV vaccination

D. Repeat cervical cytology testing in 3 years

E. Repeat cervical cytology testing in 5 years

38. A 42-year-old woman presented with a 6-month history of increased abdominal weight gain and generalized muscle weakness. She had been found to have HIV 8 years previously when she was diagnosed in pregnancy. She was initially treated with zidovudine/lamivudine and lopinavir/ritonavir during pregnancy and continued it until the previous year when she switched to tenofovir disoproxil fumarate/emtricitabine/cobicistat/elvitegravir for ART simplification. She also had a history of seasonal allergies and a sporting injury to her right knee. In addition to ART, she was taking OTC antihistamines, intranasal fluticasone spray, and ibuprofen.

What is the most likely diagnosis?

A. Lipodystrophy syndrome

B. Obesity from inactivity

C. Toxicity from antihistamine

D. Toxicity from ibuprofen

E. Toxicity from nasal spray

39. A 26-year-old man presented with a 4-day history of pleuritic chest pain and shortness of breath. He denied a history of trauma, smoking, or chronic lung disease. He was known to have HIV with a history of nonadherence to his HIV medications and antibiotic prophylaxis. He also had a sulfa drug allergy.

On physical exam, there were decreased breath sounds over the right upper lung fields with hyperresonance to percussion.

Investigations:

CXR: no pulmonary infiltrates seen; moderate-sized pneumothorax on the right lung

CD4 count 122 cells/μL

HIV viral load 2300 copies/mL

Lactate dehydrogenase 560 U/L (122–222)

1,3-beta-D-glucan >500 pg/mL (<60)

Qualitative serum cytomegalovirus (CMV) PCR-positive

What is the most appropriate treatment?

A. Amphotericin B deoxycholate plus flucytosine

B. Ceftriaxone plus azithromycin

C. Clindamycin plus primaquine

D. Fluconazole

E. Ganciclovir

40. A 53-year-old man presented with a 2-week history of fevers and worsening skin lesions. The patient had noted progressive development of three distinct purplish nodular lesions on his right arm. He had a history of hypertension, asthma, and HIV. He did not take any regular medications and had no known allergies. The patient lived in Dallas, Texas, with one dog and three cats as pets. He had not had any recent travel overseas and had spent no time in prison or homeless. The patient was sexually active with three partners in the past 6 months.

Investigations:

CD4 count 25 cells/μL

HIV viral load 35,150 copies/mL

Syphilis EIA positive

Rapid plasma reagin (RPR) titer 1:2

T. *pallidum* antibodies (TPHA) positive

Lesion biopsy: silver stain showed clumps of dark-staining rods in endothelial cells lining blood vessels

What pathogen is most likely to be responsible?

A. *Bartonella henselae*

B. *Bartonella quintana*

C. Kaposi sarcoma-associated herpesvirus

D. *Legionella pneumophila*

E. *Treponema pallidum*

41. A 50-year-old woman presented with a 2-week history of nausea, diarrhea, and abdominal pain. She had received a deceased donor kidney transplant for polycystic kidney disease 3 months prior. She had received antithymocyte globulin for induction and was on tacrolimus, mycophenolate, and prednisone for maintenance immunosuppression. She rapidly developed a purpuric rash and respiratory failure and required intubation. Gross hematuria was seen on urinary catheterization.

Bronchoscopy: diffuse hemorrhage seen.

She was started on broad-spectrum antibiotics.

In addition to supportive critical care, what is the best therapeutic intervention?

A. Ganciclovir IV

B. Intravenous immunoglobulin IV

C. Ivermectin per NG

D. Liposomal amphotericin B IV

E. Voriconazole and micafungin IV

42. A 45-year-old man presented with a 1-week of fever and right-sided pleuritic chest pain. He was not dyspneic but had noticed night sweats, weight loss, and a nonproductive cough without hemoptysis. He had been diagnosed with B-cell acute lymphocytic leukemia 2 months previously and had had a prolonged neutropenia. He was taking levofloxacin, fluconazole, valaciclovir, and trimethoprim–sulfamethoxazole prophylaxis.

On examination, his temperature was 102°F (38.8°C), his blood pressure was 120/60 mmHg, heart rate was 110 beats/minute, respiratory rate 22 breaths/minute with oxygen saturations 95% on room air. He was pale but in no acute distress except for discomfort from right-sided chest pain. His lung sounds were clear bilaterally without wheezes, rales, or crackles. There was no pedal edema, but there were some scattered petechiae on his lower extremities.

Investigations:

Total white cell count 0.1×10^9/L

Absolute neutrophil count 0.2×10^9 /L

Hemoglobin 6 g/dL

Platelets 67×10^9 /L

Urea, creatinine, and electrolytes were within normal limits

Blood cultures: no growth at 48 hours

CT chest revealed numerous nodules clustered in the right lower lobe, with surrounding halos.

What is the most likely diagnosis?

A. Cytomegalovirus pneumonitis

B. Streptococcal pneumonia

C. *Pneumocystis* pneumonia (PCP)

D. Pulmonary aspergillosis

E. Pulmonary septic emboli

43. A 30-year-old woman was seen with recurrent skin abscesses since childhood, not accompanied by surrounding redness, warmth, or tenderness. She had also had three episodes of pneumonia, which healed, leaving air-filled cavities.

On physical examination she had joint hypermobility, scoliosis, and a wide nasal base.

Investigations:

Absolute eosinophil count 3000/μL

What is the most likely diagnosis?

A. DOCK8 deficiency

B. Hyper IgD syndrome

C. Hyper IgE syndrome

D. Hyper IgM syndrome

E. Wiskott–Aldrich syndrome

44.

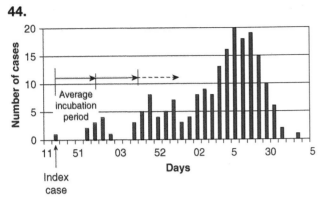

What type of outbreak is represented in the epidemic curve?

A. Common intermittent source
B. Common persistent source
C. Common point source
D. Intermittent outbreak
E. Propagated progressive source

45. A 28-year-old woman sought medical advice 48 hours after a significant chickenpox exposure. She was 32 weeks pregnant with no personal history of chickenpox. She had not received the varicella vaccine.

Investigations:
   Varicella IgG negative.
   She was treated with VZV immunoglobulin (VZIG).

What is the most appropriate definition of her treatment?

A. Active immunization
B. Natural immunization
C. Partial immunization
D. Passive immunization
E. Vaccine immunization

46. A 26-year-old man with bilateral profound hearing loss due to otosclerosis was referred for a cochlear implant.

What vaccination would be most appropriate?

A. *Haemophilus influenzae* type b
B. Meningococcal ACWY
C. Meningococcal B
D. Pneumococcal PPV23
E. Seasonal influenza

47. A 22-year-old woman presented with a 5-day history of an itchy rash on her leg. She had returned 2 weeks earlier from a holiday in the Caribbean.

On exam:

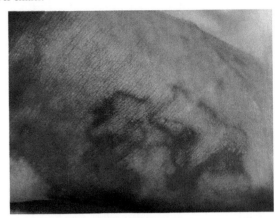

What is the most likely diagnosis?

A. Cutaneous larva migrans
B. Gnathostomiasis
C. Larva currens
D. Myiasis
E. Phytophotodermatitis

48. Dr. Jones has moved to San Francisco for her fellowship and has performed a study looking at risk factors for the development of infection with *Cryptococcus*. She created a retrospective cohort of all patients admitted to her institution and compared those with cryptococcosis and those without. While analyzing the demographics, she calculated that male patients have 2.1-fold (95% CI 1.7, 2.4) higher odds of developing cryptococcosis than women. Very excitedly, she shows the data to her advisor, who points out that HIV is more prevalent in men who have sex with men, and that HIV also predisposes for cryptococcosis. When adjusting for the diagnosis of HIV, Dr. Jones found no effect.

In this situation, HIV is behaving as a(n):

A. Confounder
B. Continuous variable
C. Independent variable
D. Ordinal variable
E. Outcome

Quiz 6

1. A 23-year-old woman was reviewed after clinically deteriorating on the ICU with increasing oxygen requirements. She had undergone multiple surgical interventions after being involved in an accident while dirt-biking at a commercial course in Kansas City, Missouri. She had sustained blunt-chest trauma and facial trauma with multiple facial bone fractures.

Investigations:

CXR: large bilateral opacities (right more than left)

CT chest: bilateral complicated pleural effusion with evidence of necrotizing pneumonia

She underwent thoracotomy with resection and chest tube placement.

Cultures from tissue grew molds. Lactophenol stain showed dark septate hyphae with alternating septate conidia (see image):

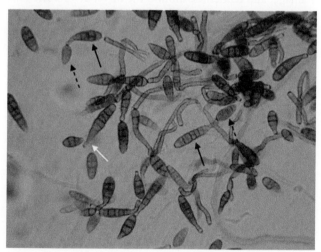

The mold was positive on Fontana–Masson stain.

What is the most likely etiologic agent?

A. *Alternaria* sp.

B. *Aspergillus fumigatus*

C. *Coccidioides immitis/posadasii*

D. *Fusarium* sp.

E. *Histoplasma capsulatum*

2. A 65-year-old woman was admitted with tachycardia and fever. She had a history of colon cancer, diabetes mellitus, acute on chronic kidney disease, and depression. She was taking citalopram and had a severe penicillin allergy (anaphylaxis).

Investigations:

Creatinine 2.9 mg/dL (baseline SCr 1.8 mg/dL)

Total white cell count 16.2×10^9/L

CXR normal

Transthoracic echocardiogram – no evidence of endocarditis

3 sets of blood cultures positive for *Enterococcus faecalis*:

ampicillin: sensitive

vancomycin: sensitive

daptomycin: sensitive

linezolid: sensitive

high-level gentamicin resistance: present

high-level streptomycin resistance: results pending

What is the most appropriate treatment?

A. Ampicillin plus ceftriaxone

B. Daptomycin

C. Linezolid

D. Quinupristin/dalfopristin

E. Telavancin

3. A 42-year-old man presented with a 3-day history of fevers, headache, and photophobia. He had no medical history of note and did not take any regular medications. He was normally resident in London. Six weeks earlier he had spent 2 weeks in Missouri, visiting relatives and camping. He had seen a tick moving on his arm but had not found any attached. His 6-year-old son had had a short-lived febrile illness 3 days before the patient developed symptoms.

On examination, there was no rash. He had photophobia and neck stiffness but was alert and oriented. He was normotensive and his heart rate was 90 beats per minute. His temperature was 38.2°C. There was no focal neurology.

A lumbar puncture was performed.

Investigations:

Peripheral white blood cell count 10.2×10^9/L

HIV Ag/Ab negative

CSF white cell count 146 ×10⁶/L; 55% lymphocytes, 45% polymorphs

CSF protein 562 mg/L

CSF/plasma glucose 3.7/4.8 mmol/L

CSF microscopy: no organisms seen

What is the most likely causative organism?

A. *Borrelia burgdorferi*

B. *Coccidioides immitis*

C. Enterovirus

D. Influenza virus

E. Mumps virus

4. A 42-year-old man presented with fluctuating headaches that had slowly worsened over the preceding month. He had lost 8 kg in weight and thought he had been having some hot flushes. His wife reported that he had started intravenous biological treatment for arthritis 3 months earlier, but she was unsure what it was. He had not recently travelled. He had been born and brought up in the UK but had spent several years working in southern Africa in his twenties.

On examination he was mildly confused. His GCS was 14/15. His temperature was 37.9°C. There was neck stiffness but no purpura. There was no focal neurology.

A CT head and lumbar puncture were performed.

Investigations:

CT head – no space-occupying lesions. Normal appearances of ventricles and brain parenchyma.

CSF white cell count 641 ×10⁶/L; 99% lymphocytes

CSF protein 1614 mg/L

CSF/plasma glucose 1.4/4.8 mmol/L

CSF microscopy: no organisms seen

HIV Ag/Ab negative

He was started on presumptive antituberculous therapy and high-dose steroids and clinically began to improve.

What biological agent is most likely to lead to infection with tuberculosis?

A. Abatacept

B. Alemtuzumab

C. Infliximab

D. Natalizumab

E. Rituximab

5. A 62-year-old man presented with a 1-month history of worsening nonproductive cough. He had chronic obstructive lung disease managed with home nebulizers. He had tried a course of a quinolone antibiotic, which resulted in little improvement in his symptoms. He had no fever, chills, or sweats. He had a 5 lb weight loss in the past 6 months. On exam, he was afebrile and had few scattered expiratory wheezes.

Investigations:

CXR: no infiltrates

High-resolution chest CT: multi-focal bronchiectasis and multiple small nodules

Expectorated sputum grew *Mycobacterium avium* complex

What is the best next step in this patient's management?

A. Hold off treatment until sensitivities are available

B. Request BAL for mycobacterial investigation

C. Send an additional expectorated sputum sample for AFB-smear and culture

D. Start therapy with ethambutol, rifampin, and clarithromycin

E. Start quadruple therapy with ethambutol, rifampin, isoniazid, and pyrazinamide

6. A 66-year-old man presented with a 1-week history of cough, pleuritic chest pain, and low-grade fevers. He was known to have chronic obstructive pulmonary disorder and had a smoking pack year history of 60 years.

Investigations:

CXR revealed a dense infiltrate in the right lower lobe

Sputum microscopy revealed numerous gram-negative cocci, many in pairs

What is the most appropriate therapy?

A. Amoxicillin/clavulanate

B. Ciprofloxacin

C. No antimicrobial therapy is required

D. Tetracycline

E. Trimethoprim–sulfamethoxazole (TMP–SMX)

7. A 35-year-old man presented with increased erythema, drainage, and tenderness around the driveline to a left ventricular assist device (LVAD). He had nonischemic cardiomyopathy and was awaiting heart transplantation.

Investigations:

Ultrasound of the exit site: small fluid collection at the site

The expressed drainage was sent for culture.

What is the most likely causative organism?

A. *Candida albicans*

B. Coagulase-negative staphylococci

C. *Cutibacterium acnes (formerly Proprionibacterium)*

D. *Klebsiella pneumoniae*

E. *Pseudomonas aeruginosa*

8. A 27-year-old businessman presented with a 14-day history of watery loose stool, bloating, and some intermittent abdominal pain. Symptoms had started on the day of his return from a 9-day business trip to Thailand. He also noted fat droplets in his stools. He had stayed in a hotel and only ventured out of the hotel on one occasion. He had enjoyed the local food served during his trip and was fond of fresh fruit, salads, and iced drinks.

What is the most likely etiologic agent?

A. *Campylobacter* spp.

B. *Cryptosporidium* spp.

C. *Giardia* spp.

D. *Vibrio* spp.

E. *Yersinia enterocolitica*

9. A 43-year-old man presented with a 2-day history of hallucinations, vertigo, and paraesthesia. He had also had a 24-hour period of diarrhea which had resolved. His symptoms started 5 hours after he had been to a local seafood restaurant. He could not recall anything unusual about his meal, which had tasted fine.

What is the most likely cause of his symptoms?

A. *Bacillus cereus*
B. *Botulinum toxin*
C. Ciguatera poisoning
D. Scombroid poisoning
E. *Staphylococcus aureus*

10. A 24-year-old woman presented with a new genital rash. The lesions were associated with mild burning. She had a history of orolabial cold sores. She and her male sex partner of 2 years reported no other concurrent sex partners. They used barrier contraception with condoms, and she was taking the combined oral contraceptive pill.

On examination, a vulvar rash was observed

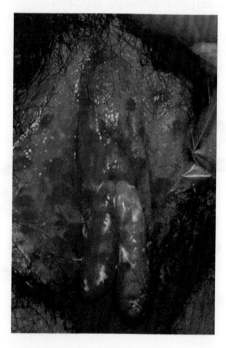

What is the most likely cause?

A. Behçet's disease
B. Latex allergy
C. New acquisition of HSV-2
D. Primary syphilis
E. Reactivation of latent HSV-1

11. A 26-year-old male presented with diarrhea. He also had some blood in his stool, tenesmus, and a mucoid discharge from his anus. He had had unprotected receptive anal intercourse 1 week earlier.

Investigations:
  4th generation HIV Ag/Ab negative
  Syphilis EIA negative
  Urine NAAT for gonorrhea and chlamydia negative
  Rectal NAAT testing positive for *C. trachomatis*, negative for *N. gonorrhoeae*

What is the most appropriate treatment?

A. Benzathine penicillin G for one dose
B. Cefixime orally in a single dose
C. Ceftriaxone IM for one dose
D. Doxycycline for 21 days
E. Doxycycline for 7 days plus one dose of azithromycin

12. A 35-year-old woman presented with jaundice, vomiting, and right upper quadrant pain. She was 22/40 weeks pregnant. She was sexually active and was not using condoms. She had received a blood transfusion for anemia 2 weeks prior to this admission. She was a nurse at a local physician's office and had received all recommended vaccinations 5 years ago when she started working.

Investigations:
  ALT 750 IU/L
  AST 2320 IU/L

What is the most likely cause of her hepatitis?

A. Cytomegalovirus
B. Erythrovirus (parvovirus B19)
C. Hepatitis B virus
D. Hepatitis G virus (GBV-C)
E. Herpes simplex virus

13. A 5-year-old child was reviewed 24 hours after a significant chickenpox exposure. She had acute myeloid leukemia and was undergoing treatment.

She had been treated with human varicella-zoster immunoglobulin (VZIG) 9 weeks previously after her varicellazoster virus (VZV) IgG was found to be negative after another significant chickenpox exposure.

What is the most appropriate action?

A. Commence aciclovir prophylaxis
B. Issue VZIG immediately
C. Reassurance only
D. Recheck VZV IgG
E. Recommend varicella vaccination

14. A 23-year-old woman presented with a 3-day history of an enlarging skin lesion and mild myalgia. She reported that she had removed an engorged tick 2 weeks previously after walking in the New Forest, UK. On examination:

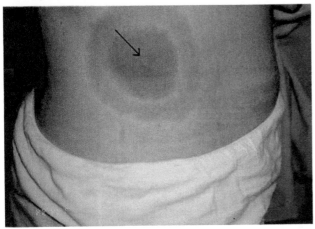

Neurologic examination was normal.

What is the most appropriate action?

A. Hold antibiotics pending serology results
B. Reassure that this is a tick bite reaction only
C. Start ceftriaxone 2 g OD for 14–21 days
D. Start ciprofloxacin 500 mg BD for 14–21 days
E. Start doxycycline 100 mg BD for 14–21 days

15. A 23-year-old man presented with a swollen, painful, and erythematous right wrist of 1-week duration. His symptoms were associated with fever, chills, and generalized malaise. Upon review of systems, he recounted painless urethral discharge in the weeks prior to his presentation. He was sexually active and reported unprotected vaginal intercourse with 3 casual partners in the last 6 months.

On examination his temperature was 100.7°F (38.2°C). His right wrist was erythematous with a small effusion and tenderness to palpation along the insertion of the tendon. There were three small vesiculopustular lesions overlying the right thenar eminence.

Investigations:
Total white cell count 12,800/mL
Two sets of peripheral blood cultures negative
X-ray of the joint did not demonstrate a fracture or erosion of the underlying bone
Joint fluid:
Macroscopic appearances: turbid synovial fluid
Microscopy: leukocyte count 42,000 cells mm³, 78% neutrophils
No organisms seen on Gram stain. No crystals seen

What is the most appropriate treatment?

A. Cefixime PO
B. Ceftriaxone IV and azithromycin PO
C. Doxycycline PO
D. None required
E. Vancomycin IV

16. A 37-year-old man presented with a 3-week history of fever, headache, and nausea with morning emesis. He was normally well and did not take any regular medications. He lived in California but recently attended a wedding on Vancouver Island, British Columbia.

On examination, vital signs were normal. The neck was supple. There was worsening of headache with passively rotating the head from side to side. The remainder of the neurologic examination was unremarkable.

Investigations:
CT head normal
Lumbar puncture: opening pressure 25 cmH$_2$O
Cerebrospinal fluid (CSF):
Visibly clear on macroscopic appearance
CSF protein 50 mg/dL (reference range: 20–40 mg/dL)
CSF glucose 50 mg/dL (reference range: 45–80 mg/dL)
300 cells/mm³ (50% lymphocytes, 30% neutrophils)
Gram stain:

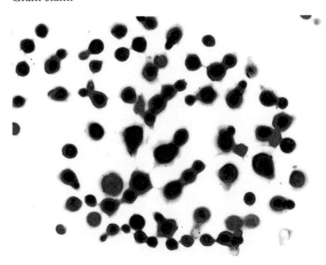

What is the most likely diagnosis?

A. *Candida albicans*
B. *Cryptococcus gattii*
C. *Cryptococcus neoformans*
D. *Pneumocystis jirovecii*
E. *Histoplasma capsulatum*

17. A 19-year-old man was admitted with a three-day history of abdominal pain and fevers. He lived in New York City, but recently traveled to visit family in Malaysia. He did not seek pretravel counseling.

On physical examination, he appeared acutely ill. His blood pressure was 108/55 mmHg, his pulse rate was 114 beats/minute, and his temperature was 40°C. He had abdominal tenderness and was dyspneic at rest, with increasing oxygen requirements.

Investigations:

Hemoglobin level 8.3 mmol/L

Platelet count 56 ×10⁹/L

Peripheral white cell 4.5 ×10⁹cells/L

Blood smear revealed the following, with parasitemia to 3.8%.

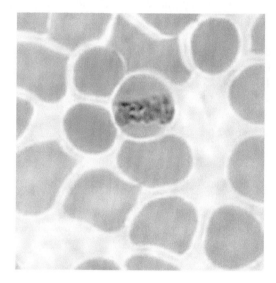

What pathogen is most likely to be responsible?

A. *P. falciparum*

B. *P. knowlesi*

C. *P. malariae*

D. *P. ovale*

E. *P. vivax*

18. A 42-year-old man presented with a 3-week history of fever associated with progressive low back pain, malaise, nausea, vomiting, and diarrhea. He had a history of asthma, for which he used regular low-dose steroid inhalers. He was not on any oral medications and had no known drug allergies. He worked in an office. He had sustained a cut to his finger 6 weeks previously while on a hunting trip that involved slaughtering, cooking, and eating wild boar. None of his friends became sick although he said that their wilderness guide had been coughing during their entire trip.

On examination, his temperature was 38.9°C. He had hepatosplenomegaly on abdominal palpation. There was some mild epididymo-orchitis on genital exam. His respiratory and cardiovascular exams were unremarkable.

Investigations:

Total white cell count 2.5 ×109/L

Hemoglobin 8.2 g/dL

Platelet count 90,000/μL

Computed tomography scan of his abdomen and pelvis demonstrated enlarged liver and spleen and also showed evidence of sacroiliitis.

What was the most likely route of acquisition of his infection?

A. Direct contact

B. Droplet inhalation

C. Ingestion

D. Sexual transmission

E. Tick bite

19. A 37-year-old woman presented with a 1-month history of reddish, painful, tender lumps on her shins. She had also noticed some fatigue and night sweats but had no other symptoms. She had a history of hypothyroidism on replacement thyroxine. She had lived in Tucson, Arizona, since birth and had not traveled outside of the state.

Exam findings:

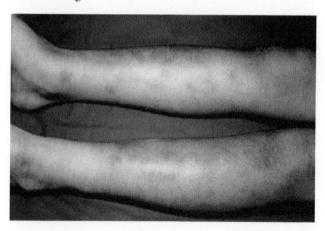

Investigations:

Moderate eosinophilia

HIV Ag/Ab negative

Interferon gamma release assay (QuantiFERON-TB gold) negative

Chest CT: bilateral hilar adenopathy but no parenchymal involvement

Skin biopsy: septal granulomatous inflammation seen, no AFB seen on ZN stain

What is the most likely cause of her symptoms?

A. Behçet's disease

B. Coccidioidomycosis

C. Oral contraceptives

D. Sarcoidosis

E. Tuberculosis

20. An outbreak of diarrhea was linked to a local water park. Before the cases were linked to a common source, patients were seen by a variety of providers, and a number of investigations performed.

Investigations:

Stool microscopy: small, round cysts seen on acid-fast stain

Colon biopsy: small cysts are seen that appear to be sitting on the surface of the colonic epithelium

What organism is most likely to be responsible?

A. *Cryptosporidium* sp.
B. *Cyclospora cayetanensis*
C. *Cystoisospora belli*
D. *Giardia duodenalis*
E. *Enterocytozoon* sp.

21. A 45-year old woman was investigated for suspected *Schistosoma* infection. Limited clinical information was provided of abdominal discomfort and intermittent diarrhea. There was no epidemiologic history available to the laboratory regarding country of origin, travel, etc.

Stool microscopy for ova, cysts, and parasites:

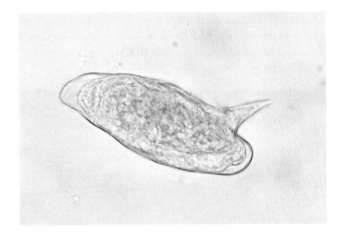

What schistosome species is responsible for her symptoms?

A. *S. haematobium*
B. *S. intercalatum*
C. *S. japonicum*
D. *S. mansoni*
E. *S. mekongi*

22. A 25-year-old woman attended clinic to discuss her birthing plans. She was 37+5 weeks gestation in her first pregnancy. She had HIV and was taking tenofovir disoproxil fumarate/emtricitabine and boosted atazanavir and reported full compliance.

Investigations:

CD4 count 456 cells/μL

HIV RNA <40 copies/mL

What delivery plan is most appropriate?

A. Elective cesarean section at 38 weeks with intravenous zidovudine commenced at least 3 hours prior

B. Elective cesarean section at 38 weeks with intravenous zidovudine commenced at least 3 hours prior plus single dose nevirapine

C. Elective cesarean section at 38 weeks without intravenous zidovudine

D. Spontaneous vaginal delivery provided obstetrically permitted with intravenous zidovudine during labor

E. Spontaneous vaginal delivery provided obstetrically permitted without intravenous zidovudine during labor

23. A 45-year-old woman presented with a 3-week history of fevers, headache, and gradually increasing confusion. The patient was known to have HIV and a history of nonadherence to her antiretroviral therapy.

On physical exam, the patient appeared somnolent but had no focal neurologic deficits. A CT head and a lumbar puncture were performed.

Investigations:

Noncontrasted CT of the head: normal appearances

CD4 count 85 cells/μL

HIV viral load 450 copies/mL

Serum cryptococcal antigen positive 1:128

Lumbar puncture:

Opening pressure 32 mmHg

CSF WBC count 4/mm³,

CSF glucose 30 mg/dL (45–80)

CSF total protein 110 mg/dL (20–40)

CSF Gram stain negative

CSF cryptococcal antigen positive 1:32

In addition to starting antifungal therapy, what therapeutic intervention is warranted?

A. Acetazolamide
B. Dexamethasone
C. Mannitol
D. Serial lumbar punctures
E. Ventriculoperitoneal shunting

24. A 35-year-old man was brought in by ambulance after being found unconscious. His partner gave a collateral history of preceding symptoms for 3 weeks of fevers, headaches, and new-onset seizures. He was known to have HIV but had not been on antiretroviral therapy or taking antibiotic prophylaxis. The patient was originally from Brazil but immigrated to the United States 2 years ago.

On physical exam, the patient was somnolent with right-sided upper and lower extremity weakness.

Investigations:

CD4 count 23 cells/μL

HIV viral load 76,850 copies/mL

Serum *Toxoplasma* IgG serologies negative

CSF EBV PCR negative

CSF VDRL negative

MRI brain: 3 discrete hypodense masses in the cerebral cortex with contrast ring enhancement

What is the most likely diagnosis?

A. Chagas brain abscess
B. Cryptococcal brain abscess
C. Primary central nervous system lymphoma
D. Syphilitic gumma
E. Toxoplasmic encephalitis

25. A 60-year-old man underwent deceased donor kidney transplant for end-stage renal disease secondary to diabetes mellitus. He received antithymocyte globulin for induction and tacrolimus, mycophenolate, and prednisone for maintenance immunosuppression.

Investigations:
    Recipient CMV IgG negative
    Donor CMV IgG indeterminate

What strategy should be recommended to prevent CMV disease?

A. Aciclovir
B. Cidofovir
C. Foscarnet
D. Ganciclovir
E. Valganciclovir

26. A 26-year-old man was diagnosed with disseminated *Mycobacterium kansasii* infection.

On examination, he had multiple warts and bilateral lymph-edema of the lower extremities.

Investigations:
    Absolute monocyte count 30/μL

What is the most likely diagnosis?

A. A defect in innate immunity due to IL-12 or IFN-gamma deficiency
B. Chronic granulomatous disease
C. DOCK8 deficiency
D. GATA2 deficiency
E. WHIM syndrome

27. A 64-year-old woman presented with a 5-day history of watery diarrhea without noticing any blood in her stool. She had not been experiencing fevers or chills. She had not had any recent international travel but had received a course of ciprofloxacin for a urinary tract infection 2 months ago.

Investigations:
    Total white cell count 14.1 ×10⁹/L
    eGFR >60 mL/min/1.73 m²
    Stool *Clostridioides difficile* EIA for toxin A/B positive, GDH positive
    She responded well to treatment with oral vancomycin.

What follow up investigation is most appropriate?

A. Cell cytotoxicity assay
B. EIA for toxin A/B and GDH
C. No follow-up necessary
D. PCR for toxigenic *C. difficile*
E. Stool culture for toxigenic *C. difficile*

28.

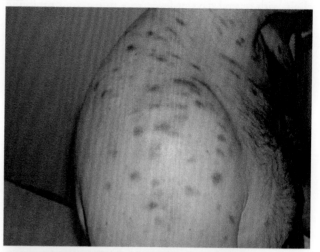

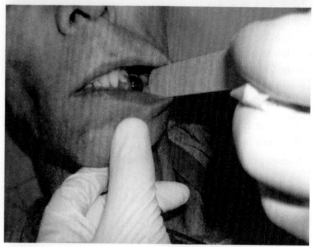

A 28-year-old man presented with a 4-month history of new skin lesions. He had no systemic symptoms. He was known to have HIV but had been lost to follow-up for 3 years and was not taking ART or any antimicrobial prophylaxis.

On examination, he was cachectic. His temperature was 36.8°C. Multiple papular lesions of varying diameter were present over his whole body and inside his mouth. The lesions were nontender. He had pitting edema of his ankles bilaterally.

Investigations:
    CD4 count 93 ×10⁶/μL

What is the most likely diagnosis?

A. Bacillary angiomatosis
B. Cutaneous T-cell lymphoma
C. Disseminated HSV
D. Eosinophilic folliculitis
E. Kaposi sarcoma

29. A 19-year-old male presented to the student health clinic with several days of fever, sore throat, and profound fatigue. He has evident tonsillitis on exam and has some palpable cervical lymphadenopathy. The provider suspected possible streptococcal pharyngitis and prescribed amoxicillin. The next day he developed a pruritic, maculopapular rash.

What is the most likely cause of his illness?

A. Adenovirus
B. Epstein–Barr virus
C. Human immunodeficiency virus
D. *Mycoplasma pneumoniae*
E. *Streptococcus pyogenes*

30. A 17-year-old male presented to the student health clinic with about a week of fevers, malaise, sore throat, oral ulcers, and one day of nonpruritic, diffuse, erythematous morbilliform rash. He is otherwise healthy and takes no medications. He is sexually active. On exam, he has non-exudative pharyngitis with stomatitis, along with palpable cervical lymphadenopathy and mild splenomegaly.

In addition to testing for infectious mononucleosis, you should also consider what diagnosis?

A. Acute HIV infection
B. Adult Still's disease
C. Herpes simplex virus infection
D. Measles
E. Parvovirus infection

31. A 4-year-old girl presented with 5 days of low-grade fevers and malaise and one day of rash on her face and trunk. Her pediatrician advised supportive care, and the rash and fevers resolved over the next few days. Her 15-year-old foster brother has sickle cell disease.

If he were to have infection with the same agent, he would be particularly at risk for what complication?

A. Aplastic anemia
B. Gastroenteritis
C. Meningoencephalitis
D. Osteomyelitis
E. Pneumonia

32. A 4-year-old girl presented to her pediatrician's office with painful ulcerative lesions on her tongue, lips, and hands. Her mother says that she started feeling ill about 1–2 days before the sores were noticed and had significant fatigue, low-grade fevers, and cough.

What is the best treatment recommendation?

A. Aciclovir
B. Amoxicillin
C. Clindamycin
D. Corticosteroids
E. Supportive care

33. A 55-year-old man presented with a 3-month history of progressive, erythematous nodules on his hand and forearm. He fishes frequently and remembers puncturing his finger with a fishhook about 2 months ago. The puncture wound healed well initially, but then he developed an erythematous nodule at the puncture site. He later noticed two new nodules on the dorsum of his hand, proximal to the initial injury. He now has another new nodule that just developed on his forearm.

What is the most likely cause of his infection?

A. *Erysipelothrix rhusiopathiae*
B. *Leishmania braziliensis*
C. *Mycobacterium marinum*
D. *Nocardia asteroides*
E. *Vibrio vulnificus*

34. What is the most likely sexually transmitted disease to be the cause of the findings in the photograph?

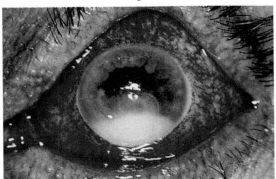

A. *Chlamydia*
B. *Gonorrhea*
C. HIV
D. Human papillomavirus
E. Syphilis

35. A 26-year-old woman with HIV, not on therapy, presents to clinic for her first visit. She has had several months of weight loss and intermittent night sweats. She has thrush. She also noted that she has had several weeks of visual changes with "floaters" and blurring of her vision bilaterally. Dilated funduscopic exam was performed, and she was found to have white, perivascular retinal infiltrates and dot-blot hemorrhages.

What is the most likely cause of these findings?

A. Bartonellosis
B. Cytomegalovirus
C. Histoplasmosis
D. Syphilis
E. Toxoplasmosis

36. A 37-year-old construction worker presented to the emergency department with fever and painful muscle spasms for 1 day. On examination, his temperature is 38.1°C, pulse 122 beats/minute, blood pressure 135/80 mmHg, and he has a small wound on his hand with surrounding erythema and induration that he says he sustained because of puncturing his hand with a nail.

What is the first-line antimicrobial of choice to inhibit further toxin production contributing to his illness?

A. Clindamycin
B. Metronidazole
C. Penicillin
D. Tetracycline
E. Vancomycin

37. A 3-month-old baby was brought to the emergency department by her parents because of lethargy and irritability. She has not been eating well and has not had a bowel movement in several days. On examination, the infant has a depressed fontanel and notably poor muscle tone and a weak sucking reflex.

How does the cause of this illness appear under Gram stain?

A. Gram-negative bacilli
B. Gram-negative diplococci
C. Gram-positive bacilli
D. Gram-positive cocci in clusters
E. Gram-positive cocci in pairs and chains

38. A patient recently started taking medication for active pulmonary tuberculosis. He has been taking his medications regularly, and his pulmonary symptoms have been improving. Unfortunately, he has begun to notice visual changes, including decreased visual acuity and disturbance in his perception of color.

Which of his medications is the most likely culprit?

A. Clarithromycin
B. Ethambutol
C. Isoniazid
D. Pyrazinamide
E. Rifampin

39. A 24-year old man is referred for evaluation of chronic pneumonia. He has had multiple courses of antibacterial therapy and still has a significant left lower lobe consolidation as seen on his chest radiograph. An HIV test is negative. On chest CT, the area of consolidation was thought to be a mass-like lesion, and he was referred for biopsy. In the interim, he also developed multiple verrucous skin plaques. He undergoes a bronchoscopy with transbronchial biopsy and the pathology shows granulomas and broad-based budding yeast forms as shown in the image.

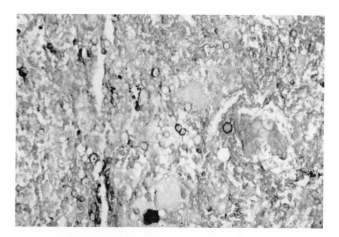

What is the most likely diagnosis?

A. Aspergillosis
B. Blastomycosis
C. Coccidioidomycosis
D. Cryptococcosis
E. Histoplasmosis

40. Three people are brought to the emergency department by ambulance from a conference at a hotel banquet hall. All had been taken ill within a short time of eating at a buffet that included fresh tuna. The patients all complained of headache, dizziness, and flushing. They were all mildly tachycardic, but none was febrile or hypotensive.

What is the most likely cause of their symptoms?

A. Bacterial infection
B. Histamine ingestion
C. Parasitic infection
D. Toxin ingestion
E. Viral infection

41. A 19-year-old man with HIV presents to clinic with a new onset rash. His RPR was 1:16 and his FTA-ABS was positive. His RPR was checked 6 months ago and at that time was nonreactive.

What is the most appropriate antibiotic treatment?

A. Azithromycin – 2 g, once
B. Ceftriaxone – 500 mg IM, once
C. Doxycycline – 100 mg PO twice daily for 2 weeks
D. Penicillin G – 2.4 million units IM, once
E. Penicillin G – 2.4 million units IM, weekly, for three doses

42. A 24-year-old woman was admitted with 2 weeks of painful finger joints and 1 week of high fevers and a rash. She described the fevers as occurring every evening, and she would have normal temperatures in the morning. The rash only appeared during febrile episodes. On direct questioning, she recalled that her symptoms had been preceded by a sore throat and some swelling of the lymph nodes in her neck.

On examination her temperature was 39.1°C, her heart rate was 96 beats per minute, and her blood pressure was 105/62 mmHg. She had a salmon-pink macular rash over her trunk, upper arms, and thighs. There was no swelling or tenderness of the small joints of the hands. Cardiovascular and respiratory examinations were unremarkable. Her spleen tip was just palpable.

Investigations:
White cell count 25.8 ×10⁹/L (4.0–11.0)
Neutrophil count 24.2 ×10⁹/L (1.5–7.0)
Platelet count 468 ×10⁹/L (150–400)
ESR 90 mm/h
CRP 12 mg/L (<10)
Albumin 24 g/L (37–49)
Ferritin 3245 µg/L (15–300)

What is the most likely diagnosis?

A. Adult Still's disease
B. Epstein–Barr virus infection
C. Familial Mediterranean fever
D. Rheumatic fever
E. Systemic lupus erythematosus

43. An 18-year-old man presented after 8 weeks of an intermittent fever, arthralgia, headache, and pruritus. He had been born and brought up in the Central African Republic, but had emigrated 5 years earlier. He had not had any foreign travel since. He did not have any other medical problems, nor did he take any regular medications. He was heterosexual but denied any unprotected sexual intercourse. He had never injected drugs.

On examination his temperature was 38.1°C. He was slim but not cachectic. He had painlessly enlarged lymph nodes in his anterior and posterior cervical chains, axillary and inguinal chains. His spleen was enlarged 2 cm below the costal margin. His liver was not palpable.

Investigations:
FBC, renal function, liver function unremarkable
HIV-1 and -2 Ag/Ab negative
Blood cultures negative after 5 days
Blood film: no parasites seen
CXR: clear lung fields
LN aspirate: numerous elongated, flagellate protozoa with posterior kinetoplasts seen on Giemsa stain
CSF:
Protein 0.32 g/L (0.15–0.45)
White cell count 15/µL (≤5)
Red cell count <5/µL (0)
No organisms seen

What is the most appropriate treatment for this man?

A. Albendazole
B. Diethylcarbamazine
C. Ivermectin
D. Nifurtimox–eflornithine
E. Pentamidine

44. A 24-year-old man returned from a 4-week volunteering expedition in the slums of Mumbai. He had been fully vaccinated prior to travel but had not taken any malaria prophylaxis. One week after his return he developed sudden onset fever, rigors, myalgia, and headache. On examination, his temperature was 38.1°C, heart rate 108 beats per minute, blood pressure 110/55 mmHg. He was alert and oriented, and there was no neck stiffness or photophobia. There was no rash or lymphadenopathy. He had profound tenderness of the calf muscles and paraspinal muscles bilaterally, and bilateral conjunctival suffusion. Examination of his cardiovascular, respiratory, and abdominal systems was unremarkable.

Investigations:
Neutrophils 8.5 ×10⁹/L (1.5–7.0)
Platelets 124 ×10⁹/L (150–400)
Serum creatinine 139 µmol/L (60–110)
Serum ALT 75 U/L (5–35)
Serum creatine kinase 455 U/L (24–195)
Malaria film x3 negative

What is the most likely diagnosis?

A. Dengue
B. Influenza A (H1N1)
C. Leptospirosis
D. Nonfalciparum malaria
E. Scrub typhus

45. An *Escherichia coli* isolate is submitted for susceptibility testing. It is resistant to ampicillin, ceftriaxone, and aztreonam, and susceptible to cefoxitin, cefepime, ertapenem, piperacillin/tazobactam, and ciprofloxacin.

This pattern is suggestive of drug resistance mediated by what mechanism?

A. AmpC
B. Cell wall modification
C. ESBL
D. PBP alteration
E. Porin production

46. The K103N mutation confers resistance to which of the following antiretroviral medications?

A. Efavirenz
B. Emtricitabine
C. Etravirine
D. Raltegravir
E. Rilpivirine

47. What is the mechanism of action of amphotericin?

A. Increased cell membrane permeability through binding to ergosterol

B. Inhibition of 1,3-β-glucan synthesis

C. Inhibition of conversion of lanosterol to ergosterol

D. Inhibition of fungal squalene epoxidase

E. Inhibition of nucleic acid synthesis

48. A 17-year-old boy returns from a trip to Argentina. He spent time hiking and on the beach and received numerous insect bites. A few weeks after he returned, he developed a gradually enlarging ulcer on his leg. The lesion began as a papule that then ulcerated. He has not had fevers or significant drainage from the ulceration. On examination, he had a 3 cm ulcer with an erythematous base and a raised border. There was no purulent drainage or surrounding cellulitis. Evaluations for bacterial and mycobacterial infections are unrevealing, and a parasitic infection is suspected. Which of the following agents would be expected to have activity against the most likely causative pathogen?

A. Albendazole

B. Artesunate

C. Ivermectin

D. Paromomycin

E. Praziquantel

49. A 10-week-old infant was admitted to the pediatric intensive care unit with severe bronchopneumonia requiring intubation and ventilation. She suffered repeated apneic attacks. She had been born at full term by normal vaginal delivery, with no instrumentation. Her APGAR scores had been 8 and 9 at 1 and 5 minutes respectively. She had received her 8-week immunizations with DTaP/IPV/HiB, PCV, meningococcal B, and rotavirus vaccines 1 week before she became unwell. She lived at home with her parents, grandmother, and two older siblings. Initial investigations revealed a lymphocytosis.

What microbiological findings would be most consistent with this infection?

A. Bisected pearl colonies on charcoal cephalexin agar

B. Blue–grey colonies on Thayer Martin agar with vancomycin, colistin, nystatin

C. Grey colonies on Hoyle's agar with potassium tellurite

D. Colonies on buffered charcoal yeast extract agar with L cysteine which fluoresce yellow–green under UV light

E. Growth around combined X+V disc only on nutrient agar

50. A 54-year-old farmer in Massachusetts became acutely unwell in late August. He had had nonspecific symptoms which came on gradually for 1 week, including fatigue, anorexia, and headache. He then developed high sustained fevers, sweats, myalgia, and dark urine. His medical history included splenectomy following a road traffic accident 15 years earlier, hypercholesterolemia, and hypertension. He was up to date with his immunizations and took amlodipine and atorvastatin. He had not traveled outside of the US in the preceding 10 years and had not left Massachusetts in the preceding 6 months. He lived with his wife and two teenage daughters, all of whom were well.

On examination, he was visibly icteric, with pale conjunctivae, and was dyspneic at rest. His temperature was 38.5°C, heart rate 124 beats per minute, blood pressure 85/50 mmHg, respiratory rate 34 breaths per minute. He had inspiratory crackles to midzones bilaterally. His liver was palpable 2 cm below the right costal margin and his spleen tip was also palpable.

Investigations:

HIV Ag/Ab negative, hepatitis C IgG negative, HBS negative

Hemoglobin 63 g/L (130–180)

White blood cell count 17.6×10⁹/L

Neutrophil count 14.3×10⁹/L

Platelet count 112×10⁹/L

Serum creatinine 213 μmol/L (60–110)

Serum alkaline phosphatase 167 U/L (45–105)

Blood film:

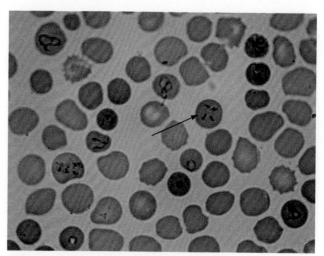

What is the most appropriate treatment?

A. Atovaquone plus azithromycin

B. Atovaquone plus proguanil

C. Chloroquine plus primaquine

D. Quinine sulfate plus clindamycin

E. Sulfadiazine plus pyrimethamine

Quiz 7

1. A 28-year-old man presented with a 2-month history of fevers, 15 lb weight loss and non-productive cough.

He was known to have HIV, complicated previously with *Pneumocystis jirovecii* pneumonia (PJP/PCP) and cryptococcal infections, and was noncompliant with his ART. He was intermittently on HAART until 6 months ago when he moved to the United States and had not set up care. He was from Vietnam, a nonsmoker, drank no alcohol, and denied any IVDU.

On examination, his temperature was 38.2°C, his heart rate was 80 beats/minute, blood pressure 110/70mmHg, and SPO_2 96% on RA. His exam showed cervical lymphadenopathy, decreased bilateral lung air-entry.
Investigations:

HIV viral load 50,090 copies/mL
CD_4 count 80/μL
CXR: interstitial infiltrates
Lymph-node biopsy: granulomas seen
LN fungal cultures grew the colony shown:

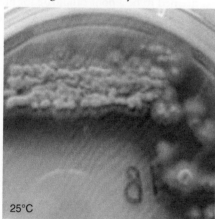

25°C

What is the most appropriate empiric therapy?

A. Amphotericin B
B. Fluconazole
C. Itraconazole
D. Posaconazole
E. Voriconazole

2. A 40-year-old man was diagnosed with endocarditis caused by viridans streptococcus. He had no known drug allergies. Pending availability of the minimum inhibitory concentration of the organism for penicillin, the patient was initiated on ceftriaxone IV plus gentamicin IV.
Investigations:

Serum creatinine 0.55 mg/dL
Total white cell count 14.5 ×10⁹/L
Normal liver function tests

What gentamicin serum concentration is in the desired range?

A. Peak concentration of 8 μg/mL
B. Peak concentration of 2.5 μg/mL
C. Trough concentration of 1.3 μg/mL
D. Trough concentration of 2 μg/mL
E. Trough concentration of 0.8 μg/mL

3. A 35-year-old man complained of new onset numbness around his mouth and face. He had been started on colistin (2.5 mg/kg ideal body weight IV q12 hours) 3 days earlier for a urinary tract infection and had clinically responded. He was paraplegic and had a long-term Foley catheter. He had no known drug allergies.

On examination, there were no appreciable lesions around his mouth. He was afebrile.
Investigations:

Total white cell count 10.1 ×10⁹/L (admission WCC 13.2 ×10⁹/L)
Serum creatinine 0.45 mg/dL (baseline serum creatinine = 0.4 mg/dL)
Admission urinalysis: 50 white blood cells/high power field; >10⁵CFU *Klebsiella pneumoniae*, resistant to meropenem, sensitive to colistin.
K. pneumoniae carbapenemase (KPC) detected

What is the most appropriate action?

A. Add ceftriaxone to colistin IV
B. Continue current colistin IV monotherapy
C. Discontinue antibiotic therapy
D. Switch colistin to ceftazidime–avibactam IV
E. Switch colistin to ceftolozane–tazobactam IV

4. A 65-year-old woman was prescribed levofloxacin, isoniazid, and ethambutol for treatment of *Mycobacterium tuberculosis*. She had a history of heartburn, which she treated with frequent calcium carbonate (TUMS®) and omeprazole.

What medication is most likely to cause a drug-drug interaction?

A. Calcium carbonate
B. Ethambutol
C. Isoniazid
D. Levofloxacin
E. Omeprazole

5. A 45-year-old woman had an acid-fast bacilli identified in her sputum culture. She had a history of diabetes mellitus, hypertension, and CKD stage III.

What medication can be given without dose adjustment for her renal impairment?

A. Amikacin
B. Ciprofloxacin
C. Doxycycline
D. Imipenem–cilastatin
E. Sulfamethoxazole–trimethoprim

6. A 3-year-old girl in Missouri was found asleep in a room with a bat. Her parents brought her to the clinic to assess the risk of rabies and to instigate management if required. She had not received rabies vaccinations prior to this.

What is the most appropriate action?

A. Check rabies antibody titers
B. Give 2 rabies vaccines (d0 and d3–7)
C. Give 4 vaccines (d0, d3, d7, d14) plus rabies immunoglobulin
D. Give 5 rabies vaccines (d0, d3, d7, d14, d28)
E. No postexposure treatment needed

7. A 24-year-old man presented with fevers, dyspnea, cough, and an erythematous rash. He was day 115 after an HLA-mismatched and T-cell-depleted allogeneic stem cell transplant for lymphoma. He had been treated at day 70 with prednisone for acute graft versus host disease.

Investigations:
Total white cell count 6.7 ×10⁹/L
CT chest: bilateral ground glass opacities
BAL cultures and stains negative
Urinalysis revealed hematuria with no bacteria on the stain
Serum cytomegalovirus PCR undetectable

What is the most likely cause?

A. Adenovirus
B. BK virus
C. Graft versus host disease
D. Herpes simplex virus
E. Varicella-zoster virus

8. A 42-year-old man presented with a 1-week history of fever and productive cough. He had a deceased donor renal transplant 7 months ago. He was taking tacrolimus, mycophenolate mofetil, and prednisone.

On exam his temperature was 38.6°C
Investigations:
CXR: left lower lobe nodule with central cavitation
Sputum microscopy revealed long, crooked, branching, beaded gram-positive filaments

What would be the most appropriate empiric therapy?

A. Ceftazidime
B. Penicillin
C. Tetracycline
D. Trimethoprim-sulfamethoxazole and imipenem
E. Tobramycin

9. A 62-year-old woman presented with subjective fevers without any localizing symptoms or signs. She had received a left ventricular assist device 6 months ago as destination strategy for chemotherapy-induced nonischemic cardiomyopathy, on a background of breast cancer.

On examination, her temperature was 38.5°C, her heart rate was 100 beats/minute, and her blood pressure was 136/80 mmHg.

Investigations:
4/4 blood cultures positive for methicillin-susceptible *Staphylococcus aureus*, resistant only to penicillin on extended susceptibility testing (sensitive to oxacillin, ceftriaxone, cefazolin, vancomycin, trimethoprim–sulfamethoxazole, doxycycline, and clindamycin)
CT chest/abdomen/pelvis: a large fluid collection surrounding the VAD pump with associated stranding and enhancement
Aspirate of collection fluid: MSSA isolated
She was deemed to be a poor candidate for open debridement and wash out, and nor was she a candidate for pump exchange.

What is the most appropriate initial treatment?

A. Cefazolin
B. Dalbavancin
C. Daptomycin
D. Linezolid
E. Vancomycin

10. A 74-year-old man presented with 2 days of watery diarrhea and 1 day of large fluid-filled skin lesions. He had a history of cirrhotic liver disease. He had recently returned from a fishing trip on the US Gulf Coast. He had been swimming in the hotel pool but not the sea. On examination he was dehydrated, his temperature was 38.3°C, blood pressure 88/52mmHg, heart rate 115 beats/minute.

Investigations:
Blood cultures: curved gram-negative rods seen on microscopy

What is the most likely infective cause?

A. *Aeromonas hydrophila*
B. *Campylobacter jejuni*
C. *Cryptosporidium parvum*
D. *Salmonella Typhi*
E. *Vibrio vulnificus*

11. A 22-year-old man presented to clinic with a "sore" on the shaft of his penis. He had noticed it 3 days earlier while showering. It was not painful. He denied dysuria or penile discharge. He returned from vacation in Panama 2 weeks ago. He reported unprotected sex with two female partners while in Panama. He had no known drug allergies.

On examination, there was a well-circumscribed firm lesion, 1 cm in diameter on the shaft of his penis.

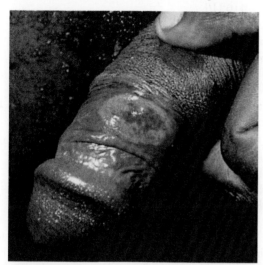

Laboratory testing was obtained, including HIV fourth-generation antibody test, urine gonorrhea and chlamydia NAAT, and a syphilis EIA.

What is the most appropriate action?

A. Administer benzathine penicillin IM for 3 doses at weekly intervals
B. Administer single dose of benzathine penicillin IM
C. Await syphilis screen and send a confirmatory anti-treponemal test if positive
D. Refer to dermatology for further evaluation
E. Start oral aciclovir

12. A 29-year-old man presented with fevers, headache, and myalgia. He had been treated 24 hours earlier with 2.4 million units of benzathine penicillin intramuscularly for a diagnosis of secondary syphilis. He reported four male sexual partners in the past 6 months, with inconsistent condom use.

On exam, he was diaphoretic, his blood pressure was 96/56 mmHg, heart rate 106 beats/minute, and his temperature was 38.2°C. He had a diffuse macular rash which included the soles of his feet and his palms. There was no meningism.

Investigations:
Syphilis EIA positive
RPR positive 1:128
Specific antitreponemal antibody positive
HIV fourth-generation Ag/Ab test failed – please send a repeat

What is the most likely explanation?

A. Coincidental influenza infection
B. Delayed anaphylaxis to penicillin
C. Inflammatory response to dying spirochetes
D. Primary HIV infection
E. Sepsis secondary to intramuscular injection

13. A 20-week pregnant woman presented to antenatal clinic 1 day after an exposure to a child with slapped cheek at the school where she works. She was asymptomatic.

Investigations:
Parvovirus B19 IgM not detected
Parvovirus B19 IgG not detected

What is the most appropriate advice?

A. Advise her that she cannot return to work
B. Reassurance only
C. Refer for serial ultrasound scan monitoring
D. Repeat parvovirus B19 serology at 4 weeks following exposure
E. Request serologic testing for toxoplasma, rubella, and CMV

14. A 35-year-old woman presented with a painless, non-healing skin lesion on her left foot, which developed over 4 weeks. She also described 2 months of fever, fatigue, and a dry cough, which had not responded to a short course of levofloxacin. She had no significant past medical history. She worked as a landscaper for the city park district in Chicago, Illinois.

Investigations:
CXR: left lower lobe infiltrate
Bronchoscopy and skin biopsy were performed (GMS stain of transbronchial biopsy shown below):

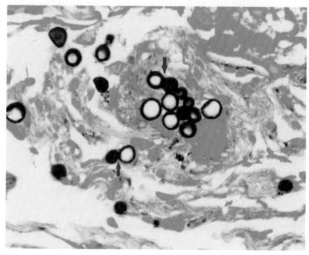

What is the most appropriate treatment?

A. Amphotericin B
B. Caspofungin
C. Itraconazole
D. Prednisone
E. Posaconazole

15. A 51-year-old woman was admitted with a 2-day history of dizziness. She had been out gardening all summer. She initially thought the dry heat was making her dehydrated, but her symptoms persisted despite water intake. She was a college professor in Connecticut and gardened every afternoon. She had not noted any tick bites or rashes. She had a history of osteoarthritis of her knees, hypertension, and raised cholesterol. She took occasional acetaminophen (paracetamol) and was taking amlodipine and atorvastatin.

Physical exam was unremarkable except for a heart rate of 47 beats/minute.

ECG:

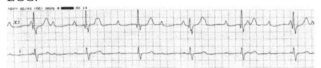

Initial enzyme-linked immunosorbent assay and a confirmatory Western blot assay were positive for *Borrelia burgdorferi*.

What is the most appropriate initial treatment?

A. Amoxicillin
B. Ceftriaxone
C. Cefuroxime
D. Doxycycline
E. Pacemaker placement

16. A 42-year-old woman developed fever and worsening confusion that evolved over 1 week. A collateral history was obtained from her partner. She worked as a zookeeper. She was usually assigned to the alligators but 2 weeks prior to presentation, she had been asked to care for the macaques as well. She had been bitten by one of the pregnant macaques and sustained a minor wound in her hand. Six months previously, she had traveled to South Africa for wilderness training related to her work. During this training, she encountered a lot of wild animals including monkeys, giraffes, lions, hyenas, and vultures. She did not take malarial and typhoid prophylaxis before the trip and had sustained multiple tick and mosquito bites.

On physical exam, she had a temperature of 40.1°C and blood pressure of 140/100 mmHg. She was disoriented and confused; there was no nuchal or muscle rigidity.

Investigations:
MRI brain: normal appearances
CSF exam: pleocytosis (lymphocyte predominant), normal glucose, and elevated total protein

What strategy could have prevented her from developing encephalitis?

A. Aciclovir prophylaxis
B. Atovaquone–proguanil prophylaxis
C. DEET-based repellents
D. Doxycycline prophylaxis
E. Tetanus immunization

17. An 80-year-old woman presented with a 5-day history of general malaise, anorexia, nausea, and two emetic episodes. She was on her fourth week of treatment with rifampin, isoniazid, ethambutol, and pyrazinamide for TB uveitis. One week earlier, she had nasal congestion and sore throat that was self-limited, for which she took acetaminophen twice a day.

Investigations:
Total white cell count 8.3 ×10⁹/L
AST 410 U/L
ALT 389 U/L
Total bilirubin 1.3 mg/dL
INR 1.1
Alkaline phosphatase 85 U/L
Albumin 42g/L

What is unlikely to have caused her drug-induced liver injury?

A. Acetaminophen
B. Ethambutol
C. Isoniazid
D. Pyrazinamide
E. Rifampin

18. A 65-year-old woman presented with 2 weeks of fever, diarrhea, and unintentional weight loss. She had a history of hypertension and migraines. She was a retired attorney and had been working with an NGO in rural Uganda (East Africa) for the past 5 months. She started to feel poorly while still in Uganda and was administered "something for malaria" by a local physician without symptomatic improvement.

On examination, her temperature was 38.3°C, and there was slight nuchal discomfort on neck flexion. Examination otherwise was unremarkable.

Investigations:
Total white cell count 7.3 ×10⁹/L
Hemoglobin 13.2 g/dL
Creatinine clearance 59 mL/min
Malaria rapid antigen test negative
Peripheral blood film: flagellated, spindle-shaped organism seen on several fields

What is the most likely agent?

A. *Giardia duodenalis*
B. *Plasmodium falciparum*
C. *Trypanosoma brucei gambiense*
D. *Trypanosoma brucei rhodesiense*
E. *Trypanosoma cruzi*

19. A 45-year-old woman presented with high fevers, severe muscle pain, tenderness, and swelling. There was no significant past medical history. There were no other symptoms reported, no recent unusual activities, although she did recall eating some undercooked pork 3 weeks previously.

On examination her temperature was 38.6°C. She was tender and had limited movement due to pain in the muscles of her shoulder girdle, upper arms, and forearms. There were numerous subungual splinter hemorrhages seen, and she had bilateral conjunctival hemorrhages. Mild hepatomegaly was palpable.

Investigations:

    Total white cell count 13.2 ×10⁹/L
    Eosinophil count 4.1 ×10⁹/L

What parasite is most likely to be responsible?

A. *Brugia malayi*
B. *Paragonimus westermani*
C. *Toxoplasma gondii*
D. *Trichinella spiralis*
E. *Wuchereria bancrofti*

20. A 55-year-old man presented with new-onset neurologic deficits. He reported having mental slowing, with poor concentration and memory loss. As an example, he reported getting lost when driving to his home of 20 years. He was known to have HIV and was taking antiretroviral therapy.

Neurologic examination was normal. A CT head and lumbar puncture were performed.

Investigations:

    CD4 count 760 cells/μL
    HIV viral load undetectable
    CT head without contrast: normal
    CSF white cell count 6 ×10⁶/L
    CSF HIV viral load 12,588 copies/mL

What is the most important diagnostic test to guide management?

A. B12, thyroid function, and syphilis screen
B. HIV genotyping of the CSF virus
C. MRI brain
D. Nerve conduction studies
E. Psychometric testing

21. A 33-year-old woman attended outpatient clinic having recently moved to the United States from Zimbabwe. She was not on antiretroviral therapy but reported receiving ART during delivery of her first child and antenatally during her second pregnancy.

Investigations:

    CD4 count 370 cells/μL
    HIV viral load 36,000 copies/mL
    HIV genotype: Y181C mutation detected

What antiretroviral agent is contraindicated with this mutation?

A. Didanosine
B. Lamivudine
C. Lopinavir
D. Nevirapine
E. Zidovudine

22. A 46-year-old man presented with a 6-week history of progressive right arm weakness and a 1-week history of increasing confusion and word-finding difficulties. He was known to have HIV, and although previously on ART he had been lost to clinical care and follow-up 3 years earlier.

On physical exam, neurologic exam was notable for 3/5 strength in the right upper extremity and an expressive aphasia.

Investigations:

    MRI of the brain: there are multiple discrete lesions in the cortical white matter and basal ganglia, which are hyperintense on the T2-weighted imaging sequences.
    CD4 count 125 cells/μL
    HIV viral load 45,200 copies/mL
    Serum RPR negative
    Serum cryptococcal antigen negative
    Toxoplasma IgG negative

What is the most appropriate treatment?

A. Aciclovir
B. Antiretroviral therapy
C. Cidofovir
D. Ganciclovir
E. Mirtazapine

23. A 43-year-old woman presented with a 2-week history of progressive dyspnea and fatigue. She had a past medical history of advanced HIV but was not taking any ART.

On physical exam, her blood pressure was 95/50 mmHg and heart rate 105 beats/min with an oxygen saturation of 95% on room air. Heart sounds were muffled, and she had elevated jugular venous distention.

Investigations:

    CXR: enlarged cardiac silhouette
    Trans-thoracic echocardiogram: large pericardial effusion
    CD4 45 cells/μL
    HIV viral load 76,850 copies/mL
    Flow cytometry of pericardial fluid: a clonal population of malignant lymphocytes, positive for CD45 and latency-associated nuclear antigen-1 (LANA-1) but negative for CD3, CD4, CD19, and CD20

What viral pathogen is most closely associated with this patient's clinical presentation?

A. Cytomegalovirus
B. Human herpesvirus 8
C. Herpes simplex virus
D. Parvovirus B19
E. Varicella-zoster virus

24. A 50-year-old man presented with left arm redness accompanied by swelling and pain. The redness had progressed to involve the entire arm and left hand. He had received a number of courses of oral antibiotics with no improvement. He had diabetes mellitus and a living unrelated kidney transplant 15 years earlier for end-stage renal disease.

A skin biopsy was performed.

Investigations:

Skin biopsy: organisms highlighted with Fontana Masson staining

What is the most likely causative organism?

A. *Blastomyces dermatitidis*
B. *Coccidioides immitis*
C. *Cryptococcus neoformans*
D. *Histoplasma capsulatum*
E. *Talaromyces (Penicillium) marneffei*

25. A 35-year-old woman presented with a 5-day history of diarrhea and shortness of breath. She had experienced bloody diarrhea and associated abdominal cramps, along with a dry cough but had not had any hemoptysis, chest pain, fevers, chills, or night sweats. She had relapsed Hodgkin's lymphoma postallogeneic stem cell transplant 2 months ago, complicated by graft versus host disease (GVHD) of the gut, skin, and lungs. She had been treated with prednisone and tacrolimus, and the GVHD was felt to be under control. She was also taking trimethoprim–sulfamethoxazole, levofloxacin, aciclovir, and voriconazole prophylaxis. She denied sick contacts and lived in an urban area.

On examination, her temperature was 37.1°C, her blood pressure was 110/58 mmHg, her heart rate was 115 beats/min, respiratory rate 24 breaths/minute, O_2 saturation 92% on 6 L/minute oxygen. She had pale conjunctivae. Respiratory examination revealed diffuse crackles bilaterally but no ronchi or wheezes. Her abdomen was soft with mild diffuse tenderness to palpation and normal bowel sounds. There was 1+ pedal edema, and hyperpigmented areas on the arms/legs at sites of prior GVHD of the skin.

Investigations:

Total white cell count 3.0×10^9 /L
Absolute neutrophil count 1.6×10^9 /L
Hemoglobin 8 g/dL
Platelets 98×10^9/L
Urea, creatinine, and electrolytes were within normal limits
Blood cultures: no growth at 48 hours
C. difficile PCR negative
Stool culture and stool ova and parasites negative
CXR: bilateral interstitial infiltrates, no consolidation, no effusions
CT abdomen/pelvis with and without contrast revealed diffuse colitis, no lymphadenopathy, no abscesses

What is the most likely pathogen?

A. *Clostridioides difficile*
B. Cytomegalovirus
C. *Pneumocystis jirovecii*
D. *Strongyloides stercoralis*
E. Varicella zoster

26. A 19-year-old man was diagnosed with chronic mucocutaneous candidiasis (CMC) after recurrent infections from the age of 5 years old. Hypoparathyroidism was diagnosed after an episode of tetanic spasms at 10 years old. At 15 years of age, he developed adrenal insufficiency.

What is the most likely diagnosis?

A. A defect in the IL-17 axis
B. APECED syndrome
C. CARD9 deficiency
D. DiGeorge syndrome
E. MCM4 deficiency

27. An outbreak of illness was reported among 50 people eating at a local restaurant. These individuals had an illness that consisted of predominately vomiting but nausea, abdominal cramps, and diarrhea were also present. Fever was present in the majority of the affected individuals. The median incubation period was 31 hours. The illness lasted approximately 48 hours. Only one person required hospitalization.

What was the most likely cause of the outbreak?

A. *Campylobacter jejuni*
B. Enterotoxigenic E. *coli* (ETEC)
C. Norovirus
D. Preformed *Staphylococcus aureus* enterotoxin
E. Shiga toxin-producing E. *coli* O157:H7 (STEC)

28. A 48-year-old man with idiopathic (immune) thrombocytopenic purpura was listed for an elective splenectomy.

What vaccination would be most appropriate?

A. BCG vaccine
B. *Haemophilus influenzae* type b vaccine
C. Hepatitis B vaccine
D. HPV vaccine
E. Varicella-zoster vaccine

29. A 9-year-old boy was reviewed with a 4-week history of mild abdominal discomfort, anorexia, and some loose stools. He was normally resident in California but had returned from 2 months living with family in Mexico 1 month prior to symptom onset.

Examination was unremarkable.

Investigations:

Stool OCP:

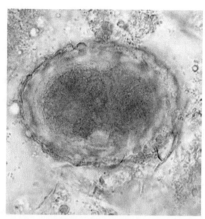

What parasite is most likely to be causing his symptoms?

A. *Ancylostoma duodenale*
B. *Ascaris lumbricoides*
C. *Enterobius vermicularis*
D. *Strongyloides stercoralis*
E. *Trichuris trichiura*

30. A 45-year-old man presents with acute unilateral vision loss. On funduscopic examination, he has significant vitreitis and retinal findings concerning for acute retinal necrosis.

What therapy should be administered?

A. Aciclovir
B. Corticosteroids
C. Foscarnet
D. Ganciclovir
E. Penicillin

31. A 50-year-old patient admitted with STEMI, now status-post CABG, and with a complicated hospital course thereafter, including prolonged respiratory failure requiring tracheostomy and gastrostomy tube placements, who also received several days of broad-spectrum antibiotics postoperatively because of shock, and concern for possible sepsis, is now having increasing supplemental oxygen requirement and fever. His chest radiograph shows diffuse pulmonary opacities, worst in the right-lower lobe. His nurse also has noted increasingly profuse and purulent tracheal secretions. He was started on linezolid and meropenem, but after 2 days he was still having fevers, and his respiratory status continued to worsen. Tracheal aspirate culture is now growing an organism that was identified as an oxidase-positive, nonfermenting gram-negative bacillus.

What is the most likely cause of his symptoms?

A. *Burkholderia cepacia*
B. *Citrobacter freundii*
C. *Escherichia coli*
D. *Serratia marcescens*
E. *Stenotrophomonas maltophilia*

32. A 42-year-old male cigarette smoker presents with several months of fever, night sweats, weight loss, cough, and hemoptysis. His chest radiograph showed bilateral pulmonary infiltrates with left upper lobe cavitary disease. Sputum samples were obtained for acid-fast stain and the stain was positive. An interferon-gamma release assay was obtained, and was also positive. PCR on the sputum sample was negative for detection of *Mycobacterium tuberculosis*.

What is the most likely cause of his symptoms?

A. *Mycobacterium bovis*
B. *Mycobacterium gordonae*
C. *Mycobacterium kansasii*
D. *Mycobacterium marinum*
E. *Mycobacterium ulcerans*

33. A 23-year-old man with HIV was admitted to the hospital with septic shock. His CD4 count was 25/µL, and he was not on antiretroviral therapy. On examination, he had diffuse rhonchi, and he was noted to have multiple papular skin lesions. His chest radiograph showed bilateral pulmonary infiltrates. He was started on broad-spectrum antibiotic therapy. Four days into his hospitalization, his blood cultures grew mold. He also had a skin biopsy done and Gomori methenamine stain of the tissue shows 2–4 µm yeast forms (see image).

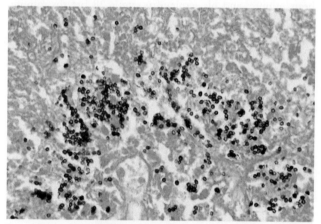

In addition to antibacterial therapy, what other antimicrobials should be instituted?

A. 5-Flucytosine
B. Amphotericin B
C. Fluconazole
D. Micafungin
E. Trimethoprim–sulfamethoxazole

34. The yeast seen in this lung biopsy specimen is most likely what organism?

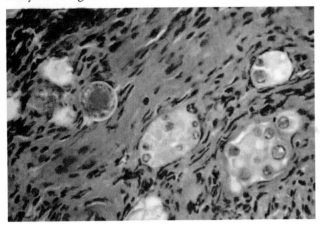

A. *Blastomyces dermatitidis*
B. *Coccidioides immitis*
C. *Cryptococcus neoformans*
D. *Histoplasma capsulatum*
E. *Paracoccidioides brasiliensis*

35. A 35-year-old man presents with a 4-week history of worsening exertional dyspnea, dry cough, and mild fever. On examination his temperature is 37.9°C, his heart rate is 110 beats/minute, and his respiratory rate is 28 breaths/minute. Oxygen saturations are 90% on room air. He has oral candidiasis and small volume lymphadenopathy in his axillary, cervical, and inguinal chains. Auscultation of his chest is unremarkable.
Investigations:

> Arterial blood gas $PO2$ ($FiO2$ room air) 7.8 kPa
> CXR: see radiograph below

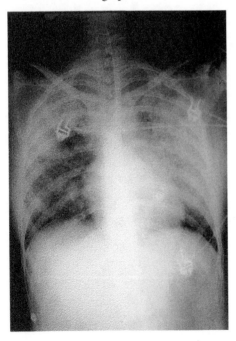

He is started empirically on intravenous trimethoprim–sulfamethoxazole (TMP–SMX) and methylprednisolone.

On the second day of treatment he develops a widespread rash consistent with erythema multiforme, including oral ulceration and eye involvement. His TMP–SMX is identified as the likely cause.

What is the most appropriate treatment choice?

A. Continue TMP–SMX at a reduced dose of 90 mg/kg per day
B. Start immediate desensitization regimen for TMP–SMX
C. Switch to dapsone plus trimethoprim
D. Switch to atovaquone
E. Switch to clindamycin plus primaquine

36. A 28-year-old woman from Zimbabwe presented with a 2-week history of increasing confusion, ataxia, headache, and fevers. She was admitted and a lumbar puncture performed after a CT scan of her head.
Investigations:

> HIV-1 Ag/Ab positive
> CD4 5 cells/μL
> HIV viral load 225 000 copies/mL
> Serum CRAG positive
> CSF: opening pressure 450 mmH$_2$O (120–250)
> Protein 0.9 g/L (0.15–0.45)
> Glucose 2.3 mmol/L (plasma glucose 7.2)
> White blood cells 0.05 ×10^9/L(50/mm^3), 90% lymphocytes
> Cryptococcal antigen positive
> CSF cultures: growth on Sab plates consistent with *Cryptococcus neoformans*

She was started on liposomal amphotericin B and 5-flucytosine.

When should she be started on antiretrovirals?

A. After 2 months of antifungals
B. After 4 weeks of antifungals
C. Immediately
D. When a repeat CSF is culture negative
E. When her serum CRAG becomes negative

37. A 28-year-old woman presented with a 5-day history of diarrhea, malaise, abdominal pain, nausea, and flatulence. She was opening her bowels on average 12 times per day. There was no blood or mucus. She attended a regular swimming class with her 9-month-old daughter, and the pool had been closed one week earlier after an outbreak of diarrhea.

Stool microscopy: multiple red oocysts, 4–6 μm diameter seen on modified acid-fast stain.

What is the most appropriate treatment?

A. Ciprofloxacin
B. Metronidazole
C. Nitazoxanide
D. Paromomycin
E. Trimethoprim–sulfamethoxazole

38. A 27-year-old man presented with 3 weeks of fever, headache, malaise, abdominal pain, and constipation. He had returned from a 6-month trip to India 2 weeks before his symptoms began. On examination, he was confused on admission but with no focal neurology or meningism. His temperature was 39.2°C, heart rate 75 beats per minute, blood pressure 110/56 mmHg. A CT scan of the head and lumbar puncture were performed, with normal CSF findings. The CT was unremarkable. He was started empirically on intravenous ceftriaxone, fluid resuscitated, and admitted to the high dependency unit. Three malaria smears at 12-hour intervals were negative. Twenty-four hours after admission he developed worsening abdominal pain, and he had peritonitis on examination. He was taken for an exploratory laparotomy (see image).

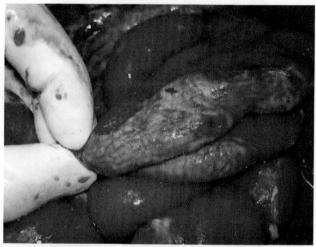

Blood cultures on admission grew gram-negative rods at 48 hours.

What part of the bowel is most likely to be involved?

A. Cecum
B. Descending colon
C. Duodenum
D. Sigmoid colon
E. Terminal ileum

39. A 47-year-old man developed fever and headache 1 week after returning from an 8-week holiday to South America. He had stayed in a retreat in the middle of the Amazon jungle. He did not seek travel advice before his travel and had not taken any malaria prophylaxis or travel vaccinations. He had stayed in a wood hut with palm leaf roof. He slept under a bednet, but he ran out of mosquito repellent. He had been well while there. His symptoms had persisted for 4 days before he sought medical attention. A fellow traveler had informed him that she had been diagnosed with malaria.

On examination he was alert and oriented. His heart rate was 88 beats per minute, blood pressure 110/74 mmHg, temperature 37.1°C. He was thin, but there was no palpable lymphadenopathy or rash. Examination of his cardiovascular, respiratory, and abdominal systems was unremarkable.

Investigations:

Hemoglobin 114 g/L (130–180)
Platelet count 137 ×10⁹/L (150–400)
Serum creatinine 74 μmol/L (60–110)
Malaria antigen positive
Malaria film: see image

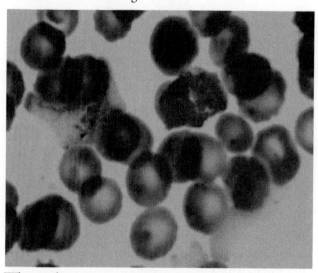

What is the most appropriate treatment?

A. Artemether–lumefantrine
B. Artesunate plus doxycycline
C. Chloroquine plus primaquine
D. Quinine plus clindamycin
E. Sulfadoxine–pyrimethamine

40. A 33-year-old Somalian man presented with a 6-month history of fever, weight loss, abdominal discomfort, and swelling. He had also noticed recurrent epistaxis. He had left Somalia 1 year before his symptoms began. On examination, he was cachectic, with bipedal edema. His spleen was palpable 8 cm below the left costal margin. There were lymph nodes palpable in both inguinal chains.

Investigations:

Hemoglobin 85 g/L (130–180)
Platelets 68×10⁹/L (150–400)
White cell count 1.8×10⁹/L (4.0–11.0)
Albumin 24 g/L (37–49)
HIV Ag/Ab negative
Bone marrow aspirate (see image):

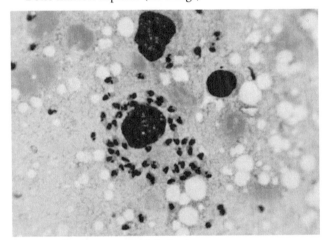

What is the treatment of choice?

A. Liposomal amphotericin B
B. Miltefosine
C. Paromomycin
D. Pentamidine
E. Sodium stibogluconate

41. A 59-year-old man was admitted with new-onset urinary retention following 72 hours of dysuria and 1 week of malaise. He had osteoarthritis of the right knee. He was not on any regular medication. He had returned from a 4-week holiday to northern Australia 2 weeks before he developed symptoms. His temperature was 38.3°C, heart rate 110 beats per minute. Blood cultures were taken. Digital rectal examination revealed a tender boggy prostate. He was given a single dose of gentamicin 5 mg/kg and started on regular co-amoxiclav, 1.2 g TDS IV.

Investigations:

Transrectal ultrasound of prostate: large prostatic abscess, maximum diameter 4.5 cm
CT scan of abdomen and pelvis: small abscess in upper pole of left kidney, maximum diameter 2.4 cm
Random glucose 17.3 mmol/L
Glycosylated hemoglobin 12.8%
Blood cultures: gram-negative rods at 14 hours
Colonies on Ashdown agar: oxidase positive; bipolar staining on Gram stain (see images)

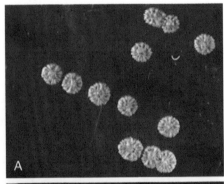

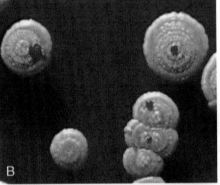

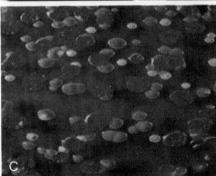

He was switched to meropenem. After 7 days he was still regularly having temperatures >38°C but was cardiovascularly stable.

What is the most appropriate management?

A. Add gentamicin
B. Continue current treatment
C. Switch to ceftazidime
D. Switch to colistin
E. Switch to trimethoprim–sulfamethoxazole

42. Which of the following antibiotics is bacteriostatic against sensitive strains of *Staphylococcus aureus*?

A. Ceftaroline
B. Daptomycin
C. Linezolid
D. Oxacillin
E. Vancomycin

43. A 45-year-old man presents with a new diagnosis of HIV and cerebral toxoplasmosis. He was started on sulfadiazine and pyrimethamine, as well as raltegravir, emtricitabine, and tenofovir. Three weeks later, he is admitted with nephrolithiasis. Which of his medications would be most likely to cause development of renal stones?

A. Emtricitabine
B. Pyrimethamine
C. Raltegravir
D. Sulfadiazine
E. Tenofovir

44. An 11-month-old boy developed a high fever. This was associated with malaise, irritability, and poor feeding. After 48 hours he developed a macular rash along his arms and legs. There was extensive confluent blistering of the perineum, but otherwise the trunk and back were spared. There were no lesions on his scalp. There were a number of perioral lesions but no lesions visible inside the mouth. Some of the lesions progressed into thin-walled vesicles containing clear fluid. There were macules on the soles of his feet. The fever resolved 24 hours after the rash appeared. The rash took 10 days to clear but left no scars. Three weeks later the skin on his feet began to desquamate. He attended a nursery for 3 days a week. He had had his vaccinations as per the UK schedule for his age. He had been born at full term and was meeting his developmental milestones. He lived at home with two older siblings.

What is the most likely pathogen?

A. Adenovirus
B. Coxsackievirus A6
C. Echovirus
D. Herpes simplex virus 1
E. Varicella-zoster virus

45. A 24-year-old pregnant woman attended her GP at 14/40 as her 2-year-old daughter had developed a rash and fever consistent with chickenpox that morning. She had been born and brought up in the UK. She was unsure of her varicella immune status.

What is the most appropriate management?

A. Ask her to re-attend if a rash illness develops
B. Check her varicella-zoster IgG
C. Give her intramuscular varicella zoster immunoglobulin
D. Give her varicella-zoster vaccine
E. Reassure her that she is likely to be immune

46. A 42-year-old man with polycystic kidney disease underwent cadaveric renal transplantation, cytomegalovirus D/R-, HLA-incompatible. His immunosuppressive regimen consisted of tacrolimus, prednisolone, and mycophenolate mofetil. He was taking trimethoprim–sulfamethoxazole for PCP prophylaxis. At 10 months after the transplantation he reported rose-colored urine. He was otherwise well.

Urinalysis: leukocytes ++, hematuria +++
Creatinine 238 μmol/L

What investigation is most likely to be diagnostic?

A. Plasma for CMV PCR
B. Renal biopsy
C. Serum galactomannan
D. Urine cytology for decoy cells
E. Urine for BK virus PCR

47. During an outbreak of West Nile virus (WNV) in late summer in northern Texas, a 44-year-old woman presented with a 4-day history of fever, headache, abdominal pain, myalgias, and anorexia. She had attended the emergency department as she had noticed difficulty in walking and twitching of her thigh muscles in the preceding 24 hours. On examination she had reduced power grade 3/5 in left hip flexion and knee extension, absent deep tendon reflexes in both lower limbs, and widespread generalized fasciculations. Sensory examination was normal.
CSF microscopy:

Total protein 0.55 g/L (0.15–0.45)
Glucose 4.1 mmol/L (3.3–4.4)
White cell count 0.34 ×10⁹/L (≤5), 70% polymorphs
CSF PCR panel HSV-1+2/VZV/enterovirus/echovirus/WNV negative
Acute serum: WNV IgM antibody positive
Convalescent serum: significantly high titer of neutralizing antibodies to WNV (1: 320)
MRI: spine ill-defined nonenhancing hyperintensity in the cervicothoracic cord

What is the likelihood that she will recover strength to near baseline?

A. 5%
B. 20%
C. 35%
D. 75%
E. 95%

48. A 24-year-old primigravida, 32+4/40 attended with a 1-day history of fever, chills, myalgia, and malaise. The pregnancy had been uncomplicated to date. She had had all her childhood vaccinations on schedule and had not been in contact with a rash illness in this pregnancy. She worked in an office. No other contacts were unwell. A single temperature measurement was 38.0°C, but otherwise there was no other abnormality. There was no meningism, no rash, and no pharyngitis. Bedside urinalysis was negative. She was kept for 6 hours' observation during which she was afebrile. She was discharged home with advice to seek help if her symptoms persisted. Three days later, her clinician was phoned by the microbiology laboratory with the following result:

Blood cultures: gram-positive rods

What are the possible consequences that should be taken into consideration?

A. Congenital glaucoma
B. Hydrocephalus
C. No increased risk of adverse outcome
D. Stillbirth
E. Thrombocytopenic purpura

49. A 23-year-old man attended the out of hours medical service and asked about postexposure prophylaxis for leptospirosis. He had fallen into a canal earlier that day, and had been fully submerged. He was taking isotretinoin for acne but was not on any other regular medication. He had no known drug allergies. He had no open grazes and had showered 1 hour after the incident.

What is the most appropriate postexposure prophylaxis?

A. Amoxicillin
B. Azithromycin
C. Doxycycline
D. No prophylaxis required
E. Trimethoprim–sulfamethoxazole

50. A 56-year-old man presented with a slow-growing painless soft tissue swelling of the perimandibular region over 2 months. It had started discharging small amounts of pus through a small opening in the skin 2 weeks earlier. It had responded temporarily to a short course of co-amoxiclav but had then relapsed. He had no weight loss, fever, chills, or other constitutional symptoms. He was otherwise in good health, worked in an office, and had a long-term male partner. He smoked 15 cigarettes a day. There was no history of recent dental work or trauma to the face or mouth.

On examination there was a firm 4×5 cm mass in right submandibular region, tender to palpate, and partially fixed on the deep tissue planes. The overlying skin was slightly bluish in color, and there was a small sinus discharging thick yellow exudate.

Investigations:

CT head/neck: ill-defined mass in the left pyriform fossa involving the perimandibular gland and platysma muscle. Mass is infiltrative, crossing tissue planes. Moderately enhancing with several low attenuating foci. No associated lymphadenopathy

A biopsy was performed:
Direct microscopy: scanty gram-positive bacilli seen; branching filaments, diphtheroids, and coccobacilli
Modified Kinyoun stain negative

Bacterial cultures: aerobic, enhanced CO_2 and anaerobic cultures negative

Fungal cultures: no growth at 25°C or 37°C

Histology: chronic inflammation with the presence of multiple granules surrounded by polymorphonuclear leukocytes; an eosinophilic fringe surrounds the PMN zone

What is the most likely diagnosis?

A. Actinomycosis
B. Mucormycosis
C. Nocardiosis
D. Nontuberculous mycobacterial infection
E. Tuberculosis

Quiz 8

1. A 34-year-old woman presented with 3 days of diarrhea and severe abdominal pain. She was living in Texas but had traveled to Mexico to visit family 2 weeks prior to presentation. The patient reported drinking raw milk routinely and had a 3-year-old daughter in daycare.

Investigations:

Multiplex gastrointestinal panel PCR: positive for Shiga toxin 2

What is the most appropriate management?

A. Monitor for development of HUS

B. Reassurance only

C. Request *Escherichia coli* O157 culture

D. Treat with azithromycin

E. Treat with ciprofloxacin

2. A 71-year-old woman presented with fevers and a discharging wound on her right calf. She had a recent right calf fasciotomy due to a popliteal thrombus and end-stage renal disease on regular thrice-weekly conventional hemodialysis. She had no known drug allergies.

On examination her temperature was 38.6°C, and there was purulent discharge from her right calf incision site.

Investigations:

Total white blood cell count 12,500 cells/mm^3

Wound swab culture: positive for methicillin-sensitive *Staphylococcus aureus* (MSSA)

2/2 blood cultures positive for MSSA

What would be most appropriate for thrice-weekly posthemodialysis dosing for treatment of this patient's infection, assuming a planned duration of therapy of 4–6 weeks?

A. Cefazolin

B. Ceftazidime

C. Linezolid

D. Oritavancin

E. Vancomycin

3. A 52-year-old man presented in status epilepticus. He was usually fit and well and had returned 1 week earlier from a 2-month visit to Taiwan to visit family. He had no history of recent hospital admission or attendance. He did not take any regular medications, nor did he use any recreational drugs.

On examination he had a temperature of 38.3°C, and his pulse was 110 beats/minute.

He was sedated, intubated, and transferred to critical care following an urgent CT scan with contrast. Empirical treatment with ceftriaxone and metronidazole was commenced.

Investigations:

White cell count 23.1 ×10^9/L (4–11)

Neutrophil count 21.8 ×10^9/L (2–7.5)

C-reactive protein 245 mg/L (0–5)

Alkaline phosphatase 197 U/L (40–129)

ALT 50 U/L (0–41)

Total bilirubin 13 μmol/L (0–21)

CT head:

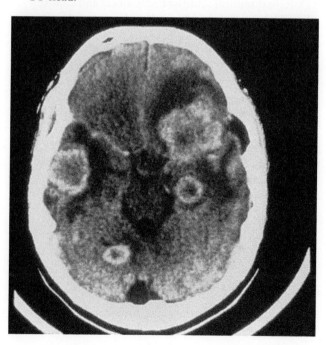

Liver USS: The liver is heterogenous and mildly enlarged. In the left lobe there is a 79 × 71 × 58mm well-circumscribed, heterogenous area with no vascularity; ? liver abscess

What is the most likely causative organism?

A. *Aspergillus fumigatus*
B. *Escherichia coli*
C. *Klebsiella pneumoniae*
D. *Nocardia asteroides*
E. *Staphylococcus aureus*

4. A 59-year-old woman was evaluated for a dry cough with moderate exertional dyspnea, which had remained stable in intensity over the past 8 months. She had occasionally been treated with antibiotics as an outpatient without any change in her symptoms. She had no systemic signs or symptoms. She was a nonsmoker and took no medications.

On physical examination, vital signs were normal. Pulmonary auscultation revealed scattered rhonchi. The remainder of the examination was normal.
Investigations:

CT lungs: nodular infiltrates, mostly confined to the right middle and bilateral upper lobes

Induced sputum: smear for acid-fast bacilli negative; culture positive at 24 days for *Mycobacterium avium* complex

What is the most appropriate action?

A. Bronchoalveolar lavage
B. Clarithromycin, ethambutol, and rifampin treatment
C. Observation
D. Repeat sputum acid-fast bacilli smear and culture
E. Video-assisted thorascopic lung biopsy

5. A 50-year-old man was admitted with a 1-week history of nasal congestion, rhinorrhea, dry cough, fever, chills, and myalgia. He was beginning to feel better until 48 hours ago when he developed recurrence of fever and chills, a productive cough with blood-streaked sputum, and right-sided pleuritic chest pain.

On physical examination, his temperature was 38.8°C, blood pressure 100/50 mmHg, pulse rate 110/minute, and respiration rate 24/minute.

CXR: right middle lobe airspace disease with a small area of cavitation as well as blunting of the right costophrenic angle.

What is the most appropriate treatment?

A. Amoxicillin and doxycycline
B. Daptomycin, oseltamivir, and azithromycin
C. Levofloxacin
D. Piperacillin/tazobactam and clarithromycin
E. Vancomycin, ceftriaxone, and azithromycin

6. A 27-year-old man presented with a 5-week history of throat pain and difficulty swallowing. The odynophagia had worsened over time, limiting oral intake. He had had a negative rapid strep test and a 2-week course of penicillin without symptomatic response. He had 1 week of night sweats but no fever or chills. He had a dry cough for 2 weeks but no dyspnea.

He had insulin-dependent diabetes mellitus and had renal transplantation 18 months prior. He had been born and brought up in Indonesia and had come to the United States for college. He had been screened for TB 4 years earlier and had had a chest X-ray then which showed a small linear opacity in the right lower lobe. Tuberculosis skin and sputum testing at that time was negative.

Current medications included prednisone 7.5 mg daily, mycophenolate 1 gram twice daily, and tacrolimus 2 mg twice daily.

On examination his temperature was 98.2°F. Tonsils and posterior pharynx were inflamed and erythematous. There were no exudates or other lesions. There were no other abnormalities on exam.
Investigations:

CXR: right lower lobe density with calcification, unchanged from previous films

HIV antibody, CMV viral load, and interferon gamma release assay for tuberculosis were negative

CT scan of the neck: thickening of the epiglottis and left piriform sinus

On endoscopy, the true vocal cords were normal in appearance. The epiglottis was thickened and the laryngeal surface of the epiglottis and supraglottic folds had irregular white friable tissue.

What is the most likely cause?

A. *Candida albicans*
B. *Haemophilus influenzae*
C. Human papillomavirus
D. Malignancy
E. *Mycobacterium tuberculosis*

7. A 27-year-old man presented with a 3-week history of intermittent fevers and pain in his right collar bone. He was an active intravenous drug user, using heroin and cocaine regularly. He had previously cleared hepatitis C infection. He was not on a methadone program. He had no known drug allergies.
Investigations:

Creatinine clearance 50 ml/min

ALT 241 U/L

4/4 blood cultures positive for methicillin-susceptible *Staphylococcus aureus*

Echocardiogram: valvular vegetations and insufficiency involving both the mitral and aortic valve

CT chest: pulmonary lesions consistent with septic emboli and fluid collection and bony erosions of the right sternoclavicular joint

What is the most appropriate treatment?

A. Cefazolin
B. Daptomycin
C. Oxacillin
D. Oxacillin plus rifampin plus gentamicin
E. Vancomycin

8. A 32-year-old woman presented with a 1-day history of fever, headaches, nausea, and watery diarrhea. Her symptoms developed 12 hours after a picnic at which she ate pate sandwiches and salad. She was concerned as she was 6 weeks pregnant.

What is the most likely diagnosis?

A. *Bacillus cereus*
B. *Clostridium perfringens*
C. *Listeria monocytogenes*
D. Norovirus
E. *Staphylococcus aureus*

9. A 25-year-old man presented with a 4-week history of a painful, hot, swollen left knee, low back pain with bilateral buttock pain, and left heel pain. There was no history of trauma. He had no fevers or other arthralgias. He had experienced some dysuria several weeks earlier without a noticeable discharge.

He was sexually active with other men and engaged in oral and unprotected anal intercourse (insertive and receptive). He had not had any recent screening.

On examination, the patient was afebrile with conjunctival injection. There was a rash on his glans penis and his feet, and a large effusion of the left knee.

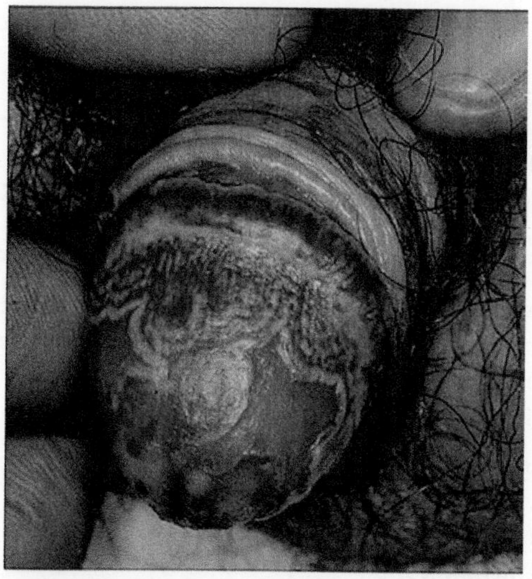

Investigations:
Total white cell count 7.3 $\times 10^9$/L
ESR 60 mm/h
CRP 20 mg/dL
Joint aspiration:
Microscopy: no crystals seen
white cell count 1000
Gram stain negative

What is the most appropriate action?

A. Refer to orthopedics for arthroscopic washout
B. Repeat arthrocentesis with cultures and P16 RNA (16S ribosomal RNA)
C. Send urine for gonococcal/chlamydia NAAT
D. Start systemic antistaphylococcal antibiotics
E. Treat empirically for secondary syphilis

10. A 27-year-old man presented with an 8-day history of a rash. He was sexually active and had receptive and insertive anal intercourse with 2 male partners in the last 30 days. He had previously had a penile ulcer which had resolved 6 months earlier.

On examination there was a diffuse, painless, macular rash involving the palms of the hands and the soles of the feet.

Investigations:
Syphilis EIA positive
RPR positive at 1:128
Specific antitreponemal antibodies positive.
The patient was treated for secondary syphilis.

How should the patient's sexual contacts be managed?

A. Advise them to seek care with their healthcare provider
B. Test for syphilis and treat if positive
C. Treat if symptomatic
D. Treat presumptively with benzathine penicillin
E. Treat presumptively with doxycycline for 2 weeks

11. A 33-year-old man presented with fatigue, malaise, abdominal pain, conjunctivitis, and myalgia. He had returned home 4 days earlier from a triathlon event in Hawaii. The myalgia was worse in his calves which he attributed to being sore after the race. In addition to participating in the triathlon, he also reported eating local food and had one unprotected sexual encounter with a fellow female athlete.

Investigations:
ALT 600 IU/L
Bilirubin 3.2 mg/dL
Creatinine 2.4 mg/dL

What is the most likely diagnosis?

A. Acute hepatitis A infection
B. Acute HIV infection
C. Dengue hemorrhagic fever
D. Leptospirosis
E. Staphylococcal toxic shock syndrome

12. A 4-year-old child had been unwell for several days with a mild fever, coryza and malaise, and flushed facies.

On examination there was a rash over both arms. It was mildly pruritic, nontender, and blanching.

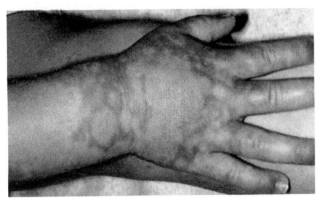

What is the most likely diagnosis?

A. Epstein–Barr virus
B. Erythema infectiosum
C. Exanthema subitum
D. Measles
E. Rubella

13. A 35-year-old man presented with a markedly swollen right knee. It was not particularly painful but examination showed a massive effusion. Two months earlier he had a rash on his back which he thought was ringworm. He had a flu-like illness at the time, which resolved. He worked as a tree surgeon in Michigan. He sustained insect bites regularly while working but did not recall a tick bite.

Investigations:

Borrelia burgdorferi IgG positive
He was started on doxycycline 100 mg BD

What is the most appropriate advice about prognosis?

A. He is likely to have long-term sequelae
B. He should expect other joints to become involved despite completing treatment
C. His symptoms should resolve in 2–4 weeks of starting therapy
D. His symptoms should resolve in several months
E. His symptoms should resolve within 48 hours of starting treatment

14. A 66-year-old man presented with an acutely painful left knee and ankle with associated swelling and the inability to bear weight. He had not experienced any fevers or chills. He had not received any recent antibiotics. He was known to have hypertension and atrial fibrillation on warfarin. He described occasional alcohol use. He had recently discontinued his naproxen secondary to gastritis.

Investigations:

Total white cell count 11,200/mL
Erythrocyte sedimentation rate 44 mm/h
C-reactive protein 2.9mg/dL
Serum uric acid 4.7 mg/dL (normal 3.4–7.0mg/dL)
INR 1.8
Left knee aspirate: 10 mL of mildly milky/opaque fluid
Synovial fluid microscopy:
    740 red blood cells (RBC)
    23,000 white blood cells (70% neutrophils)
Crystal microscopy pending
Cultures pending

What is the most likely diagnosis?

A. Crystalline arthropathy
B. Hemarthrosis
C. Osteoarthritis
D. Reactive arthritis
E. Septic arthritis

15. A 61-year-old woman presented with dyspnea associated with nonproductive cough. She rapidly progressed to acute hypoxemic respiratory failure, requiring endotracheal intubation and mechanical ventilation.

She had received an orthotopic liver transplant 3 months previously for cirrhosis due to autoimmune hepatitis. The donor was a 28-year-old man who died after a motor vehicle accident in Minneapolis. Granulomas were noted on histopathology of the transplanted liver.

Investigations:

CXR: diffuse, bilateral pulmonary infiltrates
Serum *Aspergillus* galactomannan positive with an index of 1.2 (cut-off for positivity ≥0.5)
BAL fluid: fungal cultures positive after 17 days. White to brown colonies with a fine cottony texture seen
The same organism was recovered from the lysis-centrifugation blood culture

What is the most likely pathogen?

A. *Aspergillus fumigatus*
B. *Aspergillus terreus*
C. *Histoplasma capsulatum*
D. *Penicillium* spp.
E. *Rhizopus* spp.

16. A 19-year-old man presented with a 2-day history of fever, weakness, and dark-colored urine. Ten days earlier he had been given a clinical diagnosis of erythema migrans for a new target-shaped lesion on his thigh. He was on day 10 of a 14-day course of doxycycline. He had no known drug allergies. He initially felt better and the lesions disappeared but then deteriorated symptomatically.

On physical examination, his temperature was 38.5°C. He was visibly jaundiced, and he had tender hepatosplenomegaly. No rashes were seen, and the remainder of the exam was normal.

Investigations:

Hemoglobin 8.7 g/dL

Bilirubin 3.5 mg/dL (60 μmol/L)

Peripheral smear:

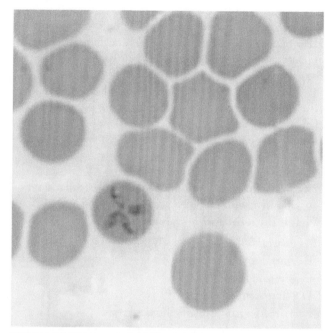

What is the best empiric therapy?

A. Artesunate

B. Atovaquone plus azithromycin

C. Ceftriaxone

D. Clindamycin plus primaquine

E. Clindamycin plus pyrimethamine

17. A 31-year-old man was admitted with a 6-week history of cough, fatigue, ~10 lb weight loss, night sweats, and fever. He had recently been diagnosed with HIV. He had been born in Thailand but moved to the United States 10 years ago. He had been in prison for 2 years and was PPD negative at that time.

Investigations:

CD4 count 312/μL

HIV VL 385, 000 copies /mL

CXR: left upper lobe infiltrates

Sputum microscopy: abundant acid-fast bacilli seen; Xpert MTB/RIF positive for both MTB and an *rpo B* gene mutation

MDR-TB was suspected; it was thought that he would need between five and seven active antituberculosis drugs during the initiation phase.

What would be the best course of action?

A. Defer TB treatment for 2 weeks and start ART now

B. Start ART within 2 weeks and start TB treatment now

C. Start both TB and ART treatment now

D. Start TB treatment now and defer ART for 2–8 weeks

E. Start TB treatment now plus steroids and defer ART for 2–8 weeks

18. A 19-year-old man was admitted with a 6-day history of fever and chills. He had also noticed some shortness of breath while walking. Ten days earlier he had arrived in the United States from Myanmar. He had no prior medical history but had been depressed for the past year.

On examination, he was awake, alert, and oriented. His temperature was 39.2°C, and his blood pressure was 110/58 mmHg. He had pale conjunctivae and some pitting edema to his ankles.

Investigations:

Hemoglobin 5.8 g/dL

Total bilirubin 3.1 mg/mL

Peripheral blood smear:

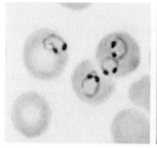 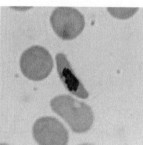

What is the most appropriate treatment?

A. Chloroquine and primaquine for 14 days

B. IV artesunate for 24 hours followed by atovaquone–proguanil for 3 days

C. IV artesunate for 24 hours followed by oral mefloquine for 3 days

D. IV artesunate to complete 3-day course of therapy

E. Oral atovaquone–proguanil for 3 days

19. A 48-year-old presented with extensive bruising on his left thigh after a minor injury 2 days earlier. Two weeks previously he had been started on rivaroxaban for a pulmonary thromboembolism and right lower extremity deep vein thrombosis. He was known to have well-controlled HIV, treated with elvitegravir/cobicistat/tenofovir/emtricitabine.

What is the most likely cause of his hematoma?

A. Drug interaction

B. Lymphoma

C. Protein C + S deficiency

D. Thrombotic thrombocytopenia purpura

E. Type 3 von Willebrand's disease

20. A 27-year-old man attended for routine follow-up. He had HIV treated with tenofovir alafenamide/emtricitabine + twice-daily raltegravir. He had been diagnosed with a peptic ulcer and had started taking lansoprazole. His brother had recently died from a drug overdose, and the patient had been drinking alcohol heavily in response. As a result he was finding it difficult to remember to take his medication.
Investigations:

	2 Weeks Before Clinic	Day of Clinic
CD4 count / μL	395	
HIV RNA copies/ml	2050	3950
HIV resistance assay		Q148R mutation detected

What is the most appropriate antiretroviral regimen?

A. Abacavir/lamivudine/dolutegravir once daily
B. Abacavir/lamivudine + raltegravir twice daily
C. Tenofovir alafenamide/emtricitabine + atazanavir/cobicistat once daily
D. Tenofovir alafenamide/emtricitabine/cobicistat/elvitegravir once daily
E. Tenofovir disoproxil fumarate/emtricitabine + ritonavir boosted darunavir once daily

21. A 62-year-old woman presented with 1 week of fevers, chills, abdominal pain, and lethargy. She was known to have advanced HIV disease on antiretroviral therapy. She also had a history of diabetes, hypertension, mild chronic kidney disease, and transient ischemic attacks. The patient lived in Dallas, Texas, and worked as a secretary at a construction job site.

On examination, her blood pressure was 85/55mmHg and her heart rate was 130 beats/minute. Pulmonary exam was normal, but there was diffuse abdominal tenderness with hepatomegaly but no peritonitis.
Investigations:
CD4 count 65 cells/μL
HIV viral load 235 copies/mL
Lactate dehydrogenase 865 U/L (122–222)
Ferritin 1550 ng/mL (20–200)
Peripheral blood smear:

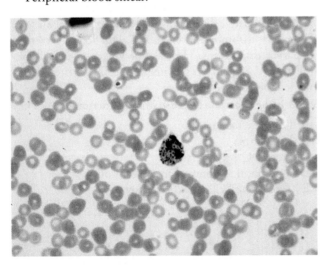

What is the most likely causative organism?

A. *Blastomyces dermatitidis*
B. *Coccidioides immitis*
C. *Cryptococcus neoformans*
D. *Histoplasma capsulatum*
E. *Talaromyces marneffei*

22. A 52-year-old man presented with a 3-week history of watery diarrhea and abdominal cramping. He reported 6–8 watery bowel movements per day, cramping abdominal pain, and 25 lb weight loss. He was known to have HIV, hypertension, type 2 diabetes, and hypercholesterolemia. He was not taking antiretroviral therapy or antibiotic prophylaxis.

On examination, there was diffuse abdominal tenderness and hyperactive bowel sounds but no peritoneal signs.
Investigations:
CD4 count 45 cells/μL
HIV viral load 145,850 copies/mL
Stool microscopy: multiple 4–6 μm oocysts that stain positive with modified acid-fast staining

What is the most appropriate treatment?

A. Albendazole
B. Antiretroviral therapy
C. Metronidazole
D. Nitazoxanide
E. Trimethoprim–sulfamethoxazole

23. A 43-year-old man presented with nausea, anorexia, and right upper quadrant pain. He was known to have co-infection with HIV and hepatitis B. He recently switched his HIV antiretroviral therapy from tenofovir/emtricitabine/efavirenz to abacavir/lamivudine and raltegravir due to concerns over worsening renal function. He was sexually active and reported 4 casual male partners in the last 6 months, without using condoms. He had not traveled outside of the United States and had never used recreational intravenous drugs.

On physical exam, he had scleral icterus and tender hepatomegaly of 3 cm.
Investigations:
CD4 count 520 cells/μL
HIV viral load <20 copies/mL
AST 1623 U/L
ALT 824 U/L
Total bilirubin 4.2 mg/dL (0.1–1.2)
Hepatitis C IgG negative
Hepatitis B surface antigen positive
Hepatitis B core IgM positive
HLAB5701 negative
Right upper quadrant sonogram demonstrated no gallstones or biliary duct dilation.

What is the most likely etiology?

A. Drug-induced liver injury from ART
B. Hepatitis B virus flare
C. Hepatitis D virus co-infection
D. HIV cholangiopathy
E. *Mycobacterium avium* complex infection

24. A 67-year-old man presented with a 2-week history of headache, nausea, vomiting, neck pain, and low-grade fever. He underwent orthotopic liver transplantation for alcoholic cirrhosis 6 months prior and was on high-dose steroids for induction and tacrolimus and mycophenolate for maintenance immunosuppression. He was on secondary prophylaxis with valganciclovir for CMV syndrome.

MRI brain: multiple rim-enhancing lesions along the frontal horns of the lateral ventricles, corpus callosum, and cerebellum.

What is the most appropriate action?

A. Check a blood CMV PCR
B. Give liposomal amphotericin B
C. Perform a brain biopsy
D. Start empirical antituberculous therapy
E. Start pyrimethamine and sulfadiazine

25. A 52-year-old woman was evaluated for nausea, anorexia, and fatigue. She underwent deceased donor kidney transplantation 6 months prior and had normal renal function with an appropriate tacrolimus level at her last follow-up. Her current medications were tacrolimus, mycophenolate, and prednisone. She reported that she took some leftover clarithromycin 5 days ago for what she thought was a tooth infection. Her vitals and physical examination were normal.

Investigations:
  Serum creatinine 4.0 mg/dL
  Urinalysis normal

What is the most likely cause of her acute kidney injury?

A. Acute cellular rejection
B. Clarithromycin-induced interstitial nephritis
C. Mycophenolate toxicity
D. Tacrolimus toxicity
E. Transplant pyelonephritis

26. A 58-year-old man presented with a 6-week history of a left buttock mass. It was nontender, and he was otherwise asymptomatic. He thought it may be related to a minor trauma when he scraped himself on a yucca plant while gardening. He had received an allogeneic stem cell transplant 9 months earlier for acute myelogenous leukemia, which had been complicated by graft versus host disease of the skin and gastrointestinal tract. He was taking prednisone 20 mg od, tacrolimus, inhaled pentamidine, and aciclovir.

On examination, his temperature was 37°C, his blood pressure was 145/73 mmHg, heart rate 88 beats/min, respiratory rate 16 breaths/min, and oxygen saturations 99% on room air. He was overweight, in no acute distress, and he had a grapefruit-sized mass on his left buttock. The rest of the exam was unremarkable.

Investigations:
  Total white cell count 8.6×10^9/L
  Hemoglobin 12.5 g/dL
  Platelets 146×10^9/L
  eGFR >60 mL/min per 1.73 m^2

Aspiration of the mass revealed gram-positive branching filamentous rods.

What is the most likely diagnosis?

A. *Listeria monocytogenes*
B. *Mycobacterium abscessus*
C. *Nocardia farcinica*
D. *Scedosporium prolificans*
E. *Stenotrophomonas maltophilia*

27. A toddler presented with *Pneumocystic jirovecii* pneumonia, following a long-standing history of diarrhea, failure to thrive, and developmental delay.

Laboratory examination revealed macrocytic anemia, leucopenia with hypersegmented neutrophils, and thrombocytopenia, as well as hypogammaglobulinemia.

What is the most likely diagnosis?

A. ADA-SCID
B. Cartilage–hair hypoplasia
C. CD40 ligand deficiency
D. Hereditary folate malabsorption
E. SP110 deficiency

28. A 45-year-old man sought medical help after learning that he had had a significant exposure to chickenpox 24 hours earlier. He had no personal history of chickenpox and had not received the varicella vaccine. He had a history of hypertension and diabetes, and was taking enalapril and metformin. He had no known drug allergies.

What is the most appropriate action?

A. Administer varicella vaccine
B. Immune globulin (IVIG) administration
C. Measure varicella antibody titer
D. Prescribe a course of valaciclovir
E. Varicella-zoster immune globulin (VariZIG/VZIG) administration

29. A 22-year-old woman sought pretravel medical advice. She planned to go to Bolivia for vacation to visit family. She had a history of liver transplantation for Wilson's disease 6 months prior and was doing well on immunosuppressants. She asked specifically about yellow fever vaccination.

What is the most appropriate action?

A. Administer yellow fever vaccine

B. Advise against future travel to Bolivia due to the risk of yellow fever

C. Counsel against the trip if visiting a high-risk area

D. Delay the travel plans until she is 2 years post-transplant

E. Mosquito bite avoidance precautions will suffice

30. A 25-year-old intravenous drug user presents to clinic with several days of fever as well as decreased visual acuity and reddening of her eye as shown.

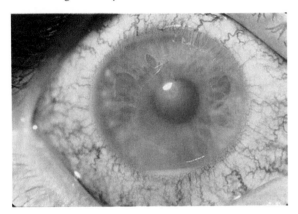

She most likely has systemic infection from what organism?

A. *Candida albicans*

B. *Haemophilus influenzae*

C. *Pseudomonas aeruginosa*

D. *Staphylococcus aureus*

E. *Staphylococcus epidermidis*

31. A 65-year-old woman presented with headache, agitation, and delirium. She had a witnessed generalized seizure in the emergency department. She was started on antiepileptic medication, and head CT was performed to evaluate for stroke. The head CT was within normal limits. Brain MRI was later performed, and it demonstrated bilateral temporal lobe enhancement.

What test would be most likely to prove the correct diagnosis?

A. Blood cultures

B. CSF Gram stain and culture

C. CSF HSV PCR

D. Serum cryptococcal antigen

E. *Streptococcus pneumoniae* antigen testing

32. A 55-year-old man is admitted in the late summer with several days of fever and headache, followed by altered mental status and progressive bilateral lower extremity weakness. On exam, he had flaccid paralysis of both legs, with some muscle fasciculations. CSF analysis showed 450 nucleated cells with 75% lymphocytes, normal glucose, and protein of 80. Brain MRI showed some T2-weighted abnormalities in his basal ganglia.

What type of virus is the most likely cause of his symptoms?

A. Bunyavirus

B. Enterovirus

C. Flavivirus

D. Herpes virus

E. Polyomavirus

33. A 51-year-old man presented with several months of rapidly progressive cognitive decline and new onset tremors. He was previously healthy and has no family history of neurocognitive disorders. Four months ago, he was able to work and function normally. He has had behavioral changes and memory impairment, and most recently has started to have gait instability and tremors. EEG showed periodic sharp waves and T2-weighted MRI showed increased activity in both thalamic nuclei. A lumbar puncture was performed and routine tests were ordered.

Which nonroutine study would you consider adding to help elucidate the most likely diagnosis?

A. Cryptococcal antigen

B. Culture for acid-fast bacilli

C. Cytology

D. HSV PCR

E. Immunoassay for 14-3-3 protein

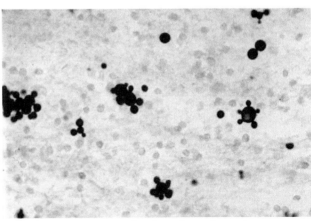

34. The yeast seen in this lymph node aspirate is most likely what organism?

A. *Blastomyces dermatitidis*

B. *Coccidioides immitis*

C. *Cryptococcus neoformans*

D. *Histoplasma capsulatum*

E. *Paracoccidioides brasiliensis*

35. A 63-year-old crab fisherman developed a painful lesion on his left ring finger. He first noticed throbbing at the tip of his finger, following which a slowly enlarging lesion developed. There was some stiffness in the index finger, but he had not noticed any swelling. He had not experienced any fevers or rigors. He felt as if the pain he was experiencing was disproportionately greater than the lesion seemed to warrant.

On examination, his temperature was 36.8°C. There was a violet-colored lesion on his left index finger of 4 cm in diameter. This had a raised border with central clearing. There was no swelling associated with the lesion, nor was there any tracking lymphangitis.

What is the most likely causative organism?

A. *Bacillus anthracis*
B. *Erysipelothrix rhusiopathiae*
C. Herpes simplex virus
D. *Mycobacterium marinum*
E. *Sporothrix schenckii*

36. A 49-year-old librarian attends the emergency department with a painful swollen right fist. She had sustained a bite injury from a stray cat 24 hours before. On examination her temperature is 38.1°C. There is an incisional wound with purulent cellulitis over the MCP joint of the ring finger on the right hand. Movement in the joint is very painful and limited. There is tracking erythema spreading up toward her elbow. Blood cultures are taken, and she is taken to theatre by the plastic surgeons for exploration and debridement of the wound.

Investigations:

Blood cultures Day 1: small gram-negative coccobacilli
Day 2: grey mucous colonies on blood agar at 37°C. No growth on MacConkey agar

What antibiotic would be active against this organism?

A. Cefalexin
B. Clindamycin
C. Erythromycin
D. Gentamicin
E. Penicillin

37. A 45-year-old male patient presented with fever, weight loss, hepatomegaly, ascites, and papular-nodular skin lesions. He was HIV-positive but had stopped antiretrovirals 3 years previously after poor adherence and intermittent clinic attendance. The lesions had developed from small red papules into large friable nodules, which easily bled on minimal trauma (see image). A skin biopsy was arranged.

What stain is most likely to confirm the diagnosis?

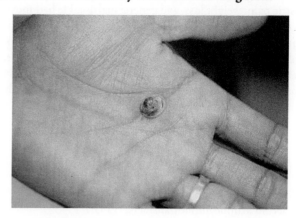

A. Giemsa
B. Iron hematoxylin
C. Methenamine silver
D. Warthin–Starry
E. Ziehl–Neelsen

38. A 41-year-old man returned from an 8-week trip to India. He had had unprotected oral and anal sex with 2 new male partners while he was traveling. Ten weeks after his return he developed dull pain in the upper abdomen and a high fever. His symptoms had started abruptly. The pain was intense and radiated to the right shoulder. He had associated rigors and profuse sweats. He also noted that his clothes had become loose and that he had a dry cough. He had not had diarrhea.

On examination, he was thin and in discomfort. His temperature was 39.9°C. He was markedly tender on palpation of the right upper quadrant and epigastrium, and his liver was palpable three fingerbreadths below the costal margin. Chest examination revealed dull percussion over the right lung base.

Investigations:

White cell count 15×10^9/L
Neutrophils 13.4×10^9/L
Eosinophil 0.2×10^9/L
Alkaline phosphatase 346 U/L (45–105)
CRP 217 mg/L (<10)
CXR: raised right hemidiaphragm; small right-sided pleural effusion with loss of the right costophrenic angle
Stool microscopy negative
Ultrasound liver: round, well-defined hypoechoic mass in the right lobe of the liver; diameter 8 cm

Blood cultures and serology are requested.

In addition to metronidazole, what therapeutic agent should he receive?

A. Albendazole
B. Ceftriaxone
C. Ciprofloxacin
D. Paromomycin
E. Praziquantel

39. A 54-year-old man presented with gradual onset epigastric pain, weight loss, and general malaise. He had moved to the UK 8 years previously. He was normally well and did not take any regular medications. He drank minimal alcohol. On examination he was afebrile and cardiovascularly stable. There was no rash or palpable lymphadenopathy. He was mildly icteric. There were several spider nevi over his torso and mild gynecomastia.

Investigations:

Neutrophil count 1.3×10^9/L (1.5–7.0)
Platelet count 115×10^9/L (150–400)
Eosinophil count 0.7×10^9/L (0.04–0.40)
Serum alkaline phosphatase 168 U/L (45–105)
Serum alanine aminotransferase 56 U/L (5–35)
Serum total bilirubin 52 μmol/L (1–22)
Serum α-fetoprotein 4 kU/L (<10)

Large low-attenuation mass in the liver with irregular margins; no clearly delineated walls visible. Central necrosis and irregular internal calcifications present within the lesion. Calcifications also visible on the surface of the liver.

What country carries the bulk of the global burden of this disease?

A. Argentina
B. China
C. Kenya
D. Peru
E. Russia

40. An 18-year-old woman presented with skin lesions on her right forearm and right cheek. They had developed gradually, from small papules which had enlarged and become nodular. She had emigrated from Afghanistan 4 months previously. She had no other known medical problems and was not taking any regular medications. A skin biopsy was taken.

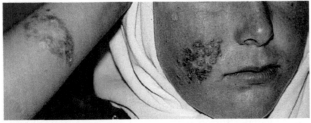

What parasitic stage is most likely to be found in the biopsy?

A. Amastigotes
B. L3 larvae
C. Merozoites
D. Nurse cell
E. Tachyzoites

41. A 34-year-old man in Kyrgyzstan presented with painless lesions on both arms. The lesions had begun as pruritic papules but had then enlarged, becoming vesicular, coalescing into bullae and developing significant local and spreading edema. He had systemic symptoms of chills and fever. The patient worked on a farm and had handled cattle 6 days earlier.

On examination there was extensive edema and hemorrhagic bullae in both arms.

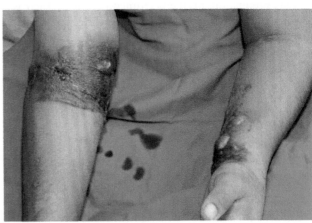

He had tender lymphadenopathy in both axillae. His temperature was 37.9°C. Swabs were taken of the vesicular fluid, and a full-thickness punch biopsy was taken. Blood cultures were also sent.

Microscopy using polychrome methylene blue stain showed blue-colored bacilli with light pink-colored capsules.

What is the most appropriate antimicrobial?

A. Benzylpenicillin
B. Ceftriaxone
C. Ciprofloxacin
D. Doxycycline
E. Streptomycin

42. A patient is admitted with cholangitis and a liver abscess. The abscess was aspirated and cultures grew *Enterobacter aerogenes*. The isolate was reported to be susceptible to ceftriaxone, and so he was started on that agent. He clinically improved over the next few days but then began to have recurrent fevers, and his liver abscess had reaccumulated when his abdominal imaging was repeated. A percutaneous drain was placed and cultures again grew *Enterobacter aerogenes*, though now resistant to ceftriaxone. What is the most likely mechanism of antibiotic resistance reflected in the different susceptibility profiles?

A. AmpC induction
B. Efflux pump
C. ESBL production
D. Metallo-β-lactamase production
E. Porin production

43. An 18-month-old boy presented with 4 days of sudden onset, severe watery diarrhea, after 2 days of being nonspecifically unwell. He was passing stool approximately 15 times/day. He had vomited for one day, but this then stopped. There was no blood in the stool. He was also noted to have a dry cough and appeared to have coryzal symptoms. He had not had a wet nappy for 24 hours. He had stopped breast feeding at 12 months old.

On examination, he was markedly dehydrated, with a temperature of 38.5°C and a tachycardia. He required aggressive fluid resuscitation.

In addition to intravenous fluids or oral rehydration solutions, what agent would improve his outcome?

A. Ascorbic acid

B. Cholecalciferol

C. Magnesium

D. Thiamine

E. Zinc

44. A 25-year-old primigravida presents at 34/40 with a 1-day history of fevers, rash, dry cough, and coryzal symptoms. She had recently moved to the UK and was uncertain of her childhood vaccinations. On examination her temperature is 39°C, and there is a generalized maculopapular rash, which is coalescent on her trunk. Some small cervical lymph nodes are palpable bilaterally. There are small white spots on the buccal membrane beside her molars. She has bilateral conjunctivitis.

She is concerned about the risk to her baby. What are the possible adverse effects that she should be made aware of?

A. Cataracts

B. Hydrops fetalis

C. Intrauterine death

D. No increased risk of fetal adverse outcome

E. Sensorineural deafness

45. A 54-year-old pet store owner presented with 4 days of fever and headache, and 2 days of a rash that had started on his face and spread outward. On examination, he had a macular rash over his face and distal extremities, with only a few lesions on his abdomen and back. His temperature was 38.3°C. He had widespread lymphadenopathy. Examination of his cardiovascular, respiratory, and abdominal examinations was unremarkable. He was admitted for observation and investigation. Over the next few days the rash evolved from macules to vesicles to pustules. The fever persisted for 8 days in total, the rash for 12 days.

Electron microscopy of lesion biopsy:

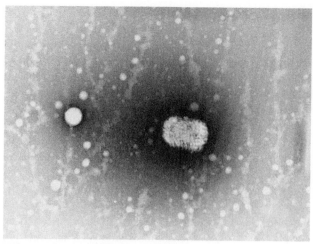

What is the most likely pathogen?

A. Herpes B virus

B. Monkeypox virus

C. *Streptobacillus moniliformis*

D. *Treponema pallidum*

E. Varicella-zoster virus

46. A 29-year-old man seeks medical attention on returning from a camping holiday in Germany. He sustained a bite wound to his left hand 4 days previously from a wild fox he had tried to feed by hand. He has not seen any other healthcare professionals. He is concerned about the risk of rabies. He has received a full course of tetanus vaccinations and the wound looks clean and dry.

What intervention is required?

A. Wound debridement and washout

B. Topical povidone-iodine

C. Five doses of IM rabies vaccine days 0, 3, 7, 14, and 28

D. Human rabies immunoglobulin infiltrated into the wound

E. Reassurance only

47. A 48-year-old Senegalese man was found to have HIV on routine screening with a fourth-generation combined p24 Ag/Ab ELISA. A confirmatory test with a second-generation ELISA for IgG to differentiate between HIV-1 and HIV-2 infection detected HIV-2 antibodies. He was negative for HIV-1 antibodies and an HIV-1 RNA viral load was negative. An HIV-2 RNA viral load was sent to the reference laboratory. His CD4 count was 458 cells/μL (mm3).

What class of antiretrovirals is HIV-2 intrinsically resistant to?

A. Chemokine receptor 5 (CCR5) antagonists

B. Integrase inhibitors

C. Nonnucleoside reverse transcriptase inhibitors

D. Nucleoside reverse transcriptase inhibitors

E. Protease inhibitors

48. A 33-year-old man attended the sexual health clinic following partner notification for gonorrhea. He was screened for rectal, urethral, and pharyngeal gonorrhea and chlamydia, and had epidemiologic treatment for gonorrhea with intramuscular ceftriaxone and oral azithromycin. Given his high-risk sexual behavior (>30 partners in the preceding 3 months, unprotected insertive and receptive anal sex, participation in chemsex parties) he requested a point of care HIV test. This was positive, and a laboratory sample confirmed HIV and hepatitis C infection. CD4 count was 525 cells/μL, HIV viral load 12,458 copies/mL. Treatment was recommended given his co-infection status and as he wanted to reduce the risk of transmission to partners. A baseline HIV resistance screen was obtained prior to starting Atripla (tenofovir, emtricitabine, efavirenz). What mutation in his resistance test would predict likely treatment failure with efavirenz?

A. M41L

B. K65R

C. N155H

D. Y181C

E. M184V

49. A 45-year-old nurse returned from voluntary work during an outbreak of Ebola virus in rural Guinea. She had been directly involved in caring for patients within the Red Zone (isolation area) in an Ebola treatment unit. Four days after her return she self-isolated and contacted her local public health unit as she had developed a fever, severe frontal headache, and a sore throat. Urine, serum, and an EDTA sample were sent urgently to the reference laboratory for an extended VHF PCR panel

What type of virus is Ebola classified as?

A. Alphavirus

B. Arenavirus

C. Bunyavirus

D. Filovirus

E. Flavivirus

50. A 22-year-old man attended clinic for review of a split-skin graft to a full-thickness burn on his left calf. The doctor was concerned about infection as there was worsening exudate and pain, with 2 cm erythema around the edges. A wound swab was taken, and the patient started on empirical flucloxacillin.

Wound swab:

1. *Staphylococcus aureus*, sensitive to methicillin
2. *Streptococcus pyogenes*
3. Gram-positive rod, identifying as *Corynebacterium diphtheriae*, awaiting confirmation

What confirmatory test on organism 3 would substantially alter the management of this patient?

A. Bacitracin sensitivity

B. Modified Elek test

C. Nagler's reaction

D. Quellung test

E. Reverse CAMP test

Quiz 9

1. A 47-year-old woman presented with a persistent productive cough and night sweats.

Investigations:

Sputum AFB stain: abundant (4+) AFBs seen; broth culture positive on day 5

What mycobacterial species can be excluded?

A. *Mycobacterium abscessus*
B. *Mycobacterium chelonae*
C. *Mycobacterium fortuitum*
D. *Mycobacterium tuberculosis*
E. None of the above

2. A 40-year-old man developed neutropenic fevers, right toe redness, and multiple skin lesions.

He had received an allogenic stem cell transplant 2 months earlier with no neutropenic recovery for relapsed acute myelogenous leukemia despite multiple chemotherapy regimens. He lived in Chicago, Illinois.

On examination, his temperature was 39.8°C. His right toe was erythematous and tender, and he had multiple tender nodular skin lesions with erythematous base scattered over his trunk and extremities.

Investigations:

MRI right toe: bone erosions

Skin biopsy culture grew fungal colonies that on lactophenol blue stain appeared as in the following image:

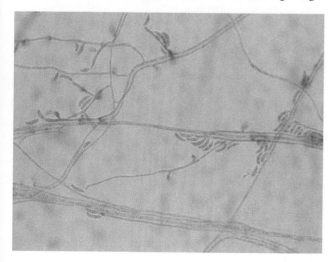

Biopsy specimen on GMS stain showed septate and branching filamentous hyphae with evidence of angioinvasion. Fungal blood cultures also grew mold.

What is the most likely causative agent?

A. *Aspergillus* spp.
B. *Blastomyces dermatitidis*
C. *Cryptococcus neoformans*
D. *Fusarium* spp.
E. *Mucor* spp.

3. A 40-year-old man was diagnosed with pneumonia caused by *Stenotrophomonas maltophilia*. He was known to have advanced HIV infection and was receiving ganciclovir for cytomegalovirus colitis and viremia. He had no known drug allergies.

Investigations:

Creatinine 0.8 mg/dL
Hematocrit 24.8
Total white cell count 2.3 ×10⁹/L
Absolute neutrophil count 1.3 ×10⁹/L
Platelet count 110 ×10⁹/L
G6PD deficiency
ECG: QTc interval 580 ms

What is the most appropriate treatment?

A. Chloramphenicol
B. Levofloxacin
C. Meropenem
D. Minocycline
E. Trimethoprim–sulfamethoxazole

4. A 60-year-old woman was admitted to the hospital with a 2-day history of fever and chills, dyspnea, and left-sided pleuritic chest pain. Five months earlier she underwent hematopoietic stem cell transplantation for myelodysplastic syndrome. She was taking trimethoprim–sulfamethoxazole, aciclovir, prednisone, and cyclosporine.

Investigations:

CXR: infiltrate in the left lower lobe

What is the most likely cause?

A. *Candida krusei*
B. Cytomegalovirus
C. *Pneumocystis jirovecii*
D. Respiratory syncytial virus
E. *Streptococcus pneumoniae*

5. A 45-year-old woman with no past medical history presented with 3 days of fever and cough. She had no known allergies.

On exam her temperature was 39.1°C.

Investigations:

CXR: patchy bilateral infiltrates

What is the most appropriate treatment?

A. Ceftaroline

B. Ceftriaxone and azithromycin

C. Clindamycin

D. Linezolid

E. Vancomycin and cefepime

6. A 26-year-old woman presented with a 4-month history of fatigue, joint aches, chills, and night sweats. She was unsure about any weight loss but thought her clothes had become looser. She denied any cough or sputum production but had noticed some dyspnea on exertion for several weeks.

She had 2 normal vaginal deliveries at full term with children now 3 and 6 years old. She had arrived in the United States 1 month earlier from Liberia, where she had been born and brought up.

On examination, her temperature was 36.9°C, her heart rate was 96 beats/minute, her blood pressure was 120/75 mmHg, and her respiratory rate was 20 breaths/minute. She had visibly bulging jugular veins and bilateral leg edema. There were no murmurs. There were decreased breath sounds on both bases on respiratory exam.

Investigations:

CXR: scattered infiltrates with bilateral pleural effusions and an enlarged cardiac silhouette

Chest CT: a thickened pericardium and a pericardial effusion are seen, in addition to the X-ray findings

Echocardiogram: limited right atrial wall motion and distended inferior vena cava with blunted respiratory variation and normal LV wall motion

A therapeutic pericardiocentesis was arranged.

What is the most appropriate empiric treatment?

A. Colchicine

B. Corticosteroids

C. Levothyroxine

D. Nonsteroidal antiinflammatories

E. Quadruple antituberculous therapy

7. A 33-year-old woman developed sudden onset profuse, watery, nonbloody diarrhea. She had initially experienced abdominal discomfort, vomiting, and noisy bowel sounds. She was assisting in an overseas medical camp in South India.

On examination, her blood pressure was 84/52 mmHg, and her heart rate was 122 beats/minute.

Investigations:

Creatinine 242μmol/L

Potassium 3.4 mmol/L

What is paramount in her management?

A. Antiemetics

B. Antimotility agents

C. Flight back to the United States

D. Fluid resuscitation

E. Surgical review

8. A 43-year-old man presented with a 2-month history of fevers, 5 kg weight loss, and increasing abdominal discomfort. During this time he had received two courses of antibiotics from his primary care physician for suspected urinary tract infections, but his symptoms persisted.

He had been diagnosed with HIV 10 years ago and was taking tenofovir, emtricitabine, and dolutegravir. His most recent viral load (taken 4 months ago) was undetectable (<40 copies/mL). He was normally compliant with HAART although he had missed two doses over the last 12 weeks because he had felt unwell.

He denied smoking, excessive alcohol consumption, or recreational drug use. He was an engineer. He grew up in Spain and emigrated to the UK 5 years ago for work. He last traveled to Spain 4 months ago to visit family during a summer vacation; this was the last time he traveled outside the UK.

On examination, he was tanned and thin. His temperature was 37.9°C. Cardiovascular and respiratory examinations were unremarkable. Abdominal examination revealed abdominal fullness: the liver edge was palpable four finger breadths below the costal margin and the spleen was palpable to the midline.

Investigations:

Hemoglobin 9.3 g/L

Total white cell count 2.1×10^9/L

Neutrophils 1.2, lymphocytes 0.4

Platelets 76×10^9/L

Bilirubin 28 μmol/L (1–22)

ALT 102 U/L

ALP 208 U/L

What is the most appropriate diagnostic test?

A. Abdominal USS

B. Blood culture

C. Bone marrow biopsy

D. HIV viral load and resistance testing

E. Triple phase MRI liver

9. A 40-year-old man presented with a history of recurrent lower urinary tract symptoms and pelvic pain. He had been diagnosed with an *Escherichia coli* UTI one month earlier. He had a prior history of treated pulmonary TB.

Examination revealed normal prostate and mild suprapubic tenderness.

Investigations:

Urine microscopy: >100 white cells/μL

What is the most likely diagnosis?

A. Bladder stones

B. Chronic bacterial prostatitis

C. Chronic pelvic pain syndrome

D. Granulomatous prostatitis

E. Ureteric reflux

10. A 22-year-old woman presented for antenatal care at 6/40 weeks pregnant. She was sexually active, with 5 casual male partners in the last year.

Investigations:

4th generation HIV Ag/Ab negative

Syphilis EIA negative

Vaginal swab NAAT negative for *Neisseria gonorrhoeae*, positive for *Chlamydia trachomatis*

One gram of azithromycin was administered orally for one dose.

What is the most appropriate action?

A. Give a stat dose of ceftriaxone IM

B. Give an additional 1 gram of azithromycin in 4 weeks

C. Give weekly suppressive azithromycin 1 gram until delivery

D. Repeat *Chlamydia* NAAT at 36/40 or before delivery

E. Repeat *Chlamydia* NAAT in 4 weeks for test of cure

11. A 3-year-old child presented with a fever and sore throat. She was previously fit and well and was up to date with her childhood vaccinations.

On examination she had superficial ulcers located on her soft palate and tongue. She was admitted to the pediatric ward due to her inability to take adequate oral fluids. While under observation she became increasingly agitated and exhibited an unsteady gait and nystagmus.

What is the most likely causative organism?

A. Enterovirus 71 (EV71)

B. Enterovirus D68 (EV-D68)

C. HIV

D. Measles virus

E. Poliovirus

12. A full-term neonate was seen on the postnatal ward and referred for an urgent neonatal consultation. Her mother had recently entered the country as a refugee and had presented in labor, having not received any antenatal care.

On examination, the baby was found to have bilateral cataracts, microcephaly, and sensorineural deafness.

What virus is most likely to be responsible?

A. Cytomegalovirus

B. Erythrovirus (parvovirus B19)

C. Measles

D. Rubella

E. Varicella-zoster virus

13. A 25-year-old man presented with 2-week history of high fevers, rigors, headaches, and muscle aches. His symptoms started the week after a 3-day fishing trip with some friends, where he slept in a wooden cabin in the forest and swam and fished on a lake. He did not recall any insect bites. None of his friends had reported similar symptoms.

His symptoms started quite abruptly, with a very high fever (39°C) and prostration. He had profuse sweating on the second night of his illness and felt better by the next day. Several days later his symptoms returned, and he had to take some time off work. He felt better again after 2 days so he did not seek medical attention. However, his fever returned so he sought medical help. He was normally well and did not take any regular medications. He had no known drug allergies. He lived in Colorado.

On examination, his temperature was 38.8°C, blood pressure was 110/75 mmHg, heart rate 100 beats/min, oxygen saturation was normal.

Clinical examination was unremarkable.

Investigations:

Total white cell count 13 ×10⁹/L

Neutrophil count 8 ×10⁹/L

CRP 103 mg/dL (<5)

Renal function and liver function tests were within range

A blood test was sent for microscopy; Wright stain of peripheral blood smear showed the following:

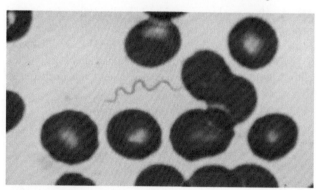

What is the most likely diagnosis?

A. Colorado tick fever

B. Leptospirosis

C. Louse-borne relapsing fever

D. Lyme disease

E. Tickborne relapsing fever

14. A 14-year-old boy presented to his primary care physician following a tick bite. The tick was unnoticed for 36 hours, and his mother was very concerned about him developing Lyme disease. Local tick infection rate with *Borrelia* is low. The boy had no relevant past medical history.

Clinical examination was unremarkable.

What is the most appropriate action?

A. Request acute and convalescent serology for Lyme disease

B. Give doxycycline 100mg stat

C. Reassure but advise the family to be vigilant for erythema migrans

D. Start 14 days of amoxicillin 500 mg TDS

E. Perform a skin biopsy at the site of the tick bite

15. A 42-year-old woman presented with progressive mid-thoracic back pain over 2 months. It woke her at night, and she was requiring opiate analgesia. She had no night sweats, but she described some mild fevers. Her weight was stable She had no medical history of note and was not taking any regular medications. She did not use any intravenous drugs, was a nonsmoker and did not drink alcohol. She had emigrated from Burma 3 years earlier. She worked as a waitress and had three school-age children.

Investigations:

MRI thoracic spine with and without IV contrast: erosive changes of the anterior vertebral bodies of T7 and T8 with relative sparing of the disc space

What is the most likely causative organism?

A. *Brucella melitensis*
B. *Klebsiella pneumoniae*
C. *Mycobacterium tuberculosis*
D. *Staphylococcus aureus*
E. Viridans group streptococci

16. A 48-year-old man attended clinic for a pretravel review. He had a history of hypertension controlled with enalapril. He had no known drug allergies. He was planning a 4-week trip to the Middle East. He had previously taken chloroquine and had tolerated it well and was keen to use that again if possible.

What country retains chloroquine sensitivity?

A. Algeria
B. Egypt
C. Lebanon
D. Sudan
E. Yemen

17. A 22-year-old man was admitted for respiratory failure, cranial nerve paralysis, and hemiplegia. He was normally well and did not take any regular medications. He had no known drug allergies.

Investigations:

CSF microscopy: mild pleocytosis with neutrophilic predominance

CSF Gram stain:

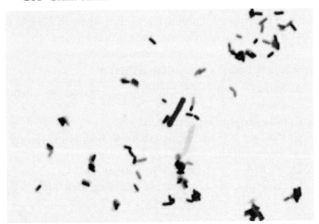

CSF/plasma glucose: normal ratio
CT head: normal appearances
MRI brain: diffuse brainstem encephalitis

What is the most appropriate treatment?

A. Ampicillin
B. Ceftriaxone
C. Levofloxacin
D. Trimethoprim–sulfamethoxazole
E. Vancomycin

18. A 29-year-old woman from Mississippi presented with a 2-week history of fever, fatigue, productive cough with traces of blood, and progressive shortness of breath. She was a smoker with a 10 pack year history. She had never been in prison or in contact with people with known TB disease, but had a prior TST read as positive 7 years earlier and never received LTBI treatment.

On examination, she was tachypneic and had bilateral leg edema with a petechial rash.

Investigations:

Hemoglobin 10.4 g/dL

Urea 9.3 mmol/L

Creatinine 3.1 mg/dL

HIV Ag/Ab negative

CXR: diffuse ground-glass opacities and nodules

Sputum microscopy: AFB negative × 3; MTB-PCR negative

What test is most likely to be diagnostic?

A. Anti-GBM antibodies
B. Hantavirus IgM and IgG
C. Interferon gamma release assay
D. Serum angiotensin-converting enzyme levels
E. Serum galactomannan levels

19. Infection prevention measures were reviewed for a 72-year-old man with noncavitary pulmonary tuberculosis. The patient initially had cough with hemoptysis and fever, but symptoms subsided. His sputum was positive for MTB by PCR, but was acid-fast bacilli negative. He had advanced HIV with CD4 of 111/µL and was taking trimethoprim–sulfamethoxazole prophylaxis. He had received 8 days of tuberculosis therapy with four drugs and discharge plans were being arranged.

What factor is most associated with TB infectivity?

A. Absence of lung cavitation
B. HIV co-infection
C. Lack of cough
D. Pleural involvement
E. Sputum induction with hypertonic saline

20. A 21-year-old man presented with a 5-month history of a progressive nonpruritic rash and a 1-month history of worsening dyspnea on exertion and a nonproductive cough. He reported that he had developed violet-colored bumps, several centimeters in diameter, on his torso and arms.

On examination he had approximately 25 skin lesions on his bilateral arms, torso, and abdomen.

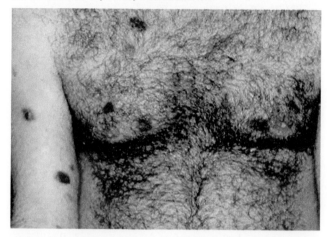

Investigations:
CXR:

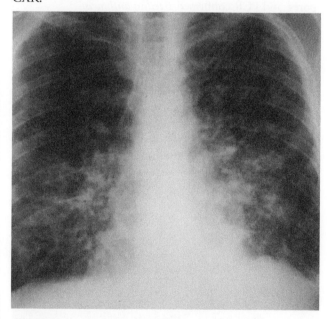

CT abdomen and pelvis: no abnormalities found
HIV Ag/Ab positive
CD4 count 46 cells/μL

In addition to starting antiretroviral therapy, what is the most appropriate treatment?

A. Antiretroviral therapy alone
B. Doxycycline and gentamicin
C. Ganciclovir
D. Liposomal daunorubicin
E. Pulsed methylprednisolone

21. A 27-year-old woman presented with a 4-day history of fever, sore throat, and a rash.

On examination she had a maculopapular rash and generalized lymphadenopathy.
Investigations:
  Creatinine 0.7 mg/dL
  AST 65 units/L
  ALT 96 units/L
  Bilirubin 1.0 mg/dL
  EBV IgM positive, IgG positive, EBNA positive
  HIV Ab/Ag test negative
  HIV viral load 1.2 million copies/mL

What is the most appropriate treatment?

A. Abacavir/lamivudine/dolutegravir
B. No treatment required
C. Tenofovir alafenamide/emtricitabine +atazanavir/cobicistat
D. Tenofovir alafenamide+cobicistat+elvitegravir
E. Tenofovir disoproxil fumarate/emtricitabine + raltegravir

22. A 43-year-old man presented with 4 weeks of worsening fatigue and dyspnea on exertion. He denied fevers, chills, weight loss, or cough. He was the primary carer for his 4-year-old nephew who had had a febrile illness with a facial rash 2 months earlier. The patient was known to have HIV and was not on antiretroviral therapy.

On examination there was conjunctival pallor but no lymphadenopathy or hepatosplenomegaly.
Investigations:
  CD4 count 45 cells/μL
  HIV viral load 14,350 copies/mL
  Total white cell count 4300 cells/μL (3500–10,500)
  Hemoglobin 7,2 g/dL (13.5–17.5)
  Reticulocyte percentage 1.2% (0.77%–2.36%)
  Haptoglobin 75 mg/dL (30–200)
  Antinuclear antibody test negative
  Direct Coombs test negative
  Bone marrow biopsy showed overall hypocellular marrow with giant pronormoblasts seen.

What is the most appropriate treatment?

A. Erythropoietin alfa
B. Intravenous immunoglobulin
C. Intravenous methylprednisolone
D. Red blood cell transfusion
E. Rituximab

23. A 55-year-old woman presented with a 2-month history of fevers, cough, and pleuritic chest pain. The symptoms were gradually progressive and accompanied by night sweats and a 15 lb weight loss. She was known to have HIV but was not taking ART. She worked as a horse trainer in Kentucky and 6 months earlier had spent a 2-week vacation in Kenya.

On examination she was cachectic and right upper lobe rales were audible on pulmonary examination.
Investigations:
CD4 count 26 cells/μL
HIV viral load 25,600 copies/mL
Sputum microscopy: neutrophils and abundant gram-positive coccobacilli seen
Sputum culture: salmon-pink mucoid colonies seen that revealed gram-positive branching filamentous rods
Sputum AFB stains positive but *Mycobacterium tuberculosis* and *M. avium-intracellulare* PCR on sputum and cultures were negative
CXR: 2 cm right upper lobe cavitary lung lesion

What pathogen is the most likely cause?

A. *Mycobacterium avium–intracellulare*
B. *Mycobacterium tuberculosis*
C. *Nocardia asteroides*
D. *Pseudomonas aeruginosa*
E. *Rhodococcus equi*

24. A 55-year-old man presented with a 4-day history of high-grade fever and chills. He had undergone liver transplantation for primary sclerosing cholangitis 3 weeks earlier. He was maintained on tacrolimus, mycophenolate, and prednisone.
Investigations:
Recipient CMV IgG negative, donor CMV IgG negative
Total white cell count 20.1 ×10⁹/L
Alkaline phosphatase 406 IU/L

What is the most appropriate management?

A. Increase immunosuppression for acute cellular rejection
B. Reduce immunosuppression for drug-induced liver injury
C. Start empirical ganciclovir for presumed CMV disease
D. Start empirical ivAB for intraabdominal infection
E. Start voriconazole for invasive aspergillosis

25. A 47-year-old woman presented with a 5-day history of shortness of breath and dry cough. There was no history of fever, hemoptysis, or coryzal symptoms. She had no sick contacts and no recent travel outside of the United States. She was 60 days postallogeneic stem cell transplant for acute myelogenous leukemia. She had previously had Stevens–Johnson syndrome due to trimethoprim–sulfamethoxazole. She was taking levofloxacin, valaciclovir, voriconazole, and inhaled pentamidine.

On examination, her temperature was 37.2°C, blood pressure was 132/65 mmHg, heart rate 105 beats/min, respiratory rate 30 breaths/minute, oxygen saturations 88% on 2LPM of O_2. Cardiovascular exam was unremarkable;

respiratory exam revealed faint bilateral crackles. There was no pedal edema, and the rest of the exam was unremarkable.
Investigations:
Total white cell count 1.4 ×10⁹/L
Absolute neutrophil count 0.8 ×10⁹/L
Hemoglobin 8.4 g/dL
Platelets 98 ×10⁹/L
eGFR >60 mL/min per 1.73 m²
LDH 340 U/L
Blood cultures: no growth at 48 hours
CXR: diffuse bilateral interstitial infiltrates

What is the most likely pathogen?

A. *Aspergillus fumigatus*
B. *Legionella pneumophila*
C. MERS coronavirus
D. *Pneumocystis jirovecii*
E. *Streptococcus pneumoniae*

26. There was a reported bioterrorist release of anthrax spores in a crowd at a professional football game in an outdoor stadium. The announcement about the release of the spores was made 3 hours after the game ended. Rapid testing confirmed contamination at the stadium with anthrax spores, and PCR confirmed *Bacillus anthracis*.

What would be the most appropriate immediate management of those who attended the game?

A. Amoxicillin prophylaxis for pregnant women
B. Anthrax immune globulin and 3 doses of anthrax vaccine
C. Hospitalization with respiratory isolation for those in contaminated seats
D. Prophylaxis with ciprofloxacin or doxycycline
E. Self-taken nasal swab to determine whether exposed

27.

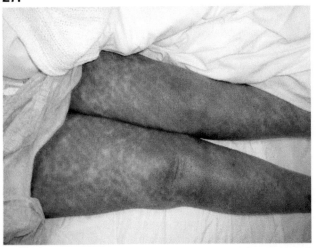

A 43-year-old woman presented with a widespread rash and facial swelling. She reported multiple lesions, which had started on her face, then spread throughout her body. She was on day 7 of trimethoprim–sulfamethoxazole for treatment of recurrent axillary community-acquired MRSA furunculosis. She was known to have diabetes mellitus and was taking metformin.

On examination, her temperature was 38.4°C, her blood pressure was 136/64 mmHg, and her heart rate was 72 beats/minute. She had facial edema and widespread erythematous maculopapular lesions.

Investigations:

Total white cell count 14.3 x10⁹/L (70% eosinophils on differential)

ALT 121 U/L

Alkaline phosphatase 145 U/L

What is the most likely diagnosis?

A. Drug reaction with eosinophilia and systemic symptoms
B. Fixed drug eruption
C. Skin lesions due to CA-MRSA sepsis and multiorgan dysfunction
D. Streptococcal toxic shock syndrome
E. Toxic epidermal necrolysis

28.

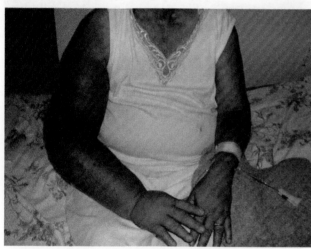

A 72-year-old woman presented with a 4-day history of worsening pain and swelling of her right arm. She had a history of hypertension, atrial fibrillation, and diet-controlled diabetes. She had a radical mastectomy and chemotherapy for invasive breast cancer 5 years prior, with an associated DVT of her right leg; and was currently undergoing investigation for unexplained iron-deficiency anemia.

What risk factor is most likely to be responsible for her current infection?

A. Chronic lymphedema postsurgery
B. Immunosuppression from an underlying malignancy
C. Inflammation due to eczema
D. Preexisting tinea pedis
E. Venous insufficiency following her DVT

29. A 14-year-old girl was reviewed with nausea and epigastric pain made worse on eating. There was no diarrhea. She had no other medical problems and did not take any

regular medications. She was normally resident in Florida but had recently returned from a 3-month stay in Costa Rica with family.

Examination was unremarkable.

Investigations:

Absolute eosinophil count 0.6 ×10⁹/L

Stool microscopy:

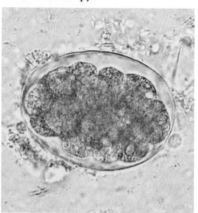

What parasite is most likely to be causing her symptoms?

A. *Ancylostoma duodenale*
B. *Ascaris lumbricoides*
C. *Enterobius vermicularis*
D. *Necator americanus*
E. *Trichuris trichiura*

30. A 42-year-old man presented to his primary care physician with 4 days of mildly pruritic rash, predominantly around his groin, and on his legs. He was otherwise feeling well. On exam, he was noted to have multiple punctate areas of erythema, surrounding hair follicles in his groin and on both legs. He had no palmoplantar lesions. He also mentioned that he had spent several hours in his hot tub the week before he noticed the rash.

What is the most likely cause of his folliculitis?

A. *Candida albicans*
B. Methicillin-resistant *Staphylococcus aureus*
C. *Mycobacterium–avium* complex
D. *Pseudomonas aeruginosa*
E. *Streptococcus pyogenes*

31. A patient presents to the emergency department with a painful left hand after being bitten by a cat. He has a deep puncture wound with some purulent drainage and surrounding cellulitis. Wound cultures are taken, and he is given broad-spectrum antibiotics and tetanus vaccination.

What bacterium is the most likely cause of his infection?

A. *Capnocytophaga canimorsus*
B. *Eikenella corrodens*
C. *Erysipelothrix rhusiopathiae*
D. *Pasteurella multocida*
E. *Pseudomonas aeruginosa*

32. A 32-year-old woman was readmitted to the hospital 3 days after having had a spontaneous abortion at 18 weeks gestation. On examination, she had a temperature of 38.1°C, pulse 132 beats/minute, blood pressure 85/60 mmHg, diffuse abdominal tenderness to palpation, and significant abdominal and lower extremity swelling. Blood cultures were obtained, and she was started on antibiotics. Within a few hours, her blood cultures were growing gram-positive rods.

What is the most likely organism?

A. *Clostridium botulinum*
B. *Clostridioides difficile*
C. *Clostridium sordellii*
D. *Clostridium striatum*
E. *Clostridium tetani*

33. A 45-year-old firefighter, just returned from working on a forest fire in California, is now presenting with malaise and progressive, ascending, bilateral lower extremity weakness. He denies having had any fever or headache. On exam, he had bilateral lower extremity hypotonia, but his sensation was intact. He went on to develop respiratory failure that required intubation and mechanical ventilation. CSF studies and imaging of his brain and spine were normal.

What is the most likely cause of his symptoms?

A. Guillain–Barré syndrome
B. Myasthenia gravis
C. Poliomyelitis
D. Tick paralysis
E. West Nile virus

34. A 5-year-old boy who recently emigrated from Mexico was brought to the doctor because of left axillary swelling. His mother said that the swelling had been gradually worsening over the last few months, but the child was otherwise feeling well and had had no fevers or discomfort related to the swelling. On examination, he was found to have a several-centimeter area of firm swelling under his left arm with some overlying ulceration.

Of the listed mycobacteria, which would be the most likely cause of his lymphadenitis?

A. *Mycobacterium abscessus*
B. *Mycobacterium fortuitum*
C. *Mycobacterium gordonae*
D. *Mycobacterium marinum*
E. *Mycobacterium tuberculosis*

35. A 23-year-old man presented to the HIV clinic complaining of painful swellings in his groin. On examination he has no genital ulcers or chancres, but he has large bilateral inguinal lymphadenopathy.

You suspect he has a sexually transmitted disease. What is the most likely diagnosis?

A. Chancroid
B. Genital herpes
C. Granuloma inguinale
D. Lymphogranuloma venereum
E. Syphilis

36. Which of the following entities is depicted here?

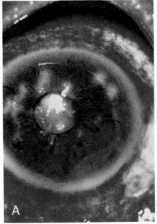 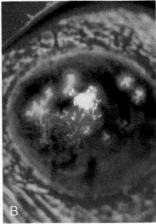

A. *Candida* endophthalmitis
B. HSV keratitis
C. Ocular histoplasmosis
D. Viral conjunctivitis
E. Zoster ophthalmicus

37. A 75-year-old man was admitted from his nursing home with several days of fever, nonproductive cough, headache, and diarrhea. The nursing staff mentioned that two other patients had also been unwell and had had fevers and respiratory symptoms. On admission, the patient had a temperature of 38.5°C, pulse of 110 beats/minute, blood pressure 98/50 mmHg, and oxygen saturation of 89% on room air. His initial laboratory evaluation was notable for a sodium of 125, creatinine of 1.6, and white blood cell count of 16,000. Chest radiograph showed bilateral, diffuse, interstitial, pulmonary opacities. Cultures were ordered, and broad-spectrum antibiotic therapy was initiated.

Of the listed antibacterials, which of the following would be most likely to be effective against the causative pathogen?

A. Amoxicillin
B. Azithromycin
C. Ceftriaxone
D. Clindamycin
E. Vancomycin

38. A 47-year-old man is sent from otolaryngology clinic for evaluation of a chronic left mandibular wound. He has poor dentition and has had multiple tooth extractions. He has, for the last 2 months, had swelling and intermittently draining sinus tracts over the angle of his mandible. Superficial wound cultures have not grown any pathogens. Imaging does not show any signs of mandibular osteomyelitis.

First-line antimicrobial therapy for patients with this condition should include treatment with an agent in which of the following antibiotic classes?

A. Aminoglycosides
B. Glycopeptides
C. Nitroimidazoles
D. Oxazolidinones
E. β-lactams

39. About 8 hours after eating a seafood dinner, a patient develops diarrhea, bradycardia, temperature-related dysesthesia and circumoral paresthesiae.

Her symptoms are most suggestive of which of the following?

A. Botulism
B. Ciguatera poisoning
C. Enterotoxigenic *Escherichia coli* infection
D. Paralytic shellfish poisoning
E. Scombroid poisoning

40. A 32-year-old woman from Jamaica has a history of chronic, watery diarrhea. Recently, she had to receive high-dose steroids for a new diagnosis of systemic lupus erythematosus. She presents now with several days of fever and headache, and her blood cultures and CSF cultures are growing *Escherichia coli*.

In addition to antibacterial therapy, what additional medications could be considered to treat her underlying condition?

A. Ivermectin
B. Niclosamide
C. Nifurtimox
D. Paromomycin
E. Praziquantel

41. A 52-year-old MSM was started on cART with efavirenz, tenofovir, and emtricitabine. He tolerated the introduction well and achieved viral suppression by 16 weeks. He was given an accelerated course of hepatitis B vaccination combined with hepatitis A. His baseline serology showed measles IgG-positive, toxoplasma IgG-positive, varicella IgG-positive, syphilis EIA-negative.

Five months after starting cART he attended the walk-in clinic as he had noticed new lesions on his feet and neck (see image).

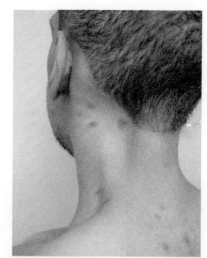
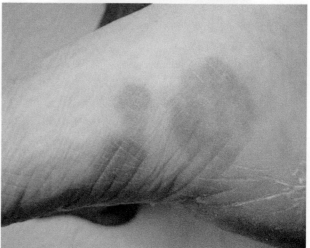

He had also developed dyspnea on exertion, orthopnea, and right-sided pleuritic chest pain. On examination his temperature was 36.9°C, heart rate regular at 88 beats/minute, respiratory rate 16 at rest, oxygen saturations 95% on room air. Chest examination was consistent with a large right-sided pleural effusion.

Following skin biopsy, a diagnosis of Kaposi sarcoma was made.

What is the most appropriate treatment strategy for him?

A. Interferon-α 2a
B. Paclitaxel
C. Pegylated liposomal doxorubicin
D. Rituximab
E. Vinblastine

42. A 46-year-old Thai woman presented with a sudden onset headache and right-sided weakness. Her temperature was 36.5°C, blood pressure 124/74 mmHg, and heart rate 88 beats/ minute. Her Glasgow Coma Score was 14/15. She was drowsy but rousable. She had a right-sided flaccid hemiparesis.

An urgent CT scan of her head was arranged.

Investigations:

Eosinophils 5.9×10⁹/L

CT scan of head:

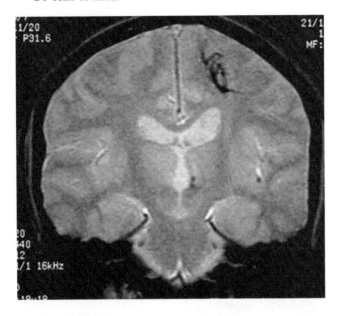

On further questioning her partner revealed that she had also had a prolonged history of recurrent superficial swellings on her arms and torso. These would last for 1–2 weeks, resolve then recur weeks to months later. She had been born and brought up in a small village in northern Thailand, but had emigrated 6 years previously. She had spent 3 months of each year since then in Thailand.

What is the most likely source of her infection?

A. Unwashed salads

B. Uncooked vegetables

C. Uncooked pork

D. Uncooked beef

E. Uncooked freshwater fish

43. A 4-year-old boy in Tanzania developed a painful lump in his left groin, preceded by systemic symptoms of fever, malaise, chills, and headache for 24 hours. The lesion rapidly expanded in size, becoming increasingly painful and tender. On examination he avoided movement of the area and was reluctant for it to be examined. There was marked edema in the tissues surrounding the lesion, but there was no obvious overlying cellulitis (see image). He appeared systemically toxic, with a tachycardia and fever.

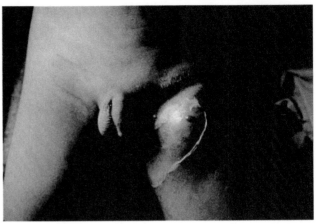

Investigations:

Peripheral white cell count: 36×10⁹/L

Platelet count: 87×10⁹/L

Microscopy of lesion aspirate: small gram-negative coccobacilli with bipolar "safety pin" staining

What vector is most likely to have transmitted this infection?

A. *Ixodes* sp. (hard tick)

B. *Leptotrombidium* sp. (red mite)

C. *Pediculus humanus* (human louse)

D. *Phlebotomus* sp. (sandfly)

E. *Xenopsylla cheopis* (rat flea)

44. Hypersensitivity to what drug can be predicted by HLAB*5701 testing?

A. Abacavir

B. Atazanavir

C. Efavirenz

D. Lamivudine

E. Nevirapine

45. A 39-year-old woman presented with mild fever, malaise, and myalgia 1 week after her 5-year-old son developed a malar rash after a few days of fever and coryzal symptoms (see image).

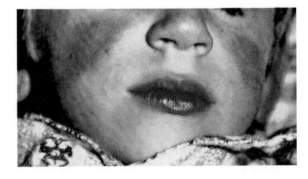

She was usually fit and well. She had an intrauterine device in situ and did not take any regular medications. She had no known allergies. She had been born and brought up in Albania and had moved to the UK at 18 years of age. **She was concerned about the possible complications. What complication is she most likely to develop?**

A. Aseptic meningitis

B. Chronic anemia

C. Myocarditis

D. Rheumatoid-like polyarthritis

E. Transient aplastic crisis

46. A 75-year-old man presented with severe left-sided otalgia, worse at night, extending into his temporomandibular joint. The pain was aggravated by chewing, and his hearing was reduced on that side. There was a purulent discharge from the ear. He had type 2 diabetes mellitus, hypertension, and end-stage renal disease requiring maintenance hemodialysis via a native fistula. He had been seen in the ENT outpatients department 3 months earlier with left otitis externa and received routine aural suction and gentamicin/hydrocortisone ear drops topically.

On examination he had a swollen erythematous external auditory canal on the left, with purulent debris and underlying granulation tissue on the floor of the canal; the right side was normal in appearance. It was not possible to visualize the tympanic membrane. There was erythema extending anteriorly over the temporomandibular joint, and posteriorly over the left mastoid process; the bony prominences and soft tissues were tender on palpation.

He had a left-sided lower motor neurone facial nerve palsy; other cranial nerves were intact.

What is the most likely causative organism?

A. *Aspergillus fumigatus*

B. *Proteus mirabilis*

C. *Pseudomonas aeruginosa*

D. *Staphylococcus aureus*

E. *Streptococcus agalactiae*

47. A 32-year-old woman presented with a 7-day history of cramping abdominal pain and bloody diarrhea. She had opened her bowels over 15 times in the preceding 24 hours. There was fresh red blood mixed in with the stool. She had vomited once and felt feverish. Her symptoms had not abated since their onset. She had returned from a family holiday with her partner and three children 2 days before onset. Nobody else was symptomatic. She had no past medical history of note.

Stool culture yielded *Campylobacter jejuni*.

In addition to fluid replacement therapy, what is the most appropriate management?

A. Azithromycin

B. Ciprofloxacin

C. Metronidazole

D. No antimicrobials needed

E. Trimethoprim–sulfamethoxazole

48. A 20-year-old man presented with fever, rigors, neck pain, and respiratory distress. He had had a sore throat for the preceding week.

On examination, his heart rate was 148 beats/minute, temperature 38.5°C, blood pressure 82/54 mmHg, SaO_2 89% on room air.

Examination of the oropharynx showed erythema over the soft palate and swollen tonsils. His neck movements were restricted, and there was tenderness and induration over the right jugular vein.

Investigations:

Peripheral white cell count 28.7×10^9/L (4.0–11.0)
Platelets 67×10^9/L (150–400)
CXR: multifocal bilateral infiltrates
CT neck:

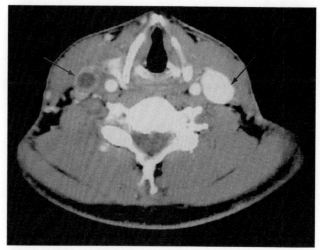

What is the most likely causative organism?

A. *Bacteroides fragilis*

B. *Eikenella corrodens*

C. *Fusobacterium necrophorum*

D. *Streptococcus dysgalactiae*

E. *Streptococcus pyogenes*

49. A 47-year-old man presented with an intensely painful ulcer of 13 days' duration over the glans penis, surrounding the urethral orifice. The lesion had started as multiple small superficial ulcers, which had then coalesced. The ulcer had distinct raised thickened erythematous edges. There was necrotic slough and a foul-smelling hemopurulent discharge. The penis was edematous, and there was bilateral tender inguinal lymphadenopathy. He had had unprotected insertive and receptive anal sex with at least 20 men in the preceding 3 months.

Investigations:

HIV: Ag/Ab negative
Syphilis: EIA negative
Direct wet mount microscopy: trophozoites containing ingested red blood cells

What is the most likely diagnosis?

A. *Balamuthia mandrillaris*
B. *Dientamoeba fragilis*
C. *Entamoeba histolytica*
D. *Giardia lamblia*
E. *Trichomonas vaginalis*

50. A 34-year-old woman presented with migratory swellings over her right arm and back. They typically lasted for 1–3 days and were hot, red, painful, and itchy. She had returned 4 weeks earlier from a 12-month job in Cameroon. A presumptive diagnosis of loiasis was made, pending investigations.

What was the most likely vector for her infection?

A. *Anopheles* mosquito
B. *Chrysops* deerfly
C. *Culex* mosquito
D. *Mansonia* mosquito
E. *Simulium* blackfly

Answers 1

1. E. *Stenotrophomonas maltophilia*
S. maltophilia is one of the few bacteria intrinsically resistant to meropenem. It is also intrinsically resistant to gentamicin. Malignancy and exposure to broad-spectrum antimicrobials, especially carbapenems, are risk factors for *S. maltophilia* infection.

Meropenem is effective against ESBLs and wild-type *B. cepacia*, *M. morganii*, and *P. aeruginosa*. Gentamicin is effective against wild-type *B. cepacia*, *M. morganii*, and *P. aeruginosa* and some ESBLs. While any of those organisms can develop resistance to meropenem, the exposure to meropenem was fairly limited, and acquired meropenem resistance is uncommon in pediatrics.

2. E. Histoplasmosis
Presence of "B-symptoms" (fevers, night sweats, weight loss) and lung nodules suggests an active fungal infection. Considering epidemiology (from Missouri) raises concern for pulmonary histoplasmosis. GMS stain showing small narrow-base budding yeast confirms *Histoplasma* sp.

Aspergillosis occurs mostly in immunocompromised hosts, and the biopsy would show septate hyphae. Travel to southwestern United States suggests coccidioidomycosis, but there are no spherules on biopsy. Biopsy results are not consistent with *Coccidioides* (spherules) or *Blastomyces* (broad-based budding) or *Cryptococcus* (round yeast with a large capsule). Despite the name, *Histoplasma capsulatum* does not have a capsule.
(Image from Kauffman CA. Histoplasmosis. *Clin Chest Med.* 2009;30(2):217–225.)

3. D. NAAT testing of the CSF for enterovirus
This patient was diagnosed with enterovirus disease. Though it is possible to culture enterovirus from the CSF, the rapid turnaround time and exquisite sensitivity and specificity of NAAT testing make it the test of choice. The CSF profile doesn't fit the typical profile for bacterial meningitis as the protein and glucose were both normal (you typically expect decreased glucose and increased protein in bacterial meningitis). NAAT testing for viruses is the appropriate method to use in most cases. One of the exceptions is West Nile virus because the level of viremia usually drops to very low, if not undetectable, levels by the time of symptom onset. Ebola virus is not realistic in this case as the patient has had no travel history.

4. E. Vancomycin
Methicillin-resistant *Staphylococcus aureus* (MRSA) must be covered empirically, pending sensitivities. Dalbavancin is not established for treatment of infections other than acute bacterial skin/skin structure infections. Linezolid should be avoided for treatment of line-related bacteremias due to inferior efficacy in that setting. Clindamycin is not as reliably active against MRSA as vancomycin and is not established as a preferred treatment for MRSA bloodstream infection. There are no apparent contraindications or concerns with using vancomycin in this case.

5. B. Ceftazidime IV
Aztreonam is best reserved for treatment of *Pseudomonas aeruginosa* infections in patients with severe beta-lactam allergy. The patient is not a candidate for oral antibiotic therapy due to recent gastrointestinal disturbances. The patient is also elderly, has renal insufficiency, and has experienced recent central nervous system pathology, each of which increases risk for carbapenem-induced seizures. Aminoglycoside therapy would be risky given the patient's renal function and is not preferred for monotherapy of serious *Pseudomonas aeruginosa* infections. Ceftazidime is a first-line therapy for treatment of *Pseudomonas* infections.

6. C. Imipenem–cilastatin
Imipenem–cilastatin is most likely to be the cause of his seizures. Within the carbapenem drug class, imipenem–cilastatin has been reported to have the highest risk of causing seizures. The other medications listed had reported no risk or minimal risk of causing seizures.

7. C. Continue itraconazole oral solution 200 mg by mouth twice daily
The patient started the itraconazole 2 weeks ago and reported 100% adherence. The itraconazole was at steady state, and the timing of the blood draw in relation to the timing of administration will not make a clinically significant difference. The patient's itraconazole level was the sum of the itraconazole (0.8 μg/mL) and hydroxyitraconazole (1.5 μg/mL). A level of 2.1 μg/mL is between the goal range of 1–10 μg/mL. Continuing the same formulation and dose is most appropriate.

The dose does not need to be increased, and doses above 200 mg are best split into multiple doses to maximize absorption.

The patient is correctly taking itraconazole solution on an empty stomach to maximize absorption, and the patient should not be advised to take itraconazole with food.

Itraconazole solution has better bioavailability than the capsule formulation, and the capsule formulation absorption will be inhibited by the omeprazole. The patient has shown clinical improvement, a therapeutic itraconazole level, and no adverse drug reactions secondary to itraconazole. There is no need to change to another agent with relatively less data and experience.

8. D. Mefloquine
A variety of neuropsychiatric side effects of mefloquine are well described. In particular, strange dreams and sensations of paranoia are among the most frequent.

9. D. Wait and observe the patient
This patient's long history of fever and unremarkable work-up puts him squarely in the diagnosis of FUO. A thorough history and baseline work-up has not suggested a source, and the patient's very mild symptoms imply that this is a patient at low risk for adverse outcomes. This makes therapeutic and aggressive diagnostic measures inadvisable due to risk of complications or unnecessary harm to the patient. These types of patients can be monitored for additional signs/symptoms and will likely have spontaneous resolution of fever.

10. C. Penicillin
Microbiology and clinical presentation are consistent with infection by *Actinomyces* sp. Penicillin is the drug of choice for actinomycosis. Surgical resection is not typically necessary for *Actinomyces* cervicofacial infections unless there is a complex abscess or unless marsupialization of a fistula were required as antibiotics alone should be curative. If an empyema were present, drainage would be indicated. Doxycycline and clindamycin would be second-line agents and are reserved for cases where the patient has penicillin allergy. TMP–SMX would be used if treating *Nocardia*, but recall that *Nocardia* is an aerobic organism. *Nocardia* would be an unlikely organism in this location unless the patient had a penetrating trauma to the area.

11. D. Trimethoprim–sulfamethoxazole
She is displaying signs of a meningoencephalitis with rhombic involvement (possible ataxia, nystagmus, and VIIth cranial nerve palsy) and is at higher risk of *Listeria* due to her age. *Listeria* are insensitive to cephalosporins. Empirical antibacterial treatment would normally consist of a third-generation cephalosporin such as ceftriaxone as well as amoxicillin/ampicillin to cover for *Listeria* in this age group; however, as there is a history of penicillin allergy, TMP–SMX (co-trimoxazole) is used for *Listeria* cover instead. Another alternative would be meropenem.

12. D. Reassurance only
The question is asking you to determine if the patient's tuberculin skin test of 8 mm of induration warrants further work-up and/or therapy for latent or active TB. CDC guidelines suggest that tuberculin skin tests should be read at 48–72 hours after administration. The reaction is measured in millimeters of the induration (NOT erythema). The classification of positive/negative depends on both the diameter of induration AND the person's risk of infection and of progression to disease if infected. The recommendations for classification of a tuberculin skin test reaction are shown below.

Induration of ≥5 mm	Induration of ≥10 mm	Induration of ≥15 mm
HIV infected persons	Recent immigrants (less than 5 years) from high-prevalence countries	Considered positive in any person
Recent contact of a person with TB	Injection drug users	
Persons with fibrotic changes on chest radiograph consistent with prior TB	Residents and employees of high-risk congregate settings	
Patients with organ transplants	Mycobacteriology laboratory personnel	
Persons who are immunosuppressed for other reasons	Children less than 4 years	
	Persons with clinical conditions that place them at high risk	
	Infants, children, and adolescents exposed to adults in high-risk categories	

The patient in this case would need an indurated area of 10 mm or greater to warrant further work-up or therapy; therefore reassurance only is the correct answer

13. E. Trimethoprim–sulfamethoxazole (TMP–SMX)
The patient in this clinical vignette presents with diffuse lung disease and is immunocompromised due to his HIV status. In addition, the patient has a silver stain that is positive, and he must be treated for pneumocystis pneumonia with TMP–SMX. The recommendation would also include administration of steroids due to the PaO_2 being less than 60.

14. D. *Staphylococcus aureus*
S. aureus is an aggressive pathogen that can cause a variety of potentially life-threatening syndromes. When recovered

from blood cultures, it should not be regarded as a contaminant. Patients with blood cultures that are positive for *S. aureus* require thorough evaluation for sites of infection, exclusion of infective endocarditis, and parenteral IV antibiotic therapy.

15. B. Continue prophylaxis until age 25
All patients with rheumatic fever should receive secondary prophylaxis independent of the presence or absence of carditis and/or residual heart disease; these will only affect the **DURATION** of prophylaxis.

The patient has known RF with carditis but no residual cardiac manifestations. In this case the recommendation is for patients to continue prophylaxis for at least 10 years from diagnosis or until age 21, whichever is longer. Since she was diagnosed at age 15, she should receive prophylaxis until age 25 which is longer than age 21.

Short term duration of prophylaxis is only recommended for patients who have RF with no evidence of cardiac involvement.

The recommendation to treat until age 40 or lifelong is for patients with RF with carditis and residual valvular disease, which this patient does not have.

She has no indication to switch to oral antibiotics, although this could be considered. The success rates of oral prophylaxis at preventing relapse are lower than parenteral prophylaxis even with 100% adherence.

Episodes of GAS pharyngitis in the patient or in household contacts should be treated promptly but not at the expense of continuing prophylaxis.

16. E. Trichinellosis
This patient most likely has trichinellosis with myocarditis as a disease manifestation. He likely acquired *Trichinella spiralis* from consumption of undercooked boar meat. Clinically relevant clues to the diagnosis include the ingestion of undercooked boar, the GI syndrome followed by intense myalgia and fever, as well as periorbital edema and conjunctivitis.

Although enteroviral and influenza myocarditis can present with a viral prodrome and malaise, the myalgias would be milder, and there would not be associated facial edema.

Although the ECG findings and elevated enzymes would fit a diagnosis of lateral wall MI, the additional symptoms and findings would not be explained by this diagnosis.

While *Brucella* is present in wild boar meat, most infections are due to skinning and meat handling, and the symptoms of myocarditis do not fit the clinical presentations of brucellosis.

17. D. Norovirus
This fulfils Kaplan outbreak criteria for an outbreak as more than two patients related in time and space have developed similar symptoms. Norovirus is highly infectious and in this case has caused an outbreak. Although loose stool could be due to underlying inflammatory bowel disease in this population, vomiting is more indicative of norovirus, and even though the patients have been in hospital for 3 weeks, norovirus can often be introduced from the community, and the involvement of staff members here is highly suggestive. Accompanying fever is also commonly seen in norovirus infection, and there is no clear ingestion of a common food source to suggest *Staphylococcus aureus* or *Bacillus cereus* infection.

Stool cultures should always be sent to exclude other enteric causes, and samples should also be tested for *C. difficile* as this can be commonly seen in patients with inflammatory bowel disease who receive multiple courses of antibiotics. Separate stool samples should be sent for norovirus as vomitus cannot be tested.

18. E. Surgical referral for nephrectomy
This question reviews the diagnosis of emphysematous pyelonephritis. Surgical management is often required, i.e., resection. Case mortality is high; diabetes mellitus and obstruction are risk factors.

19. D. Send serum for VZV IgG testing
The patient's history suggests that she may be naïve to VZV infection, and therefore although she is in the 3rd trimester and the fetus is not at risk of congenital varicella syndrome, she is at risk of severe varicella disease if infection occurs. There is also a risk that delivery may occur around the time of clinical illness if she is infected, risking perinatal transmission to the neonate.

As she has sought medical attention promptly following exposure, it is appropriate to assess her preexisting immunity by checking her VZV IgG status before ordering the administration of VZIG, which is effective if given within 10 days of exposure. Varicella vaccine is a live attenuated vaccine and therefore is not appropriate in pregnancy. Aciclovir/valaciclovir prophylaxis is also not recommended to avert clinical illness in pregnant women exposed to chickenpox.

20. D. Metronidazole 500 mg BD for 7 days
This patient meets all four of Amsel's criteria for bacterial vaginosis: homogeneous, thin, white discharge that smoothly coats the vaginal walls, clue cells on microscopic examination, pH of vaginal fluid of >4.5, and a fishy odor of vaginal discharge before or after addition of 10% KOH solution. Bacterial vaginosis is most commonly a polymicrobial infection related to *Prevotella* spp., *Mobiluncus* spp., or *Gardnerella vaginalis*. Treatment is with a 7-day course of metronidazole 500 mg BID. The 2-gram dose of metronidazole is intended for trichomoniasis therapy. Fluconazole would be appropriate for vulvovaginal candidiasis. Doxycycline and ceftriaxone are used to treat common causes of cervicitis.

21. A. Ceftriaxone 250 mg IM stat plus doxycycline 100 mg BID
In patient with the above clinical constellation, a low threshold to treat empirically for pelvic inflammatory

disease should be maintained. Empiric outpatient therapy should cover *Gonorrhea*, *Chlamydia*, and anaerobic organisms. Current recommendations are to initiate therapy with one dose of ceftriaxone 250 mg IM plus doxycycline 100 mg every 12 hours with follow-up in 3 days for repeat evaluation.

Other therapeutic regimens would not adequately cover likely culprit organisms.

22. B. Give single-dose HAV vaccination.
Postexposure prophylaxis is warranted as the index case was in a childcare center, caring for children likely to still be in diapers.

Food handlers and close household/sexual contacts of a confirmed case would also be advised to receive PEP.

For healthy persons aged 12 months to 40 years, single-antigen hepatitis A vaccine at the age-appropriate dose is preferred to immunoglobulin because of the vaccine's advantages, including long-term protection and ease of administration, as well as the equivalent efficacy of vaccine to immunoglobulin.

Adults ≥40 or with immunocompromised or chronic liver disease also required HAV immunoglobulin.

For more information, see https://www.cdc.gov/hepatit is/hav/havfaq.htm.

23. A. Chikungunya virus
Parvovirus B19, chikungunya, and rubella are all associated with arthritis, most commonly of the small joints such as hands and wrists. The arthritis associated with rubella usually lasts up to a few weeks. Chronic arthritis is rare in rubella but is described in both parvovirus and notably chikungunya, in which reportedly up to 35% of cases may develop chronic joint symptoms. Chikungunya was found for the first time in the Americas as recently as 2013 but has since been responsible for hundreds of thousands of cases in North, Central, and South America.

24. E. *Treponema pallidum* subsp. *pertenue*
The case describes the typical clinical presentation of yaws, endemic treponematosis caused by *T. pallidum* subsp. *pertenue*. This typically occurs in children from rural communities in tropical areas. Clinical picture shows raised cutaneous lesions (daughter yaws) consistent with early infection.

Bejel and pinta, the other endemic treponematoses have different geographical distribution. The clinical story does not suggest venereal syphilis; positive treponemal serology together with a clinical response to penicillin makes cutaneous leishmaniasis unlikely.

(Image from Ferine PL, Hopkins DR, Niemel PLA, et al. *Handbook of Endemic Treponematoses*. Geneva: World Health Organization; 1984.)

25. E. Piperacillin–tazobactam, vancomycin, clindamycin
Necrotizing soft tissue infection calls for empiric antibiotic coverage of Gram-positive (including methicillin-resistant *Staphylococcus aureus*, MRSA), gram-negative, and anaerobic bacteria. Clindamycin is added to inhibit toxin production. Piperacillin–tazobactam, vancomycin, clindamycin provides the most appropriate coverage, including that of MRSA.

26. C. Pentamidine
This patient has severe pneumocystis pneumonia (PCP). PCP is associated with a variety of immunocompromising conditions. It is a potential complication of most immunosuppressants, including TNF-α-antagonists like infliximab.

He has a history of severe allergy to sulfasalazine, a sulfa agent, and thus TMP–SMX should be avoided. His history also hints at possible G6PD deficiency (he developed hemolytic anemia after taking rasburicase).

His clinical findings of hypoxia and bilateral reticular opacification suggest the diagnosis. His disease is classified as severe based on $PaO2$ <70 mmHg.

Atovaquone is not indicated for use in severe PCP. It can only be used in mild PCP.

Clindamycin and primaquine are appropriate alternatives to TMP–SMX in severe PCP, but G6PD deficiency should be ruled out before use of primaquine given the patient's history which raises concern for this disorder.

TMP + dapsone are not indicated in severe PCP. Additionally, G6PD deficiency should be ruled out before use of dapsone given the patient's history.

(Image from Kumar P, Clark M. *Kumar & Clark's Cases in Clinical Medicine*. 3rd ed. Elsevier; 2013.)

27. A. *Madurella mycetomatis*
Eumycetoma (Madura foot) is a chronic subcutaneous skin and soft tissue infection usually affecting the lower extremity (typically single foot). Areas exposed to trauma are most commonly affected. The disease presents with nodular lesions and sinus tracts draining macroscopic grains. The condition may evolve over years.

Trichophyton rubrum is an agent of dermatophytosis. Talaromycosis typically presents with diffuse papular lesions that demonstrate central umbilication. *Talaromyces marneffei* (formerly *Penicillium marneffei*) is endemic in Southeast Asia and is predominantly affecting patients with AIDS. The chronicity of the disease is not consistent with *P. aeruginosa* or *S. aureus* infection.

28. E. Yellow fever immunization
This is yellow fever, within the first viremic stage of infection. This will be followed by a period of remission for up to 48 hours, and then a proportion of patients will develop the third life-threatening stage of intoxication.

Yellow fever vaccine is recommended for patients (above the age of 9 months) who will travel to the Americas and sub-Saharan Africa. This live attenuated vaccine is not recommended for immunocompromised patients. Booster doses after 10 years are recommended to a subset of individuals who may be at continued risk. Malaria, viral hepatitis, and leptospirosis should be considered in the differential but the rash, the platelet count, and the normal renal function make them less likely than yellow fever. Antibiotic or antiparasitic prophylaxis may be recommended on certain geographic regions, but would not protect him against yellow fever. Hepatitis A, typhoid, and hepatitis B immunizations would all be appropriate to recommend to this man, but would not have protected him.

29. A. Floodwater exposure
Although the differential diagnoses for his clinical presentation are broad (and hence must be ruled out carefully), the most likely diagnosis is leptospirosis. The following clues in his history and exam point to this diagnosis: jaundice, calf tenderness, and the elevated total bilirubin that is out of proportion to the mildly elevated aspartate aminotransferase and alanine aminotransferase levels (rarely >200 U/L). Note that acute hepatitis A (from contaminated food consumption) presents similarly except for the profoundly elevated aspartate aminotransferase and alanine aminotransferase levels.

30. B. Change to RIF, EMB, PZA
Given his history of treatment for latent tuberculosis with INH for 5 months, while having symptoms consistent with TB disease, INH monoresistance should be a concern. INH as preventive therapy while the patient has TB disease has been associated with INH resistant in several studies. However, outcomes are no different between INH-monoresistant TB and pansensitive TB, thus this patient could be treated with a three-drug regimen. Getting sputum samples for AFB smear and culture could also be done, as they may occasionally be positive even in the context of normal chest imaging and could yield additional information, especially in this case with respect to susceptibility testing. As with any other patient with TB disease, an HIV test should also be done.

31. E. *Mycobacterium kansasii*
Clinical features are compatible with *M. kansasii*, but other nontuberculous mycobacteria (NTMs) may also have a similar presentation. Rapid growers are expected to grow faster, usually within 7 days. So the fact that the culture took 3 weeks to show growth eliminates *M. abscessus*, *M. fortuitum*, and *M. chelonae*. Between the two slow growers left, *M. kansasii* is a photochromogen, and the colonies are yellow in color when grown in light, while MAC is nonchromogenic.

32. A. Atovaquone and azithromycin PO for 7 days
The most likely explanation is a co-infection with babesiosis. *Ixodes scapularis* is the vector for Lyme disease, human anaplasmosis, and babesiosis. It is likely that he was appropriately diagnosed with early Lyme disease (given classic bull's-eye skin rash). Although he initially responded, he had a deterioration which is classic for co-infection with babesiosis. *Babesia* has a slightly longer incubation period

and tends to occur later. In contrast to anaplasmosis, *Babesia* is not covered by doxycycline. Chloroquine has no activity against *Babesia* either. The current recommended therapy is atovaquone and azithromycin for 7–10 days.

33. E. *Trichuris trichiura*
The most likely organism here is *Trichuris trichiura*. Rectal prolapse is a known complication of this infection. Trichuris ova are typically 50 × 20 μm in size and are barrel-shaped. They have a smooth wall with a hyaline plug at both ends. Egg numbers usually correlate with adult worm burden.
(Image from Bogitsh B, Carter C, Oeltman T, eds. *Human Parasitology*. 5th ed. Elsevier; 2019.)

34. C. Receptive anal intercourse.
Receptive anal intercourse carries a significantly higher risk of HIV transmission than any other sexual activity.

35. D. Tenofovir alafenamide/emtricitabine + boosted darunavir
Rilpivirine is not recommended in patients who have a HIV RNA >100,000 copies/mL or CD 4 T cell count <200 cells/μL at the start of treatment. Similarly abacavir is only recommended for treatment in patients with HIV RNA >100,000 copies/per mL if it is combined with dolutegravir. In practice INSTI-based regimens are preferred and NNRTI-based regimens are now considered alternative. However if an INSTI cannot be used then boosted darunavir, rilpivirine or efavirenz can be considered in combination with TDF or TAF.

36. C. 4 weeks
Due to the potential for immune reconstitution inflammatory syndrome (IRIS), timing of ART initiation in patients with tuberculosis infection may need to be delayed until effective anti-TB therapy has been instituted. Based on available evidence for nonmeningeal TB infections, current HIV treatment guidelines recommend that ART be started within 2 weeks for patients with a CD4 count <50 cells/μL and between 2 and 8 weeks for patients with a CD4 count >50 cells/μL.

37. B. Fluconazole
The patient's presentation with clinical symptoms suggestive of esophagitis and oral candidiasis (thrush) is most consistent with candida esophagitis, which is treated with fluconazole. Nystatin would be inadequate for esophageal involvement. Herpes simplex virus and cytomegalovirus can also cause esophagitis but would be less common, particularly given the concomitant thrush. Pantoprazole, used for reflux esophagitis, would be a diagnosis of exclusion after infectious causes were ruled out.

38. C. Colonoscopy with biopsies

In an advanced HIV/AIDS patient presenting with symptoms concerns for possible CMV colitis, colonoscopy with biopsies for histopathology and immunohistochemical staining for CMV is the diagnostic modality of choice. Serum or plasma serum PCR is neither sensitive nor specific enough to exclude or confirm a diagnosis of CMV colitis. Serology can demonstrate whether the patient has had exposure but is not useful for diagnosis of active disease which is typically due to reactivation. CT scan may demonstrate colitis but is nonspecific, and viral stool culture is not able to confirm tissue invasive disease.

39. E. Viridans group streptococci

Viridans group streptococci have been well described as virulent pathogens in neutropenic patients. The source of bacteremia is typically from the upper GI track, and often patients will have significant mucositis. It can cause a GNR-like sepsis picture clinically as well as acute respiratory distress syndrome (ARDS). Breakthrough infections on fluoroquinolone prophylaxis can occur, especially with ciprofloxacin due to the poor antistreptococcal activity.

40. C. BK virus nephropathy

BK virus nephropathy is asymptomatic and should be suspected when there is an unexplained rise in serum creatinine in kidney transplant recipients. The diagnosis is confirmed by the identification of decoy cells in urine cytology and detection of BK virus nucleic acid in urine and blood. Other options listed are typically symptomatic.

41. C. Dihydrorhodamine (DHR) test

Chronic granulomatous disease (CGD) is seen mainly in boys (most common cause is X-linked), and the spectrum of infection is distinct, including *Serratia marcescens*, *Nocardia*, and *Burkholderia*, The DHR test is diagnostic and measures the superoxide production in neutrophils via the NADPH oxidase complex.

42. B. Continue standard precautions

Neisseria meningitidis is transmitted person-to-person by respiratory droplets, which travel about 3–6 feet before being removed from the air by the force of gravity. Patients with suspected bacterial meningitis are placed on droplet precautions. After 24 hours of effective therapy, patients with meningitis due to *N. meningitidis* are no longer considered contagious. In this case, the patient had been treated for greater than 24 hours, and precautions were no longer indicated.

43. E. Take a 6–9 month course of isoniazid

Treatment of latent TB infection (LTBI) is essential to controlling and eliminating TB in the United States because it significantly reduces the risk that TB infection will progress to TB disease.

There are different PPD cutoffs for LTBI treatment:

≥5 mm: HIV, recent contact of a TB case, organ transplant recipients, immunosuppression

≥10 mm: IVDU, persons from high prevalence countries, HCW, children <4 years old

≥15 mm: no known risk factors

Based on the above, treatment for LTBI is appropriate as additional testing would not change treatment course. In the United States, 9 months is the preferred course of therapy if feasible; in the UK, either 6 months of isoniazid, or 3 months of rifampicin/isoniazid combination is offered. She is asymptomatic, and her chest radiograph is negative, so she does not require treatment for active TB infection. BCG vaccine would not be recommended for her as she has a positive Mantoux test.

44. E. Two doses of hepatitis B immunoglobulin (HBIG) 1 month apart

The healthcare worker has no immunity to hepatitis B and has sustained a significant exposure to a patient who is HBsAg+ and thus requires immediate intervention. The CDC recommend that nonresponders should preferably receive two doses of HBIG 1 month apart as postexposure prophylaxis. Adequate protection against infection would not be provided by the alternative options. If the recipient's anti-HBsAb status is unknown, then the CDC recommend a single dose of HBIG and commencing a course of HBV vaccination.

45. C. MMR

Vaccinations should be tailored to the patient based on previous vaccinations, specific trip, and risks. HAV and typhoid are endemic in India and should be given. The risk for Japanese encephalitis and rabies should be mentioned and discussed (mosquito precautions, avoidance of contact with animals), but the risk is very small in short-lasting trips limited to urban areas. HBV is endemic in India (intermediate/high prevalence) so vaccination should be considered, but is only recommended for those whose activities or medical history put them at increased risk (for example, healthcare workers, IDU, those who may have unprotected sex).

For patients from the United States, MMR is indicated in those born in 1957 or later, without evidence of immunity or two doses of the live vaccine. MMR was given as a single dose before the 1990s, so in this case it is very likely that the patient has not received a second MMR dose. In the UK, individuals born before 1970 are likely to have had measles naturally, but MMR should be offered if they are considered to be at high risk of exposure, such as travel to areas with high incidence; those born between 1970 and 1979 should be offered MMR wherever feasible.

46. B. Chickenpox

The characteristic rash, with vesicles affecting the trunk as opposed to extremities, and easy to slough off, indicates chickenpox as the likely diagnosis. He could have been exposed to monkeypox in Nigeria as there are ongoing outbreaks, but the rash in monkeypox largely affects the face and extremities. He is also a postal worker, an occupational risk factor for exposure to bioterrorist acts, but the rash distribution, and the lesions at differing stages of development are against a diagnosis such as smallpox.

47. C. Familial Mediterranean fever
FMF is the most likely diagnosis in an 18-year-old of Turkish descent, with fever, peritonitis, and previous laparotomy, suggesting recurrence of symptoms. Erysipelas-like lesions on the lower legs may be experienced by 15%–20% of patients.

There is a very low risk of malaria in Turkey, and antimalarial prophylaxis is not recommended. Malaria would not be expected to cause a skin rash.

Yersinia enterocolitica and *Yersinia pseudotuberculosis* may cause acute yersiniosis. This usually manifests as fever, abdominal pain, and diarrhea, which have often been present for at least 1 week before the patient seeks help.

Bartonella henselae infection would typically present either with skin changes at the primary inoculation site or with regional lymphadenopathy. It can manifest as a fever of unknown origin or with abdominal pain secondary to granulomatous involvement of the liver and/or spleen.

48. D. Randomized controlled trial
Randomized controlled trial is the correct answer because it is the strongest design in terms of establishing causation, since participants are randomized to treatment. Due to randomization, measured and unmeasured confounders should be equally distributed among the groups.

An ecological study is the weakest design in terms of causation, because no inferences can be made about individuals from this design which involves aggregate data. Case–control and prospective cohorts are observational studies, and as such at risk for confounding and selection bias since treatment was not randomized. Meta-analyses combine the results of multiple studies and thus are not used to analyze data from individuals in order to establish causation.

49. D. Nodular granulomatous perifolliculitis (Majocchi's granuloma)
Nodular granulomatous perifolliculitis (Majocchi's granuloma) occurs when dermatophytes invade hair follicles leading to granulomas and/or suppuration. The same organisms which are responsible for tinea corporis and/or pedis (*Trichophyton rubrum*, *T. mentagrophytes*, *Epidermophyton floccosum*, etc.) are involved. Occlusion, trauma to skin (e.g., shaving), use of topical steroids on unsuspected tinea, and immunocompromised states increase risk.

It presents as subacute to chronic nodular lesions that progressively increase in size and number after dermatophyte invasion of hair follicles. Look for cluster(s) of pustules/papules/nodules within erythematous scaling plaques, that may resemble bacterial furuncles or carbuncles. Treatment requires systemic antifungals.

This page intentionally left blank

Answers 2

1. C. Modified acid-fast

The Gram stain shows filamentous beaded gram-positive rods, indicative of an aerobic actinomycete, most closely resembling *Nocardia*. A modified acid-fast stain would be positive for *Nocardia*. A positive modified acid-fast stain result would not provide a definitive diagnosis since other aerobic actinomycetes can be modified acid-fast positive. However, based on the other factors, it supports the diagnosis of nocardiosis while waiting for the organism to grow in culture.

The acid-fast stain is for *Mycobacterium* spp. *Nocardia* will stain negative with the acid-fast stain, as it uses a stronger decolorizing agent. Giemsa, periodic acid–Schiff, and Warthin–Starry are histopathology stains that are unrelated to the diagnosis of aerobic actinomycetes.

2. C. *Legionella* culture on BAL

The *Legionella* urine antigen test only detects *L. pneumophila* serogroup 1. Although *L. pneumophila* serogroup 1 is the most common cause of infection and the urine antigen test has a fast turnaround time, a negative urine antigen does not effectively rule out *Legionella*. Culture and some PCRs detect all species of *Legionella* and should be ordered in addition to the urine antigen.

BAL is not an appropriate specimen for anaerobic culture, and an anaerobic infection is low on the differential. If anaerobic cultures were desired, a bronchial brushing or lung biopsy should be performed.

C. psittaci does not fit since there is no bird exposure. It is diagnosed by serology rather than PCR/NAAT.

Serology is not the preferred test for diagnosis of *M. pneumoniae*. The correct test would be PCR/NAAT.

WNV antibodies are not found in CSF without also being found in serum. Since the serum serology was negative, the CSF serology will also be negative.

3. B. CSF cryptococcal antigen

His clinical presentation is consistent with meningitis. He has high-risk sexual behavior that increases probability of HIV. High opening pressure with predominantly mononuclear cells and normal CT imaging raise concern for possible cryptococcal meningitis with undiagnosed HIV.

CSF cryptococcal antigen, which is highly specific and sensitive for cryptococcal meningitis, should be performed to establish the diagnosis.

A normal CT and no encephalopathy make HSV less likely.

Epidemiology is concerning for CNS coccidioidomycosis, but the high opening pressure is more suggestive for cryptococcosis. Additionally the definitive test in patients with presumed HIV would be CSF antigen for coccidioidomycosis, not the antibody.

Syphilis is always a possibility, especially in patients with high-risk sexual behavior, and should be ruled out. However, this case presentation is unlikely to be due to syphilis, and the VDRL alone has a low sensitivity.

Histoplasmosis is possible due to his exposure (cleaning and painting the old bridge will involve exposure to aerosolized bird droppings), however he is outside of the endemic area, and meningitis with a high opening pressure would be a rare presentation of the disease.

4. D. Telavancin

The possible agents listed have variable coverage against MRSA, with linezolid and telavancin being most established for treatment of serious systemic MRSA infections. Clindamycin, minocycline, linezolid, and tigecycline do not require dosage adjustment in the setting of renal insufficiency. Therefore serum concentrations of these agents would not be expected to accumulate in this patient as a result of renal insufficiency. Telavancin is eliminated primarily by the kidneys and is also recognized as potentially nephrotoxic. This agent can accumulate in patients with renal insufficiency and increased risk of adverse effects.

5. A. Audiology exam

Aminoglycosides, including amikacin, can cause ototoxicity. Thus baseline and serial audiograms are recommended until 2 months after the final dose of an aminoglycoside.

6. C. Itraconazole oral solution 200 mg by mouth once daily

Itraconazole is the recommended treatment of disseminated histoplasmosis during the maintenance phase of therapy. The itraconazole oral solution formulation is preferred over the capsule formulation due to increased bioavailability. Itraconazole doses greater than 200 mg should be split into multiple doses to help optimize absorption. Itraconazole is a major substrate of CYP450 3A4. Cobicistat/darunavir is a strong CYP450 3A4 inhibitor, which will decrease the metabolism of itraconazole, resulting in increased itraconazole levels. Itraconazole inhibits the metabolism of cobicistat/darunavir, resulting in an increase in darunavir. The interaction is clinically significant. The usual, i.e., in the setting of no drug–drug interactions, itraconazole maintenance dose is 200 mg by mouth twice daily. With these drug–drug interactions in place, the recommendation is to reduce the itraconazole dose to 200 mg once daily, and then check itraconazole levels.

7. B. IV foscarnet

The patient is likely infected with a thymidine kinase (TK)-deficient virus, and the virus is resistant to high-dose aciclovir, valaciclovir, famciclovir, ganciclovir, or valganciclovir. **Foscarnet** is the drug of choice in thymidine kinase-deficient HSV. Alternatively, cidofovir can also be used, but it is much more nephrotoxic than foscarnet. Topical compound cidofovir creams can also be used, but this is not commercially available. Ribavirin has no activity against the herpes viruses.

8. B. Artesunate hemolysis

Delayed postartesunate hemolysis is likely the result of the clearance of previously infected erythrocytes by the spleen. Artesunate kills parasites while not affecting the erythrocytes themselves; however, their ultimate lifespan is shortened. This generally happens 7–14 days after treatment initiation.

9. E. Refer patient for guided drainage tube placement

This patient is septic due to a perforated diverticulitis. He remains persistently septic and hypotensive despite broad spectrum antibiotic therapy. While some may take this as a sign of additional infection, or failure of antibiotic therapy, the more likely cause is that antibiotics alone are insufficient to gain control over a closed source infection such as an abscess. The only way to gain source control over an infection of this type is physical removal of the infected fluid, which can be done either through surgical debridement and washout, or through placement of a drain (which is more likely in this case due to the patient's hemodynamic instability).

10. D. Vaccinia immunoglobulin and topical trifluridine

The patient has vaccine-associated preseptal cellulitis and conjunctivitis from contact with the military recruit who had recent smallpox immunization. It is important to remember that patients who receive smallpox vaccination may shed live virus while the vaccination site is healing. This typically lasts until separation of the scab which is usually 2–3 weeks after the vaccination. Vaccinia immunoglobulin and topical trifluridine are the treatment of choice. More

severe cases warrant immunoglobulin, and it does help decrease shedding of virus. While vancomycin and a cephalosporin would be reasonable for the preseptal cellulitis, it would not address the conjunctivitis in this case. The vesicle points toward a viral etiology. Azithromycin would be for suspected *Chlamydia*; however, the clinical scenario is not consistent with such given the vesicle and recent contact with a contact of a recently vaccinated person.

11. D. HSV-2

Aseptic meningitis may be caused by HSV, enterovirus, CMV, and *B. burgdorferi*; however, the recurrent nature of the episodes of meningitis make this much more likely to be HSV-2. Recurrent meningococcal infections are recognized and occur due to a terminal complement deficiency; however, the CSF profile does not fit, she is older than would be expected for an inherited complement deficiency, and she has no risk factors for an acquired deficiency. Neuroborreliosis may present with an acute or chronic meningitis, but recurrent episodes would be unusual.

HSV-2 meningitis may present in the absence of genital lesions; humans are the only known reservoir, but the vast majority of genital HSV infections are unrecognized (approx. 85%–90%). The first episode of HSV-2 meningitis usually occurs within 2 weeks of primary genital HSV infection. It is more common in women than men. The incidence of recurrent meningitis is reported to be around 30%. Lack of prior HSV-1 infection may predispose to more symptomatic HSV-2 infection, both genital and meningeal.

12. B. Adenosine deaminase measurement

The patient presents with a new pleural effusion after returning from an endemic area for tuberculosis. The concern is for a tuberculous effusion and an LDH, pH, or Gram stain would not help diagnose tuberculosis. An AFB stain would be low yield, and therefore the correct answer is an adenosine deaminase. An adenosine deaminase would be expected to be high in the setting of a tuberculous effusion, and of the choices listed would be the most helpful for establishing the diagnosis.

13. A. Cefazolin

This patient has MSSA bacteremia, and there should be some concern that she may also have endocarditis. According to the guidelines, recommended agents in this circumstance would include cefazolin or an antistaphylococcal penicillin (nafcillin or oxacillin). Alternative agents may be employed based on individual circumstances (e.g., vancomycin in the setting of β-lactam allergy).

14. A. She does not require prophylaxis because she does not have a high-risk cardiac condition.

High-risk cardiac conditions include prosthetic valves, previous endocarditis, congenital heart disease with unrepaired cyanotic defects, repaired defects with prosthetic materials in the first 6 months postrepair, repaired congenital defects with residual defects next to a prosthetic material, and cardiac transplant recipients with valvulopathy of the transplanted heart.

MVP is not a high-risk condition, so she does not require antibiotic prophylaxis. If she were a candidate for prophylaxis and had a reliable history of penicillin allergy, clindamycin, azithromycin, or clarithromycin would be reasonable alternatives.

A tonsillectomy is a high-risk procedure which involves incision of the respiratory mucosa. If she had one of the high-risk cardiac conditions mentioned above, then in the United States she would be a candidate for prophylaxis for tonsillectomy. In the UK, NICE guidance currently does not advise routine antibiotic prophylaxis against endocarditis, even in patients with cardiac conditions that are at higher risk of developing infective endocarditis. This is because the clinical effectiveness of antibiotic prophylaxis is not proven, it is not cost-effective, and there may be more deaths due to anaphylaxis than are prevented.

An echocardiogram is not indicated.

15. D. Send stool for enteric pathogens (culture/NAAT)

This patient has enterohemorrhagic *E. coli* (EHEC, also called Shiga toxin-producing *E. coli* or STEC) causing bloody diarrhea following contact with a petting farm. This has caused hemolytic uremic syndrome (HUS) with renal failure, thrombocytopenia, and microangiopathic anemia. HUS can occur in 6%–9% of EHEC infections, and this patient also has neurologic symptoms. EHEC is also a rare cause of pseudomembranous colitis when culture-negative for *Clostridioides difficile*.

Antibiotic treatment is contraindicated pending stool culture results and may make symptoms worse. Hence supportive treatment is advised. There are also likely to be other patients on the excursion who may be affected, and this should be further investigated as part of a possible outbreak.

16. B. Atherosclerotic disease

The patient is likely to have acquired *Salmonella* spp. infection from her reptiles, which can act as a reservoir for infection. Patients younger than 12 months have a high risk of neurologic infection and mortality and often may not appear unwell. It is recommended that children <5 years and immunocompromised patients should avoid contact with reptiles. Invasive disease occurs in those who are immunosuppressed and in those aged over 50 years where due to atherosclerotic disease they have a high risk (10%) of endovascular infection if bacteremia develops. Persistent fever, hospital admission, and cardiac or other valvular disease are also risk factors. This patient may also have disseminated *Salmonella* infection and osteomyelitis of her leg should be excluded.

17. E. *Strongyloides stercoralis* hyperinfestation

Strongyloides hyperinfestation is the most likely condition. *Strongyloides* are nematodes (roundworms) that may be acquired from dogs and other companion animals, but also from soil or other materials contaminated with human feces. Countries in South America (particularly Peru) have a high prevalence of *Strongyloides* infection, and consequently latent asymptomatic infection is common. Hyperinfestation illness can occur in patients with underlying asymptomatic disease who become immunosuppressed, as in this case with high-dose steroids. Consider asking patients about clinical manifestations of initial infection (rash, respiratory symptoms). *Strongyloides*-associated pancreatitis is a recognized feature of hyperinfestation illness but remains an infrequent cause of acute pancreatitis, particularly in immunocompetent hosts.

The patient's total leucocyte count and neutrophil count is raised. Neutrophilia commonly reflects bacterial infection, but it should be noted that steroids cause an accelerated release of neutrophils from the bone marrow. As a result neutrophilia is commonly seen in patients receiving steroid therapy. In this scenario the total leucocyte count is not completely accounted for by neutrophils, lymphocytes, or monocytes. This suggests that another leucocyte is raised, such as eosinophils, which would fit with tissue-migratory helminth infection.

Acute cholangitis is a common condition although the patient does not have classic risk factors, clinical features, or radiologic findings. Of note, the absence of gallstones or inflammation on USS does not entirely rule this out but does make this condition less likely. The chest X-ray reveals bilateral pulmonary infiltrates, which are seen in SIRS, but can also be seen in other conditions including atypical pneumonia and hyperinfestation illness.

Community-acquired pneumonia caused by mycoplasma can present as severe shortness of breath with extrapulmonary features such as pancreatitis. Despite this, the clinical situation is atypical for mycoplasma infection as it is most common in patients <40 years old, symptoms crescendo over 2–3 weeks, and are commonly associated with cough and headaches (absent in the patient). Blood tests can also reveal a hemolytic anemia (again absent).

Adult-onset asthma is plausible, particularly as he has a history of atopy, but this is uncommon, and the association of other features (pancreatitis) makes this unlikely.

Acute HIV classically presents as an infectious mononucleosis-type illness with fever, rash, sore throat, and lymphadenopathy. Atypical presentations with involvement of different body systems can occur but as the patient does not have clear risk factors (although these should be clarified) and lymphocyte count is normal, this would make acute HIV unlikely. An HIV test should still be performed.

(Image from Wang Y, Ma Y, Xu Y, et al. *Strongyloides stercoralis* disseminated infection in a patient misdiagnosed with chronic asthmatic bronchitis. *J Microbiol Immunol Infect.* 2016;49(1):154–156.)

18. B. Cephalexin

Treatment is indicated as asymptomatic bacteriuria is associated with a greater risk of subsequent pyelonephritis and consequent preterm delivery. Depending on local resistance rates, the organism may not be reliably susceptible to amoxicillin, and many labs may not test its susceptibility. Fluoroquinolones are not recommended in pregnancy. Trimethoprim–sulfamethoxazole would be ok earlier in pregnancy but in later pregnancy is associated with greater risk of kernicterus and hyperbilirubinemia in the newborn.

19. D. *Mycoplasma genitalium*

M. genitalium should be considered in men with persistent urethritis especially after treatment with doxycycline. Azithromycin 1 g orally as a single dose should be administered in men initially treated with doxycycline. However, azithromycin resistance is also reported in *M. genitalium*. *C. trachomatis* and *N. gonorrhoeae* are less likely causes based upon the negative NAAT. HSV can cause urethritis, but typically symptoms would resolve even in the absence of treatment. The absence of dermatologic findings makes contact dermatitis less likely.

20. E. Tenofovir alafenamide, emtricitabine, and dolutegravir

In a patient co-infected with HBV and HIV, treatment should include tenofovir to cover both viruses. Only A and E include fully active antiretroviral regimens, and only E includes tenofovir. Although lamivudine has activity against HBV, resistance develops quickly. Regimen B would be unconventional and would cover HIV but has no HBV coverage, and ledipasvir alone will not treat HCV. Regimen D includes a single drug for HBV, HIV, and HCV. Both HIV and HCV require more than one active antiviral for efficacy. Given the risk of HBV reactivation with treatment of HCV, in the setting of all three infections, most would recommend controlling HIV and HBV first before starting HCV therapy.

21. D. Measles virus

Postexposure prophylaxis with MMR vaccine is recommended for susceptible individuals exposed to proven cases of measles. Immunoglobulin is available for protection postexposure in those who are unable to have MMR, such as immunocompromised children or adults and pregnant women. Prophylactic regimens are not available postexposure to CMV, rubella, parvovirus B19, or HSV although specific testing and follow-up may be indicated.

22. C. *Borrelia garinii*

Borrelia afzelii and *Borrelia garinii* are both part of the *Borrelia burgdorferi* sensu lato group. *B. afzelii* is found in Europe and is associated with acrodermatitis chronica atrophicans whereas *B. garinii*, which is also found in Europe, is associated with neurologic presentations of Lyme disease.

Babesiosis is also a tickborne disease. It is a parasitic infection affecting red blood cells, but neurologic disease is not described.

Tickborne encephalitis virus is a member of the family *Flaviviridae*. It is a viral infection with acute onset of symptoms (incubation 7–14 days), and rash is not described.

Treponema pallidum may cause neurosyphilis with an aseptic meningitis, but the rash is not typical for syphilis, nor would a tick bite be related.

23. C. Incision and drainage at the bedside

A carbuncle of this size is likely to respond well to bedside incision and drainage. Antibiotics alone are unlikely to address the infection, and surgical debridement of the carbuncle and/or hospitalization to receive intravenous antibiotics for a lesion of this size is not indicated, particularly given that the patient does not have any systemic signs of infection (e.g., fevers, chills). Superficial skin cultures are likely to grow commensal flora; abscess cultures are preferred to guide antibiotic therapy.

24. E. Two-stage exchange

Given the presence of a late prosthetic joint infection (onset >24 months after surgery), prolonged duration of symptoms, and presence of sinus tract on physical exam, a DAIR would not be recommended given the risk for relapse of infection, especially in the setting of MRSA infection. With DAIR and one-stage exchange, a period of oral antibiotic suppression is required following completion of parenteral therapy. The patient as described above does not have any viable oral antibiotic options given the isolate's susceptibility pattern and his allergy history. While the isolate is sensitive to linezolid, it is not an ideal antibiotic for long-term use given the potential for hematologic toxicity associated with >14 days of therapy (most commonly, thrombocytopenia) as well as rare adverse events (lactic acidosis, optic neuritis, and peripheral neuropathy). Additionally, the patient has a history of depression, to which selective serotonin reuptake inhibitors (SSRIs), and tricyclic antidepressants (TCAs) can pose significant drug–drug interactions with linezolid use. Given the nature of his infection, the patient's allergy history, and comorbidities, a two-stage exchange would be ideally employed in this scenario.

25. A. *Candida auris*

Candida auris is an emerging multidrug-resistant pathogen that causes otomycosis and invasive candidiasis. It is an important nosocomial pathogen, especially in some parts of the world where it has already established endemicity. Healthcare-associated outbreaks have been reported in the United States.

C. auris will be misidentified by commercial identification systems. The Vitek-2 will usually misidentify *C. auris* as *Candida haemulonii* and sometimes as *Candida famata*; the API-20C system will misidentify *C. auris* as *Rhodotorula glutinis*, *Candida sake*, or *Saccharomyces cerevisiae*. The correct identification can be made through DNA sequencing or with matrix-assisted laser desorption ionization-time of flight (MALDI-TOF).

26. B. Blood culture on Sabouraud dextrose with olive oil

This is a case of disseminated *Malassezia* infection. Risk factors in this case include CVC and lipid infusions (TPN).

Malassezia spp. are intrinsically resistant to echinocandins, thus a response to micafungin is not expected.

Malassezia spp. are lipophilic, and all species but *M. pachydermatis* require exogenous lipids for growth. *M. furfur* is the most common pathogen involved in disseminated disease. Recovery from standard blood cultures is low unless the media is enriched with fatty acids, i.e., with olive oil, palmitic acid, Tween, etc., or with Dixon's agar, which contains glycerol mono-oleate.

Serum 1,3-β-D-glucan is a nonspecific biomarker of fungal disease. It is not particularly helpful in making a diagnosis.

Panfungal PCR is not useful on blood because of the low burden of organisms in the total circulation.

Serum CrAg is used for the diagnosis of cryptococcosis (including subclinical disease). It also can cross react with *Trichosporon* spp. in disseminated disease, although a negative result does not exclude the diagnosis. Trichosporonosis has been reported in neonates but is less likely than *Malassezia* disease.

27. A. Dengue

The patient has signs and symptoms of dengue fever and recently traveled to a highly endemic area. Think of dengue in any febrile traveler returning from endemic regions. For your boards, remember key differences between yellow fever (more transaminitis and jaundice, lack of immunization prior to travel), chikungunya (more joint disease, less plasma leakage), and leptospirosis (water exposure, conjunctival suffusion).

Disease	Dengue	Chikungunya	Yellow Fever	Leptospirosis
What to look for:	Febrile illness, mosquito exposure Thrombocytopenia Shock	Febrile illness, mosquito exposure Joint pains Milder disease than dengue	Febrile illness, mosquito exposure Transaminitis, jaundice, no vaccine prior to travel	Febrile illness, water exposure Hyperbilirubinemia out of proportion to transaminitis Conjunctival suffusion

28. E. *Yersinia pestis*

The pneumonic form of plague, caused by *Yersinia pestis* infection, occurs via inhalation of aerosols from an infected person (i.e., during close contact with a person). Person-to-person transmission does not occur in Q fever, tularemia, or anthrax and is exceedingly rare in brucellosis.

29. A. Isoniazid and rifapentine weekly for 3 months

With the exception of option E, all of the above are valid LTBI treatment regimens. However, shorter courses, like the combination of INH plus RPT once a week for 3 months (A) or 4 months of daily RIF have higher completion rates (>80%) compared to longer regimens. INH/RPT weekly for 3 months (3HP) has also shown high completion rates when self-administered for LTBI treatment.

30. C. *Mycobacterium genavense*

Mycobacterium avium complex is the most common cause of disseminated NTM infection in AIDS patients. *M. genavense*, on the other hand, can present in a similar way in AIDS patients and should be considered when patient presents with classic picture of disseminated MAC infection, but the routine AFB cultures remain negative. Incubation of the culture at lower temperature can assist in the recovery of this organism.

31. D. *Entamoeba histolytica*

This is an example of amoebic colitis caused by *Entamoeba histolytica*. The trophozoites are present in the ulcer and have ingested red blood cells, which is a classic finding in invasive cases. *Giardia lamblia* is a flagellate protozoan, resides in the small intestine, and does not cause ulcers. *Balantidium coli* (or *Neobalantidium*) can cause disease similar to amoebiasis but is a ciliate protozoan. *Blastocystis hominis* may cause diarrhea but does not ingest red blood cells or cause ulcers.

32. A. Albendazole

The history of chronic abdominal pain, microcytic anemia, mild eosinophilia, and epidemiologic exposure is most likely to be explained by a hookworm infection. Albendazole (or mebendazole) is used most frequently as first-line treatment. Iron replacements may be used, but anemia will recur without specific treatment to clear the parasites. Pyrantel is a good alternative; ivermectin has poor activity against hookworm. There is no indication for DEC.

33. D. p24 antigen

The fourth-generation HIV test is an ELISA testing for both HIV-1/HIV-2 antibodies as well as the p24 antigen (a capsid protein of the virus). Because the p24 antigen is detectable before HIV antibodies, fourth-generation tests can detect HIV infection earlier than tests that only detect HIV antibodies (third-generation tests).

34. B. Continue current ART and routine monitoring

HIV-infected pregnant women established on ART who present for care during the 1st trimester should continue treatment during pregnancy, provided the regimen is tolerated and effective in suppressing viral replication. Women who become pregnant on efavirenz-containing regimens who are virally suppressed and tolerating it should continue their current regimens. In the past efavirenz was linked with teratogenicity based on animal studies; however, increased teratogenicity has not been seen in the babies of mothers exposed to efavirenz in the 1st trimester in registry studies and meta-analyses. Therefore guidelines recommend continuing treatment: http://aidsinfo.nih.gov/contentfiles/lvguidelines/PerinatalGL.pd. There is no data on cobicistat in pregnancy, therefore for present protease inhibitors should be ritonavir-boosted.

35. B. Addition of a nonsteroidal antiinflammatory

This presentation would be most consistent with an immune reconstitution inflammatory syndrome (IRIS) from the TB lymphadenitis in a setting of rise in CD4 count and drop in HIV viral load with initiation of ART. Recommendations in most cases of TB IRIS are to continue ART and anti-TB therapy. In moderate to severe cases of IRIS, nonsteroidal antiinflammatory drugs or corticosteroids can be added. The development of drug-resistant TB would be less likely at this time point, and surgical excision would not be recommended for a likely reversible and non-life-threatening situation.

36. E. Indefinite

Due to high relapse rates in meningeal and CNS coccidioidomycosis in HIV patients, secondary prophylaxis with oral azole therapy is recommended indefinitely, regardless of CD4 count recovery.

37. D. Stop natalizumab and consider plasma exchange

Based on risk factors and clinical presentation, the diagnosis is most likely to be progressive multifocal leukoencephalopathy (PML). The recommended treatment is to immediately stop the natalizumab, and some experts also recommend plasma exchange.

38. C. Positron emission tomography scan

A large retrospective study performed at a referral center in France showed that PET scan was superior to ultrasound, CT scan, and MRI for the detection of infected cysts.

39. D. *Fusarium solani*

Fusarium are species of mold that may cause disseminated disease in immunocompromised patients. It tends to be more resistant to the azole antifungals than *Aspergillus* species but sensitive to amphotericin. Disseminated fusariosis may be identified through positive blood cultures. The typical clinical picture is as described in a patient with prolonged (>10 days) neutropenia, persistent fevers, widespread skin lesions that evolve rapidly, and blood cultures growing a mold. Unlike aspergillosis, blood cultures are commonly positive. Mortality rates are high even with appropriate antifungals and immunotherapy such as G-CSF.

Because the pathogen identified is a mold, *Candida tropicalis*, *Histoplasma capsulatum*, and *Cryptococcus neoformans* would not be the answer, as they appear as yeast forms in the human body. However, these pathogens can cause disseminated nodular skin lesions in immunocompromised patients. *Aspergillus fumigatus* is not the correct answer, as voriconazole is usually effective prophylaxis against invasive aspergillus infections, and aspergillus rarely is identified in blood cultures.

40. B. CH50

Recurrent *Neisseria* infections are a red flag for complement deficiencies, and the past medical history of SLE is another clue toward this diagnosis. The best screening test is CH50. This is a screening test for deficits in either the classic or terminal complement pathways. It tests the functional ability of complement components to lyse antibody-coated sheep red blood cells and is sensitive to a decrease, absence, or inactivity of components in the pathway.

41. A. 2 doses of rabies vaccine

This patient who was previously vaccinated for rabies has now had a potential rabies exposure. She should receive two intramuscular doses of the vaccine. The first dose should be given immediately and a second dose 3 days later. The rabies immune globulin does not need to be given in this case because the woman was previously vaccinated. If she had never been vaccinated or had not received the full vaccine series, the rabies immune globulin would be indicated.

42. B. Perform an interferon gamma release assay

This new staff member is from a low-incidence TB setting and has no history of BCG vaccine. He needs an IGRA to confirm exposure to TB and will then need a medical assessment and chest X-ray to determine whether he has latent or active TB infection. Treatment options will depend on this. He should not be given the BCG vaccine as he has a positive Mantoux. There is no benefit in repeating the PPD test in this scenario.

43. E. Mefloquine

Pregnancy is a risk factor for severe disease in malaria, and pregnant women are advised to avoid travel to malarious areas. However, if travel cannot be avoided, then prophylaxis for malaria should be offered to all patients traveling to areas at risk.

Although chloroquine is safe in all trimesters of pregnancy, resistance in *Plasmodium falciparum* is widespread, and mefloquine is the only other medication shown to be safe for use during pregnancy and that remains active in most areas.

Doxycycline and atovaquone–proguanil should not be used in pregnancy.

44. A. *Burkholderia mallei*

Clinically, this patient has glanders. She has the potential for occupational exposure, and the nasal involvement and tracheobronchial ulceration reflect likely inhalational transmission of *Burkholderia mallei* from one of her equine patients. The biphasic illness may also be characteristic. Treatment options are limited by the facultative intracellular nature of *B. mallei*, as well as multiple antimicrobial resistance mechanisms. First-line options are ceftazidime, imipenem, or meropenem, with or without trimethoprim–sulfamethoxazole (co-trimoxazole).

45. D. Periodic fever, aphthous stomatitis, pharyngitis, adenitis syndrome

The regular periodicity of fevers suggests either cyclic neutropenia or PFAPA. This patient's WBC count is elevated, therefore cyclic neutropenia is unlikely.

46. E. 75% and 60%

The data from this comparison is shown below in table format, based on the information provided:

Test Result	EIA/Western Blot +	EIA/Western Blot −
Positive	60	40
Negative	20	880

Based on these results the sensitivity = 60/80 = 75%.
The positive predictive value = 60/100 = 60%.

47. A. Crusted scabies

The correct answer is crusted scabies. While scabies can affect anyone, groups of people at higher risk for crusted scabies include the elderly, those with a psychiatric disorder or intellectual disability, HTLV-1 infection, and patients who are immunosuppressed (HIV/AIDS, diabetes, steroid use, etc.).

Scabies typically involves dozens of mites that cause itching nodules and burrows primarily in the trunk/extremities, genital areas, web spaces, and wrists/ankles.

In crusted scabies, thousands to millions of mites cause itching (50% of cases), lesions may involve the whole body and include crusting (see feet in picture) and may present as erythroderma (like the lesions in the more proximal lower extremity in the picture).

Treatment of crusted scabies requires a combination of oral (e.g., ivermectin) and topical (e.g., permethrin) therapy.

48. E. Psoriasis

Genital psoriasis can cause significant distress and is often confused with sexually transmitted infections. It has been estimated that the first presentation of psoriasis is genital in as many as 2%–5% of cases, making it a diagnosis that Infectious Disease clinicians may encounter.

The lesions develop due to the Koebner phenomenon or "isomorphic response," which describes the development of skin lesions in sites of skin trauma (in this case friction associated with coitus) that may be seen in psoriasis.

There is no history of latex allergy in the setting of likely prior contact ("works in a laboratory," no history of food allergies), nor are the lesions or time course a good fit for primary syphilis, HIV, or HSV.

49. C. *Corynebacterium minutissimum*

The description is consistent with a diagnosis of erythrasma, caused by *Corynebacterium minutissimum*. There is an increased risk of erythrasma in immunocompromised adults (diabetes, elderly, etc.). It may also occur in healthy adults, rarely in children. *Corynebacterium minutissimum* proliferates in areas of moisture and occlusion (obesity, hyperhidrosis, living in tropical climate, etc.). Coral red fluorescence on Wood's lamp examination is a classic finding in erythrasma and is due to porphyrin production by *C. minutissimum* (note test can be false-positive if patients bathed washing away porphyrins prior to exam). In addition to affecting intertriginous areas (groin, axillary, inframammary) *C. minutissimum* is the number 1 cause of bacterial interdigital infection of the feet. It is clinically indistinguishable from dermatophyte and fungal infections, in this case the only differentiator was the failure of prior topical and oral antifungal therapy. The clinical course and exam findings make CA-MRSA less likely.

This page intentionally left blank

Answers 3

1. E. Susceptibility can be inferred

Oxacillin is an indicator drug for determining MSSA vs. MRSA. Breakpoints do not exist for other beta-lactam drugs for staphylococci, and testing other beta-lactams can lead to inaccurate results. Oxacillin-susceptible staphylococci are susceptible to nafcillin, cephalosporins, beta-lactam/beta-lactamase inhibitor combinations, and carbapenems. Because the isolate is susceptible to oxacillin, it can be inferred that it is also susceptible to ceftriaxone.

2. A. *Blastomyces dermatitidis*

Epidemiology (from Wisconsin), skin involvement, and a culture positive for a mold is highly suggestive of disseminated blastomycosis. Skin lesions are a common presentation, commonly misidentified as squamous cell cancer on histopathology. The phenomenon is called pseudoepitheliomatous hyperplasia (PEH).

His exposure (chiropterologist – study of bats) increases risk for histoplasmosis. However, skin lesions together with the presence of PEH are not consistent with it.

Coccidioidomycosis is a likely possibility due to recent travel, but skin lesions in coccidioidomycosis are mostly on extremities and resemble erythema nodosum. It is also not a common cause of PEH.

Skin findings are not consistent with *Candida* or *Cryptococcus*.

3. C. Increased measles IgG in the serum and CSF

The patient in this case has subacute sclerosing panencephalitis (SSPE). The patient was not vaccinated. Additionally, molecular testing as well as culture of the CSF for bacterial and viral pathogens is negative. The symptoms, imaging, and progression are consistent with SSPE. SSPE is a fatal complication resulting from persistent infection of the CNS with the measles virus. The typical presentation is 7–10 years after the initial measles infection, though this can vary. SSPE is typically seen in the pediatric population between 8 and 10 years old, though numerous cases with adult onset have been reported. SSPE typically progresses through four stages beginning with failure to learn at work and school coupled with personality changes and overall odd behavior. The second stage consists of myoclonic jerks, seizures, and dementia while the third stage progresses to unresponsiveness and rigidity. Finally, coma and autonomic failure make up the final stage. SSPE can progress rapidly with stages being indistinguishable or more slowly with a prolonged first stage. It affects males more often than females in the pediatric and adult populations. Ultimately SSPE results in the death of the patient. The diagnosis of SSPE is made by demonstrating elevated IgG to measles in the CSF and serum coupled with clinical signs and symptoms and a combination of other tests such as pathology, MRI and EEG which shows periodic complexes. SSPE is fatal in 95% of cases.

4. E. Double the infusion time of subsequent vancomycin doses

Tigecycline achieves marginal serum concentrations and is not suitable for bloodstream infections. The current vancomycin dose of 1250 mg q12 hours provided a therapeutic trough concentration of 16.1 μg/mL and should not be reduced. Daptomycin is inactivated in pulmonary surfactant and is ineffective for pneumonia. Linezolid should be avoided in combination with selective serotonin reuptake inhibitors due to risk of serotonin syndrome. This patient is likely experiencing red-man syndrome with vancomycin, which can typically be controlled by extending the length of each vancomycin infusion and/or premedicating with diphenhydramine.

5. B. Ferrous sulfate

Atorvastatin would not be expected to interact with the planned antibiotic regimen. Ciprofloxacin can significantly increase serum concentrations of theophylline, tizanidine, and warfarin and should be avoided in combination with these agents. Polyvalent metallic cations, such as ferrous sulfate, can adsorb oral fluoroquinolone doses and dramatically reduce systemic exposure and clinical effects of the fluoroquinolone.

6. B. Electrocardiogram

Azithromycin can cause QTc prolongation, especially if it is concomitantly prescribed with another QTc prolonging agent. Thus an electrocardiogram (ECG) should be routinely monitored.

7. D. Liposomal amphotericin B 350 mg IV once daily and flucytosine 2000 mg by mouth four times daily.

The recommended regimen for the treatment of cryptococcal meningitis begins with an induction phase consisting of a combination of liposomal amphotericin B 4 mg/kg per day IV and flucytosine 50–150 mg/kg per day divided into 4 doses and given by mouth every 6 hours for patients with normal renal function. For this patient, correct doses would be liposomal amphotericin B 350 mg and flucytosine 2000 mg by mouth four times daily.

Echinocandins like caspofungin have no activity against *Cryptococcus*. Fluconazole is the recommended medication for the treatment of cryptococcal meningitis during the consolidation and maintenance phases of treatment. It may also be used during the induction phase of therapy but as an alternative to liposomal amphotericin B and flucytosine. This patient does not have a contraindication to the use of these agents. Voriconazole is not the recommended medication for the treatment of cryptococcal meningitis but may be considered for salvage therapy.

8. B. Peginterferon alfa 2B

The patient is refusing HIV treatment at this time. The concern is that using an agent for her hepatitis that also has activity against HIV would lead to the development of HIV resistance. Entecavir, lamivudine, tenofovir, and emtricitabine are all active against both HIV and HBV. Only peginterferon alfa 2B alone will not lead to HIV-resistance. Remember that interferon therapy has many disadvantages, multiple side effects (i.e., influenza-like syndrome, myalgias, depression, fatigue, etc.) and is only given IM.

If the patient would have accepted treatment for both HIV and HBV, then combination therapy with tenofovir, emtricitabine, and dolutegravir would have been the optimal choice. This regimen offers three active drugs against HIV as recommended by the DHHS guidelines and at the same time would offer two active drugs against hepatitis B (tenofovir and emtricitabine).

9. B. Ivermectin

While both ivermectin and albendazole have activity against *Strongyloides*, ivermectin has a better reported efficacy. Pentamidine, praziquantel, and suramin have no role in the treatment of strongyloidiasis.

10. D. Lumbar puncture

Lumbar puncture (LP) is indicated to evaluate for neurosyphilis if ocular syphilis is present. All patients with ocular syphilis require HIV testing and LP. *Neisseria* may cause a keratoconjunctivitis and typically has very purulent discharge. *Chlamydia* may cause conjunctivitis that can progress to keratitis but does not typically cause posterior uveitis. The patient should have pain if the cornea is involved.

11. A. Delay in initiating aciclovir therapy

Herpes encephalitis carries a high morbidity and mortality even with prompt diagnosis and appropriate treatment. A multivariate analysis identified two factors associated with a poorer outcome. These were a high "simplified acute physiology score" at admission and a delay of longer than 2 days between admission and starting aciclovir therapy.

12. B. Isoniazid

Isoniazid has excellent CSF penetration (90%–95%) and has early potent bactericidal efficacy. Rifampin penetrates the CSF less well, but its importance has been demonstrated in the higher mortality of rifampin-resistant TB infections. There is no conclusive evidence that pyrazinamide improves outcomes of TBM, but it has good CSF penetration. There is also little evidence to support which fourth drug to use. Both streptomycin and ethambutol have poor CSF penetration and can have significant adverse reactions.

13. A. Bronchoscopy for AFB culture

The patient in this vignette presents with constitutional symptoms as well as a major risk factor for reactivation of tuberculosis (i.e., silicosis). The patient should be worked up for infection due to *Mycobacterium tuberculosis*. Lung biopsy and high-resolution CT of the chest would be used to help with diagnosing interstitial lung disease, but the patient's pulmonary function testing has not changed in the past year making interstitial lung disease unlikely. Prednisone would not be recommended for treatment at this time.

14. D. Ganciclovir

The bone marrow transplant recipient is at risk for CMV-associated syndromes. Other risk factors for CMV disease in hematopoietic transplant recipients are the presence of graft versus host disease, CMV seropositivity, and older age. Cultures can be falsely negative, and results can take several days to return. Cytomegalic cells isolated from open lung biopsy are the pathologic hallmark of CMV infection, and they are characterized by a large size and the presence of intranuclear inclusions that are centrally placed. Ganciclovir would be the recommended therapy. CMV immune globulin has been used in combination with medical treatment for CMV pneumonitis but would not be recommended as the sole treatment. Letermovir is an antiviral drug that inhibits the CMV–terminase complex. It may have a role in the prophylaxis of CMV reactivation and disease in recipients of allogeneic hematopoietic stem cell transplants but not in treatment of CMV disease.

15. D. *Pseudomonas aeruginosa*

Pseudomonas infections are commonly considered as important causes of neutropenic fever. This patient presented also with skin lesions, which could be consistent with ecthyma gangrenosum, of which *Pseudomonas* is an important cause. The other gram-negative bacteria listed can certainly cause BSI but would be less likely in this scenario.

16. E. Urgent transthoracic echocardiogram, but AICD will require removal independent of results

This patient is presenting with sepsis and an occult source of bacteremia in the setting of a recent AICD exchange. This is a common presentation for cardiac implanted electronic device-related infection. Whenever a device-related infection is suspected in a bacteremic patient, the next step in evaluation would be to obtain an echocardiogram to evaluate for the presence of valvular or wire-related endocarditis. Although the absence of vegetations on echocardiogram would not preclude the need for removal of the device, it would potentially affect the duration of antimicrobial therapy, need for valvular surgery, and timing to re-implantation of the device.

Even if the transthoracic echocardiogram is negative, the patient has evidence of device infection. In this setting device removal is always recommended due to the high rates of relapsed infection with device retention.

Even though it is true that the device should be removed independent of the echo results, these can affect the duration of antimicrobial therapy, need for valvular surgery, and time to re-implantation of the device.

Transesophageal echocardiogram is incorrect because the right-sided chambers are actually in the anterior portion of the heart. Therefore the distance traveled by ultrasound waves in a thin patient can be shorter than those from a transesophageal approach. As a result, the images can be just as good if not better, obviating the need for a transesophageal echocardiogram in all patients.

17. D. Transthoracic echocardiogram
This patient is presenting with acute congestive heart failure after a viral prodrome and evidence of myocardial involvement suggestive of myocarditis. Although endomyocardial biopsy is considered the gold standard for diagnosis, it is a test with low sensitivity and reserved only for cases where results of biopsy may alter the treatment course. The best initial test to assess overall cardiac function and involvement of myocardium is a transthoracic echocardiogram.

Transthoracic echocardiogram is the best initial test to assess cardiac function and complications from myocardial involvement. Cardiac MRI is reserved for more detailed noninvasive evaluation once the suspicion of myocarditis is confirmed.

Serial enzymes would be useful to follow disease course and response, but they will not be of additional help in confirming the suspected diagnosis.

Although hypothyroidism can cause myocarditis leading to heart failure, however, it would not account for previous viral prodrome. The initial hyperthyroidism of Hashimoto's thyroiditis could explain subjective fevers but not upper respiratory symptoms.

18. A. Bone marrow culture
This patient has a suspected diagnosis of *Salmonella* Typhi, acquired in India, and has constipation, rather than diarrhea, seen in about 30% of patients. He has developed hepatosplenomegaly and may have bacteremia.

Blood and stool cultures should be requested; blood cultures are positive in 40%–80%, stool culture positivity is 30%–40% and although not often performed, bone marrow may have additional yield >90% in more complicated

cases or if unresponsive to treatment and can remain positive for >5 days after antibiotic initiation.

19. B. Polymicrobial bacterascites (PMBA)
This man has clinical evidence of decompensated chronic liver disease. He complains about sweating, which could be due to underlying infection. An alternative explanation is alcohol withdrawal, as evidenced by being housebound for one week and being tremulous on examination.

A low ascitic protein count does increase his risk of infection. Whilst the WCC is >250 PMNs, there are a large number of RBCs which need to be corrected for. Using the appropriate formula (deduct one WCC for every 250 RBCs) the corrected WCC is 211. As <250, this is unlikely to represent current infection by standard definitions.

SBP or primary peritonitis is a risk in this patient, but this is unsupported by the clinical history, normal glucose (usually raised), WCC <250, and sterile blood cultures.

Secondary or tertiary peritonitis is unlikely as there is no clinical or radiologic evidence of GI (or other) pathology, and the ascitic WCC is <250.

That leaves MNBA and PMBA. While both are plausible, MNBA is commonly monomicrobial, and the high RBC suggests trauma. PMBA related to a traumatic tap is most likely given the mixed microscopy and cultures.

While it was appropriate to empirically treat the patient with broad-spectrum antibiotics, there needs to be clinical assessment about on-going need. Many clinicians try to stop therapy when there is no evidence of overt infection, but due to risk of progression to peritonitis, some advocate completing treatment.

20. C. Miscarriage
This patient has bacterial vaginosis (BV), given the clinical presentation of malodorous, thin discharge and microscopy results. BV is associated with preterm labor and miscarriage. Treatment is therefore advised during pregnancy.

21. C. Reassurance only
There is no indication to treat asymptomatic candiduria in this clinical context. Pyuria is not an indication for treatment.

22. C. Meropenem
This man has acute prostatitis and is systemically unwell. He has a history of recurrent catheterization-associated urinary tract infection and will not tolerate FLQ. In addition, he may be at risk of a drug-resistant *Pseudomonas* species, and so a carbapenem is a reasonable initial regimen. Ertapenem will not cover *Pseudomonas*. Treatment for STI is not appropriate as first line in this clinical context. Also considering the patient's age and background history, a focus on Enterobacteriaceae and *Pseudomonas* is more appropriate.

23. C. Parvovirus B19
Several of the options could cause fever and a rash; however, measles and rubella are now rare in routine clinical practice

due to vaccination. These would be possible diagnoses, particularly if the woman were unvaccinated, had traveled overseas, or there was an epidemiologic link to a measles outbreak. Secondary syphilis could cause a rash and fever but not upper respiratory symptoms. Acute Q fever would more usually be associated with cough and myalgia rather than coryza and does not typically cause a rash. Parvovirus B19 is a ubiquitous infection which is frequently asymptomatic but can cause these symptoms. Moreover, identifying acute parvovirus infection in this context is important because of the associated risk of hydrops fetalis.

24. D. Vaccinate with three-dose series
HPV vaccination is recommended for adolescents age 11 or 12 years. Vaccination is also recommended for females between the ages of 13 and 26 and for males between the ages of 13 through 21 who were not adequately vaccinated previously. HPV vaccination is also recommended for gay, bisexual, and other men who have sex with men, transgender people, and those with some immunocompromising conditions between ages 22 and 26 years, if inadequately vaccinated in the past. The vaccine should be administered regardless of history of exposure.

25. C. Co-infection with HBV and HDV
The timing is most consistent with co-infection with HBV and HDV, which is more likely to present with worsening liver disease. The serologies are not consistent with acute infection with either HAV or HCV but are consistent with acute HBV infection, which initially improved. Acute HIV infection does not cause a fulminant hepatitis, although it can raise transaminases.

26. D. VZV PCR of lesion
This patient is relatively immunocompromised on long-term steroids. The distribution of rash suggests the possibility of herpes zoster, or shingles. Subsequent widespread development of vesicular lesions indicates the possibility of disseminated zoster. In the presence of clinical uncertainty, the most definitive investigation would be PCR of vesicular fluid to confirm virus.

27. D. Leptospirosis
The case describes a presentation of leptospirosis (Weil's disease) with fever, acute kidney injury, and hepatitis following exposure to fresh water in the state with the highest incidence of this disease. Diagnosis is usually confirmed by serology. MAT is one of the most widely used essays. Severe leptospirosis is often treated with IV beta-lactam agents such as penicillin or ceftriaxone; milder cases can be managed with oral doxycycline.

Tularemia is unlikely in this clinical scenario given the 10–12-day incubation period (3–5 days is more common for tularemia), and it is not known to be present in Malaysia. It is only seen in the northern hemisphere; cases in the United States are most commonly reported from Arkansas, Missouri, South Dakota, and Oklahoma. It is endemic in most European countries, China, and Japan.

iGAS would be in the differential diagnosis; however, no clues are given in the question to lead you to this diagnosis (prior sore throat, signs/symptoms of skin/soft tissue infection).

CCHF is not yet reported in Malaysia, although it has been reported from over 30 countries in Africa, the Middle East, Asia, and Europe. The incubation period, clinical features, and lab would be a good explanation otherwise.

Acute hepatitis E may cause a fulminant infection with acute hepatic failure and encephalopathy in a small proportion of individuals, but there are usually risk factors such as pregnancy, malnourishment or preexisting liver disease.

28. E. *Staphylococcus aureus*
Gram-positive bacteria (*Staphylococcus*, *Streptococcus*) are the most common organisms associated with burn wound infections immediately following injury. The shift to gram-negative bacteria (e.g., *Pseudomonas aeruginosa*, *Acinetobacter* spp.) and fungi occurs several days later, particularly with prolonged hospitalization and broad-spectrum antibiotic exposure.

29. C. *Histoplasma capsulatum*
The presence of fever and a chronic wasting illness associated with adenopathy, splenomegaly, pancytopenia, mild transaminitis, and reticulonodular infiltrates suggests an opportunistic infection in the setting of advanced HIV infection. While HIV itself could account for some of the symptoms and findings, fever, reticulonodular infiltrates (miliary pattern), and splenomegaly support a concomitant infection. Blood cultures grew yeast and peripheral smear shows small intracellular organisms. The yeast do not have the appearance of *Cryptococcus*, which is a large round cell with a surrounding capsule. Given that the patient lives in an endemic region, the likeliest diagnosis is disseminated histoplasmosis associated with advanced HIV infection.

(Image from Bibbo M, Wilbur DC. *Comprehensive Cytopathology*. 4th ed. Elsevier; 2015.)

30. E. Switch to voriconazole
Scedosporium apiospermum is resistant to amphotericin B and the echinocandins. Voriconazole is the treatment of choice. Posaconazole may be used as an alternative agent.

In contrast to *Scedosporium apiospermum*, *Scedosporium prolificans* (now called *Lomentospora prolificans*) is resistant to all antifungals. Combination treatment with amphotericin B and echinocandins or terbinafine may be of benefit due to the potential synergistic activity in *L. prolificans* infection.

31. A. *Francisella tularensis*
Ulceroglandular tularemia is the most likely diagnosis, as it fits clinically and epidemiologically. Tularemia has been reported from all US states except Hawaii. All of the choices provided are differential diagnoses for eschar formation with regional lymphadenopathy except *Streptobacillus moniliformis*. However, geographically *Spirillum minus* is limited to Asia, and

recluse spiders (leading to loxoscelism) are not found in northern California; *Rickettsia conorii* is found around the Mediterranean and causes Mediterranean spotted fever.

(Image from Cox JA, Visser LG. A family with African tick bite fever. *Travel Med Infect Dis.* 2015;13(3):274–275.)

32. C. Pyrazinamide
BCG is a live-attenuated strain derived from *Mycobacterium bovis*, both of which are intrinsically resistant to PZA; thus this agent is not indicated as part of the treatment regimen of disseminated BCG disease. QuantiFERON-TB Gold is negative in this case; IGRA tests are based on detection of a T-cell immune response to TB antigens (ESAT-6 and CFP-10) encoded by genes in the region of difference-1 (RD1), which is present in *M. tuberculosis* complex, but absent in *M. bovis*, Bacillus Calmette-Guérin (BCG), and most non-tuberculous mycobacteria (NTM).

33. B. *Mycobacterium chelonae*
This is a case of disseminated *M. chelonae* infection. It is the most common rapid-growing mycobacteria to cause disseminated skin infection in immunocompromised hosts. The organism grew in 5 days after incubation indicating that this might be a rapid grower. *M. chelonae* is the only rapid grower in the list. While the patient did have a fish tank at home, which is a classic risk factor for *M. marinum* infection, he did not have direct contact with it, plus *M. marinum* is a slow grower that also needs special culture conditions to grow and less likely to grow in 5 days.

34. A. *Diphyllobothrium latum*
Diphyllobothrium latum infection can cause vitamin B_{12} deficiency with a megaloblastic anemia.

35. A. Eastern and Southern Africa
Eastern and Southern Africa has an estimated HIV prevalence of 7% according to 2016 UNAIDS data. Western and Central Africa has an estimated prevalence of 2%, Eastern Europe and Central Asia has an estimated prevalence of 0.9%, Latin America has an estimated prevalence of 0.5%, and Western and Central Europe and North America has an estimated prevalence of 0.3%.

36. A. Abacavir/lamivudine/dolutegravir + entecavir
The presence of a hyperchloremic nonanion gap metabolic acidosis, hypokalemia, hypophosphatemia, glucosuria, and proteinuria suggest that this patient has tenofovir-induced Fanconi's syndrome; therefore tenofovir should be discontinued. Although raltegravir has been associated with rhabdomyolysis the other laboratory findings are suggestive of Fanconi's syndrome. This patient has hepatitis B co-infection, and therefore an optimal treatment regimen should cover both viruses. Discontinuation of agents with anti-HBV activity can result in serious hepatocellular damage following reactivation of HBV. Lamivudine has activity against HBV; however, resistance develops quickly, and therefore dual therapy is recommended.

37. A. Hepatitis B virus vaccine
The patient has isolated hepatitis B virus (HBV) core antibody positivity but no evidence of chronic HBV or immunity to HBV based on negative HBV DNA and HBV surface antibody. Therefore HBV vaccination is indicated at this time even though the response rate may be lower given the low CD4 count. The patient's CD4 count <200 cells/mm^3 is a contraindication to live attenuated vaccines including herpes zoster (shingles), varicella (chickenpox), and measles, mumps, rubella (MMR) vaccines. HPV vaccine is indicated for women through the age of 26 based on the licensing studies and since sexually active patients above this age are more likely to already have acquired HPV infection.

38. E. Rifampin
Due to significant drug interactions between boosted protease inhibitors and certain anti-TB drugs, modified regimens are often required. Rifampin, which is a potent CYP3A4 inducer, is contraindicated in the treatment of TB with patients on protease inhibitor-based HIV regimens. Rifabutin is a less potent CYP3A4 inducer so it can be used, with dose modification, in protease inhibitor-based regimens.

39. C. Meningococcal ACWY and menB
There is a boxed warning on the eculizumab due to meningococcal infections which may be fatal or life-threatening. Eculizumab recipients are 1000–2000× increased risk of meningococcal infections compared to healthy individuals. Therefore there is a strong recommendation to vaccinate against meningococcus at least 2 weeks prior to the initiation of eculizumab. If they cannot be vaccinated 2 weeks prior, they should receive antibiotic prophylaxis until 2 weeks after vaccination. Patients are also at risk for infections due to other encapsulated organisms, and the patients are likely to have chronic renal failure, so other vaccinations that should be considered are influenza, Hib, and pneumococcal vaccines, but meningococcal vaccine is imperative.

40. D. Sulfadiazine
High-dose sulfonamides can cause crystalluria. Some antiretroviral agents can also cause crystalluria, most notably indinavir and atazanavir. Aciclovir is another drug that can be associated with crystalluria.

41. B. A defect in the IL-12 or interferon-gamma pathway
Inherited defects of innate immunity of the IL-12 or IFN-gamma pathways present with disseminated mycobacterial and *Salmonella* infections. In countries where Bacillus Calmette-Guérin (BCG) vaccination against tuberculosis is recommended, a common presentation of this disorder is disseminated BCG infection. Defects in the IL-17 pathway lead to chronic mucocutaneous candidiasis, while defects in the IL-21 pathway lead to hepatobiliary cryptosporidiosis.

42. E. Standard precautions only

These materials used as drum heads can be contaminated with anthrax spores. The patient is not at risk to those around him and therefore requires only standard precautions. The exposure does need to be pursued, and there may be family and friends that require chemoprophylaxis. The healthcare workers that came into contact with him do not need immunization or chemoprophylaxis.

43. E. Schistosomiasis

Based on the incubation period and symptoms, the most likely diagnosis of the options provided is acute schistosomiasis. Acute schistosomiasis (Katayama fever) is a hypersensitivity response to the start of egg production by the adult worms and manifests with a variety of symptoms, including fever, dry cough, diarrhea, urticaria, and angioedema. Measles, dengue, and Marburg (one of the hemorrhagic fevers) would not present this late. Malaria is not associated with a rash.

(Image from James WD, Elston DM, McMahon PJ. Parasitic infestations, stings, and bites. In *Andrews' Diseases of the Skin Clinical Atlas.* Elsevier; 2018.)

44. D. Gentamicin and ciprofloxacin

The clinical findings and the occupation of the patient should prompt consideration of a diagnosis such as anthrax or pneumonic plague. Anthrax may cause pleural effusions but is commonly associated with a widened mediastinum and may have clear lung fields; plus the Gram stain does not fit. Both the clinical, radiographic and microscopy results are consistent with infection by *Yersinia pestis*, the cause of plague. D (gentamicin and ciprofloxacin in combination) is the correct treatment for pneumonic plague. Answer A (benzylpenicillin + meropenem + linezolid) would be the correct treatment for pulmonary anthrax.

45. E. Sweet syndrome

This patient with immune neutropenia is likely on granulocyte colony-stimulating factor (G-CSF) as her WBC count is very elevated. Sweet syndrome is the typical cause of painful nodules in a patient on G-CSF.

46. A. Kawasaki syndrome

Measles is less likely in a vaccinated child. Rubella and parvovirus infection do not involve conjunctiva. SJS would progress with more extensive cutaneous disease. Kawasaki disease typically presents with the above features.

47. D. Prevalence

Prevalence is the correct result because the 1000 individuals were surveyed in the community, so this represents both new (incident) and preexisting HCV infection, and therefore prevalence. Incidence is not correct because an assay would have to be done to identify only newly infected individuals, which was not the case. Positive predictive value, sensitivity, and positive likelihood ratio are characteristics of diagnostic tests and therefore incorrect.

Answers 4

1. C. *Mycobacterium kansasii*

Although IGRAs were developed for detection of *M. tuberculosis*, infection with other mycobacterial species can cause false-positive results. False-positive results are most commonly seen with, but not limited to, *M. kansasii*, *M. marinum*, and *M. szulgai*. *M. kansasii* is the most concerning of the three as it can cause tuberculosis-like illness. If the causative agent in this case was *M. tuberculosis*, the Xpert MTB/RIF PCR should have been positive, due to the high sensitivity (97%–99%) of smear-positive specimens. Although the sensitivity is <100%, which leaves room for rare false-negatives, *M. kansasii* also fits the clinical picture. *M. kansasii* primarily affects middle-aged white males, although patients of any sex, age, or race can be affected. Central and southern US states have the highest incidence of *M. kansasii* pneumonia. COPD, previous mycobacterial disease, malignancy, and alcoholism are risk factors for *M. kansasii* disease, but approximately 40% of patients have no identifiable predisposing conditions.

2. A. CSF coccidioidal antibodies

Endemic exposure (travel), biphasic presentation with initial respiratory illness that resolves spontaneously followed by dissemination to extrapulmonary sites (brain/bone/skin) raises suspicion for coccidioidal meningitis. Considered to have high specificity and sensitivity in coccidioidal meningitis, CSF coccidioidomycosis serologies should be performed to establish the diagnosis.

Cryptococcosis is less likely considering normal opening pressure and absence of underlying immune condition. Some patients with *Cryptococcus* are immunonormal, but that is more common with *Coccidioides*.

Blastomycosis can have similar presentation with dissemination, but CNS involvement is usually with brain abscess, not meningitis. Histoplasmosis rarely affects the CSF.

3. B. EBV

The serologic results and heterophile antibody test support the diagnosis of EBV infection. IgM and IgG antibodies to the viral capsid antigen (VCA) are usually positive at the onset of symptoms, as are IgG antibodies to the early antigen (EA). EBNA antibodies, however, appear weeks later and then persist. They should be negative in the early stages of clinical illness, as they are here. Exudative pharyngitis in EBV can be confused for *S. pyogenes*, though rapid testing is negative. Of note a back-up culture or NAAT test should be performed to confirm the rapid test. CMV IgM is most likely a cross-reaction as IgM can cross-react with EBV VCA.

4. B. Cefepime

While each of the beta-lactam antibiotics listed has the potential to cause neurotoxicity, cefepime is most associated with the development of this adverse effect. A US Food and Drug Administration safety alert for cefepime identified age >50 and inadequate renal dosing adjustments as risk factors for neurotoxicity.

5. A. Clindamycin

Adding clindamycin introduces a 2nd agent with an alternative mechanism of action. Clindamycin acts on the ribosome, interrupting protein synthesis, and hence toxin production. IDSA recommend that dual therapy with penicillin and clindamycin is used for *S. pyogenes* necrotising fasciitis. Doxycycline does not provide adequate coverage of *Streptococcus pyogenes* and would not be indicated in this case. Since *S. pyogenes* are reliably sensitive to penicillin, gentamicin would not be expected to help control pathogenicity of this infection. There is no evidence of an anaerobic component to this infection, making the addition of metronidazole unnecessary. Penicillin G is considered to be the most active antibiotic against *S. pyogenes*. The addition of vancomycin would not be expected to further control the pathogenicity of this infection, given the fact that there is no evidence of beta-lactam-resistant organisms in this case.

6. E. Rifampin and warfarin

The most clinically significant drug–drug interaction would be rifampin and warfarin. Rifampin induces the metabolism of warfarin thus requiring a significant increase in warfarin dose to maintain appropriate INR levels. Pyrazinamide may enhance the hepatotoxic effects of rifampin, but the rifampin and warfarin drug–drug interaction is more clinically significant.

7. C. Change to posaconazole DR tablets 300 mg once daily

Voriconazole is the only azole known to carry the risk of photosensitivity reactions, including an association with skin cancers. Voriconazole is at steady state after 1 week of therapy, and the timing of the level (trough) is appropriate. The level is therapeutic (between 2 and 5.5 μg/mL). However, the adverse drug reaction is most likely attributed to voriconazole, and with other available treatment options, it would be best to use another agent. Continuing the voriconazole as is and decreasing the voriconazole are not the best options. Fluconazole does not have activity against *Aspergillus*. While echinocandins have activity against *Aspergillus*, anidulafungin monotherapy is inappropriate. Changing voriconazole to posaconazole is the most appropriate option.

8. E. Valaciclovir 1 gram PO every 8 hours for 2 weeks

This question relates to the risk of herpes B virus infection. There is a small risk for transmission, but herpes B virus infection can cause fatal encephalomyelitis in humans after bites and scratches. In humans, herpes B virus prophylaxis is indicated to avoid disease, especially in a deep wound like this. Long courses of postexposure prophylaxis are recommended for high-risk exposures like the patient above. It is reasonable to consider an individual uninfected if symptom-free and seronegative at 12 weeks. Valaciclovir 1 gram PO every 8h for 2 weeks is the recommend prophylaxis. Alternative options include aciclovir and valganciclovir. There is no known advantage to using either cidofovir or foscarnet, both of which are more toxic than valaciclovir and must be given IV. Treatment of established disease: IV aciclovir or IV ganciclovir. Ribavirin is used as PEP for Lassa fever and CCHF but has no efficacy against herpes B virus.

9. E. Praziquantel

While both praziquantel and bithionol have activity against paragonimiasis, praziquantel is a better tolerated agent and therefore the more appropriate first-line therapy.

10. B. Voriconazole

Voriconazole or fluconazole would be the best option as they penetrate the eye well, unless there are concerns for resistance. Her case is describing the natural course of endophthalmitis rather than treatment failure, and *C. parapsilosis* should be azole-sensitive. While amphotericin will penetrate the eye, she could avoid the toxicity by using an azole. The echinocandins have very poor penetration into the eye.

11. E. Tonsil biopsy for PrP^{SC} immunostaining

PrP^{sc} immunostaining of tonsillar tissue is both sensitive and specific for vCJD and avoids more invasive procedures such as a brain biopsy.

EEG changes and CSF 14-3-3 protein may be negative in vCJD; they are more useful in classic CJD. MRI changes in vCJD tend to show bilateral pulvinar hyperintensity. Cortical ribboning is seen with classic CJD.

Genotyping for codon 129 of the *PrP* gene confirming methionine/methionine homozygosity would be interesting but would not confirm the diagnosis of vCJD.

12. D. Tetanus

Tetanus is the most likely diagnosis due to risk factors (gender and age mean she is unlikely to have completed a vaccination course; gardening injuries are a recognized route of entry) and to the clinical features of excessive muscle spasm and sympathetic activity. Generalized tetanus is commonly a descending pattern after a nonspecific prodrome of fever, malaise, and headache. Patients are usually cognitively intact.

Neuroleptic malignant syndrome is most commonly associated with drugs affecting dopamine activity, within 1–4 weeks of initiating or changing dose; it is also usually associated with an altered mental status. She has had no history of exposure to rabies, nor are the classic clinical features of rabies present, such as hydrophobia or insomnia. She has no features of cognitive impairment or confusion that would be expected with a herpes encephalitis.

13. B. *Legionella* and *Streptococcus pneumoniae* urine antigen assays

The patient in this clinical vignette has presented with a severe pneumonia requiring admission to the intensive care unit for mechanical ventilation. The recommendation for patients presenting with a severe community-acquired pneumonia is to have *Legionella* and *S. pneumoniae* urine antigen testing in addition to blood and sputum cultures.

14. A. Bronchiectasis

Bronchiectasis is an abnormal permanent dilation of the bronchi, typically on the basis of chronic destruction and inflammation caused by recurrent infections or other chronic diseases. Immune deficiencies, such as common variable immunodeficiency and cystic fibrosis, can lead to dilated bronchi. This disorder can lead to purulent sputum production and recurrent cough as well as hemoptysis. The chest imaging findings can demonstrate cystic spaces caused by bronchiectasis or the parallel linear opacities or rings as in this vignette.

15. E. Vancomycin

Central-line associated infections are most commonly caused by gram-positive organisms, most notably *Staphylococcus* and *Streptococcus* spp. MRSA is sufficiently prevalent to warrant empiric coverage with vancomycin or another effective agent, and parenteral therapy should be considered until bacteremia is excluded.

16. A. Ampicillin plus ceftriaxone

For patients with enterococcal endocarditis with susceptible strains the preferred treatment regimens include ampicillin or penicillin G as these are rapidly cidal agents. For patients with normal renal function these agents should be combined with 2 weeks of aminoglycoside such as gentamicin.

In patients with contraindications to aminoglycosides, an alternate regimen of ampicillin and ceftriaxone should be used.

Linezolid and daptomycin should be reserved for patients with resistant enterococci not amenable to treatment with rapidly cidal beta-lactams. Vancomycin should be reserved for patients with penicillin-resistant enterococci, and beta-lactams should be used whenever possible. In this patient with a very limited creatinine clearance, vancomycin should also be avoided to prevent further damage to his renal function.

17. D. Surgical intervention for wash out, operating room culture sampling, and targeted antibiotics
This patient is presenting with post-CABG mediastinitis, with evidence of sternal osteomyelitis and involvement of hardware. In this case, the best strategy to control the source and have better chance of treatment success is with OR revision, wash out, removal of hardware, and debridement of bone. OR cultures would be most definitive to identify the organism and target antimicrobial therapy. The duration of therapy will vary depending on organisms, extent of infection, and response.

The patient has purulent discharge and evidence of infected fluid in the deep tissue planes/bone, which would need source control and antimicrobial therapy for proper wound healing to occur in the surface. Wound care alone would be insufficient.

Bedside debridement would only be superficial and surface cultures may not accurately represent the organisms causing deep tissue infection.

Although aspirate may be useful for culture and organism identification, it will have limited ability to perform source control given the presence of hardware and infected bone that require debridement.

18. E. *Yersinia enterocolitica*
Erythema nodosum and reactive arthritis can be seen following infection with *Yersinia enterocolitica* which can be acquired through consumption of undercooked meat, especially pork products. Postinfectious immunologic sequelae (e.g., reactive arthritis and erythema nodosum) can develop 2 weeks after the diarrheal illness.

Twenty percent of patients may present with pharyngitis, which is not seen in other causes of gastroenteritis. Throat cultures may also yield positive growth for *Y. enterocolitica*. Although *Yersinia* does not cause thyroiditis, it shares antigens that resemble TSH and hence cross-react with antibodies in Graves' disease.

19. B. *Clostridium perfringens*
Clostridial necrotizing enterocolitis (also known as pigbel disease in Papua New Guinea and "Darmbrand" in Germany) presents with segmental necrosis of the jejunum and ileum, severe abdominal pain, distension, and dilated loops of bowel. *C. perfringens* should be clinically suspected when a patient presents with a history of ingesting poorly cooked

or stored meat or meat products (8–16 hours after). Both stool and food should be tested for toxin and cultured if possible and surgery to remove ischemic gut is required.

20. A. Emphysematous cholecystitis
This scenario demonstrates an older man who fails to respond to treatment for acute cholecystitis. Urgent abdominal X-ray reveals air within the gallbladder which is diagnostic of emphysematous cholecystitis (EC). In addition, the patient has risk factors for this condition including his age (mean age of EC is 59 years) and diabetes. EC complicates 1% acute cholecystitis and is caused by gas-forming organisms (including clostridia). Definitive management is urgent cholecystectomy.

Dual agents (with different mechanisms of action) were chosen as empirical treatment. It is plausible that non-susceptible organisms are involved with this infection and broadening cover might be appropriate. However, in light of the radiologic findings, emphysematous cholecystitis is a more likely diagnosis, and surgery is the definitive treatment.

Mirizzi syndrome is a rare complication where a gallstone impacts the cystic duct or neck of the gallbladder, compressing the common bile duct or common hepatic duct, leading to obstruction and jaundice. There are no pathognomonic signs or symptoms, and this is usually diagnosed on USS.

Gallstone ileus is a rare cause of small bowel obstruction where a gallstone enters intestinal lumen (thought to be through a cholecystoenteric fistula) and obstructs the distal ileum. Diagnosis includes pneumobilia (air in the biliary tree), evidence of small bowel obstruction, and radioopaque gallstone on abdominal X-ray. In addition to the imaging, normal bowel sounds would go against obstruction.

Gallbladder perforation is a possibility but one would expect evidence of gas within the peritoneal cavity.

(Image from Dalrymple NC, Leyendecker JR, Oliphant M. *Problem Solving in Abdominal Imaging.* Mosby; 2009.)

21. E. *Ureaplasma urealyticum*
Chorioamnionitis is usually an ascending polymicrobial infection. All of the options have been implicated in the pathogenesis of chorioamnionitis. However, the most common causative organism is *Ureaplasma urealyticum*, which causes 47% of cases.

22. B. Ciprofloxacin + stat aminoglycoside
This male patient has a complicated UTI until proven otherwise thus requiring investigation for evidence of obstruction, especially if slow to resolve. He requires antibiotic selection that will provide good serum levels. You may even consider a stat dose of third-generation cephalosporin while awaiting sensitivities, but this is not given as an option. Nitrofurantoin and fosfomycin are only appropriate for lower urinary tract infection whereas this patient is systemically unwell so more likely to have upper tract infection. Gram-positive cover might be required in the context of *Staphylococcus aureus* (hematogenous spread) pyelonephritis/renal abscess, but the stem might give additional information

regarding risk factors for *S. aureus* bacteremia, e.g., intravenous drug use history. First-line treatment should focus on more common uropathogens: Enterobacteriaceae. This patient is systemically unwell with upper urinary tract signs and significantly abnormal labs; sexually transmitted infection with *Neisseria gonorrhoeae* or *Chlamydia trachomatis* is not the likely cause.

23. B. Urine and rectal screening by NAAT for *N. gonorrhoeae* and *C. trachomatis*, oropharyngeal screening by culture for *N. gonorrhoeae* plus syphilis serology

This patient has high risk for exposure to STI. In this case, STI screening is recommended at 3- or 6-month intervals. Screen urethral (urine) and rectal sites by NAAT for *N. gonorrhoeae* and *C. trachomatis*. Oropharyngeal screening for *C. trachomatis* is not recommended. NAAT or culture can be used for oropharyngeal screening for *N. gonorrhoeae*. Note that some NAAT for *N. gonorrhoeae* are less sensitive because they cross react with other *Neisseria* spp. found in the oral environment.

24. D. Metronidazole × 1 dose

This is *Trichomonas* infection, as confirmed by the flagellated protozoan organism on microscopy. *Trichomonas vaginalis* should be treated with metronidazole 2 g for one dose. Alternative regimens include metronidazole 500 mg twice daily for 7 days. Rescreening should be performed in 3 months because reinfection is common.

(Image from Gardella C, Eckert LO, Lentz GM. Genital tract infections. In Lobo RA, Gershenson DM, Lentz GM, Valea F, eds. *Comprehensive Gynecology*. 7th ed. Elsevier; 2017.)

25. E. Reactivation of HBV

Reactivation of HBV in a patient with co-infection with HBV and HCV has been reported in patients being treated for HCV. A patient responding to HCV treatment who has a flare of hepatitis, but still with undetectable HCV viral loads, should be evaluated for HBV. Drug reaction is possible but rarely causes transaminases this elevated.

For more information, see https://www.hhs.gov/hepatitis/blog/2017/1/17/hbv-reactivation-during-hcv-treatment.html

26. A. *Aedes* mosquito

This is most likely to be Zika infection, but could easily be dengue or chikungunya. *Aedes aegypti* is the main vector in transmission of all three viruses, but *Aedes albopictus* is also responsible for spreading disease. The mosquito feeds largely during the day but may still bite at night. The principal method of protection is bite avoidance with the use of personal protective measures, such as insect repellents and attempts to remove potential breeding sites for mosquitos in urban areas.

27. A. *Treponema carateum*

Treponema carateum is the treponemal species that causes pinta.

28. A. *Capnocytophaga canimorsus*

Capnocytophaga canimorsus, commonly found in canine oral flora, can cause bacteremia and fulminant sepsis in humans, particularly those with asplenia or underlying liver disease. All of the organisms may be involved in bite injury infections, whether human, dog, or cat bite.

29. B. *Coccidioides immitis*

The patient presents with a community-onset pneumonia. However, important diagnostic clues are the subacute presentation, recent travel to the southwestern United States, and a CBC that reveals peripheral eosinophilia. The likeliest diagnosis is acute pulmonary coccidioidomycosis, which he likely acquired through inhalation of aerosolized spores during his bike trip through the Arizona desert. The incubation period is about 2 weeks, which fits with his presumed environmental exposure and onset of symptoms. For most otherwise healthy patients with no underlying immunodeficiency, the acute infection may resolve spontaneously without treatment and close clinical monitoring. For those with moderate to severe, or prolonged symptoms, multilobar infiltrates, or high anti-coccidioides complement fixation titers (>1:16) a course of oral fluconazole (minimum dose 400 mg daily) given for 3–6 months may be offered.

30. E. Itraconazole

The most likely diagnosis in this case is sporotrichosis, notably the fixed cutaneous form as there is no mention of the typical lymphangitic pattern of nodules along the ipsilateral limb. Although she does occasionally clean her son's fish tank (consider *Mycobacterium marinum*) and owns a cat (consider *Bartonella henselae* or cat scratch disease) the most important clue is the history of the wooden splinter that she removed from her finger one month prior to this, suggesting direct inoculation with *Sporothrix*. It is also possible, and often more common, for cats to transmit *Sporothrix* with a scratch (particularly cats that spend time outdoors with soil contamination of their claws); although still plausible, there is no mention of a cat scratch. The prolonged duration of symptoms and findings argue against this being a pyogenic (e.g., staphylococcal) infection. Sporotrichosis does not resolve without treatment. A skin biopsy for histopathology and fungal culture should confirm the diagnosis. Treatment with itraconazole is recommended for a total duration of 3–6 months until all lesions have fully resolved for at least 2–4 weeks.

(Image from Cohen BA. Nodules and tumors. In *Pediatric Dermatology*. 4th ed. Elsevier; 2013.)

31. D. *Ehrlichia chaffeensis*

HME, or ehrlichiosis, is caused by *Ehrlichia chaffeensis*, an intracellular pathogen that infects monocytes. The image shows morulae within monocytes. This is diagnostic for HME.

32. B. Drug adverse effect

The clinical presentation of tingling in stocking glove distribution is consistent with INH-induced neurotoxicity. Her pregnancy could be the result of decreased levels of oral contraceptives due to pharmacologic interaction with rifampin. The vignette does not mention whether the patient is receiving pyridoxine, but pregnancy puts her at higher risk for pyridoxine deficiency.

33. C. Chloroquine

Malaria prophylaxis is indicated as Haiti is considered at moderate risk for acquisition of malaria. Although *Plasmodium falciparum* accounts for almost all cases of malaria in Haiti, resistance is exceedingly rare. In addition, the patient is pregnant, and the only medication that is considered safe from the above list is chloroquine. Atovaquone–proguanil, artemether–lumefantrine, and doxycycline are contraindicated regardless of the trimester. Mosquito bite avoidance is extremely important, and suitable precautions must be discussed. She should also be advised that national recommendations (both CDC and the PHE Advisory Committee on Malaria Prevention) are that pregnant women should avoid all nonessential travel to malarious areas due to the increased risk of severe malaria and death or serious adverse outcomes such as stillbirth and miscarriage.

34. A. *Acanthamoeba* sp.

This is a case of *Acanthamoeba* keratitis associated with improper contact lens care. *Entamoeba histolytica* is an amoebic parasite but would be very unusual as a cause of keratitis. *Giardia lamblia* is a flagellate protozoan and not known to cause keratitis. *Balamuthia* is a free-living ameba similar to *Acanthamoeba* but typically causes CNS or cutaneous disease and not keratitis. *Dientamoeba* is only associated with GI disease.

35. B. Drug–drug interaction with statin

This patient is suffering from a drug–drug interaction from being on an antiretroviral therapy regimen with cobicistat and initiation of a statin. Because of the association of HIV with dyslipidemia, it is recommended to screen all new patients for hyperlipidemia at their first HIV Clinic appointment. If hyperlipidemia is found, then statins should be initiated, and lipid panels should be monitored within 1–3 months and then every 6–12 months thereafter. However, guidelines for initiation of a cholesterol-lowering agent are the same as the general population for persons living with HIV. It is contraindicated to start statins metabolized by CYP3A in patients on protease inhibitors, including simvastatin and lovastatin. For patients on a ritonavir-boosted protease inhibitor regimen, it is recommended to start pitavastatin and, for patients on all other regimens, it is recommended to start atorvastatin at 10 mg daily. A lower dose is recommended because atorvastatin is partially metabolized by CYP3A. Pravastatin is not recommended any longer, because it is not as potent as the other two mentioned above. Now with the advent of antiretroviral regimens containing cobicistat, which is also an inhibitor of CYP 3A4, it is also contraindicated to initiate statins that are highly metabolized by CYP3A. While rosuvastatin

is not metabolized by CYP3A4, five- to sevenfold increases in rosuvastatin levels are seen when co-administered with a boosted protease-inhibitor regimen or a regimen including cobicistat; therefore it is recommended to start rosuvastatin at a lower dose of 10 mg daily.

Hepatitis B co-infection can be adequately treated with tenofovir alafenamide with no resistance seen in studies where patients are compliant. Therefore this patient should not be developing transaminitis due to viral hepatitis. A hepatitis D superinfection is possible, but unlikely.

Primary biliary cholangitis is an autoimmune disease of the small intralobular bile ducts that characteristically leads to drastic elevation in alkaline phosphatase levels, which was not seen in this case. However, there are biliary tract disorders that are more common among persons living with HIV, including acalculous cholecystitis and AIDS cholangiopathy.

ACE-I are not known to cause hepatic impairment. In patients with renal impairment, decreased elimination of ACE-I can be seen leading to increased serum creatinine levels.

36. E. Tenofovir disoproxil fumarate/emtricitabine/efavirenz once daily

Rifampicin is a strong CYP3A inducer and causes significant decreases in concentrations of protease inhibitors, thus co-administration is contraindicated. Although INSTIs can be co-administered, both raltegravir and dolutegravir require twice-daily dosing. Rifampin decreases the concentrations of elvitegravir and cobicistat significantly, and therefore this combination is not recommended. TAF is contraindicated with all rifamycins.

37. B. Tenofovir alafenamide/emtricitabine/cobicistat/elvitegravir + darunavir

Guidelines recommend that antiretroviral regimens should contain three active agents where possible. M184V mutation causes loss of susceptibility to lamivudine and emtricitabine as well as reduced susceptibility to abacavir. Additionally, the maraviroc regime only contains two active agents as the patient is dual tropic for X4 and R5 co-receptors. Unboosted darunavir should not be used.

38. B. Atovaquone PO once daily

Given the patient's CD4 count <200 cells/μL, prophylaxis against *Pneumocystis* pneumonia is indicated. The history of severe sulfa allergy and evidence of G-6-PD deficiency are contraindications to the use of trimethoprim–sulfamethoxazole or dapsone therapy. The patient's history of asthma and travel plans limiting ability to return monthly for treatments also make the use of aerosolized pentamidine less attractive. Therefore atovaquone is the most appropriate option. The patient does not have an indication for *Mycobacterium avium* complex or *Toxoplasma* primary prophylaxis with the CD4 count at the current level.

39. C. Clarithromycin, ethambutol, and rifabutin

The most likely infection to cause this clinical presentation of fevers, diarrhea, and wasting in an advanced AIDS patient with positive AFB blood cultures is disseminated *Mycobacterium avium* complex disease. The recommended treatment is a macrolide (azithromycin or clarithromycin), ethambutol, plus an optional third agent in severe cases or patients failing ART (typically rifabutin).

40. E. Piperacillin–tazobactam
Empiric treatment for patients with febrile neutropenia and abdominal pain should include an antimicrobial regimen active against enteric GNRs, *Pseudomonas aeruginosa*, sensitive GPCs, and anaerobes. MRSA or VRE do not need to be covered unless previous cultures indicate.

41. D. Oral typhoid vaccine
Immunosuppressed patients should not receive live vaccines such as BCG, MMR, oral polio, and oral typhoid vaccine. Inactivated vaccines such as influenza, hepatitis A or B, pneumococcal, and adsorbed tetanus vaccine are permitted, although these are less likely to be effective in immunocompromised hosts. Both oral and inactivated polio vaccine offer excellent individual immunity, but the oral vaccine is live and therefore contraindicated in this patient. Routine polio immunizations in both the UK and the United States are given as inactivated polio vaccine (IPV).

42. A. Chediak–Higashi syndrome
Although both Chediak–Higashi syndrome and Griscelli syndrome can present with silvery hair, immunodeficiency, and neurologic involvement, only Chediak–Higashi syndrome presents with giant inclusions in polymorphonuclear cells.

43. B. Chemoprophylaxis
The meningococcal conjugate vaccine only provides protection against serogroups A, C, Y, W135. Chemoprophylaxis is necessary for contacts of patients with invasive meningococcal disease. If this is identified to be an outbreak due to meningococcal serogroup b, vaccination against serogroup b may be recommended at that point but does not have a role in immediate postexposure prophylaxis. Options for prophylaxis include rifampin, ceftriaxone, azithromycin, and ciprofloxacin.

44. E. Varicella-zoster vaccine
Live-attenuated virus vaccines, such as VAR vaccine, are contraindicated in pregnancy. Influenza and pertussis containing vaccines such as DTap/IPV are indicated in pregnancy. Hepatitis A and hepatitis B vaccines may be safely administered if indicated in pregnancy.

45. E. Stop antibiotics and consider temporal artery biopsy
In a stable patient with FUO, antibiotics should be stopped. Endocarditis is unlikely as TTE is normal and blood cultures are negative, so a TOE is not indicated. In an older adult with fever, headache, and raised inflammatory markers, giant cell arteritis needs to be ruled out.

46. B. Type I
Type I error is the type of error that occurs when the null hypothesis is incorrectly rejected (in reality there was no association, but by chance a positive result was found). Alpha is the significance level, the probability of making a type I error. Type II error (also called β) is the opposite – the null hypothesis of no association was accepted, but there truly was a difference in results. Confounding bias is due to an additional factor that distorts the relationship between an outcome and exposure.

47. A. Acute generalized exanthematous pustulosis (AGEP)
Acute generalized exanthematous pustulosis (AGEP) is an eruption commonly related to drugs (90%). Commonly associated drugs include antibiotics (penicillins and other beta-lactams commonly) as well as calcium channel blockers and other drugs. This pattern has also been reported postviral illness (e.g., enterovirus, adenovirus, EBV, CMV, HBV, etc.).

Typically there is an acute onset after drug exposure (within 1–2 days), and the rash starts with pustules on an erythematous base (often begin on face or intertriginous areas), accompanied by fever and neutrophilia (due to IL-8 secretion by T cells and keratinocytes). Symptoms resolve with discontinuation of the offending drug, and skin will desquamate in the subsequent 4-10 days.

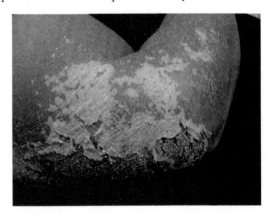

48. D. Lobular capillary hemangioma (pyogenic granuloma)
Pyogenic granuloma is a misnomer as this lesion is neither pyogenic nor granulomatous. It is a rapidly growing benign vascular growth, better referred to as a lobular capillary hemangioma (LCH). LCH presents as a solitary red papule or nodule (skin, face, or gingiva), that is friable, ulcerates easily, and grows fast (in weeks). There are many associations reported, including medications (e.g., retinoids, protease inhibitors, chemotherapeutic agents, etc.), pregnancy (second or third trimester gingival lesions – granuloma gravidarum), and trauma (physical, after laser therapy, etc.). Treatment focuses on removal. Recurrences are common, and the inciting factor needs recognition and removal.

Longitudinal melanonychia consists of longitudinal bands of pigment (e.g., lines) that are a constant diameter throughout the length of multiple nails. It must be differentiated from acral lentiginous melanoma which typically affects one nail and has diffuse asymmetric discoloration throughout the length of the nail. Acral lentiginous melanoma accounts for <5% of melanoma subtypes, but it occurs in all races and is the most common subtype in darker-complexioned individuals.

A glomus tumor is a rare, small benign hamartoma that may be found in nail beds.

While the appearance of Kaposi sarcoma can be nodular, the time course, single lesion, and clinical status of his HIV do not favor this diagnosis.

49. E. *Pseudomonas aeruginosa*

This is a picture typical of ecthyma gangrenosum. Ecthyma gangrenosum is classically associated with *Pseudomonas*

aeruginosa bacteremia in the setting of immunocompromise. It can also (but less commonly) develop with *Staphylococcus aureus*, *Streptococcus pyogenes*, and *Candida albicans* among others, especially gram-negatives. It is usually due to hematogenous dissemination of the pathogen, with subsequent invasion of small vessel walls, leading to ischemia and necrosis distally. Typically lesions start as painless macules which evolve rapidly into indurated bullae which then become necrotic.

Multiple molds can invade the vascular endothelium causing necrotic skin lesions as well as systemic involvement, such as *Aspergillus*, *Fusarium*, and *Mucor*.

In the setting of neutropenia and necrotic skin lesions, additional imaging seeking thoracic and abdominal lesions due to angioinvasive molds would also be appropriate.

This page intentionally left blank

Answers 5

1. A. *Leptospira* culture of blood

Leptospira culture of blood and/or CSF should be performed during the first week of symptoms. After the first 7–10 days of symptoms, *Leptospira* culture of urine is preferred. *Leptospira* does not grow on routine bacterial culture media. For *Leptospira* serologic testing, only IgM should be tested, but it is insensitive during the first 7–10 days of illness.

2. E. *Trichosporon* sp.

Neutropenic fevers in immunocompromised patients have broad differential, including bacterial as well fungal etiologies.

Line-associated sepsis with blood culture positive for yeast could represent *Candida, Rhodotorula, Trichosporon,* or *Cryptococcus*.

Pseudohyphae with barrel-shaped arthroconidia and pleomorphic budding yeast favors *Candida* or *Trichosporon*. *Cryptococcus* are round yeast with no budding or pseudohyphae.

The positive cryptococcal antigen is likely to be a false-positive (*Cryptococcus* sp. would grow as a yeast) and raises the concern for infection with *Trichosporon*.

Management includes line removal and antifungal with amphotericin or voriconazole.

(Image from Lee W-S, Yu F-L, Ou T-Y. Breakthrough *Trichosporon asahii* fungemia during caspofungin therapy. *J Exp Clin Med.* 2014;6(3):108–109.)

3. A. Acute hepatitis B

Hepatitis C and Hepatitis A testing are both negative. Hepatitis B surface antigen (HBsAg) is a marker for active replication signifying that the patient is infectious. It is present in high amounts during the acute phase of infection. It can also be present during the chronic phase of infection if the immune system fails to clear the virus effectively. If HBsAg is present at all the patient should be considered contagious. If it is present for 6 months or more the patient is considered to have chronic hepatitis B.

Differentiation between chronic replicating and chronic, nonreplicating is the presence of hepatitis B e antigen (HBeAg) and anti-HBe antibodies. In chronic, replicating hepatitis B the patient will be positive for HBeAg; during chronic, nonreplicating infection anti-HBe antibodies will

be present. In both chronic conditions the total core antibody (anti-HBc) will be positive while anti-HBc IgM will be negative. If NAAT testing is performed during this time the amount of HBV DNA will be higher during chronic, replicating hepatitis B.

This person is in the acute phase of infection as the HBsAg is positive and no antibodies to the surface antigen have been generated. In addition, the total and IgM core (HBc) antibodies are present, as is the case in acute hepatitis B.

4. E. Meropenem

While cefotetan, a cephamycin, is active against many ESBL-producing Enterobacteriaceae, it is not established for central nervous system infections and is vulnerable to treatment-emergent resistance with these strains. Ceftriaxone is not considered reliably active against ESBL-producing organisms. Gentamicin IV poorly penetrates the central nervous system and is not appropriate for monotherapy of central nervous system infections. Imipenem is reliably active against most ESBL-producing strains but is relatively inactive against *Proteus mirabilis* and should be avoided for treatment of serious infections caused by this organism. Imipenem is also widely believed to be the most epileptogenic carbapenem, which could be a concern in this case. Meropenem is active against ESBL-producing strains and is clinically established for treatment of central nervous system infections.

5. C. Imipenem–cilastatin

Neither sulbactam or tazobactam reliably inhibit AmpC beta-lactamases that *Citrobacter freundii* is known to produce. Ertapenem is inactive against enterococci, and meropenem possesses only marginal activity against *Enterococcus faecalis*. Imipenem–cilastatin is stable to AmpC beta-lactamases produced by *Citrobacter freundii* and is also reliably active against *Enterococcus faecalis*.

6. E. Ceftriaxone

Cefazolin does not adequately penetrate the blood–brain barrier and is not appropriate for treatment of central nervous system infections. Cefepime and ceftazidime are established treatments for gram-negative central nervous system infections but offer no advantage over ceftriaxone for coverage of viridans group streptococci. Cefotetan is not established for treatment of central nervous system infections. Ceftriaxone is considered a therapy of choice for central nervous system infections caused by viridans group streptococcus.

7. E. Skin discoloration
Clofazimine can cause reddish-black or orange skin discoloration within weeks of therapy and can discolor hair and bodily fluid. This side effect is dose-related and is slowly reversible upon discontinuation.

8. B. Micafungin
Due to this patient being critically ill and the possibility of azole-resistant *Candida*, when *Candida* speciation and susceptibilities are unknown, empiric coverage with an echinocandin-like micafungin is recommended. Additionally, micafungin is not known to prolong the QTc interval. All of the azoles, except for isavuconazole, have a risk of prolonging the QTc interval. Terbinafine does not have a role in the treatment of disseminated candidiasis.

9. D. Stop citalopram
The combination of tremor and fever, in the context of recent initiation of a serotonergic agent (citalopram), makes the hyperthermic reaction of serotonin syndrome the most likely diagnosis. Treatment for serotonin syndrome primarily revolves around stopping the inciting agent.

10. D. *Staphylococcus aureus*
S. aureus is the most common cause of suppurative parotitis. Diabetic and elderly patients are at higher risk for developing parotitis. An antistaphylococcal agent would be indicated as empiric coverage.

11. E. Tubular obstruction by crystal precipitation
Nephrotoxicity is well recognized as a complication of aciclovir therapy, especially at the high doses required for treatment of herpes encephalitis and in patients with preexisting kidney disease. Aciclovir is usually rapidly excreted into the tubules. Toxicity is related to the formation of intratubular crystals, which cause tubular obstruction. Renal function tends to deteriorate within 24–48 hours of starting treatment. Birefringent needle-shaped crystals may be visible on urine microscopy. Toxicity may be prevented by ensuring volume repletion and slower infusions.

12. B. Consumption of undercooked snails
The infective organism is most likely to be *Angiostrongylus cantonensis*, the rat lungworm. This is due to the geographical exposure (SE Asia), the incubation period (average 10 days), the clinical features (excruciating progressive headache), and the eosinophilic meningitis without raised red cells. The commonest source of *A. cantonensis* is consumption of raw or undercooked snails.

13. A. *Actinomyces* spp.
Pathogens can enter the lung by way of aspiration of oropharyngeal contents. In a chronic alcoholic with greater risk of aspiration, aspiration pneumonia must be considered. The question is asking you to decide which of the organisms listed could cause a cavitary lesion in a lower lobe. *Streptococcus pneumoniae*, *Mycoplasma pneumoniae*, and *Haemophilus influenzae* are less likely to cause a cavitary lung lesion. Cavities associated with *Mycobacterium tuberculosis* would be more likely to be present in the upper lobe. The lesion in this case is found in a dependent area of the lungs and would be consistent with an oral anaerobe, such as *Actinomyces*.

14. B. Observation
The patient has sinusitis. The most likely cause of this syndrome is a virus and would not warrant antibiotic therapy. The exception would be if the patient has an extended duration of symptoms (normally >7 days). The patient does not present with evidence of complications of sinusitis, such as severe headaches, visual disturbances, or neurologic deficits that would warrant ENT consultation or additional imaging. The best answer to the question would be just observation at this time.

15. B. Nontunneled femoral CVC
Risk of bloodstream infection from IV access varies based on type of catheter and site of placement. Non-tunneled CVCs (central venous catheters) have higher rates of infections than tunneled catheters, PICCs (peripherally inserted central catheters), and peripheral IVs. Femoral placement confers a higher risk of central line-associated bloodstream infection (CLABSI) than internal jugular and subclavian insertions.

Type of catheter: Peripheral IV < PICC < Tunneled central venous catheter (CVC) < Nontunneled CVC

Site of CVC: Subclavian < Internal jugular < Femoral CVC

16. E. *Staphylococcus epidermidis*
IDSA guidelines suggest that long-term CVCs should be removed in the circumstance of a CLABSI from all of the organisms listed, apart from *S. epidermidis*. Catheter removal, however, in this circumstance can shorten the needed antibiotic duration and can reduce the risk of relapsed BSI from any residual biofilm formation.

17. A. Cefazolin
For deep LVAD infections, especially with associated bacteremia with an aggressive organism such as MSSA, it is best to initiate treatment with an IV agent with cidal activity for at least 6 weeks followed by suppression with an oral agent. This is done due to concern for biofilm formation and the inability to control the source of the infection.

Vancomycin, daptomycin, dalbavancin, and linezolid should not be used first-line for MSSA infection.

18. B. Scombroid poisoning
Food poisoning associated with seafood is known as scombroid poisoning. It is commonly misdiagnosed as a seafood allergy. Poisoning is acquired through seafood consumption,

especially dark meat of finfish from the Scombridae and Scomberesocidae families, such as tuna, mackerel, skipjack, and bonito; other fish such as dolphin fish, tilapia, salmon, swordfish, trout, sardines, and anchovies have been implicated.

Symptoms are due to histamine reaction occurring within 1 hour of consumption. Fish may appear to have "honey-combed" scales and taste "peppery," "bubbly," or "spicy." Elderly patients and those taking medication which prevent the breakdown of histamine such as monoamine oxidase inhibitors or isoniazid are likely to have more severe and prolonged symptoms as compared with those taking antihistamines.

19. D. Oral vancomycin
This patent has *Clostridioides difficile* secondary to recurrent courses of antibiotics and hospital exposure, and he has markers of severity with his raised white cell count and serum creatinine. He should be started on therapy as soon as possible with oral vancomycin, which achieves high levels within the bowel lumen compared to systemic therapy. Imaging should be arranged to ensure he does not have toxic megacolon, requiring a surgical opinion and intervention. Imaging may show signs of toxic megacolon or bowel perforation in addition to bowel mucosa and submucosa edema.

If lower GI endoscopy is performed to exclude other causes, pseudomembranes may be visible as raised patches of yellow and white, 2 cm in diameter, on the mucosa, but endoscopy carries a risk of perforation and should not be performed early on in disease.

20. E. *Klebsiella pneumoniae*
K. pneumoniae (K1 capsular serotype) is an emerging pathogen causing liver abscesses in the absence of hepatobiliary disease. It is found in SE Asia, in particular Malaysia. *K. pneumoniae* are oxidase-negative, lactose fermenting organism. The hypermucoviscous variant grows as very mucoid colonies and can be identified by a positive string test (stretching colonies forms a "string" of >5mm).

E. coli is a common causes of liver abscess, and the culture results would fit (although most *E. coli* are indole positive) but in the absence of hepatobiliary pathology and sterile blood cultures this would be unlikely.

E. histolytica commonly presents as an indolent infection and is endemic in rural areas of Malaysia. Against this diagnosis is no preceding colitis (one third) and *Entamoeba* do not grow on blood or MacConkey agar as they require supplemented media (usually egg yolk).

Melioidosis, caused by *B. pseudomallei*, is a condition causing large abscesses. *B. pseudomallei* is an environmental saprophyte found in aquatic environments and when cultured grows as mucoid colonies. Going against this as a diagnosis is that infections are most prevalent following the rainy season (rather than summer months when the patient traveled). Also, while it can be found in Malaysia is it more prevalent in Thailand and North Australia. Furthermore, *B. pseudomallei* are oxidase-positive.

Streptococcus intermedius is one of the *S. milleri* group, which are well recognized as causing deep-seated abscesses such as this. However, the colonial appearances on blood agar are not consistent with *S. intermedius*, and MacConkey agar does not support its growth.

(Image (*left*) reprinted with permission from Elsevier. The Lancet. From Prokesch BC, et al. Primary osteomyelitis caused by hypervirulent *Klebsiella pneumoniae*. *Lancet Infect Dis.* 2016;16(9):e190–e195. Image (*right*) from Rath S, Padhy RN. Prevalence of two multidrug-resistant *Klebsiella* species in an Indian teaching hospital and adjoining community. *J Infect Public Health.* 2014;7(6):496–507.)

21. E. Preterm delivery
This patient has asymptomatic bacteriuria as evidenced by the positive urinalysis without any symptoms. Asymptomatic bacteriuria is associated with preterm delivery which is why guidelines suggest routine screening in pregnancy, with treatment and test of cure if found. Screening should be by urine culture rather than by urine dipstick as sensitivity is greater. Two consecutive specimens with the same organism are required to confirm the diagnosis. Pregnant women with asymptomatic bacteriuria also have a 20–30-fold increased risk of developing pyelonephritis and to have infants of low birthweight.

22. E. Urine CMV DNA PCR
Neonatal serology is unhelpful as this will only reflect transplacental maternal antibody transfer. The mother is already known to be CMV IgG positive. Urine (or saliva) CMV DNA PCR are the recommended first-line investigations in screening for congenital CMV infection as they are more sensitive than plasma CMV DNA PCR, and the clinical specimens are easily obtained. A positive urine/saliva result should be confirmed with a second sample from any site, and plasma CMV DNA PCR, if positive, may be used to monitor the response to treatment. Lumbar puncture would not routinely be performed on a well infant as a screening test for CMV infection, although CSF CMV DNA PCR might be performed as part of the assessment of an infant found to have congenital CMV infection.

23. B. Ceftriaxone 250 mg IM stat and azithromycin 1 gram stat
Gonococcal urethritis can be reliably diagnosed via Gram stain performed on samples obtained in office. The presence of gram-negative diplococci in the setting of neutrophils is highly suggestive of gonococcal urethritis. Ceftriaxone 250 mg plus azithromycin 1 g is the recommended regimen for uncomplicated urethritis, cervicitis, and proctitis.

NAAT tests should be sent on this patient, but treatment should not be delayed until results return. Ceftriaxone 125 mg intramuscularly was used to treat gonorrhea in the past but is no longer recommended. The higher dose of ceftriaxone plus the addition of azithromycin is recommended to reduce the development of resistant *Neisseria gonorrhoeae*. Ciprofloxacin and other fluoroquinolones were recommended for the treatment of gonorrhea in the past, but because of high rates of resistance, their use is no longer recommended.

(Image from Braverman PK. Urethritis, vulvovaginitis, and cervicitis. In Long SS, Prober CG, Fischer M, eds. *Principles and Practice of Pediatric Infectious Diseases.* 5th ed. Elsevier; 2018.)

24. A. Perform a treponemal antibody test
Falsely reactive RPR testing can occur in autoimmune diseases such as SLE. The RPR is based upon antigen synthesized from lecithin, cholesterol, and cardiolipin and reacts with antibodies produced in response to *Treponema pallidum* subsp. *pallidum* infection. Similar antibodies can be formed in the setting of autoimmune diseases leading to a false-positive RPR. All reactive RPRs should be confirmed with a treponemal-specific test.

Repeating an RPR will offer no diagnostic value. Dark field microscopy is not performed on blood samples but rather on specimens collected from chancres. In the absence of active lesions (primary or secondary syphilis) and with the concern for a false-positive result, therapy should be withheld until confirmatory results are available.

25. E. Hepatitis E virus
Although all of these viruses can cause hepatitis in patients, hepatitis E is unique in that it more commonly causes a fulminant hepatitis in pregnant women. Pregnant travelers should be warned to protect themselves against this fecal–oral transmitted virus.

26. C. Vitamin A supplements
Most deaths attributable to measles occur in low-resource settings in children with poor access to healthcare and who have poor nutrition. Children with vitamin A deficiency appear to be at greater risk of severe measles resulting in increased mortality and morbidity. Vitamin A supplements have been shown to reduce overall mortality by up to 30% in children under the age of 5, with preexisting vitamin A deficiency and have been shown to have protective benefit in those complicated by pneumonia.

27. E. *Leptospira icterohaemorrhagiae*
Leptospirosis is typically transmitted by contact with water or soil contaminated with animal urine. It is classically described as a biphasic illness with leptospiremic and leptospiuric phases. Acute renal failure and hepatitis are common complications in the context of leptospirosis; diagnosis is usually confirmed by serology.

The other pathogens are all potentially acquired by exposure to rodents but leptospirosis is by far the commonest.

28. D. Aciclovir
Monkey bites involving macaques carry the risk for transmission of B virus, a herpesvirus that can cause fatal encephalomyelitis in humans. Postexposure prophylaxis with either aciclovir or valaciclovir is appropriate.

29. E. Switch to liposomal amphotericin B
The microscopic finding of nonseptate hyphae is consistent with an agent of mucormycosis. Rhizoids (rootlike hyphae) are typically produced by *Rhizopus* spp. Voriconazole has no activity against *Rhizopus*. Breakthrough infections while on voriconazole prophylaxis have been reported. Renal failure requiring hemodialysis is a risk factor for the disease. Hospital outbreaks have been associated with the use of contaminated linen which may have been the source in this case.

Amphotericin B in combination with adequate surgical debridement is the treatment of choice. Treatment can be stepped down to posaconazole or isavuconazole after clinical improvement. However, initial therapy with an azole as a single agent is not recommended. *Lomentospora prolificans* (formerly *Scedosporium prolificans*) is inherently resistant to all antifungals. *Lomentospora* forms septate hyphae with branching similar to *Aspergillus* spp.

30. B. *Fusarium solani*
The patient has disseminated fusariosis, a disease that can be encountered in patients with prolonged neutropenia after induction chemotherapy or bone marrow transplant. In a study of HSCT recipients, metastatic skin lesions were encountered in 75%. Fungemia is present in 44% of patients. Radiographic findings are similar to other invasive mold infections (nodules, halo sign, cavitation). The patient has traveled to the Dominican Republic, an area endemic for histoplasmosis. However, *Histoplasma* is a dimorphic fungus that grows slowly. Agents of mucormycosis (*Rhizopus, Lichtheimia*) form nonseptate hyphae and are morphologically distinct from *Fusarium*. In contrast to invasive aspergillosis, fusariosis is much more likely to be associated with fungemia. *Fusarium* can in many cases (although not in this one) begin with onychomycosis and localized cellulitis.

31. E. Mefloquine
Mefloquine is the drug of choice for prophylaxis in the setting of pregnancy. Clindamycin is not an adequate drug for malaria chemoprophylaxis. Hydroxychloroquine and doxycycline should not be used during pregnancy due to teratogenic effects. Atovaquone–proguanil has emerging data for use during pregnancy, but mefloquine remains the drug of choice for chemoprophylaxis during pregnancy. If travel is essential, the risk of any prophylactic drug in pregnancy has to be weighed against the risk of contracting malaria. However, do not forget that pregnant women should be advised to avoid traveling to malarial areas; pregnant women are at higher risk of severe malaria, and malaria increases the risk of adverse fetal outcomes, including premature birth and stillbirth.

32. D. Start 14 days doxycycline
Early Lyme with erythema migrans or disseminated erythema migrans is a clinical diagnosis. Serologies may be falsely negative in early infections. Serology is only sent for atypical or difficult cases.

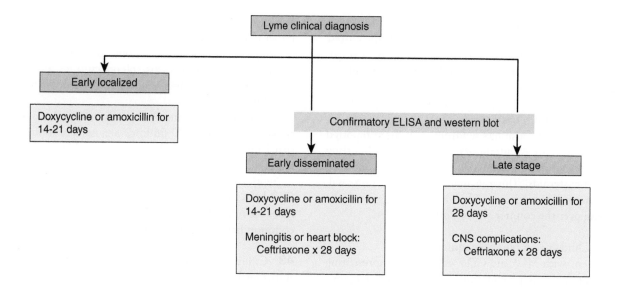

33. B. Hantavirus

The clinical picture of a rapidly progressing respiratory failure associated with diffuse pulmonary edema, fever, leukocytosis with left shift and atypical lymphocytosis, thrombocytopenia, and elevated hematocrit, in the correct epidemiologic setting (Utah, Colorado, Arizona, New Mexico) and exposure history (rodents), is consistent with hantavirus pulmonary syndrome (Sin Nombre virus).

(Image from Shandro JR, Jauregui JM. Wilderness-acquired zoonoses. In Auerbach PS, Cushing TA, Harris NS, eds. *Auerbach's Wilderness Medicine.* 7th ed. Elsevier; 2017.)

34. A. Do a chest X-ray to rule out pulmonary involvement

Clinical presentation is most consistent with intestinal TB. *Mycobacterium bovis* is usually transmitted via consumption of unpasteurized dairy products and is intrinsically resistant to PZA. However, a diagnosis of pulmonary TB in infants is typically made through gastric aspiration given the inability to get sputum samples; assessment for pulmonary involvement, however, is obviously important. GI symptoms in this case could also have many other different etiologies, i.e., cow's milk colitis, other acquired infections, etc.

35. C. *Mycobacterium chimaera*

This is a case of *M. chimaera*-related endocarditis following a valve replacement surgery. High level of suspicion is needed to make the diagnosis and to send the appropriate cultures. Incubation period for symptom presentation can be as long as 5 years. Slow rate of growth and absence of underlying immunodeficiency can help you eliminate the other options.

36. D. *Leishmania mexicana*

This is a case of cutaneous leishmaniasis acquired from the bite of an infected sandfly. The amastigotes of *Leishmania* will be seen in histiocytes while those of *Trypanosoma cruzi* will be seen in somatic cells (i.e., cardiac myocytes). Histoplasma can be seen in histiocytes as a small budding yeast but will not have a kinetoplast. *Candida* also does not have a kinetoplast and will show budding forms and possibly pseudohyphae depending on the species. *Acanthamoeba* is a free-living ameba that will have cysts and trophozoites when seen in tissues.

37. D. Repeat cervical cytology testing in 3 years

Cervical cancer is considered an AIDS-defining illness, because of the higher rates seen among persons infected with HIV with advanced disease. The etiology for this is likely due to more difficulty in clearing HPV infection due to immunosuppression among those infected.

Current guidelines for screening HIV-infected women are based upon age. It is recommended that all women undergo screening upon initiation of care.

For women less than 30 years of age (as with this patient), it is recommended to screen at 12-month intervals for 3 years if results remain normal and then every 3 years thereafter.

If atypical squamous cells of undetermined significance (ASCUS) are seen with positive HPV testing, colposcopy is recommended with repeat cytology at 6–12 months.

If low-grade squamous epithelial lesions (LSIL) and higher, colposcopy should be performed.

Co-testing is not recommended in this age group for HPV.

For women 30 years and older, cervical cytology with or without co-testing with HPV should be done every 12 months for 3 consecutive years and, if normal, then every 3 years thereafter.

For ASCUS results with positive HPV testing, management is the same as above. For LSIL and higher, recommendations are the same as above.

However, for women who receive co-testing where cytology is negative and HPV is positive, it is recommended to repeat co-testing in 1 year (unless genotypes 16/18, in which colposcopy is recommended). If either of the co-test is abnormal at 1 year, then colposcopy should be performed.

HPV vaccine is recommended for young women only up until age 26.

38. E. Toxicity from nasal spray
Cases of iatrogenic Cushing's syndrome have been reported in patients who are co-administered antiretroviral boosting agents ritonavir or cobicistat with cytochrome 3A metabolized corticosteroids. This can include inhaled, intranasal, and intraarticular corticosteroids, which the patient may be acquiring over the counter or from other providers.

39. C. Clindamycin plus primaquine
In a patient with HIV and CD4 <200 cells/μL presenting with a spontaneous pneumothorax, a presumed diagnosis of *Pneumocystis* pneumonia (PCP) is strongly suspected. Given the sulfa drug allergy, clindamycin plus primaquine would be the appropriate treatment. The elevated LDH and 1,3-beta-D-glucan would also be consistent with PCP while this presentation would be less likely due to bacterial or endemic fungal pneumonias treated by the other answer choices. Although the CMV PCR was positive in the serum, CMV pneumonitis in HIV-infected patients (which would require ganciclovir) is very rare compared to PCP and usually requires lung biopsy for diagnosis.

40. A. *Bartonella henselae*
The clinical presentation (fevers, purplish nodular skin lesions) in an advanced AIDS patient with characteristic skin biopsy findings is diagnostic for bacillary angiomatosis caused by *Bartonella* spp. *B. henselae* is the most common cause in the United States and is typically associated with cat exposure; *B. quintana* is more commonly seen in Latin America and associated with human body lice and homelessness. The skin biopsy findings would not be consistent with Kaposi sarcoma or syphilis lesions due to *Treponema pallidum.*

41. C. Ivermectin per NG
The patient has *Strongyloides* hyperinfection syndrome. Light microscopy of urine showed larvae consistent with *Strongyloides.*

42. D. Pulmonary aspergillosis
Pulmonary aspergillosis is one of the most common invasive fungal infections in patients with hematologic malignancies, especially in those with prolonged neutropenia. Fluconazole unfortunately does not provide adequate prophylaxis. Voriconazole or posaconazole are recommended prophylaxis. The pulmonary nodules with surrounding halos are consistent and should raise suspicion for this infection.

PCP is incorrect, because trimethoprim–sulfamethoxazole prophylaxis is extremely effective for the prevention of *Pneumocystis*, he is not hypoxemic, and usual CT imaging findings with PCP consist of bilateral interstitial infiltrates rather than nodules with halo sign.

Streptococcal pneumonia would be unusual in patients on levofloxacin prophylaxis, blood cultures are negative, and the imaging findings are not consistent with streptococcal pneumonia.

Cytomegalovirus pneumonitis is rare and would be a consideration, but CT findings are not consistent. Interstitial infiltrates are usually seen rather than nodules with halos.

Septic pulmonary emboli may manifest as nodules on CT chest, especially at the periphery, but the surrounding halos are not consistent, and blood cultures are negative for common bacterial pathogens.

43. C. Hyper IgE syndrome
Autosomal dominant hyper IgE syndrome manifests with recurrent skin abscesses and recurrent respiratory infections healing with pneumatoceles, as well as eczema and eosinophilia. Nonimmune manifestations include joint laxity, scoliosis, fractures, and a wide nasal tip. DOCK8 deficiency is also associated with hyper IgE and frequent infections but not with skeletal manifestations. Wiskott–Aldrich syndrome also has eczema but is X-linked and is thus mainly seen in males.

44. E. Propagated progressive source
An epidemic curve is a visual display of the onset of illness during an outbreak. Point source epidemics involve a common source and occur over a brief period. Common persistent courses rise and fall, but the cases do not occur within a single incubation period. Propagated progressive sources occur when there is an initial wave of infections followed by second or third waves. There are successively larger peaks. Intermittent outbreaks are separated by periods without evidence of infection.

45. D. Passive immunization
This is an example of passive immunization, that is, the induction of immunity by transfer of antibodies to the nonimmune host. Vaccine immunization describes a method of immunization; partial immunization occurs when a person becomes ill with an infection but is not susceptible to severe illness or death; natural immunization is induction of immunity in a host who is exposed to the live pathogen; active immunization is the induction of immunity by antigen exposure, usually by vaccination.

46. D. Pneumococcal PPV23
Children with cochlear implants have a substantially higher risk of developing pneumococcal meningitis than their peers. Extrapolating from this, all children and adults having cochlear implants are advised to receive pneumococcal vaccination. There is no evidence that people with cochlear implants are more likely to get meningococcal meningitis.

47. A. Cutaneous larva migrans

The rash is characteristic and diagnostic of cutaneous larva migrans (CLM), pruritic, serpiginous, located in lower extremities.

CLM is a result of infection by animal hookworm larvae, most commonly *Ancylostoma braziliense* or *A. caninum*. These are found worldwide, but infection is commoner in tropical and subtropical regions. The larvae can penetrate the skin but cannot pass through the basement membrane of the epidermis. They migrate slowly at a few centimeters/day, causing an inflammatory response along their track. This manifests as an intensely pruritic, red, raised, serpiginous lesion, usually on a lower extremity, or any part of the body exposed to contaminated sand. The actual larvae are a centimeter or two ahead of the lesion. Lesions normally resolve within 2–8 weeks.

Gnathostomiasis can cause localized lesions, but these are associated with edema and pain as well as itching and erythema. Most cases are reported from Asia (especially Thailand and Japan) as well as Mexico.

Larva currens is caused by infection with *Strongyloides stercoralis*. It is also a serpiginous eruption, but the tracks are less defined. They are much faster moving than CLM lesions, at approximately 5 cm/hour, but only last a few hours.

Phytophotodermatitis is caused by topical exposure to certain plant substances; commonly lime juice. Irregular itchy blisters and erythematous patches develop on sun-exposed skin. Linear lesions are common. Lesions appear 24 hours after sun exposure, are not pruritic, but may be painful.

(Image from Kincaid L, Klowak M, Klowak S, Boggild AK. Management of imported cutaneous larva migrans: a case series and mini-review. *Travel Med Infect Dis.* 2015;13(5):382–387.)

48. A. Confounder

Confounder is the correct answer, because in this example cryptococcal infection was associated with HIV infection, and HIV is more prevalent in men who have sex with men. While it initially appeared that the infection was associated with male sex, the relationship was distorted by the third variable (confounder), which is HIV infection. The dependent variable (outcome) in this example is cryptococcosis. HIV infection is a yes/no variable and thus not an ordinal variable (categorical variable with order) nor is it a continuous variable (quantitative).

This page intentionally left blank

Answers 6

1. A. *Alternaria* sp.

Traumatic inoculation of dematiaceous mold is common in motor-vehicle accident or combat wound. In the above case, development of delayed necrotizing pneumonia with positive Fontana–Masson stain (stains melanin found in dematiaceous molds) is highly consistent with dematiaceous mold, likely *Alternaria* sp.

None of the other species would stain positively with the Fontana–Masson stain.

(Image from Rifai N, et al., eds. T*ietz Textbook of Clinical Chemistry and Molecular Diagnostics*. 6th ed. Elsevier; 2018.)

2. B. Daptomycin

Quinupristin/dalfopristin is not active against *E. faecalis*. While telavancin is active against vancomycin-susceptible enterococci, the patient has AKI/CKD, which makes this agent undesirable from a safety standpoint. While the strain is ampicillin-susceptible, the patient has a severe penicillin allergy, which precludes ampicillin. Linezolid should be avoided for routine use in combination with selective serotonin re-uptake inhibitors. Daptomycin is active against this strain of *Enterococcus faecalis*, and there is no evidence of pulmonary involvement based on lack of pulmonary/respiratory symptoms and negative chest X-ray.

3. C. Enterovirus

All of the options can cause an aseptic meningitis; however, the most likely in this case is enterovirus. Enterovirus may be associated with a diffuse maculopapular exanthema, but its absence does not preclude the diagnosis. Up to 2/3 of patients with enteroviral meningitis may have polymorphs in the CSF if taken early in the illness. He is likely to be immune to mumps, whether via childhood illness or immunization, and he has no geographical risk for *Coccidioides*. Enterovirus meningitis is much commoner than Lyme meningitis in the UK, and there is no Lyme reported in the Midwest United States.

4. C. Infliximab

Infliximab is a chimeric mAb directed against TNF. All biologics targeting TNF-α carry a risk of reactivation of tuberculosis. The risk is higher with infliximab and adalimumab than with etanercept. Most cases are likely to be due to reactivation of LTBI, but newly acquired infection is responsible for a number of cases in areas of low TB prevalence. Screening for LTBI should be done before initiating therapy with anti-TNF agents.

Abatacept prevents CD28 binding, inhibiting T-cell costimulation. It carries an increased risk of severe infection but not opportunistic infections or TB.

Alemtuzumab (otherwise known as Campath) carries a risk for *Pneumocystis jirovecii* (*carinii*) pneumonia (PCP), herpes, and CMV infections.

Natalizumab blocks binding of VLa4 on VCAM1, reducing migration of activated white cells. It is associated with a risk of JC virus infection leading to progressive multifocal leukoencephalopathy (PML).

Rituximab is a B cell-depleting monoclonal anti-CD20 antibody and requires consideration of HBV reactivation, prophylaxis for PCP, and JC virus infection leading to PML.

5. C. Send an additional expectorated sputum sample for AFB-smear and culture

The patient has risk factors for infection due to *M. avium* complex (MAC) but requires additional testing to make the official diagnosis with a sputum sample for AFB smear and culture. The medications contain toxicities, and it would be best to provide further work-up to diagnose MAC lung disease before beginning treatment with multidrug therapy. He does not need a bronchoscopy as he is able to expectorate sputum.

6. A. Amoxicillin/clavulanate

In addition to *Haemophilus influenzae* and *Streptococcus pneumoniae*, *Moraxella catarrhalis* is a common cause of exacerbations of COPD. The Gram stain depicts gram-negative cocci in pairs, typical of *Moraxella catarrhalis*. The best answer choice would be amoxicillin/clavulanate due to increasing resistance noted to TMP–SMX and tetracyclines for *Moraxella*. Amoxicillin/clavulanate would be preferred over a quinolone.

7. B. Coagulase-negative staphylococci

Approximately 50% of all LVAD and MCS (mechanical circulatory support) infections are due to gram-positive organisms including coagulase-negative staphylococci, *Staphylococcus aureus*, and enterococcal species. In the case of driveline infections, these are more likely to be introduced as ascending infection from the exit site in the abdomen.

Although Enterobacteriaceae and *Pseudomonas* are important causes of infection, these are not epidemiologically more likely than gram-positive infections. *Cutibacterium* can be seen as a cause of infection in MCS, especially in pacers and AICD infections, but these are not close in frequency to staphylococcal infections. *Candida* species are found only rarely to be associated with driveline infections.

8. C. *Giardia* spp.

The exposure to iced drinks even in a hotel setting along with fresh salads, likely to have been washed in local water, is suggestive of *Giardia* infection. The development of symptoms with watery diarrhea at 7–14 days is typical of *Giardia* infection.

9. C. Ciguatera poisoning

Fish with ciguatera toxin do not look, smell, or taste any different, unlike with scombroid poisoning. Caribbean ciguatera poisoning is not life-threatening and presents with gastrointestinal symptoms followed by neurologic signs without altered mental status. Neurologic signs (weakness, paresthesia, headache, vertigo, pruritus, hallucinations) develop within 3–72 hours after consumption, with abnormalities persisting for several weeks to months (20%).

Ciguatera poisoning should be notified to the local health protection unit and regional poison center to identify the source and affected reef.

10. C. New acquisition of HSV-2

Symptoms associated with HSV-2 infection vary wildly. Primary episode outbreaks are associated with initial infection and are typically more severe than recurrences. Nonprimary first episode of genital herpes (i.e., in a patient who already has oral herpes as this patient does) may be less severe or asymptomatic. Typically there are fewer lesions and fewer systemic symptoms.

In patients presenting with lesions concerning for genital herpes, HSV-2 and HSV-1 NAAT or culture should be performed on specimens obtained from the lesion(s). Concurrently serologic testing should be performed. Positive culture or NAAT without antibody is consistent with recent infection. Positive culture with antibody is consistent with longer infection. Testing her current partner might be helpful but if he were positive, it would not delineate whether she acquired HSV from him. The rash will spontaneously resolve. However, it may recur. Latex allergies are less likely to present with localized findings like this. *T. pallidum* is possible but typically presents with one ulcer and most often without itching or pain.

(Image from Patel R. Genital herpes. *Medicine*, 2014;42(7),354–358.)

11. D. Doxycycline for 21 days

LGV can result in proctitis and proctocolitis. This may manifest as tenesmus, rectal bleeding, and mucoid discharge from the rectum. Laboratory diagnostics to distinguish LGV serovars of *C. trachomatis* are not widely available. The patient should be treated for LGV based upon the clinical presentation and positive *C. trachomatis* by NAAT. Treatment course for LGV proctitis is doxycycline 100 mg BD for 21 days.

12. E. Herpes simplex virus

Both hepatitis B and herpes simplex virus infection can cause a fulminant hepatitis. She is unlikely to get HBV as she is vaccinated. Herpes simplex has been described to more commonly cause fulminant hepatitis in pregnancy. Hepatitis G virus (GBV-C) is transmitted by transfusion but does not cause any known disease. CMV can cause a mild hepatitis, but HSV would more commonly cause fulminant hepatitis.

13. D. Recheck VZV IgG

This is to assess her immune status and re-administer VZIG as soon as possible if found to be varicella susceptible.

Where possible, immune status should be tested in immune compromised individuals prior to the administration of VZIG. VZIG offers no additional protection to individuals who have VZV antibody. Patients may still develop chickenpox, however, following administration of VZIG, and therefore advice to commence antivirals should lesions develop is essential. A proportion of patients will seroconvert in the absence of clinical disease. For this reason, repeat testing for immune status is indicated, as in this case. If an exposure occurs after 3 weeks a further dose of VZIG is required if the individual is still varicella susceptible.

14. E. Start doxycycline 100 mg BD for 14–21 days

The lesion shown is erythema migrans and is typical for early Lyme disease. It is a clinical diagnosis and serology may initially be negative. Guidelines state that treatment with doxycycline should be given for 14–21 days. (Image from Nadelman RB. Erythema migrans. *Infect Dis Clin North Am.* 2015;29(2):211–239.)

15. B. Ceftriaxone IV and azithromycin PO

The patient is a young sexually active male with gonococcal arthritis with concern for disseminated gonococcal infection (DGI) with associated purulent arthritis given systemic symptoms, tenosynovitis, and vesiculopustular lesions noted on physical exam. With this entity, distal joints are commonly affected (knees, ankles, wrists). Lyme arthritis, while often monoarticular, tends to affect larger joints, such as the knee. He is young for a crystal arthropathy; and while staphylococcal arthritis must be considered, he is unlikely to have an MRSA joint infection, and ceftriaxone would safely cover an MSSA infection.

Patients with DGI may have evidence of asymptomatic infection at other sites (oropharynx, genitourinary, or rectal) and testing from these sites is recommended. Cultures obtained may or may not be positive. Gonorrhea and chlamydia nucleic acid amplification test (NAAT) from urogenital and extragenital sites can be sent in order for indirect confirmation of infection. Some laboratories may offer NAAT testing of synovial fluid. Initial therapy recommended is dual antibiotic therapy with intravenous ceftriaxone daily for at least 1 week in addition to a one-time dose of azithromycin given increasing rates of resistance.

16. B. *Cryptococcus gattii*

Cryptococcus gattii is endemic to parts of British Columbia (including Vancouver Island), the Pacific Northwest, and Australia.

The Gram stain in this case demonstrated narrow-based budding yeasts of variable size with thick capsules, suggesting *Cryptococcus*. Gram stain is not typically the stain of choice – India Ink enables visualization of the capsules. Cryptococcal antigen of CSF has replaced India Ink in many clinical laboratories of the diagnostic of choice for cryptococcal meningitis.

The clinical picture and investigations are not suggestive of *Candida albicans*. *Candida* spp. can cause meningitis, but it is unusual and typically occurs in medically and surgically compromised patients. The yeasts of *C. albicans* are 5–8 μm and usually demonstrate pseudohyphae.

Cryptococcus neoformans is possible in this case, but it is less likely than *C. gattii* in an immunocompetent host from an endemic area. *C. gattii* can be distinguished from *C. neoformans* by canavanine-glycine-bromthymol blue medium, which turns blue for the former but not the latter. They can also be distinguished by molecular analysis.

CNS pneumocystosis is reported, but it is very uncommon and occurs exclusively in immunocompromised hosts. *Pneumocystis jirovecii* is more commonly associated with pneumonia in immunocompromised patients. The cytopathology is not consistent with *P. jirovecii*, which does not bud.

There is overlap in the cytopathologic and histopathologic appearance of *Histoplasma* and *Cryptococcus* spp. They overlap in size, and both demonstrate narrow budding. A thick capsule can be demonstrated for *Cryptococcus* with mucicarmine stain. Despite its name, *H. capsulatum* does not have a capsule. However, a thin clearing around the nucleus can appear like a capsule, which resulted in the name.

(Image from Murray PR, Rosenthal KS, Pfaller MA. *Medical Microbiology*. 8th ed. Elsevier; 2016.)

17. B. *P. knowlesi*

The patient has manifestations of severe malaria, with high parasitemia and end-organ damage. *P. falciparum* is the most common cause of severe malaria. However, you are shown a band trophozoite on peripheral smear. This is consistent with *P. knowlesi*. Another clue is geographic. This patient is in an area where *P. knowlesi* is present. It is important, especially for your boards, to be able to differentiate between malaria species.

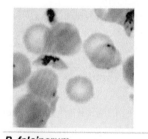

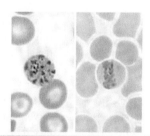

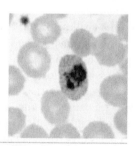

P. falciparum	*P. malariae*	*P. ovale*
Banana	Band trophozoite	Round or oval
Severe disease	Mild disease	Can have Schuffner dots

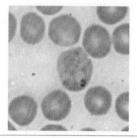

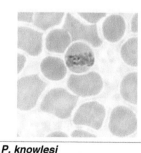

P. vivax	*P. knowlesi*
Schuffner dots	Band trophozoite
	Severe disease

18. A. Direct contact

This is a two-stage question, requiring you first of all to identify what the infection is most likely to be and then how the patient has acquired it. This is a case of acute brucellosis, compatible with the exposure history and clinical findings of fever/sacroiliitis/hepatosplenomegaly and pancytopenia. Genitourinary symptoms may also be seen. The incubation period is usually a week to a month but may be much longer. *Brucella* spp. may be found worldwide, and on average 100–200 cases are reported annually in the United States. The highest number of cases are reported from California, Texas, Arizona, and Florida. Brucellosis has multiple routes of acquisition: direct contact, inhalation of aerosol from an infected animal, ingestion of unpasteurized milk, blood transfusion, and organ transplantation. There is no person-to-person transmission. Infection also does not occur after an arthropod bite or ingestion of cooked meat.

Hunters may be particularly at risk through coming into contact with the blood and organs of the hunted animals, such as wild boar, elk, moose, and deer. Vets and slaughter-house workers may also be exposed occupationally.

19. B. Coccidioidomycosis

This is erythema nodosum. Coccidioidomycosis is the most common cause of erythema nodosum in the North American southwest. The concomitant presence of systemic symptoms, eosinophilia, and hilar adenopathy support the diagnosis. Without this epidemiologic background, sarcoidosis would be the commonest cause of erythema nodosum with these clinical features.

20. A. *Cryptosporidium* sp.

Cryptosporidium is the smallest of the coccidian parasites that are acid fast. While *Cryptosporidium* is an intracellular parasite it often appears to be sitting on the surface of the epithelium. *Cyclospora* is also acid fast but is twice the size of *Cryptosporidium* and will be in the cytoplasm of enterocytes. *Cystoisospora* is the largest of the coccidian parasites and will also be in the cytoplasm of enterocytes. *Giardia* is not acid fast and is a parasite of the small intestine where the trophozoites are attached to the mucosal surface but are not intracellular. *Enterocytozoon* is smaller than *Cryptosporidium*, is intracellular, but is not acid fast.

21. D. *S. mansoni*

There is a clear lateral spine present on diagnostic faecal sample, consistent with a diagnosis of *S. mansoni*.

(Image from McPherson RA, Pincus MR. *Henry's Clinical Diagnosis and Management by Laboratory Methods*. 23rd ed. Elsevier; 2017.)

22. E. Spontaneous vaginal delivery provided obstetrically permitted without intravenous zidovudine during labor

Intravenous zidovudine should be administered to women with HIV RNA >1000 copies/mL (or unknown HIV RNA) near delivery but is not required for women receiving ART regimens who have HIV RNA ≤1000 copies/mL during late pregnancy and near delivery and no concerns regarding adherence to the ART regimen. Scheduled cesarean delivery at 38 weeks' gestation (compared to 39 weeks for most indications) is recommended for women who have HIV RNA >1000 copies/mL near delivery. https://aidsinfo.nih.gov/contentfiles/lvguidelines/PerinatalGL.pdf

23. D. Serial lumbar punctures

The patient has presented with cryptococcal meningitis and evidence of elevated intracranial pressures (ICP). Unlike some other causes of elevation in the ICP, pharmacologic management with either acetazolamide, dexamethasone, or mannitol is not effective in cryptococcal meningitis. The first-line treatment is serial large-volume lumbar punctures to reduce the elevated ICP. Neurosurgical interventions such as lumbar drain placement, ventriculostomy, or VP shunting are reserved for refractory cases or in patients with evidence of imminent herniation.

24. A. Chagas brain abscess

In patients from endemic regions, *Trypanosoma cruzi* can cause acute or reactivation disease, particularly in patients with advanced AIDS. The most common presentation is CNS reactivation leading to meningoencephalitis or brain abscesses, which presents very similarly to *Toxoplasma* with ring-enhancing lesions on MRI imaging. The negative serum *Toxoplasma* serologies and EBV PCR in the CSF make other causes such as toxoplasmic encephalitis or primary CNS lymphoma less likely while the patient's country of origin in South America is endemic for Chagas disease.

25. E. Valganciclovir

Since the donor had indeterminate CMV serology, and the recipient was CMV seronegative, clinicians should assume that the donor was CMV seropositive since this is the higher-risk possibility and administer prophylaxis accordingly. The standard for CMV D+/R– patients is to administer valganciclovir for 6 months. Valganciclovir is rapidly metabolized to active ganciclovir in the GI tract and liver and may be taken once daily. Use of oral ganciclovir has very low bioavailability and would have a very high pill burden. Foscarnet and cidofovir are only available IV, and their role is for CMV prophylaxis when first-line treatments are contraindicated, or there is resistance. Aciclovir is not active against CMV.

26. D. GATA2 deficiency

Although patients with deficiencies of the IL-12 and IFN-gamma axis and with CGD can present with disseminated mycobacterial infections, while patients with WHIM syndrome (CXCR4 deficiency) and DOCK8 deficiency can present with disseminated warts, patients with GATA2 deficiency also have monocytopenia and lymphedema.

27. C. No follow-up necessary

No follow-up testing should be done after successful completion of *Clostridioides difficile* infection. Detection of *C. difficile* toxins is possible even after successful completion of treatment but has no prognostic significance for recurrent disease.

28. E. Kaposi sarcoma

Kaposi sarcoma (KS) is a malignancy of endothelial vascular cells (vascular tumor) associated with human herpesvirus 8 (HHV8), also known as Kaposi sarcoma herpes virus (KSHV). Four forms that are morphologically and histologically indistinguishable: AIDS-related (considered an AIDS-defining illness), endemic or African, organ transplant associated (thought to be associated with chronic immunosuppression), and classic (indolent disease affecting older Mediterranean men and Jewish origin). The most common presentation is cutaneous KS. Whereas classic KS favors lower extremity involvement, AIDS-associated KS may affect multiple locations. Varied colors (deep red, brown, purple, pink) and morphology (patches, plaques, nodules, fungating) on lower extremities, face, oral mucosa, and genitalia. Lesions are not painful, pruritic, or necrotic. Lymphedema may occur in area of lesion distribution (obstructive lymphadenopathy and cytokines associated with KS pathogenesis contribute). KS can also involve visceral sites, most frequently reported in oral cavity (palate then gingiva most commonly affected), GI tract, and respiratory system. In addition to ART, visceral KS may require concomitant chemotherapy.

29. B. Epstein–Barr virus

This patient most likely has infectious mononucleosis caused by EBV. He has tonsillitis with prominent adenopathy and fatigue. Splenomegaly may also be identified on exam, and laboratory evaluation can show atypical lymphocytosis, thrombocytopenia, and hepatitis. Patients with active EBV infection may develop drug eruptions when prescribed penicillins.

30. A. Acute HIV infection

Acute HIV can present with fever, pharyngitis, lymphadenopathy, and exanthematous rash and should be considered in the differential diagnosis when a patient presents with a mononucleosis-like syndrome.

31. A. Aplastic anemia

In patients with hemoglobinopathies, parvovirus can cause pure red cell aplasia by driving persistent lysis of red blood cell precursors. Pregnant women are also particularly at risk for severe complications with parvovirus infection, including miscarriage, intrauterine fetal death, and hydrops fetalis.

32. E. Supportive care

This patient likely has hand, foot, and mouth disease, which is typically caused by *Enteroviridae*, most commonly coxsackie A16. The illness is usually mild and self-limited. Analgesics may be helpful for symptomatic relief.

33. C. *Mycobacterium marinum*

This patient had an aquatic inoculation injury to his hand and then developed nodular lesions with proximal sporotrichoid spread. He most likely developed infection with *Mycobacterium marinum*.

34. E. Syphilis

The image shows significant keratitis and hypopyon as seen with anterior uveitis. Syphilis can have a variety of ocular manifestations including anterior uveitis, which is most commonly seen during secondary syphilis, posterior uveitis and retinitis, and interstitial keratitis that is a late sequela of congenital infection. Herpes simplex virus could also be considered in the differential diagnosis.

(Image from Assessments. In Cohen J, Powderly W, Opal S, eds. *Infectious Diseases*. 4th ed. Elsevier; 2017.)

35. B. Cytomegalovirus

CMV is the most common ocular infection in patients living with HIV. It is most common in patients who have CD4 counts <50/μL, and patients often present with complaints of "floaters" and blurred vision. Examination shows necrotizing, full-thickness retinitis, often with some associated hemorrhage, which creates a "brush fire" or "ketchup and cottage cheese" appearance.

36. B. Metronidazole

Treatment with metronidazole, along with tetanus immune globulin, should be administered. Metronidazole is recommended as first-line antimicrobial therapy for tetanus. The other antibiotics listed are recommended as second-line agents.

37. C. Gram-positive bacilli

Clostridium botulinum is an anaerobic, gram-positive bacillus. This patient has infant botulism caused by toxin production from this organism.

38. B. Ethambutol

The most important complication of ethambutol therapy is optic neuritis, which can manifest as decreased visual acuity, restriction of visual fields, and disturbance of color vision. Other important side effects of antituberculous medications include hepatotoxicity, peripheral neuropathy, hypersensitivity reactions, bone marrow suppression, and orange discoloration of bodily fluids.

39. B. Blastomycosis

Blastomycosis appears as broad-based budding yeast in tissue. Pulmonary blastomycosis can present as nonresolving pneumonia, cavitary pneumonia, or a mass-like lesion that can be confused with multiple other entities, including tuberculosis and lung cancer. Cutaneous lesions are the most common extrapulmonary manifestation of blastomycosis and typically appear as well-demarcated plaques or ulceronodular lesions.

(Image from Assessments. In Cohen J, Powderly W, Opal S, eds. *Infectious Diseases*. 4th ed. Elsevier; 2017.)

40. B. Histamine ingestion

These patients have scombroid poisoning, which is caused by excess histamine production from bacterial overgrowth in poorly cleaned or stored fish. It is most commonly seen with oily fish, including tuna and mackerel. Symptoms include flushing, vomiting, diarrhea, dizziness, and palpitations, and patients typically become symptomatic within an hour of ingesting the contaminated seafood.

41. D. Penicillin G - 2.4 million units IM, once
This patient has early secondary syphilis, as manifested by the diffuse, morbilliform rash and RPR conversion in less than a 6-month period. The recommended treatment is one IM dose of penicillin G. Doxycycline for 2 weeks or azithromycin can be considered as alternative regimens. Three doses of IM penicillin G would be appropriate for late latent syphilis.

42. A. Adult Still's disease
There is no definitive laboratory test for adult Still's disease, but it is the most common rheumatologic cause of fever of unknown origin. The diagnosis is largely clinical and includes criteria such as the characteristic evanescent salmon-pink rash, fevers over 39°C, and a neutrophilia. Markedly elevated ferritin levels are a key clue.

43. D. Nifurtimox-eflornithine
This is first-line therapy for second-stage *Gambiense* human African trypanosomiasis and has been included in the WHO's Essential Medicines List. It has been a milestone improvement in the treatment and outcomes for HAT.

44. C. Leptospirosis
This is a classic case of leptospirosis, given the conjunctival suffusion, calf and paraspinal muscle tenderness, and elevated creatine kinase. Contaminated floodwater in urban rodent-infested slums is the likely route of exposure to the leptospires. The clinical manifestations are highly variable, with many subclinical while a few are severe and potentially fatal. Conjunctival suffusion is useful in distinguishing leptospirosis from other common causes of fever.

45. C. ESBL
Extended-spectrum β-lactamases confer resistance to third-generation cephalosporins but not cephamycins or drugs containing β-lactamase inhibitors.

46. A. Efavirenz
K103N is the most common mutation associated with efavirenz resistance. This mutation also confers resistance to delavirdine and nevirapine, but not rilpivirine and etravirine.

47. A. Increased cell membrane permeability through binding to ergosterol
Amphotericin is a polyene macrolide antibiotic that acts through binding ergosterol, a prominent component in the cell membranes of most fungi. It leads to the formation of ion channels, composed of AmB multimers, that causes cell death.

48. D. Paromomycin
This patient likely has cutaneous leishmaniasis. Therapeutic options include observation, local treatment with cryotherapy or paromomycin, and systemic therapy with azoles, miltefosine, amphotericin, pentavalent antimonials, or pentamidine.

49. A. Bisected pearl colonies on charcoal cephalexin agar
This would be consistent with *Bordetella pertussis*, the likely pathogen in this infant (see image).

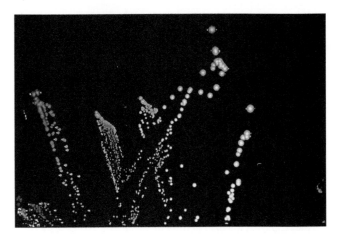

Perinasal swabs with a Dacron Tip or nasopharyngeal aspirates are the specimens of choice and should be plated at the bedside or placed in charcoal transport medium. PCR is more sensitive, especially later in the presentation and after antibiotics. The highest rates of disease in the UK are in infants under 3 months. It is highly contagious, with up to 90% of unimmunized household contacts developing the disease. Public health should be notified as contacts may need assessment, chemoprophylaxis, and vaccination (households with other infants <4 months old, pregnant women, and healthcare workers).
(Image from Assessments. In Cohen J, Powderly W, Opal S, eds. *Infectious Diseases.* 4th ed. Elsevier; 2017.)

50. D. Quinine sulfate plus clindamycin
In asplenic patients infection with *Babesia microti* can be severe, with intense hemolysis leading to severe anemia, jaundice, and renal failure. DIC, ARDS, and noncardiac pulmonary edema are described. Diagnosis is by microscopic examination of a Giemsa-stained thin blood film. The blood film shows a typical tetrad of merozoites within an erythrocyte ("Maltese cross") as well as multiple ring forms.

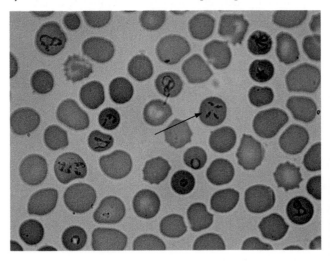

First-line treatment for severe babesiosis or infection in immunosuppressed patients is with quinine and clindamycin. Treatment is recommended for at least 6 weeks. Blood transfusion and intensive care support may be required.
(Image from Assessments. In Cohen J, Powderly W, Opal S, eds. *Infectious Diseases.* 4th ed. Elsevier; 2017.)

Answers 7

1. A. Amphotericin B

Talaromyces marneffei (formerly *Penicillium marneffei*) is an endemic dimorphic fungus in Southeast Asia. Common clinical presentation includes B-symptoms and lymphadenopathy.

There is a higher prevalence in patients with newly diagnosed or poorly controlled HIV.

Cultures grow unique colonies with a reddish-yellow base.

The drug of choice is amphotericin B induction followed by itraconazole. The other azoles might have a role in salvage therapy but are not appropriate as first-line therapy.

(Image reprinted with permission from Elsevier. The Lancet. Limper AH, Adenis A, et al. *Lancet Infect Dis.* 2017;17(11):e334–e343.)

2. E. Trough concentration of 0.8 μg/mL

The desired gentamicin serum trough concentration range for synergistic therapy of gram-positive infections is <1 μg/mL, in order to preserve activity and minimize risk of aminoglycoside toxicity. The desired gentamicin peak concentration range for synergistic treatment of endocarditis caused by viridans *streptococcus* is 3–4 μg/mL. When used for treatment of serious gram-negative infections, a typical gentamicin peak concentration range to target is 4–10 μg/mL.

3. D. Switch colistin to ceftazidime–avibactam IV

The patient is likely experiencing colistin-induced neurotoxicity, warranting discontinuation of colistin. Ceftazidime–avibactam is active against KPC-producing *Klebsiella pneumoniae* and would be an appropriate agent to switch to. Ceftriaxone would not be expected to provide coverage of KPC-producing Enterobacteriaceae strains. Ceftolozane–tazobactam does not provide activity against KPC-producing strains. Discontinuing therapy for a complicated urinary tract infection at day 3 of therapy is not appropriate.

4. A. Calcium carbonate

The bioavailability of fluoroquinolones is significantly decreased by chelation with divalent cations. These interactions can be minimized by administering the oral quinolone at least 2 hours before or 6 hours after exposure to the medication/food that contains polyvalent cations.

5. C. Doxycycline

Doxycycline does not require dose adjustment due to renal impairment. Amikacin, imipenem–cilastatin, ciprofloxacin, and sulfamethoxazole–trimethoprim would all require dose adjustments for renal impairment.

6. C. Give 4 vaccines (d0, d3, d7, d14) plus rabies immunoglobulin

Bats are a potential source of rabies-related viruses. Bat bites are usually felt rather than seen. However, 50% of human cases with bat-variant rabies virus in the United States have resulted from unrecognized bat bites.

Guidelines differ currently between the US and UK. ACIP guidance for the US in this situation advises 4 doses for postexposure prophylaxis and rabies immunoglobulin.

Current Public Health England guidance is that where there is uncertain physical contact, such as with a young child, then treatment should be initiated with vaccine. If the patient is non- or partially immune, this should be with 4 doses. RIG (rabies immunoglobulin) is only additionally required for nonimmune patients in direct contact with bats, or patients who are immunosuppressed.

7. A. Adenovirus

The patient in this case is immunocompromised and at risk for many opportunistic infections, but the T-cell-depleted graft and graft versus host disease are both risk factors for disseminated adenovirus infection. The hematuria in the case suggests adenovirus or BK virus, but BK virus would not cause the pneumonitis. HSV and VZV would be unusual causes of hematuria and diagnostic testing for CMV was negative.

8. D. Trimethoprim-sulfamethoxazole and imipenem

The patient is immunocompromised due to his transplantation and presents with a cavitary lung lesion. He is at risk for many opportunistic pathogens but has Gram stain findings suggestive of infection due to *Nocardia*. Two-drug therapy with sulfamethoxazole and imipenem would be recommended empirically and the patient will likely require a minimum of 6 months of treatment.

9. A. Cefazolin

For deep LVAD infections, especially with associated bacteremia with an aggressive organism such as MSSA, it is best to initiate treatment with an IV agent with cidal activity for at least 6 weeks followed by suppression with an oral agent. This is done due to concern for biofilm formation and the inability to control the source of the infection.

Vancomycin, daptomycin, dalbavancin, and linezolid should not be used first-line for MSSA infection.

10. E. *Vibrio vulnificus*
This patient has acquired systemic *Vibrio vulnificus* infection following the ingestion of seafood in the US Gulf coast. Patients with cirrhosis or hemochromatosis are particularly susceptible to systemic infection and have a high mortality rate, ranging from 40% to 90%. They can present with fever and hypotension, developing bullous lesions and cellulitis. This patient is bacteremic with *Vibrio* as evidenced by the curved gram-negative rods indicative of *Vibrio vulnificus* and other *Vibrio* spp.

Patients with a presumptive diagnosis of *V. vulnificus* septicemia should be started immediately on antibiotic therapy and managed aggressively in an intensive care unit. A tetracycline plus a third-generation cephalosporin is recommended.

11. A. Administer single dose of benzathine penicillin IM
Although appropriate testing should be performed, a patient with symptoms or signs of primary or secondary syphilis should be empirically treated at the time of presentation. Note also that syphilis serologic testing (either treponemal or nontreponemal tests) may not be immediately positive in primary syphilis. When suspicion is high, empirically treat (even when tests are negative). 2.4 million units of benzathine penicillin is the treatment of choice for both primary and secondary syphilis. Evaluation of lesions for HSV-2 or HSV-1 is appropriate in this situation. However, the lesions are painless and empirical aciclovir is not indicated. Referral to dermatology could be considered if STI work-up and treatment did not result in recovery.

(Image from Cox DJ, Ballard RC. Syphilis. In Morse SA, et al., eds. *Atlas of Sexually Transmitted Diseases and AIDS.* 4th ed. Saunders; 2010.)

12. C. Inflammatory response to dying spirochetes
The patient has developed a Jarisch–Herxheimer reaction after treatment of his syphilis. This syndrome is characterized by release of lipoproteins, cytokines, and immune complexes shortly after treatment. This reaction is characterized by fevers, chills, headaches, and myalgias. NSAIDs are recommended for treatment for these symptoms, and the reactions are usually self-limited.

13. D. Repeat parvovirus B19 serology at 4 weeks following exposure
Serologic testing shows the patient to be susceptible to parvovirus B19. A significant proportion of infections with parvovirus B19 are asymptomatic; therefore guidance recommends re-testing at 4 weeks postcontact. If her serologic tests at this time remain negative she can be reassured that she has not had the infection. However, she should be advised that she remains susceptible to infection.

14. C. Itraconazole
The patient lives in the Midwest and presents with chronic pneumonia and a skin lesion. She works as a landscaper with likely extensive soil exposure and potential for inhalation of fungal spores. The GMS stain shows large broad-based budding yeast forms consistent with *Blastomyces dermatitidis*. This patient has disseminated blastomycosis (pulmonary infection with cutaneous dissemination). She is clinically stable with no symptoms or signs noted that would be concerning for severe infection or CNS involvement. If she had severe infection a course of amphotericin B, preferably a lipid formulation, would be warranted. Itraconazole is the treatment of choice for mild to moderate forms of blastomycosis including nonsevere, disseminated infection. Fluconazole and the echinocandins are poorly active. Posaconazole has *in vitro* activity against *Blastomyces*, but clinical data are limited, and first-line therapy with this drug is not recommended. Prednisone should be avoided.

15. B. Ceftriaxone
The patient has AV block from Lyme disease. Treatment of Lyme disease depends on stage and severity. For heart block which requires hospitalization, parenteral ceftriaxone is the initial treatment of choice. Doxycycline may be used to complete the course, or for a full course of treatment in ambulatory patients with cardiac Lyme disease.

16. A. Aciclovir prophylaxis
Fever, confusion, and a cerebrospinal fluid exam that shows lymphocytic-predominant pleocytosis with normal glucose suggest viral encephalitis. A recent history of a bite from a macaque should raise the suspicion for herpes B virus (also called B virus) infection, which is essentially the homologue of herpes simplex virus infection in macaques. B virus causes human encephalitis that is indistinguishable from other causes of viral encephalitis. Aciclovir postexposure prophylaxis after a macaque bite is recommended to prevent B virus infection.

Although the patient should have received appropriate advice on using antimosquito repellent and prophylaxis for malaria prior to her trip, malaria and tick-associated illnesses would have manifested earlier after her return from South Africa. Her clinical presentation is also not consistent with tetanus.

17. B. Ethambutol
Acetaminophen is a common known cause of drug-induced liver injury. The most common antituberculosis drugs to be associated with liver toxicity are INH > PZA > RIF. EMB is not a common cause of hepatotoxicity.

18. D. *Trypanosoma brucei rhodesiense*
This is most likely *T. brucei rhodesiense*, the cause of East African sleeping sickness. The acute presentation and geographic location of the patient's travels support this over *T. b. gambiense*. *T. cruzi*, the cause of Chagas disease, is found in the Americas. *G. duodenalis*, which a flagellate, is an intestinal pathogen and unlikely to cause this type of severe systemic presentation. *P. falciparum*, while high on the differential for fever in a traveler, is not a flagellated parasite.

19. D. *Trichinella spiralis*

The most likely diagnosis is infection with *Trichinella spiralis*, a tissue nematode. It is transmitted through ingestion of raw or undercooked contaminated meat (encysted larvae). Muscle stage develops when intestinal adult-derived larvae disseminate hematogenously (or via lymphatics) and invade striated muscle.

20. B. HIV genotyping of the CSF virus

CNS viral escape syndrome is an uncommon condition that can be seen in patients with HIV on ART. It is defined by presence of CNS HIV replication in CSF despite viral suppression or low-grade viremia. New-onset neurocognitive symptoms may range from HIV-associated dementia to focal neurologic deficits. CSF pleocytosis is often present with a CD8 predominance. Clinical management should include assessment of the CSF genotype due to compartmentalized resistant virus that may be present in the CSF. If found, ART regimens should be changed based on CSF genotype results.

A nerve conduction study would be used to evaluate for neuropathies. HIV-associated peripheral neuropathies are common in persons with advanced disease (CD4 cell counts <200 cells/μL). They are usually distal symmetrical neuropathies. Several drugs may also be associated with development of peripheral neuropathies, particularly older protease inhibitors (i.e., indinavir, saquinavir, and ritonavir). This may also be caused by drugs used to treat opportunistic infections and AIDS-defining illnesses, like dapsone, vincristine, isoniazid, and ethambutol. Initiation of ART is recommended to reduce the risk of developing distal symmetric polyneuropathy, but it is unclear if it can reduce severity of already present disease. Symptomatic management with pharmacotherapy is recommended such as gabapentin and potentially second-line regimens like a tricyclic antidepressant and topical capsaicin.

MRI are typically recommended to evaluate patients where HIV-associated dementia is a concern with severe deficits to rule out other common neurologic disorders like neoplasms or infections. Also, while MRI is typically included in the evaluation of a patient with neurocognitive decline and suppressed viral load, it would not guide management in this case. HIV-associated dementia almost exclusively is seen in persons who have not initiated ART with advanced disease (CD4 cell count <200 cells/μL). Lumbar punctures may also be done when evaluating a patient with advanced disease and neurocognitive deficits to rule out other etiologies. However, CSF HIV RNA levels would not be diagnostic of HAD, and typically an elevated CSF protein and red blood cells may be seen.

B12 deficiency, thyroid function, and syphilis should all be considered in a patient with dementia but are unlikely to have been undetected in a patient who has been under routine HIV care for a prolonged period.

21. D. Nevirapine

Y181C is selected in patients treated with nonnucleoside reverse transcriptase inhibitors. It is the signature mutation for nevirapine and causes high-level reduction in nevirapine susceptibility, intermediate-level reduction in rilpivirine and etravirine susceptibility, and low-level reduction in efavirenz susceptibility.

22. B. Antiretroviral therapy

The most likely diagnosis given the clinical syndrome and characteristic findings on MRI of the brain is progressive multifocal leukoencephalopathy (PML) caused by JC virus. The recommended treatment for PML is immediate initiation of ART to achieve immune reconstitution. Treatments such as cidofovir, cytarabine, and 5HT2a serotonin reuptake inhibitors such as mirtazapine have been tested but have shown no or inconclusive clinical benefit. The antivirals aciclovir and ganciclovir do not have activity against JC virus.

23. B. Human herpesvirus 8

The clinical presentation is most consistent with primary effusion lymphoma (PEL), which is most closely associated with HHV-8. Rather than presenting as a discrete mass, PEL presents in advanced HIV/AIDS as a "liquid tumor" as effusion of pleural, pericardial, or abdominal spaces. Diagnosis is typically made by fluid cytology showing high-grade malignant B lymphocytes, which typically have a null phenotype (CD45 + but negative for B- and T-cell markers). The diagnosis is confirmed with positive immunohistochemical staining of the malignant lymphocytes for HHV-8 (or associated markers such as a LANA-1).

24. C. *Cryptococcus neoformans*

The Fontana-Masson stain highlights melanin, which is an important component of cryptococcal cell wall. *Cryptococcus neoformans* can present atypically in transplant recipients, which leads to delayed diagnosis and treatment. An Alcian Blue stain highlights polysaccharide.

25. B. Cytomegalovirus

Varicella may cause pneumonitis with hypoxemia in immunocompromised patients and may also cause gastrointestinal manifestations. However, the patient is on aciclovir, which is effective prophylaxis for varicella.

Cytomegalovirus (CMV) causes both colitis and pneumonitis, among other manifestations. Infiltrates on imaging are usually interstitial, and diagnosis is made via CMV PCR of the blood in addition to bronchoscopy with positive transbronchial biopsy. CMV colitis may be associated with negative CMV PCR, so diagnosis would be through sigmoidoscopy with biopsy of the colon to look for CMV viral inclusions or positive immunostain on pathology. Aciclovir is not effective at preventing CMV.

Strongyloides can cause both pneumonitis and gastroenteritis in immunocompromised patients, but the stool ova and parasite test is negative, and it is less common in transplant recipients who are not foreign-born or who reside in urban areas.

Clostridioides difficile may cause colitis, but *C. difficile* PCR test is negative and has a very high sensitivity. In addition, *C. difficile* does not cause pneumonitis.

Pneumocystis jirovecii may cause hypoxemia with interstitial pulmonary infiltrates in immunocompromised patients but does not cause colitis. In addition, this patient is on trimethoprim–sulfamethoxazole prophylaxis, rendering pneumocystis pneumonia even less likely.

26. B. APECED syndrome

Autoimmune Polyendocrinopathy–Candidiasis–Ectodermal Dystrophy (APECED) or autoimmune polyendocrine syndrome type 1 is characterized by the triad of CMC, hypoparathyroidism, and Addison disease. CARD9 deficiency and IL-17 deficiencies can also present with CMC but lack the endocrinopathies. Patients with MCM4 deficiency, on the other hand, also present with adrenal insufficiency, while patients with DiGeorge syndrome also have hypoparathyroidism.

27. C. Norovirus

The illness fits criteria for a norovirus outbreak. Vomiting predominated, the incubation period was between 24 and 48 hours, and the illness lasted between 12 and 60 hours. This is not STEC because if STEC was the cause of such an outbreak, hospitalization and hemolytic–uremic syndrome would have been seen. Bloody diarrhea was not mentioned in the stem. Vomiting would not have predominated for infection due to *Campylobacter*, and the illness would have lasted longer. ETEC typically causes more of a watery diarrhea but not prominent vomiting. The incubation period is too long for staphylococcal food poisoning, which is between 2 and 7 hours.

28. B. *Haemophilus influenzae* type b vaccine

Hib, meningococcal ACWY vaccine, meningococcal B vaccine, and influenza vaccines should be administered ideally ≥2 weeks before the procedure or delayed until 2 weeks afterward.

29. B. *Ascaris lumbricoides*

The egg seen is that of *Ascaris lumbricoides*. Stool OCP (ova, cysts, and parasites) microscopy is usually positive in *Ascaris* infection due to the huge numbers of eggs that are produced and shed. Fertilized eggs are rounded with a thick bumpy outer shell, often stained brown. Abdominal symptoms are often absent or nonspecific unless an adult worm is passed in the stool. It takes around 6–8 weeks after egg ingestion for abdominal symptoms to develop.

(Image from Maguire JH. Intestinal nematodes (roundworms). In Bennett JE, Dolin R, Blaser MJ, eds. *Mandell, Douglas, and Bennett's Principles and Practice of Infectious Diseases*. Updated 8th ed. Elsevier; 2015.)

30. A. Aciclovir

Acute retinal necrosis is most often caused by varicella zoster virus, and therapy with aciclovir should be administered. Corticosteroids may be used to decrease ocular inflammation but should not be given until after antiviral therapy is initiated.

31. E. *Stenotrophomonas maltophilia*

This patient has hospital-acquired pneumonia and did not demonstrate clinical improvement on broad-spectrum antibiotic therapy. He has multiple risk factors for development of drug-resistant pathogens, including his prolonged ICU stay and antecedent antibiotic therapy. Linezolid and meropenem would provide more than adequate activity against most gram-positive and gram-negative pathogens, including those that would produce extended-spectrum β-lactamases. *Stenotrophomonas* can be a cause of HAP, is intrinsically resistant to the antibiotic agents that he has been receiving, and is a nonfermenting gram-negative bacillus that is oxidase-positive. Other nonfermenting, oxidase-positive gram-negative bacilli include *Pseudomonas*, *Acinetobacter*, *Achromobacter*, and *Burkholderia*, among others.

32. C. *Mycobacterium kansasii*

Sensitivity of PCR detection of *M. tuberculosis* is high on smear-positive samples. Positive interferon gamma release assays have been reported in association with *M. kansasii* infection. *M. kansasii* infection can present with insidious pulmonary and constitutional symptoms and is frequently associated with hemoptysis and cavitary lung disease. Disseminated infection may also be seen in patients with HIV.

33. B. Amphotericin B

This patient has disseminated histoplasmosis, which can cause a sepsis syndrome in patients with HIV. He should receive amphotericin. Caution should also be taken to look for additional opportunistic processes as with his degree of immunocompromise he is at risk of having more than one disease process.

(Image from Assessments. In Cohen J, Powderly W, Opal S, eds. *Infectious Diseases*. 4th ed. Elsevier; 2017.)

34. B. *Coccidioides immitis*

This specimen shows several *Coccidioides* spherules containing endospores.

(Image from Assessments. In Cohen J, Powderly W, Opal S, eds. *Infectious Diseases*. 4th ed. Elsevier; 2017.)

35. E. Switch to clindamycin plus primaquine

This is the correct answer as the patient has presented with features of severe PCP and has developed a severe (grade 4) reaction to first-line treatment with TMP–SMX.

(Image from Assessments. In Cohen J, Powderly W, Opal S, eds. *Infectious Diseases*. 4th ed. Elsevier; 2017.)

36. B. After 4 weeks of antifungals

Cryptococcosis is one of the few opportunistic infections for which early initiation of antiretroviral therapy (less than 2 weeks) is associated with increased mortality. It is generally recommended to delay ART initiation to at least 4 weeks after start of antifungal therapy to avoid severe immune reconstitution syndrome.

37. C. Nitazoxanide
The pathogen here is *Cryptosporidium*; first-line treatment is with nitazoxanide.

38. E. Terminal ileum
Gastrointestinal perforation, usually at the terminal ileum, is the most serious complication of typhoid infection. It manifests as an acute abdomen or as worsening of abdominal pain accompanied by shock. Perforation is associated with a high mortality risk and needs urgent surgical intervention.
    (Image from Assessments. In Cohen J, Powderly W, Opal S, eds. *Infectious Diseases*. 4th ed. Elsevier; 2017.)

39. C. Chloroquine plus primaquine
This is the recommended treatment of choice for *P. vivax* infection currently according to Public Health England. Primaquine is required to clear the hypnozoite stage of infection in order to prevent relapse.
    (Image from Assessments. In Cohen J, Powderly W, Opal S, eds. Infectious Diseases. 4th ed. Elsevier; 2017.)

40. A. Liposomal amphotericin B
Liposomal amphotericin B is rapidly effective against visceral leishmaniasis and relatively nontoxic. It is the drug of choice for ill patients with visceral leishmaniasis as it is the best tolerated, and patients show a rapid response (afebrile within 1 week, and normalization of clinical signs and laboratory abnormalities within 2 weeks).
    (Image from Assessments. In Cohen J, Powderly W, Opal S, eds. *Infectious Diseases*. 4th ed. Elsevier; 2017.)

41. B. Continue current treatment
Melioidosis is characterized by difficulty in eradicating the causative organisms. Fever clearance is often slow (median fever clearance time of 9 days) and without evidence of clinical deterioration is not normally sufficient to indicate the need for a change in therapy. A patient who has clinical deterioration or persistently positive blood cultures should be viewed as failing treatment, at which stage the need for imaging, drainage of collections, and change in antimicrobial therapy should be considered.
    (Image from Assessments. In Cohen J, Powderly W, Opal S, eds. *Infectious Diseases*. 4th ed. Elsevier; 2017.)

42. C. Linezolid
Linezolid is a protein synthesis inhibitor and while bactericidal against *Streptococcus* spp., it is bacteriostatic against enterococci and staphylococci.

43. D. Sulfadiazine
High-dose sulfonamides can cause crystalluria. Some antiretroviral agents can cause crystalluria as well, most notably indinavir and atazanavir. Aciclovir is another drug that can be associated with crystalluria.

44. B. Coxsackievirus A6
This is a case of hand, foot, and mouth disease (HMFD), most commonly caused by Coxsackieviruses A10, A6, A16, and enterovirus A71. Outbreaks are commonly associated with daycare centers among others, and in infants and children under the age of 5.

45. B. Check her varicella-zoster IgG
She may require VZIG to reduce the risk of severe maternal disease and to reduce the risk of fetal varicella syndrome, but as it is a human product and there is time, she should have her immunity checked first, as she may be immune already.

46. B. Renal biopsy
This is a case of BK virus nephropathy. The definitive diagnosis of BKVN requires a renal biopsy showing polyomavirus-induced cytopathic changes in tubular or glomerular epithelial cells.

47. C. 35%
Among patients with acute flaccid paralysis, about one-third recover strength to near baseline, one-third have some improvement, and one-third have little or no improvement. Treatment of WNV infection is supportive. Several investigated therapeutic approaches, including ribavirin, steroids, IVIG, and monoclonal antibodies, have failed to demonstrate efficacy.

48. D. Stillbirth
This is a case of maternal listeriosis. The risks of this in late pregnancy include death in utero or premature delivery of an infected infant if the infection progresses untreated. The classic description is of a biphasic illness, in which the first phase is a nonspecific acute influenza-like illness. Blood cultures at this point are invaluable in providing an early diagnosis. If unnoticed or untreated, premature labor or death in utero may follow within 2–14 days of the acute presentation. This can be prevented by early antibiotic treatment

49. D. No prophylaxis required
The role of postexposure prophylaxis for leptospirosis is debatable, with local guidelines varying. Current UK guidelines are that postexposure management is limited to advice on showering promptly after water exposure, to minimize the swallowing of water, and to thoroughly clean abrasions caused during the water exposure. The contraindication to doxycycline in this patient due to his isotretinoin treatment means that the most appropriate option is no antimicrobial prophylaxis but heightened awareness and self-monitoring for fever and flu-like symptoms.

50. A. Actinomycosis
Actinomycosis is most commonly caused by *Actinomyces israelii*, which may be a component of normal oropharyngeal flora. This chronic, invasive infection mimics malignancy as it may invade local muscle and bone if left untreated. Sinus tracts may occur. Oral cervicofacial actinomycosis is the commonest presentation, but thoracic and abdominopelvic infections are also seen. Diagnosis is usually by demonstration of gram-positive branching filamentous bacilli and sulfur granules; cultures are rarely positive if broad-spectrum antibiotics have been taken.

This page intentionally left blank

Answers 8

1. A. Monitor for development of HUS

Although *E. coli* O157 is the serotype most commonly associated with HUS, any serotype can cause HUS. There is no reason to rule out O157 since the patient should be monitored for HUS regardless of serotype.

The presence of Shiga toxin 1 or Shiga toxin 2 is indicative of Shiga toxin-producing *E. coli* (STEC), not *Shigella*. If *Shigella* was present, it would have been detected as *Shigella*. A *Shigella*-specific target is part of all currently available GI panels.

Antimicrobial treatment of STEC has historically been associated with worse outcomes. There are some newer data that refute this dogma, but the standard practice is still to avoid antimicrobials for STEC.

2. A. Cefazolin

Ceftazidime is only marginally active against MSSA and would not be appropriate. Linezolid dosing is unaffected by renal insufficiency or dialysis and should not be given just postdialysis. Oritavancin is not established for treatment of MSSA bacteremia nor for treatment courses of 4–6 weeks in length. Vancomycin has been found to be clinically inferior to beta-lactams (including cefazolin) for MSSA infection in patients with end-stage renal diseases on regular thrice-weekly hemodialysis. Cefazolin postdialysis dosing has been shown to be effective for MSSA bacteremia in patients with end-stage renal disease.

3. C. *Klebsiella pneumoniae*

The patient has both cerebral abscesses (ring-enhancing lesions) and a liver abscess. There is a systemic inflammatory response with fever, neutrophilia, and raised C-reactive protein. There is a recognized association of primary liver abscesses caused by *Klebsiella pneumoniae* with hematogenous spread leading to cerebral abscesses. The travel history should be elicited as there is a higher incidence in SE Asia.

(Image from Prayson RA, Neuropathology, 2nd ed. Saunders; 2012.)

4. D. Repeat sputum acid-fast bacilli smear and culture

The patient requires a repeat acid-fast bacilli smear and culture before treatment is initiated. Nontuberculous mycobacteria (NTM) are easily recovered from the environment,

and when they are isolated from nonsterile sites, results require interpretation within the context of the patient's clinical syndrome to avoid treating colonization. Along with symptoms and CT findings, this patient requires a second positive MAC culture that can be obtained from sputum sample, bronchial wash or lavage, or a histopathologic specimen so that official diagnosis can be established.

5. E. Vancomycin, ceftriaxone, and azithromycin

This patient has a classic presentation for a postinfluenza or viral illness with initial flu-like symptoms progressing to worsening fever, productive cough, and imaging findings suggestive of a pleural effusion. Although the infection could be due to *Streptococcus pneumoniae*, there is concern for postinfluenza *Staphylococcus aureus* pneumonia, and the patient requires empiric coverage for MRSA. Although daptomycin does provide MRSA coverage, it is inactivated in the lung by surfactant and would be a poor choice in this clinical scenario.

6. E. *Mycobacterium tuberculosis*

The patient presents with a chronic epiglottitis, on a background of immunocompromise due to immunosuppression for renal transplantation. Granulomatous diseases and malignancy must be considered in the differential diagnosis. Due to the patient's history of being born in Indonesia, along with the radiographic abnormalities, tuberculosis is the likely diagnosis in this case.

7. A. Cefazolin

This patient has infective endocarditis (IE) due to MSSA with evidence of septic complications. Ideal therapy for native valve endocarditis (NVE) due to MSSA includes oxacillin, nafcillin, or cefazolin. Baseline abnormalities in his LFTs mean that avoiding oxacillin is advisable, as it can frequently be associated with hepatotoxicity, and instead use cefazolin give its proven efficacy and safe adverse effects profile.

Although vancomycin is an alternative treatment for patients with MSSA IE intolerant to penicillins and cephalosporins, beta-lactam therapy is preferred whenever feasible and should be selected over vancomycin.

There is no role for rifampin or aminoglycoside therapy in NVE due to MSSA.

8. C. *Listeria monocytogenes*
The history is consistent with a diagnosis of *Listeria monocytogenes* gastroenteritis and although *Staphylococcus aureus* and *Bacillus cereus* can also cause infection following consumption of infected food within a short period of time, *S. aureus* infection presents with vomiting 1–6 hours following ingestion; fever is rare, and symptoms usually resolve within 24–48 hours. Vomiting is the predominant symptom in all the other diagnoses listed.

Listeria monocytogenes is more likely to cause invasive disease in pregnant patients and can lead to possible fetal loss in severe disease.

9. C. Send urine for gonococcal/chlamydia NAAT
Reactive arthritis can have multiple presentations beyond the common findings described in medical textbooks such as conjunctivitis, monoarticular arthritis, and urethritis. This particular patient is a sexually active young male engaging in high-risk sexual behavior, and in this case sexually transmitted infectious etiologies are more likely etiologic agents of reactive arthritis.

Clinical findings such as keratoderma blennorrhagicum can be found on the soles of the feet and less commonly on the palms of the hand. It is most commonly due to skin thickening. Circinate balanitis can also occur with a distinct serpiginous annular dermatitis of the glans penis.

Empiric therapy for secondary syphilis should not immediately be considered in this case given findings of conjunctivitis, urethritis, and a monoarticular arthritis. Testing for syphilis would not be incorrect in this situation, however.

Repeat arthrocentesis testing is not warranted in this case given negative Gram stain and negative culture result from the arthrocentesis fluid. Orthopedic evaluation is not warranted in this situation given the relatively benign appearance of arthrocentesis fluid studies.

(Image from Wu IB, Schwartz RA. Reiter's syndrome: the classic triad and more. J Am Acad Dermatol 59:113-21, 2008.)

10. D. Treat presumptively with benzathine penicillin
Persons exposed to patients with primary, secondary, or early latent syphilis should be evaluated clinically and serologically, but those who have had sexual contact with a patient with primary, secondary, or early latent syphilis within 90 days preceding diagnosis should be treated presumptively for early syphilis, even if serologic testing is negative.

11. D. Leptospirosis
The clinical picture is most consistent with leptospirosis, given his exposure to animal-contaminated water in Hawaii and constellation of symptoms, including calf pain, conjunctivitis, abdominal pain, and lab findings.

12. B. Erythema infectiosum
Erythema infectiosum or parvovirus B19 is usually diagnosed clinically in children with the classic appearance of malar rash: the slapped cheek rash. In some cases, a further rash develops predominantly on the arms and legs, which is described as lacy in appearance and may take several weeks to resolve fully. The rash of rubella, measles, and human herpesvirus 6 (exanthem subitum) are characteristically widespread, generalized maculopapular exanthems.

(Image from Kadambari S, Segal S. Acute viral exanthems. *Medicine.* 2017;45(12):788–793.)

13. C. His symptoms should resolve in 2–4 weeks of starting therapy
Ninety percent of patients show symptom resolution within 2–4 weeks of commencing therapy.

14. A. Crystalline arthropathy
Basewd on the preliminary results of the synovial fluid cell count and differential, an inflammatory arthritis appears to be present and most likely due to crystalline arthropathy. Effusion due to osteoarthritis is clear, with minimal WBC noted (<2000 white cells) with <25% neutrophils. Given the lack of antecedent antibiotic, we would anticipate turbid synovial fluid and a more robust cell count and differential (septic arthritis is defined as WBC >20,000 cells but can often average ~50,000 cells and >75% neutrophils) if a septic arthritis was present. While the patient is on anticoagulation on warfarin, we could possibly note reddish synovial fluid if hemarthrosis was present and an elevated RBC relative to WBC. Based on our initial results from the arthrocentesis and patient history of naproxen discontinuation, a crystalline arthropathy would be the most likely diagnosis and would be confirmed by crystal analysis and negative synovial fluid cultures.

15. C. *Histoplasma capsulatum*
The patient has disseminated histoplasmosis, a disease endemic in the midwestern United States. The presence of granulomas in the transplanted liver suggests donor-derived disease which typically occurs in the early posttransplant period as in this case. Galactomannan, a polysaccharide present in the cell wall of several fungi, is released during host infection. Serum galactomannan can be detected in invasive aspergillosis, histoplasmosis, fusariosis, and penicilliosis (but not mucormycosis). In contrast to *Aspergillus*, *Histoplasma* may be recovered from blood cultures in cases of disseminated disease.

16. B. Atovaquone plus azithromycin
The patient has babesiosis and was co-infected with Lyme disease. The image shows Maltese crosses in a patient with active symptoms and risk factors for babesiosis. Asymptomatic disease does not require treatment. For mild disease, atovaquone plus azithromycin for 7–10 days is the treatment of choice. Remember the co-infections that can occur: babesiosis and Lyme disease. A phrase to help you remember: "**Anna** gives **lime** juice to her **babies**" (anaplasmosis, Lyme, babesiosis).

17. D. Start TB treatment now and defer ART for 2–8 weeks

Tuberculosis treatment should always be started once the clinician determines the diagnosis. In HIV-TB co-infection, ART should be initiated within 2 weeks only if CD4 count is <50/μL. In all other cases with CD4 count ≥50 initiation of ART should be started within 8 weeks, with exception of TB involving the CNS, where ART should be delayed for the first 8 weeks.

18. B. IV artesunate for 24 hours followed by atovaquone–proguanil for 3 days

The peripheral smear shows the presence of a *Plasmodium falciparum* gametocyte, classically described as "banana-shaped" and ring trophozoites. Although the patient is hemodynamically stable, he has signs of severe malaria, including a hemoglobin <7 g/dL and a bilirubin >3 mg/mL. For that reason, the most appropriate therapy is IV therapy with artesunate followed by an oral agent. The IV therapy should be continued for a minimum of 24 hours and should be transitioned to an oral regimen to complete a full course of therapy. They also need to have a second agent to ensure eradication of parasites. The patient has a prior history of depression and mefloquine would be contraindicated as it is associated with neuropsychiatric disturbances. Given the emergence of resistance in the South Asian continent, chloroquine is no longer an acceptable option for this region.

(From Garcia LS. Malaria. *Clin Lab Med.* 2010;30(1):93–129.)

19. A. Drug interaction

This patient is suffering from a drug–drug interaction between his rivaroxaban and the cobicistat in his antiretroviral therapy. Cobicistat is an inhibitor of CYP 3A4 and would lead to higher plasma concentrations of the rivaroxaban, which could lead to hemorrhagic events. Therefore, it is not recommended to start rivaroxaban in patients on an ART regimen with cobicistat.

Non-Hodgkin's lymphoma (NHL) is considered an AIDS-defining illness and is typically seen in patients with advanced disease (CD4 cell count <100 cells/μL). Primary CNS lymphoma and primary effusion lymphoma may also be seen in patients with advanced disease. The most common NHL seen in patients with HIV is B-cell lymphoma, followed by Burkett's lymphoma. Plasmablastic lymphomas are rare but are also more common in people with HIV. The clinical presentation is also not characteristic, with no B-type symptoms, growing masses, lymphadenopathy, or hepatosplenomegaly.

This patient does not have any other clinical features suggesting a thrombotic microangiopathy, thrombocytopenic purpura, or hemolytic uremic syndrome with signs of systemic organ dysfunction, which are all more common in patients infected with HIV.

Protein C and S deficiencies are usually seen in patients with advanced disease and co-infection with an opportunistic infection. Protein C and S deficiency usually result in hypercoagulability manifesting as venous thromboembolism or arterial thrombosis. There have been case reports of patients developing warfarin-induced skin necrosis with protein C and S deficiency.

Von Willebrand disease is the commonest inherited bleeding disorder. Mild type 1 WBD may well manifest later in life when uncovered by antiplatelet medications; however, type 3 WBD usually presents in infancy or early childhood with bleeding provoked by minor trauma.

20. E. Tenofovir disoproxil fumarate/emtricitabine + ritonavir boosted darunavir once daily

Q148R is a mutation that reduced susceptibility to both raltegravir and elvitegravir. Alone, there is evidence that Q148R confers low-level resistance to dolutegravir, and therefore if dolutegravir is used it should be dosed twice daily. Co-administration of atazanavir with a proton pump inhibitor is not recommended.

21. D. *Histoplasma capsulatum*

The patient's clinical presentation is most consistent with progressive disseminated histoplasmosis caused by *Histoplasma capsulatum* seen in advanced HIV disease. This endemic fungi is seen in the Ohio and Mississippi river valley extending down into the South as far as Texas. Typical presentations include fevers, hepatosplenomegaly, and multiorgan involvement that can progress to septic shock. Marked elevations in LDH and ferritin can be seen although these are nonspecific. The peripheral blood smear may show characteristic intracellular, 2–4 μm yeast forms in the WBCs, as seen in the image. The geographic epidemiology, clinical presentation and peripheral smear findings are not compatible with the other endemic fungi listed.

(Image from Singh NK, Nagendra S. *Histoplasma capsulatum* peripheral blood smear. BMJ Case Reports. https://doi.org/10.1136/bcr.05.2009.1877.)

22. B. Antiretroviral therapy

The patient's clinical presentation is consistent with diarrhea associated with *Cryptosporidium*, which is identified by modified acid-fast staining of stool demonstrating 4-6 μm oocysts. Because there is no proven effective treatment for this disease, immediate antiretroviral therapy (ART) is imperative to achieve immune restoration. Nitazoxanide is an effective treatment in immunocompetent patients and may offer some benefit but only as an adjunct to ART initiation. The other treatments are not active against this pathogen.

23. B. Hepatitis B virus flare

In this patient with HIV–HBV co-infection, the most likely cause of the acute hepatitis is a flare of the chronic hepatitis B precipitated by the change from a tenofovir-based ART to one containing lamivudine. Monotherapy with lamivudine for HBV is not recommended due to the risk of drug resistance and an acute flare in HBV. This is also supported by the positive HBV core IgM which often is seen in flares. Drug-induced liver injury from the current ART is less likely and fails to explain the hepatitis B virus serologies. Hepatitis D virus is most closely associated with IVDA or travel to areas of endemicity such as the Mediterranean basin. HIV cholangiopathy and MAC are primarily seen in patients with advanced AIDS and CD4 <50–100.

24. C. Perform a brain biopsy

The differential for this presentation is too broad, and empiricism may lead to bad outcomes. The patient underwent a stereotactic needle biopsy of the right frontal lesion. Pathology showed diffuse large B-cell lymphoma that was CD20-positive. In situ hybridization was positive for EBV-encoded small RNA (EBER). A PET scan showed no activity outside of the CNS. This was a case of posttransplant primary CNS lymphoma, which carries a dismal prognosis.

25. D. Tacrolimus toxicity

Macrolide antibiotics such as erythromycin and clarithromycin, and azoles such as posaconazole and fluconazole can decrease the metabolism of cyclosporine and tacrolimus leading to markedly increased levels and toxicity. Physicians and patients should be aware of interactions among antibiotics and immunosuppressive medications.

26. C. *Nocardia farcinica*

Nocardia farcinica is an opportunistic pathogen found in soil and water, which can cause skin and soft tissue infections when it gets into open wounds or cuts. The typical appearance on Gram stain is as gram-positive branching filamentous rods. Treatment of choice is trimethoprim–sulfamethoxazole. *Mycobacterium abscessus* is a nontuberculous mycobacterium which would appear as acid-fast bacilli on acid-fast staining. It can cause nodular and ulcerative lesions in areas of trauma. *Stenotrophomonas maltophilia* is a multidrug-resistant gram-negative pathogen that can cause ventilator-associated pneumonia. *Scedosporium prolificans* is an opportunistic fungus that can cause infections in immunocompromised patients and would not appear as a gram-positive filamentous rod. *Listeria monocytogenes* would appear as a gram-positive rod on Gram stain, not filamentous, and causes meningitis in immunocompromised patients.

27. D. Hereditary folate malabsorption

All these conditions can present with pneumocystis pneumonia. Cartilage–hair hypoplasia can also present with macrocytic anemia and short stature, but it lacks the other features of the disease (in particular, diarrhea and neurologic involvement). CD40L deficiency is accompanied by elevated IgM concentrations, while SP110 deficiency exhibits hepatic veno-occlusive disease.

28. A. Administer varicella vaccine

The chickenpox (varicella) vaccine would be recommended for all healthy adults who are exposed to chickenpox and do not know their immune status. Reasons for this are twofold. There is some evidence that vaccine may be effective in preventing chickenpox if given within 3 days of exposure. It is also an opportunity to protect the patient against future varicella exposures if they do not contract chickenpox on this occasion, so should be given irrespective of the interval since exposure. Varicella-zoster immune globulin (VariZIG/VZIG) is recommended for susceptible pregnant women and immunosuppressed individuals who have had a significant exposure. Intravenous immune globulin is not recommended. Valaciclovir is not indicated as prophylaxis for healthy adults but could be used to protect immunosuppressed individuals. Measuring titers may not provide an answer in time to give the vaccine and is not considered cost effective.

29. C. Counsel against the trip if visiting high-risk area

This is an immunocompromised patient planning an elective trip to a country that has yellow fever. Yellow fever is a live vaccine that could cause significant side effects in immunosuppression. Areas with risk for yellow fever are geographically restricted and thus avoided. A review of the specific destinations can inform if the patient will be exposed to yellow fever or not.

30. A. *Candida albicans*

This patient likely has fungal endophthalmitis caused by *Candida albicans*. On examination, she has hypopyon and also has "fungal balls" visible near the periphery of her iris. IV drug users are at particular risk to develop endogenous endophthalmitis. Initial evaluation and management should include blood cultures and systemic and intravitreal antibiotic therapy, as well as echocardiography to assess for infective endocarditis.

(Image from Assessments. In Cohen J, Powderly W, Opal S, eds. *Infectious Diseases*. 4th ed. Elsevier; 2017.)

31. C. CSF HSV PCR

This patient likely has HSV-1 encephalitis. Disproportionate enhancement of the temporal lobes, as demonstrated on her MRI, is characteristic. Behavioral abnormalities and new-onset seizures are also common.

32. C. Flavivirus

This patient most likely has infection with West Nile virus. He is presenting with meningoencephalitis with prominent peripheral neurologic sequelae. Other *Flaviviridae*-associated diseases include St. Louis encephalitis virus, dengue, Japanese encephalitis virus, and yellow fever virus.

33. E. Immunoassay for 14-3-3 protein

This patient likely has Creutzfeldt–Jakob disease. He has had rapidly progressive cognitive decline with extrapyramidal symptoms. Classic EEG pattern with CJD includes periodic sharp-wave activity. Brain MRI showed the "pulvinar sign" with increased thalamic activity bilaterally. Elevated levels of 14-3-3 protein in the CSF would be supportive of a diagnosis of CJD, though it can be elevated in a variety of other conditions, including other viral encephalitides and stroke.

34. E. *Paracoccidioides brasiliensis*
This image shows the typical "pilot's wheel" appearance of *Paracoccidioides*.

(Image from Assessments. In Cohen J, Powderly W, Opal S, eds. *Infectious Diseases*. 4th ed. Elsevier; 2017.)

35. B. *Erysipelothrix rhusiopathiae*
Erysipelothrix rhusiopathiae is a gram-positive bacillus that is ubiquitous in nature. Humans usually develop a local infection through direct contact with an infected animal or animal product. At particular risk are butchers and fishermen handling crabs, but also farmers, abattoir workers, and veterinarians. There is no documented human-to-human transmission.

36. E. Penicillin
The organism is most likely to be *Pasteurella multocida*, given the history of a penetrating cat bite, the aggressive nature of the infection manifest in the speed of onset, the associated bacteremia, and the likely tenosynovitis. The microbiology findings are consistent with this epidemiologic and clinical suspicion. Penicillin sensitivity is used within the laboratory to distinguish *Pasteurella* species from other gram-negative bacilli.

37. D. Warthin-Starry
The Warthin–Starry stain is the diagnostic stain for demonstrating *Bartonella* organisms within a biopsy specimen.

(Image from Assessments. In Cohen J, Powderly W, Opal S, eds. *Infectious Diseases*. 4th ed. Elsevier; 2017.)

38. D. Paromomycin.
This is a case of amebic liver abscess. This is generally managed with a tissue amebicide such as metronidazole and a luminal agent such as paromomycin.

39. B. China
This is a case of hepatic alveolar echinococcosis, an infection with the larval stage of *Echinococcus multilocularis*. It can cause severe hepatic disease and, rarely, metastatic disease. *E. multilocularis* is restricted to the northern hemisphere. The European endemic area has expanded, but the global burden of disease lies in China. It is estimated that 91% of new cases globally each year occur in China. Cases usually become symptomatic after an incubation period of 5–15 years.

40. A. Amastigotes
In cutaneous leishmaniasis, amastigotes multiply in dermal macrophages near the site of inoculation.

(Image from Assessments. In Cohen J, Powderly W, Opal S, eds. *Infectious Diseases*. 4th ed. Elsevier; 2017.)

41. A. Benzylpenicillin
Penicillin is the drug of choice in naturally occurring anthrax. This can either be oral or intramuscular in mild uncomplicated cutaneous anthrax or intravenous in complicated or severe cutaneous anthrax. Penicillin is used in combination with other antimicrobials such as clindamycin and ciprofloxacin in inhalational anthrax or with streptomycin in gastrointestinal infection.

(Image from Assessments. In Cohen J, Powderly W, Opal S, eds. *Infectious Diseases*. 4th ed. Elsevier; 2017.)

42. A. AmpC induction
Some bacteria, most notably some *Enterobacteriaceae*, have chromosomally determined ampC β-lactamases that can be expressed at high levels after exposure to β-lactams. This can cause clinical failure even if an isolate initially seems susceptible *in vitro*.

43. E. Zinc
This is a case of rotavirus infection. There is no specific antiviral treatment. However, zinc, given for 10–14 days during and after a diarrheal episode, has been shown to decrease diarrhea mortality by 23%. Additionally, vitamin A supplementation reduces all-cause diarrhea mortality by 30% in children aged 6–59 months.

44. C. Intrauterine death
This is measles, as evidenced clinically by the 3 Cs – cough, coryza, conjunctivitis – and the Koplik spots. Measles infection in pregnancy is associated with higher rates of premature delivery and intrauterine death.

45. B. Intrauterine death
The diagnosis of monkeypox infection requires clinical (rash), epidemiologic (equatorial Africa), and laboratory (the presence of genomic DNA or brick-shaped virions in scab material) findings.

(Image from Assessments. In Cohen J, Powderly W, Opal S, eds. *Infectious Diseases*. 4th ed. Elsevier; 2017.)

46. E. Reassurance only
Western Europe (including Germany) is free of rabies in terrestrial animals. As such, even though a bite that penetrates skin is high risk, the epidemiology means that rabies postexposure prophylaxis is not warranted. If this had been a bat bite, this would not be the case.

47. C. Non-nucleoside reverse transcriptase inhibitors
The NNRTI binding pocket is structurally different in HIV-2, conferring innate resistance onto this class of drugs. They should not be used in the treatment of HIV-2.

48. D. Y181C
Amino acid substitutions such as K103N or Y181C prevent NNRTIs binding.

49. D. Filovirus
Ebola and Marburg are both filoviruses. They have a distinctive filamentous morphology under the electron microscope with a nonsegmented, negative-stranded RNA genome. They have a lipid envelope derived from host cell plasma membrane.

50. B. Modified Elek test

The Elek immunoprecipitation test confirms the production of diphtheria toxin. PCR tests are now also available to demonstrate presence of the diphtheria toxin genes. Diphtheria toxin production requires enhanced public health management of both the patient and their close contacts.

Answers 9

1. E. None of the above

M. abscessus and *M. chelonae* are rapidly-growing mycobacteria (RGM) while *M. tuberculosis* is a slowly-growing species (SGM). However, the classification of RGM vs. SGM is determined by the growth rate after subculture, not the growth rate in primary culture. Rapid-growers with grow within 7 days after subculture, while slow-growers require 7 or more days to grow after subculture. Growth on day 5 from primary culture does not provide any information about whether the organism is a rapid-grower or a slow-grower because the growth rate from the primary culture depends more on infectious burden.

2. D. *Fusarium* spp.

Fevers with disseminated skin lesions in neutropenic patients, especially hematologic malignancy, raise concern for disseminated infection (bacterial and fungal).

Considering poor prognosis, prompt diagnosis and administration of antifungals is critical.

Biopsy and stain showing septate hyphae with canoe-shaped macroconidia are consistent with *Fusarium* infection. These infections often start as onychomycosis in the toes. Treatment will include empirical amphotericin B and voriconazole until further speciation is performed.

Epidemiology is concerning for *Blastomyces*, but the stain rules out other fungal etiologies, and the skin biopsy would show yeast not hyphae.

Aspergillus should be considered in neutropenic patient with fevers. However multiple skin lesions, toe infection, and stain are not consistent with it.

Mucormycosis is associated with invasive sinusitis in an immunocompromised host, but dissemination to skin is not common, and the biopsy is more consistent with hyaline hyphomycete than a zygomycete.

Presence of mold rules out *Cryptococcus*.

(Image from Narayanan G, Nath R. *Mayo Clinic Proc.* 2016;91(4):542–543. © 2016.)

3. D. Minocycline

Stenotrophomonas maltophilia is intrinsically resistant to carbapenems (meropenem). Chloramphenicol would be considered risky given the patient's pancytopenia. The patient's prolonged QTc interval makes levofloxacin a suboptimal choice. Trimethoprim–sulfamethoxazole poses a risk of

hemolytic anemia given the underlying G6PD deficiency. Minocycline provides activity against many strains of *Stenotrophomonas maltophilia* and has no apparent safety concerns precluding its use in this case.

4. E. *Streptococcus pneumoniae*

The patient is 5 months out from a stem cell transplant and presents with a lobar pneumonia. Although she is immunocompromised, she is on *Pneumocystis* prophylaxis and does not present with interstitial lung disease. CMV pneumonia would also be unlikely without a diffuse pneumonitis on imaging, and she would require histopathology with positive CMV staining to make the diagnosis. RSV pneumonia would normally present with bilateral asymmetric infiltrates and *Candida* spp. rarely cause pneumonia. The correct answer is therefore pneumococcal pneumonia as this patient is at risk for pneumococcal pneumonia, and a lower lobe infiltrate would fit the classic description.

5. B. Ceftriaxone and azithromycin

The patient presents in the setting of community-acquired pneumonia. The only answer choice with a guideline-recommended regimen for CAP is ceftriaxone and azithromycin. The patient has no past medical history or risk factors warranting pseudomonal coverage and does not present with evidence of a pleural effusion after a viral illness that would be concerning for MRSA infection.

6. E. Quadruple antituberculous therapy

This patient has insidious constitutional symptoms, with a constellation of findings suggestive of pulmonary TB with associated constrictive pericarditis and right heart failure. This is in the setting of appropriate exposure to TB as the patient is coming from an endemic region. Because of the constrictive findings and HF, pericardiocentesis is likely to be diagnostic and therapeutic and should be performed as soon as possible. In addition to pericardiocentesis, the patient may require pericardiectomy if her symptoms persist. For management of her underlying infection she would also require adequate antituberculous therapy.

NSAIDS and colchicine are only adequate for patients with idiopathic or viral pericarditis. In the setting of TB pericarditis, the patient should receive targeted therapy.

Although she may benefit from corticosteroids due to early signs of constriction, the best next step in management would be for pericardiocentesis and anti-TB treatment.

Hypothyroidism may present with a number of cardiac symptoms, including bradycardia, edema, exertional dyspnea, and pericardial effusion. However, levothyroxine should not be started without confirmatory thyroid function tests.

7. D. Fluid resuscitation

This patient has *Vibrio cholerae*, and fluid resuscitation is paramount to her survival (as she is already demonstrating fluid and electrolyte loss). Antibiotic treatment is also important as it can shorten the duration of diarrhea, reduce the volume of stool losses, and decrease the duration of *V. cholera* shedding.

Options for cholera include macrolides, fluoroquinolones, and tetracyclines based on local resistance profile.

8. C. Bone marrow biopsy

This man has visceral leishmaniasis characterized by darkening of skin with fever, weight loss, hepatosplenomegaly, and pancytopenia. Hypergammaglobulinemia is also common. He has risk factors including HIV and travel to Spain, where leishmaniasis is endemic. He may have acquired infection during his last trip (which fits in with traditional incubation periods), but due to HIV, either atypical infections or reactivation of latent infections can occur. In addition, the patient is noted to be tanned although he has not traveled outside the UK in 4 months. Darkening of the skin can occur in visceral leishmaniasis through melanocyte stimulation (kala-azar = black skin).

The diagnosis of visceral leishmaniasis is made by tissue biopsy. Samples can be stained and evaluated under light microscopy for *Leishmania* amastigotes and undergo PCR to confirm speciation. Hence biopsy is the diagnostic test of choice in this instance. Bone marrow biopsy is usually chosen over splenic biopsy due to high sensitivity and low risk of hemorrhage. Other tissue samples include liver and lymph nodes. Culture is available in some centers although this requires special media and is slow (4 weeks). Serologic antibody testing provides supportive evidence of infection, although the sensitivity is lower in HIV-positive individuals.

Abdominal ultrasound and cross-sectional imaging would be useful to characterize the extent of visceral involvement but are unlikely to be diagnostic.

Blood culture would be appropriate if concerned about secondary bacterial infection but will not detect leishmaniasis.

The patient has been well controlled on HIV treatment with a recent undetectable viral load. Missing two doses is unlikely to impact on the viral load significantly over such a short period of time.

9. B. Chronic bacterial prostatitis

Pelvic pain and relapsing UTI suggest a deep-seated infection. Prostate exam is normal in chronic bacterial prostatitis and urine tends to be inflammatory with bacteriuria. Prior treatment for TB is a distractor – granulomatous prostatitis is a histologic diagnosis after work-up for an abnormal prostate exam. Chronic pelvic pain syndrome is a diagnosis of exclusion, and the recent diagnosis of a UTI with relapse is more suggestive of chronic bacterial prostatitis.

10. E. Repeat *Chlamydia* NAAT in 4 weeks for test of cure

Test of cure for *Chlamydia* is recommended during pregnancy. This recommendation was put in place to prevent the severe sequelae that can occur in mothers and neonates if infection persists. Repeat screening in the 3rd trimester may be warranted based upon patient risk. However, it is not the best of the options.

11. A. Enterovirus 71 (EV71)

Enterovirus 71 is one of the principal causes of hand, foot, and mouth disease (HFMD) but has been associated with severe neurologic complications, particularly in young children. These may arise in isolation or in association with skin or mucosal lesions. EV71 has been associated with large epidemics in Southeast Asia but has been reported also in the United States and Europe. Brainstem encephalitis, aseptic meningitis, and acute flaccid paralysis (AFM) are all recognized complications. Enterovirus D68 has been associated with neurologic symptoms such as aseptic meningitis and AFM but is not a cause of HFMD. EV-D68 is more commonly associated with severe respiratory illness.

12. D. Rubella

The greatest risk of severe congenital disease occurs if the mother acquires rubella in the 1st trimester of pregnancy. Other features of the congenital rubella syndrome include cardiac defects, hepatomegaly or hepatitis, bone lesions, and developmental delay. Congenital varicella syndrome is rare but usually occurs in neonates whose mother acquired infection in the 2nd trimester and is characterized by cicatricial skin lesions (scars), limb hypoplasia, and ocular defects. Parvovirus B19 is associated with fetal hydrops, although most intrauterine parvovirus infections are not adversely affected. Evidence of parvovirus as a teratogen is lacking. CMV is asymptomatic at birth in 90% of children born with congenital CMV; although microcephaly, deafness, and visual loss due to chorioretinitis are associated with CMV, cataracts are not typical and suggest an alternative etiology. Measles is not associated with congenital disease.

13. E. Tickborne relapsing fever

The case describes a pattern of recurrent fevers with spirochetemia on a patient with consistent epidemiologic exposure (sleeping in wood cabins in an endemic area) with tickborne relapsing fever (TBRF).

The typical recurrent febrile episodes make TBRF more likely than Leptospirosis or Lyme disease.

The epidemiologic history does not fit with louseborne relapsing fever, which is endemic in the Horn of Africa.

Peripheral blood smear shows spirochetes, hence option A is incorrect, as Colorado tick fever is a viral illness.

(Image from Rhee KY, Johnson WD. *Borrelia* species (relapsing fever). In Mandell GL, Bennett JE, Dolin R, eds. *Principles and Practice of Infectious Diseases*. 6th ed. Churchill Livingstone; 2005.)

14. C. Reassure but advise the family to be vigilant for erythema migrans

There is no evidence of infection. Serology is not advised simply following a tick bite. Prophylaxis is not advised in this scenario when the local tick infection rate with *Borrelia* is low. Skin biopsy is not indicated.

15. C. *Mycobacterium tuberculosis*

Brucellosis is endemic to the Middle East and Mediterranean regions. When involved in vertebral osteomyelitis, there is a predilection for the lumbosacral spine, or it can manifest as a sacroiliitis. Routine bacterial organisms are well known to cause discitis/osteomyelitis but tend to infect the disc space first with subsequent spread to adjacent vertebral bodies, *opposite* to that of *Mycobacterium tuberculosis*, which spreads to the disc later in the disease process. Given this and her history of emigration from an endemic region, Pott's disease should be given further diagnostic consideration.

16. B. Egypt
Know the countries with chloroquine-sensitive malaria.

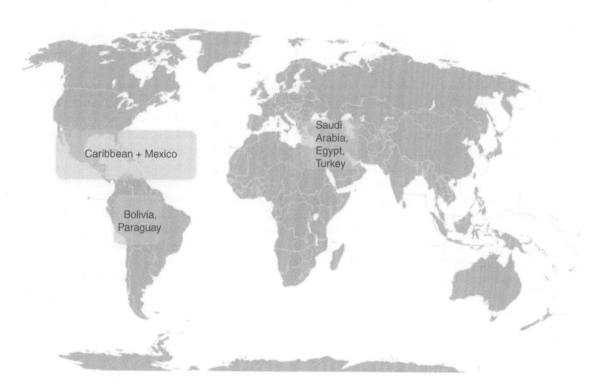

17. A. Ampicillin
Be aware of *Listeria monocytogenes* (gram-positive bacilli as shown in the image) rhombencephalitis (brainstem-predominant encephalitis) that occurs more commonly in immunocompetent patients (as opposed to regular *Listeria*-associated meningitis in immunocompromised patients). Ampicillin is the drug of choice for *Listeria* infection.

(Image from Murray PR, Rosenthal KS, Pfaller MA. *Medical Microbiology*. 8th ed. Elsevier; 2016.)

18. A. Anti-GBM antibodies
This patient has a renopulmonary syndrome, and the presence of fever and a petechial rash also raise concern for a possible concomitant vasculitis. There are several possible diagnoses in this case, but of the listed options, anti-GBM antibodies would be probative for Goodpasture's syndrome.

If this patient did have LTBI in the past, her IGRA would not be helpful.

19. E. Sputum induction with hypertonic saline
Factors associated with tuberculosis infectivity include the presence of cough, lung cavitation, acid-fast bacilli on smear, TB involving the airways (larynx, lungs, etc.), not on TB treatment or on it for <2 weeks, positive sputum cultures, undergoing cough-inducing procedures (i.e., bronchoscopy, sputum induction, and administration of aerosolized medications). This patient has been on adequate treatment for less than 2 weeks, thus is still considered infectious despite having improved his symptoms (lack of cough) and not having other factors associated with increased infectiousness. (CDC TB infection prevention guidelines.)

20. D. Liposomal daunorubicin

Kaposi sarcoma (KS) is an AIDS-related low-grade vascular tumor associated with human herpesvirus 8 with treatment guided by staging of disease. Staging is based on extent of tumor, immune status, and severity of illness. Extent of tumor involvement is based on oral cavity and visceral disease. Patients with CD4 cell counts less than 200 cells/μL are considered to have advanced disease.

Illness severity is either S1 (a history of opportunistic infection, thrush, or B symptoms) or S0 (patients without any of these factors).

Evaluation of visceral involvement is necessary when considering treatment options. To assess for gastrointestinal involvement, an occult stool can be used as a screening tool. Chest X-ray is useful to screen for pulmonary involvement. More invasive testing such as endoscopy or bronchoscopy may be pursued if screening tests are positive.

Initiation of antiretroviral therapy is always recommended.

Local symptomatic therapy, including intralesional chemotherapy with vinblastine or topical alitretinoin is recommended for small lesions.

In patients with greater than 25 lesions, extensive edema, symptomatic visceral involvement, immune reconstitution syndrome, or extensive cutaneous disease not responsive to local therapy, systemic chemotherapy is recommended in addition to antiretroviral therapy. First-line therapy includes liposomal anthracyclines like pegylated liposomal doxorubicin or liposomal daunorubicin. Second-line regimens may include taxanes like paclitaxel.

Steroids are not recommended to treat KS and, in fact, regression of KS lesions can be seen when steroids are stopped in patients infected with HIV.

Doxycycline and gentamicin are used for the treatment of bacillary angiomatosis which may present with similar lesions, but the duration of onset, the lung involvement, and the lack of fever do not support this diagnosis.

(Clinical photograph from Wick MR, Patterson JW, et al. *Practical Skin Pathology: A Diagnostic Approach*. Elsevier; 2013. Radiograph from Grainger RF, Allison DJ, Adam A, Dison AK, eds. *Grainger & Allison's Diagnostic Radiology*, 4th ed. Harcourt; 2001.)

21. C. Tenofovir alafenamide/emtricitabine +atazanavir/cobicistat

Initiation of ART in symptomatic acute HIV reduces symptoms and is now recommended. As a HLA B*5701 result is not available, abacavir-based regimens should be avoided. In the setting of acute infection, resistance assays may not be readily available, as in this case. In the absence of a resistance assay a protease-based or dolutegravir-based regimen is recommended pending results. Tenofovir alafenamide+cobicistat+elvitegravir is incorrect as it is an incomplete regimen.

22. B. Intravenous immunoglobulin

The presentation of severe anemia without evidence of hemolysis and an inappropriately low reticulocyte count is suggestive of pure red cell aplasia. In advanced AIDS patients, parvovirus B19 is a well-recognized cause of this condition, with characteristic bone marrow findings as in this case. Parvovirus B19 causes Fifth disease in children, usually manifesting with febrile illness and slapped cheek rash. Diagnosis is usually confirmed with parvovirus B19 PCR, and the treatment of choice for pure red cell aplasia in advanced AIDS is IVIG.

23. E. *Rhodococcus equi*

An unusual opportunistic infection that can cause cavitary pulmonary disease in advanced HIV disease is *Rhodococcus equi*.

This pathogen is a gram-positive coccobacillus or diphtheroids on Gram stain but can be seen as branching rods from liquid media. It can also be AFB-positive on stains, but the negative MTB and MAI PCRs make these pathogens much less likely. There is an association of this pathogen with exposure to horses and other livestock although only about 50% of patients recall this specific exposure history.

24. D. Start empirical ivAB for intraabdominal infection

Intraabdominal and biliary complications after liver transplant range from biliary leaks and bilomas to ascending cholangitis and liver abscess from biliary strictures resulting from hepatic artery thrombosis. These patients can present without right upper quadrant pain or tenderness because of allograft denervation. CMV disease is unlikely given leukocytosis and D–/R– status, and invasive aspergillosis is unlikely given early presentation posttransplant and the absence of neutropenia. Surgical complication or intraabdominal infection should be suspected, empiric broad-spectrum antibiotics started, and the abdomen imaged.

25. D. *Pneumocystis jirovecii*

Legionella and *Streptococcus pneumoniae*, although can cause pneumonia in transplant recipients, would be unlikely given the levofloxacin prophylaxis, which is effective treatment for both of these pathogens. Typical findings on X-ray would be consolidations. Pulmonary aspergillosis would be unusual given the patient is on voriconazole prophylaxis, and typical findings on chest X-ray tend to be cavitations with air-crescent sign or nodules rather than interstitial infiltrates. MERS coronavirus can cause hypoxemia and interstitial infiltrates on chest radiography; however, the patient has not traveled to a part of the world affected by MERS coronavirus, such as the Middle East. Although the patient is receiving inhaled pentamidine for pneumocystis prophylaxis, this is not as effective as trimethoprim–sulfamethoxazole, and breakthrough infections have been reported. Thus the correct answer is *Pneumocystis jirovecii*.

26. D. Prophylaxis with ciprofloxacin or doxycycline

Nasal swabs are not indicated in this setting as everyone at the stadium would be presumed to have been exposed. Although ciprofloxacin and doxycycline are contraindicated in pregnancy and in children, they are both recommended as prophylaxis for anthrax exposure. If sensitivities of *B. anthracis* return as penicillin-susceptible, the regimen can then be changed to amoxicillin. Hospitalization is not required unless symptomatic. Anthrax immune globulin is indicated for the treatment of inhalational anthrax. Anthrax vaccine may be indicated for exposure in a mass-incident exposure such as this, but not in combination with immune globulin.

27. A. Drug reaction with eosinophilia and systemic symptoms

Drug reaction with eosinophilia and systemic symptoms (DRESS) presents in a broad spectrum of clinical manifestations typically 1–8 weeks after the start of an offending medication. The triad of fever, rash, and internal organ involvement (renal, hematologic, and liver involvement most common) is suggestive. Current treatment recommendations include treatment with corticosteroids. Mortality can be as high as 10%, mostly due to liver failure. Many medications have been associated with DRESS including antibiotics (sulfonamides, minocycline, etc.), anticonvulsants, and other drugs.

With no sepsis and stable vital signs both streptococcal toxic shock and sepsis with multiorgan dysfunction due to CA-MRSA infection are unlikely.

Fixed drug eruption does not cause systemic repercussions and typically leads to more focalized lesions. The liver abnormalities and eosinophilia are part of the presentation for DRESS not TEN.

28. A. Chronic lymphedema postsurgery

All of the options (skin barrier disruption or inflammation, immunosuppression, preexisting skin infections, and edema) can be risk factors for the development of cellulitis. However, in this particular instance, it is her arm that is affected, and the risk of lymphedema following axillary node dissection (ANC) and radiotherapy for breast cancer is high (roughly 40% if both ANC and radiotherapy). Onset of lymphedema is insidious and progressive. Patients with lymphedema have an increased risk of infection in the affected area (up to 70×); over a quarter of patients will have at least one infection annually.

29. D. *Necator americanus*

This is a hookworm egg. It is not possible to distinguish between *Ancylostoma duodenale* and *Necator americanus* on microscopy (that requires the larval stage), but geographically this is more likely to be *Necator americanus*.

(Image from Maguire JH. Intestinal nematodes (roundworms). In Bennett JE, Dolin R, Blaser MJ, eds. *Mandell, Douglas, and Bennett's Principles and Practice of Infectious Diseases*. Updated 8th ed. Elsevier; 2015.)

30. D. *Pseudomonas aeruginosa*

This patient likely has hot tub folliculitis, which is most commonly caused by *Pseudomonas aeruginosa*. This infection is usually self-limited and does not require systemic antibiotic therapy.

31. D. *Pasteurella multocida*

Gram-negative anaerobes, including Pasteurella, are commonly associated with both cat and dog bites.

32. C. *Clostridium sordellii*

Clostridium sordellii infections can develop following childbirth or after gynecologic procedures and can also be seen with contaminated lacerations or in intravenous drug users. Patients may not present with high fevers but may have significant leukemoid reaction and hemoconcentration, as well as edema on examination.

33. D. Tick paralysis

Tick paralysis causes an ascending, flaccid paralysis that can progress to respiratory failure and can be associated with cranial nerve involvement. Level of consciousness and sensation typically remain intact. Fever and headache are not typically seen, and the CSF studies are normal. Symptoms typically improve rapidly once the tick is found and removed.

34. E. *Mycobacterium tuberculosis*

Of the listed species of mycobacteria, *M. tuberculosis* would be the most likely cause of lymphadenitis. Among the atypical mycobacteria, *Mycobacterium–avium* complex and *M. scrofulaceum* are also important considerations. *M. bovis* can also cause lymphadenitis but is typically associated with cervical lymphadenitis and in the context of ingestion of unpasteurized dairy products.

35. D. Lymphogranuloma venereum.

The photograph below depicts the "groove sign" of Lymphogranuloma venereum (LGV), wherein groups of enlarged inguinal lymph nodes are cleaved by the inguinal ligament.

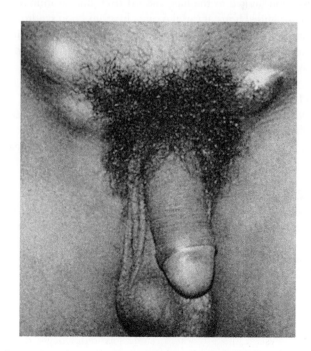

(Image from Assessments. In Cohen J, Powderly W, Opal S, eds. *Infectious Diseases*. 4th ed. Elsevier; 2017.)

36. B. HSV keratitis

The image demonstrates dendritic keratitis associated with HSV. Branching epithelial lesions are seen on examination.

(Image from Assessments. In Cohen J, Powderly W, Opal S, eds. *Infectious Diseases*. 4th ed. Elsevier; 2017.)

37. B. Azithromycin

This patient is presenting with a syndrome compatible with atypical pneumonia. It is also noteworthy that there was a cluster of sick patients at his nursing home, which could be suggestive of a spreading respiratory viral infection or *Legionella*, which has been associated with hospital and nursing home-related outbreaks because of contaminated water sources. Hyponatremia, acute renal failure, abnormal liver function tests, and gastrointestinal symptoms may be seen with legionellosis. Other causes of atypical pneumonia can include *M. pneumonia* and *C. pneumonia*, which can also be treated with azithromycin.

38. E. β-lactams

Cervicofacial actinomycosis is most often treated with penicillins. A variety of other agents have been used with success, including cephalosporins, carbapenems, clindamycin, tetracyclines, erythromycin, and chloramphenicol.

39. B. Ciguatera poisoning

She most likely has ciguatoxin poisoning. Early symptoms can include abdominal cramps, diarrhea and circumoral paresthesiae. Later neurologic symptoms can include a sensation of reversal of hot and cold perception.

40. A. Ivermectin

This patient likely has infection with *Strongyloides stercoralis*, which is more common in tropical countries. It typically causes infection limited to the lung and GI tract, but, in immunocompromised hosts, it can also cause hyperinfection syndrome that can present as gram-negative bacteremia and meningitis because of parasite-driven translocation of enteric bacteria. Treatment of choice for strongyloidiasis is ivermectin.

41. C. Pegylated liposomal doxorubicin

Doxorubicin given as Caelyx™ or Doxil™ is the treatment of choice.

(Image from Assessments. In Cohen J, Powderly W, Opal S, eds. *Infectious Diseases*. 4th ed. Elsevier; 2017.)

42. E. Uncooked freshwater fish

This is a clinical case of gnathostomiasis, evidenced by the recurrent cutaneous swellings, the epidemiologic risk factors associated with Thailand, and the investigative findings. *Gnathostoma spinigerum* is acquired by eating undercooked infected poultry, snake, or freshwater fish, or by drinking water contaminated with infected Cyclops crustaceans.

(Image from Assessments. In Cohen J, Powderly W, Opal S, eds. *Infectious Diseases*. 4th ed. Elsevier; 2017.)

43. E. *Xenopsylla cheopis* (rat flea)

This is a case of bubonic plague, as typified by the acute onset of systemic symptoms with an exquisitely tender bubo (nonfluctuant lymph node) with associated edema. The microbiologic and hematologic findings are characteristic of *Yersinia pestis* infection. Flea bites are the most common source of human *Y. pestis* infection. Antimicrobial prophylaxis may be offered to household contacts because of likely flea exposures.

(Image from Assessments. In Cohen J, Powderly W, Opal S, eds. *Infectious Diseases*. 4th ed. Elsevier; 2017.)

44. A. Abacavir

Abacavir hypersensitivity can be predicted by testing for the HLAB*5701 allele. The syndrome can be life-threatening and can manifest with fever and other constitutional symptoms, rash, nausea, vomiting, diarrhea, cough, and dyspnea.

45. D. Rheumatoid-like polyarthritis

Accompanying joint symptoms are rare in children but may be severe in adults, more often in women. These consist of an acute, symmetric, rheumatoid-like polyarthritis which usually improves within 2 weeks but occasionally may persist for months.

(Image from Assessments. In Cohen J, Powderly W, Opal S, eds. *Infectious Diseases*. 4th ed. Elsevier; 2017.)

46. C. *Pseudomonas aeruginosa*

This is a case of malignant (necrotizing) otitis externa, which is an aggressive infection of the external auditory canal that may be fatal. The majority of cases are caused by *P. aeruginosa*. Other organisms implicated less frequently include *Staphylococcus aureus*, *Aspergillus fumigatus*, and *Proteus mirabilis*. Elderly people with diabetes mellitus are particularly at risk. As the infection progresses it may spread to cause an osteomyelitis of the base of the skull and the temporomandibular joint.

47. A. Azithromycin

This is the first choice antibiotic for *Campylobacter enteritis*, as resistance is low for macrolide antibiotics.

48. C. *Fusobacterium necrophorum*

Lemierre's syndrome is characterized by thrombosis and suppurative thrombophlebitis of the internal jugular vein. It is associated with disseminated septic emboli to the lungs and other sites. The most common pathogen is *Fusobacterium necrophorum*, but other organisms implicated include *Eikenella*, *Bacteroides*, and streptococcal species. Organisms may be isolated from blood cultures and from infective metastases.

(Image from Assessments. In Cohen J, Powderly W, Opal S, eds. *Infectious Diseases*. 4th ed. Elsevier; 2017.)

49. C. *Entamoeba histolytica*
Primary infection of the skin by *Entamoeba histolytica* can be acquired by direct contact with an infected subject during vaginal or anal intercourse. Identification of trophozoites containing ingested red blood cells is consistent with a clinical picture of amebic infection. Biopsy may be necessary to demonstrate trophozoites and to exclude other diagnoses such as squamous cell carcinoma. PCR may be useful in confirming the diagnosis.

(Image from Assessments. In Cohen J, Powderly W, Opal S, eds. *Infectious Diseases*. 4th ed. Elsevier; 2017.)

50. B. *Chrysops* deerfly
This is the vector responsible for the transmission of *Loa loa*, with the female of the species biting during the day, especially in the wet season.

Printed and bound by CPI Group (UK) Ltd, Croydon, CR0 4YY

08/05/2025

01864792-0001